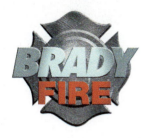

KIRK'S FIRE INVESTIGATION

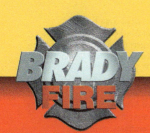

KIRK'S FIRE INVESTIGATION

Eighth Edition

David J. Icove, Ph.D., P.E., F.SFPE
Board Certified, Fellow, National
Academy of Forensic Engineers (NAFE)
The University of Tennessee

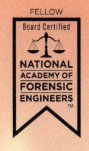

Gerald A. Haynes, M.S., P.E., SFPE
Board Certified, Member, National
Academy of Forensic Engineers (NAFE)
Haynes and Associates, LLC

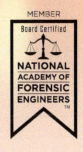

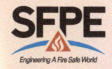

Engineering A Fire Safe World

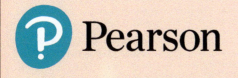

330 Hudson Street, NY, NY 10013

Vice President, Health Science and TED: Julie Levin Alexander
Director of Portfolio Management: Marlene McHugh Pratt
Portfolio Manager: Derril Trakalo
Development Editor: Carol Lazerick
Portfolio Management Assistant: Lisa Narine
Vice President, Content Production and Digital Studio: Paul DeLuca
Managing Producer, Health Science: Melissa Bashe
Project Monitor: Rhonda Aversa, SPi Global
Operations Specialist: Mary Ann Gloriande
Managing Producer, Digital Studio, Health Science: Amy Peltier
Digital Content Team Lead: Brian Prybella

Digital Content Project Lead: Lisa Rinaldi
Vice President, Product Marketing: David Gesell
Field Marketing Manager: Brian Hoehl
Full-Service Project Management and Composition: iEnergizer Aptara®, Ltd.
Inventory Manager: Vatche Demirdjian
Cover Design: Carie Keller, Cenveo
Cover Photo: Detective Aaron L Allen, Knox County Sheriff's Office, Knoxville, Tennessee
Printer/Binder: LSC Communications, Inc.
Cover Printer: LSC Communications, Inc.

Credits and acknowledgments borrowed from other sources and reproduced, with permission, in this textbook appear on appropriate pages within text.

Many of the designations by manufacturers and sellers to distinguish their products are claimed as trademarks. Where those designations appear in this book, and the publisher was aware of a trademark claim, the designations have been printed in initial caps or all caps.

Note: A portion of this book was prepared by David J. Icove, a former employee of the US Tennessee Valley Authority (TVA) and Federal Bureau of Investigation (FBI). The views expressed in this book are the views of Dr. Icove and his coauthors. They are not necessarily the views of TVA or the United States government. Reference in this book to any product, process, or service by trade name, trademark, manufacturer, or otherwise does not necessarily constitute its endorsement or recommendation by TVA or the United States government.

Disclaimer: The authors and Pearson Education make no warranty, expressed or implied, to the readers of *Kirk's Fire Investigation*, and accept no responsibility for its use. The readers assume sole responsibility for determining the appropriateness of its suggested use in any particular methodology, calculation, or fire modeling application; for any conclusions drawn from the results of its use; and for any actions taken or not taken as a result of analyses performed using these tools.

Readers are warned that this textbook is intended for use only by those competent in the fields including, but not limited to, fire investigation, fluid dynamics, thermodynamics, combustion, and heat transfer; and the textbook is intended only to supplement the informed judgment of the qualified user. This textbook provides methodologies that may or may not have predictive capability when applied to a specific set of factual circumstances. Lack of accurate predictions by any particular methodology, calculation, or fire modeling application could lead to erroneous conclusions with regard to fire safety. All results should be evaluated by an informed user.

Throughout this document, the mention of products or commercial software does not constitute endorsement by the authors or Pearson Education, nor does it indicate that the products are necessarily those best suited for the intended purpose.

Library of Congress Cataloging-in-Publication Data

Names: Icove, David J., 1949- author. | Haynes, Gerald A. (Firefighter),
     author. | based on (work): Kirk, Paul L. (Paul Leland), 1902-1970. Kirk's fire investigation.
Title: Kirk's fire investigation / David J. Icove, Ph.D., P.E., board
     certified, fellow, National Academy of Forensic Engineers, The University
     of Tennessee, Gerald A. Haynes, M.S., P.E., board certified, fellow,
     National Academy of Forensic Engineers, Forensic Fire Analysis, LLC.
Other titles: Fire investigation.
Description: Eighth edition. | NY, NY : Pearson, [2018] | Revised edtion of:
     Kirk's fire investigation / John D. DeHaan, David J. Icove. 2012. | Includes bibliographical references and index.
Identifiers: LCCN 2017030182| ISBN 9780134237923 (hardcover) | ISBN 0134237927 (hardcover)
Subjects: LCSH: Fire investigation.
Classification: LCC TH9180 .K5 2018 | DDC 363.37/65—dc23 LC record available at https://lccn.loc.gov/2017030182

4 2020

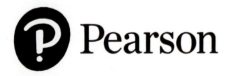

ISBN 10:   0-13-423792-7
ISBN 13: 978-0-13-423792-3

DEDICATION

The authors dedicate this eighth edition of Kirk's Fire Investigation to Dr. Vytenis (Vyto) Babrauskas, Fire Science and Technology Inc., San Diego, California.

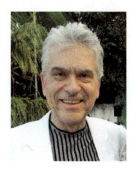

Dr. Babrauskas has his Bachelor's degree from Swarthmore College in Physics followed by an M.S. degree in Structural Engineering and a Ph.D. degree in Fire Protection Engineering from the University of California, Berkeley. He was the first person ever to be awarded a Ph.D. degree in Fire Protection Engineering.

A Principal Member of the *NFPA 921* and *NFPA 901* Committees, Dr. Babrauskas single handedly has contributed much to the field of fire and explosion investigation. His keynote textbook, the Ignition Handbook, is a must-have reference in the field.

The authors recognize Dr. Babrauskas for his past, present, and continuing contributions.

CONTENTS

Chapter 2 The Basic Science and Dynamics of Fire 59

Chapter 3 Chemical Fires and Explosions 173

Chapter 7 Fires by Property Type 440

Part 1: General Principles 441

Chapter 9 Fire Modeling 604

Chapter 10 Fire Testing 628

More has changed in the last year in the field of fire investigation than in all the years since the 1969 publication of the first edition of *Fire Investigation* by Dr. Paul L. Kirk and the 2004 publication of the first edition of *Forensic Fire Scene Reconstruction*. Dr. Paul L. Kirk was a professor of biochemistry and criminalistics at the University of California at Berkeley, but it was his specialty of microchemistry that focused his attention on physical evidence and its analysis. In 1953, he wrote the landmark text, *Crime Investigation*, and maintained a private criminalistics consulting practice where he became involved in a wide variety of fire and explosion cases. He published *Fire Investigation* in 1969 as the first textbook on fire investigation written by a scientist rather than a fire investigator. Dr. Kirk remained in charge of the criminalistics program at Berkeley until his death in 1970 and launched the careers of many criminalists who now practice around the world. His concern with using science to solve the puzzles of fires and explosions presaged the current emphasis on using the scientific method to investigate fires by more than 30 years. It is in honor of Dr. Kirk's pioneering work in bringing science to fire investigation that his name remains included in the title, *Kirk's Fire Investigation*, and the spirit, of this text. No longer is the investigation of fires just limited to inspecting the ruins, asking questions of the witnesses, and applying basic common sense and observations to determine the fire's origin and cause. Fire investigators must now keep in step with the rapid changes in the forensic sciences, the innovations in fire scene documentation, and challenges in the court stressing precise defensible expert testimonies.

Dr. John D. DeHaan became the author of **Kirk's** in 1980, at the request of the then publisher, John Wiley & Sons. His involvement with international fire, explosion, and forensic professional organizations provided a wide variety of knowledge and the opportunity to share techniques and information with many renowned experts. His Ph.D. research was on the development of layers of flammable liquid vapors (University of Strathclyde, 1995). After more than 30 years however, Dr. DeHaan felt it was time for a newer generation of authors with skills in the engineering applications required of today's investigators to take the lead.

The eighth edition of *Kirk's Fire Investigation* blends the seventh edition of *Kirk's* with the third edition of *Forensic Fire Scene Reconstruction*. The design of this new textbook meets the emerging forensic challenges. *Kirk's* still ranks as the foremost authoritative text for training as well as an expert treatise for fire investigation professionals. It also serves as a bridge textbook providing interoperation of the concepts presented in the latest editions of the National Fire Protection Association (NFPA) *Guide for Fire and Explosion Investigation* (NFPA 921), *Standard for Professional Qualifications for Fire Investigator* (NFPA 1033), and related standards of care.

The premier aspect of *Kirk's* is that it maintains its role as the leading peer-reviewed and widely cited expert treatise in the fire investigation field. Concepts and investigative techniques presented are supported by peer-reviewed references and have already gained general acceptance in the fire and explosion investigation field. Notwithstanding, *Kirk's* ability to assimilate and interpret emerging techniques typically outpaces the publication of *NFPA 921* and other standards of care, and can be safely relied upon by expert witnesses.

Because forensic fire scene documentation is emerging as the cornerstone in nearly all judicially contested investigations, modest reconstructive efforts such as repositioning furniture and other post-fire artifacts into pre-fire positions no longer suffice. Therefore, during scene documentation, today's fire investigator must possess skill in scientifically based fire pattern analysis and must employ analytical methodologies based on expert interpretation of discernible patterns and fire dynamics principles.

Delving deeply into the forensic fire protection engineering field, this eighth edition of *Kirk's* covers engineering calculations and fire modeling, and features several exhaustive case studies that leverage the current technology explained in depth throughout the text. Several specialized topic areas also are covered, including use of scanning and panoramic photography, preparation of comprehensive reports, the ignition matrix, expert testimony, and computer modeling and laser imaging. Also included is an advanced discussion of tenability.

Paving the way for those investigators who seek to take their forensic investigation skills to the next level, this new edition emphasizes the need to use the scientific method and details the need-to-know information behind developing a working hypothesis. Readers are also thoroughly prepared for the courtroom with this guide, which teaches investigators how to form and authoritatively present their expert testimony.

Kirk's eighth edition is the most in-depth textbook in the field of fire investigation on the subject of arson crime scene analysis and examining motive as it relates to fire setting. For investigators seeking to gain a deeper and more advanced understanding of fire protection engineering concepts, technology, and analysis in the field of fire investigation, *Kirk's* takes readers to the next level of expertise.

About This Book

Forensic fire investigations go well beyond establishing what furnishings were present and where they were originally placed. Fire scene analysis and reconstruction involves identification and documentation of all relevant features of the fire scene—materials, dimensions, location, and physical evidence—that help identify fuels and establish human activities and contacts. This information, placed in context with principles of fire engineering and human behavior, is used to evaluate various scenarios of the origin, cause, and development of the fire and the interaction of people with it.

This textbook is intended for use by a broad range of both public and private sector individuals in the investigative, forensic, engineering, and judicial sectors. Intended users include the following:

- Public safety officials charged with the responsibility of investigating fires;
- Prosecutors of arson and fire-related crimes who seek to add to their capabilities of evaluating evidence and presenting technical details to a nontechnical judge and jury;
- Judicial officials seeking to better comprehend the technical details of cases over which they preside;
- Private-sector investigators, adjusters, and attorneys representing the insurance industry who have the responsibility of processing claims or otherwise have a vested interest in determining responsibility for the start or cause of a fire;
- Citizens and civic community service organizations committed to conducting public awareness programs designed to reduce the threat of fire and its devastating effect on the economy; and
- Scientists, engineers, academicians, and students engaged in the education process pertaining to forensic fire scene reconstruction.

A thorough understanding of fire dynamics is valuable in applying forensic engineering techniques. This book describes and illustrates the latest interpretations of systematic approaches for reconstructing fire scenes. These approaches apply the principles of fire protection engineering along with those of forensic science and behavioral science.

Using historical fire cases, both in the textbook, the authors provide new lessons and insight into the ignition, growth, development, and outcome of those fires. All documentation in the case examples follows or exceeds the methodology set forth by the NFPA in both the 2017 edition of *NFPA 921: Guide for Fire and Explosion Investigations* and its companion standard, the 2014 edition of *NFPA 1033: Standard for Professional*

Qualifications for Fire Investigator. This text includes the real-world case examples to illustrate the concepts that shed new light on the forensic science, fire engineering, and human factor issues. Each example is illustrated using the guidelines from *NFPA 921* and *Kirk's Fire Investigation*. In cases where fire engineering analysis or fire modeling is applicable, these techniques are explored.

The authors acknowledge the numerous essential references from the Society of Fire Protection Engineers (SFPE) that form the basis for much of the material included in this textbook. These essential references, ranging from core principles of fire science to human behavior, include the *SFPE Handbook of Fire Protection Engineering* and many of SFPE's engineering practice guides.

New to This Edition

The eighth edition is one of the most adventurous editions over the last decade. Fully updated and streamlined from the previous edition, the eighth edition of *Kirk's* offers the latest information on investigative technologies and innovative documentation techniques.

The following highlights are changes to this edition that set it apart from previous ones:

- Meets the FESHE guidelines for Fire Investigation and Analysis, with correlations to the 2017 Edition of *NFPA 921 and* the 2014 Edition of *NFPA 1033*.
- Emphasizes and cross-references the critical Job Performance Requirements (JPRs) of *NFPA 1033* for fire investigators.
- Provides background for *NFPA 1033*'s "Basic Sixteen" knowledge requirements.
- Includes the latest information on applying the scientific method to fire investigations, particularly with the use of *Bilancia Ignition Matrix*™.
- Nearly all photos are now in color, making interpretation by the reader easier.
- Updated, in-depth case examples demonstrate the use of forensic fire investigation and analysis approaches.
- Comprehensive glossary of terms used throughout the textbook provides the latest definitions of common forensic fire investigation terminologies.
- The textbook is included in required and supplemental fire investigation professional training and certification programs by the National Fire Academy, the International Association of Arson Investigators (IAAI), and the National Association of Fire Investigators (NAFI).
- Provides the essential information required in preparing for the International Association of Arson Investigator's (IAAI) *Fire Investigation Technician (IAAI-FIT)* and *Evidence Collection Technician (IAAI-ECT)* Examinations.
- Provides websites for both instructors and students, including problem sets from NIST, NFPA, US Department of Justice, and the US Chemical Safety and Hazard Assessment Board.

Hallmark Features

- Describes a systematic approach to reconstructing fire scenes in which investigators rely on the combined principles of fire protection engineering along with forensic and behavioral science.
- Describes the scientific underpinnings of how fire patterns are produced and how they can be used by investigators in assessing fire damage and determining a fire's origin.
- Details the systematic approach needed to support forensic fire analysis and reports.
- Reviews the techniques used in the analysis of arsonists' motives and intents.
- Discusses the use of various mathematical, physical, and computer-assisted techniques for modeling fires, explosions, and the movement of people.

- Provides an in-depth examination of the impact and tenability of fires on humans.
- Reviews the applicable standard forensic laboratory and fire testing methods that are important to fire scene analysis and reconstruction.

Scope of the Book

Kirk's Fire Investigation is divided into the following chapters, which flow logically and build on one another:

Chapter 1, "Principles of Fire Investigation," describes the foundation and background of the rapidly developing field of determining origin and cause of fires. It presents a systematic approach to reconstructing fire scenes in which investigators rely on the combined principles of fire protection engineering along with forensic and behavioral science. Using this approach, the investigator can more accurately document a structural fire's origin, intensity, growth, direction of travel, and duration as well as the behavior of the occupants.

Chapter 2, "The Basic Science and Dynamics of Fire," provides the investigator with a firm understanding of the phenomenon of fire, heat release rates of common materials, heat transfer, growth and development, fire plumes, and enclosure fires.

Chapter 3, "Chemical Fires and Explosions," provides the fire investigator with a thorough coverage of the interrelationships of chemical fires and explosions, hazard classification systems. Significant contributions to this chapter were provided by Dr. Elizabeth Buc, an internationally recognized expert in the field.

Chapter 4, "Sources of Ignition," explores existing and new methodologies of investigating and identifying competent sources of ignition. This approach uses the Bilancia Ignition Matrix™ method to ensure that exhaustive hypotheses are systematically generated per the scientific method.

Chapter 5, "Fire Scene Examination," describes the science and engineering underpinnings of how fire patterns are used by investigators in assessing fire damage and determining a fire's origin. Fire patterns are often the only remaining visible evidence after a fire is extinguished. The ability to document and interpret fire pattern damage accurately is a skill of paramount importance to investigators when they are reconstructing fire scenes.

Chapter 6, "Fire Scene Documentation," details a systematic approach needed to support forensic analysis and reports. The purpose of forensic fire scene documentation includes recording visual observations, emphasizing fire development characteristics, and authenticating and protecting physical evidence. The underlying theme is that thorough documentation produces sound investigations and courtroom presentations. The chapter includes commentaries on new technologies useful in improving the accuracy and comprehensiveness of documentation.

Chapter 7, "Fires by Property Type," describes the principles of fuels, ignition, and fire behavior with which investigators should be reasonably familiar before undertaking the probe of a fire. This chapter covers structural, wildland, motor vehicle, and ship fires. It also discusses the necessity of having a clear understanding of the purposes and goals of the investigation and a rational, orderly plan for carrying it out to meet those purposes, as well as the value and limitations of post-fire indicators and the basic physical processes that create them.

Chapter 8, "Forensic Laboratory Services," describes the role of laboratory services in fire and explosion investigation and the types of examinations that can be requested. These include not only fire debris analysis but the application of a wide range of physical, chemical, optical, and instrumental tools on a variety of substances.

Chapter 9, "Fire Modeling," discusses the use of various mathematical, physical, and computer-assisted techniques for modeling fires, explosions, and the movement of people. Numerous models are explored, along with their strengths and weaknesses. Several case examples are also presented.

Chapter 10, "Fire Testing," describes how despite governmental regulations, fires in which fabrics are the first materials to be ignited are still a very common occurrence. The chapter discusses the nature of common fabrics and upholstery materials and their contributions to both ignition hazard and fuel load in current studies.

Chapter 11, "Arson Crime Scene Analysis," reviews the techniques used in the analysis of arsonists' motives and intents. It presents nationally accepted motive-based classification guidelines along with case examples of the crimes of vandalism, excitement, revenge, crime concealment, and arson-for-profit. The geography of serial arson is also examined, along with techniques for profiling the targets selected by arsonists.

Chapter 12, "Fire Deaths and Injuries," provides an in-depth examination of the impact and tenability of fires on humans. The chapter examines what kills people in fires, namely their exposure to by-products of combustion, toxic gases, and heat. It also examines the predictable fire burn pattern damage inflicted on human bodies and summarizes postmortem tests and forensic examinations desirable in comprehensive death investigations.

The **Appendices** contain a short refresher lesson on scientific notations and calculations.

Peer Reviewers

Peer review is important for ensuring that a textbook is well balanced, useful, authoritative, and accurate. The following individuals, agencies, institutions, and companies provided invaluable support during the peer-review process in the present and past editions of *Kirk's Fire Investigation* and *Forensic Fire Scene Reconstruction*.

Dr. Vytenis (Vyto) Babrauskas, Fire Science and Technology Inc., San Diego, California

John Bailot, MPA, IAAI-CFI, EMT-P, Adjunct Faculty, St. Louis Community College – Forest Park, St. Louis, Missouri

David M. Banwarth, P.E., Fire Protection Engineer, David M. Banwarth Associates, LLC, Dayton, Maryland

Richard L. Bennett, Associate Professor of Fire Protection & Emergency Services, The University of Akron, Akron, Ohio

Dr. Elizabeth C. Buc, P.E., CFI, Fire and Materials Research Lab, LLC, Livonia, Michigan

Dr. John L. Bryan, Professor Emeritus, University of Maryland, Department of Fire Protection Engineering, College Park, Maryland (deceased)

Charlie Butterfield, M. Ed., NRP, CFO, Professor, Fire Service Administration Program, Idaho State University, Pocatello, Idaho

Brian Carlson, MS, Fire Science, University of Cincinnati, Ohio

Guy E. "Sandy" Burnette, Jr., Attorney, Tallahassee, Florida

Steven W. Carman, MS, Fire Protection Engineering, IAAI-CFI, Owner, Carman & Associates Fire Investigation, Grass Valley, California

Jody Cooper, IAAI-CFI, CVFI, Owner/investigator, JJMA Investigations LLC, and Instructor, Oklahoma State University, Poteau, Oklahoma

Carl E. Chasteen, BS, CPM, FABC, Chief of Forensic Services, Florida Division of State Fire Marshal, Havana, Florida

Robert F. Duval, National Fire Protection Association, Quincy, Massachusetts

Mark Fyffe, MPA, BS, Fire and Safety Engineering, Adjunct Professor, University of Cincinnati, Ohio

Christopher Gauss, IAAI-CFI, Captain, Baltimore County Fire Investigation, Towson, Maryland

Dr. Gregory E. Gorbett, MScFPE, CFEI, IAAI-CFI, Associate Professor/FPSET Program Coordinator, Eastern Kentucky University, Richmond, Kentucky

Kristopher Grod, Professional License, Higher-Ed Instructor, Certified Firefighter 1 & 2, Northcentral Technical College, Wausau, Wisconsin

Gary S. Hodson, Utah Valley University, Utah Fire and Rescue Academy, Utah

William Jetter, Doctorate, Higher-Ed Instructor, Fire Safety Management, Hazardous and Solid Waste, Health and Safety, Fire Science, Cincinnati, Ohio

Patrick M. Kennedy (deceased), National Association of Fire Investigators, Sarasota, Florida

Frederick J. Knipper, Fayetteville State University, Durham, North Carolina

Chris W. Korinek, P.E., Synergy Technologies, LLC, Arbor Vitae, Wisconsin

Richard E. Korinek, P.E., Synergy Technologies, LLC, Arbor Vitae, Wisconsin

Daniel Madrzykowski, Underwriters Laboratories, Gaithersburg, Maryland

John E. "Jack" Malooly, Bureau of Alcohol, Tobacco, Firearms and Explosives, Chicago, Illinois (retired)

Michael Marquardt, Bureau of Alcohol, Tobacco, Firearms and Explosives, Grand Rapids, Michigan

J. Ron McCardle, Bureau of Fire and Arson Investigations, Florida Division of State Fire Marshal (retired)

Irvin Miller, Masters, Stanford Certified Project Manager, Graduate certificate Homeland Security, Fire Prevention management and Organization, Texas A & M University San Antonio, Texas

C. W. Munson, Captain, Long Beach Fire Department, California (retired)

Bradley E. Olsen, BS, Fire Science Management, Southern Illinois University; Fire Captain, City of Madison Fire Department, Madison, Wisconsin

Robert R. Rielage, former State Fire Marshal, Ohio Division of State Fire Marshal, Reynoldsburg, Ohio

James Ryan, Investigator, New York State Office of Fire Prevention & Control, New York

Dr. Robert Svare, Isanti, Minnesota.

Michael Schlatman, Fire Consulting International Inc., Shawnee Mission, Kansas

Nathan Sivils, BS, Industrial Distribution, Director of Fire Science, Blinn College, Brenham, Texas

Carina Tejada, BA, Mathematics QAS, Marietta, Georgia

Robert K. Toth, Iris Fire, LLC, Parker, Colorado

Luis Velazco, Bureau of Alcohol, Tobacco, Firearms and Explosives, Brunswick, Georgia, (retired)

Dr. Qingsheng Wang, P.E., ASSE, SFPE, Higher-Ed Instructor, Oklahoma State University, Stillwater, Oklahoma

ACKNOWLEDGMENTS

We have many people to thank for both their help on and their inspiration for this and past editions of this book, including the many individuals and present and past employees at the following institutions and agencies.

David M. Banwarth Associates, LLC, Dayton, Maryland: David M. Banwarth, P. E.

Bureau of Alcohol, Tobacco, Firearms and Explosives (ATF): Steve Carman (retired), Steve Avato, Dennis C. Kennamer (retired), Dr. David Sheppard, Jack Malooly (retired), Wayne Miller (retired), Michael Marquardt, Luis Velaszco (retired), John Mirocha (retired), Ken Steckler (retired), Brian Grove, John Allen, and Jeffrey E. Theodore.

J. H. Burgoyne & Partners (UK): Robin Holleyhead and Roy Cooke

Chambliss, Banner & Stophel, P.C., Chattanooga, Tennessee: Jeffrey, G. Granillo, Richard W. Bethea, William Dearing, and John G. Jackson

Donan Engineering, LLC: Sandra K. Wesson, James Enos, James Caton, and Thomas R. May

Eastern Kentucky University: Dr. Gregory E. Gorbett, James L. Pharr, Dr. Andrew Tinsley, and Ronald L. Hopkins (retired)

Federal Bureau of Investigation (FBI): Richard L. Ault (retired), Dr. Stephen R. Band, S. Annette Bartlett, James E. Bentley, Jr. (retired), Dr. John Henry Campbell (retired), Theodore E. Childress (deceased), R. Joe Clark (retired), Dr. Roger L. Depue (retired), Jon Eyer (retired), William Hagmaier (retired), Joseph A. Harpold (retired), Robert "Roy" Hazelwood (deceased), Timothy G. Huff (retired), Edwin Kelly (deceased), Sharon A. Kelly (retired), John L. Larsen (retired), Dr. James A. O'Connor (retired), John E. Otto (retired), Rex W. Ownby (retired), Robert K. Ressler (deceased), Dr. William L. Tafoya (retired), Dr. Howard "Bud" Teten (retired), Scott A. Wenger, Arthur E. Westveer (deceased), and Eric Witzig (retired)

Fire and Materials Research Lab, LLC.: Dr. Elizabeth C. Buc, P.E., Livonia, Michigan

Mark A. Campbell, Fire Forensic Research, Colorado.

Fire Safety Institute: Dr. John M. "Jack" Watts, Jr.

Fire Science and Technology: Dr. Vyto Babrauskas

Forensic Fire Analysis: Lester Rich

Gardiner Associates: Mick Gardiner, Jim Munday, and Jack Deans

Goodson Engineering, Denton, Texas: Mark Goodson, P.E. and Lee Green, P.E.

Rodger H. Ide

Iris Fire, LLC, Parker, Colorado: Robert K. Toth

Israel National Police, Jerusalem: Shalom Tsaroom (retired), Arnon Grafit, Dr. Dan Muller, Ran Shelef, Dana Sonenfeld, and Myriam Azoury

Kent Archaeological Field School, UK: Dr. Paul Wilkinson and Catherine Wilkinson

Knox County (Tennessee) Sheriff's Office: Carleton E. Bryant, IV; Knox County Fire Investigation Unit: Det. Michael W. Dalton (retired); Inv. Shawn Short; Inv. Greg Lampkin; Det. Aaron Allen; Inv. Michael Patrick; Inv. Daniel Johnson; Kathy Saunders, Knox County Fire Marshal

Knoxville Fire Department, Tennessee: Asst. Chief Danny Beeler

Leica Geosystems: Rick Bukowski and Tony Grissim

Mesa County Sheriff's Office, Colorado: Benjamin J. Miller

Metropolitan Police Forensic Lab, Fire Investigation Unit, London (UK): Roger Berrett (retired)

McKinney (Texas) Fire Department: Chief Mark Wallace

Murder Accountability Project: Thomas K. Hargrove and Eric Witzig

National Academy of Forensic Engineers: Michael D. Leshner, P.E.

National Institute of Standards and Technology (NIST): Richard W. Bukowski, Dr. William Grosshandler (retired), Dan Madrzykowski (retired), and Dr. Kevin McGrattan

National Museum of Bermuda: Dr. Edward C. Harris

New Hampshire State Fire Marshal's Office: J. William Degnan, Donald P. Bliss (retired)

New South Wales Fire Brigades: Ross Brogan (retired)

Nistico, Crouch & Kessler, P.C.: Kathleen Crouch and Rachel Wall

Novato Fire Protection District: Assistant Chief Forrest Craig

Ohio State Fire Marshal's Office, Reynoldsburg: Eugene Jewell (deceased), Charles G. McGrath (retired), Mohamed M. Gohar (retired), J. David Schroeder (retired), Jack Pyle (deceased), Harry Barber, Lee Bethune, Joseph Boban, Kenneth Crawford, Dennis Cummings, Dennis Cupp, Robert Davis, Robert Dunn, Donald Eifler, Ralph Ford, James Harting (retired), Robert Lawless, Keith Loreno, Mike McCarroll, Matthew J. Hartnett, Brian Peterman, Mike Simmons, Rick Smith, Stephen W. Southard, and David Whitaker (retired)

Panoscan: Ted Chavalas

Precision Simulators, Inc.: Kirk McKenzie

Quist, Fitzpatrick & Jarrard, PLLC, Knoxville, Tennessee: Michael A. Durr

Richland (Washington) Fire Department: Glenn Johnson and Grant Baynes

Sacramento County (California) Fire Department: Jeff Campbell (retired)

Saint Paul (Minnesota) Fire Department: Jamie Novak

Santa Ana (California) Fire Department: Jim Albers (retired) and Bob Eggleston (retired)

Seneca College School of Fire Protection Engineering Technology: David McGill

Tarrant County (Texas) Office of the Medical Examiner: Dr. Nizam Peerwani, Ronald L. Singer.

Tennessee State Fire Marshal's Office: Richard L. Garner (retired), Robert Pollard, Eugene Hartsook (deceased), and Jesse L. Hodge (retired)

Tennessee Valley Authority (TVA): Carolyn M. Blocher, James E. Carver (retired), R. Douglas Norman (retired), Larry W. Ridinger (retired), Sidney G. Whitehurst (retired), and Norman Zigrossi (retired)

Texas State Fire Marshal's Office: Chris Connealy

Underwriters Laboratories(UL): Dr. J. Thomas Chapin, Dr. Pravinray D. Gandhi, P.E., and Dan Madrzykowski, P.E.

University of Arkansas, Department of Anthropology: Dr. Elayne J. Pope, now at Office of the Chief Medical Examiner Tidewater District, Norfolk, Virginia

University of Edinburgh, Department of Civil Engineering: Professor Emeritus Dr. Dougal Drysdale

University of Maryland, Department of Fire Protection Engineering: Dr. John L. Bryan (Emeritus), Dr. James A. Milke, Dr. Frederick W. Mowrer (Emeritus), Dr. James G. Quintiere (Emeritus), Dr. Marino di Marzo, and Dr. Steven M. Spivak (Emeritus)

University of Tennessee: Dr. A. J. Baker, Dr. William M. Bass, Dr. Wayne Davis, Samir M. El-Ghazaly, Dr. Rafael C. Gonzalez, Sonja Hill, Dr. Michael Langston, Dr. Evans Lyne, Dr. Matthew M. Mench, Lindsey K. Miller, Dr. Masood Parang, Dr. Leon Tolbert, Dr. M. Osama Soliman, Dr. Dawnie Wolfe Steadman, Dr. Jerry Stoneking (deceased), and the many students in the Fire Protection Engineering concentration courses.

US Attorney's Office: Jack B. Hood, Jason R. Cheek, and Gary Brown

US Consumer Products Safety Commission: Gerard Naylis (retired) and Carol Cave

US Fire Administration, Federal Emergency Management Agency (FEMA): Edward
J. Kaplan, Kenneth J. Kuntz (retired), Robert A. Neale (retired), Dr. Denis
Onieal, Lester Rich
US Nuclear Regulatory Commission: Mark Henry Salley, P.E.

Our sincere, heartfelt thanks go to everyone who reviewed the early manuscripts,
addressed technical questions, and made many beneficial suggestions as to the format and
content of this textbook.

A very special mention goes to our development editor Carol Lazerick; our copyeditor,
Bret Workman; proofreader Karen Jones; and Lisa Narine, Portfolio Management Assistant.

Also, special thanks go to our families and close friends over the years for their patient
support.

ABOUT THE AUTHORS

This textbook is coauthored by two of the most experienced forensic fire protection engineers in the United States. Their combined talents total more than 100 years of experience in the fields of fire service, behavioral science, fire protection engineering, fire behavior, investigation, criminalistics, and crime scene reconstruction.

An internationally recognized forensic fire engineering expert with more than 45 years of experience, Dr. Icove is coauthor of *Kirk's Fire Investigation,* 7th ed., *Forensic Fire Scene Reconstruction*, both leading treatises in the field, and *Combating Arson-for-Profit,* the leading textbook on the crime of economic arson. Since 1992 he has served and maintained an appointment as a principal member of the *NFPA 921 Technical Committee on Fire Investigations.* He is also chair of *NPFA 901 – Committee on Fire Reporting.*

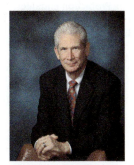

David J. Icove, PhD, PE, CFEI-NAFI, CFI-IAAI, F. SFPE, F. NAFE
Photo courtesy of the University of Tennessee, College of Engineering.

As a retired career federal law enforcement agent, Dr. Icove served as a criminal investigator on the federal, state, and local levels. He is a Registered Professional Engineer, a Certified Fire Investigator (CFI) from the International Association of Arson Investigators, a Certified Fire and Explosion Investigator (CFEI) from the National Association of Fire Investigators, a Fellow in the Society of Fire Protection Engineers, and a Board Certified Diplomat and Fellow in the National Academy of Forensic Engineers (NAFE).

He retired in 2005 as an Inspector in the Criminal Investigations Division of the US Tennessee Valley Authority (TVA) Police, Knoxville, Tennessee, where he was assigned for his last 2 years to the Federal Bureau of Investigation (FBI) Joint Terrorism Task Force (JTTF). In addition to conducting major case investigations, Dr. Icove oversaw the development of advanced fire investigation training and technology programs in cooperation with various agencies, including the Federal Emergency Management Agency's (FEMA's) US Fire Administration.

Before transferring to the US TVA Police in 1993, he served 9 years as a program manager in the elite Behavioral Science and Criminal Profiling Units at the FBI, Quantico, Virginia. At the FBI, he implemented and became the first supervisor of the Arson and Bombing Investigative Support (ABIS) Program, staffed by FBI and ATF criminal profilers. Prior to his work at the FBI, Dr. Icove served as a criminal investigator at arson bureaus of the Knoxville Police Department, the Ohio State Fire Marshal's Office, and the Tennessee State Fire Marshal's Office.

His expertise in forensic fire scene reconstruction is based on a blend of on-scene experience, conducting of fire tests and experiments, and participation in prison interviews of convicted arsonists and bombers. He has testified as an expert witness in civil and criminal trials, as well as before US congressional committees seeking guidance on key arson investigation and legislative initiatives.

Dr. Icove holds BS and MS degrees in Electrical Engineering and a PhD in Engineering Science and Mechanics from the University of Tennessee. He also holds a BS degree in Fire Protection Engineering from the University of Maryland–College Park. He is currently the UL Professor of Practice in the Department of Electrical Engineering and Computer Science at the University of Tennessee, Knoxville; serves on the faculty of the University of Maryland's Professional Master of Engineering in Fire Protection program; and serves as an Investigator in the Knox County Fire Investigation Unit and as a Reserve Deputy Sheriff for the Knox County Sheriff's Office, Knoxville, Tennessee.

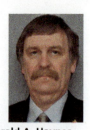

**Gerald A. Haynes,
PE, DFE, CFPS, CFEI, CVFI
Fire Protection Engineer
Haynes and Associates,
LLC**

*Photo courtesy of Gerald
A. Haynes, PE.*

Gerald A. Haynes is a registered Professional Engineer with more than 40 years of experience in the field of Fire Protection. He holds both Bachelor of Science and Masters of Science degrees in Fire Protection Engineering from the University of Maryland—College Park. He is currently the President of Haynes and Associates, LLC and serves as an adjunct lecturer for the Office of Advanced Engineering Education at the University of Maryland.

Mr. Haynes' experience includes work at the U.S. Department of Justice, Bureau of Alcohol, Tobacco, Firearms and Explosives and the U.S. Department of Commerce, National Institute of Standards and Technology Building and Fire Research Laboratory. His experience is multi-dimensional, including municipal fire service, fire and explosion investigations, complex case analysis and engineering support, and military service. He has provided testimony as an expert witness in state and federal courts in cases related to fire cause and fire testing protocols. He has conducted numerous presentations in the U.S. and internationally in the areas of fire dynamics, fire modeling and forensic fire engineering analysis. He currently is a member of numerous professional organizations, including the Society of Fire Protection Engineers (SFPE), the National Academy of Forensic Engineers (NAFE), the National Society of Professional Engineers (NSPE), the National Fire Protection Association (NFPA), the International Association of Arson Investigators (IAAI), the National Association of Fire Investigators, (NAFI) and ASTM International. He is a former member of the technical committees of NFPA 921 Guide for Fire and Explosion Investigations, and NFPA 1033 Standard for Professional Qualifications for Fire Investigator.

COURSE DESCRIPTION

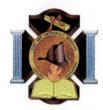

This course examines the technical, investigative, legal, and social aspects of arson, including principles of incendiary fire analysis and detection, environmental and psychological factors of arson, legal considerations, intervention, and mitigation strategies.

The National Fire Academy–developed Fire and Emergency Services Higher Education (FESHE) curriculum serves as a national training program guideline that is a requirement for many fire service organizations and training programs. The following grid outlines Fire Investigation and Analysis course requirements and where specific content can be located within this text.

Course Requirements	Chapter												
	1	2	3	4	5	6	7	8	9	10	11	12	13
Demonstrate a technical understanding of the characteristics and impacts of fire loss and the crime of arson necessary to conduct competent fire investigation and analysis.	X	X	X	X	X	X	X	X	X	X	X	X	X
Document the fire scene, in accordance with best practice and legal requirements.	X				X	X	X	X	X	X	X	X	X
Analyze the fire scenario utilizing the scientific method, fire science, and relevant technology.	X	X	X	X	X	X	X	X	X	X	X	X	X
Analyze the legal foundation for conducting a systematic incendiary fire investigation and case preparation.	X				X	X	X	X	X	X	X	X	X
Design and integrate a variety of arson related intervention and mitigation strategies.	X						X				X	X	X

Professional Levels of Job Performance for Fire Investigators as Cited in *NFPA 1033*, 2014 Edition

General Requirements for a Fire Investigator	**4.1.2** Employ all elements of the scientific method as the operating analytical process **4.1.3** Complete site safety assessments on all scenes **4.1.4** Maintain necessary liaison with other interested professionals and entities **4.1.5** Adhere to all applicable legal and regulatory requirements **4.1.6** Understand the organization and operation of the investigative team and incident management system
Scene Examination	**4.2.1** Secure the fire ground **4.2.2** Conduct an exterior survey **4.2.3** Conduct an interior survey **4.2.4** Interpret fire patterns **4.2.5** Interpret and analyze fire patterns **4.2.6** Examine and remove fire debris **4.2.7** Reconstruct the area of origin **4.2.8** Inspect the performance of building systems **4.2.9** Discriminate the effects of explosions from other types of damage
Documenting the Scene	**4.3.1** Diagram the scene **4.3.2** Photographically document the scene **4.3.3** Construct investigative notes
Evidence Collection and Preservation	**4.4.1** Utilize proper procedures for managing victims and fatalities **4.4.2** Locate, collect, and package evidence **4.4.3** Select evidence for analysis **4.4.4** Maintain a chain of custody **4.4.5** Dispose of evidence
Interview	**4.5.1** Develop an interview plan **4.5.2** Conduct interviews **4.5.3** Evaluate interview information
Post-Incident Investigation	**4.6.1** Gather reports and records **4.6.2** Evaluate the investigative file **4.6.3** Coordinate expert resources **4.6.4** Establish evidence as to motive and/or opportunity **4.6.5** Formulate an opinion concerning origin, cause, or responsibility for the fire
Presentations	**4.7.1** Prepare a written report **4.7.2** Express investigative findings verbally **4.7.3** Testify during legal proceedings **4.7.4** Conduct public informational presentations

Source: NFPA 1033: Standard for Professional Qualifications for Fire Investigator. Published by National Fire Protection Association, © 2014.

CHAPTER 1

Principles of Fire Investigation

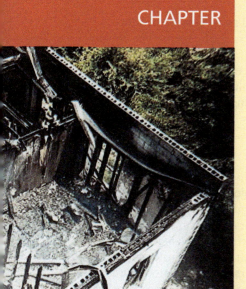

Courtesy of David J. Icove, University of Tennessee.

OBJECTIVES

After reading this chapter, you should be able to:

- Describe the role of fire investigators in their determination of the origin, cause, and development of a fire or explosion.
- Identify the major peer-reviewed publications in the field of fire investigation.
- Explain the impact of *NFPA 921* and *NFPA 1033* on scientific fire investigations and expert testimony.
- Explain scope and impact in the field of fire investigation of job performance responsibilities (JPR) expected from both public and private sector investigators.
- Explain the problem of the reporting of fire loss statistics in the United States and the United Kingdom, particularly in the estimation of incendiary fires.

- Discuss the levels of confidence as applied to expert opinions in fire and explosion investigations.
- Explain the need for science in fire investigation and scene reconstruction.
- Demonstrate an understanding of how to apply the scientific method in fire and explosion investigations.
- List the seven basic steps used in the systematic process of the scientific method.
- Describe the foundations of expert testimony as applied to fire scene investigation.
- Explain the concept of developing alternative working hypotheses.

1.1 Fire Investigation

origin ▪ The general location where a fire or explosion began (NFPA 2017, pt. 3.3.133).

fire ▪ A rapid oxidation process, which is a chemical reaction resulting in the evolution of light and heat in varying intensities; uncontrolled combustion (NFPA 2017, pt. 3.3.66).

explosion ▪ The sudden conversion of potential energy (chemical or mechanical) into kinetic energy with the production and release of gases under pressure, or the release of gas under pressure. These high-pressure gases then do mechanical work such as moving, changing, or shattering nearby materials (NFPA 2017, pt. 3.3.56).

cause ▪ The circumstances, conditions, or agencies that brought about or resulted in the fire or explosion incident, damage to property resulting from the fire or explosion incident, or bodily injury or loss of life resulting from the fire or explosion incident (NFPA 2017, pt. 3.3.26).

arson ▪ The crime of maliciously and intentionally, or recklessly, starting a fire or causing an explosion (NFPA 2017, pt. 3.3.14).

This text focuses on the field of fire investigation, which is the formal process of determining the **origin**, cause, and development of a **fire** or **explosion**. Often called a **fire origin and cause** (O&C) investigation, the probe is launched after a fire or explosion is extinguished and investigators strive to determine what circumstances caused or contributed to the incident. Due to the complex nature of the event, where a fire often distorts or destroys the evidence, fire investigation is among the most difficult of the forensic sciences to practice. Not knowing whether the fire was **incendiary** or **arson**, investigators must prove or disprove any allegations or suspicions and piece together the pre- and post-fire events. If the investigation indicates that a fire was deliberately set, reasonable **accidental fire** causes must be evaluated and eliminated.

The latest edition of *Kirk's Fire Investigation* is considered the leading authoritative text and legal expert treatise in the field. The text is used both for training and as the basis for certification in many jurisdictions. A majority of the overall methodology of fire investigation relies upon *Kirk's*, as well as on the following three peer-reviewed sources:

- The third edition of *Forensic Fire Scene Reconstruction*, published in 2013, is also considered a leading forensic text that serves as a bridge textbook, tying the concepts of fire engineering analysis to fire investigations (Icove, DeHaan, and Haynes 2013).
- The National Fire Protection Association's *NFPA 921: Guide for Fire and Explosion Investigations*, approved by the NFPA Standards Council on November 12, 2013, and issued with an effective date of November 11, 2016 (NFPA 2017). The 2017 edition of *NFPA 921* supersedes all previous issues and is considered by practitioners and judicial authorities the standard of care for conducting fire and explosion investigations. *NFPA 921* was approved as an American National Standard on December 1, 2016.
- The National Fire Protection Association's *NFPA 1033: Standard for Professional Qualifications for Fire Investigator*, approved by the NFPA Standards Council on May 28, 2013, with an effective date of June 17, 2013 (NFPA 2014). The 2014 edition of *NFPA 1033* supersedes all previous issues and was approved as an American National Standard on June 17, 2013.

Fire investigators must possess and maintain broad and up-to-date **requisite knowledge** and **skills** in their field. Standard professional qualifications, also known also as **job performance requirements**, mandate that fire investigators have and maintain basic working knowledge of 16 essential areas beyond a high school educational level (NFPA 2014, pt. 1.3.7).

The process of **fire scene investigation and reconstruction** determines the most likely development of a fire using a science-based methodology. Reconstruction begins with an understanding of the conditions and actions just prior to the fire and follows the fire from ignition to extinguishment. It explains aspects of the fire and smoke development, the role of fuels, effects of ventilation, the impact of manual and automatic extinguishment, the performance of the building, life safety features, and the manner of injuries or death.

TABLE 1-1	Professional Levels of Job Performance for Fire Investigators as Cited in *NFPA 1033*, 2014 Edition

CATEGORY	JOB PERFORMANCE REQUIREMENT
4.1 General Requirements for a Fire Investigator	4.1.1 Shall meet the job performance requirements defined in Sections 4.2 through 4.7 4.1.2 Shall employ all elements of the scientific method as the operating analytical process throughout the investigation and for the drawing of conclusions 4.1.3 Site safety assessments shall be completed on all scenes and regional and national safety standards shall be followed and included in organizational policies and procedures 4.1.4 Shall maintain necessary liaison with other interested professionals and entities 4.1.5 Shall adhere to all applicable legal and regulatory requirements 4.1.6 Shall understand the organization and operation of the investigative team within an incident management system
4.2 Scene Examination	4.2.1 Secure the fire ground 4.2.2 Conduct an exterior survey 4.2.3 Conduct an interior survey 4.2.4 Interpret effects of burning characteristics on materials 4.2.5 Interpret and analyze fire patterns 4.2.6 Examine and remove fire debris 4.2.7 Reconstruct the area of origin 4.2.8 Inspect the performance of building systems 4.2.9 Discriminate the effects of explosions from other types of damage
4.3 Documenting the Scene	4.3.1 Diagram the scene 4.3.2 Photographically document the scene 4.3.3 Construct investigative notes
4.4 Evidence Collection and Preservation	4.4.1 Utilize proper procedures for managing victims and fatalities 4.4.2 Locate, collect, and package evidence 4.4.3 Select evidence for analysis 4.4.4 Maintain a chain of custody 4.4.5 Dispose of evidence
4.5 Interview	4.5.1 Develop an interview plan 4.5.2 Conduct interviews 4.5.3 Evaluate interview information
4.6 Post-Incident Investigation	4.6.1 Gather reports and records 4.6.2 Evaluate the investigative file 4.6.3 Coordinate expert resources 4.6.4 Establish evidence as to motive and/or opportunity 4.6.5 Formulate an opinion concerning origin, cause, or responsibility for the fire
4.7 Presentations	4.7.1 Prepare a written report 4.7.2 Express investigative findings verbally 4.7.3 Testify during legal proceedings

From NFPA 1033: Standard for Professional Qualifications for Fire Investigator. Published by National Fire Protection Association, © 2014.

accidental fire ■ Involves all fires for which the proven cause does not involve an intentional human act to ignite or spread fire into an area where the fire should not be (NFPA 2017, pt. 20.1.1).

fire investigator ■ An individual who has demonstrated the skills and knowledge necessary to conduct, coordinate, and complete a fire investigation (NFPA 2014, pt. 3.3.7).

requisite knowledge ■ Fundamental knowledge one must have in order to perform a specific task (NFPA 2014, pt. 3.3.10).

requisite skills ■ The essential skills one must have in order to perform a specific task (NFPA 2014, pt. 3.3.11).

job performance requirement ■ A statement that describes a specific job task, lists the items necessary to complete the task, and defines measurable or observable outcomes and evaluation areas for the specific task (NFPA 2014, pt. 3.3.9).

fire scene investigation and reconstruction ■ The process of recreating the physical scene during fire scene analysis investigation or through the removal of debris and the placement of contents or structural elements in their pre-fire positions (NFPA 2017, pt. 3.3.76).

NFPA 1033 (2014) identifies the professional level of job performance requirements for fire investigators. This standard specifies the minimum job performance requirements for service as a fire investigator in both the private and public sectors. Job performance requirements for each duty are the tasks an investigator must be able to perform to successfully carry out that duty. These tasks are summarized in Table 1-1.

Not only must fire investigators refer to and rely on *Kirk's Fire Investigation*, *Forensic Fire Scene Reconstruction*, *NFPA 921*, *NFPA 1033*, and expert treatises, they also must conduct their investigations using a systematic and scientifically guided approach. In addition to documenting the scene investigation, the investigator must collect physical and testimonial evidence, conduct a post-incident investigation, and prepare a comprehensive written report in anticipation of civil or criminal litigation.

In cases of **incendiary fires**, in addition to determining the origin and cause of the fire, the investigator has the added responsibility of identifying the person who set the fire and providing proof to a trier of fact. Incendiary fires represent a significant percentage of all fires and, because they are set specifically with the intent of destroying property, an inordinately high percentage of dollar losses.

A majority of the fire investigators who testify as expert witnesses have certification by one or more internationally recognized professional organizations. To be effective, the work products and results of fire investigators must be able to pass the eventual and rigorous scrutiny of **peer review** through cross-examinations, sworn depositions, hearings, challenges, and courtroom testimony. In summary, the test of a comprehensive fire investigation is that when peer-reviewed by a non-involved expert fire investigator, they would reach similar, if not the same, opinions and conclusions.

incendiary fire ■ A fire that is intentionally ignited in an area or under circumstances where and when there fire should not be a fire (NFPA 2017, pt. 3.3.116).

peer review ■ A formal procedure generally employed in prepublication review of scientific or technical documents and screening of grant applications by research-sponsoring agencies. Carries with it connotations of both independence and objectivity. Peer reviewers should not have any interest in the outcome of the review (NFPA 2017, pt. 4.6.3).

1.2 The Fire Problem

Internationally, fire continues to be the most costly of all public safety problems. Losses in human lives and injuries due to fires and explosions continue to occur. Fire-caused property losses far exceed those caused by all classes of crime and rival those produced by hurricanes and earthquakes. There is a major problem in identifying and quantifying the issues surrounding the fire problem due to the failure to obtain accurate incident data.

1.2.1 FIRE STATISTICS IN THE UNITED STATES

In the United States, fire incident data are collected by the Federal Emergency Management Agency's US Fire Administration (FEMA/USFA). In coordination with the National Fire Information Council, submitting agencies use the National Fire Incident Reporting System (NFIRS) on a voluntary basis. Shrinking state budgets have often resulted in the downgrading of the priorities of fire incident data collection programs.

Uniform Crime Reporting (UCR) statistics are amassed through the Federal Bureau of Investigation's (FBI's) National Incident-Based Reporting System (NIBRS), but arson incident data are collected only when a fire or police investigator actually submits a report into NIBRS. Subsequently, arson cases go unreported when fire departments fail to pass along and fill out a separate police report on intentionally set fires.

Although the National Fire Protection Association (NFPA) collects data on fire incidents, its estimates are based on data that the association receives from fire departments that respond to its National Fire Experience Survey. Since 1977, this annual sample enables the NFPA to compile national fire problem statistics that include the fires that local fire departments attend, and the resulting deaths, injuries, and property losses (Haynes 2015).

The NFPA estimated that public fire departments in the United States responded to a total of 1,298,000 fires in 2014, causing $11.6 billion in property damage. Of these, an estimated 494,000 were structure fires, which represented an increase of 1.3 percent from the number in 2013. The total monetary property loss for structure fires was $9.8 billion, an increase of 3.4 percent over the previous year's total. The average overall loss per structure fire was $19,931, an increase of 2 percent from the 2013 average. Residential fires accounted for about 74 percent of all structure fires, estimated at 367,500, a slight decrease of 0.5 percent from the previous year. The NFPA study estimated in 2014 that there were approximately 167,500 vehicle fires and 610,500 outside fires, increases of 2.1 and 8.1 percent, respectively (Haynes 2015).

No accounting can accurately reflect the loss in lives and injuries that result from fires. In 2014, the NFPA estimated that 53,275 civilians died as a result of fires, and

15,775 suffered injuries. Home fires were responsible for 2,745 deaths and 11,825 injuries, while vehicle fires caused 310 deaths and 1,275 injuries (Haynes 2015). The National Safety Council reports that accidental fire-related burn injuries are the sixth leading cause of all accidental deaths (NSC 2008).

The NFPA estimates that there were 3,275 civilian fire deaths and 15,775 civilian fire injuries in 2014, an increase from 2013 totals of 1.1 percent and a 0.9 percent decrease, respectively. An estimated 2,745 civilians perished and 11,825 were injured in residential fires. Another 310 civilians died and 1,275 were injured in highway vehicle fires (Haynes 2015).

NFPA statistics recorded 64 on-duty firefighter deaths in the United States in 2014 and 68 deaths in 2015, representing a decrease from 97 deaths in 2013. By contrast, in 2014, the largest multiple-death incidents were two double-fatality fires, both in apartment buildings. The annual average number of deaths over the past decade is 83 (Fahy, LeBlanc, and Molis 2015). During the previous year in 2013, 65,880 firefighter injuries occurred in the line of duty, along with 7,100 exposures to infectious diseases and 17,400 to hazardous conditions (Karter and Molis 2014).

In addition to these direct losses are the incalculable indirect fiscal costs. The actual dollar property losses previously listed probably represent only 10 percent of the total costs. There are inestimable losses due to lost business income, unemployment, reduced property values, and reduced tax bases as a result of nearly every major fire. In a 2005 *Fire Protection Engineering* article, Frazier estimated that the total cost of fire in the United States is on the order of $130–$250 billion per year (Frazier 2005). In the suppression of every fire, personnel and equipment costs are incurred and historic structures are lost forever. Wildland fires destroy watersheds, timber, and wildlife, which cannot be replaced at any cost.

The latest NFPA statistics (Hall 2014) show that the total cost of fire in the United States is a combination of the direct losses caused by fire combined with funding spent on fire prevention, protection, and mitigation. For 2011, that total cost is estimated at $329 billion, more than 2 percent of US gross domestic product. The NFPA arrives at this estimate by including economic loss due to property damage ($14.9 billion), insurance coverage ($20.2 billion), career fire departments ($42.3 billion), new building costs ($31.0 billion), other ($48.9 billion), donated time from volunteer firefighters ($139.8 billion), and civilian and firefighter deaths and injuries due to fire ($31.7 billion) (Hall 2014).

1.2.2 FIRE STATISTICS IN THE UNITED KINGDOM

The United States is not alone in the problem of fire loss. In 2009, the fire and rescue authorities in the United Kingdom adopted an electronic Incident Recording System (IRS), replacing its predecessor, the Fire Data Report system. The Department of Communities and Local Government (CLG) in the United Kingdom collects, maintains, and analyzes the UK fire statistics.

Statistics in Great Britain from April 2013 to March 2014 show the fire service responding to 212,500 fires, which continues a generally downward trend of the past decade. Nearly 19 percent of the fires were dwellings, and 68 percent were outdoor fires consisting of refuse, road vehicles, grasslands, and heathlands (Crowhurst 2015).

During this time period, there were 322 fire-related deaths, the lowest recorded figure in 50 years. Dwelling fires account for 80 percent of the fatalities, with individuals over 80 years old at four times the fatality rate. Gas, smoke, and toxic fumes impact 41 percent of the victims, with burns accounting for 20% of the fatalities (Crowhurst 2015).

1.2.3 ROLE OF THE FIRE INVESTIGATOR IN ACCURATELY REPORTING THE CAUSES OF FIRES

What role does the fire investigator play in these tragedies? By accurately and efficiently identifying the causes of fires, whether accidental or incendiary, investigators can make a substantial contribution to reducing these terrible losses. Fewer lives have been lost because in the 1960s investigators identified the danger of flammability of clothing and bedding, in the 1970s tracked down the problems with instant-on televisions, and in the 1980s identified the danger of coffeemakers and portable heaters. In the 1990s scores of potential victims in several large cities were saved when serial arsonists were caught and incarcerated. Saving lives and preventing injuries are the real reasons fire investigators spend long hours searching a fire scene or doing laboratory analysis and fire research.

The role that thorough fire investigation plays in the regulatory and code-making process is also significant. Advances made in improving life safety and fire safety codes have resulted in reducing the frequency of fires and fire deaths. Although these codes are written on the basis of the best predictive models, the only way to be sure they have the desired effect and do not create other, unanticipated risks is to document the effects of fire in code-compliant buildings and transport. In the early 1900s builders were proud of fire-resistant buildings constructed with stone, concrete, steel, and glass. It was not until major tragedies like the Triangle Shirtwaist fire in 1911 that people realized that building contents and not just the structures were major factors in fires, and having adequate means of escape was critical to survival (Von Drehle 2003). Manual alarm and firefighting systems were also found to be woefully inadequate.

1.3 The Detection of Incendiary Fires

Few other investigations are as daunting as that of a fire scene. Because a fire scene has to be investigated before it can be established whether the crime of arson has been committed, every fire scene must be considered a possible crime scene from the standpoint of scene security, processing, and evidence collection. As a crime scene, the typical fire scene is the antithesis of the ideal.

There has been wholesale destruction of the physical material and substance of the scene, first by the fire itself and second by fire suppression and overhaul by the firefighters. This destruction affects evidence of both accidental and incendiary causes.

Vehicles, personnel, equipment, hoses, and large quantities of water contaminate the scene. Scene security and control of unauthorized persons are difficult because of the attraction fire offers to the public and the press, and may be further complicated by the large area involved in many fire scenes.

Often, the scene investigation is carried out days or weeks after the incident, after weathering and vandals may have further compromised whatever evidence remains. Considering these negative factors, it is not surprising that police and fire personnel have often let fire investigation fall through the cracks of responsibility. As a result, it is surprising that fire causes are ever accurately determined, and civil and criminal cases successfully brought to trial.

1.3.1 REPORTING ARSON AS A CRIME

The *Uniform Crime Reports (UCR),* published by the FBI of the US Department of Justice (DOJ), provides enlightening statistics on arson in the United States. Statistics for 2014, published in 2015, are used in this chapter. Annually, the FBI publishes *Crime in the United States*, which catalogs the entire crime picture of the United States. *UCR* reported in 2013 that the number of arson offenses decreased 13.5 percent compared with those reported in 2012 (FBI 2015).

The FBI's UCR Program defines arson as

> *any willful or malicious burning or attempting to burn, with or without intent to defraud, a dwelling house, public building, motor vehicle or aircraft, personal property of another, etc.*

The FBI collects data only on the fires that through investigation were determined to have been willfully set. Fires whose cause are labelled as "suspicious" or are "unknown or undetermined" are not included in the data.

The FBI points out that arson rates are calculated based on data received from all law enforcement agencies that provide the UCR Program with data for 12 complete months. Unlike other national reporting systems, UCR Program data collection does not include any estimates for arson because the level of reporting arson offenses varies from agency to agency.

According to the 2014 *UCR,* 15,324 law enforcement agencies (providing 1–12 months of arson data) reported 42,934 arsons, which was a 4 percent decrease from 2013. Of those agencies, 14,646 provided expanded offense data on about 40,268 arsons. These data show that arsons involving structures (residential, storage, public, etc.) accounted for 17,790 fires, or 44.2 percent of the total number of arson offenses. Mobile property was involved in 23.2 percent of arsons, and other types of property (such as crops, timber, fences, etc.) accounted for 31.5 percent of arsons (FBI 2015). See Table 1-2 for a detailed breakdown of the 2014 statistics for FBI Uniform Crime Reporting reported by 14,750 agencies representing an estimated population of 262,342,126 persons.

The 2014 FBI statistics showed that the average dollar loss per incident due to arson was $16,055. Arsons of industrial/manufacturing structures resulted in the highest average dollar losses (an average of $167,545 per arson incident). Regarding arson rates, the 2014 *UCR* data showed that nationwide, the rate of arson was 14.2 offenses for every 100,000 inhabitants in the United States (FBI 2015).

The NFPA noted in its 2008 report that in Version 5.0 of the NFIRS the classification of arson was changed to "intentionally set" from the previous "incendiary" category. NFIRS no longer carries a **suspicious** fire category in its reporting system (Karter 2009).

The NFPA statistics for the years 2007–2011 estimated that 282,600 intentionally set fires reported by fire departments in the United States resulted in 420 deaths and

suspicious ■ Fire cause has not been determined, but there are indications that the fire was deliberately set and all accidental fire causes have been eliminated.

TABLE 1-2	Arson in the United States by Type of Property, 2014						
PROPERTY CLASSIFICATION	NUMBER OF ARSON OFFENSES	PERCENT DISTRIBUTION[1]	PERCENT NOT IN USE	AVERAGE DAMAGE	TOTAL CLEARANCES	PERCENT OF ARSONS CLEARED[2]	PERCENT OF CLEARANCES UNDER 18
Total	39,174	100.0		$16,055	8,555	21.8	25.5
Total structure:	17,854	45.6	14.6	$29,779	4,577	25.6	25.6
Single occupancy residential	8,630	22.0	14.9	$27,742	2,109	24.4	18.2
Other residential	3,071	7.8	10.1	$26,786	848	27.6	15.2
Storage	1,113	2.8	18.9	$11,341	233	20.9	41.6
Industrial/ manufacturing	141	0.4	29.8	$167,545	35	24.8	14.3
Other commercial	1,594	4.1	16.7	$56,592	370	23.2	23.2
Community/public	1,513	3.9	14.9	$15,948	579	38.3	63.0
Other structure	1,792	4.6	14.6	$33,161	403	22.5	27.0
Total mobile:	9,154	23.4		$7,716	1,051	11.5	10.4
Motor vehicles	8,608	22.0		$7,416	937	10.9	9.4
Other mobile	546	1.4		$12,458	114	20.9	18.4
Other	12,166	31.1		$2,189	2,927	24.1	30.6

[1] Because of rounding, the percentages may not add to 100.0.
[2] Includes arsons cleared by arrest or exceptional means.
FBI Uniform Crime Reporting offenses reported during 2014 by 14,750 agencies with an estimated population of 262,342,126

TABLE 1-3	Annual Averages of Intentional Fires by Incident Type							
INCIDENT TYPE	FIRES		CIVILIAN DEATHS		CIVILIAN INJURIES		DIRECT PROPERTY DAMAGE (IN MILLIONS)	
Outside or unclassified fires	211,500	(75%)	20	(4%)	150	(11%)	$60	(5%)
Outside trash or rubbish fires	126,300	(45%)	0	(1%)	40	(3%)	$10	(0%)
Outside or unclassified fires (excluding trash or rubbish fires)	85,200	(30%)	10	(4%)	110	(8%)	$50	(4%)
Structure fires	50,800	(18%)	370	(92%)	1,150	(84%)	$1,050	(86%)
Vehicle fires	20,400	(7%)	30	(8%)	70	(5%)	$180	(14%)
Total	282,600	(100%)	420	(100%)	1,360	(100%)	$1,290	(100%)

Source: Reprinted with permission from NFPA's report, "Annual Averages of Intentional Fires by Incident Type" Copyright © 2014, National Fire Protection Association.

1,360 injuries to civilians, along with $1.3 billion in direct property damages. Of these fires, only 18 percent involved structures, 7 percent involved vehicles, and 75 percent involved outside or unclassified incidents (Campbell 2014). See Table 1-3 for a detailed breakdown of the 2007–2011 statistics.

These estimates are almost certainly very low, since some US jurisdictions may not always report arson incidents (structural or vehicular) to law enforcement incident collection systems. In addition, arsons classified as vandalism may also be underreported.

A recent audit survey of selected jurisdictions by Scripps Howard News Service and the University of Tennessee reveal that many investigators think that the total of intentionally set structure fires is closer to 40 percent of all fires (Icove and Hargrove 2014). These statistics may be further compromised as departments facing budget reductions devote larger portions of their resources to other emergency services and less to fire investigation.

1.3.2 PROBLEMS ASSOCIATED WITH ESTIMATING INCENDIARY FIRES

The US estimates are on the conservative side, since many fires are never properly investigated because of lack of time, or are misidentified inadvertently as accidental fires due to lack of experienced investigators, or intentionally to avoid the complications that arise from identifying a fire as a criminal act. These complications can range from administrative, such as requiring more investigative time or involving another public agency, to political, such as generating negative publicity about the community. The sharp contrast between the UK estimates and the NFPA estimates that only 6.1 percent of the reported structure fires were incendiary demonstrates a systematic problem with the NFPA's data gathering and statistical processing.

Recent NFPA estimates indicate that the incidence of intentionally set fires has fallen since 1980. Total intentional fires have declined 69 percent from a high of 859,800 in 1980 to 269,900 in 2011. These estimates include the decrease of intentionally set structure fires by 76 percent, vehicles by 77 percent, and outside and unclassified fires by 65 percent (Campbell 2014).

One significant reason offered for this decrease is that the NFIRS changed its categories in 2003, eliminating the outmoded "suspicious" causation category. Only fires specifically determined to be intentionally set are now reported in the "incendiary" category. In the past, estimates of half of "suspicious" and "undetermined" fires were added to the "incendiary" total. Fire investigators across the United States suspected that even the old percentage (15 percent) was far below the reality of actual investigations.

Lack of evidence, lack of time and resources, and limited cooperation of other public agencies make the selection of **undetermined** or even **accidental** causation the expedient solution. These problems have recently been exacerbated. Budgeting problems at all levels of state and local governments have severely curtailed or even cut fire investigation services in both fire and police agencies. Consequently, the decision-making process has reverted to fire company officers who may or may not be trained or prepared to identify evidence supporting an incendiary cause.

In 2000, the National Institute of Justice published *Fire and Arson Scene Evidence: A Guide for Public Safety Personnel* for first responders in police, fire, and medical services (NIJ 2000). The NIJ hoped that by educating these professionals with the basics of fire-related investigation and physical evidence, a higher percentage of them could contribute toward successful prosecutions. With the cutbacks in public services experienced across the United States, it is not known whether this guide has been successfully utilized. From the small percentages of fires actually reported as intentional via NFIRS, it would appear not.

The situation is made even more critical by the law enforcement agencies that find themselves unable to cope with the onslaught of criminal cases of homicide, rape, assault, and drug-related activity and decide to ignore arson as a crime. This practice is conveniently expedited by categorizing arson as a property crime so that it can be allotted reduced priority and less tactical support than the more urgent crimes against persons.

It must be recognized that arson is a crime against people. It is aimed against people where they live, where they work, and where they do business or go to church. Fire is just as much a weapon as a gun, a knife, or an axe. When aimed at persons, fires may be set directly on them or, more often, set deliberately to trap the victims in a structure or vehicle. Every set fire is a crime against the personnel of fire and police agencies who are obligated to respond to and enter fires in lifesaving efforts.

Successful fire investigation, culminating in an accurate determination of cause, is the only way to minimize these terrible losses. Accidental fires can be prevented by the identification and elimination of hazardous products and processes or careless practices, as well as the development and enforcement of better building codes and fire safety practices. As the recent British experience with vehicle arsons has shown, incendiary fires can be reduced by recognizing them, identifying those responsible, and prosecuting them (ODPM 2005).

With such massive losses involved, it is not surprising that fire losses are one of the most common subjects of civil litigation. Yet, for all its economic and legal importance, fire remains one of the most difficult areas of investigation. It is challenging because the destruction of the fire and, sometimes, its suppression create difficulties in reaching firm and unassailable conclusions as to the fire's cause. It is the investigator's responsibility not only to identify the origin and cause of the fire but also to be prepared to defend their conclusions in a rational, logical manner supported by scientifically valid data. In the absence of rational reconstruction or scientific data, conclusions cannot be substantiated, and successful prosecution for arson is virtually impossible. Civil cases, even with their reduced requisite of proof, are made more difficult to decide fairly without such scientific analysis.

As Sherlock Holmes pointed out, "It is a capital mistake to theorize before one has data. One begins to twist facts to suit theories instead of theories to suit facts." (Doyle 1891) From the standpoint of public safety and economic considerations, it is important that investigative methods for accurately determining the causes of fires be understood and applied to the fullest extent possible. There should be no presumption that a fire is either accidental or incendiary. It is vital that the investigator not prejudge any fire as to cause without evaluating all the collected evidence. If an investigator decides that a fire is arson before collecting any data, then only data supporting that premise are likely to be recognized and collected.

The same caution is necessary for those who decide that all fires are accidental, no matter what their true cause may be. Although fire has been known since prehistoric times, it is still poorly understood by many people, including some firefighters, fire investigators, and others whose services depend on such understanding.

undetermined ■ The final opinion is only as good as the quality of the data used in reaching that opinion. If the level of certainty of the opinion is only "possible" or "suspected," the fire cause is unresolved and should be classified as "undetermined" (NFPA 2017, pt. 19.7.4).

accident ■ An unplanned event that interrupts an activity and sometimes causes injury or damage or a chance occurrence arising from unknown causes; an unexpected happening due to carelessness, ignorance, and the like (NFPA 2017, pt. 3.3.3).

1.4 The Need for Science in Fire Investigations

1.4.1 INTERNATIONAL CONFERENCE ON FIRE RESEARCH FOR FIRE INVESTIGATION

The need for science in fire investigations is not a newly raised issue within the forensic sciences and many of the same principles and methods are as pertinent today as outlined at the 1997 International Conference on Fire Research for Fire Investigation. For example, the international conference in November 1997 assessed the current state of the art and identified technical gaps in fire investigation (Nelson and Tontarski 1998). The conference concluded that many scientific gaps existed in the methodologies and principles used to investigate and reconstruct fire scenes.

This conference cited research, development, training, and education needs, including the following:

- *Fire incident reconstruction:* laboratory methods for testing ignition source hypotheses
- *Fire and burn pattern analysis:* methods for validation of and training in the evaluation of patterns on walls and ceilings, and patterns resulting from liquids on floors, and comparison with patterns generated by radiant heat from solid fuels
- *Burning rates:* determination of burning rates for different items, and development of a burning rate database
- *Electrical ignition:* validation of means of identifying electrical faults as an ignition source
- *Flashover:* impacts of flashover on fire patterns and other indicators
- *Ventilation:* effects of ventilation on fire growth and origin determination
- *Fire models:* methods for validation of, training in, and education on the use of fire models
- *Health and safety:* methods for evaluating fire investigator occupational health and safety
- *Certification:* development of training and certification programs for investigators and laboratory personnel
- *Train-the-trainers:* methods for teaching training objectives and expertise to groups of qualified trainers

The primary goal of the conference was to encourage the development and use of scientific principles by fire investigators and to determine what methodologies could improve investigations by public sector investigators. Post-conference work resulted in the issuance of a white paper under the auspices of the Fire Protection Research Foundation (FPRF 2002). That study concluded that many methods in use lack a basic scientific foundation for identifying the area of origin and the cause of fires. The study listed complex types and forms of burning materials, building geometry, ventilation, and firefighting actions as contributing effects that complicate these determinations.

1.4.2 NATIONAL RESEARCH COUNCIL REPORT

In 2009, the Committee on Identifying the Needs of the Forensic Sciences Community of the National Research Council issued a report published through the National Academies Press (NAP 2009) titled "Strengthening Forensic Science in the United States: A Path Forward." The study addressed challenges facing the forensic science community, including those of fire investigation.

The study specifically stated:

By contrast, much more research is needed on the natural variability of burn patterns and damage characteristics and how they are affected by the presence of various accelerants. Despite the paucity of research, some arson investigators continue to make determinations about whether or not a particular fire was set. However, according to testimony presented to the committee, many of the rules of thumb that are typically assumed to indicate that an accelerant was used (e.g., "alligatoring" of wood, specific char patterns) have been shown not to be true. Experiments should be designed to put arson investigations on a more solid scientific footing.

The National Research Council report addressed the need for integrated governance of crime scene investigation, the forensic science system, laboratories, research funding, and professional associations. Finally, the report recommended improving methods, practice, and performance in forensic science, accreditation, proficiency testing, training, education, medical examiner/coroner systems, automated fingerprint identification systems, and homeland security.

There is a natural tendency for everyone to be impressed by the magnitude and violence of the fire itself and the degree of destruction that results from a large fire. In the case of insurance investigators, this tendency is aggravated by the fact that they are expected to assess this damage and possibly pay a claim for it. For the accurate investigation of fires, this preoccupation with the magnitude and results of the fire is detrimental. Cause, not extent, should be the investigator's concern, and too much attention to extent will obscure and complicate the search for the origin and cause.

1.4.3 THE NFPA 1033'S "BIG SIXTEEN"

Because of the difficulty and complexity of a complete and accurate fire investigation, and preconceptions, there is a need for every investigator to develop a comprehensive analytical approach to the task. This analytical approach recognizes that to be a successful fire investigator, a person must understand and master numerous facets of fires, fuels, people, and investigative procedures. The investigator must really understand how a fire burns, what factors control its behavior, and that all fires do not necessarily behave in a precisely predictable fashion. Such deviations from typical or expected **fire dynamics** must be correlated with the fire conditions and their causes established. These causes usually involve the nature of the fuel involved or the physical circumstances and environment of the fire.

In response to the minimum educational requirements for fire investigators, *NFPA 1033: The Standard Professional Qualifications for Fire Investigators* mandated a series of educational subject areas of competency. The *NFPA 1033* 2009 edition required 13, to which the 2014 edition added 3 additional areas.

NFPA 1033 (2014, pt. 1.3.7) states that the fire investigator shall have and maintain at a minimum an up-to-date basic knowledge beyond the high school level of the following 16 topics. Note the cross-referenced chapters in *NFPA 921* (2017) that address each of these areas.

(1) Fire science (See: *NFPA 921*, 2017 edition, Chapter 5)
(2) Fire chemistry (See: *NFPA 921*, 2017 edition, Chapter 5)
(3) Thermodynamics (See: *NFPA 921*, 2017 edition, Chapter 5)
(4) Thermometry (See: *NFPA 921*, 2017 edition, Chapter 5)
(5) Fire dynamics (See: *NFPA 921*, 2017 edition, Chapter 5)
(6) Explosion dynamics (See: *NFPA 921*, 2017 edition, Chapter 23)
(7) Computer fire modeling (See: *NFPA 921*, 2017 edition, Chapter 22)
(8) Fire investigation (See: *NFPA 921*, 2017 edition, Chapter 4)
(9) Fire analysis (See: *NFPA 921*, 2017 edition, Chapters 4 and 22)
(10) Fire investigation methodology (See: *NFPA 921*, 2017 edition, Chapter 4)
(11) Fire investigation technology (See: *NFPA 921*, 2017 edition, Chapter 22)
(12) Hazardous materials (See: *NFPA 921*, 2017 edition, Chapter 13)
(13) Failure analysis and analytical tools (See: *NFPA 921*, 2017 edition, Chapter 22)
(14) Fire protection systems (See: *NFPA 921*, 2017 edition, Chapter 8)
(15) Evidence documentation, collection, and preservation (See: *NFPA 921*, 2017 edition, Chapter 29)
(16) Electricity and electrical systems (See: *NFPA 921*, 2017 edition, Chapter 9)

fire dynamics ■ The detailed study of how chemistry, fire science, and the engineering disciplines of fluid mechanics and heat transfer interact to influence fire behavior (NFPA 2017, pt. 3.3.70).

This eighth edition of *Kirk's Fire Investigation* addresses each of these areas. Notations throughout this text cross-reference the 2014 editions of *NFPA 921* and *NFPA 1033*, as well as other associated standards.

1.4.4 THE NEGLECTED 17TH AREA OF FIRE INVESTIGATION

ventilation ■ Circulation of air in any space by natural wind or convection or by fans blowing air into or exhausting air out of a building; a fire-fighting operation of removing smoke and heat from the structure by opening windows and doors or making holes in the roof (NFPA 2017, pt. 3.3.199).

The concept of **ventilation** is one of the most important, yet often neglected, areas of fire investigation. An adequate understanding of the fundamental properties of the fuels involved is necessary, along with the impact of ventilation. These properties, which include the chemistry, density, thermal conductivity, and heat capacity of the fuel, determine the ignitability and flame spread characteristics of the fuel. These, in turn, control the nature of ignition as well as events that follow.

These properties are determined primarily by the chemistry of the fuel, and the investigator should have a thorough knowledge of the relevant chemistry and what happens in the reaction. Different ignition sources, whether glowing, flaming, or electric arc, will affect fuels differently; therefore, the investigator must rely on scientific data about the interaction of such sources with the first fuel ignited to help establish whether a particular source is even competent to accomplish ignition and what time factors may be involved. The focus tends to be simply on identifying fuels in fire scenes, but ventilation factors are equally important (because without air, there won't be much of a fire to investigate). Investigators need to document and evaluate the sizes of rooms, windows, and doors, and changes in their condition during the fire.

Ventilation factors must be considered as carefully as fuel factors. The fundamental requirements for a fire are the presence of fuel (in suitable form), oxygen, and heat (in suitable quantities), all linked by a self-sustaining chemical reaction. Investigators must take these factors into account when evaluating every stage of a fire's development from ignition to extinguishment. The physical principles of heat transfer and effects on surfaces must also be understood because they are fundamental to fire spread and to the production of fire patterns on which investigators rely after the fire.

combustion ■ A chemical process of oxidation that occurs at a rate fast enough to produce heat and usually light in the form of either a glow or flame (NFPA 2017, pt. 3.3.35).

Combustion plays an important role. Investigators involved in fire cases, whether criminal or civil, need to be familiar with the same areas of chemistry. An attorney who has no understanding of what happens in chemical reactions and the results of those reactions may not recognize facts crucial to a correct decision when questioning lay and technical witnesses. Such knowledge can also influence the decision whether to try a case or settle it on the best available terms. Thus, it is advantageous for the investigator to have a basic understanding of the simple chemistry of fuels, fire, and combustion and the physical laws that control the production of post-fire indicators.

Because most fires investigated involve either residential or industrial structures, there is a tendency to think of fires only in those terms. This error becomes apparent when a forest or wildland fire is under investigation. Although wildland fires involve the same basic combustion of fuel in air, the dynamics of fire spread and the analysis and interpretation of diagnostic signs of fire behavior are quite different from those for structural fires. Factors such as weather, topography, and fuel density must be assessed in such fires.

Today we commonly face the problems of investigating fires in the urban/wildland interface, where houses and trees coexist. Whenever the fire is of a highly local but very specialized nature, such as a fire in an industrial facility, the investigator must carefully analyze what is found and seek technical assistance if the issues are even marginally in doubt. Such fires are increasingly common when dealing with new products or complex processes of modern technology, with which even experienced investigators have no familiarity.

Investigators must also understand that explosions, like the fires that sometimes accompany them, can be accidental or intentional in cause. The interrelation and distinction between these two types of chemical events must be clearly understood so that the combined event is correctly interpreted when it occurs. The explosion that accompanies a fire is usually quite different from that produced by a bomb, commercial explosive, or a premixed fuel–air mixture, although all involve the rapid exothermic oxidation of a fuel or starting material. That distinction is sometimes lost both in the investigative and legal phases of subsequent actions. The investigation of a bombing may be very different in character from that of a fire-related explosion, but both rely on systematic collection and analysis of data and careful formulation of accurate conclusions.

1.5 The Scientific Approach to Fire Investigation

The scientific approach to fire investigation extends not only to the review of the entire case but also to the examination of the scene, where patient, thorough, and systematic evaluation of the scene and its contents will usually disclose information critical to the case. In some cases, the destruction of some scenes can be so complete due to prolonged burning that virtually nothing can be ascertained reliably from the ashes regarding the origin, cause, and development of the fire. There can be virtually no reliable interpretation of burn patterns to establish direction or duration of fire exposure. However, even compromised scenes offer information about the contents of the structure, which can reveal fraud.

There is a curious tendency for some investigators to show an inherent bias as to cause. These investigators appear to believe that all fires have a single cause, for example, electrical appliances or smoking materials; they then expend a vigorous effort to prove that the fire had this cause, rather than spend the time seeking the true cause. Adhering to a systematic scientific approach will minimize the unfortunate effects of such prejudicial tendencies.

There is also an inclination to extrapolate observations about fuels and combustion in small-scale fires to full-blown incidents without knowing whether they are, in fact, appropriate or accurate. By applying data from fire engineering and fire dynamics studies, the investigator will understand the conditions and limitations of extrapolated information.

1.5.1 THE SCIENTIFIC METHOD

Although he began his professional career as a barrister, Francis Bacon (1561–1626) is best known for establishing and popularizing the method of **inductive logic or reasoning** for conducting critical scientific inquiries. Using this method, Bacon constructed and evaluated propositions or principles that were abstractions of observations of a series of specific events. The method of inductive logic extracts knowledge through observation, experimentation, and testing of hypotheses.

The underpinning of forensic fire scene reconstruction is the use and application of relevant scientific principles and research in conjunction with a systematic examination of the scene. This is particularly important for cases that later require expert witness opinions.

ASTM International, formerly the American Society for Testing and Materials, succinctly defines a **technical expert** as "a person educated, skilled, or experienced in the mechanical arts, applied sciences, or related crafts" (ASTM International 1989). A properly trained and qualified fire investigator who applies and practices the principles of fire science can clearly be considered a technical expert under the ASTM definition. These and related definitions unfortunately do not appear in the 10th edition of the *ASTM Dictionary of Engineering Science and Technology* (ASTM International 2005).

The basic concepts of the **scientific method** are simply to observe, document, hypothesize, test, reassess, and conclude. The scientific method, which embraces sound scientific and fire protection engineering principles combined with peer-reviewed research and testing, is considered the best approach for conducting fire scene analysis and reconstruction. Recently, the National Academy of Sciences published its third edition of the *Reference Manual on Scientific Evidence,* which cites the major impact of the use of the scientific method, particularly in the forensic and engineering sciences (NAP 2011).

inductive logic or reasoning ■ The process by which a person starts from a particular experience and proceeds to generalizations. The process by which hypotheses are developed based on observable or known facts and the training, experience, knowledge, and expertise of the observer (NFPA 2017, pt. 3.3.117).

technical expert ■ A person educated, skilled, or experienced in the mechanical arts, applied sciences, or related crafts (ASTM International 1989).

scientific method ■ The systematic pursuit of knowledge involving the recognition and definition of a problem; the collection of data through observation and experimentation; analysis of the data; the formulation, evaluation and testing of a hypothesis; and, when possible, the selection of a final hypothesis (NFPA 2017, pt. 3.3.160).

NFPA 921 (NFPA 2017, pt. 3.3.160) defines the application of the scientific method as

the systematic pursuit of knowledge involving the recognition and definition of a problem; the collection of data through observation and experimentation; analysis of the data; the formulation, evaluation, and testing of hypotheses; and, when possible, the selection of a final hypothesis.

Furthermore, present job performance requirements under *NFPA 1033* (NFPA 2014, pt. 4.1.2) specify the requirement for the use of the scientific method in every case:

The fire investigator shall employ all elements of the scientific method as the operating analytical process throughout the investigation and for the drawing of conclusions (emphasis added).

NFPA 921 (2017, pt. 1.3.2) also makes this requirement:

As every fire and explosion incident is in some way unique and different from any other, this document is not designed to encompass all the necessary components of a complete investigation or analysis of any one case. The scientific method, however, should be applied in every instance (emphasis added).

When utilizing the scientific method, a fire investigator continuously refines and explores a working hypothesis until he or she reaches a final expert conclusion or opinion, as illustrated in Figure 1-1. An important concept in the application of the scientific method to fire scene investigations is that the investigator should approach all fire scenes without a presumption of the cause. Until sufficient data have been collected in the examination of the scene, no specific hypothesis should be formed (NFPA 2017, pt. 4.3.6).

The following list outlines the seven-step systematic process, as expanded upon by the authors, for applying the scientific method to fire investigation and reconstruction. Properly applied, this systematic process addresses how to correctly formulate, test, and validate a hypothesis.

1. ***Recognize the need.*** A paramount responsibility of first responders is to protect a scene until a full investigation can be started. After initial notification, the investigator should proceed to the scene as soon as possible and determine the resources needed to conduct a thorough investigation. It is necessary to determine not only the origin and cause of this event but also whether future fires, explosions, or loss of life can be prevented through new designs, codes, or enforcement strategies. In public safety sectors, determination of the origin and cause of every fire is often a statutory requirement. The identification of unsafe products related to the cause of the fire can also result in recalls and prevention of future incidents.

2. ***Define the problem.*** Devise a tentative investigative plan to preserve and protect the scene, determine the cause and nature of the loss, conduct a needs assessment, formulate and implement a strategic plan, and prepare a report. Also determine who has the primary responsibility and authority to interview witnesses, protect evidence, and review preliminary findings and documents describing the loss.

data ■ Facts or information to be used as a basis for a discussion or decision (ASTM International 1989).

3. ***Collect data.*** **Data** are "facts or information to be used as a basis for a discussion or decision" (ASTM International 1989). Collect facts and information about the incident through direct observations, measurements, photography, evidence collection, testing, experimentation, historical case histories, and witness interviews. All collected data are subject to verification of how it was legally obtained, its chain of custody, and confirmation of its reliability and authoritative nature. Data collection should include the comprehensive documentation of the building, vehicle, or wildlands involved; construction and occupancy; fuel or fire loading; the processing and layering of the debris and evidence as found; examination of the fire (heat and smoke) patterns; char depths, calcination, and the application of electrical arc mapping surveys where relevant.

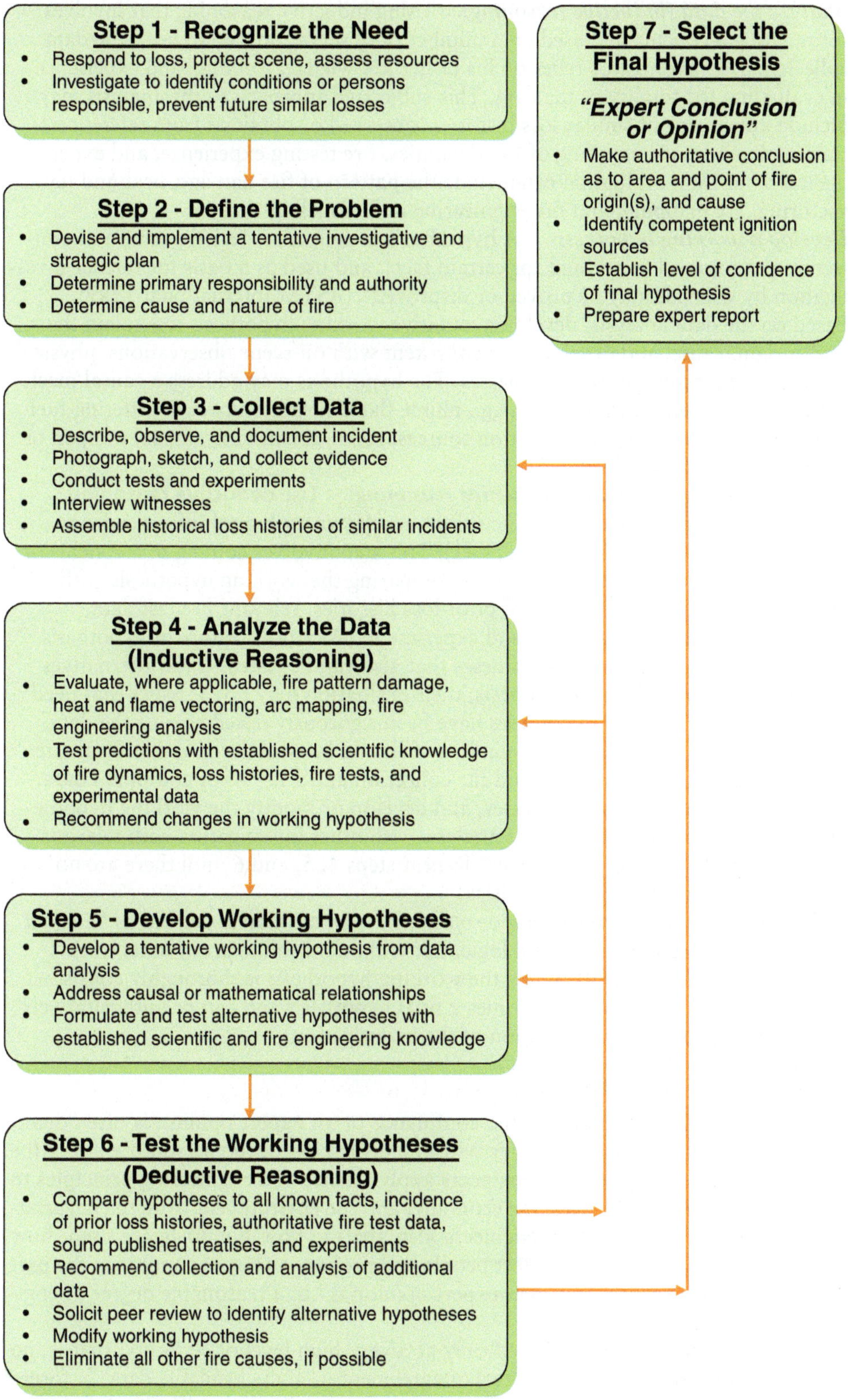

Step 1 - Recognize the Need
- Respond to loss, protect scene, assess resources
- Investigate to identify conditions or persons responsible, prevent future similar losses

Step 2 - Define the Problem
- Devise and implement a tentative investigative and strategic plan
- Determine primary responsibility and authority
- Determine cause and nature of fire

Step 3 - Collect Data
- Describe, observe, and document incident
- Photograph, sketch, and collect evidence
- Conduct tests and experiments
- Interview witnesses
- Assemble historical loss histories of similar incidents

**Step 4 - Analyze the Data
(Inductive Reasoning)**
- Evaluate, where applicable, fire pattern damage, heat and flame vectoring, arc mapping, fire engineering analysis
- Test predictions with established scientific knowledge of fire dynamics, loss histories, fire tests, and experimental data
- Recommend changes in working hypothesis

Step 5 - Develop Working Hypotheses
- Develop a tentative working hypothesis from data analysis
- Address causal or mathematical relationships
- Formulate and test alternative hypotheses with established scientific and fire engineering knowledge

**Step 6 - Test the Working Hypotheses
(Deductive Reasoning)**
- Compare hypotheses to all known facts, incidence of prior loss histories, authoritative fire test data, sound published treatises, and experiments
- Recommend collection and analysis of additional data
- Solicit peer review to identify alternative hypotheses
- Modify working hypothesis
- Eliminate all other fire causes, if possible

**Step 7 - Select the
Final Hypothesis**

*"Expert Conclusion
or Opinion"*
- Make authoritative conclusion as to area and point of fire origin(s), and cause
- Identify competent ignition sources
- Establish level of confidence of final hypothesis
- Prepare expert report

FIGURE 1-1 A flowchart outlining the scientific method as it applies to fire scene investigation and reconstruction. Derived from *NFPA 921* [NFPA editions 2008, 2011, and 2014, pt. 4.3]. *Source: Icove, D. J., and J. D. DeHaan. 2009.* Forensic Fire Scene Reconstruction. *2nd ed. Upper Saddle River, NJ: Pearson Brady Publications.*

4. *Analyze the data (inductive reasoning).* Using inductive reasoning that involves formulating a conclusion based on a number of observations, analyze all the data collected. The investigator relies on his or her knowledge, training, and experience in evaluating the totality of the data. This subjective approach to the analysis may include knowledge of similar loss histories (observed or obtained from references), training in and understanding of fire dynamics, fire testing experience, and experimental data. Data evaluation can include the pattern of fire damage, heat and flame vectoring, arc mapping, and fire engineering and modeling analysis.

5. *Develop a working hypothesis.* A **hypothesis** is defined as "a supposition or conjecture put forward to account for certain facts, and used as a basis for further investigation by which it may be proved or disproved" (ASTM International 1989). Based on the data analysis, develop a tentative working hypothesis to explain the fire's origin, cause, and development consistent with on-scene observations, physical evidence, and testimony from witnesses. The hypothesis may address a causal mechanism or a mathematical relation (e.g., plume flame height, impact of differing fuel loads, locations of competent ignition sources, room dimensions, impact of open or closed doors and windows).

6. *Test the working hypothesis (deductive reasoning).* Use **deductive reasoning**, which is "the process by which conclusions are drawn by logical inference from given premises" (NFPA 2017, pt. 3.3.41). This step involves coming to a conclusion based on previously known facts, while comparing the working hypothesis with all other known facts, the incidence of prior loss histories, relevant fire test data, authoritative published treatises, and experiments. A critical feature of hypothesis testing is creating alternative hypotheses that also can be tested. If the alternatives are counter to the working hypothesis, their evaluation may reveal issues that need to be addressed. After all hypotheses have been rigorously tested against the data, those that cannot be conclusively eliminated should be considered viable. Evaluate all working hypotheses, recommend the collection and analysis of additional data, seek new information from witnesses, and develop or modify the working hypothesis. This may involve reviewing the analysis with other investigators with relevant experience and training (peer review). Repeat steps 4, 5, and 6 until there are no discrepancies with the working hypothesis.

7. *Select final hypothesis (conclusion or opinion).* An **opinion** is defined as "a belief or judgment based upon facts and logic, but without absolute proof of its truth" (ASTM International 1989). When the working hypothesis is thoroughly consistent with evidence and research, it becomes a final hypothesis and can be authoritatively presented as a conclusion or opinion of the investigation.

hypothesis ■ A supposition or conjecture put forward to account for certain facts, and used as a basis for further investigation by which it may be proved or disproved (ASTM International 1989).

deductive reasoning ■ The process by which conclusions are drawn by logical inference from given premises (NFPA 2017, pt. 3.3.42).

opinion ■ A belief or judgment based on facts and logic, but without absolute proof of its truth (ASTM International 1989).

1.5.2 LEVELS OF CERTAINTY

Upon selection of a final hypothesis, the confidence of an expert opinion is often determined. Levels of certainty may also vary with the profession of the person preparing the report. For example, fire protection engineers apply science and engineering principles to protect people, homes, workplaces, the economy, and the environment from the devastating effects of fires. Fire protection engineers also analyze how buildings are used, how fires start and grow, and how fires affect people and property. They commonly in the past stated in their written reports that their expert opinion is "to a reasonable degree of engineering certainty."

Forensic opinions should be offered only at a very high level of certainty; that is, no other logical solutions offer the same level of agreement with the available data. In forensic origin and cause determination, the investigator applies scientific knowledge to re-create the path of spread of the fire, trace it back to its origin, and, there, establish the cause of the fire. Such opinions have often been expressed "to a reasonable degree of scientific certainty."

However, recent guidelines published September 6, 2016, by the USDOJ state that forensic scientists in DOJ labs can no long use terms such as "reasonable scientific certainty" or "reasonable [forensic discipline] certainty" in their reports or testimony. This change was in direct response to recommendations to the DOJ by the National Commission on Forensic Science (NCFS). The DOJ directive also states, "Department prosecutors will abstain from use of these expressions when presenting forensic reports or questioning forensic experts in court unless required by a judge or applicable law." In addition, the DOJ labs are required to post internal validation studies online, and forensic scientists will be expected to uphold a 16-part "Code of Professional Responsibility for the Practice of Forensic Science" (DOJ 2016).

When various hypotheses about the cause of the fire or explosion are tested, if only one hypothesis fits the available data and others are conclusively eliminated, the opinion can be expressed to a reasonable degree of scientific certainty (within the limitations of the available data). All scientific conclusions are subject to continual retesting or re-evaluation if new reliable data are presented. For example, early observational data led the ancients to believe that Earth was at the center of the universe. Later data showed that belief to be wrong and suggested a heliocentric universe. Modern data, of course, show our entire solar system to be circulating in an enormous galaxy moving across the universe.

If two (or more) hypotheses about the origin or cause of a fire or explosion exist and neither can be demonstrated to be false, the degree of certainty or confidence is reduced to "possible" or "suspected," and the conclusion should be undetermined. The posing of alternative hypotheses is, in the US adversarial judicial system, a fair way of testing the strength or certainty of expert conclusions.

An expert opinion should be expected to withstand the challenges of a reasonable examination by peer review or through cross-examination in the courtroom, according to *NFPA 921* (NFPA 2017, pt. 19.6). *NFPA 921* currently discusses only two levels of certainty with respect to opinions—probable and possible. This is not always realistic since there is no mention of a "conclusive" opinion. A "conclusive" opinion can be offered when all the available data fit the final hypothesis and all the reasonable alternatives can be tested and have been conclusively accepted or rejected. Obviously, if there is not a conclusive opinion, but the weight of available data suggests one alternative is vastly more likely than the others, a "probable" opinion can be offered. If two or more hypotheses are equally likely, then a "possible" opinion is justified.

A **probable** opinion ranks at a level of certainty of being more likely true, or the likelihood that the hypothesis is true is greater than 50 percent. A **possible** opinion ranks at the level of certainty of being feasible, but not probable, particularly if two or more hypotheses are equally likely.

If the level of certainty of the opinion is only "possible" or "suspected," the **fire cause** is unresolved and a single final hypothesis cannot be determined, then the cause should be classified as undetermined. *NFPA 921* (NFPA 2017, pt. 4.5.2 and pt. 20.1.4) notes that the decision as to the level of confidence in data collected in the investigation or of any hypothesis drawn from an analysis of the data rests solely with the investigator.

NFPA 921 currently does not include such a characterization in its hierarchy. In criminal cases, such opinions are scrutinized under the same "beyond a reasonable doubt" standard as are the ultimate decisions of the triers of fact. In civil cases, opinions may rest on an evaluation as to whether the event was more likely than not. An opinion is expected to withstand the challenges of a reasonable examination by peer review or a thorough cross-examination in the courtroom (NFPA 2017, pt. 19.7).

1.5.3 THE WORKING HYPOTHESIS

The concept of the working hypothesis is central within the framework of the scientific method. In the case of fire scene reconstruction, the working hypothesis is based on how an investigator describes or explains the fire's origin, cause, and subsequent development.

probable ■ This level of certainty corresponds to being more likely true than not. At this level of certainty, the likelihood of the hypothesis being true is greater than 50 percent (NFPA 2017, pt. 4.5.1).

possible ■ At this level of certainty, the hypothesis can be demonstrated to be feasible but cannot be declared probable (NFPA 2017, pt. 4.5.1).

fire cause ■ The circumstances, conditions, or agencies that bring together a fuel, ignition source, and oxidizer (such as air or oxygen) resulting in a fire or a combustion explosion (NFPA 2017, pt. 3.3.69).

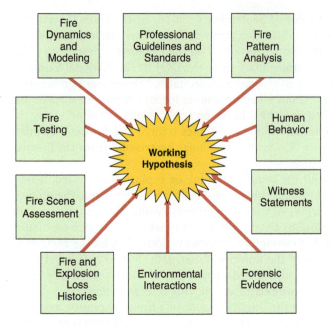

FIGURE 1-2 Sources of information that may contribute to a working hypothesis. *Courtesy of David J. Icove, University of Tennessee.*

The working hypothesis is subject to continuous review and modification and is not the final conclusion.

As shown in Figure 1-2, the investigator molds a working hypothesis, then modifies and refines it by drawing on and examining many sources of information, including past investigative experiences. The working hypothesis may include technical reviews by other qualified investigators, who bring institutional knowledge and experiences. Alternative hypotheses should be created and tested. See *NFPA 921* (NFPA 2017, pt. 4.6.2) for a detailed discussion of technical reviews.

New hypotheses are often built on their predecessors, particularly when the knowledge base of a discipline broadens. When an accepted working hypothesis cannot explain new data, investigators strive to construct a new hypothesis and in some cases generate completely new insight into the problem.

One of the underpinnings of the scientific method is the concept of reproducibility, whereby facts from a preceding hypothesis can be independently tested and verified again. Even when a working hypothesis agrees with all known experimental evidence, it may, nevertheless, be disproved through subsequent experimentation or an emergent discovery. For example, experimental evidence brought new insights to the interpretation of fire patterns (Shanley 1997; Hopkins 2008; Hopkins, Gorbett, and Kennedy 2009; Icove and DeHaan 2006). Certain classes of fire pattern damage once thought to be produced solely by accelerants at fire scenes have been disproved by new principles, practice, and testing (DeHaan and Icove 2012; NFPA 2017). These include, for example, spalling of concrete, collapsed furniture springs, and crazed glass (DeHaan and Icove 2012; Lentini 1992; Tobin and Monson 1989).

Knowledge of the application of fire dynamics and fire modeling may differentiate expert fire investigators from novices based upon their appreciation of complexities of the underlying science. Although the basic tenets of fire spread are based on the established principles of fire dynamics, the understanding of fire dynamics is improving steadily, specifically by modeling actual fire situations. Because investigators apply fire science in their profession, the use of consistent terminology, descriptions of the scene, and interpretations are important in developing and communicating the working hypothesis and in conducting peer review.

The development of hypotheses is built on professional guidelines and standards, particularly those that are authoritative. Engineering handbooks in wide use include the *Fire Protection Handbook* (NFPA 2008); the *SFPE Handbook of Fire Protection Engineering* (SFPE 2008); and the *Ignition Handbook: Principles and Applications to Fire Safety Engineering, Fire Investigation, Risk Management, and Forensic Science* (Babrauskas 2003). Widely recognized guides include *NFPA 921: Guide for Fire and Explosion Investigations* (NFPA 2017); the National Institute of Justice's *Fire and Arson Scene Evidence: A Guide for Public Safety Personnel* (NIJ 2000); *Kirk's Fire Investigation*, 7th ed. (DeHaan and Icove 2012); and *Combating Arson-for-Profit: Advanced Techniques for Investigators*, 2nd ed. (Icove, Wherry, and Schroeder 1998). Other NIJ national guidelines cover such topics as general crime scenes, death investigations, eyewitness identification, bombings, digital images, and electronic evidence. ASTM has several standard practices applicable to fire investigations, which are discussed later in this chapter.

The Society of Fire Protection Engineers (SFPE) publishes a series of engineering guides, many of which are directly applicable to better understanding fire and human behavior and to making realistic assessments. These publications include the *SFPE Engineering Guide for Assessing Flame Radiation to External Targets from Pool Fires, Predicting 1st and 2nd Degree Skin Burns, Piloted Ignition of Solid Materials under Radiant Exposure, Performance-Based Fire Protection Analysis and Design of Buildings, Human Behavior in Fire, Fire Exposures to Structural Elements, Evaluation of the Computer Fire Model DETACT-QS, Fire Risk Assessment in Fire Protection Design, Peer Review in the Fire Protection Design Process,* and *Substantiating Whether a Computer Model Is Appropriate for a Given Application*. The SFPE offers these references and other publications for a nominal fee through its website, www.sfpe.org.

Fire pattern is an important aspect of interpreting the impact of the fire plume on the structure and contents of the building, vehicle, wildland, other property, or the victim. Because liquid accelerants are frequently used by arsonists, authoritative fire testing expands the body of knowledge to include fire pattern analysis, particularly in comparing burn patterns produced by flammable liquids and combustible liquids with those produced by ordinary combustibles (DeHaan 1995; DeHaan and Icove 2012; Putorti, McElroy, and Madrzykowski 2001; Shanley 1997).

fire patterns ■ The visible or measurable physical changes, or identifiable shapes, formed by a fire effect or group of fire effects (NFPA 2017, pt. 3.3.74).

An understanding of human behavior is paramount when evaluating the movement and tenability of persons involved in fires. Not all people respond to perceptions of fire danger in the same way. The investigator must be able to understand and describe how occupants may respond to smoke and fire conditions that change in time and location, resulting in either their successful escape or their death from exposure to various byproducts of combustion. The evaluation should include not only behavior patterns of individuals but also interactions with their primary group (family) or with strangers. This understanding should include gender-based differences of persons in their response to the interpretation of the fire cues, decision making, decisions, and resulting coping actions. For additional information on this topic, see the *Engineering Guide: Human Behavior in Fire,* published by the SFPE (2003).

Witness statements giving accounts of actions taken prior to, during, and after the fire are important to include when developing and testing the working hypothesis. Often, witnesses may need to be interviewed a second time to elicit details left out of the initial statements given to authorities. This information may include observations seen by a witness prior to the fire and as the fire was discovered and progressed.

Forensic science can add additional information to a working hypothesis. Examples include the use of traditional forensic examinations of fire debris, the analysis of impression and trace evidence, and, lately, the increased use of DNA in cases of death investigations. Knowledge of environmental interactions of the initial temperature, humidity, wind speed, and direction on the developing fire may play an important role in developing the working hypothesis. For example, in a high-rise building fire, the environmental

forensic science ■ The application of science to answer questions of interest to the legal system (NFPA 2017, pt. 3.3.90).

factors of wind and temperature, along with information about the location of the fire, such as whether it occurred above or below the neutral plane, may affect the initial discovery of odors, smoke, and fire development or the spread or intensity of the fire (Madrzykowski and Kerber 2009; SFPE 2008). Lightning strikes are an environmental interaction and potential cause for ignition that should be considered. US meteorological studies identify Louisiana and Florida as the leading states for the highest density of lightning strikes, followed by the adjacent states of Tennessee, Mississippi, and Kentucky (Orville and Huffines 1999).

Fire and explosion loss histories are significant to the development of any working hypothesis. The knowledge of similar case histories may offer another perspective helpful in developing the hypotheses that should be tested before selecting the final hypothesis. Such statistical data should not be relied on to prove the cause of a particular fire under investigation; rather, they can help to formulate, examine, or refine the working hypotheses.

Many public and private organizations collect fire data for statistically profiling occupancies to develop risk assessment and fire prevention strategies. Table 1-4 is a profile of average annual fire losses in eating and drinking establishments by cause for the years 2004–2008 (Evarts 2010).

The NFPA also profiles fires in residences and publishes statistics on the forms of material first ignited, data that are essential when developing hypotheses (Rohr 2001, 2005). Other industry sources of fire loss experience data are also available, such as the periodically issued FM Global "Property Loss Prevention Data Sheets" (FM Global 2015).

These loss histories may also be included in the investigator's experience of fire scene assessments while he or she is working on, reviewing, or reading about similar cases. The investigator may draw on heuristic knowledge, training, and experience, combined with professional investigative guidelines and standards, during the development of a working hypothesis. Such statistical histories are useful for developing alternative hypotheses to be tested but not for eliminating a cause for a specific fire because it does not appear on the list.

The combination of generally accepted scientific principles and research, when supported by empirical fire testing, can yield valuable insight into fire scene reconstruction. Scientifically conducted test results can normally be reproduced and their error rates validated. Such results are considered to be objective—neither prejudiced nor biased by the researcher. Accepted fire testing procedures are developed and maintained by the Committee on Fire Standards (E05) of ASTM International.

TABLE 1-4	Profile by Cause for Average Annual Fire Losses in Eating and Drinking Establishments, 2004–2008	
FIRE CAUSE	**NO. OF LOSSES**	**PERCENTAGE**
Cooking equipment (stove, fryer, grill)	4410	54
Electrical distribution (lights, lamps, wiring)	620	8
Arson	410	5
Heating equipment	830	10
Smoking materials	610	7
Clothes dryer or washer	130	2
Other	1150	14
Total losses	8160	100.0

Source: Data from Evarts, B. 2010. U.S. Structure Fires in Eating and Drinking Establishments. Quincy, MA: National Fire Protection Association.

1.5.4 TESTING THE WORKING HYPOTHESIS

It is vital for every experienced investigator to become proficient in the development of the working hypothesis. Proficiency can be accomplished by consistently documenting and evaluating evidence from the fire scene, recording observations and behaviors of witnesses to the fire, comparing similar case histories, reading the fire literature, actively participating in authoritative fire testing, and writing and publishing peer-reviewed research.

The scientific method as it applies to forensic fire scene reconstruction provides fundamental principles for developing a modifiable (working) hypothesis about a fire, testing the hypothesis, and deriving a sound theory as to its origin, development, damage, and cause. Through an iterative process, the working hypothesis is revisited, revised, and reformulated until it is reconciled with all the available data. At that point, the hypothesis becomes a final theory and can be presented as a conclusive opinion of the investigation.

Struggling with the concept of alternative hypotheses is not new in fire investigations. Case Study 1-1 illustrates the many hypotheses that arose during the investigation of the 1942 Cocoanut Grove Night Club fire. Some of the theories appeared far-fetched, but investigators examined each one during the case. This is an example of how the scientific method can be used to discount those theories that cannot be supported by analytical data, fire protection principles, and witness observations.

Hypothesis Testing

CASE STUDY 1-1

The Cocoanut Grove Night Club fire of November 28, 1942, in Boston cost the lives of 492 people, with many others seriously injured, including 131 treated at nearby hospitals. The fire was first discovered in the basement area called the Melody Lounge. It spread quickly through the lounge and up the stairs to the entrance lobby at street level.

Investigating authorities probing the fire were flooded with publicly expressed opinions explaining how the fire started and progressed. Even though the exact source of ignition is still disputed today, many of the publicly expressed opinions had to be addressed in the report. The major issues were the use of combustible decorations, the rapid rate of fire spread, the lack of adequate exits, and the cause of so many post-fire deaths. What is known is that witnesses first reported that the fire originated in the lounge, ignited adjacent combustible decorations and cloth-covered ceilings and walls, and progressed up the stairs, thereby blocking the only visible means of exiting the building.

Many of the theories on the fire's origin, cause, and rapid spread were reported in the official NFPA (1943) report issued January 11, 1943. Even though the published report does not go into sufficient technical detail on these theories, it still serves as an example of a working hypothesis in fire scene reconstruction and analysis. The initial NFPA report listed the following theories and eliminated some based on their improbability and others on the lack of supporting physical evidence.

Ordinary Fire Theory. The ordinary fire theory stated that the cloth and paper decorations on the ceiling and walls, and other available combustible materials, generated an abundance of smoke and carbon monoxide and a means for rapid fire spread. The report noted the possibility of another unexplained element that could have accelerated the growth of the fire. The report did not further discuss the unexplained element. In retrospect, the high number of deaths—hours after the fire—of some who had initially survived led to suspicion of unusual factors in the toxicity of the smoke.

Alcohol Theory. The alcohol theory suggested that vapors from the mouths of heavy drinkers contributed to the rapid fire spread. This included the proposal that warm alcohol evaporating from drinks on tables could also have contributed to the fire. This theory was discounted as a possibility because the concentration of such vapors would be far too low to enhance flame spread.

Pyroxylin Theory. The pyroxylin (nitrocellulose) theory suggested that the extensive use of artificial leather on the walls of the building caused the rapid fire spread and production of nitrous by-products of combustion, accounting for the numerous fatalities. A scientific assessment led to the elimination of this theory. These materials contained only a small percentage of pyroxylin, which was insufficient to contribute to the fire spread or to the number of fatalities.

Motion Picture Film Theory. The motion picture film theory was raised when it was determined that the building had previously been used as a motion picture film exchange. The theory suggested that a quantity of decomposing scrap nitrocellulose film might have remained in a hidden storage area and was ignited by a source of ignition. The observations of witnesses did not support this theory.

Refrigerant Gas Theory. The air conditioning supplying the Melody Lounge was located in a false corner wall. Historically, air-conditioning systems used ammonia or sulfur dioxide as refrigerant. These refrigerant gases are combustible and toxic. A theory suggesting that these refrigerant gases ignited was discounted. Ammonia is a flammable gas but at concentrations far above the tolerable level for human exposure. Also, survivors did not report ammonia odors. Furthermore, the refrigerant gas ran in copper tubing, which would have needed to be thermally or mechanically breached to release the gas during the initial stages of the fire.

Flameproofing Theory. The flameproofing chemicals theory was based on the suggestion that additives to the combustible decorations may have given off ammonia and other gases when heated. The investigation failed to determine whether any flame retardants were ever applied to the decorations, and the surviving victims did not report any symptoms associated with this type of exposure. Fire inspectors at the time routinely exposed the edge of a portion of the decorative fabric to a match flame as a field test. Decorations tested prior to the fire reportedly passed this limited test.

Fire Extinguisher Theory. The fire extinguisher theory came about when investigators learned that fire extinguishers were used on an incipient fire in an artificial palm tree and that the extinguishing liquid may have emitted toxic gases. The investigation found no supporting evidence for this theory.

Insecticide Theory. The insecticide theory emerged when investigators learned that insecticides were used in the basement kitchen. They suggested that if flammable vapors had collected in concealed wall spaces, the vapors might have caused the reported initial flash fire. There was no information as to whether the insecticide used contained an ignitable liquid, and there were no indications of excess quantities of any insecticide.

Gasoline Theory. The gasoline theory was suggested when investigators determined that the building had previously been used as a garage and that gasoline tanks still existed under the basement floor. The theory that gasoline vapor emerged from these tanks was discounted, since such fumes are heavier than air and would have remained at floor level. Furthermore, the physical scene examination proved that there was no source to create an adequate concentration of vapors to support the flame spread seen in this fire. Occupants would have detected vapors by their odor at levels far below ignitable concentrations.

Electric Wiring Theory. The electric wiring theory came about when investigators learned that an unlicensed electrician had installed part of the wiring in the building. The theory suggested that the heated insulation on overloaded wiring was responsible for forming flammable and toxic vapors. No evidence was found that could support the theory of overloading or that an electrical failure was responsible for ignition.

Smoldering Fire Theory. The smoldering fire theory was suggested when investigators learned that witnesses reported that several walls were hot to the touch and that a smoldering fire went undetected. Investigators physically examining the fire scene found no physical evidence to support this theory.

As a postscript to these theories, more than half a century later the cause of the fire is still listed as "undetermined." Some witnesses reported that the initial fire was in an artificial tree, where an errant flame from a match, lighter, or candle could have started it. Hypotheses are still being tested as to the cause of the Cocoanut Grove fire. Reviews of the investigation by the NFPA begun in 1982 along with the latest reviews suggest that fire modeling combined with the use of the scientific method may shed new insights into this case (Beller and Sapochetti 2000; Grant 1991; Reinhardt 1982). For further reading, see Schorow (2005) and Esposito (2005).

1.5.5 BENEFITS OF USING THE SCIENTIFIC METHOD

There are numerous benefits to using the scientific method to examine fire and explosion cases, including the following:

- Acceptance of the methodology in the scientific community
- Use of a uniform, peer-reviewed protocol of practice, such as *NFPA 921*
- Improved reliability of testimony from opinions formed using the scientific method

First, the use of the scientific method is well received in both the technical and research communities. An investigation conducted using this approach is more likely to be embraced by those who would tend to doubt a less thoroughly conducted probe.

Second, the scientific method is a generally accepted protocol of practice in the literature. Those persons ignoring or deviating from recommended practices will be subject to closer scrutiny of their reports and opinions. Modern fire investigation texts endorse the application (DeHaan and Icove 2012).

The NIJ's (2000) *Fire and Arson Scene Evidence: A Guide for Public Safety Personnel* repeatedly cites the scientific method. The guide notes that actions taken at the scene of a fire or arson investigation can play a pivotal role in the resolution of a case. A thorough investigation is key to ensuring that potential physical evidence is neither tainted nor destroyed, nor potential witnesses overlooked.

Third, and most important, expert testimony in fire and explosion cases relies more heavily on opinions formed using the scientific method. Recent US Supreme Court decisions underscore these principles, with many state courts following the trend. Section 1.6 discusses at length many issues surrounding expert testimony.

1.5.6 ALTERNATIVES TO THE SCIENTIFIC METHOD

There are alternative approaches to the scientific method that use other forms of logic apart from inductive and deductive reasoning. For example, **abductive reasoning** involves the process of reasoning to the best explanations for a phenomenon. An example of using abductive reasoning to explain an observation might be, "If it rains, the grass is wet." This abductive rule explains why the grass is wet. An alternative explanation might answer the question: Can the grass be wet if it has not rained? Yes, the lawn sprinklers were used, or the dew was heavy. In this approach, the reasoning starts with a set of given facts and derives their most likely explanations or hypotheses. Such reasoning leads to testable alternatives and is therefore key to proper application of the scientific method to origin and cause determination.

abductive reasoning ■ The process of reasoning to the best explanations for a phenomenon.

Modern-day applications of abductive reasoning include artificial intelligence, fault tree diagnosis, and automated planning. For a thorough discussion on the comparison of inductive, deductive, and abductive reasoning, see the National Defense Intelligence College paper titled "Critical Thinking and Intelligence Analysis" (Moore 2007). The admissibility of abductive reasoning and inference has been discussed but has not yet been included in *NFPA 921*, but it has been cited in fire symposiums (Brannigan and Buc 2010).

1.5.7 LEGAL OPINIONS REGARDING SCIENCE IN INVESTIGATION

Some of the most significant changes in fire investigation in the past 15 years have been the result of legal interpretations of the *Daubert, Kumho Tire, Joiner,* and *Benfield* decisions. Today's fire investigator must demonstrate to the court that he or she has the training and qualifications to offer an opinion about the fire, has data (information) to support the conclusion drawn from the data, has followed an appropriate protocol in the investigation and decision-making process, and has followed, in general, the scientific method of inquiry.

Data collection through a uniform protocol is important in fire and explosion investigations. Examples of basic protocols include the one outlined in the NIJ *Guide* described earlier. More detailed protocols are discussed in *Forensic Fire Scene Reconstruction* (Icove, DeHaan, and Haynes 2013) and *NFPA 921: Guide for Fire and Explosion Investigations* (NFPA 2017). A commercially available protocol for documenting fire investigations is available for use in all forms of inclement weather (Rite-in-the-Rain 2016). Note that a protocol is not a cookbook with all the steps laid out in mandatory order, but it is merely an outline of a systematic, comprehensive data gathering and preservation approach to scene investigation.

The complexities encountered in fire investigation can be overwhelming to the investigator, but patience and adherence to fundamental scientific principles of combustion, fire behavior, and heat transfer will usually result in a reasonable and defensible diagnosis of the fire if there are sufficient reliable data.

1.6 Foundations of Expert Testimony

Under NFPA 1033, 2014 ed., pt. 4.7.3, fire investigators should be experienced and able to testify as an expert. The investigator may also be called upon to present their findings in public presentations, per NFPA 1033, 2014 ed., pt. 4.7.4.

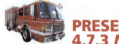

PRESENTATION STANDARD: 4.7.3 *NFPA 1033*, 2014 EDITION

TASK:

Testify during legal proceedings, given investigative findings, contents of reports, and consultation with legal counsel, so that all pertinent investigative information and evidence is presented clearly and accurately and the investigator's demeanor and attire is appropriate to the proceeding.

PERFORMANCE OUTCOME:

The investigator will testify and be cross-examined in a mock courtroom.

CONDITIONS:

Given investigative findings, 30 minutes to review information, and consultation with prosecution legal counsel.

TASK STEPS:

1. Review provided information within 30 minutes
2. Ask questions of the prosecutor before testifying
3. Answer questions from the prosecutor before testifying
4. Testify in court to prosecutor's questions without error
5. Testify in court to cross-examination by defense counsel without error
6. Demonstrate appropriate court room demeanor:
   a. Posture
   b. Mannerisms
   c. Composure
   d. Confidence
7. Demonstrate appropriate communication skills:
   a. Respond to questions appropriately
   b. Maintain objectivity
   c. Use appropriate professional language
   d. Avoid using jargon/idiomatic expressions and profanity
   e. Accurately convey facts
   f. Testimony is consistent with documented facts

Source: Derived and updated from Washington State Patrol, Form No. 3000-420-081 (Sept. 2014) Fire Protection Bureau, Standards and Accreditation, Olympia, Washington http://www.wsp.wa.gov/fire/docs/cert/fire_invest.pdf

PRESENTATION STANDARD: 4.7.4 *NFPA 1033*, 2014 EDITION

TASK:

Conduct public informational presentations, given relative data, so that information is accurate, appropriate to the audience, and clearly supports the informational needs of the audience.

PERFORMANCE OUTCOME:

The investigator will conduct a public informational presentation within 5 minutes.

CONDITIONS:

Given an investigation report, a briefing from the Incident Commander, information on the type of audience, and a 5-minute time frame.

(Continued)

1.6.1 FEDERAL RULES OF EVIDENCE

For the purposes of this text, emphasis is placed on testimony given primarily in the federal court system. The *Federal Rules of Evidence* (FRE 2012) clearly state who may offer testimony in federal court. Although federal guidelines do not apply to all state courts or international situations, many state courts model their guidelines on the federal rules.

The following amendments to the *FRE*, which were effective December 1, 2011, address the admissibility of evidence and opinion testimony under *Rules 701, 702, 703, 704,* and *705:*

Rule 701. Opinion Testimony by Lay Witnesses

If the witness is not testifying as an expert, the witness' testimony in the form of opinions or inferences is limited to those opinions or inferences which are (a) rationally based on the perception of the witness, (b) helpful to a clear understanding of the witness' testimony or the determination of a fact in issue, and (c) not based on scientific, technical, or other specialized knowledge within the scope of Rule 702.

Rule 702. Testimony by Experts

If scientific, technical, or other specialized knowledge will assist the trier of fact to understand the evidence or to determine a fact in issue, a witness qualified as an expert by knowledge, skill, experience, training, or education may testify thereto in the form of an opinion or otherwise, if (1) the testimony is sufficiently based upon reliable facts or data, (2) the testimony is the product of reliable principles and methods, and (3) the witness has applied the principles and methods reliably to the facts of the case.

Rule 703. Bases of Opinion Testimony by Experts

The facts or data in the particular case upon which an expert bases an opinion or inference may be those perceived by or made known to the expert at or before the hearing. If of a type reasonably relied upon by experts in the particular field in forming opinions or inferences upon the subject, the facts or data need not be admissible in evidence in order for the opinion or inference to be admitted. Facts or data that are otherwise inadmissible shall not be disclosed to the jury by the proponent of the opinion or inference unless the court determines that their probative value in assisting the jury to evaluate the expert's opinion substantially outweighs their prejudicial effect.

Rule 704. Opinion on Ultimate Issue

(a) Except as provided in subdivision (b), testimony in the form of an opinion or inference otherwise admissible is not objectionable because it embraces an ultimate issue to be decided by the trier of fact.

(b) No expert witness testifying with respect to the mental state or condition of a defendant in a criminal case may state an opinion or inference as to whether the defendant did or did not have the mental state or condition constituting an element of the crime charged or of a defense thereto. Such ultimate issues are matters for the trier of fact alone.

Rule 705. Disclosure of Facts or Data Underlying Expert Opinion

The expert may testify in terms of opinion or inference and give reasons therefor without first testifying to the underlying facts or data, unless the court requires otherwise. The expert may in any event be required to disclose the underlying facts or data on cross-examination.

1.6.2 SOURCES OF INFORMATION FOR EXPERT TESTIMONY

In general, experts normally base their opinions on four major sources of information (Kolczynski 2008):

1. Firsthand observations

Examples of firsthand observations include those observed at a fire scene, in a laboratory examination or fire test, or from evaluation of evidence under *FRE 703*. It is important that experts try to visit the fire scene and not merely rely on sketches and photographic evidence taken by another party. Although valuable, it is not always required or possible to visit the scene, particularly if the scene has been considerably altered or destroyed. If photographic documentation is sufficiently comprehensive and can be documented or validated by other means, the expert can rely on it (*United States v. Ruby Gardner* 2000).

2. Facts presented to experts prior to trial

Experts usually critically review the case and gain insight and knowledge of facts prior to trial. This knowledge may be based on facts gleaned from reports of other experts, scientific manuals, learned treatises, or results of historical testing. Examples include information learned through expert treatises such as *NFPA 921, Kirk's Fire Investigation,* and the *SFPE Handbook.*

Rule 701 allows for lay witnesses to offer non-expert opinion testimony as evidence. These opinions might include the state of intoxication, a vehicle's speed, and the memory of an identifiable odor of gasoline. For example, firefighters who are not experts in fire investigation may be allowed to testify that they detected a strong odor of gasoline when they entered a certain room of a burning structure.

Rule 702 requires that the expert's testimony must assist the trier of fact, and its admissibility depends in part on the connection between the scientific research or test to be presented and the particular disputed factual issues in this case [(*In re Paoli Railroad Yard PCB Litigation* (1994) citing *United States v. John W. Downing* (1985)]. Furthermore, each step in the expert's analysis must reliably connect the work of the expert to that particular case.

A lay witness may also offer expert testimony under *Rule 702* when the opinion is based on an accepted evaluation method, as long as the witness is qualified to make this evaluation. Examples of accepted evaluation methods include the guidelines in *NFPA 921* and various ASTM standards.

Since its enactment in 1975, *Rule 703* allowed experts to form an opinion based on facts, whether or not in evidence, as long as those facts were necessary to form professional judgments from a non-litigation point of view. Just because an expert witness uses information to form an opinion, its use does not automatically make that information admissible in court. Under *FRE 703*, experts may also rely on the hearsay statements, such as those of other witnesses. For example, the expert may use information from the persons who witnessed the fire, testimony of other witnesses, documents and reports, videotapes of the fire in progress, and related written reports submitted in the case, to help form an opinion (*United States v. Ruby Gardner* 2000).

3. Facts supplied in court

Facts supplied in court may also be a basis for expert witness testimony. These facts may include information from testimony of other witnesses and evidence presented. The expert witness may also be asked a hypothetical question. For example, an expert may be asked, "Assume that three separate gasoline-filled plastic jugs with partially burned wicks were found in separate rooms of the house. What would be your conclusions based on these facts and your 25 years of experience as a fire investigator?"

4. Testing of alternative hypotheses

The testing of alternative hypotheses is an important concept in expert witness testimony, whether it be physical laboratory tests or critical reviews of other reasonable hypotheses raised in a case. In *ASTM E620-11,* (ASTM International 2011a, pt. 4.3.2), the expert is required to document in his or her report the logic and reasoning used to reach each of the opinions and conclusions. In a recent case, an expert did not undertake a process to eliminate another possible cause of a fire that might otherwise seem on par with his hypothesis. The court found that although the expert was qualified in fire research, his testimony lacked objective, evidence-based support for his conclusions (*Wal-Mart Stores, Petitioner, v. Charles T. Merrell, Sr., et al.* 2010).

1.6.3 DISCLOSURE OF EXPERT TESTIMONY

The following is an excerpt regarding guidelines on the requirement to disclose expert testimony in civil cases from *Rule 26(a)(2)(B)* of the *Federal Rules of Civil Procedure* (FRCP 2010) effective December 1, 2010, as amended.

---

2. Disclosure of Expert Testimony

    A. *In General.* In addition to the disclosures required by Rule 26(a)(1), a party must disclose to other parties the identity of any witness it may use at trial to present evidence under Federal Rule of Evidence 702, 703, or 705.

    B. *Witnesses Who Must Provide a Written Report.* Unless otherwise stipulated or ordered by the court, this disclosure must be accompanied by a written report—prepared and signed by the witness—if the witness is one retained or specially employed to provide expert testimony in the case or one whose duties as the party's employee regularly involve giving expert testimony. The report shall contain:

        (i) a complete statement of all opinions the witness will express and the basis and reasons for them;

        (ii) the facts or data considered by the witness in forming them;

        (iii) any exhibits that will be used to summarize or support them;

        (iv) the witness's qualifications, including a list of all publications authored in the previous 10 years;

        (v) and a list of all other cases in which, during the previous 4 years, the witness has testified as an expert at trial or by deposition; and

        (vi) a statement of the compensation to be paid for the study and testimony in the case.

    C. *Witnesses Who Do Not Provide a Written Report.* Unless otherwise stipulated or ordered by the court, if the witness is not required to provide a written report, this disclosure must state:

        (i) the subject matter on which the witness is expected to present evidence under Federal Rule of Evidence 702, 703, or 705; and

        (ii) a summary of the facts and opinions to which the witness is expected to testify.

    D. *Time to Disclose Expert Testimony.* A party must make these disclosures at the times and in the sequence that the court orders. Absent a stipulation of a court order, the disclosures must be made:

        (i) at least 90 days before the date set for trial or for the case to be ready for trial; or

        (ii) if the evidence is intended solely to contradict or rebut evidence on the same subject matter identified by another party under Rule 26(a)(2)(B) or (C), within 30 days after the other party's disclosure.

    E. *Supplementing the Disclosure.* The parties must supplement these disclosures when required under Rule 26(e).

FRE Rule 705 addresses the disclosure of facts or underlying data on which an expert forms his or her expert opinion. The expert may testify as to an opinion without first introducing the underlying facts or data used to develop that opinion, unless otherwise directed by the court. However, the expert may be required to later disclose the underlying facts or data used during a cross-examination.

Under *FRCP Rule 26(a)(2)(B)*, experts are required to provide a written expert witness report. This report, which must be prepared and signed by the expert witness, must contain the following:

- Complete statement of all opinions to be expressed along with the basis for these opinions
- Data or information considered by the expert used in forming the opinions

- Exhibits planned to be used in summarizing or supporting the opinions
- Qualifications of the expert witness, including a list of all publications authored within the preceding 10 years
- Compensation to be paid for the report and testimony
- Listing of all cases in which the expert has testified in trial or deposition within the preceding 4 years

The outlined format of written expert disclosure reports varies. Table 1-5 is an example of an outline for a summary disclosure letter or report sent by an expert to an attorney. Table 1-6 lists areas to cover when qualifying as a fire expert (Beering 1996).

1.6.4 DAUBERT CRITERIA

Fire and explosion investigation is being considered more as a science and less as an art. This is particularly true when the scientific method is combined with relevant engineering principles and research in providing expert witness testimony (Kolar 2007; Ogle 2000). In its recent decisions, the US Supreme Court has continued to define and refine the admissibility of expert scientific and technical opinions, particularly those concerning scene investigations. These decisions affect how expert testimony is interpreted and accepted.

A judge has the discretion to exclude testimony that is speculative or based on unreliable information. In the case *Daubert v. Merrell Dow Pharmaceuticals* (1993), the Court placed the responsibility on a trial judge to ensure that expert testimony was not only

TABLE 1-5	Suggested Headings in an Expert Disclosure Report

1. Disclosure and scope of engagement

2. Personal background and qualifications

3. Summary of professional opinion(s)

4. Description of the property destroyed

5. The standard of care and methodology used in fire investigations

6. The fire incident (include names, table of events)

7. An analysis of other investigations
   - Training and experience in fire investigations
   - Postsecondary education
   - Knowledge and certification
   - Expertise in applying a reliable methodology
   - Qualifications

8. Impact of spoliation (if present)
   - Definition, responsibility, and documentation
   - Realization timeframe of potential litigation
   - Notification of interested parties
   - Loss and destruction of critical evidence
   - Timeframe of spoliation of evidence

9. Impact of conducting an independent fire investigation

10. Executive summary of opinions with signature/seal

Appendix A – List of information reviewed

Appendix B – Professional qualifications, past testimony

Appendix C – Compensation received

Appendix D – Supplementary data

Appendix E – Program listings (computer models)

TABLE 1-6	Areas to Address When Qualifying as a Fire Expert

CATEGORY	EXAMPLE
Identification—Who is the expert and how long has he or she worked in the field?	Name
	Title, department
	Employment—current and previous
Education and training—What formal specialized training has the expert received?	Formal education
	Fire training academies
	National Fire Academy
	FBI Academy
	Federal Law Enforcement Training Center
	Annual international and state seminars
	Specialized training
Certifications—Is the expert licensed, certified, or otherwise credentialed in his or her field?	Fire investigator
	Police officer
	Fire protection specialist
	Professional engineer
	Instructor
Experience—How has the expert acquired firsthand knowledge and experience about fire?	Fire suppression
	Fire investigations
	Fire testing
	Laboratory
Prior testimony—Has the expert given prior testimony?	Criminal, civil, and administrative courts
	Lay and expert witness
	Jurisdictions (state, federal, international)
Professional associations—Of which professional associations is the expert a member, and in what standing (e.g., fellow, life member)?	Professional fire investigation
	Fire and forensic engineering
Teaching experience—Has the expert delivered certified and credible training to others in the field?	Local, state, federal, international schools and organizations
	National academies
	Colleges and universities
Professional publications—Has the expert written and published peer-reviewed quality articles?	Peer-reviewed articles, technical papers
	Books
	National standards
Awards and honors—What significant honors and awards has the expert received?	Local, state, federal, and international professional organizations and societies

Source: Data from Summarized and updated from Beering, P. S. 1996. Verdict: Guilty of Burning—What Prosecutors Should Know about Arson. Insurance Committee for Arson Control. Indianapolis, IN.

relevant but also reliable. The judge's role is to serve as a gatekeeper who determines the reliability of a particular scientific theory or technology. As a result of *Daubert v. Merrell Dow Pharmaceuticals*, the Court defined four criteria to be used by the gatekeeper to determine whether the expert's theory or underlying technology should be admitted. These

TABLE 1-7	Criteria and Pertinent Issues Examined by *Daubert*

CRITERIA	PERTINENT ISSUES EXAMINED
Testing	Has the methodology, theory, or technique been tested?
Peer review and publication	Has the methodology, theory, or technique been subjected to peer review and publication?
Error rates and professional standards	What are the known or potential error rates of this methodology, theory, or technique?
	Does the methodology, theory, or technique comply with controlling standards, and how are those standards maintained?
General acceptance	Is the methodology generally accepted in the scientific community?

criteria, known as the *Daubert* criteria, examine testability, peer review and publication, error rates and professional standards, and general acceptability, as explained in Table 1-7.

Daubert allows the judge to gauge whether the expert testimony aligns with the facts of the case as presented. The central issue is often whether the expert has followed an identified, accepted, and peer-reviewed method as the basis for his or her conclusion.

In a more recent decision, *Kumho Tire Co. Ltd. v. Carmichael* (1999), the Court applied the *Daubert* criteria to determine whether the expert testimony was based on science or experience. In short, expert testimony must rely on a balance of valid peer-reviewed literature, testing, and acceptable practices and a demonstration that the courts followed those practices if they considered the testimony credible.

A federal case citing *Daubert* and *Rules 702* and *703* allowed the expert testimony of Dr. John DeHaan pertaining to the origin and cause of an arson fire based on his review of case materials relied on by other experts (*United States v. Ruby Gardner* 2000). Dr. DeHaan relied on a review of reports, photographs, and third-party observations, some of which may not have been directly admissible as evidence.

The court determined that this procedure was reliable and appropriate, confirming the conviction. Furthermore, the court drew a parallel to other testimony, including hearsay and third-party observations used by an arson investigation expert in forming an opinion on the ability of a psychiatrist to testify as an expert by relying only on staff reports, interviews with other doctors, and background information.

In *United States v. John W. Downing* (1985), a Third Circuit case, both *Daubert* and *Downing* factors were used in determining whether an expert's methodology was reliable. *Downing* factors consider (1) the relationship of the technique to methods that have been established to be reliable, (2) the qualifications of the expert witness testifying based on methodology, and (3) the non-judicial issues to which the method has been put.

1.6.5 FRYE STANDARD

At present, 16 states and the District of Columbia (Giannelli and Imwinkelried 2007, 1–15) rely on the *Frye* test (or a local variant of it, such as the *Kelly-Frye* test in California, *Reed-Frye* in Maryland, and *Davis-Frye* in Michigan) as the standard for admissibility of expert testimony instead of the *Daubert* standard. The original *Frye* decision was reached in 1923 over the issue of admissibility of the (then) new scientific discipline of polygraph examinations, for which a limited number of adherents maintained its reliability in the face of general skepticism. The US Court of Appeals for the District of Columbia stated:

Just when a scientific principle or discovery crossed the line between experimental and demonstrable stages is difficult to define. Somewhere in this twilight zone, the evidential force of the principle must be recognized and, while courts will go a long way in admitting expert testimony deducted from a well-recognized scientific principle or discovery, the thing from which the deduction is made must be sufficiently established to have gained general acceptance in the particular field in which it belongs (Frye v. United States 1923).

Similar to the *Daubert* decision, the *Frye* decision recognized the judge as the gatekeeper responsible for excluding junk science. It has been suggested (Graham 2009) that the reasoning behind the *Frye* standard or general acceptance test is to assist the trier of fact in six ways:

1. Promote a degree of uniformity of decision across the judiciary
2. Avoid the interjection of a time-consuming and often misleading determination of the reliability of a scientific technique during litigation
3. Assure that the scientific evidence introduced will be reliable and thus relevant
4. Ensure that a pool of experts exists who can critically examine the validity of a scientific determination
5. Provide a preliminary screening to protect against the natural inclination of the jury to assign significant weight to scientific techniques presented as evidence where the trier of fact is in a poor position to evaluate the reliability of that evidence accurately
6. Impose a threshold standard of reliability for scientific expert testimony in new areas when cross-examination by opposing counsel may be unable or unlikely to bring inaccuracies to light

The *Frye* standard is a conservative one, when strictly applied, requiring new technologies or techniques to have been in use long enough for them to have been tested by a number of practitioners. It is the offering party's burden to prove the concept of general acceptance. There are no methods suggested in *Frye* by which a judge should determine general acceptance. The testimony of a single expert, particularly one who might have a bias or vested interest, is rarely acceptable. Presentations of multiple peer-reviewed, published papers; testimony of an independent expert retained by the court; and testimony of multiple experts have all been used.

"The trial judge determines whether the *Frye* test has been satisfied under a rule comparable to *Federal Rules of Evidence 104(a)*. The 'preponderance' standard applies" (Giannelli and Imwinkelried 2007, 1–5). Some courts have applied *Daubert*-type considerations to determine whether techniques such as independent peer review, thorough testing, establishing error rates, or promulgation of objective standards applicable to the technique are acceptable. One measure is that general acceptance is met if the use of the technique is supported by a clear majority of the scientific community.

Another major issue with *Frye* is the difficulty in establishing in which field the technique falls. Fire investigation and reconstruction both rely on multiple fields—fire dynamics, fire engineering, chemistry, and, in some cases, human behavior. They do not fall within a single academic discipline or professional discipline. The judge may turn to the published fire investigation literature or to resources in fire engineering, fire safety, or chemistry (including local college instructors who may or may not have the necessary familiarity with the concepts).

Some courts have extended the *Frye* standard beyond the reliability of the technique to considerations of the underlying theory or theories on which the technique is based. That extension can create real problems for fire investigators if called on to prove the validity of underlying theories for events such as V patterns, spalling, failure of glass, flashover, or halo or ring patterns whose underlying theories, if known, are couched in the fire dynamics and materials science disciplines.

Other courts have avoided the *Frye* issue by deciding that some evidence does not fall within the scientific realm but is simply demonstrative evidence (physical models, photographs, X-rays, and the like). In those cases, the jury does not have to place blind faith in the assurances of a testifying expert but can verify the results by their own observations.

For a detailed discussion of these concepts, see Case Studies 1-2, 1-3, 1-4, 1-5, and 1-6.

The debate over the application of *Daubert* to fire scene investigations has intensified and focused on whether origin and cause determination is to be considered scientific evidence or nonscientific technical evidence. The advocates of the strict scientific approach bristle at the suggestion that fire scene investigation is in any way non-scientific, pointing to the many misconceptions previously used by fire investigators (spalling, floor penetrations, etc.) that were corrected by fire scientists only in recent years. They advocate the use of *Daubert* in fire scene analysis as the only means of preventing a return to the improper fire scene methodologies employed by unqualified investigators lacking proper scientific training.

In contrast, the technicians argue that fire scene investigation has never been a pure science like chemistry or physics because it employs elements of both disciplines. The term *nonscientific* in the context of *Daubert* is a legal distinction, rather than a scientific one. That is not to say that fire investigation is *un*scientific or devoid of any application of scientific principles. Instead, it is a recognition of the objective and subjective components that form a part of every fire scene investigation, more precisely, the human component in examining, analyzing, and, ultimately, interpreting fire scene evidence to reach a conclusion about the fire's origin and cause.

Early on in *Daubert*'s history, the US Court of Appeals for the Tenth Circuit directly addressed the testimony of a fire investigator in an arson case. In *United States v. Markum* (1993), the court found the admission of a fire chief's testimony that a fire was the result of arson to be proper based primarily on his extensive experience in fire investigations. The court said:

> *Experience alone can qualify a witness to give expert testimony. See* Farner v. Paccar, Inc., *562 F. 2d 518, 528–29 (8th Cir. 1977);* Cunningham v. Gans, *501 F. 2d 496, 500 (2nd Cir. 1974).*
>
> *Chief Pearson worked as a firefighter and Fire Chief for 29 years. In addition to observing and extinguishing fires throughout that period, he attended arson schools and received arson investigation training. The trial court found that Chief Pearson possessed the experience and training necessary to testify as an expert on the issue of whether the second fire was a natural rekindling of the first fire or was deliberately set. That finding was not clearly erroneous (*United States v. Markum *1993, 896).*

Another case that directly addressed the application of *Daubert* to fire investigation was *Polizzi Meats, Inc. (PMI) v. Aetna Life and Casualty* (1996). In that case, the Federal District Court of New Jersey ruled:

> *PMI's counsel argues that because of a lack of "scientific proof" of the fire's causation, none of Aetna's witnesses may testify at trial. This astounding contention is based on a seriously flawed reading of the United States Supreme Court's decision in Daubert v. Merrell Dow Pharmaceuticals, Inc. Daubert addresses the standards to be applied by a trial judge when faced with a proffer of expert scientific testimony based upon a novel theory or methodology. Nothing in Daubert suggests that trial judges should exclude otherwise relevant testimony of police and fire investigators on the issues of the origins and causes of fires (*Polizzi Meats, Inc. v. Aetna Life and Casualty *1996, 336–37; citations omitted).*

These two decisions were the only reported cases considering *Daubert* in the specific context of fire investigation until the Eleventh Circuit announced its decision in the *Joiner* case, which took an entirely different view on the process of fire scene investigation.

The *Markum* case analysis was provided courtesy of Guy E. Burnette, Jr., Tallahassee, Florida (2003).

As courts from various jurisdictions continued trying to shed light on the full meaning of *Daubert*, the US Supreme Court took up the issue again and provided some guidance and insights. In *General Electric Company v. Joiner* (1997), the Court reviewed a case in which the trial judge had entered summary judgment in favor of the defendant in a lawsuit alleging that the plaintiff had contracted cancer as the result of exposure to PCB chemicals. The scientific evidence in support of the plaintiff's claim was derived from laboratory studies of mice that had been injected with massive doses of PCB chemicals and certain limited epidemiological studies suggesting a causal connection between PCB chemicals and cancer in humans. The trial judge ruled that the evidence offered by the plaintiff failed to satisfy the requirements of *Daubert*, describing the evidence offered by the plaintiff's experts as "subjective belief or unsupported speculation." It was noted that *Joiner* failed to present any credible scientific evidence of a direct causal connection between exposure to PCB chemicals and cancer.

On appeal, the ruling was reversed by the US Court of Appeals for the Eleventh Circuit, which held that the evidence should have been presented to the jury for a decision. The appellate court observed that the *Federal Rules of Evidence* favor the admissibility of expert testimony as a general rule. Furthermore, the appellate court applied a more stringent standard of review of the trial court's ruling, since the ruling was "outcome determinative" (i.e., resolved the entire case).

The US Supreme Court overturned the decision of the Eleventh Circuit and reinstated the ruling of the trial court. In doing so, the Court reiterated and clarified some of the points made in the *Daubert* decision. First, the role of the trial judge as gatekeeper was reaffirmed. In particular, the trial judge not only was allowed to draw his own conclusions about the weight of evidence offered by an expert witness but was expected to do so. It was noted that this had been a function of the trial judge long before the *Daubert* decision itself. Since this was a proper role of the trial judge, the decision to accept or reject expert testimony would not be subject to a more stringent standard of review on appeal. The decision of the trial judge would be given deference on appeal and it would require showing an "abuse of discretion" for the decision of the trial judge to be overturned.

The Supreme Court held that the application of *Daubert* to expert testimony is not merely a review and approval of the methodology employed but also includes scrutiny of the ultimate conclusions reached by the expert witness based on the methodologies and data employed to reach those conclusions. Notably, the Court did not clarify the controversy over scientific evidence versus technical evidence. The Court did not address the issue in *Joiner* because it was clearly a "scientific evidence" case. That remains a major part of the controversy in construing *Daubert* and the admissibility of expert testimony. The *Benfield* decision did directly address this issue and demonstrated a new perspective on this critical aspect of fire investigation.

This case history was provided courtesy of Guy E. Burnette, Jr., Tallahassee, Florida (2003).

The *Benfield* Case

In *Michigan Miller's Mutual Insurance Company v. Benfield* (1998), the US Court of Appeals for the Eleventh Circuit applied the *Daubert* analysis to a fire scene investigation. This case has attracted great attention within the fire investigation community and has become a focal point of the *Daubert* controversy.

In January 1996, the *Benfield* case was tried in federal district court in Tampa, Florida. The case involved a house fire for which the insurance company, Michigan Miller's Mutual, refused to pay on the policy based, in part, on the fire's being incendiary and on the apparent involvement of an insured party in setting the fire. As a part of the insurer's case, a fire investigator with more than 30 years of experience in fire investigations was called as an expert witness to present his opinion as to the origin and cause of the fire. He testified that the fire was started on top of the dining room table where some clothing, papers, and ordinary combustibles had been piled together. He examined the fire scene primarily by visual observation and concluded that the fire was incendiary based on the absence of any evidence of an accidental cause, along with other evidence and factors noted at the scene. After cross-examining the investigator, the plaintiff moved to exclude the testimony under *Daubert*. The trial court agreed. In the trial court's ruling striking the expert's testimony, the judge specifically found that the witness

> cites no scientific theory, applies no scientific method. He relies on his experience. He makes no scientific tests or analyses. He does not list the possible causes, including arson, and then using scientific methods exclude all except arson. He says no source or origin can be found on his personal visual examination and, therefore, the source and origin must be arson. There is no question but that the conclusion is one to which *Daubert* applies, a conclusion based on the absence of accepted scientific method.
>
> And finally, it must be noted that [his] conclusion was not based on a scientific examination of the remains, but only on his failure to be able to determine a cause and origin from his unscientific examination. This testimony is woefully inadequate under *Daubert* principles and pre-*Daubert* principles, and his testimony will be stricken and the jury instructed to disregard the same (*Michigan Miller's Mutual Insurance Company v. Benfield*, 140 F.3d 915, 1998, *Daubert* motion hearing transcript at 124–26).

Interestingly, the court in *Benfield* initially found the expert to be qualified to render opinions in the area of origin and cause of fires and allowed him to testify, based on his qualifications and credentials as a fire investigator. However, the judge struck the expert's testimony after it was presented based on his methodologies in conducting the particular fire scene investigation in that case. Having stricken the expert's testimony, the judge then found that, as a matter of law, arson had not been proved by Michigan Miller's and directed a verdict against them on the arson issue.

The evidence was undisputed that the area of origin was on top of the dining room table. Therefore, the only issue was the cause of the fire. The expert testified that while he was conducting his investigation, he spoke with Ms. Benfield, who told him that when she was last in the house before the fire there was a hurricane lamp and a half-full bottle of lamp oil on the top of the table. He further testified that he examined photographs taken by the fire department before the scene was disturbed and observed an empty, undamaged bottle of lamp oil lying on the floor with the cap removed (also undamaged), indicating that it had been opened and moved from the table prior to the setting of the fire. He also explained his observations at the fire scene that enabled him to rule out all possible accidental causes. He concluded that the fire was incendiary using the elimination method, long recognized as a valid method of determining fire origin and cause. He could not, however, determine the source of ignition for the fire. More important, he did not "scientifically document" his findings on various points and relied primarily on his 30 years of experience as a fire investigator, even as he held himself out as an expert in fire science adhering to the scientific method in conducting his investigation.

On cross-examination by Ms. Benfield's attorney, the expert was asked to define the scientific method and was asked the "scientific basis" for the taking of certain photographs apparently unrelated to the fire itself. The cross-examination continued by attacking each piece of evidence used by the expert that could not be said to be scientifically objective and scientifically verified. The investigator's determination of the smoldering nature of the fire and the time he estimated it burned before being discovered were discredited as not being based on scientific calculations of heat release rate and fire spread, but merely the investigator's observations of the smoke damage and other physical evidence. The court noted those points from the cross-examination in finding that the expert's methodology was not in conformity with the scientific method, relying instead almost exclusively on the expert's own training and experience, which it held to be inadmissible under *Daubert*.

On May 4, 1998, the Eleventh Circuit issued its ruling in the *Benfield* case. Contrary to the Tenth Circuit decision in *Markum* and the federal district case in *Polizzi Meats*, the court found the investigator's fire scene analysis to be subject to the *Daubert* test of reliability. In reaching this conclusion, the court noted that the investigator in *Benfield* held himself out as an expert in the area of "fire science" and claimed that he had complied with the "scientific method" under *NFPA 921*. Thus, by his own admission he was engaged in a "scientific process," which the court held to be subject to *Daubert*.

Under the *Daubert* test of reliability, the appeals court upheld the decision of the trial judge striking the expert's testimony. Noting that it is within the trial court's discretion to admit expert testimony, such a decision will be affirmed on appeal absent a showing of an abuse of discretion or that the decision was "manifestly erroneous." Under such a daunting standard, the trial judge is effectively given the final word on whether both the qualifications and findings of an expert witness will be considered sufficient and reliable enough to be presented to the jury. It is not simply a matter of having the power to decide whether a witness is qualified to testify as an expert; the substance of the expert's testimony and his or her professional conclusions first have to meet the approval of the trial judge before they can be presented to the jury. The trial judge acting as gatekeeper can summarily reject the findings and conclusions of an expert witness, preempting the jury from making that decision.

In the *Benfield* decision, various scientifically unsupported and scientifically undocumented conclusions of the investigator were cited as grounds for the determination that his observations and findings failed the *Daubert* reliability test. A chandelier hanging over the dining room table where the fire started showed no signs of having caused the fire, but the investigator had not conducted any tests or examinations to eliminate it scientifically as a potential cause of the fire. His observations alone were held inadequate. Similarly, his opinion that the fire had likely been accelerated with the lamp oil contained in the bottle was rejected under *Daubert*, since he could not scientifically prove that there had been oil in the bottle before the fire and he had not taken any samples from the fire debris to prove scientifically its presence or absence at the time the fire was ignited. These and other observations of the investigator were held to demonstrate that there was no scientific basis for his conclusions, only his personal opinion from experience in investigating other fires.

It was not that the investigator was found to be "wrong" in the *Benfield* case. Indeed, there was never any evidence of an accidental cause of the fire. Ironically, although the appeals court upheld the decision of the trial judge to strike the testimony of the insurance investigator, it granted a new trial for Michigan Miller's on the arson defense. The appeals court felt that a prima facie case of arson had been shown at trial through the fire department investigator, who initially classified the fire only as suspicious (with virtually no challenge to the scientific documentation of his opinion), and the many incriminating circumstances surrounding the fire itself.

Circumstances included the fact that Ms. Benfield claimed that she had not locked the deadbolts when she left the house, yet the deadbolts were locked when she returned to discover the fire. Ms. Benfield and her daughter (who had been out of town) had the only keys to those locks. Her assertion that her boyfriend extinguished the fire with a garden hose was refuted by the observations of the responding firefighters. Her insurance claim appeared to be significantly inflated. She had tried to sell the house and could not do so. She was trying to convince her estranged husband to transfer the house to her but could not do so. Ms. Benfield had given conflicting and contradictory accounts of her activities immediately before the fire.

In listing all these reasons, the appeals court found that there was compelling evidence of arson even as it discredited the findings of the insurance investigator that the fire was incendiary. The critical point in the case appears to be the distinction between the insurance investigator's testifying as an expert in fire science and the fire department representative's testifying as an expert in fire investigation.

This case history was provided courtesy of Guy E. Burnette, Jr., Tallahassee, Florida (2003).

A decision of the US Court of Appeals for the Tenth Circuit underscored the importance of properly evaluating and presenting expert testimony in fire litigation cases. *Truck Insurance Exchange v. MagneTek, Inc.* (2004) not only demonstrated the application of the *Daubert* standard for the admissibility of expert testimony but effectively contradicted a long-standing principle of fire science that had been used in a significant number of cases to prove the cause of a fire.

The *MagneTek* case involved a subrogation action filed by Truck Insurance Exchange against the manufacturer of a fluorescent light ballast that was alleged to have caused a fire that destroyed a restaurant in Lakewood, Colorado. Responding to the alarm, the fire department first found heavy smoke in the restaurant but no open flames. The fire subsequently broke through the kitchen floor in the restaurant from the ceiling of a storage room in the basement. Before the fire could be controlled and extinguished, it destroyed the restaurant and caused damages in excess of $1.5 million.

Investigations by both the local fire protection district and a private fire investigation firm hired by the insurer determined that the fire had started in a void space between the basement storage room ceiling and the kitchen floor. In the basement, the investigators found the remains of a fluorescent light fixture that had been mounted to the ceiling of the storage room. They determined the light fixture had been located in the area of origin of the fire and concluded that the fire had been caused by an apparent failure of the ballast in the light fixture.

The investigators and a physicist examined the remains of the fluorescent light fixture. They determined that MagneTek manufactured the ballast. They observed oxidation patterns on the light fixture indicating an internal failure, along with discoloration of the heating coils of the ballast suggesting it had shorted to cause overheating, which resulted in the fire. The ballast contained a thermal protector designed to shut off power to the fixture when the internal temperature exceeded 111°C (232°F). The thermal protector in the ballast appeared to function properly, even after the fire. However, the investigators remained convinced that the ballast had somehow failed, overheated, and started the fire.

Tests were conducted with similar ballasts manufactured by MagneTek, which showed that at least one of the exemplar ballasts when shorted would not cut off power to the fixture until the internal temperatures had reached at least 171°C (340°F) and would continue to provide power to the fixture even when the ballast maintained constant temperatures of 148°C (300°F) or more.

The investigators theorized that the heat from the ballast had caused pyrolysis to occur in the adjacent wood structure of the ceiling, causing pyrophoric carbon to form over a prolonged time, which would be capable of ignition at temperatures substantially below the normal ignition range of 204°C (400°F) or more for the fresh whole wood. The phenomenon of pyrolysis in the formation of pyrophoric carbon has been the subject of a number of studies, reviews, and articles by fire investigators and fire scientists. It has been cited as the cause of a number of fires having no other apparent explanation, often linked to heated pipes in structures within walls, ceilings, and floor areas. As the MagneTek court case would note, however, the validity of this phenomenon has been discussed and debated by fire investigators and fire scientists for a number of years.

The investigators in this case acknowledged that electrical wiring ran through the ceiling area of the storage room near the fluorescent light fixture but discounted the possibility of a failure in the electrical wiring. They reported finding no evidence of arcing or shorting in the electrical wiring, although the fire at the restaurant resulted in the destruction of much of the electrical wiring and other evidence in the area. Because the investigations concluded the fire had originated in the immediate area of the light fixture, they concluded the only source of ignition for the fire was the light fixture and its ballast.

Pyrolysis and the formation of pyrophoric carbon was the foundation of the plaintiff's case against MagneTek. The ballast in the light fixture showed no signs of failure in the thermal protector, which would have limited the heat generated by the ballast to about 111°C (232°F). Even with the exemplar ballast whose thermal protector failed to perform as it had been designed, the temperatures generated did not exceed 171°C (340°F). The investigators admitted the ignition temperature of fresh whole wood is typically at least 204°C (400°F), and the temperatures from the ballast alone would not have been sufficient to cause ignition. Their theory that the ballast had caused the fire depended on the concept of pyrolysis to allow ignition to occur at a lower temperature within the range of the temperatures generated by the ballast.

Following discovery in the case, MagneTek filed a *Daubert* motion to exclude the testimony of the experts that the ballast had caused the fire. MagneTek asserted that the theory of pyrolysis was not sufficiently reliable and scientifically verifiable to be offered by the experts in support of their conclusion for the cause of the fire. It was a challenge to the reliability of the experts' theory, which required a consideration of whether the reasoning or methodology underlying the testimony was scientifically valid, as mandated by *Daubert* and *FRE Rule 702*.

The Supreme Court in *Daubert* had outlined a number of factors that, although not an exclusive list of considerations for a trial court, should be examined in making the determination of reliability (see Table 1-4).

In proving the scientific validity of an expert's reasoning or methodology, the Court noted that "the plaintiff need not prove that the expert is indisputably correct or that the expert's theory is 'generally accepted' in the scientific community. Instead, the plaintiff must show that the method employed by the expert in reaching the conclusion is scientifically sound and that the opinion is based on facts which sufficiently satisfy *Rule 702*'s reliability requirements." See also *Mitchell v. Gencorp Inc.* (10th Cir. 1999).

The Tenth Circuit applied the standard of appellate review for a trial court ruling on a *Daubert* issue: the showing of an abuse of discretion demonstrating that the appellate court has "a definite and firm conviction that the lower court made a clear error of judgment or exceeded the bounds of permissible choice in the circumstances" (*United States v. Ortiz* 1986). The court then looked to the ruling of the trial judge finding that the testimony of the experts failed to satisfy the reliability standard under *Rule 702* and the *Daubert* decision. The physicist testifying on behalf of Truck Insurance Exchange was a highly credentialed expert with an advanced degree in physics from Oxford University and more than 20 years of experience in the study of fire and explosion incidents. Both the trial court and the appellate court observed that this expert was unquestionably qualified to testify as an expert witness under *Rule 702*. However, his hypothesis of pyrolysis and pyrophoric carbon as the cause of ignition of the wood in the area surrounding the light fixture could not be considered a reliable basis for the admission of his expert testimony on the cause of the fire.

The reliability standard under *Daubert* applies to both the theory offered and its application to the facts of the case. The court focused on the first component of these reliability criteria. In support of the theory of its experts, the insurer had introduced into evidence three publications on the theory of pyrolysis and pyrophoric carbon. Those articles were written by some of the most respected fire scientists in the world, but those articles and case studies acknowledged that the process of pyrolysis occurs over an undefined period of time described as "a period of years" or "a very long time" with no specific parameters for the timing and sequence of events involved in pyrolysis. One of those articles acknowledged that there are "a number of things not known about the process" and that "it may be many decades before it will be solved by sufficiently improving theory." The article concluded by stating "the phenomenon of long-term, low-temperature ignition of wood has neither been proven nor successfully disproven at this time."

The plaintiff's engineer had stated in his deposition that the process of pyrolysis "depends on a lot of factors, as yet quantitatively unidentified." He went on to testify "you would have to have a good theory of pyrophoric carbon and formation and the chemical kinetics of that; and there isn't one . . ." The other experts testifying for the plaintiff in this case based their theory of pyrolysis and pyrophoric carbon on their experience in the investigation of fires without any reference to a specific scientific basis for that theory.

The court noted that under *NFPA 921* an investigator offering the hypothesis of an appliance fire must first determine the ignition temperature of the available fuel in the area and then must determine the ability of the appliance or device to generate temperatures at or above the ignition temperature of the fuel. In that regard, the experts failed on both counts. The ignition temperature of the fuel (wood) exposed to the fixture in this case could not be scientifically proved to be below the 204°C (400°F) threshold for the ignition of most types of wood, and the tests of the ballasts had shown that even with a failed thermal protector, a ballast could not generate temperatures anywhere near that range. Their hypothesis would have to be based on either an unreliable theory (pyrolysis) or unsubstantiated assumptions and speculation about the temperature of the ballast that contradicted their own test results. As such, their testimony could not be admitted.

The appellate court affirmed the ruling of the trial court that the testimony of all the experts had been shown to be not sufficiently reliable to be admitted under the standards of the *Daubert* decision. Without the testimony of the experts, Truck Insurance Exchange could not make a prima facie case for establishing the cause of the fire. Accordingly, the trial court entered a summary judgment in favor of MagneTek, and the appellate court affirmed.

This decision has significant implications for the litigation of fire cases everywhere. It demonstrates the importance of developing sound and scientifically verifiable theories for proving the cause of a fire as required by the standards of the *Daubert* decision. Moreover, it provides a compelling example of how a theory that has not been validated and generally recognized by others in the scientific community may not withstand a *Daubert* challenge in court.

The lessons from this decision are many. First and foremost, experts must be prepared to prove the reliability of their investigative methodologies and theories to the satisfaction of the trial court. Experience alone is not sufficient. Even a theory that appears on the surface to be a reasonable and logical theory for the cause of a fire must be shown to be scientifically verifiable. Without a foundation in science, even the most experienced investigator will never be allowed to testify in court. Parties hiring investigators in their cases must be aware of the requirements for proving a case using investigative methodologies and theories that will meet the reliability standards of the *Daubert* decision, to guide them in both the selection of the expert used to investigate the fire and the decision to litigate the case. Attorneys handling cases must be aware of these issues to successfully litigate that case at trial. The investigator, the client, and the attorney all have a responsibility to ensure that cases are properly investigated and properly litigated. The *MagneTek* case is a striking example of the consequences of not doing so.

This case history was provided courtesy of Guy E. Burnette, Jr., Tallahassee, Florida (2003).

A scientific analysis and assessment of the *MagneTek* case decision indicates that the court may not have understood several important aspects of fire science, including pyrolysis, which is not newly discovered or scientifically disputed. In the *MagneTek* case, the court rejected under *Daubert* the pyrolysis theory of long-term, low-temperature ignition as being unreliable. Fire investigators who wish to explain this phenomenon in court must be prepared to make clear and convincing arguments using authoritative treatises and clearly defined definitions.

In the *Ignition Handbook* (Babrauskas 2003, p. 18), pyrolysis is clearly defined as "the chemical degradation of a substance by the action of heat." This definition includes both oxidative and non-oxidative pyrolysis, taking into account the cases where oxygen plays a role. Pyrolysis is a process that has been studied for many decades. Without pyrolysis to break down their molecular structures, most solid fuels will not burn. Unfortunately, the published court decision declares pyrolysis to be inadequately studied and documented (presumably intending to refer to the pyrophoric process). It is unclear what effect this misstatement of the court will have on future deliberations.

The scientific method states that a description of the conditions under which ignition can take place (1) may use a scientific theory, test, or calculation or (2) refer to authoritative data on the substance. For example, in the second case, the peer-reviewed literature (Babrauskas 2004, 2005) could have been used to show that the ignition temperatures of wood exposed to long-term, low-temperatures are documented as low as 77°C (170°F). Excluding other competent sources of energy, it could have been substantiated in the *MagneTek* case that a heat-producing product in excess of 77°C (170°F) in contact with wood for an extended period of time created a potential risk. Some substances have spontaneous combustion models. Unfortunately for the fire investigator, there does not exist at this time a model that predicts ignition of wood by pyrolysis with time/temperature curves that would allow the accurate prediction of necessary conditions, primarily owing to the complex chemical nature of wood as a fuel and the wide variability in the physical nature of the types and forms of wood.

Even more problematic, the court effectively denied the existence of any ignition due to self-heating because it declared that ignitable substances have a "handbook" ignition temperature, and a hot object below that temperature will not be a competent source of ignition. In actual fires, self-heating substances do not have a unique ignition temperature. Furthermore, if a substance (e.g., wood) can ignite owing to external, short-term heating or to a prolonged process involving self-heating, the minimum temperature for the latter has no relation to the published ignition temperatures for the former.

Finally, in the future, fire investigators who testify as to pyrophoric (i.e., low-temperature) ignition of wood should be prepared to discuss the phenomenon by referring to this collected set of observations on the topic and the hard scientific data. In addition to the *Ignition Handbook*, there exist ample peer-reviewed publications and case studies on the ignition process of wood. Also, additional information is available on the charring rate and ignition of wood (Babrauskas 2005; Babrauskas, Gray, and Janssens 2007).

This scientific case analysis is primarily based on information courtesy of Dr. Vytenis Babrauskas, Fire Science and Technology, Inc., Issaquah, Washington. For additional information, Zicherman and Lynch (2006) and Babrauskas (2004) also address the technical merits of this case.

1.7 Impact of *NFPA 921* on Science-Based Expert Testimony

NFPA 921 has been cited along with *Daubert* as a crucial element of expert testimony since it establishes guidelines for reliable and systematic investigations and the analysis of fire and explosion incidents (Campagnolo 1999; DeHaan and Icove 2012). Federal court opinions and rules cluster into the following areas:

- Use of investigative protocols, guidelines, and peer-reviewed citations
- Methodological explanations for burn patterns
- Qualifications to testify

As new protocols evolve and methodologies improve, ongoing professional education to keep abreast of relevant fire, engineering, and legal publications is critical for all professional fire investigators. As with science, today's knowledge may change with new developments and impact the reviews of an established hypothesis.

1.7.1 REFERENCES TO *NFPA 921*

In 1997, a federal judge upheld a motion by a defendant insurance company in a civil case barring the plaintiff's expert fire investigator from mentioning *NFPA 921* during his testimony.

NFPA 921 was first published in 1992, well after the November 16, 1988, fire in question. The judge requested that the plaintiffs provide him a copy of *NFPA 921*. The judge found that under *Rule 703* of the *Federal Rules of Evidence,* any reference to *NFPA 921* would have little probative value and would confuse the jury (*LaSalle National Bank et al. v. Massachusetts Bay Insurance Company et al.* 1997). This ultraconservative finding has not been widely accepted. In fact, most court decisions since then have acknowledged the value of *NFPA 921.*

For example, following a November 18, 1999, motor vehicle accident, an individual was trapped for approximately 45 minutes in the front passenger seat after the car in which he was riding collided with a utility pole. Eyewitnesses reported a bluish flickering and fire that engulfed the vehicle's interior and severely burned the trapped passenger. A product liability lawsuit against the vehicle's manufacturer alleged a defective design, since a proposed safety device would have disconnected the battery after the collision (*John Witten Tunnell v. Ford Motor Company* 2004). The plaintiffs alleged that the energized wiring harness suffered a high-resistance fault, which could have caused a fire without blowing a fuse. The judge reviewed and overruled motions to exclude the testimony of fire origin experts and repeatedly cited the applicability of the *NFPA 921* methodology to the case.

1.7.2 INVESTIGATIVE PROTOCOLS

In a 1999 federal criminal case, the defendant moved that the court exclude a state fire marshal's testimony on the incendiary nature of a fire, arguing that the testimony did not meet the standards for admissibility under *Daubert* (*United States v. Lawrence R. Black Wolf, Jr.* 1999). The defendant argued that the testimony should be excluded because the investigator did not arrive at the scene until 10 days after the fire occurred and did not take samples for laboratory analysis; the theory of the fire's origin and cause had not been subject to accurate and reliable peer review; and no scientific methods or procedures were used to reach the conclusions. The defendant's Exhibit A was the 1998 edition of *NFPA 921.*

The federal magistrate reviewing this dispute determined that the investigator's proffered testimony was reliable, since he had indeed used an investigative protocol consistent with the basic methodologies and procedures recommended by *NFPA 921,* and he passed the requisite scrutiny demanded of fire origin and cause experts (Figure 1-3).

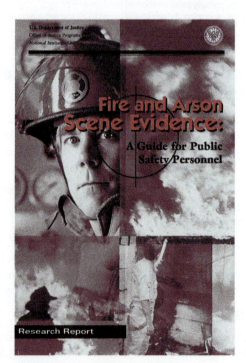

FIGURE 1-3 An investigator's proffered testimony may be deemed reliable if it is in accordance with an investigative protocol, such as the one published by the US Department of Justice that cites methodologies and procedures recommended by *NFPA 921. Courtesy of US Department of Justice, www.usdoj.gov.*

Regarding the relevancy test, the magistrate determined that the investigator's testimony would help a jury understand the circumstances surrounding the fire's origin and cause. The magistrate further found that *Rule 703* had been met, since the investigator's proffered testimony relied on facts and data normally collected by experts when forming opinions as to the fire's origin and cause. The magistrate concluded that the defendant would have ample opportunity to address the expert's opinion during cross-examination, through presentation of contrary evidence, and in instructions to the jury.

1.7.3 CASE EXAMPLES OF THE USE OF GUIDELINES AND PEER-REVIEWED CITATIONS

In a case involving a November 16, 1994, residential fire, a number of independent investigators attempted to determine the exact origin and cause of the fire. One investigator, an electrical engineer, offered the opinion that a television set located in the basement family room caused the fire. The plaintiffs sued the manufacturer of the television, alleging product liability, negligence, and breach of warranties (*Andronic Pappas et al. v. Sony Electronics, Inc. et al.* 2000).

A federal judge adjudicating the case held a two-day *Daubert* hearing and concluded that the one investigator's causation testimony was inadmissible. The judge cited that the primary concern with the testimony stemmed from the second *Rule 702* factor, that an expert's opinion should be based on a reliable methodology. The judge noted that the investigator did not use a fixed set of guidelines in determining the cause of the fire. Notably, the investigator did confirm that even though he was aware of the existence of established guidelines in *NFPA 921* and *Kirk's Fire Investigation,* he relied on his own experience and knowledge. During the hearing, the plaintiffs did not submit any books, articles, or witnesses on proper fire causation techniques other than the testimony of one investigator. The judge specifically commented on the fact that the one investigator referred to his reliance on a burn pattern inside the television set. No citations were made to peer-reviewed sources to support this opinion.

In a product liability case arising from a fire on July 16, 1998, which destroyed a business, the plaintiff's only expert placed the origin of the fire at a product manufactured by the defendant (*Chester Valley Coach Works et al. v. Fisher-Price Inc.* 2001). Based on testimony and arguments received at a *Daubert* hearing held June 14, 2001, the court excluded the expert's testimony and his opinion regarding the fire's origin and cause. At the hearing, the expert indicated his conclusions were based primarily on his experience and education and not based on any testing, experimentation, or generally accepted texts or treatises. Several of the steps he undertook in his investigation were contrary to the *NFPA 921* guidelines.

In a federal court decision on April 16, 2003, a plaintiff's *Daubert* motion to exclude the testimony of a defendant's expert witness was overruled (*James B. McCoy et al. v. Whirlpool Corp. et al.* 2003). The plaintiffs alleged that a dishwasher caused a fire at their residence on February 16, 2000, and argued that the expert's report on the origin and cause of the fire did not explicitly cite the methodology set forth in *NFPA 921*. In its decision, the court noted that the expert did not need to cite *NFPA 921*, since he had adequately provided a complete statement of all opinions and a substantive rationale for the basis of these opinions.

1.7.4 PEER REVIEW OF THEORY

In a case involving a residence fire that occurred around December 22, 1996, an insurance company hired an investigator to determine the cause of the fire, which all parties agreed had originated in an area to the right of a fireplace firebox. The defendants disputed the cause of the fire and filed a motion to exclude the testimony of the plaintiff's expert (*Allstate Insurance Company v. Hugh Cole et al.* 2001).

Even though the plaintiff filed his complaint on December 21, 1998, prior to the December 1, 2000, effective date of the amended *Rule 702*, the judge applied the amended *Rule 702* to the admissibility of the testimony (FRCP 2010). The plaintiff asserted that in his trial testimony the investigator would rely on data from *NFPA 921* to support his opinion.

The opinion of the plaintiff's investigator was that heat from a metal pipe ignited adjacent combustibles. The judge noted that the theory, based on principles embodied in *NFPA 921,* had already been subjected to peer review, was generally accepted in the scientific community, and met the sufficient reliability guidelines to satisfy the admissibility requirements of *Rule 702*. Peer review can also include consultation with other qualified fire experts, both scientific and investigative.

1.7.5 METHODOLOGY NEEDED

On September 13, 1996, a residential fire started in the corner of a kitchen containing a dishwasher, toaster oven, and microwave oven. The municipal fire marshal concluded that the fire was caused by the microwave oven, whereas in a federal civil case, the plaintiff's expert asserted that a defective toaster oven caused the fire (*Jacob J. Booth and Kathleen Booth v. Black and Decker, Inc.* 2001).

A senior federal judge held a *Daubert* hearing in which evidentiary and testimonial records were reviewed. He ruled that the opinion of the plaintiff's investigator was not admissible under *Rule 702* because the plaintiff's investigator did not provide sufficient reliable evidence to support the methodology for investigating the cause of the fire. The judge also noted that the comprehensive nature of *NFPA 921* contained a methodology that could have supported the opinion and could have been utilized as a basis for testing the hypothesis for the fire's cause.

On December 8, 1999, a circuit court judge in the State of Michigan granted a plaintiff's motion *in limine* to exclude the testimony of the defendant's expert witness (*Ronald Taepke v. Lake States Insurance Company* 1999). In testimony and written reports, the defendant's expert admitted the authoritative nature of *NFPA 921* yet admitted that he did not follow its accepted methodology. Furthermore, the methodology used to conclude that the fire was arson is not recognized in any reliable source of literature in the fire investigation field. In other areas, the expert admitted that he speculated that high-temperature accelerants were used without a reliable evidentiary basis for the opinion.

In a federal civil case opinion issued on March 28, 2002, involving automobile ignition switch fires, a federal judge examined the proposed use of a statistical vehicle fire loss database in litigation. The judge also examined in detail the importance of reliance on *NFPA 921* in fire investigations when forming a hypothesis using the scientific method (*Snodgrass et al. v. Ford Motor Company and United Technologies Automotive, Inc.* 2002). Since this court case was within the Third Circuit, a determination of whether an expert's methodology was reliable used the combined *Daubert* and *Downing* factors.

In *United States v. John W. Downing* (1985), the court considered the admissibility of expert testimony concerning the reliability of eyewitness identification. The court held that in appropriate cases, an eyewitness expert can indeed assist the trier of fact, and thus the expert's testimony is admissible under the *Federal Rules of Evidence*. An expert's opinion testimony is considered helpful to the jury because many of the factors the expert will testify to go beyond common knowledge, at times may directly contradict common sense, and may be able to refute jurors' erroneous assumptions about eyewitness reliability.

In a state court of appeals opinion decided on June 16, 2005, the court ruled that the testimony of the appellee's independent fire investigator was correctly permitted by the trial court under *Daubert* as to the origin and cause of the fire (*Abon Ltd. et al. v. Transcontinental Insurance Company* 2005). The court noted that the independent investigator followed the *NFPA 921* methods and principles to reach his opinion as to the incendiary nature of the fire's origin and cause.

In a fatal apartment fire on October 23, 2000, personal representatives and relatives of the decedent brought an action against the manufacturer of an electric blanket, alleging it had a defective safety circuit that caused the deadly fire (*David Bryte v. American Household Inc.* 2005). The fire marshal who determined the origin and cause of the fire was not certified as a fire investigator, yet he had attended training in the fire and explosion investigation field. He traced the fire's path to the deceased's left side, took photographs, made a fire scene sketch, and took oral statements from witnesses. While he did not inspect the electrical wiring or take any evidence, he noted an electrical cord draped across the victim's body and concluded the cause of the fire to be the improper use of an electric blanket. During the trial on December 8, 2003, a *Daubert* analysis was conducted in which the court disallowed the fire marshal and another expert from providing expert testimony because they did not have a sufficiently reliable basis for their testimony.

In a federal court of appeals ruling in a product liability case concerning a fire-related death, both the magistrate judge and district court concluded that pursuant to the *Daubert* and *Federal Rules of Evidence* standards, the methodologies employed by the plaintiff's expert witnesses were too unreliable to serve as the basis for admissible testimony (*Bethie Pride v. BIC Corporation, Société BIC, S.A.* 2000). The case alleged that the death of a 60-year-old man who sustained burns on 95 percent of his body was caused by an explosion of a disposable lighter he was carrying while inspecting a pipe behind his house. The court noted that the plaintiff's experts failed to conduct timely, replicable laboratory experiments demonstrating how the explosion was consistent with a manufacturing defect in the lighter. One of the plaintiff's experts testified he began a laboratory experiment to test his hypothesis but "chickened out and shut the experiment down."

In a federal case in which an insurance company attempted to recover in subrogation for fire damage to the property of one of its insureds, the defendant construction company filed a motion to preclude the trial testimony of the plaintiff's fire expert on origin and cause (*Royal Insurance Company of America, as Subrogee of Patrick and Linda Magee v. Joseph Daniel Construction, Inc.* 2002). The plaintiff's insureds had hired a construction company to work on a garage on their property on December 14, 1998. The work involved the use of an acetylene torch to install new beams above the second floor. During the operation of the torch, two fires occurred and were extinguished. Approximately 14 hours after the construction company left, a fire was discovered in the garage, which sustained damage.

Approximately one year after the fire, the plaintiffs hired an expert to investigate the origin and cause of the fire. Based on his investigation, the expert concluded that the fire was caused by the careless use of the welding and cutting equipment by the construction company employees. The court noted that the expert conducted the investigation in accordance with methodology set forth by *NFPA 921*. To develop his hypothesis that the garage fire occurred as a result of molten slag dropped by careless construction workers, the investigator used data consisting of information gleaned from copies of photographs, insurance investigative and engineering reports, reviews of depositions, and his own witness interviews. He also eliminated other common causes for the fire. Citing the *Daubert* standard, the court ruled that the expert's testimony was relevant in establishing a direct relationship between the proffered theory concerning the carelessness of the defendant with regard to molten slag and the cause of the fire.

An unpublished case from the US Court of Appeals for the Third Circuit concluded that a district court did not err in granting and excluding the testimony of a plaintiff's expert witness (*State Farm and Casualty Company, as Subrogee of Rocky Mountain and Suzanne Mountain v. Holmes Products; J.C. Penney Company, Inc.* 2006). On April 5, 1999, a fire destroyed a residence. The insurance company's investigator placed the fire's area of origin at a halogen lamp that lacked a safety guard to prevent contact between the high-temperature portions of the lamp and nearby curtains, clothing, or other flammable materials. After eliminating all other potential causes, the investigator concluded that the fire was caused by nearby draperies' coming into contact with the defective energized lamp. The investigator further hypothesized that the dog belonging to the residence's owners might have accidentally pulled the window draperies over the energized lamp or knocked the lamp into contact with the draperies. The judge concluded that the fire investigator's testimony did not satisfy *Daubert* because the conclusion on causation was based on assumptions and was not supported by any methodology.

In a subrogation lawsuit, an insurance company brought an action against a clothes dryer manufacturer to recover damages in connection with 23 fires allegedly caused by a design defect (*Travelers Property and Casualty Corporation v. General Electric Company* 2001). A *Daubert* hearing was necessary when the defendant manufacturer moved to prevent the testimony of the plaintiff's expert, who had written and issued a three-page report alleging that accumulated lint in an undetectable location could be ignited by the dryer's heating elements. The judge overruled the motion, finding that the expert's proffered opinion testimony met the requirements of both *Rule 702* and *Daubert,* that the opinion was consistent with the principles of *NFPA 921* and the scientific method, and the expert's qualifications were sufficient. However, the judge found that the plaintiff's three-page expert disclosure report amounted to bad faith, and he ordered the plaintiff to reimburse the defendant for one-third of its costs and expenses for taking the first 12 days of the expert's deposition and permitted up to 2 more days of depositions.

1.7.6 METHODOLOGICAL EXPLANATIONS FOR BURN PATTERNS

In the case of an April 23, 1997, building fire, a federal magistrate denied the plaintiff's motion to bar opinion testimony at the time of trial as to the origin and cause of the fire (*Eid Abu-Hashish and Sheam Abu-Hashish v. Scottsdale Insurance Company* 2000). In this case, both a municipal fire department investigator and a private insurance investigator concluded from their examinations of the scene that the fire was incendiary in origin. No physical evidence was taken for laboratory examination.

The plaintiff argued that these investigators were not reliable and their testimonies were inadmissible under *Rule 702* because they did not use the scientific method as outlined in *NFPA 921* and relied only on physical evidence observed at the scene. The case also contained parallels with the *Benfield* case (*Michigan Miller's Mutual Insurance Company v. Benfield* 1998), where the Eleventh Circuit upheld the trial court's decision to exclude an expert witness who testified on fire causation that the fire in the Benfield home was intentionally set. In denying the plaintiff's motion, the magistrate noted that the investigators were able to provide an adequate methodological explanation for the analysis of burn patterns that led to how they reached their conclusion as to the fire's incendiary origin (Figure 1-4).

In a product liability case arising from a fire on October 16, 2000, which destroyed a video rental store, two of the plaintiff's fire causation experts determined the origin and cause of the fire to be a copier machine (*Fireman's Fund Insurance Company v. Canon USA, Inc.* 2005). The two experts relied on burn patterns inside the copier and testing of an exemplar heater assembly for the copier. A federal appeals court upheld the district court's ruling that documentation of the experimentation by the plaintiff's experts did not meet the standards of *NFPA 921* and was unreliable and potentially confusing to a jury. The court found that tests must be carefully designed to replicate actual conditions, conducted properly, and documented thoroughly.

A state civil court opinion and order entered February 1, 2006, precluded *in limine* the testimony of the defendant's expert, who proposed to testify regarding the incendiary nature of a fire he investigated (*Marilyn McCarver v. Farm Bureau General Insurance Company* 2006). On August 16, 2003, a fire damaged the plaintiff's residence. A report authored August 23, 2003, by the defendant insurance company's expert concluded that the fire was incendiary in origin after visiting and viewing the remains of the residence, taking photographs, taking samples for laboratory examination, and performing other techniques. The state court noted that although the defendant's expert stated that his investigation complied with *NFPA 921*, he did not follow procedure in several areas. The expert failed to document

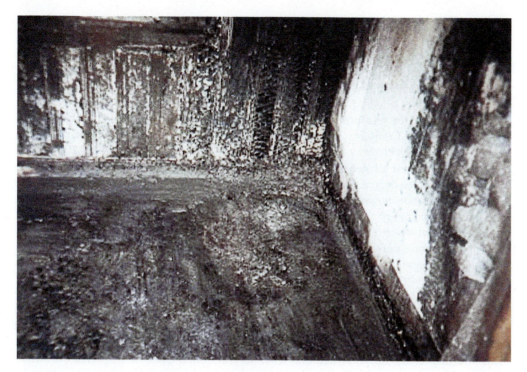

FIGURE 1-4 Investigators should be able to provide adequate and methodical explanations of the fire pattern analysis methods they use to reach conclusions as to the origin of a fire. *Courtesy of David J. Icove, University of Tennessee.*

any depth-of-char physical measurements; failed to document his vector analysis, which formed the basis for flame patterns; and failed to retrieve samples submitted for chemical testing, which resulted in their destruction. After a *Daubert* hearing, the court concluded that the fatal flaw of the expert's failure to collect and record depth-of-char data undermined his methodology for determining the origin and cause of the fire.

1.7.7 METHODOLOGY AND QUALIFICATIONS

In the case of a residential fire on July 1, 1998, which resulted in a federal lawsuit for product liability, the judge granted the defendant's motion to exclude the testimony of the electrical engineer, citing *Daubert, Rule 702,* and *Rule 704* (*American Family Insurance Group v. JVC America Corp.* 2001). In this case, an insurance company investigator called on an electrical engineer to remove and examine the charred remains of a bathroom exhaust fan, clock, lamp, timer, compact disc player, computer with printer and monitor, ceiling fan, power receptacle, and power strip. The engineer came to an opinion that a defect in the compact disc player caused the fire. His observations were based on burn patterns in the room, on appliance remains, and on his experience, education, and training. In his ruling, the judge noted that the training and experience of the engineer did not qualify him to offer an analysis of burn patterns and theory of fire origin. Furthermore, the judge noted that the engineer did not use the scientific method recommended by *NFPA 921* to form a hypothesis from the analysis of the data, nor did he satisfy the requirements for expert testimony under *Daubert.*

In a fire on March 1, 2001, originating in a building's janitorial closet, the plaintiff alleged that the fire was caused by a short circuit in a contaminated electrical bus duct (*103 Investors I, L.P. v. Square D Company* 2005). The plaintiff retained a licensed mechanical engineer who was also a certified fire investigator to investigate the origin and cause of the fire. The engineer testified that he investigated the fire in accordance with the scientific method protocol set forth in *NFPA 921*. In an opinion dated May 10, 2005, a federal judge ruled that the engineer's testimony could include that the short circuit resulted from the presence of contaminants. However, since the engineer failed to follow established methods of inquiry for hypothesis testing of how the contamination actually occurred, he could not testify that the fire specifically resulted from short-circuiting in the bus duct.

In a case before a federal magistrate, the magistrate denied a third-party defendant's motion to exclude the testimony of the plaintiff's expert on the origin and cause of a vehicle fire (*TNT Road Company et al. v. Sterling Truck Corporation, Sterling Truck Corporation, Third-Party Plaintiff v. Lear Corporation, Third-Party Defendant* 2004). The third-party defendant alleged that the witness was not qualified to render an expert opinion, lacked a college degree, was not a certified fire investigator, was not a licensed private investigator, did not interview every conceivable witness, quickly came to his conclusion, relied heavily on theory and circumstantial evidence, had testified only once as an expert witness, and that his investigation was too faulty to be admissible under *FRE Rule 702*.

The magistrate noted that the witness had demonstrated sufficient knowledge, skill, training, and education to qualify as an expert and that his methodology appeared reliable. The judge decided that the witness's investigation substantially complied with *NFPA 921* because with the vehicle's owners he had systematically examined and photographed the scene and all the components that may have been potential causes of the fire. He also obtained and reviewed the maintenance records, systematically removed and photographed the fire debris, formed no immediate opinions as to the cause of the fire, and narrowed his focus to a suspected ignition switch only after several hours. Once he suspected the switch may have been the cause of the fire, the expert suspended his investigation to preserve the evidence until other interested parties could be available to also inspect the vehicle.

On February 15, 2001, a fire broke out in the kitchen of a residence near a coffeemaker, causing extensive fire, smoke, and water damage. The insurance company paid the claim and pursued subrogation against the manufacturer of the coffeemaker (*Vigilant Insurance v. Sunbeam Corporation* 2005). The testimonies of several witnesses were limited based on a *Daubert* hearing on March 1, 2004. The testimony of the fire investigator was found inadmissible under *Rule 702* because his opinion was not based on data that he might have gleaned from testing the coffeemaker and toaster cords, safety devices, or the fluorescent light. He was able to testify under *Rule 701* as a lay witness as to his personal observations that the coffeemaker was at the base of the V burn pattern. During the hearing, the court found that another witness's burn test was simply a reenactment of the kitchen fire and was not substantially similar owing to differences in the heat applied to the coffeemaker, the amount of water in the coffeepot, and the thickness of the countertop. A jury trial held from March 2, 2005, to March 17, 2005, resulted in a verdict in favor of the plaintiff's insurance company.

In a federal civil lawsuit, the plaintiffs sought to hold the defendant, the manufacturer of a freezer, liable for damages stemming from a fire that allegedly originated in the freezer (*Mark and Dian Workman v. AB Electrolux Corporation et al.* 2005). Despite using *NFPA 921* to guide his investigative process, the investigator for the plaintiff's insurance company failed to determine what caused the fire. The investigator then arranged for a mechanical engineer, who conducted a further destructive examination and determined that the fire originated inside the freezer as the result of a short circuit in the evaporator compartment. The court's review of the engineer's testimony based on the criteria set forth in *Daubert* and *Rule 702* found the engineer's testimony reliable. However, the engineer did not mention or describe a defect in the freezer.

In a federal civil lawsuit, a June 1, 2001, fire damaged the home, garage, and property of the plaintiffs (*Theresa M. Zeigler, individually; and Theresa M. Zeigler, as mother and next friend of Madisen Zeigler v. Fisher-Price, Inc.* 2003). The fire allegedly originated in a toy vehicle parked in the garage and plugged into a charger. Two expert witnesses looked into the causation of the fire. The court determined that the insurance company investigator followed *NFPA 921* and an appropriate and generally accepted methodology, and found that his opinions were reliable. The second investigator was an engineer who did not perform an origin and cause analysis but had an opinion that the fire's ignition source was located on a connector to the toy vehicle. The court ruled that the engineer could not give an opinion as to the manufacturer's record keeping, or the origin or cause of the fire.

1.7.8 AUTHORITATIVE SCIENTIFIC TESTING

The *Daubert* criteria list testability as one of the primary considerations in evaluating and demonstrating the reliability of a scientific theory or technique. In fire investigations, the scientific theory relies heavily on established and proven aspects of nature, such as those demonstrated in the science of fire dynamics. The combination of generally accepted scientific principles and research, when supported by empirical fire testing, can yield valuable insight into fire scene reconstruction. Much of the accumulated knowledge of fire scene reconstruction is impossible for individual investigators to gain from personal experience alone, regardless of the skill and diligence with which their analyses are conducted.

There are cases demonstrating that reliance on tests conducted prior to the event is less likely to be biased. Some experts develop opinions based solely on the results of tests conducted specifically to support expert testimony. The *Daubert II* (*Daubert v. Merrell Dow Pharmaceuticals, Inc.* 1995) court placed greater weight on testimony based on pre-existing research that used the scientific method because it is considered more reliable (Clifford 2008).

Scientifically conducted test results can normally be reproduced and their error rates validated or estimated. Such results are considered to be objective, neither prejudiced nor biased by the researcher. An example of peer-reviewed published guidelines is incorporated in the accepted fire testing procedures developed and maintained by the Committees on Fire Standards (E05) and Forensic Sciences (E30) of ASTM International.

It is important to understand the hierarchy of the interrelationships of these ASTM standards and guidelines, especially *NFPA 921* as shown in Figure 1-5. Table 1-8 lists the main ASTM testing and forensic standards applicable to fire investigations, particularly when civil or criminal litigation is anticipated. The capstone standard is *ASTM E1188-11* (ASTM International 2011b), which lists the physical standards on the left-hand side and the informational standards on the right-hand side. The number appended to the right of each standard indicates its year of last issuance. For example, *ASTM E620-11* was last issued in 2011.

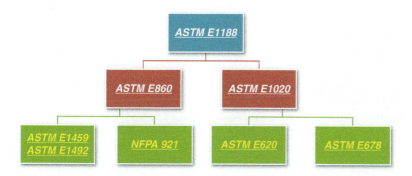

FIGURE 1-5 ASTM standards cited when civil or criminal litigation is anticipated. *Icove, D. J., and B. P. Henry. 2010. "Expert Report Writing: Best Practices for Producing Quality Reports." ISFI 2010, International Symposium on Fire Investigation Science and Technology, University of Maryland, College Park, Maryland, September 27–29.*

TABLE 1-8	Testing Standards Applicable to Fire Investigations	
TECHNIQUE	**INSTRUCTION**	**STANDARD**
Reporting	Standard Practice for Reporting Opinions of Scientific or Technical Experts	ASTM E620
	Standard Practice for Evaluation of Scientific or Technical Data	ASTM E678
	Standard Practice for Examining and Preparing Items That Are or May Become Involved in Criminal or Civil Litigation	ASTM E860
	Standard Practice for Reporting Incidents That May Involve Criminal or Civil Litigation	ASTM E1020
	Terminology of Technical Aspects of Products Liability Litigation	ASTM E1138
	Standard Practice for Collection and Preservation of Information and Physical Items by a Technical Investigator	ASTM E1188
	Standard Guide for Physical Evidence Labeling and Related Documentation	ASTM E1459
	Standard Practice for Receiving, Documenting, Storing, and Retrieving Evidence in a Forensic Science Laboratory	ASTM E1492
Laboratory Testing	Debris Samples by Steam Distillation	ASTM E1385
	Debris Samples by Solvent Extraction	ASTM E1389
	Debris Samples by Gas Chromatography	ASTM E1387
	Debris Samples by Headspace Vapors	ASTM E1388
	Debris Samples by Passive Headspace	ASTM E1412
	Debris Samples by GC-MS	ASTM E1618
Flash and Fire Point	Tag Closed Tester	ASTM D56
	Cleveland Open Cup	ASTM D92
	Pensky-Martens Closed Tester	ASTM D93
	Tag Open Cup Apparatus	ASTM D1310
	Setaflash Closed Tester	ASTM D3278
	Ignition Temperature of Plastic	ASTM D1929
Autoignition Temperature	Liquid Chemicals	ASTM E659
Heat of Combustion	Hydrocarbon Fuels by Bomb Calorimeter	ASTM D2382
Flammability	Apparel Textiles	ASTM D1230
	Apparel Fabrics by Semi-restraint Method	ASTM D3659
	Finished Textile Floor Covering	ASTM D2859
	Aerosol Products	ASTM D3065
	Chemical Concentration Limits	ASTM E681
	Standard Methods of Fire Tests for Flame Propagation of Textiles and Films	NFPA 701
	Recommended Practice for a Field Flame Test for Textiles and Films	NFPA 705
Cigarette Ignition	Mockup Upholstered Furniture Assemblies	ASTM E1352
	Upholstered Furniture	ASTM E1353
Surface Burning	Building Materials	ASTM E84

TABLE 1-8	Testing Standards Applicable to Fire Investigations (*Continued*)

TECHNIQUE	INSTRUCTION	STANDARD
Fire Tests and Experiments	Roof Coverings	ASTM E108
	Floor/Ceiling, Floor/Roof; Walls, Columns	ASTM E119
	Room Fire Experiments	ASTM E603
	Measurement of Gases Present or Generated	ASTM E800
	Windows	ASTM 2010
	Doors	ASTM 2074
Critical Radiant Flux	Floor Covering Systems	ASTM E648
Release Rates	Heat and Visible Smoke	ASTM E906
	Heat and Visible Smoke Using an Oxygen Consumption Calorimeter	ASTM E1354
Rate of Pressure Rise	Combustible Dusts	ASTM E1226
Electrical	Dielectric Withstand Voltage	ASTM D495
	Insulation Resistance	MILSTD202F
	Investigation of Electrical Incidents	ASTM E2345
Self-Heating	Spontaneous Heating Values of Liquids and Solids (Differential Mackey Test)	ASTM D3523
		UN N.1, N.4

ASTM E1188-11, Standard Practice for Collection and Preservation of Information and Physical Items by a Technical Investigator presents an outline of evidence documentation and preservation implemented in good crime scene practices that establish a defensible chain of custody for any physical evidence recovered.

The first-tier physical evidence standard on the left is *ASTM E860-02* (ASTM International 2013b). It governs the second-tier standards *ASTM E1459-13* (ASTM International 2013d), *ASTM E1492-11* (ASTM International 2011c), and *NFPA 921: Guide for Fire and Explosion Investigations* (NFPA 2017).

ASTM E860-07(2013)e1, Standard Practice for Examining and Preparing Items That Are or May Become Involved in Criminal or Civil Litigation is the leading standard practice addressing the examination and testing of items that are or may become involved in litigation. The standard explains the necessary actions that need to be taken if the testing methods will alter or destroy the evidence in any way. Destructive testing may limit how additional testing may occur. The standard recommends documenting the condition of the evidence prior to and after any examination or testing and establishing the chain of custody. If proposed tests are expected to alter the item, procedures are outlined for notifying the client and other interested parties, giving them the opportunity to respond, or to attend the proposed tests.

ASTM E1459-13, Standard Guide for Physical Evidence Labeling and Related Documentation (ASTM International 2013d) sets procedures for producing a traceable audit trail so that any item of physical evidence will have documentation of its origin, past history, treatment, and analysis. The guide also describes methods for labeling physical evidence collected during field investigations as it is received in a forensic laboratory or derived from other items submitted for laboratory examination. The guide points out that some physical evidence may be hazardous; therefore, personnel handling this evidence must be properly trained and outfitted to handle this task.

ASTM E1492-11, Standard Practice for Receiving, Documenting, Storing, and Retrieving Evidence in a Forensic Laboratory (ASTM International 2011c) describes the appropriate procedures and techniques that must be in place in a forensic laboratory to protect and document the integrity of physical evidence.

The information in standard *ASTM E1020-13e1* (ASTM International 2013c) governs *ASTM E620-11* (ASTM International 2011a) and *ASTM E678-07* (ASTM International 2013a). Thorough documentation of all phases of testing will help the courts evaluate the reliability and admissibility of the test results.

ASTM E1020-13e1, Standard Practice for Reporting Incidents That May Involve Criminal or Civil Litigation (ASTM International 2013c) is a guide to the information that should be included in reports of accidents or events that may become the subject of an investigation or litigation. Its provisions are very similar to the content of fire incident report forms such as those reprinted in Appendix H of *Kirk's Fire Investigation* (DeHaan and Icove 2012).

ASTM E620-11, Standard Practice for Reporting Opinions of Scientific or Technical Experts (ASTM International 2011a) outlines the content that should be included in a typical report of a technical expert: names and addresses of authors, descriptions of items examined, date and location of exam, scope of activities performed, pertinent facts relied on and sources for them, all opinions and conclusions rendered, logic and reasoning of the expert by which each of the conclusions was reached, and signature of the expert with affiliations. These requirements follow *FRCP Rule 26(a)*.

ASTM E678-07, Standard Practice for Evaluation of Scientific or Technical Data (ASTM International 2013a) is essentially a description of the scientific method. It recommends including the definition of the problem or issue addressed, identification and explanation of hypotheses addressed (including alternatives), a description of the data collected and analyzed (and sources for that data), an estimation of the reliability of data used, and the opinion reached. Conclusions expressed must be consistent with known facts and accepted scientific principles.

1.7.9 PEER REVIEW AND PUBLICATIONS

A credible, reliable theory must take into account the body of research that has been compiled, verified, and published by experts in the field. The need for credibility underscores the advantages of using the scientific method. Recently, there has been a tendency for courts to hold experts to the same standards that scientists use in evaluating each other's work, sometimes referred to as peer review (Ayala and Black 1993).

NFPA 921 provides investigators with professional guidelines as to the methodology, protocols, and data for conducting origin and cause investigations. The document also provides guidance on definitions for the following three levels of peer review.

Peer Review. Peer review is a formal procedure generally employed in prepublication review of scientific or technical documents and screening of grant applications by research-sponsoring agencies. Peer review carries with it connotations of both independence and objectivity. Peer reviewers should not have any interest in the outcome of the review. The author does not select the reviewers, and reviews are often conducted anonymously. As such, the term *peer review* should not be applied to reviews of an investigator's work by coworkers, supervisors, or investigators from agencies conducting investigations of the same incident. Such reviews are more appropriately characterized as *technical reviews*, as described below (NFPA 2017, pt. 4.6.3).

Administrative Review. An administrative review is one typically carried out within an organization to ensure that the investigator's work product meets the organization's quality assurance requirements. An administrative reviewer will determine whether all of the steps outlined in an organization's procedure manual, or required by agency policy, have been followed and whether all of the appropriate documentation is present in the file, and may check for typographical or grammatical errors (NFPA 2017, pt. 4.6.1).

Technical Review. A technical review can have multiple facets. If a technical reviewer has been asked to critique all aspects of the investigator's work product, then the technical reviewer should be qualified and familiar with all aspects of proper fire investigation and should, at a minimum, have access to all of the documentation available to the investigator whose work is being reviewed. If a technical reviewer has been asked to critique only specific aspects of the investigator's work product, then the technical reviewer should be qualified and familiar with those specific aspects and, at a minimum, have access to all documentation relevant to those aspects. A technical review can serve as an additional test of the various aspects of the investigator's work product (NFPA 2017, pt. 4.6.2).

Peer review is common among respected journals that publish the results of theories, testing, and methodology. The common approach to peer review in technical journals is to use reviewers who are familiar with the published scientific data and methodologies to determine whether the author's views are of the quality of these publications and whether the data presented support the conclusions of the author. Peer-reviewed journals useful in the field of forensic fire investigation include *Fire Technology, Journal of Fire Protection Engineering, Fire and Materials, Fire Safety Journal, Combustion and Flame,* and *Journal of Forensic Sciences.* Another valuable resource is the *Fire & Arson Investigator,* a journal produced by the International Association of Arson Investigators.

The SFPE's "Guidelines for Peer Review in the Fire Protection Design Process" (2002) cover the scope and standard of care related to a peer review, the confidentiality of the results of a peer review, and the manner in which the results should be reported. Although these guidelines concentrate on the design of fire protection systems, they include concepts with significant parallels to the fire investigation field.

Investigators can participate in a technical peer review when their cases are submitted to supervisors for review (*NFPA 921,* 2014 ed., pt. 4.6.2). *NFPA 921* cautions that a technical review can have multiple facets and that the reviewer should be qualified and familiar with all aspects of proper fire investigation and have access to all the documentation available to the investigator whose work is being reviewed (NFPA 2017, pt. 4.6.2).

In cases in which a technical reviewer is asked to critique only specific aspects of the investigator's work product, the technical reviewer should be qualified and familiar with those specific aspects. For example, an engineer may be asked to conduct a technical peer review of another engineer's report of investigation. In some states this type of technical peer review is considered the practice of engineering and may require registration as a licensed professional engineer.

NFPA 921 cautions that although technical review may add value to an investigation, the reviewers might have a bias or an interest in the outcome of the case. These interests, conscious or subconscious, may introduce confirmation bias (NFPA 2017, pt. 4.3.9) or expectation bias (NFPA 2017, pt. 4.3.8). Either of these biases may result in the failure of both the investigator and the reviewer to consider alternative hypotheses, thus undermining the case under review. In law enforcement, the primary function of supervisory review is to assure that all questions, logical investigative leads, laboratory examinations, and plausible theories are addressed. Private investigation companies working in civil cases often have their own supervisors peer-review fire reports. Some corporations use qualified experts to peer-review fire investigation reports when their companies are too small or do not have an established peer-review process. Other equally qualified employees in the same agency or company often carry out peer review.

In these instances, it must be stressed that the initial investigator still has the primary responsibility to collect and report relevant information in a manner consistent with the scientific method. The investigator, not the peer reviewer, will still be the primary witness in any litigation.

Peer review also applies to establishing the credibility of published information (Icove and Haynes 2007). Several recommended peer-reviewed textbooks and references in both conducting and assessing complex fire investigations are listed in Table 1-9. These texts, written by prominent credentialed fire scientists and engineers, are widely cited in scholarly publications, are used and distributed in the fire investigation community, are

TABLE 1-9	Expert Peer-Reviewed Treatises in the Fire Investigation Field

- Babrauskas, V. 2003. *Ignition Handbook: Principles and Applications to Fire Safety Engineering, Fire Investigation, Risk Management, and Forensic Science.* Issaquah, WA: Fire Science Publishers, Society of Fire Protection Engineers.

- Babrauskas, V., and S. J. Grayson. 1992. *Heat Release in Fires.* Basingstoke, UK: Taylor and Francis.

- Beveridge, A. D. 2012. *Forensic Investigation of Explosions.* 2nd ed. Boca Raton, FL: CRC Press/Taylor and Francis.

- Brannigan, F. L., and G. P. Corbett. 2007. *Brannigan's Building Construction for the Fire Service.* 4th ed. Sudbury, MA: National Fire Protection Association; Jones and Bartlett.

- Cole, L. S. 2001. *The Investigation of Motor Vehicle Fires.* 4th ed. San Anselmo, CA: Lee Books.

- Cooke, R. A., and R. H. Ide. 1985. *Principles of Fire Investigation.* Leicester, UK: Institution of Fire Engineers.

- DeHaan, J. D., D. J. Icove, and G. A. Haynes. 2017. *Kirk's Fire Investigation.* 8th ed. Upper Saddle River, NJ: Pearson-Prentice Hall.

- Drysdale, D. 2011. *An Introduction to Fire Dynamics.* 3rd ed. Chichester, West Sussex, UK: Wiley.

- Icove, D. J., J. D. DeHaan, and G. A. Haynes. 2013. *Forensic Fire Scene Reconstruction.* 3rd ed. Upper Saddle River, NJ: Pearson/Prentice Hall.

- Icove, D. J., V. B. Wherry, and J. D. Schroeder. 1998. *Combating Arson-for-Profit: Advanced Techniques for Investigators.* 2nd ed. Columbus, OH: Battelle Press.

- Iqbal, N., and M. H. Salley. 2004. *Fire Dynamics Tools (FDTs): Quantitative Fire Hazard Analysis Methods for the US Nuclear Regulatory Commission Fire Protection Inspection Program.* Washington, DC: US Nuclear Regulatory Commission.

- Janssens, M. L., and D. M. Birk. 2000. *An Introduction to Mathematical Fire Modeling.* 2nd ed. Lancaster, PA: Technomic.

- Karlsson, B., and J. G. Quintiere. 2000. *Enclosure Fire Dynamics.* Boca Raton, FL: CRC Press.

- Lentini, J. J. 2013. *Scientific Protocols for Fire Investigation.* 2nd ed, Protocols in forensic science series. Boca Raton, FL: Taylor & Francis.

- Quintiere, J. G. 1998. *Principles of Fire Behavior.* Albany, NY: Delmar.

- Quintiere, J. G. 2006. *Fundamentals of Fire Phenomena.* Chichester, West Sussex, UK: Wiley.

included in association publication lists, are cited in court cases, and have often been reviewed by forensic journals.

These texts have become, or have the potential to become, expert or learned treatises in the field of fire investigation. Learned treatises are those texts that rise to the level of authoritative acceptance, so that they can be admitted as evidence in court to support or rebut the testimony given by an expert witness. Furthermore, authoritative references are those that the fire investigator frequently uses as a reference or guide because they have been found to be reliable. When asked in court what they consider to be an authoritative text, some fire investigators will list only those that have a legal or administrative impact on their work.

1.7.10 NEGATIVE CORPUS

The use of the **negative corpus**, or arson by default approach (the process of ruling out all accidental causes for a fire without sufficient scientific and factual basis to determine what did cause the fire), is rarely an acceptable methodology for determining that a fire was intentionally set. The term *negative corpus* has no recognized definition but its use is obvious. It implies that the **corpus delicti** of the event (not necessarily of a crime) has not been proven.

The latest guidance by *NFPA 921* regarding negative corpus is as follows:

> **19.6.5* Appropriate Use.**   The process of elimination is an integral part of the scientific method. Alternative hypotheses should be considered and challenged against the facts. Elimination of a testable hypothesis by disproving the hypothesis with reliable evidence is a fundamental part of the scientific method. However, the process of elimination can be used inappropriately. The process of determining the ignition source for a fire, by eliminating all ignition sources found, known, or believed to have been present in the area of origin, and then claiming such methodology is proof of an ignition source for which there is no supporting evidence of its existence, is referred to by some investigators as negative corpus. Negative corpus has typically been used in classifying fires as incendiary, although the process has also been used to characterize fires classified as accidental. This process is not consistent with the scientific method, is inappropriate, and should not be used because it generates untestable hypotheses, and may result in incorrect determinations of the ignition source and first fuel ignited. Any hypotheses formulated for the causal factors (e.g., first fuel, ignition source, and ignition sequence) must be based on the analysis of facts. Those facts are derived from evidence, observations, calculations, experiments, and the laws of science. Speculative information cannot be included in the analysis (NFPA 2017, pt. 19.6.5).

The logic of negative corpus cause determination was examined in great detail by Smith (2006). He pointed out that if it has any application at all, it is only where the origin is "clearly defined" or is identified as the "exact point of origin" (DeHaan and Icove 2012). Until the 2011 edition of *NFPA 921*, there was the allowance of determination of cases where area of origin was "clearly defined." However, this terminology has been eliminated (Lentini 2013).

The US Court of Appeals for the Eleventh Circuit applied *Daubert* and excluded the testimony of a fire investigator in the *Benfield* case (*Michigan Miller's Mutual Insurance Company v. Benfield* 1998). In that case, the investigator was not able to articulate the methodology he used to eliminate possible ignition sources and had no scientific basis for his opinion. The court held that the investigation of fires is science-based and that the *Daubert* criterion applies.

It is argued that if the fire damage is severe, the surrounding materials will be too degraded, and a clearly defined point of origin cannot be determined. This may be true when post-fire burn patterns are the entirety of the evidence of origin location. However, when a reliable witness or several witnesses observe an established fire in only one area and can view other nearby areas and reliably conclude there was no observable fire there, then that should be taken as strong evidence that an ignition occurred in that location.

negative corpus ■ The process of determining what caused a fire by eliminating each possible cause, one by one, until only one possible cause remains.

corpus delicti ■ Literally, the body of the crime. The fundamental facts necessary to prove the commission of a crime.

Sometimes, color and density of smoke or height of flames will offer a clue as to the nature of the first fuel package involved, further narrowing the area of interest. In many fires that have caused great destruction, surveillance cameras have recorded the area, or even the point of first ignition. Once a narrow area of origin can be established, then possible sources of heat can be identified. An origin determination is a hypothesis that requires testing, like any other inductive conclusion. This testing involves careful physical examination of the area for remains of either fuel packages or processes known to have been in that vicinity.

Before possible ignition sources are blindly pursued only within a defined area, the scientific method demands testing by posing and testing alternatives. Such efforts could take the form of asking, "This looks like the origin, but I have a heat source over there. Could the damage I'm seeing (or the events a witness saw) have been the result of something (wall covering, drapery, cabinet) igniting from that and falling into this area?" Smith (2006) points out that the better the knowledge base of the investigator, the more likely he or she will be to see (and test) these alternatives. The poorly prepared investigator is far more likely to seize on an apparent point of origin based on burn pattern and then look for heat sources only in that area, never considering that his or her hypothesis concerning the area of origin is wrong.

All aspects of origin and cause determination should be subjected to comprehensive and repetitive analysis through hypothesis testing by all means available, including the formation and testing of alternatives—both consistent and contrary ones. The cause of a fire is a determination of the first fuel ignited (not necessarily an identification of the cause), the source of heat, and the circumstances that brought them together. The determination of first fuel ignited can rely on laboratory tests (ignitable liquid or chemical incendiary residues), physical remains, or witness observations. In a criminal case, where the standard of proof is very high, circumstantial evidence of first fuel or even heat source may not be adequate. In a civil case, where the standard of proof may be "preponderance of evidence" or "more likely than not" (NFPA 2017, pt. 12.5.5), circumstantial exclusion of all but one competent ignition source and one susceptible fuel may be adequate (NFPA 2017). The tests for "competent" and "susceptible" are part of the fire engineering analysis conducted as part of the scientific method of fire investigation.

Presently, the only reference to negative corpus appears in *NFPA 921* (2014a, pt. 19.6.5). If pursued vigorously and within bounded known experimental limits, the scientific method can be used to demonstrate successfully that the only mechanism for ignition had to be deliberate by demonstrating that all relevant accidental mechanisms were specifically evaluated, tested, and eliminated, and that deliberate ignition (and its expected aftermath) fits all the available data. If new data are presented, the conclusion must be reevaluated, possibly resulting in a different conclusion. For a more detailed discussion on negative corpus, see Smith (2006).

1.7.11 ERROR RATES, PROFESSIONAL STANDARDS, AND ACCEPTABILITY

Under *Daubert*, a court may consider the known or potential rate of error and the existence of acceptable professional standards for the techniques used by the expert. Error rates from repeated tests are available for many equations, relationships, and models used to describe fire and explosion dynamics. These error rates are evaluated during fire test development, such as those listed in Table 1-5. Error rates have not yet been established for the entire process of origin and cause determination.

ASTM E860-02(2013)e1, Standard Practice for Examining and Preparing Items That Are or May Become Involved in Criminal or Civil Litigation (ASTM International 2013b) has a broad impact on investigators. This practice covers evidence (actual items or systems) that may have future potential for testing or disassembly and are involved in litigation, including:

- Documentation of evidence prior to removal and/or disassembly, testing, or alteration
- Notification of all parties involved
- Proper preservation of evidence after testing

This practice also stresses the importance of safety concerns associated with testing and disassembly of evidence, which is particularly important when dealing with energized equipment or evidence containing potentially hazardous chemicals. The ASTM E30 committee has jurisdiction over these standards and is presently revising them to make them suitable for all litigation, both civil and criminal.

Summary

This chapter introduced the application of the scientific method formed by validated principles and research (fire testing, dynamics, suppression, modeling, pattern analysis, and historical case data) to fire investigation and reconstruction. This approach relies on combined principles of fire protection engineering, forensic science, and behavioral science. In using the scientific method, the investigator can more accurately estimate a fire's origin, intensity, growth, direction of travel, and duration, as well as understand and interpret the behavior of the occupants.

Fire scene reconstruction can also bring in additional fire testing and similar cases to support the final theory. In addition to *NFPA 921,* the fire investigator should become familiar with other authoritative references and sources of data and information such as the job performance requirements of *NFPA 1033*. It should be remembered that *NFPA 921* is a summary of practices, extracted and developed from thousands of research efforts, some extending back over a century. There is a universe of reliable information available to fire investigators that is not included in *NFPA 921*.

The strengths of this approach make a thorough examination of many hypotheses more effective. The reliability of the result of a specific method of investigation is a function of the number of alternative hypotheses that have been tested and eliminated. Fire engineering analysis also offers many advantages. In particular, it allows the investigator to evaluate the potential of several scenarios without repeated full-scale fire testing. A sensitivity analysis can also extend the analysis to different ranges of conditions.

Review Questions

1. Obtain an adjudicated case from your local fire marshal's office involving the conviction of an arsonist who pleaded guilty to setting a fire. Analyze the fire investigator's opinion as to the origin and cause of the fire. Demonstrate how it did or did not meet the guidelines for the scientific method.

2. Obtain a photograph of a fire plume against a wall. Trace the lines of demarcation for char, scorching, and smoke deposition onto a plastic overlay. What can you learn from this exercise?

3. Search the Internet or current published periodical fire investigation literature and list three examples of peer-reviewed fire testing research.

4. Search the Internet or current published periodical fire investigation literature and list three federal and state court cases mentioning *NFPA 921* and *Daubert*.

5. Identify scientific treatises that describe pyrolysis. What is the earliest date?

6. Review recent fire investigation publications and find five references to the scientific method. What is the described impact on the investigations?

References

ASTM International. 1989. *E1138-89, Terminology of Technical Aspects of Products Liability Litigation.* (Withdrawn 1995). West Conshohocken, PA: ASTM International.

———. 2005b. *ASTM Dictionary of Engineering Science and Technology.* 10th ed. West Conshohocken, PA: ASTM International.

———. 2011a. *E620-11, Standard Practice for Reporting Opinions of Scientific or Technical Experts.* West Conshohocken, PA: ASTM International.

———. 2011b. *E1188-11, Standard Practice for Collection and Preservation of Information and Physical Items by a Technical Investigator.* West Conshohocken, PA: ASTM International.

———. 2011c. *E1492-11, Standard Practice for Receiving, Documenting, Storing, and Retrieving Evidence in a Forensic Science Laboratory.* West Conshohocken, PA: ASTM International.

———. 2013a. *E678-07(2013), Standard Practice for Evaluation of Scientific or Technical Data.* West Conshohocken, PA: ASTM International.

———. 2013b. *E860-07(2013)e1, Standard Practice for Examining and Preparing Items That Are or May Become Involved in Criminal or Civil Litigation*. West Conshohocken, PA: ASTM International.

———. 2013c. *E1020-13e1(2013), Standard Practice for Reporting Incidents That May Involve Criminal or Civil Litigation*. West Conshohocken, PA: ASTM International.

———. 2013d. *E1459-13, Standard Guide for Physical Evidence Labeling and Related Documentation*. West Conshohocken, PA: ASTM International.

Ayala, F. J., and B. Black. 1993. "Science and the Courts." *American Scientist* 81: 230–39.

Babrauskas, V. 2003. *Ignition Handbook: Principles and Applications to Fire Safety Engineering, Fire Investigation, Risk Management, and Forensic Science*. Issaquah, WA: Fire Science Publishers, Society of Fire Protection Engineers.

———. October 2004. "*Truck Insurance v. MagneTek*: Lessons to Be Learned Concerning Presentation of Scientific Information." *Fire & Arson Investigator* 55: 2.

———. 2005. "Charring Rate of Wood as a Tool for Fire Investigations." *Fire Safety Journal* 40, no. 6: 528–54. doi: 10.1016/j.firesaf.2005.05.006.

Babrauskas, V., B. F. Gray, and M. L. Janssens. 2007. "Prudent Practices for the Design and Installation of Heat-producing Devices near Wood Materials." *Fire and Materials* 31: 125–35.

Babrauskas, V., and S. J. Grayson. 1992. *Heat Release in Fires*. Basingstoke, UK: Taylor & Francis.

Beering, P. S. 1996. "Verdict: Guilty of Burning—What Prosecutors Should Know about Arson." *Insurance Committee for Arson Control*. Indianapolis, IN.

Beller, D., and J. Sapochetti. 2000. "Searching for Answers to the Cocoanut Grove Fire of 1942." *Fire Journal* 94, no. 3: 84–86.

Beveridge, A. D. 2012. *Forensic Investigation of Explosions*. 2nd ed. Boca Raton, FL: CRC Press/Taylor & Francis.

Brannigan, F. L., and G. P. Corbett. 2007. *Brannigan's Building Construction for the Fire Service*. 4th ed. Sudbury, MA: National Fire Protection Association; Jones and Bartlett.

Brannigan, V. M., and E. C. Buc. 2010. "The Admissibility of Forensic Fire Investigation Testimony: Justifying a Methodology Based on Abductive Inference under *NFPA 921*." Paper presented at the ISFI 2010 International Symposium on Fire Investigation Science and Technology, College Park, Maryland, September 27–29.

Burnette, G. E. 2003. "Fire Scene Investigation: The *Daubert* Challenge." Personal communication.

Campagnolo, T. Fall 1999. "The Fourth Amendment at Fire Scenes." *Arizona Law Review* 41: 601–50.

Campbell, R. 2014. "Intentional Fires." In *Fire Analysis and Research Division*. Quincy, MA: National Fire Protection Association.

Clifford, R. C. 2008. *Qualifying and Attacking Expert Witnesses*. Costa Mesa, CA: James Publishing.

Cole, L. S. 2001. *The Investigation of Motor Vehicle Fires*. 4th ed. San Anselmo, CA: Lee Books.

Cooke, R. A., and R. H. Ide. 1985. *Principles of Fire Investigation*. Leicester, UK: Institution of Fire Engineers.

Crowhurst, E. 2015. "Fire Statistics: Great Britain April 2013 to March 2014." London, UK: Department for Communities and Local Government.

DeHaan, J. D. 1995. "The Reconstruction of Fires Involving Highly Flammable Hydrocarbon Liquids." PhD diss., University of Strathclyde.

DeHaan, J. D., and D. J. Icove. 2012. *Kirk's Fire Investigation*. 7th ed. Upper Saddle River, NJ: Pearson-Prentice Hall.

DOJ. September 2016. "Recommendations of the National Commission on Forensic Science." Memorandum for Heads of Department Components from the Attorney General. Washington, DC: US Department of Justice.

Doyle, A. C. 1891. "A Scandal in Bohemia." *The Strand*.

Drysdale, D. 2011. *An Introduction to Fire Dynamics*. 3rd ed. Chichester, West Sussex, UK: Wiley.

Esposito, J. C. 2005. *Fire in the Grove: The Cocoanut Grove Tragedy and Its Aftermath*. Cambridge, MA: Da Capo Press.

Evarts, B. 2010. *US Structure Fires in Eating and Drinking Establishments*. Quincy, MA: National Fire Protection Association.

Fahy, R. F., P. R. LeBlanc, and J. L. Molis. 2015. "Firefighter Fatalities in the United States, 2015." Edited by Fire Analysis and Research Division. Quincy, MA: National Fire Protection Association.

FBI. 2015. "Arson." In *Crime in the United States*. Washington, DC: Federal Bureau of Investigation.

FM Global. 2015. "FM Global Property Loss Prevention Data Sheets." Retrieved September 30. www.fmglobaldatasheets.com.

FPRF. 2002. "The Recommendations of the Research Advisory Council on Post-fire Analysis: A White Paper, IV." Quincy, MA: Fire Protection Research Foundation.

Frazier, P. 2005. "Total Cost of Fire." Fire Protection Engineering 26: 22–26.

FRCP. 2010. *Federal Rules of Civil Procedure*. www.law.cornell.edu/rules/frcp.

FRE. 2012. *Federal Rules of Evidence*. Arlington, VA: Federal Evidence Review. www.federalevidence.com.

Giannelli, P. C., and E. J. Imwinkelried. 2007. *Scientific Evidence*. 4th ed. Newark, NJ: LexisNexis.

Graham, M. H. 2009. *Cleary and Graham's Handbook of Illinois Evidence*. 9th ed. Austin, TX: Aspen Publishers.

Grant, C. C. 1991. "Last Dance at the Cocoanut Grove." *Fire Journal* 85, no. 3: 74–80.

Hall Jr., J. R. 2014. "The Total Cost of Fire in the United States." Quincy, MA: National Fire Protection Association.

Haynes, H. J. G. 2015. "Fire Loss in the United States during 2014." In *Research and Reports*. Quincy, MA: National Fire Protection Association.

Hopkins, R. L. 2008. "Fire Pattern Research in the US: Current Status and Impact." Richmond, KY: TRACE Fire Protection and Safety.

Hopkins, R. L., G. E. Gorbett, and P. M. Kennedy. 2009. "Fire Pattern Persistence and Predictability during Full-scale Comparison Fire Tests and the Use for Comparison of Post-fire Analysis." Paper presented at Fire and Materials 2009, 11th International Conference, San Francisco, California, January 26–28.

Icove, D. J., and J. D. DeHaan. 2006. "Hourglass Burn Patterns: A Scientific Explanation for Their Formation." Paper presented at the International Symposium on Fire Investigation Science and Technology, Cincinnati, Ohio, June 26–28.

Icove, D. J., J. D. DeHaan, and G. A. Haynes. 2013. *Forensic Fire Scene Reconstruction*. 3rd ed. Upper Saddle River, NJ: Pearson Education, Inc.

Icove, D. J., and T. K. Hargrove. 2014. "Project Arson: Uncovering the True Arson Rate in the United States." Paper presented at International Symposium on Fire Investigation Science and Technology, College Park, Maryland, September 22–24.

Icove, D. J., and G. A. Haynes. 2007. "Guidelines for Conducting Peer Reviews of Complex Fire Investigations." Paper presented at Fire and Materials 2007, 10th International Conference, San Francisco, California, January 29–31.

Icove, D. J., V. B. Wherry, and J. D. Schroeder. 1998. *Combating Arson-for-Profit: Advanced Techniques for Investigators*. 2nd ed. Columbus, OH: Battelle Press.

Iqbal, N., and M. H. Salley, 2004. *Fire Dynamics Tools (FDTs): Quantitative Fire Hazard Analysis Methods for the US Nuclear Regulatory Commission Fire Protection Inspection Program*. Washington, DC: Nuclear Regulatory Commission.

Janssens, M. L., and D. M. Birk. 2000. *An Introduction to Mathematical Fire Modeling*. 2nd ed. Lancaster, PA: Technomic.

Karlsson, B., and J. G. Quintiere. 2000. *Enclosure Fire Dynamics*. Boca Raton, FL: CRC Press.

Karter Jr., M. J. August 2009. "Fire Loss in the United States, 2008." Quincy, MA: National Fire Protection Association Report, Fire Analysis and Research Division.

Karter Jr., M. J., and J. L. Molis. 2014. "US Firefighter Injuries, 2013." Edited by Fire Analysis and Research Division. Quincy, MA: National Fire Protection Association.

Kolar, R. D. Spring 2007. "Scientific and Other Expert Testimony: Understand It; Keep It Out; Get It In." *FDCC Quarterly*: 207–35. Tampa, FL: The Federation of Defense & Corporate Counsel, Inc.

Kolczynski, P. J. 2008. *Preparing for Trial in Federal Court*. Costa Mesa, CA: James Publishing.

Lentini, J. J. 1992. "Behavior of Glass at Elevated Temperatures." *Journal of Forensic Sciences* 37, no. 5: 1358–62.

———. 2013. *Scientific Protocols for Fire Investigation*. 2nd ed. Protocols in forensic science series. Boca Raton, FL: Taylor & Francis.

Madrzykowski, D., and S. Kerber. 2009. "Fire Fighting Tactics under Wind-driven Conditions: Laboratory Experiments." Gaithersburg, MD: National Institute of Standards and Technology.

Moore, D. T. 2007. "Critical Thinking and Intelligence Analysis." Occasional paper no. 14, 2nd printing with rev. Washington, DC: Center for Strategic Intelligence Research, National Defense Intelligence College.

NAP. 2009. *Strengthening Forensic Science in the United States: A Path Forward*. Washington, DC: National Academy of Sciences, National Academies Press.

———. 2011. *Reference Manual on Scientific Evidence*. 3rd ed. Washington, DC: National Academy of Sciences, National Academies Press.

Nelson, H. E., and R. E. Tontarski. 1998. "Proceedings of the International Conference on Fire Research for Fire Investigation." HAI Report 98-5157-001. Washington, DC: Department of Treasury, Bureau of Alcohol, Tobacco & Firearms.

NFPA. 1943. "The Cocoanut Grove Night Club Fire, Boston, November 28, 1942." Quincy, MA: National Fire Protection Association.

———. 2008. *Fire Protection Handbook*. 20th ed. Quincy, MA: National Fire Protection Association.

———. 2014. *NFPA 1033: Standard for Professional Qualifications for Fire Investigator*. Quincy, MA: National Fire Protection Association.

———. 2017. *NFPA 921: Guide for Fire and Explosion Investigations*. Quincy, MA: National Fire Protection Association.

NIJ. 2000. "Fire and Arson Scene Evidence: A Guide for Public Safety Personnel." Washington, DC: Technical Working Group on Fire/Arson Scene Investigation (TWGFASI), Office of Justice Programs, National Institute of Justice.

NSC. 2008. *Report on Injuries in America*. Itasca, IL: National Safety Council.

ODPM. 2005. "Economic Cost of Fires in England and Wales—2003." London, UK: Office of the Deputy Prime Minister.

Ogle, R. A. 2000. "The Need for Scientific Fire Investigations." *Fire Protection Engineering* 8: 4–8.

Orville, R. E., and G. R. Huffines. 1999. "Annual Summary: Lightning Ground Flash Measurements over the Contiguous United States: 1995–97." *Monthly Weather Review* 127: 2693–2703.

Putorti Jr., A. D., J. A. McElroy, and D. Madrzykowski. 2001. "Flammable and Combustible Liquid Spill/Burn Patterns." Rockville, MD: National Institute of Standards and Technology.

Quintiere, J. G. 1998. *Principles of Fire Behavior*. Albany, NY: Delmar.

———. 2006. *Fundamentals of Fire Phenomena*. Chichester, West Sussex, UK: Wiley.

Reinhardt, W. 1982. "Looking Back at the Cocoanut Grove." *Fire Journal* 76, no. 11: 60–63.

Rite-in-the-Rain. 2016. Accessed April 14. www.riteintherain.com/contact.

Rohr, K. D. 2001. "An Update to What's Burning in Home Fires." *Fire and Materials* 25, no. 2: 43–48. doi: 10.1002/fam.757.

————. 2005. "Products First Ignited in US Home Fires." Quincy, MA: National Fire Protection Association.

Schorow, S. 2005. *The Cocoanut Grove Fire.* Beverly, MA: Commonwealth Editions.

SFPE. 2002. "Guidelines for Peer Review in the Fire Protection Design Process." Bethesda, MD: Society of Fire Protection Engineers.

————. 2003. *Engineering Guide: Human Behavior in Fire.* Bethesda, MD: Society of Fire Protection Engineers.

————. 2008. *SFPE Handbook of Fire Protection Engineering.* 4th ed. Quincy, MA: National Fire Protection Association, Society of Fire Protection Engineers.

Shanley, J. H. 1997. "Report of the United States Fire Administration Program for the Study of Fire Patterns." Washington, DC: Federal Emergency Management Agency, USFA Fire Pattern Research Committee.

Smith, D. W. 2006. "The Pitfalls, Perils, and Reasoning Fallacies of Determining the Fire Cause in the Absence of Proof: The Negative Corpus Methodology." Paper presented at the International Symposium on Fire Investigation Science and Technology, Cincinnati, Ohio, June 26–28.

Tobin, W. A., and K. L. Monson. 1989. "Collapsed Spring Observations in Arson Investigations: A Critical Metallurgical Evaluation." *Fire Technology* 25, no. 4: 317–35.

Von Drehle, D. 2003. *Triangle: The Fire That Changed America.* New York: Atlantic Monthly Press.

Zicherman, J., and P. A. Lynch. 2006. "Is Pyrolysis Dead?—Scientific Processes vs. Court Testimony: The Recent 10th Circuit Court and Associated Appeals Court Decisions." *Fire & Arson Investigator* 56, no. 3: 46–52.

Legal References

103 Investors I, L.P. v. Square D Company. Case No. 01-2504-KHV, 372 F.3d 1213 (US App. 2004). LEXIS 12439, US Dist. LEXIS 8796, 10th Cir. Kan., 2004. Decided May 10, 2005.

Abon Ltd. et al. v. Transcontinental Insurance Company. Docket No. 2004-CA-0029, 2005 Ohio 302 (Ohio App. 2005). LEXIS 2847. Decided June 16, 2005.

Allstate Insurance Company, as Subrogee of Russell Davis v. Hugh Cole Builder Inc. Hugh Cole individually and dba Hugh Cole Builder Inc. Civil Action No. 98-A-1432-N, 137 F. Supp. 2d 1283 (US Dist. 2001). LEXIS 5016. Decided April 12, 2001.

American Family Insurance Group v. JVC American Corp. Civil Action No. 00-27 (DSD-JMM) (US Dist. 2001). LEXIS 8001. Decided April 30, 2001.

Andronic Pappas et al. v. Sony Electronics, Inc. et al. Civil Action No. 96-339J, 136 F. Supp. 2d 413 (US Dist. 2000). LEXIS 19531, CCH Prod. Liab. Rep. P15,993. Decided December 27, 2000.

Bethie Pride v. BIC Corporation, Société BIC, S.A. Civil Case No. 98-6422; 218 F.3d 566 (US App. 2000). LEXIS 15652; 2000 FED App. 0222P (6th Cir.); 54 Fed. R. Serv. 3d (Callaghan) 1428; CCH Prod. Liab. Rep. P15,844. Decided July 7, 2000.

Chester Valley Coach Works et al. v. Fisher-Price Inc. Civil Action No. 99-CV-4197 (US Dist. 2001). LEXIS 15902, CCH Prod. Liab. Rep. P16,18. Decided August 29, 2001.

Cunningham v. Gans. 501 F.2d 496, 500 (2nd Cir. 1974).

Daubert v. Merrell Dow Pharmaceuticals Inc. 509 US 579 (1993); 113 S. Ct. 2756, 215 L. Ed. 2d 469.

Daubert v. Merrell Dow Pharmaceuticals Inc. (Daubert II). 43 F.3d 1311, 1317 (9th Cir. 1995).

David Bryte v. American Household Inc. Case No. 04-1051, CA-00-93-2, 429 F.3d 469 (4th Cir. 2005; 2005 US App.). LEXIS 25052. Decided November 21, 2005.

Eid Abu-Hashish and Sheam Abu-Hashish v. Scottsdale Insurance Company. Case No. 98 C4019, 88 F. Supp. 2d 906 (US Dist. 2000). LEXIS 3663. Decided March 16, 2000.

Farner v. Paccar Inc. 562 F.2d 518, 528–29 (8th Cir. 1977).

Fireman's Fund Insurance Company v. Canon USA, Inc. Case No. 03-3836, 394 F.3d 1054 (US App. 2005). LEXIS 471; 66 Fed. R. Evid. Serv. (Callaghan) 258; CCH Prod Liab. Rep. P17,274. Filed January 12, 2005.

Frye v. United States. 293 F.1013 (DC Cir. 1923).

General Electric Company v. Joiner. 66 USLW 4036 (1997).

In re Paoli Railroad Yard PCB Litigation. 35 F.3d 717 (US App. 1994). LEXIS 23722; 30 Fed. R. Serv.3d (Callaghan) 644; 25 ELR 20989; 35 F.3d at 743. Filed August 31, 1994.

Jacob J. Booth and Kathleen Booth v. Black and Decker Inc. Civil Action No. 98-6352, 166 F. Supp. 2d 215 (US Dist. 2001). LEXIS 4495, CCH Prod. Liab. Rep. P16, 184. Decided April 12, 2001.

James B. McCoy et al. v. Whirlpool Corp. et al. Civil Action No. 02-2064-KHV; 214 F.R.D. 646 (US Dist. 2003). LEXIS 6901; 55 Fed. R. Serv. 3d (Callaghan) 740.

John Witten Tunnell v. Ford Motor Company. Civil Action No. 4:03CV74; 330 F. Supp. 2d 731 (US Dist. 2004). LEXIS 24598 (W.D. Va., July 3, 2004). Decided July 2, 2004.

Kumho Tire Co. Ltd. v. Carmichael. 119 S. Ct. 1167 (1999). US LEXIS 2199 (March 23, 1999).

LaSalle National Bank et al. v. Massachusetts Bay Insurance Company et al. Case No. 90 C 2005. (US Dist. 1997). LEXIS 5253. Decided April 11, 1997. Docketed April 18, 1997.

Marilyn McCarver v. Farm Bureau General Insurance Company. Case Number 2004-3315-CKM, State of Michigan, County of Berrien. Decided February 1, 2006.

Mark and Dian Workman v. AB Electrolux Corporation et al. Case No. 03-4195-JAR (US Dist. 2005). LEXIS 16306. Decided August 8, 2005.

Michigan Miller's Mutual Insurance Company v. Benfield. 140 F.3d 915 (11th Cir. 1998).

Mitchell v. Gencorp Inc. 165 F.3d 778, 780 (10th Cir. 1999).

Polizzi Meats, Inc. v. Aetna Life and Casualty. 931 F. Supp. 328 (D.N.J. 1996).

Ronald Taepke v. Lake States Insurance Company. Fire No. 98-1946-18-CK, Circuit Court for the County of Charlevoix, State of Michigan. Entered December 8, 1999.

Royal Insurance Company of America, as Subrogee of Patrick and Linda Magee v. Joseph Daniel Construction, Inc. Civil Action No. 00-Civ.-8706 (CM); 208 F. Supp. 2d 423 (US Dist. 2002). LEXIS 12397. Decided July 10, 2002.

State Farm and Casualty Company, as Subrogee of Rocky Mountain and Suzanne Mountain, v. Holmes Products; J.C. Penney Company. Case No. 04-4532 (3rd Cir. 2006). LEXIS 2370. Argued January 17, 2006. Filed January 31, 2006. (Unpublished).

Teri Snodgrass, Robert L. Baker, Kendall Ellis, Jill P. Fletcher, Judith Shemnitz, Frank Sherron, and Tamaz Tal v. Ford Motor Company and United Technologies Automotive Inc. Civil Action No. 96-1814 (JBS) (US Dist. 2002). LEXIS 13421. Decided March 28, 2002.

Theresa M. Zeigler, individually; and Theresa M. Zeigler, as mother and next friend of Madisen Zeigler v. Fisher-Price Inc. No. C01-3089-PAZ (US Dist. 2003). LEXIS 11184; Northern District of Iowa. Decided July 1, 2003. (Unpublished).

TNT Road Company et al. v. Sterling Truck Corporation, Sterling Truck Corporation, Third-Party Plaintiff v. Lear Corporation, Third-Party Defendant. Civil No. 03-37-B-K (US Dist. 2004). LEXIS 13463; CCH Prod. Liab. Rep. P17,063 (US Dist. 2004). LEXIS 13462 (D. Me., July 19, 2004). Decided July 19, 2004.

Travelers Property and Casualty Corporation v. General Electric Company. Civil Action No. 3; 98-CV-50(SRU); 150 F. Supp. 2d 360 (US Dist. 2001). LEXIS 14395; 57 Fed. R. Evid. Serv. (Callaghan) 695; CCH Prod. Liab. Rep. P16,181. Decided July 26, 2001.

Truck Insurance Exchange v. MagneTek, Inc. (US App. 2004). LEXIS 3557 (February 25, 2004).

United States v. John W. Downing. Crim. No. 82-00223-01 (US Dist. 1985). LEXIS 18723; 753 F.2d 1224, 1237 (3d Cir. 1985). Decided June 20, 1985.

United States v. Lawrence R. Black Wolf Jr. CR 99-30095 (US Dist. 1999). LEXIS 20736. Decided December 6, 1999.

United States v. Markum. 4 F.3d 891 (10th Cir. 1993).

United States v. Ortiz. 804 F.2d 1161 (10th Cir. 1986).

United States v. Ruby Gardner. No. 99-2193, 211 F.3d 1049 (US App. 2000). LEXIS 8649, 54 Fed. R. Evid. Serv. (Callaghan) 788.

Vigilant Insurance v. Sunbeam Corporation. No. CIV-02-0452-PHX-MHM; 231 F.R.D. 582 (US Dist. 2005). LEXIS 29198. Decided November 17, 2005.

Wal-Mart Stores, Petitioner, v. Charles T. Merrell, Sr. et al. Supreme Court of Texas, No. 09-0224, June 2010.

The Basic Science and Dynamics of Fire

Courtesy of NIST

KEY TERMS

After reading this chapter, you should be able to:

- Describe the basis of how elements can combine with other atoms to form molecules by chemical interaction.
- Explain simple oxidation reactions involving carbon, carbon monoxide, or sulfur with oxygen.
- Describe four items formed during the thermal decomposition of wood (pyrolysis).
- List and describe three physical states of fuel.
- Describe different modes by which fuel vapors are generated from a solid fuel.
- Demonstrate a clear understanding of the combustion properties of wood, paper, plastics, paint, metals, and coal.
- Explain the importance of dust particle size and concentration in dust explosions.
- Explain how the flammability limits of a vapor/air mixture are affected as a function of initial temperature.
- Describe how the heat of combustion of a fuel is of importance to the fire investigator.
- Describe the behavior of liquid pools on porous and nonporous surfaces.
- Describe the distribution and effects of radiant heat from a burning pool of an ignitable liquid.

Fire is a chemical reaction that produces physical effects. As a result, the fire investigator should have some familiarity with the simpler chemical and physical properties and processes involved. Because fire consists of a number of chemical reactions occurring simultaneously, it is important to understand first what a chemical reaction is and how it is involved in a fire.

The body of fire dynamics knowledge as it applies to fire scene reconstruction and analysis is derived from the combined disciplines of physics, thermodynamics, chemistry, heat transfer, and fluid mechanics, many of the subjects required under *NFPA 1033* (2014, pt. 1.3.7). Accurate determination of a fire's origin, intensity, growth, direction of travel, duration, and extinguishment requires that investigators rely on and correctly apply all principles of fire dynamics. Investigators must realize that variability in fire growth and development is influenced by a number of factors such as available fuel load, ventilation, and physical configuration of the room.

PART 1: Basic Fire Science

2.1 Elements, Atoms, and Compounds

All matter is composed of elements or combinations of elements called compounds. An element is a substance that cannot be decomposed into simpler substances by chemical or physical treatment. There are 92 naturally occurring elements, along with a number of unstable, synthetic elements that are never encountered outside the laboratory. In descriptions of chemical reactions, each element is represented by a symbol, usually the first letters of an element's English or Latin name. For example, hydrogen is represented as H, oxygen as O, carbon as C, lead (plumbum) as Pb, and iron (ferrum) as Fe.

atom ■ The smallest particle of an element that can exist either alone or in combination with an atom of hydrogen.

Elements are composed of **atoms**. All atoms of a single element have the same size, weight, and chemical properties, but the atoms of one element are different from those of every other element. Although the atom is not the indivisible block of matter that it was once thought to be, in a chemical reaction like fire, it does not break up into its component particles. The atom is the smallest unit of an element that takes part in a chemical reaction.

The atoms of nearly every element can combine with other atoms to form molecules by chemical interaction. A molecule is the smallest unit of an element or compound that retains the chemical characteristics of the original substance. For example, the atoms of hydrogen, the simplest and lightest element, like those of most other elements, do not exist for very long as single or free atoms. They prefer to be in combination with other atoms. If the hydrogen is pure, two atoms of hydrogen will combine with each other to form a relatively stable **diatomic** (having two atoms) molecule of hydrogen gas, represented by the chemical formula H_2. The letter H represents the hydrogen atoms, with the subscript 2 meaning that there are two hydrogen atoms in that molecule.

Every atom consists of a central core of subatomic particles called protons (positively charged) and neutrons (neutral or uncharged) in various numbers, surrounded by a cloud of negatively charged electrons circulating about the nucleus like planets around our sun. It is these electrons and the ease with which they are shared with other atoms that determine the chemical reactivity of the element. This chemical reactivity tells us how easily the atom will break the bonds or ties that hold it in its molecule and how easily it will form bonds with other elements. The electrons surrounding the nucleus of each atom determine how that atomic element will prefer to combine with other atoms in particular ratios.

For example, at normal temperatures oxygen, which constitutes about 21 percent of the air, is a diatomic gas represented by the formula O_2. Occasionally, oxygen will combine as a triatomic molecule, O_3. This compound is called ozone and is produced most often by a high-voltage electrical arc in an oxygen environment. The ozone molecule is not very stable and will readily give up its extra atom to form a stable oxygen molecule, O_2. The free atomic oxygen produced then very quickly reacts with other atoms in the vicinity to form oxides or with another free oxygen atom to form additional O_2 molecules. Oxygen is the most critical component of all ordinary fires because it is essential for common combustion. Eliminating it will extinguish nearly all fires.

2.2 The Oxidation Reaction

Fire is not only a number of simultaneous chemical reactions, but also, a series of oxidative reactions. Atoms in the fuel are being oxidized, that is, combining with the oxygen of the air. There are many kinds of chemical reactions, but the ones of most interest in a **flame** are oxidations (Gardiner 1982).

It is interesting to see what happens in a very simple **oxidation**, common to most fires. When hydrogen, an excellent fuel, is oxidized, two diatomic molecules of hydrogen combine with one diatomic molecule of oxygen to form two molecules of water. The chemical formula for that reaction can be written as

$$2H_2 + O_2 \rightarrow 2H_2O$$

Because water is a more stable compound than the gases that form it, the reaction occurs with great vigor and the output of much **heat** and is called an **exothermic** (heat-producing) reaction. If the gases are mixed before being ignited, a violent explosion will result upon ignition. When they are combined in a flame, a very hot flame is produced.

Because hydrogen is found in almost all fuels, even in the complex molecules that make up wood, plastic, or oil, the burning of virtually any common fuel results in the production of water vapor in large quantities. This water **vapor** sometimes condenses on the cold glass windows of a burning structure. The conversion of chemically bound hydrogen in the fuel into water vapor during the fire also invariably leads to the production of much heat, although less than what is produced when pure hydrogen is burned. The net energy content of complex fuels is less than that of pure hydrogen or pure carbon because some of the energy is consumed in breaking the chemical bonds that hold the oxidizable atoms in their molecular structure.

diatomic ▪ Molecules made up of two atoms.

flame ▪ A body or stream of gaseous material involved in the combustion process and emitting radiant energy at specific wavelength bands determined by the combustion chemistry of the fuel. In most cases, some portion of the emitted radiant energy is visible to the human eye (NFPA 2017d, pt. 3.3.80).

oxidation ▪ Reaction with oxygen either in the form of the element or in the form of one of its compounds (NFPA 2016d).

heat ▪ A form of energy characterized by vibration of molecules and capable of initiating and supporting chemical changes and changes of state (NFPA 2017d, pt. 3.3.101).

exothermic ▪ A reaction or process accompanied by the release of heat.

vapor ▪ The gas phase of a substance, particularly of those that are normally liquids or solids at ordinary temperatures (NFPA 2017d, pt. 3.3.196; *see also* pt. 3.3.96, Gas).

Compounds may be represented by their numerical or empirical formulas, such as H_2O, CO_2, and O_2, or by structural or molecular formulas in which lines are used to represent the sharing of electrons by the atoms of a molecule. In this way water, H_2O, is represented as

$$\underset{H}{\diagdown}\overset{O}{}\underset{H}{\diagup}$$

and carbon dioxide, CO_2, is

$$O = C = O$$

The lines represent the forces or bonds between the atoms of elements making up the molecule. A single line indicates that one pair of electrons is shared, two lines indicate two pairs shared, three lines mean three pairs, and so on. In this way, the chemist shows not only how many atoms are in a molecule but in what order they are arranged and the nature of the chemical bonds between them, giving a great deal of information in a small space.

2.3 Carbon Compounds

flammable (same as inflammable) ■ Capable of burning with a flame (NFPA 2017d, pt. 3.3.83).

Carbon, represented chemically as C, is, like hydrogen, another element usually found in fuels. In fact, it is the element around which most of the **flammable** compounds are built.

Some materials, such as diamonds and graphite, are pure carbon in crystalline forms that are very difficult to burn. When diamond does burn, it produces the same products (CO_2 and CO) and energy as any other form of carbon. High-temperature crucibles are often made from graphite since when it burns, it is consumed slowly. Charcoal and coke are both industrial products consisting primarily of carbon, but quite impure carbon. These materials do not ignite easily. However, when afire, they produce considerable heat and are consumed at a slow rate. The chemical equation applied to the oxidation of carbon is

$$C(solid) + O_2(gas) \rightarrow CO_2(gas)$$

Carbon dioxide (CO_2) is always produced in fires involving carbonaceous fuels. It is an end product of nearly all combustions, including those that occur in the animal body. Exhaled breath is markedly enriched by carbon dioxide formed by oxidation of foodstuffs in the tissues. This is an oxidation like that which occurs in a fire, although the foodstuffs are not carbon alone but compounds of carbon with other elements. In all fires, another reaction may occur. This reaction may be secondary or may become primary depending on the supply of oxygen. This reaction produces carbon monoxide (CO), a gas known to produce an asphyxiating effect. Although CO invariably accompanies combustion reactions involving any carbonaceous fuel, it will not reach dangerous proportions in a properly adjusted gas appliance. Its production rate is dependent on fire conditions: generally low in free-burning fires but high in smoldering fires and high-temperature low-oxygen concentration burning.

The equation applied to the production of CO is

$$2C(solid) + O_2 \rightarrow 2CO$$

The three reactions producing H_2O, CO_2, and CO indicate the basis of the final combustion products and do not define the complex mechanisms by which the products are actually formed; however, they constitute the three most basic reactions of the fire. Water and carbon dioxide are the major products of nearly all fires, with carbon monoxide in somewhat lower concentrations in the effluent gases. Some fuels, notably those of coal or petroleum origin, are composed almost entirely of carbon and hydrogen and have only small amounts of other elements. A possible exception is sulfur, which is an impurity in most raw fuels. It also is oxidized, to form sulfur dioxide, according to the simple reaction

$$S(solid) + O_2 \rightarrow SO_2$$

Sulfur dioxide (SO_2) is a very sharp smelling gas often noted around metal smelters and other industrial operations.

Other Elements

Numerous other elements are found in the fuels most commonly encountered by fire investigators. Nitrogen, for example, does not burn in the sense of generating an exothermic reaction. Its role in a fire is complex, and yet it is inconsequential as a fuel. The nitrogen in air (~78 percent by volume) absorbs heat and expands proportionally. Nitrogen may be encountered when it is part of a molecule such as a nitrate, which provides oxygen to reactions.

Other elements present in wood—sodium, silicon, aluminum, calcium, and magnesium—are the constituents (in the form of their respective oxides) that form the white or gray ash that remains after wood is burned. They do not contribute significantly to the combustion itself.

2.4 Organic Compounds

Most of the compounds we have discussed fall into the class of molecules called the **inorganics**. They are the combinations of sulfur, lead, chlorine, iron, and, in fact, all elements except carbon. The compounds based on carbon are numerous and vital to life processes. They are considered a branch of chemistry themselves. The chemistry of carbon-containing compounds is called **organic** chemistry. Most of the fuels involved in structure and wildland fires are organic compounds. For the fire investigator, hydrocarbons and carbohydrates are the most significant organic compounds.

inorganic ■ A material made from or containing material that does not come from plants or animals.

organic ■ Of, relating to, or derived from living organisms.

2.5 Hydrocarbons

Many types of compounds form good fuels. **Hydrocarbons**, compounds composed solely of carbon and hydrogen, are the most common. Methane (CH_4), the chief component of natural gas, is the simplest compound.

Written structurally,

hydrocarbon ■ An organic compound consisting entirely of hydrogen and carbon.

$$\begin{array}{c} H \\ | \\ H-C-H \\ | \\ H \end{array}$$

the formula indicates the important fact that carbon has four valences, or combining points, on each atom. Hydrogen has only one, which means that four hydrogen atoms can combine with a single atom of carbon. The complete combustion of methane yields CO_2 and H_2O as final combustion products, but even this seemingly simple reaction goes through numerous intermediate reactions. The combustion of methane in oxygen is thought to involve about 100 such elementary reactions (Gardiner 1982, 110–25). These reactions involve the loss of hydrogen atoms and then various recombinations that produce ethene and acetylene within the flame as well as unstable molecular species such as —OH, —CH_2O, and —CHO.

These unstable species are called free radicals. The more complex the molecule, the more pathways the intermediate reactions can follow and the greater the variety of free radicals that are produced. In hydrocarbon combustion, the —CHO and —OH free radicals (as well as CO) combine with O and H to form H_2O and CO_2. Free radicals can exist only at relatively high temperatures, but as they cool they can condense and form the pyrolysis products such as the brown varnish or oily residues that are seen adhering to surfaces after a fire.

In addition, carbon is somewhat unique in that its atoms have a very strong capacity to combine with one another to form chains, rings, and other complex structures. This capacity to form chains can be illustrated by the compound butane, which is packaged as a liquid petroleum gas, with the formula C_4H_{10}, written structurally as

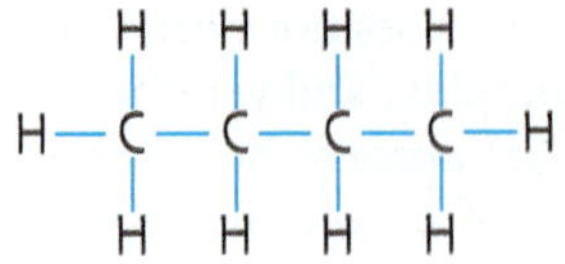

$$
\begin{array}{ccccccccc}
 & H & & H & & H & & H & \\
 & | & & | & & | & & | & \\
H - & C & - & C & - & C & - & C & - H \\
 & | & & | & & | & & | & \\
 & H & & H & & H & & H & \\
\end{array}
$$

These straight-chain compounds, called normal hydrocarbons or *n*-alkanes, can be extended almost indefinitely and can branch out to produce more complex structures including only the elements carbon and hydrogen. Because there are many possibilities for the location of such branching, many compounds may exist that have the same empirical formula but different structures. For example, the compound isobutane has the same empirical formula as butane but the structure

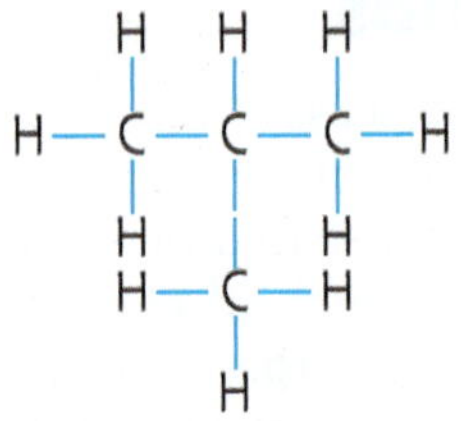

$$
\begin{array}{ccccccc}
 & H & & H & & H & \\
 & | & & | & & | & \\
H - & C & - & C & - & C & - H \\
 & | & & | & & | & \\
 & H & & | & & H & \\
 & & & H - C - H & & & \\
 & & & | & & & \\
 & & & H & & & \\
\end{array}
$$

Here the prefix *iso-* indicates a branched structure. Both chain length and point of branching can vary almost indefinitely, so there are many possible compounds. All these compounds are called **aliphatic** or **paraffinic** (meaning they have the maximum number of hydrogen atoms attached to carbon atoms with no double bonds) and are named according to the number of carbon atoms in the longest carbon chain in the molecule.

Another important class of hydrocarbons has a six-membered ring of carbon atoms as part of its structure. The simplest such compound is benzene (C_6H_6):

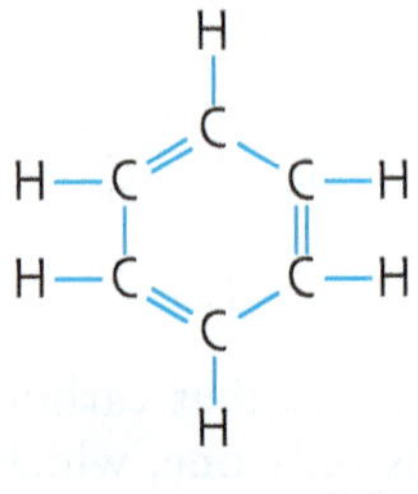

Note that there is an alternating sequence of double and single bonds between the carbons in the benzene ring. Many of these ring structure compounds have a characteristic smell and are called **aromatics**. One or more of the hydrogen atoms of a ring compound can be replaced with any number of chemical structures, some of which can be very large and complex. The simplest of the substituted benzene-ring or aromatic hydrocarbons is toluene (C_7H_8), with the structural formula

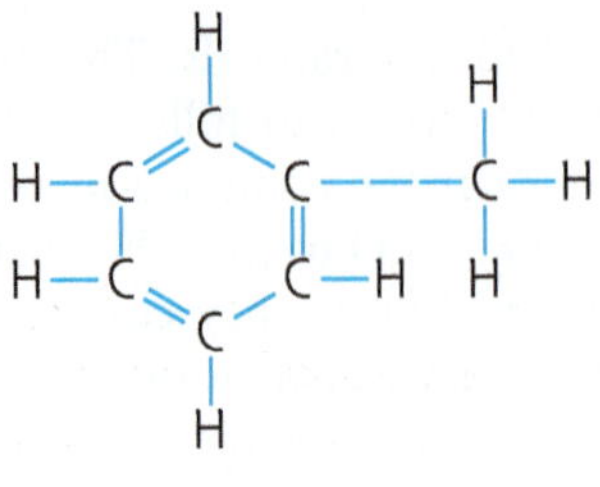

Thus far, the aliphatic compounds listed are all **saturated**, or lacking double bonds, but not all aliphatic compounds are in this category. For example, the gas eth*e*ne (not eth*a*ne, which is saturated) is C_2H_4, written structurally as

$$\begin{array}{ccc} H & & H \\ \diagdown & & \diagup \\ & C = C & \\ \diagup & & \diagdown \\ H & & H \end{array}$$

saturated ■ A hydrocarbon that has no double or triple bonds, and containing the greatest possible number of hydrogen atoms.

while propene (C_3H_6) is

$$\begin{array}{ccccc} & H & H & & \\ & | & | & & H \\ H - & C - & C = & C & \diagup \\ & | & & & \diagdown \\ & H & & & H \end{array}$$

Another category of unsaturated hydrocarbons involves triple bonds between adjacent carbons. Such compounds are usually designated by the suffix *–yne*, as in pentyne (or 1-pentyne to designate the carbon atom to which the triple bond attaches):

$$\begin{array}{ccccc} & & H & H & H \\ & & | & | & | \\ H - C \equiv C - & C - & C - & C - H \\ & & | & | & | \\ & & H & H & H \end{array}$$

The most common triple-bond hydrocarbon encountered in fire investigation is ethyne (C_2H_2), or, as it is more commonly known, acetylene:

$$H - C \equiv C - H$$

Another class of hydrocarbons commonly encountered in fuels has rings consisting of five, six, or seven carbons but without the combination of single and double bonds that characterize the aromatics. These cycloparaffins, as they are called, appear as in cyclohexane (C_6H_{12}):

$$\begin{array}{c}
\text{H} \quad \text{H} \\
\text{H} \qquad \diagup\diagdown \qquad \text{H} \\
\backslash \qquad C \qquad \diagup \\
\text{H} - C \qquad\qquad C - \text{H} \\
| \qquad\qquad | \\
\text{H} - C \qquad\qquad C - \text{H} \\
\diagup \qquad C \qquad \diagdown \\
\text{H} \qquad \diagup\diagdown \qquad \text{H} \\
\text{H} \quad \text{H}
\end{array}$$

2.6 Petroleum Products

Generally, hydrocarbons are good fuels, but few are used commercially as pure compounds. It can be very expensive to isolate any single compound from petroleum or coal tar mixtures in a pure state. Once isolated, the pure compounds might not have the desired physical or chemical properties and would have to be blended with another compound in any event. Virtually all commercial fuels are mixtures of relatively large numbers of individual compounds with similar chemical structure that provide the desired combustion properties.

2.6.1 PETROLEUM DISTILLATES

Petroleum products are first separated from one another by heating raw petroleum and collecting the vapors as they distill off at various temperatures. Such products are labeled petroleum distillates. Each of these fractions, or cuts, will contain a mixture of all the compounds that boil off between two set temperatures. For example, petroleum ether is a cut of distillates that boil off at temperatures between 35°C and 60°C (95°F–140°F), while kerosene contains distillates that boil off between 150°C and 300°C (300°F–572°F) (ASTM International 2013a). Most of the compounds found in these two fractions are aliphatic straight-chain or branched alkanes, and most are saturated—that is, with no double bonds. Some aromatics will also be present.

Cycloparaffins and aromatics have better characteristics as motor fuels, and their proportions are enhanced through chemical processing of the crude oil by such processes as cracking and reforming. They are then blended with various distillate cuts into fuels such as gasoline with the desired combustion properties. Gasoline is not a true petroleum distillate but rather a blended product that typically covers the boiling point range from 40°C to 190°C (100°F–375°F).

Because all these common petroleum products are complex mixtures of hydrocarbons, not all their components evaporate or burn at the same rate. Their evaporation starts with the lightest and most **volatile** compounds and generally progresses to heavier compounds as the temperature rises. Petroleum products that have undergone progressive partial evaporation are sometimes referred to as weathered. Stauffer, Dolan, and Newman (2008) address the forensic impact of weathered petroleum distillates commonly found in fire scene debris.

During combustion, the evaporation process has the same progression but occurs at a much faster rate, as radiation from the flames causes the temperature of the liquid pool of fuel to rise. As a result, the residues of partially burned petroleum products found in fire debris have different chemical and physical properties (vapor pressure, flash point, **specific gravity**, viscosity, etc.) from those of the original fuel. At the same time, the flammability properties of the fresh or unburned fuel are determined in large part by the lighter, more easily vaporized components of the mixture. Winter-blend gasolines, for instance, may contain 6 to 10 percent by weight methyl butane and 5 to 6 percent *n*-pentane, while summer-blend gasolines may contain 4 to 8 percent methyl butane and 4 to 5 percent *n*-pentane to maintain the same bulk properties of vapor pressure and flash point at very different temperatures (DeHaan 1995).

Hydrocarbons with carbon backbone (chain) lengths greater than C_{24} are waxes at room temperatures. In general, the longer the chain length, the higher the melting and boiling points of the compound will be. Mixtures of various high boiling point hydrocarbons will be encountered as petrolatum (petroleum jelly) or paraffin wax. The heaviest (longest chain) hydrocarbons are found in asphalt.

2.6.2 NONDISTILLATES

A number of petroleum products are not true petroleum distillates but are used in a variety of consumer and industrial products that will be encountered in fire debris. One class of compounds consists of blends of isoparaffinic (branched hydrocarbon chain) compounds used in insecticide solvents, hand cleaners, lamp oils, and some lighter fuels. Isoparaffinic compounds have good solvent properties but little of the odor commonly associated with petroleum solvents. Another class of petroleum products is **naphthenics**. Found in solvents and torch fuels, naphthenics have the aromatic and paraffinic components stripped out (by catalytic reactions or absorption/elution methods). These products consist largely of cyclohexane and cycloheptane with various substitutions. Others are blends of aromatics in various volatility ranges used in insecticides and adhesives for their specific solvent properties. There are also products that consist entirely of *n*-alkanes (sometimes just one or two, such as *n*-dodecane and *n*-tridecane) intended for use in liquid fuel candles. All these product types constitute possible volatile fuels but are synthesized products and not true petroleum distillates.

volatile ■ A liquid having a low boiling point, typically less than 68°F (20°C), that is readily evaporated into the vapor state.

specific gravity ■ (air) (vapor density). The ratio of the average molecular weight of a gas or vapor to the average molecular weight of air (NFPA 2017d, pt. 3.3.176).

naphthenics ■ Relating to or derived from naphthene.

2.7 Carbohydrates

The most important type of organic compound involved in combustion processes is in a different group: carbohydrates. Carbohydrates are the primary ingredient of wood, the most common fuel of structural fires. They differ from the hydrocarbons in very significant ways. Here the molecules are very large and complex. More significantly, they contain a relatively high content of oxygen; that is, they are already partially oxidized. The process of burning wood is simply a completion of the oxidation that started in the natural synthesis of the fuel itself.

Carbohydrates are so named because their chemical formulas include the elements carbon, hydrogen, and oxygen in multiples of the simple formula

$$-CH_2O-$$

which is a combination of a carbon with water (hydrate). Actually, the simplest carbohydrate has the formula

$$C_2H_{12}O_6$$

which is the empirical formula for several sugars, of which the most common are glucose (or dextrose), the sugar found in the blood; and fructose, which is obtained from grapes and other fruit. Cellulose, the major constituent of wood, is made up of many units of glucose attached to one another in chains. Because cellulose is simply an infinite replication of glucose units (a natural polymer), the main reaction that occurs on burning cellulose is the same as that for burning glucose:

$$\text{Glucose:} \quad C_6H_{12}O_6 + 6O_2 \rightarrow 6CO_2 + 6H_2O$$

$$\text{Cellulose:} \quad C_6H_{10}O_5 + 6O_2 \rightarrow 6CO_2 + 5H_2O$$

Ordinarily, as with other fuels, not all of the carbon is oxidized to carbon dioxide. In most fires, less oxygen is available and some CO is produced instead of CO_2. The hydrogen originally present is not as effective a fuel as it is in hydrocarbons, since it has already been partially oxidized in forming the original molecule. This partial oxidation accounts in part for the fact that wood fires do not readily achieve the high heat output of fires burning many other fuels.

Fats are a form of carbohydrates and can be significant fuels in some fires. Whether they are vegetable oils (such as cotton, corn, or linseed) or animal fats, they are carbohydrates (called fatty acids) with the characteristic molecular structure that they are straight-chain or branched hydrocarbons at one end and —COOH groups at the other, and are, in turn, substituted onto a glycerol backbone, as shown here:

Glycerol (Glycerin)   Linoleic acid ($C_{18}H_{32}O_2$)

Because of their largely carbon–hydrogen makeup, fats can burn readily and yield significant amounts of heat.

The amount of heat that any fuel can produce when burned is called its **heat of combustion**, and it is a measure of the number of **joules** or **Btus** (British thermal units) of heat released per kilogram (or pound) of fuel. The heat of combustion is a means of estimating how much total heat a given amount of fuel can produce; it is not a measure of the

heat of combustion ■ The total energy released as heat when a substance undergoes complete combustion with oxygen under standard conditions.

joule ■ The preferred SI unit of heat, energy, or work. A joule is the heat produced when one ampere is passed through a resistance of one ohm for one second, or it is the work required to move a distance of one meter against a force of one newton. There are 4.184 joules in a calorie, and 1055 joules in a British thermal unit (Btu). A watt is a joule/second (NFPA 2017d, pt. 3.3.122; *see also* pt. 3.3.22, British Thermal Unit (Btu), and pt. 3.3.25, Calorie).

British Thermal Unit (Btu) ■ The quantity of heat required to raise the temperature of one pound of water 1°F at the pressure of 1 atmosphere and temperature of 60°F; a British thermal unit is equal to 1055 joules, 1.055 kilojoules, and 252.15 calories (NFPA 2017d, pt. 3.3.22).

rate at which the heat can be released, or of the flame temperature a fuel will produce. Heat of combustion is measured by calorimetry techniques. Heat of combustion is represented by the symbol ΔH_c, where Δ (delta) represents change, H represents heat (enthalpy), and the subscript c denotes combustion. Other constituents of wood, such as resins, not only have a higher heat of combustion than cellulose, but their chemistry produces a higher flame temperature. Therefore, resinous woods such as pine or fir are more likely to produce hotter fires than are nonresinous woods such as birch or balsa.

2.8 State of the Fuel

The three physical states of matter of interest to the fire investigator are solids, liquids, and gases. The state in which a fuel exists is related to its combustion properties.

A solid is a substance in which molecules are held in a fixed, three-dimensional relationship to one another by molecular forces. Therefore, a solid has fixed volume and shape. Some solid fuels like candle wax melt to a liquid, which then evaporates to form a vapor. Some solids, like naphthalene, evaporate directly to a vapor state (a process called sublimation). Many solids do not melt but decompose by pyrolysis.

A liquid has no fixed three-dimensional shape but assumes the shape of the portion of any container it occupies and has a specific volume. Gasoline, like other liquid fuels, does not burn when in the liquid state. Liquid fuels are, however, easy to vaporize. The vapor that is formed burns like a gas mixing with oxygen and combusting as a flame. Because the molecular bonds in liquids are typically not as strong as those in solids, less heat is required to break these bonds in liquids compared with those in solids.

The molecules in a gas have only very weak forces between them because the molecules are generally very far apart (depending on temperature and pressure). Thus, a gas will expand to fill any available volume and diffuse (more or less) freely in air. Although there are relatively few gaseous fuels at room temperature, many materials become gaseous at the temperatures that occur in a fire, and virtually all materials can be converted to gases by applying sufficiently high temperatures. Another hydrocarbon, paraffin wax, requires much higher temperatures first to melt it, then to vaporize it to a form whose vapors will burn in the familiar form of a candle flame.

The classification of liquids, solids, and gases is far from absolute. They are to a large extent interchangeable. The conversion from one state to another is a function of the temperatures and pressures that exist during a particular fire. A change in physical state (such as from a bulk liquid to a finely divided aerosol when hydraulic fluid leaks under high pressure) can dramatically change the ignitability of the fuel and the size of the resulting fire. In general, the physical state of the fuel controls, in many ways, the ignitability of the fuel, its burning rate once ignited, and the quantity and nature of combustion products that result.

A number of materials in hydrocarbons are difficult to classify as gases or liquids. The liquid petroleum gases, for instance, of which propane and butane are the prime examples, can exist briefly in both states at ordinary temperature and pressure. Because they are so very volatile, when exposed they readily vaporize, leaving no liquid residue. Propane, with a boiling point of –42°C, vaporizes much more rapidly than butane, which is heavier (longer carbon chain) and has a higher boiling point (–0.6°C) (Perry and Green 1997). When vapors such as these are placed under pressure, they condense to form liquids.

By definition, a vapor can be condensed to a liquid by the application of pressure, whereas a gas is above its critical temperature and pressure and cannot be condensed by pressure alone. Commercial-grade butane and propane, a mixture often called liquefied petroleum gas (LPG), is stored and transported in tanks, largely in liquid form. On release of the pressure, as when the overlying gas in the tank is fed to a burner, more of the liquid vaporizes and maintains the same pressure (critical pressure) in the tank until all the fuel has evaporated.

GASES AND THE IDEAL GAS LAW

Hydrogen, methane, ethane, propane, and acetylene are the most common gaseous fuels. Like other gases, these gases generally obey the ideal gas law, which relates the amount of gas to its pressure, volume, and temperature.

The ideal gas law relationship is

$$pV = nRT$$

Where:

p = pressure
V = volume
n = number of moles of gas
T = temperature (**absolute temperature**, measured in Kelvin)*
R = universal gas constant

Increasing the temperature increases the volume if pressure is held constant or increases pressure if the volume is held constant. It is the heat-driven expansion of gases (or liquids) that gives rise to buoyancy. The same number of molecules occupying a larger volume produces a lower density.

If the amount of gas present is measured in moles (one mole of any material is equal in weight to its molecular weight and always contains the same number of molecules (Avogadro's number, or 6.023×10^{23}). One mole of oxygen (O_2) then weighs 32 g, and one mole of butane (C_4H_{10}) weighs 58 g. At standard temperature and pressure [0°C, 760 mmHg (1 atm)], one mole of gas will always occupy 22.4 L (liters).

*Temperature above absolute zero (0°C = 273 K).

■ **absolute temperature**
A temperature measured in Kelvins (K) or Rankines (R) (NFPA 2017d, pt. 3.3.1).

2.9 Solid Fuels

Solid fuels, as a rule, do not burn as solids. When a solid is burning, a portion of its surface may be smoldering, even glowing. Yet when a nonglowing solid fuel is surrounded by flames, we say that it is burning. This is not strictly true; the flames are the result of gas combustion. The gaseous pyrolysis products, not the solid fuel, mix with air to produce the flames. The smoldering phase generally follows when the thermal decomposition of the solid has slowed to the extent where some oxygen can reach the hot solid surface. Very porous solid fuels may allow diffusion through the fuel as well. If the surface is hot enough, a gas–solid interaction can take place that we observe as a glowing combustion. In a wood fire, the turbulence of the flames or the presence of a strong draft often makes it possible for glowing and flaming combustion to occur at the same time.

Solids burn by direct combination of oxygen with their surface (smoldering combustion), as volatilized materials that have melted and vaporized, or as complex fuels that pyrolyze to form combustible gases and vapors and leave a noncombustible solid residue. Reactive metals, such as magnesium, sodium, potassium, or phosphorus, and carbonaceous fuels, such as charcoal, burn only at their surface, as a glowing fire. If the vapors being pyrolyzed from common solid fuels are disregarded, most of the properties just mentioned do not apply to solids. Nonpyrolyzable solids have no flash point in the strict sense, no vapor density, and no single ignition temperature. They have a flammable mixture range only when they are finely divided and stirred into air as a combustible dust suspension. The physical properties that control their flammability are such factors as density, conductivity, and thermal capacity. Their porosity and melting point will also influence their performance as fuels under some conditions. The chemical properties of a solid fuel will determine the nature of volatile pyrolysis products and the rate at which they are generated.

Very finely divided solid fuels (such as wood dust or grain dust) can burn very quickly, even to the point of creating explosive forces, because the small volume of the individual particles permits rapid heating and decomposition into combustible products, and the large surface area permits rapid mixing with surrounding air.

The ignition and combustion of solid fuels are more complex than that of liquid or gaseous fuels because solid ignition usually depends on pyrolyzing enough of the material into a combustible fuel and having those products mix with the correct amount of air to be ignited. The ignition of any solid fuel is a surface phenomenon, which means that the temperature of the surface is the critical factor, not the bulk temperature. The ignition of a typical solid fuel depends on the fuel's density, thermal conductivity, and thermal capacity, as well as its rate of heat absorption. Ignition has been defined as the initiation of a self-sustaining combustion (Babrauskas 2003). Because combustion can be either flaming or smoldering, when we examine ignition processes we have to be aware of the difference between those processes. As Babrauskas has pointed out, some ignition temperature data are the surface temperatures of fuels as they ignite into flames, and others are the temperature of an oven into which the object is placed that results in smoldering combustion (Babrauskas 2003).

Reasonably pure cellulose is rare in nature, occurring in substances like cotton or linen fiber. Thus, an undyed cotton dress or linen shirt is fairly pure cellulose. A wooden beam is composed largely of cellulose, but with a different structural arrangement and many additional complex organic substances.

Most solid fuels, when heated, undergo heat decomposition or pyrolysis with the production of simpler molecular species that have definite properties. Precise values are not often available because in some instances the pyrolysis of solid materials has been inadequately studied and because the pyrolysis of a single solid material gives rise to a great many simpler products. The resulting complex mixture varies with the thermal and environmental conditions and has physical and chemical properties unlike those of any pure compound.

2.9.1 PYROLYSIS

Except for the simplest hydrocarbon fuels that merely need to evaporate to produce molecules simple enough to combine directly with oxygen in a flame, all fuels have molecules that have to be broken into small enough "pieces" to undergo combustion. The primary effect of heat on wood or other solid fuel is to decompose, or pyrolyze, it. The words *pyrolyze* or *pyrolysis* stem from the Greek words *pyro* (meaning fire) and *lysis* (meaning decompose or decay). Therefore, **pyrolysis** can be defined as the decomposition of a material into simpler compounds brought about by heat.

Similarly, in chemistry, pyrolysis is defined as the decomposition of a material brought on by heat in the absence of reactions with oxygen. In fires, pyrolysis of fuel also includes thermal decomposition that takes place in the presence of oxygen. Oxidation by-products are therefore common in real-world combustion products. To understand what occurs during the pyrolysis of fuel, it is necessary to remember that all practical fuels are organic in nature; that is, they are complex compounds based on carbon.

Pyrolysis of wood, for example, yields

- burnable gases such as methane;
- volatile liquids such as methanol (methyl alcohol) in the form of vapors;
- **combustible** oils and resins, which may be as vapors of their original forms or pyrolyzed from more complex structures; and
- a great deal of water vapor, leaving behind a charred residue, which is primarily carbon or charcoal.

The gases and vapors generated diffuse into the surrounding air to burn via **flaming combustion**. The charcoal then burns with a considerably greater heat output on a

pyrolysis ■ A process in which material is decomposed, or broken down, into simpler molecular compounds by the effects of heat alone; pyrolysis often precedes combustion (NFPA 2017d, pt. 3.3.150).

combustible ■ Capable of undergoing combustion (NFPA 2017d, pt. 3.3.31).

flaming combustion ■ Combustion of the gaseous vapors produced from pyrolysis.

weight-for-weight basis than does the original wood, since the noncontributing oxygen has been driven off, largely as water. The carbon combines directly with the oxygen in the air in contact with it to support heat output of the reaction. They also have different characteristics with respect to the temperature at which they ignite, the quantities of oxygen used per unit of fuel, the rate at which they will oxidize, and other properties related to their physical state.

The most significant part of all flaming fires is the flame itself, in which the combustion reaction takes place solely between gases. This remains true even though the fuel feeding the flame is a solid like wood, cloth, plastic, paper, or even coal. How then does a solid fuel maintain a gaseous reaction in the flames that burn around it? There are several routes by which this can occur.

Some solid fuels can evaporate directly to vapors, by a process called sublimation. Naphthalene, a flammable solid formerly used as mothballs, and methenamine, used for ignition tests, sublime at room temperatures. Other solid fuels, such as candle waxes, melt and then evaporate. Thermoplastics melt, decompose into smaller molecular species, and then evaporate. Another class, such as polyurethane, decomposes when heated to form volatile liquid products, which evaporate. The final category includes wood, paper, other **cellulosic** products, and most **thermosetting resins** that decompose when heated to yield both volatile products and a charred matrix. The key to most of these mechanisms is the phenomenon of pyrolysis, which occurs within the solid fuel as a result of its being strongly heated.

cellulosic ■ Plant-based materials based on a natural polymer of sugars.

thermosetting resin ■ Polymer that decomposes or degrades as it is heated rather than melts.

Nearly all fuels of importance to the fire investigator are vegetable in origin or are derived by decomposition, bacterial action, or geologic processes from "living" material, both animal and vegetable. This is true of oil and coal as well as of natural gas. Wood, the most common fuel in ordinary fires, is the direct result of life processes in which very complex organic structures are synthesized by natural processes within living cells. To date, no one can write a complete structural formula for wood, although it is well known that its major constituent is cellulose, a very large molecule synthesized from many glucose (sugar) molecules in long chains of undetermined length. In addition to cellulose, there are many other compounds in wood: hemicellulose and lignin are the most prevalent (up to about one quarter each), and there are various resins, pitches, oils, and other substances in various quantities. Certain softwoods, such as pine, have large quantities of volatile oils called terpenes and oleoresins (the source of commercial rosin), while most hardwoods contain little or no resin and only low concentrations of some of the terpenes.

Organic compounds (including the constituents of wood) when heated are subject to complex degradations to simpler compounds that are more volatile and more flammable. It is these compounds that oxidize in the flame. If a sample is pyrolyzed by heating it electrically in an inert atmosphere, the decomposition products may be separated by gas chromatography, identified by mass spectrometry, and studied by a variety of tests. Such studies have been important in recent years in understanding the mechanism of heat decomposition.

Pyrolysis products from wood include water vapor, methane, methanol, and acrolein. It is not important for the fire investigator to understand the exact mechanism of pyrolysis or all the intermediate products that result. However, it is important to understand the basic concept of heat decomposition because it is at the heart of understanding the basic nature of solid fuel combustion.

There is a zone just below the surface where pyrolysis occurs, and beneath (or behind) there is a region where no pyrolysis has yet occurred. Recent work by Stauffer has demonstrated that polyethylene pyrolyzes into a homologous series of alkanes, alkenes, and dienes; polystyrene forms aromatic products while burning; and polyvinyl chloride first releases noncombustible hydrogen chloride (HCl) gas and then subsequently yields burnable organic fragments (Stauffer 2004). Animal fats pyrolyze into homologous series of alkenes, aldehydes, and alkanes (DeHaan, Brien, and Large 2004).

Nonpyrolyzing Fuels

Not all solid fuels undergo pyrolysis before they burn. Reactive metals like sodium, potassium, phosphorus, and magnesium combust in air when oxygen combines directly in contact with the exposed surface. The resulting heat vaporizes the fuel and produces hot gases and incandescent oxides (ash), but the fuel does not first pyrolyze into simpler compounds. A few solid fuels like asphalt and wax melt and vaporize when heat is applied, and these vapors burn. Carbon (as charcoal) can undergo combustion without flames (smoldering combustion) as a solid–gas interaction on its myriad surfaces as oxygen diffuses into it.

2.9.2 COMBUSTION PROPERTIES OF WOOD

Wood is burned as fuel in structural and outdoor fires more often than any other solid material. Thus, its properties as a fuel, in regard to its behavior during combustion, are generally of greater importance to the fire investigator than those of any other solid combustible material.

Components of Wood

The term *wood* is generic and covers a wide variety of materials, natural and man-made, whose chief component is vegetable in origin. The major constituent of wood is cellulose (~50 percent), while numerous other constituents are present: hemicellulose (~25 percent) and lignin (~25 percent), with resins, salts, and water making up variable percentages (Drysdale 1999). Wood comes from a variety of trees, some resinous, some not; some dense, others light. Woods vary greatly in their water content, volatile components, and chemical properties.

Wooden materials are altered by manufacturing processes with treatments and finishes. Wood products include manufactured boards and panels, formed items such as furniture, and paper and cardboard products manufactured from wood pulp.

Ignition and Combustion of Wood

Wood is a chemically and physically complex cellulosic fuel. Each of the major constituents has a different temperature at which it undergoes pyrolysis: hemicellulose at 200°C to 260°C (400°F to 500°F), cellulose at 240°C to 350°C (460°F to 660°F), and lignin at 280°C to 500°C (536°F to 930°F) (Drysdale 1999). The thermal conductivity of wood varies with orientation, as does its permeability to air, both being significantly higher in the direction of the grain than across it. This will affect the ignitability of a wood mass or surface, for some portions will be more easily ignited than others. Heat must penetrate the wood to initiate pyrolysis and charring, as illustrated in Figure 2-1. The production of volatile oils and resins is also faster along the grain than at right angles to it, adding further variation.

Wood discolors and chars relatively quickly at temperatures above 200°C to 250°C (400°F to 480°F), as shown in Figure 2-2, but prolonged heating at temperatures above 107°C (225°F) will have the same effect (Drysdale 1999). [There are limited data on long-term (days or weeks) exposure to lower temperatures, but it appears that destructive pyrolysis can occur very slowly at temperatures down to 85°C (175°F).] As wood **chars**, its absorptivity of incident heat flux becomes higher due to the darker surface and the lower thermal inertia ($k\rho c$) of the char, so its temperature begins to increase faster once charring begins. All this means that wood does not have a fixed ignition temperature; it varies with the rate and manner in which heat is applied to it. When heated, a wood surface has one temperature at which it generates enough volatiles that can be ignited by the application of a pilot (external) flame (**piloted ignition**), and another much higher temperature at which the vapors themselves will ignite without any external pilot flame (nonpiloted ignition). The nature of the heating (radiant or convective) will influence both piloted and nonpiloted ignition temperatures. Other variables such

char ■ Carbonaceous material that has been burned or pyrolyzed and has a blackened appearance (NFPA 2017d, pt. 3.3.29).

piloted ignition ■ The initiation of combustion by means of contact of gaseous material with an external high-energy source, such as a flame, spark, electrical arc, or glowing wire.

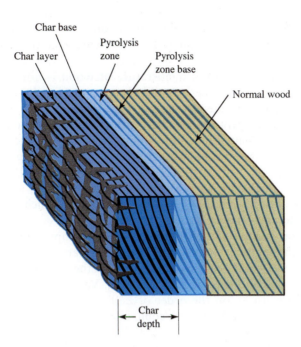

FIGURE 2-1 Normal combustion of wood resulting in progressive formation of char and pyrolysis zones. *Courtesy of the USDA Forest Service, Forest Products Laboratory, Madison, WI.*

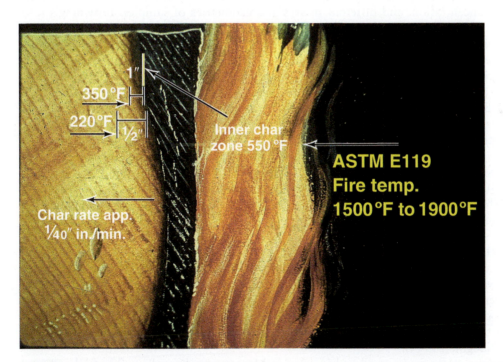

FIGURE 2-2 When Douglas fir and similar softwoods are exposed to a fire temperature of 700°C to 900°C (1500°F to 1900°F), the pyrolysis and accompanying charring occur at temperatures of approximately 177°C to 288°C (350°F to 550°F), as shown. The depth of the pyrolysis is dependent on the moisture content, density of the wood, and intensity of the approaching fire. Note that the char rate is only approximated even under these idealized laboratory test conditions. *Courtesy of the USDA Forest Service, Forest Products Laboratory, Madison, WI.*

as moisture content, size and thickness of the sample, orientation (vertical or horizontal), oxygen concentration, and duration of heat exposure will also impact ignition temperatures.

Due to its complexity, the ignition temperature of wood is not a single, clearly defined value for all woods and thermal conditions, as evidenced by the scattering of temperatures reported here. It is generally agreed that even with fresh (undecomposed) woods, the piloted ignition temperature will vary with the species of wood, the size and form of the sample itself, the ventilation, and the intensity, manner, and period of heating. The autoignition temperature is similarly variable. It might be thought to be dependent on the ignition temperatures of the pyrolysis products formed in the wood, but the major species—methane, methanol, and carbon monoxide—all have autoignition temperatures on the order of 450°C to 600°C (850°F to 1100°F), which are much higher than some observed autoignition temperatures for wood.

Clearly, other factors not yet identified are involved, perhaps the glowing combustion of surface char. The ignition temperature is closely related to the temperature at which the oxidation of the wood becomes sufficiently exothermic to raise the temperature of the surrounding fuel and become self-sustaining. Various authors have reported autoignition temperatures to be on the order of 230°C to 260°C (440°F to 500°F). Browning reported that ignition temperatures could be as low as 228°C (442°F) for some woods, and temperatures ranging from 192°C (378°F) to 393°C (740°F) have been reported elsewhere in the literature, but it is not clear whether they were observing flaming ignition or self-sustaining smoldering combustion (Brown 1934; Browning 1951; Fleischer 1960; NFPA 2008).

The reported variabilities may be due to the effects of different test methods, oxygen concentration, and different masses and geometries of samples. Browning's tests were of small wood chips embedded with thermocouples in a heated chamber. His criterion for ignition was the oven temperature at which the wood chip temperature exceeded that of the environment. Many of these earlier studies did not discriminate between smoldering and flaming combustion, so it is not surprising that reported results vary widely.

Babrauskas has assembled the results of numerous studies and concluded that values around 250°C to 260°C (480°F) represent a defensible surface temperature for piloted or nonpiloted ignition of fresh whole wood in a reasonably short period of time (Babrauskas 2003). Piloted ignition temperatures measured in tests where loose specimens were in open air being heated by a **radiant heat** source were typically 300°C to 400°C (570°F to 750°F). For smoldering ignition, surface temperatures under 300°C are typical. Higher temperatures favor gasification and flaming combustion (Babrauskas 2003).

Ignition Variables

Dry wood is more readily ignited than wood with a higher moisture content. Continuous or even recurrent exposure to raised temperatures will dry wood, resulting in somewhat lower ignition temperatures. However, there is not a significantly increased hazard as the wood dries until the temperatures reach 275°C to 280°C (527°F to 536°F), by which point both paint and wood are thoroughly charred (Forest Products Laboratory 1945; McNaughton 1944).

One recent study of piloted ignition of Masson pine by radiant flux (in horizontal specimens 10 cm × 10 cm) revealed surface ignition temperatures of 301°C to 405°C (574°F to 761°F) (Xiang and Cheng 2003). The higher the moisture content of the sample (0–30 percent MC), the higher the ignition temperature (301°C at 0 percent MC to 368°C at 30 percent MC, for example). Janssens reported that the ignition temperature is increased by 2°C for every 1 percent moisture increase (Babrauskas 2003). Hemicellulose has the lowest ignition temperature and lignin the highest. Softwoods, with less

radiant heat ■ Heat energy carried by electromagnetic waves that are longer than light waves and shorter than radio waves; radiant heat (electromagnetic radiation) increases the sensible temperature of any substance capable of absorbing the radiation, especially solid and opaque objects (NFPA 2017d, pt. 3.3.152).

hemicellulose and more lignin, have slightly higher autoignition temperatures (349°C to 364°C; 660°F to 687°F) than do hardwoods (300°C to 311°C; 572°F to 592°F) under the same test protocol (Xiang and Cheng 2003).

Some woods, like pine, will ignite into flames more readily and burn vigorously because they contain resinous materials that easily produce volatile flammable vapors when heated. Ease of ignition of wood is correlated with the content of pitch and other components that readily decompose to generate combustible vapors. Some woods, like pitch pine and slash pine, contain so many combustible components that they may easily be ignited with a match flame and will burn furiously, as if soaked in kerosene.

Other than volatile resins found in many species of wood, the main fuel component is cellulose. Cellulose is a derivative of glucose, and is already partly oxidized, and therefore has proportionately less fuel (per unit weight) available for oxidation in fire ($\Delta H_c \sim 16$ kJ/g). The total heat output is less on a weight-for-weight basis than that of fuels with a higher percentage of hydrogen such as coal or petroleum ($\Delta H_c = 46$ kJ/g). Thus, fires that have only wood for fuel *may* be somewhat less intense than those that are fed by hydrocarbon liquids.

Decomposed Wood

The ignition temperatures of fresh, undecomposed wood measured in the laboratory may not be important to the fire investigator, since fresh, new wood is not always involved in a structure fire. Of more interest is the effect of organic decomposition (decay) and thermal decomposition (pyrolysis) on the ignitability of wood. Angell reported that the ignition temperature of southern pine, measured at 205°C (400°F) when sound, dropped to 150°C (300°F) when decayed (Angell 1949). These values seem far too low for autoignition and may represent values for piloted ignition or sustained smoldering, possibly as a result of self-heating.

The minimum radiant heat flux for ignition of wood has been measured at ~12 kW/m² for piloted ignition and 20 to 40 kW/m² for autoignition (depending on time of exposure and test protocol). These samples were small (0.5 in. × 2 in.) and exposed to convective, short-term heating. Ignition times were recorded as 427 seconds for the sound wood and 105 seconds for the rotted wood (Babrauskas 2003). The relationship between applied heat flux and piloted ignition has been studied by Janssens. The higher the heat flux and the lower the thermal inertia, the faster ignition will occur. Because different woods have different densities and thermal conductivities, the ignition time will depend on the variety of wood involved.

Regarding time to ignition, Babrauskas's data offered the empirical correlation

$$t_{ig} = \frac{130\rho^{0.73}}{(\dot{q}_e'' - 11.0)^{1.82}} \tag{2.1}$$

where ρ = density of the wood (kg/m³), and $\dot{q}_e''$ is the radiant heat flux to which the (thick) wood is exposed (over the range 20–40 kW/m²) (Babrauskas 2003). The lower the density or the higher the radiant heat flux, the shorter the ignition time. There is a relationship between environmental (immersion) temperature and ignition time for wood. Data published by the NFPA show that longleaf pine, for instance, does not produce piloted ignition at 157°C (315°F) even after exposure for 40 minutes, yet piloted ignition can occur after 14.3 minutes at 180°C (360°F), 11.8 minutes at 200°C (390°F), 6 minutes at 250°C (480°F), 2.3 minutes at 300°C (570°F), or 0.5 minute at 400°C (750°F) (NFPA 2008).

Low Temperature Ignition of Wood

Fire investigators are often concerned with the effects of slow, prolonged heating of wood, which dehydrates and then decomposes the wood by pyrolytic action. The normal combustion of wood is a progressive process with zones of char and pyrolysis that progress inward from surfaces exposed to heat, as illustrated in Figure 2-2. At temperatures between 100° (212°F) and about 280°C (540°F), wood loses weight slowly as moisture and volatile oils are released gradually, and a large percentage (~40 percent) of the wood is turned to charcoal (Drysdale 1999). At temperatures above about 180°C (360°F), the pyrolysis of all three major solid constituents (i.e., cellulose, hemicellulose, and lignin) reaches its maximum rate, leaving a smaller percentage (10 to 20 percent by weight) as char. If the heat being accumulated by the char is retained, and there is an adequate supply of oxygen, the temperature of the mass can rise to the point at which combustion can take place [ignition temperatures of about 300°C (570°F)].

The retention of heat depends on the amount of thermal insulation available and the amount of heat that is being lost to convective and conductive processes. If there is too much insulation, the supply of oxygen becomes inadequate to sustain combustion, although smoldering combustion can be sustained even at very low oxygen levels. It is for these reasons that the formation of charcoal by slow heating of wood can play a significant role in the initiation of some accidental smoldering fires (Babrauskas 2003) as depicted in Figure 2-3.

Failure of the insulation around metal chimneys or fireboxes can expose wooden building components to such temperatures, while the failure of the integrity of metal or masonry flues may allow flames or sparks to provide piloted ignition. Direct flame exposure from an opening in a flue or chimney will lead to relatively rapid ignition of exposed wood. There is also a relationship between incident heat flux, piloted ignition temperature, and time to ignition. Yudong and Drysdale demonstrated that the higher the heat flux (between 15 and 32 kW/m^2), the lower the observed ignition temperature and the shorter the time to ignition (Yudong and Drysdale 1992).

Although whole wood itself may not ignite at low temperatures, it is well known that prolonged exposure to heat at temperatures below 120°C (248°F) over an extended period of time can cause wood to degrade to charcoal by the distillation and pyrolysis process described (Drysdale 1999). Shaffer calculated that exposure to temperatures as

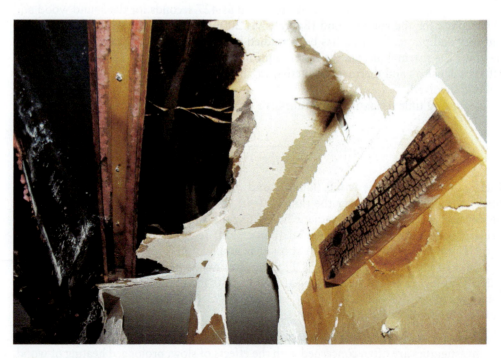

FIGURE 2-3 Charring in ceiling from prolonged contact with electric radiant-heat ceiling panels. *Compliments of Robert K. Toth, IAAI-CFI® - IRIS Fire Investigations Inc.*

low as 150°C (300°F) for long periods can decompose finely divided cellulosics to charcoal, which then may ignite (Shaffer 1980). This charcoal has been referred to as pyrophoric carbon or pyrophoric charcoal, alluding to the properties of activated (laboratory) charcoal to oxidize with room air even at modestly elevated temperatures. It has been argued that pyrophoric is a misnomer, since the US Department of Transportation defines **pyrophoric materials** as those that can ignite spontaneously within five minutes of exposure to air. [The Chemical Manufacturers Association defines pyrophoric as a material that will ignite spontaneously in dry or moist air at a temperature of 54.4°C (130°F) or below (Babrauskas 2001)].

Bowes, in his comprehensive study of self-heating mechanisms, points out that activated charcoal is made by heating a carbonaceous fuel (often, coconut hulls for laboratory use) under reducing conditions (in the absence of all oxygen). Although this material is capable of self-heating when exposed to air, especially when warm, exposure to air over a long period of time simply permits oxidation of the carbon (Bowes 1984). If a wooden surface is exposed to a radiant heat source when air is freely available, the pyrolysis products will distill away, but the activated form of charcoal will not be formed in bulk. The resulting char may not be susceptible to self-heating, and flames could not be supported because the required volatiles have already dissipated. Bowes's examination of the problem showed, however, that if a heated cylinder such as a flue or pipe runs through a massive wood member with minimal clearance, the conditions will be appropriate for the formation of a charcoal that can self-heat to smoldering combustion if the temperatures are high enough.

Bowes offered the opinion that the temperatures produced by ordinary steam pipes would not be adequate to create this condition but that superheated steam pipes or flues might. He commented, however, that if a suitably hot source (i.e., one with adequately high radiant heat output) was close to a wood surface overlaid with a noncombustible layer of sheet metal, tile, or similar barrier to oxygen, a reducing atmosphere could be produced, as shown in Figure 2-4. The failure of the barrier or some other change that

pyrophoric material ■ Any substance that spontaneously ignites upon exposure to atmospheric oxygen (NFPA 2017d, pt. 3.3.151).

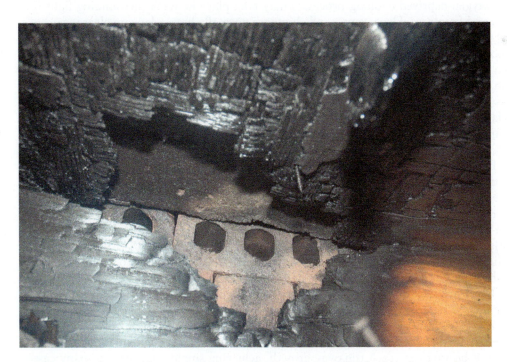

FIGURE 2-4 Fire in a wood floor under the hearth of an improperly installed fireplace. *Courtesy of Greg Lampkin, Knox County Sheriff's Office, Tennessee, Fire Investigation Unit.*

would suddenly bring the heated charcoal into contact with fresh air could then result in flaming combustion. Bowes presented the thermodynamic argument that to accomplish this, the temperature of the source would have to be considerably hotter than steam pipes operating at normal pressures.

Degradation to Char

Recent work by Cuzzillo and Pagni has explored a number of factors associated with heating or cooking at temperatures well below normal ignition temperatures of wood (Cuzzillo and Pagni 1999, 2000). Their findings show that the degradation of wood to char over a long period of time decreases the thermal conductivity and dramatically increases the porosity of wood. Cracking of the char makes it even more accessible to atmospheric oxygen. When wood is heated at low temperatures even in the presence of air, charcoal is formed. If enough char is produced to be a critical mass for self-heating and is sufficiently porous to permit diffusion of oxygen through the mass, the heated material can be ignited as a self-sustaining, smoldering combustion. If conditions promote a sufficient increase in heat release rate (HRR), there can be a transition to flaming combustion in adjoining masses of wood that have not been degraded completely.

Cuzzillo's work showed that self-heating of the char formed by low-temperature cooking is a likely mechanism leading to runaway self-heating when the conditions are right. It has to be realized that runaway self-heating of such char does not necessarily lead to flaming combustion because so much of the volatile content has been cooked out of the char. But a change in ventilation (such as shrinkage of wood timbers, failure of a metal or tile covering, or even a shift in the direction and intensity of ambient wind) could be the factor to push the combustion process into flames. The processes that prompt transition from smoldering to flaming are not well understood. Flaming may be triggered by better ventilation that causes a higher HRR (above a critical threshold), or the creation of hot spots in the char that cause piloted ignition.

Oxygen-deprived cooking processes may take place in areas surrounding light fixtures and fireplaces. Flues, vents, and chimneys normally have adequate clearances built into them because they are recognized sources of heat, but untreated cellulose insulation (wood shavings, sawdust, or paper pulp) can inadvertently be brought into contact with such heat sources. Pipes carrying steam under pressure can reach temperatures of more than 150°C (300°F) and should be well ventilated with adequate clearances where they pass through wooden structural members. Typically, any heat source that can create surface temperatures on wood members in excess of 77°C (170°F) must be properly separated or insulated (as UL recommended years ago). In fact, that is a requirement of the City of New York Building Code (Babrauskas, Gray, and Janssens 2007).

Babrauskas revealed numerous well-documented cases in which low-temperature ignition issues (i.e., cellulosic materials including sawdust, wood boards, and timber) were ignited by sources between 90°C and 200°C (196°F to 390°F) (Babrauskas 2001). Charring of wood is known to take place at temperatures as low as 105°C to 107°C (221°F to 225°F). Wood charred at such low temperatures exhibits similar exothermic oxidation as char produced at very high temperatures (>375°C; 700°F). Moisture and cyclic heating and cooling may play roles in making charred wood susceptible to self-heating.

There are well-documented fire cases where *massive* wood timbers in a residence were ignited by prolonged contact with steam heating pipes whose surface temperatures never exceeded 120°C (250°F), as illustrated in Figure 2-5. As with other self-heating materials, if there is a sufficient reactive mass, adequate oxygen, insulation, and time, such self-heating can reach runaway growth, achieving smoldering that, in many cases, can transition to open flame.

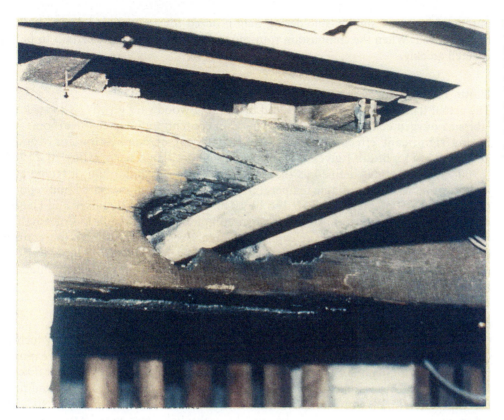

FIGURE 2-5 Massive floor timbers more than 80 years old ignited by hot-water pipes. Residents smelled smoke for two weeks prior to detecting smoldering fire. *Courtesy of Thomas Goodrow, Fire/Explosives Technical Specialist, ATF (retired).*

In the 2004 *MagneTek* court decision, several scientific errors were validated by the published decision (*Truck Insurance Exchange v. MagneTek, Inc.* 2004). These included a claim that pyrolysis is just a theory that is not suitably supported by scientific data. Pyrolysis has been known for more than 200 years to be part of the combustion process, and thousands of papers support and prove its mechanisms. Somehow the court became convinced that wood has a fixed ignition temperature of 400°F (195°C) and that any ignition has to be caused by a source with at least that temperature.

The court failed to note that wood is a very complex fuel that undergoes numerous chemical and physical changes as it is heated. The various forms created by these processes have different chemical and physical properties, some of which include an increased propensity to self-heat. Even though the term *pyrophoric* is misapplied to wood and charcoal (and that is presumably the term the court meant to discredit), the mechanisms of self-heating are well known.

There is no tested and published formula that can accurately predict the relationship between heat (or temperature) exposure and time to ignition for such a complex and multivariate problem as low-temperature ignition of wood; however, that does not mean that scientifically defensible hypotheses cannot be offered and tested in fire investigation. Designed to capture the energy of the sun's heat radiation, some solar water heaters can produce temperatures above 150°C (300°F) both in the heat-collecting element and in the pressurized transfer medium (if any). When the circulating pumps for these heaters fail, charring of underlying wood structures and roof fires have reportedly resulted.

Investigators tend to associate the time of discovery with the time of first ignition. This assumption may introduce serious errors into the fire analysis. Due to its slow output of heat and smoke, smoldering may proceed for an extended period without being noticed. When the combustion transitions to flame, it is almost certain to be discovered quickly.

Flame Temperatures

The actual flame temperatures produced by burning wood vary greatly, with such variables as oxygen content, forced-air draft, resin content, and degree of carbonization having significant effects. Using a typical net heat of combustion for wood of 18 MJ/kg (7755 Btu/lb.) gives a calculated adiabatic flame temperature of 1590°C (2900°F). **Adiabatic** is defined as the ideal conditions of equilibrium of temperature and pressure. The actual flame temperature of wood has been measured and reported as being some 500°C less (estimated to be 1040°C, or 1900°F) (Lightsey and Henderson 1985). The combustion of wood is so complex that a calculation of adiabatic flame temperature is of little relevance. It merely serves to illustrate the contrast between such calculated values and observed flame temperatures. It should also be remembered that measurements of turbulent flame temperatures produce time averages of rapidly fluctuating temperatures.

Char Rates

Once ignited, the rate at which wood will char is dependent on the heat flux to which the wood is exposed, its material, and its physical form (Figure 2-6). The standard exposure for wall and floor materials uses the E119 furnace, whose temperature and heat flux rise from near ambient to a maximum after 60 to 90 minutes. Under these test conditions, the char rate for plywood ranged from 1.17 mm/min. to 2.53 mm/min. (0.05 to 0.1 in./min.). For ½ in. (12.7 mm) plywood, burn-through times were 10 to 12 minutes. For ¾ in. plywood (18–19 mm), burn-through times were 7.5 to 17.6 minutes. For boards with tongue-and-groove edges or no gaps, burn-through times were 10.5 minutes for 19.8 mm pine, 14.17 minutes for 20.6 mm oak, and 24.3 minutes for 38 mm boards (Babrauskas 2004). The presence of gaps dramatically decreased burn-through times,

adiabatic ■ The ideal conditions of equilibrium of temperature and pressure. The actual flame temperature of wood has been measured and reported as being some 500°C less (estimated to be 1040°C, or 1900°F) (Lightsey and Henderson 1985).

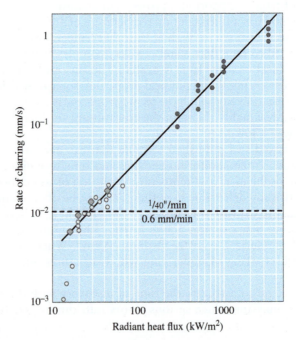

FIGURE 2-6 Variation of charring rate of wood with radiant heat flux. Note the log/log scale and sharp decrease below 20 kW/m². *From Butler, C. P. 1971. "Notes on Charring Rates in Wood." Fire Research Note No. 896. Reproduced in Drysdale, D. 1985. An Introduction to Fire Dynamics. New York: John Wiley & Sons: 182.*

reducing them to half that of tightly fitted boards of the same thickness. These rates are in accordance with results reported for jet fires against softwoods and for higher-temperature fires than the E119 protocol, in which for exposures to mild fluxes (~20 kW/m^2) the char rates are on the order of 0.6 to 1.1 mm/min. (0.02 to 0.04 in./min.) (White and Nordheim 1992).

Charcoal and Coke

Although wood contains oxygen in its structure and could be considered partially oxidized, one of its main combustion products, charcoal, contains no significant oxygen and is therefore an entirely carbonaceous fuel. Charcoal is an excellent fuel, having a heat of combustion of 34 MJ/kg. Charcoal is formed by pyrolyzing and destructively distilling the volatile materials out of the wood, leaving behind the nonvolatile constituents, chiefly carbon, as shown in Figures 2-1 and 2-2. Charcoal is correspondingly difficult to ignite and, lacking volatile materials, gives little flame. The small blue flames associated with its burning result from the formation of carbon monoxide (CO) gas, which burns rapidly, close to the surface of the charcoal from which it was generated, to form carbon dioxide (CO$_2$). A charcoal fire is largely a smoldering fire, that is, one without flame, but intensely hot. Here the solid is reacting with gaseous oxygen to produce combustion on and slightly below the surface of the fuel.

Coke, formed similarly from coal or petroleum, displays burning characteristics much like those of charcoal and for the same reasons.

2.9.3 WOOD PRODUCTS

There are a large variety of manufactured wood products used in building construction. These products may be used as structural elements, roofing, flooring, and interior finishes. The ignition and burning characteristics of these materials may differ from those of the wood from which they are derived.

Adhesives used in manufactured wood products can affect the wood product's burning characteristics. Often, the adhesive is less readily combustible than the wood layers. The resins used in oriented strand board (OSB) have the same ignition and combustion properties as the bulk solid timber, so burn-through times are reported as similar (Babrauskas 2003).

Plywood and Veneer Board

Plywood and veneer board are common examples of manufactured wood product. Both are made from thin sheets of wood laminated to one another with layers of adhesive. The nature of the adhesive determines the suitability of the product for interior (dry conditions only), exterior (some weather exposure), or marine (extended exposure to water) use. Standard plywood is largely made from fir, with cheaper, imperfect sheets and pieces in the interior layers.

Veneer board generally is made with a top layer of hardwood laminated to less expensive base layers. Plywood and veneer board delaminate as they burn. The thin laminate layers can contribute to rapid flame spread as they separate from the main sheet.

Particleboard or Chipboard

Particleboard or chipboard is made from small chips and sawdust from wood and paper mills bonded together under great pressure with a suitable adhesive. Particleboard is very dense but cheaper to make than plywood and is widely used in floors, cabinets, and furniture where appearance is not of importance. Particleboard has very limited strength under wet conditions and tends to swell and crumble when exposed to water for any length of time. Both plywood and particleboard are often finished with a thin vinyl covering that can be combustible.

OSB, or chipboard, is widely used for exterior sheathing and manufactured structural components. OSB is manufactured using large splinters, shards, and thin fragments of wood oriented so that their grain is roughly parallel. These materials are then glued together under great pressure and heat using formaldehyde resins. OSB is generally stronger than particleboard and less expensive than plywood because it can be made from wood processing waste materials.

Exterior Deck Materials

There are a number of manufactured wood products used on exterior decks as alternatives to natural or treated wood. These consist of cellulose materials (wood flour, wood fiber, or ground paper) blended with a polyethylene or polypropylene binder. They can vary from 41 to 65 percent wood fiber, with 31 to 50 percent plastic and ash (Quarles, Cool, and Beall 2003). The individual members may be solid in cross section, hollow, or channeled. These products have been tested for ignitability by burning brand and for fire performance when ignited by an underdeck burner, or in a cone calorimeter. These composite materials may produce a higher HRR than a comparable solid wood material (Stark, White, and Clemons 1997). They may also drip molten plastic as they burn, increasing the chances of spreading fire down onto combustibles below, and can rapidly fail structurally without warning (increasing risk of injury to firefighters) (Quarles, Cool, and Beall 2005).

Other Cellulosic Building Materials

Other cellulosic building materials, not necessarily made from wood but similar in their combustion properties, include Celotex, Masonite, and similar boards made from compressed and bonded fibrous cellulosic materials. Low-density products (such as Celotex), formerly used as acoustical tiles to cover ceilings, are now used in large sheets, as insulation, floor underlayment, or for other such purposes.

Several new building materials have been introduced for use as exterior decks, railings, and fences. These are basically extruded plastic (reinforced or nonreinforced), often made entirely from recycled polyethylene, PVC, or ABS (Quarles, Cool, and Beall 2005), as seen later in Figure 2-9. These materials have been shown to be easily ignited with a match or other small open flame to produce a rapidly growing fire, with molten burning material dripping or running off as it burns. The result can be a large pool fire of the molten material, or rapid ignition of other combustibles located below. Such rapid combustion also leads to loss of structural strength (Albers 1999).

Tests show that some of these materials can support rapid flame spread across their surfaces and are subject to a smoldering fire along their edges or, occasionally, in their interiors. In a large surrounding fire, they burn well and contribute much fuel. Thus, it is common to see that in a room fire, all the acoustical tiles have fallen and burned on the floor. They fall readily because they are generally glued into place, and the heat softens the adhesive.

This was common in older construction (glued tiles), but is not normally used in modern construction. Also, the ceiling tile materials have changed substantially, such that they are not as combustible as the cellulose tiles that were glued previously.

The high-density products (Masonite) have similar properties but are more ignition resistant.

flame retardant ■ Materials that are chemically treated to be slow burning or self-extinguishing when exposed to an open flame.

Blown-in ceiling insulation can be shredded or macerated paper with a **flame retardant** added. A similar product is also made for application by being blown in while wet for use in walls, where the dried mass is more resistant to mechanical disturbance and fire penetration. Blown-in insulation can also be mineral fiber, which is noncombustible. Both types of products are typically gray in color, and careful examination and laboratory analysis may be required to identify the product.

Loose blown-in cellulose insulation is a triple threat when it comes to accidental ignition for the following reasons:

- ■ Its insulative properties minimize heat loss from even small heat sources buried in it.
- ■ Its loose texture means it can be moved or can fall into contact with heat sources.

- Its fire retardance can be compromised by moisture or mechanical separation, making it susceptible to smoldering.
- Some brands of cellulose insulation have been formulated with fire retardants that can be corrosive to metals.

Proper flame-retardant treatment will make the bulk material resistant to both flaming and smoldering combustion. Samples of structural, decorative, or insulation materials related to ignition or significant fire spread should be retained for laboratory analysis.

2.9.4 PAPER

The basic ingredient of all paper is cellulose, the same material basic that is in cotton and is a major constituent of wood. Cellulose is readily combustible, but not all the constituents of paper are. "Slick" papers have a high clay content, which is not combustible. Many writing papers also have a high clay content. The differences in the combustion properties of various papers are readily demonstrated by burning a piece of newspaper, which leaves a small and very light ash, followed by burning a piece of heavy, smooth, slick magazine paper, which leaves a very heavy ash. The ash in most instances is the clay, although many specialty papers also contain such constituents as titania (titanium dioxide), barium sulfate, and other noncombustibles.

Because paper is a cellulosic product like wood, its ignition properties are not easily measured. Graf found the ignition temperature of a variety of papers to be between 218°C and 246°C (425°F and 475°F). At 150°C (300°F) most papers appeared to be unchanged during the duration of his tests. Many papers tanned in the range up to 177°C (350°F), went from tan to brown by about 204°C (400°F), and if not ignited, went from brown to black at about 232°C (450°F). Such events are affected by the rate of heating, manner of ignition, nature of heat exposure, and ventilation; therefore, a precise ignition temperature cannot be cited (Graf 1949). Smith's data (as reported in the *Ignition Handbook*) indicate that most uncoated papers ignited at surface temperatures of 260°C to 290°C (500°F to 550°F) (Babrauskas 2003). Long-term ignition was reported to occur in paper wrapped around a pipe maintained at 200°C (400°F).

Paper ignites easily because it has a low thermal inertia so its surface temperature goes up rapidly, and it is thermally thin, allowing rapid heating of its entire thickness. The minimum heat flux for ignition of various paper products is from 20 to 35 kW/m^2 (Mowrer 2003). If paper is exposed as a single sheet rather than compressed in a stack, its large surface area and low mass allows rapid burning, and a high, but brief, HRR. When paper is stacked, it no longer acts as a thermally thin material, and a pile of stacked papers is more difficult to burn.

A stack of paper can support smoldering fire within its mass. Once burning at a steady rate, cardboard cartons (flats) have been measured to yield a maximum mass flux of 14 g/m^2/s compared with that of wood cribs, 11 g/m^2/s (Quintiere 1998).

In the interpretation of a fire, it is not the presence of paper that is significant but its distribution in terms of exposed surface. Sometimes, the presence of a stack of papers is taken as the origin of a general fire. Although it is possible to burn a stack of folded newspapers to completion over an extended time, it is surprisingly difficult to do because of the limited surface area exposed to the air. In contrast, a pile of loosely crumpled sheets of the same paper is not only easy to ignite but also quickly raises the temperature of nearby combustibles to their ignition points and thus initiates a fast-growing, very destructive fire.

2.9.5 PLASTICS

Investigators find plastics, universal in modern structures and vehicles, burned in nearly all fires. Thus, fire investigators need a working knowledge of the kinds of plastics, their applications, and their burning behaviors.

General Characteristics

There are many kinds of plastics, with a variety of physical and chemical properties. Some, like Teflon (tetrafluoropolyethylene), are not readily combustible and will exhibit heat damage only at extremely high temperatures. Others, such as nitrocellulose, are readily ignitable and violently flammable. Most of the commonly used plastics range between these two extremes.

Plastics are called **synthetics** as a class because they are not natural products but are usually manufactured from petroleum feedstocks. Most plastics are readily combustible. Many laboratory tests of the ignition and combustion properties of plastics are used to identify and classify them as to fire hazard. Nearly all plastics are made from long chains of hydrocarbons linked together in various ways. Sufficient heat input will rupture the chemical bonds holding the chains together, and the plastic will pyrolyze to simpler, more volatile compounds.

These pyrolysis products may be very toxic, as in the case of styrene monomer and cyanogens; extremely flammable, as in the case of CO and the short-lived radicals CH and CH_2; or may be susceptible to further pyrolysis. Some plastics and rubbers create pyrolysis products that can have serious consequences in the fire environment. Polyvinyl chloride releases hydrochloric acid (HCl), and Teflon releases hydrogen fluoride (HF) and fluorine (F_2) when it decomposes due to heating. Some rubbers generate hydrocyanic acid (HCN) during combustion.

Thermoplastic polymers will melt and flow, sometimes dripping onto a fire fueling it and sometimes collecting into a pool of burning plastic, which can burn fiercely. As with laboratory tests of other solid fuels, the fire behavior of plastics is largely dependent on their degree of molecular cross-linking, physical form (sheet, rod, fiber, etc.), test conditions, and presence of inorganic fillers and fire retardants.

The chemistry of plastics is similar to that of petroleum products, and they tend to produce similar sooty flames when burning in air. The open-flame temperatures produced by burning plastics are similar to those of common petroleum distillates. The flame temperatures produced by some plastics can be quite high. Polyurethane is one example for which flame temperatures up to 1300°C (2400°F) have been measured (Damant 1988). These mass fluxes can be used to approximate the HRR per area of a horizontal plastic fuel surface. Multiplying the mass flux rate by the heat of combustion for the fuel of interest results in a HRR per unit area. These HRRs are similar to those of common **ignitable liquids**.

The combustion of many polymers contributes largely to the formation of the greasy or sticky dense **soot** found at many fire scenes and is responsible for dense black smoke frequently noted during the early stages of structure fires. The dense smoke that many polymers produce is rich in flammable vapors, and the ignition of dense clouds of these vapors can quickly involve an entire room. Only polyethylene, polypropylene, and polyoxymethylene (Delrin) generally burn with a clear flame and little soot. Polyethylene and polypropylene also produce a candle-wax smell, since upon heating, they pyrolyze into much the same components as wax, with the resulting similar behavior.

The autoignition temperatures of plastics are generally 330°C to 600°C (650°F to 1100°F), but their universal applications in packaging, utensils, furnishings, wall coverings, windows, walls, and even exterior structure panels provide many opportunities for them to come into contact with temperatures of this magnitude (Babrauskas 2003).

Behavior of Plastics

Plastics that undergo reversible melting without appreciable chemical degradation are called **thermoplastics**. Plastics that do not melt but rather decompose and leave behind a solid char are called thermosetting plastics. There is a small group of plastic materials that

PLASTIC	MINIMUM IGNITION TEMPERATURE		
		°C	°F
Polyethylene	365*	488	910
Polyisocyanate		525	977
Polymethyl methacrylate	310*	467	872
Polypropylene	330*	498	928
Polystyrene	360*	573	1,063
Polytetrafluoroethylene		660	1,220
Polyurethane foam (flexible)		456–579	850–1,075
Polyurethane foam (rigid)		498–565	925–1,050
Polyvinyl chloride		507	944

Sources: NFPA. 2003. *Fire Protection Handbook*. 19th ed. Quincy, MA: National Fire Protection Association, Table A-6.

*Babrauskas, V. 2003. *Ignition Handbook*. Issaquah, WA: Fire Science Publishers, 244.

decompose into volatile materials that are not rigid and are sometimes called elastomers; these include polyurethane rubber. Minimum autoignition temperatures of common plastics are shown in Table 2-1.

Polyvinyl Chloride

The behavior of a particular plastic in a fire is the result of many factors, all of which should be kept in mind when evaluating its potential contributions to the fire. Vinyl (polyvinyl chloride—PVC) may burn slowly when tested in solid form in a laboratory but has been observed to burn rapidly and contribute greatly to flame spread when present as a thin film on wall coverings. PVC wire insulation softens and melts when heated but chars when exposed to a flame.

Nylon

One of the first synthetic fibers, nylon is widely used in carpets. Most nylon-fueled flames tend to be self-extinguishing, but under intense radiant heat flux, nylon fiber carpet has been shown to burn with some enthusiasm.

Polyurethane and Polystyrene Foams

Unless it is properly treated with fire retardants, polyurethane foam is very flammable because it is readily ignited with any open flame. It produces a hot, smoky flame that progressively decomposes more and more of the foam, with the melt joining the burning substance at the bottom of the crater. Rigid (and flexible) polyurethane foam and polystyrene foam are used as thermal insulation in equipment and in structures and have contributed to the rapid spread of many destructive and often-fatal fires.

The 2003 tragic nightclub fire in West Warwick, Rhode Island, killed 100 of the 400 patrons present when stage pyrotechnics ignited the unprotected urethane foam sound insulation covering the stage walls. The fire growth was captured on videotape and shows progression from localized flashover in the drummer's alcove into the main room ($\sim$10 m $\times$ 15 m) in less than three minutes as the fire spread across the walls with extreme rapidity (Madrzykowski et al. 2004). Plastic foams in foam-core steel structural sandwich panels have become more commonly used in constructing commercial buildings (Cooke 1998a, 1998b). Polystyrene foam–filled panels are especially susceptible to failure at joints and seams. Others have been seen to delaminate, exposing the melting plastic foam to external flames (Shipp, Shaw, and Morgan 1999). Recent advances in this technology have improved the fire performance of some sandwich panels, with some being resistant to both ignition and melting (Fire 1985; Fire 2005). Investigators should take a sample of any polymeric filler for analysis before reaching conclusions about sandwich panel contribution to fire spread.

Latex or Natural Rubber

Largely replaced by polyurethane foams, latex or natural rubber foam products are still encountered in older furnishings and carpet pads, and on high-end custom mattresses. Although latex foam products sometimes physically resemble high-density urethane foams, their flammability properties are very different. Urethane foams can be ignited by an open flame (Figure 2-7) or intense radiant heat from an external source, but most cannot be ignited by direct contact with a glowing cigarette unless they are covered with a susceptible fabric or are in contact with a sustained heat source (Holleyhead 1999).

Unlike urethane foams, latex foams can be ignited by a small glowing ignition source (such as a cigarette) and once ignited will sustain a smolder and are capable of rekindling into a flaming fire many hours after suppression of flaming combustion. Latex foams are also capable of self-heating to **spontaneous ignition** if preheated to a modest level, whereas finished urethane foams do not self-heat. The chemical reaction that creates the foamed elastomer, however, is exothermic, and incompletely cured blocks of foam and waste products can self-heat to ignition. Like urethane foams, latex foams can be ignited by a flaming source and will generate a dense, toxic smoke when burning.

spontaneous ignition ■ Initiation of combustion of a material by an internal chemical or biological reaction that has produced sufficient heat to ignite the material (NFPA 2017d, pt. 3.3.180).

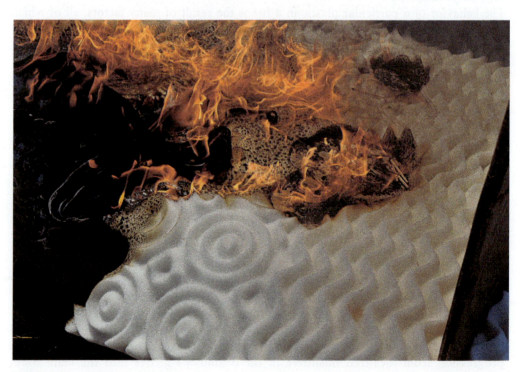

FIGURE 2-7 Polyurethane foam mattress topper burns readily after match flame ignition. *Courtesy of John Jerome and Jim Albers.*

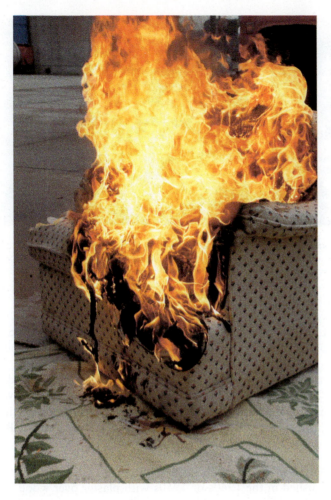

FIGURE 2-8 Burning synthetic upholstery melts as it burns. Burning droplets ignite the carpet below and the lower portion of the vertical upholstery face. *Courtesy of Jamie Novak, Novak Investigations and St. Paul Fire Dept.*

Thermoplastics

Thermoplastics are molten at the temperatures of the burning fuel surface, so they will run and drip as they burn, as pictured in Figure 2-8. If the droplets are on fire as they fall to floor level, they can ignite new flames along the vertical upholstered surfaces of sofas. Plastic skylights, lampshades, and light fixture diffusers can be ignited by the heated gases and flames at the ceiling in a room fire. As these articles burn, they soften and sag, sometimes falling onto combustibles below, producing patterns that may appear to be isolated, discrete points of origin.

During postfire examination, some investigators have been misled by these numerous separate fires, suspecting an incendiary cause. The investigator should be careful to attempt to correlate all unusual fire patterns with the fuels involved. Plastics are being used increasingly as a substitute for glass in windows, particularly in schools where vandalism is a problem. These plastics have been ignited by matches or lighters and gone on to ignite major structural fires. Large polypropylene waste bins, if not flame retardant, are easily ignited to produce very large, sustained pool fires, especially when empty. Examples of extruded plastic deck planking and resulting fire behavior are illustrated in Figures 2-9A and B.

2.9.6 CHANGES IN MATERIALS

Years ago, televisions, radios, and other small appliances were constructed with wood or metal housings, which would often contain the small flames of internal fires. Now these

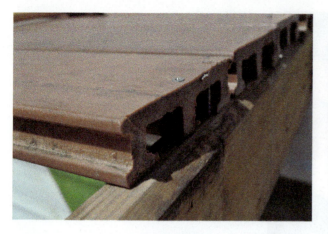

FIGURE 2-9A Plastic decking ignited with a match. *Courtesy of John Jerome and Jim Albers, Barona Fire Dept.*

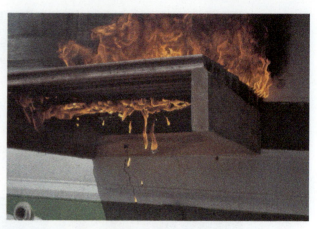

FIGURE 2-9B Dripping flaming plastic with rapidly growing flames above. *Courtesy of Jim Albers and John Jerome, Barona Fire Dept.*

items may be made of synthetics that can fuel the initial fire and may help spread it. Some but not all plastic appliance housings include fire retardants and will resist modest internal fire exposure.

When the fire investigator is faced with reconstructing a fire, these considerations of fuel type are critical. The materials that make up the bulk of the fuels involved in most structure fires have changed dramatically over the past 30 or 40 years, affecting the way in which fires ignite and spread, the combustion products they create, the HRRs and temperatures they produce, and the residues they leave behind.

Post–World War II Finishes and Furnishings

A typical house was finished in the 1940s or 1950s with plaster over wood lath or wire mesh, painted or covered with heavy paper or cloth wallpaper. Floors were bare wood or linoleum with wool carpets and rugs. Window coverings were heavy cotton (brocade) or wool fabrics (or steel-and-wood window blinds). Furniture was often bare wood. When it was upholstered, it was usually with cotton velour, wool mohair, or leather over padding of horsehair or cellulosic (vegetable) fibers (cotton, coir, kapok, Spanish moss, etc.). Latex foam rubber was found in some cushions and pillows, and mattresses were stuffed with cotton or other vegetable fiber, or even feathers. Rooms were usually poorly insulated, and glass windows were single glazed.

Such furnishings were all combustible, but how readily? Most of the materials just listed were susceptible to smoldering ignition sources such as a dropped cigarette, but, with a few exceptions, most would not be readily ignited (to a self-sustaining fire) by a short-lived flame source such as a common match. Ignition of all but latex foam and kapok took many seconds or even minutes of exposure, and all produced large quantities of smoke prior to ignition to flames. Once ignited, they would burn slowly, often reluctantly, producing small flames, preferring to smolder instead. HRRs would be very low (300–400 kW being typical for a cotton sofa), so spread to other fuels would require direct flame contact. See Figure 2-10 for an example. Although the localized flame temperatures would be "normal" [i.e., 800°C to 900°C (1700° to 1800°F)], because the HRRs were so low (and room insulation so poor), overall hot gas layer temperatures would usually remain below the 600°C (1200°F) range.

Progression to flashover would therefore be rare and would take a long time to develop when it did occur. Combustion products included carbon monoxide (CO), soot,

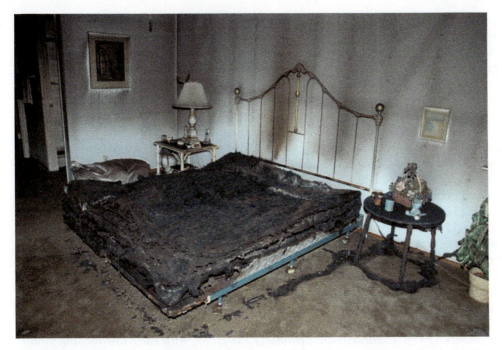

FIGURE 2-10 Traditional cotton mattress burned over a period of hours (unobserved). Heat release rate was never sufficient to ignite nearby combustibles except for tablecloth on nearest table. *Courtesy of Kyle Binkowski, Fire Cause Analysis.*

acrolein (from wood), and hydrogen cyanide (HCN) (from wool). Carpets and floors burned only with reluctance and only after a lot of radiant heat had been applied. Postfire residues of liquid accelerants were relatively easy to identify based on odor and, later, by simple gas chromatography (GC), because the furnishings offered little in the way of interfering pyrolysis products.

Changing Contemporary Finishes and Furnishings

By the 1960s and 1970s, things were changing. Wall coverings tended to be paint or vinyl wallpapers over gypsum wallboard (Sheetrock; drywall), with its better durability under fire exposure. Floor coverings were often wall-to-wall carpet of nylon or polyester face yarns with jute fiber backings over a pad of butyl rubber or mixed fiber. Furnishings were often polyurethane (PU) foam or cotton padding covered by cotton or cotton/synthetic upholstery fabric (or vinyl). Window coverings were cotton or synthetic, or sometimes fiberglass fabrics. After 1972, mattresses were more commonly combinations of a cotton core with a polyurethane foam layer to improve resistance to smoldering sources (cigarettes). Thermal insulation in rooms became more common, and double glazing appeared.

As a result, fire behavior began to change. Synthetic fabrics and PU foam added smolder resistance to furnishings but made them more susceptible to ignition by short-lived open-flame sources. Fires became hotter, and HRRs increased as more synthetics became involved. Fire growth was more rapid in this new style of furniture, and rooms could approach flashover more readily and in a shorter period of time. Numerous researchers have confirmed these results (Krasny, Parker, and Babrauskas 2001).

Carpets, however, and many other furnishings resisted ignition even by radiant heating. When carpets did ignite, the face yarns tended to burn off, but the heavy jute backings would burn slowly and remain in place to protect the rubber pad beneath. Vinyl products could resist ignition and slow the progress of the fire, but when they finally became involved, could contribute hydrogen chloride (HCl) vapors to the fire gases. Gas chromatography could discriminate flammable liquid residues from all the pyrolysis patterns, thanks to improved chromatography, because the peak patterns produced by these pyrolysis products were easily distinguished from the patterns from common flammable liquids (DeHaan and Bonarius 1988).

By the late 1980s, floor coverings still consisted of various synthetic face yarns, but the backing came to be made of polypropylene due to its lower cost and better resistance to odors and mildew. Polyurethane foam carpet padding (new or rebond) completely replaced latex rubber or fiber padding. Under severe radiant heating, face yarns could melt and even ignite, as could the backing, exposing the combustible PU foam underlay beneath. Such carpets would tend to resist localized flame and heat sources, but once alight could burn more completely than before and create much more heat and floor-level damage than ever before. Combustion products now included a wide range of aldehydes, ketones, and toxic intermediates known as free radicals.

Furnishings became made almost exclusively of polyurethane foam padding (rarely with flame retardants) with synthetic covering—very difficult to ignite with a smoldering cigarette, but readily ignited by even a small flame. Once furnishings were ignited, flames could spread quickly and engulf all of a large chair or sofa in flames in less than five minutes (Albers 1999). Thermoplastic upholstery materials, with their low melting points, melt as they burn, producing molten, burning droplets of materials that fall to the base of the furniture and institute rapidly growing vertical-face fires on the sides of the furniture, as well as drop-down damage to floors and carpets beneath (see Figure 2-8). Ignition of a modern mattress and comforter is shown in Figures 2-11 and 2-12.

Calorimetry tests have revealed that modern queen-size mattresses are capable of producing a HRR of more than 3 MW (Nurbakhsh 2006). Since 2007, all mattresses and futons sold in the United States (even for residential use) are required to pass a stringent ignition test, *16 CFR 1633*. This test involves exposing the side of the mattress to a sustained 18 kW gas burner flame and mandates the maximum HRR and total heat released after removal of the burner (CPSC 2006). This requirement will significantly

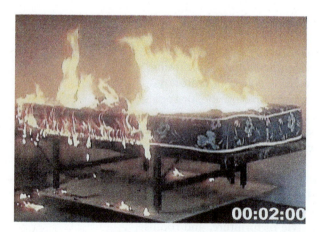

FIGURE 2-11 Open-flame ignition by small gas burner causes rapidly growing fire on (a) common polyurethane mattress set. *Courtesy of Bureau of Electronics & Appliance Repair, Home Furnishings.*

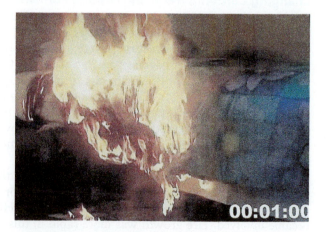

FIGURE 2-12 Polyester/cotton comforter. (Ignition with a match flame would add less than one minute to these development times.) *Courtesy of Bureau of Electronics & Appliance Repair, Home Furnishings.*

reduce the ignitability and size of any resulting fire originating from new mattresses. Sadly, this standard does not apply to foam mattress toppers or other bedding, and imported mattresses with forged approval labels have already been seen in the marketplace.

Except for "high-end" mattresses, for which latex foams are being offered once again (due to their better breathability and reduced moisture buildup), polyurethane foams are nearly universal in mattresses and furniture cushions. Such PU foams are very resistant to smolder ignition but are still easily ignited with a match. The acquisition of comparison samples of upholstery fabrics, padding (fillers), and floor coverings has become more important to the fire investigator than previously.

New regulations for mattresses do not imply a similar improvement for upholstered furniture. The Consumer Product Safety Commission has recently proposed new regulations for upholstered furniture flammability, but these would do little more than enforce existing voluntary industry efforts to make furniture cigarette-resistant. Flaming-ignition behavior would not be regulated. Flaming-ignition behavior has been regulated in California for more than three decades by the California Bureau of Home Furnishings. However, these regulations have not resulted in consumer furniture that is difficult to ignite from flames, nor furniture with improved HRR characteristics. It is apparent, however, that the simple inclusion of a barrier layer of PVC, aluminized fabric, wool, or even fiberglass can dramatically improve all types of fire resistance at a very modest increase in cost (Holleyhead 1999).

Polypropylene carpets will pass the methenamine tablet test (originally *DOC FF 1-70*, now known as *16 CFR 1630*) (meaning that a dropped match or similar flame of ~50W HRR will not ignite the carpet to a self-sustaining fire) and are therefore legal for use in residences. Unfortunately, exposure to a slightly larger fire (such as a burning crumpled sheet of paper) with its higher heat flux can initiate a self-sustaining fire that spreads at about 1 m^2/hr (10 ft^2/hr) with very small flames of 5 to 8 cm (2 to 3 in.) in height along the margins (i.e., a very low HRR) (DeHaan and Nurbakhsh 1999). If the fire starts in an unoccupied building, it can burn for hours, consuming entire rooms of carpet without running out of oxygen, due to its very low rate of combustion. In addition, because of its low critical incident heat flux, polypropylene carpet is more readily ignitable by radiant heat even at some distance away from a large fire (such as a chair fire). As the face yarn burns, the polypropylene backing melts and shrinks (as shown in Figure 2-13), exposing the combustible PU foam underlay, which can now ignite and sustain the spread of fire through and across the carpet. The rate of spread is dependent on the interaction between the carpet and the pad and can be affected by such variables as whether the carpet is stretched tightly and securely fastened or is lying loosely atop the pad with plenty of air between the two.

Urethane foam carpet pads (particularly rebond) and all-synthetic carpets produced complex "stews" of pyrolysis products that can sometimes be quite difficult to distinguish from some non-distillate-type petroleum products. Comparison samples of unburned carpet and pad are very important evidence.

Today's furniture is markedly improved in its resistance to the most common type of accidental ignition, e.g., a dropped cigarette or other forms of glowing sources (electric heaters, glowing electrical connections, etc.), but the significant disadvantage is little or no resistance to flaming sources. Once alight, furnishings can be completely involved in 3 to 5 minutes and be reduced to a charred frame in 10 minutes while producing high temperatures in excess of 1000°C (2000°F) in the flame plume and enormous HRRs (2 to 3 MW is common for a sofa or recliner today) (Krasny, Parker, and Babrauskas 2001). Such performance virtually ensures that the average-size furnished room with an open door will be completely engulfed in a post-flashover fire within 3 to 10 minutes of first established flame. The intensity of these fires can obliterate traces of ignition sources,

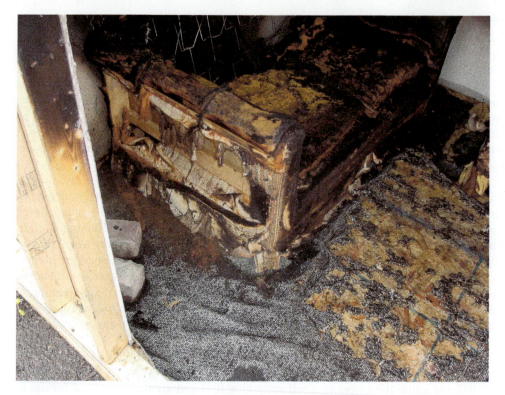

FIGURE 2-13 Synthetic carpet melted by radiant heat from chair fire. *Courtesy of David J. Icove, University of Tennessee.*

obscure fire patterns (if sustained for more than 5 minutes), induce the speed of spread and kind of damage once thought possible only for accelerated fires, and make the recovery and identification of possible accelerant traces very difficult. Gas chromatography/ mass spectrometry is now needed to discriminate possible accelerant traces from pyrolysis products. Further changes for the future include **flame resistant** performance standards for bed covers and household furnishings. As these products appear, fire growth will be affected.

The best the investigator can do is to be aware of the contributions furnishings can make to the ignition and growth of a fire and to take whatever steps necessary to document the kind of furnishings present (new or old? cellulosic or synthetic fabrics and padding?) and, especially, to collect comparison samples of carpet, pad, upholstery, and padding whenever possible for later identification in the forensic lab (even partially burned samples are better than no samples at all). This may be the only way to accurately reconstruct the train of events of a fire.

Paint

The newer water-based paints are generally emulsions of latex, polyvinyl acetate, or acrylics in water when applied and form a plastic-like polymer coating when they dry. Their properties are similar to the plastics on which they are based. Varnishes, shellacs, and lacquers tend to be more combustible, since they are often based on naturally occurring resins or on combustible plastic polymer equivalents.

Historically, paint consisted of a drying oil (such as linseed or tung oil) in which mineral-based pigments were suspended. The mixture was then thinned using turpentine or a petroleum distillate. The thinner evaporates shortly after application, and plays an important part in the flammability of the paint only while it is still wet. The drying oils

flame resistant ■
Materials that are inherently nonflammable. These materials have flame resistance built into their chemical structures.

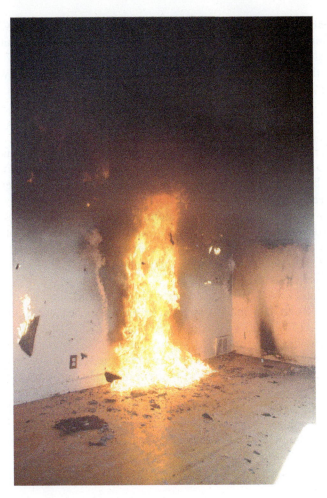

FIGURE 2-14 Test fire of gasoline and diesel caused ignition of paint on walls, which peeled off and fell as flaming sheets. *Courtesy of Jamie Novak, Novak Investigations and St. Paul Fire Dept.*

and other resins present are combustible even after the paint has dried and constitute the major fuel contribution of many paints.

The mineral powders once used universally as pigments were not combustible and so tended to retard the combustion of the paint itself. This is no longer the case. The cost and environmental hazards posed by most inorganic pigments have caused them to be replaced in large part by cheaper organic dyes and fillers, which will burn.

Most paints and coatings will add slightly to the fuel present in a structure and can aid the spread of flames from one part of a room to another. In some cases the paint layers have been seen to soften and peel off the wall or ceiling as they ignite and thus aid the spread of fire, as pictured in Figure 2-14. This is especially true if there are many layers of paint. Then, even noncombustible surfaces of painted steel or gypsum board can contribute to the fire's spread.

There are also numerous coatings intended to protect the substrate from fire effects. These coatings, called **intumescents**, swell and bubble when heated, providing a noncombustible layer of thermal insulation that slows the incursion of heat into the substrate (Jackson 1998). Intumescents are widely used to protect steel structural members as well as combustible surfaces.

Whether a paint or other coating will aid or retard the flames of a small, growing fire cannot be generalized without testing the specific product. The professional investigator must consider the contribution of layers of paint to the fuel load of an ordinary structure.

intumescent coating ▪ A coating used to increase the fire endurance of structural steel or other materials. These coatings appear as paints during normal conditions, but when heated intumesce, or swell, forming an insulation around the steel (NFPA 2017d, pt. 7.5.1.4).

Tests by McGraw and Mowrer revealed that at applied heat fluxes of 50 kW/m², multiple layers of latex paint on gypsum wallboard did not support flame spread but doubled the HRR (from paper alone) to ~111 kW/m² (of wall area). At heat fluxes of 75 kW/m², fire spread was modestly accelerated, and the HRR rose to 134 kW/m² (of wall area) (McGraw and Mowrer 1999).

2.9.7 METALS

Metals, as fuels, are so rarely of importance that they may be overlooked. Actually, most metals can be burned, and many metals, when finely divided, are susceptible to combustion in air. Others can burn when they are in relatively massive form, but generally only in a very hot environment. Some metals are pyrophoric, meaning they can burn spontaneously in air when finely divided. A metal like uranium, for example, is extremely hazardous when finely divided because of its tendency to oxidize in air. The heat of the slow spontaneous oxidation may be sufficient to ignite a larger quantity of stored uranium powder. Iron powder is, to a considerable extent, pyrophoric, although without the special hazard that characterizes some other metals.

Iron in the form of steel wool or fine powder will burn readily and requires only a modest ignition source, such as a match, sparks, or electrical heating. Ignition temperatures are as low as 315°C (600°F) (for powder) and 377°C (710°F) (for fine steel wool). Very fine iron powder is pyrophoric (Babrauskas 2003). The important qualification of the dangers associated with metal combustion is the state of subdivision. The finer the metal powder, the more likely it is to ignite, but rarely without supplemental ignition.

The danger associated with the burning of metals is confined almost exclusively to industrial plants, especially those in which the metals are handled in a finely divided state. Chemical laboratories or manufacturing facilities may contain enough reactive metals like sodium, potassium, or phosphorus to cause special fire hazards.

Magnesium

Magnesium is not readily ignited unless it is finely divided—in the form of ribbons, chips, shavings, filings, or dust. In a large fire, massive magnesium castings, such as wheels and aircraft components, can burn producing an intense hot fire. When water is sprayed on hot magnesium and some other metals, large quantities of hydrogen gas can be generated, which can explode or increase the fire intensity.

In a fire where large magnesium pieces have burned, it is likely that the magnesium was ignited by a strong surrounding fire. The reported ignition temperature of magnesium ranges from 520°C (968°F) (powder) to 623°C (1153°F) (solid). Magnesium/aluminum alloys with more than 10 percent magnesium have ignition temperatures in the 500°C to 600°C (930°F to 1112°F) range (Babrauskas 2003).

Aluminum

Aluminum is more difficult to ignite than magnesium because of its tendency to form a fine adherent film of oxide on the surface. In structural fires, it is common to find much aluminum that has melted but not burned. Under special test conditions, ignition temperatures have been measured from 1500°C to 1750°C (2822°F to 3182°F) (Babrauskas 2003). Residential fires typically are hot enough to exceed the melting point of aluminum (660°C; 1220°F). This temperature can be reached in the hot gas layer during fire growth, directly in a flame plume, and even at floor level during post-flashover fire conditions. Thin aluminum roofing or sheathing may oxidize to white aluminum oxide ash in commercial structures or mobile homes where aluminum sheathing is common.

2.9.8 COAL

Coal ranks high as a fuel widely used in industrial power production and general heating purposes. Although there is progressively less use of coal for heating structures than in the past, it is of increasing industrial importance as a fuel because of new low-pollution combustion techniques. Both the mining and storage of coal are hazardous due to the combustibility of coal. For example, under proper conditions, both stored and unmined coal is subject to self-heating to the point of spontaneous ignition (Hodges 1963). Large masses of coal and long time frames are typically needed, as well as both oxygen and moisture, to initiate and sustain self-heating (Babrauskas 2003). The dimensions of piles of coal are critical to self-heating, with deep piles more susceptible (Babrauskas 2003).

Coal is highly carbonaceous, being an organic fuel made up of approximately 80 to 90 percent carbon, 4 to 5 percent hydrogen, and 12 percent oxygen, nitrogen, sulfur, and other elements in (usually) trace quantities. The presence of these other elements suggests that coal contains a variety of compounds that can undergo pyrolysis. Coal differs from most other organic fuels in that the proportion of such pyrolyzable fuels is relatively small. The more readily pyrolyzable compounds that are present in a fuel, generally the easier it is to ignite. Coal requires considerable input of heat from an ignition source to initiate a self-sustaining, flaming combustion (in a bulk solid) because of the small quantities of pyrolyzable compounds. Coke is made by heating coal in the absence of oxygen to drive off light fractions and impurities to increase its heat content.

Explosions involving coal dust can occur in mines and in coal-handling equipment (such as conveyors) in mines, power plants, and railroad facilities. Smaller quantities and dry conditions are involved in such explosions. Reported autoignition temperatures range from 200°C to 600°C (400°F to 1120°F) depending on grade (lignite being the lowest) (Babrauskas 2003).

2.9.9 COMBUSTION OF SOLID FUELS

Flame Color

The color of the flame, especially in the very early stages of a fire, can be significant but rarely remembered or recorded with accuracy. It may be captured in videos or photos of the fire. In most fires the flame color is not likely to have great significance because most structural, as well as outdoor, fires involve only cellulosic material such as wood and some other organic construction materials such as asphalt, paint, and similar supplemental substances. For these materials, the flame will be more or less yellow or orange in color, and only the amount and color of smoke given off will be related to the character of the fuel and the adequacy of the oxygen supply. Flame color, when not complicated by special elements that produce unusual colors, is related to the flame temperature, which is, in turn, generally related to the oxygen admixture with the fuel. Thus, the color of the flame is indicative of burning conditions as well as of the actual temperature of the flame.

However, unusual colors of flame are sometimes seen in fires and require consideration. For example, the simpler alcohols burn with a relatively blue or purple flame. If such a flame was observed *immediately after the fire started,* it could well indicate the use of this type of material as an accelerant. It would also rule out hydrocarbon accelerants, which burn with a yellow flame. Natural gas (if not premixed), like liquid hydrocarbons, generally burns with a yellowish flame, tending to be blue in the periphery. If adequate air is mixed with it, as is done in a heating burner, the flame is colorless to blue. Hydrocarbon gases or vapors properly mixed with air burn with blue flames. Without the proper air mixture, they become yellow and smoky due to incomplete combustion.

One gas that is of special interest relative to flame color is carbon monoxide, which is extremely flammable. Most of it is produced by oxygen-deficient flames in which the combustion is not complete, and the gas escapes before it is consumed by further oxidation. CO also burns with a blue flame. In a confined space, if the amount of carbonaceous fuel involved greatly exceeds the amount of air available to combine with it, there will be strong generation of CO. The CO may escape to a region richer in oxygen, where it may be reignited and ring the primary fire with blue flames. This situation will provide insight into the combustion of excess fuel with limited air in the initial fire area.

Kirk reported that the most intense part of a large hotel fire was in a subbasement fed by hydrocarbons. Firefighters noted blue flames coming from a sidewalk entrance to the basement while black smoke was emerging elsewhere. The blue flames were at a significant distance from the subbasement, and there was as yet little fire in the intervening space. The reasons for the existence of the bluish flame were not immediately perceived, and the only explanation that fit the facts was a secondary burning of CO produced in the basement fire because of limited ventilation (Kirk 1969).

Other special flame colors may also be significant. Colored flames have long been generated for pyrotechnical purposes by adding certain metallic salts that produce spectral colors at flame temperature. Traces of sodium, present in most fuel, yield a yellow flame, making it difficult to distinguish from the yellow produced in flames by glowing carbon particles. Strontium salts give the bright red color used in many flares and decorative flame and explosion effects. Copper halides impart an intense green color to the flame, potassium salts give violet, and barium salts a yellowish green. Brilliant white flames will accompany the burning of magnesium/alloy components (as previously shown in Figure 2-14). Many other variations of color will be characteristic either of the elements or of certain of their compounds (Conkling 1985).

Unusual colors of flame will occasionally be significant in investigation of fires. For instance, if there is an intense fire in the interior of a motor vehicle, this fire might be due to various types of fuel material and ignition sources, one of which could have been road flares. If a brilliant red color was noted in the early part of the fire, this information could assist in locating the early fuel as flares. Yellow flames could indicate more conventional fuels such as synthetic upholstery. The investigator who is aware of the potential value of flame color in the interpretation of fire will be alert for any color that is unusual or not explainable in the most obvious hypothesis, and this awareness could lead to more accurate appraisal of the cause and sequence of many fires. The firefighters who were first on the scene should be interviewed to determine any unusual flame conditions on their arrival.

Smoke Production

Observation of smoke may be helpful in obtaining an indication of the type of the fuel. Smoke color, especially colors other than the neutral white, gray, or black, may give indications of special types of fuel being combusted if they are present in large amounts. Smoke that has an unusual hue, such as red-brown or yellow, may indicate the presence of materials other than conventional building materials and furnishings.

When complete combustion occurs, most materials produce little or no visible smoke. Under these ideal conditions, all carbon is burned to carbon dioxide, a colorless gas.

Incomplete combustion of carbon leads to carbon monoxide, also colorless and odorless but having very toxic properties. Incomplete combustion of carbonaceous materials also produces various highly carbonaceous compounds that are opaque, such as soot, which is largely carbon.

Hydrogen, present in all organic materials, burns to water vapor, a major constituent of all combustion gases. It does not contribute to the smoke characteristics, although it may at times be recognized as steam. Other elements often present in organic materials, such as nitrogen, sulfur, and halogens, contribute gases to the combustion products. However, only under very special conditions do these alter the color of the smoke. They may contribute strongly to its odor when present in larger-than-ordinary amounts. Such effects may be encountered in industrial fires but rarely in residential ones.

The color of smoke is almost entirely determined by the character and type of fuel and the availability of oxygen for complete combustion. Most materials, including all hydrocarbons, will never burn completely even in the presence of excess air, without premixing of the fuel with air. This is true of natural gas when burning in large volumes.

As the hydrocarbon molecules become larger, such as those in petroleum oils, more air is required, and it becomes more difficult to completely mix the fuel with air. Thus, in an ordinary fire, materials such as petroleum distillates tend to produce a large quantity of dense black smoke. Therefore, the presence of much black smoke *may* indicate the burning of a highly carbonaceous material like the petroleum products sometimes used as accelerants. Dense black smoke, however, is usually more indicative of the amount of ventilation and the stage of development at which the fire is burning. For example, fire burning in a restricted space without adequate and complete ventilation will always form more smoke and darker smoke than when the same fire is well ventilated.

The early stages of a developing structure fire may be dominated by the incomplete combustion and partial pyrolysis of fuels present. These products of incomplete combustion are often characterized by dense clouds of dark smoke that form until flashover occurs, windows break, and the flammable vapors freely combust. At this point, the smoke becomes a lighter color and less opaque, sometimes almost transparent. If the initial fuel is cellulosic, the smoke will be light colored from the outset due to the release of water vapor and absence of soot.

Oxygenated organic materials, such as cellulosics, burning freely in the presence of air often produce little or no colored smoke. Alcohols, for example, are in this category. If used as accelerants, they will not be detected by observing the smoke. The same is true of wood and most cellulosic building materials that produce either a white or light gray smoke, except when the supply of air is greatly restricted. Even under these circumstances, they will not produce the heavy black smoke that follows the burning of heavier hydrocarbons. Asphalt-like materials, also common in building construction, and materials such as tar paper, some paints, sponge rubber upholstery, adhesives, sealing compounds, and most floor coverings will generally produce a black smoke. These are more likely to burn late in a fire, so that the production of heavy black smoke late in a fire is not ordinarily an indication of the use of accelerant. Many plastics, especially polystyrenes and polyurethane, produce thick black smoke when burned in large quantities in air.

The optical density of smoke produced during oxygen-depletion calorimetry is measured by a standardized light-path method in the exhaust duct. The value obtained can be used to predict the visibility factors that affect tenability and escape paths for people in the fire room. Once again, if comparison samples of suspected fuels are available, tests can be conducted to assess their contributions.

2.10 Liquid and Gaseous Fuels

Combustion properties have different significance, or at times perhaps no significance, when applied to various types of fuel. Thus, the concept of flash point is essential information when studying liquids, is rarely ever used for solids, and would have no meaning if applied to gases. The relationship between the type of fuel and the type of property is clarified later.

2.10.1 PHYSICAL PROPERTIES OF FUELS

Vapors from liquids are the materials that directly support the flame over a liquid fuel. For the liquid/vapor combination, vapor pressure, flash point, and, to a lesser degree, boiling point are all important considerations. Ignition temperature, range of flammable concentrations of vapor/air mixtures, and vapor densities are critical properties of the vapors themselves. Liquids themselves do not undergo combustion, except in exotic cases; instead, it is the vapors emanating from liquids that can ignite and burn as flames.

Physical properties of fuels of particular interest to the fire investigator include vapor pressure, flammability or explosive limits, flash point, flame point/fire point, ignition temperature, ignition energy, boiling points, vapor density, and heat of combustion.

Vapor Pressure

Any liquid exposed to air will evaporate as molecules escape its surface. If this process occurs in a sealed system, an equilibrium state will be reached in which the vapor reaches saturation, and there is no further evaporation. The partial atmospheric pressure exerted by the vapor at this stage is called the saturated vapor pressure, most often measured in millimeters of mercury (mmHg) (atmospheric pressure is 760 mmHg) or kilopascals (kPa), where 1 atmosphere (atm) is 101.32 kPa. The vapor pressure is a direct measure of the volatility of a liquid and is determined by its molecular weight, its chemical structure, and the temperature (see Figure 2-15). The higher the temperature, the more liquid will evaporate and the higher the vapor pressure. Table 2-2 displays several pressure equivalents.

As seen in Figure 2-16, the relationship between temperature and vapor pressure is not linear but is a logarithmic function with controlling constants that are different for each liquid. For a given class of compound (alkane, alcohol, branched alkane), the lower the molecular weight, the higher the vapor pressure. Because the vapor pressure of an aromatic or a normal alkane is lower than that of a branched alkane of the same molecular weight at the same temperature, a branched (iso) alkane will have a lower **flash point** than an alkane of the same molecular weight. For example, benzene (molecular weight 78): flash point, −11°C; hexane (MW = 82): flash point, −22°C; isohexane (MW = 82): flash point, −29°C.

Vapor pressure is a fundamental physical property that has a great influence on the flammability of liquid fuel. When the vapor pressure of a liquid reaches 760 mmHg, the

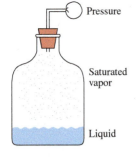

Pressure

Saturated vapor

Liquid

FIGURE 2-15 Vapor pressure is the pressure created by a liquid (or solid) evaporating to saturation in a sealed vessel.

flash point ■ The lowest temperature of a liquid, as determined by specific laboratory tests, at which the liquid gives off vapors at a sufficient rate to support a momentary flame across its surface (NFPA 2017d, pt. 3.3.88).

TABLE 2-2	Pressure Equivalents				
kPa	**mmHg**	**psi**	**atm**	**Bar**	**in. w.c.**
689.2	5170	100	6.80	7	—
101.32	760	14.7	1	1.013 (1013 mbar)	406.7
6.89	51.7	1	0.068	0.07 (70 mbar)	27.67
0.69	5.2	0.1	0.007	0.007 (7 mbar)	2.77

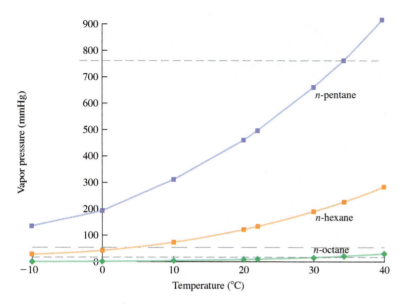

FIGURE 2-16 Calculated saturation vapor pressure (in mmHg) as a function of temperature (°C) for three common hydrocarbons: *n*-pentane, *n*-hexane, and *n*-octane. Upper dashed line is atmospheric pressure (760 mmHg). Middle (long-dashed) line corresponds to the upper explosive limit (UEL) (8 percent in air, 61 mmHg) for *n*-alkanes. The lowest dashed line corresponds to the lower explosive limit. Note that at all temperatures above 5°C, pentane and hexane are above their UEL at saturation.

liquid is at its boiling point and is recorded as its boiling temperature. When the temperature of a liquid fuel is such that its vapor pressure reaches the percentage of 760 mmHg that is equivalent to the lower flammability limit of the fuel, the fuel is said to be at its flash point, as discussed later in this section.

The vapor pressure is also dependent on the contour of the surface of the liquid, being higher for a convex surface than for a flat surface at the same temperature. This partly explains why an aerosol of small droplets or a liquid distributed on the fibers of a porous wick is often easier to ignite than a pool of the same liquid. Also playing a critical role in such ignitions is that the larger total surface area and small size of the aerosol droplets allows them to absorb heat more quickly from their surroundings. A thin film of liquid on a fiber of a wick can absorb heat very quickly from applied heat flux as well as from the surrounding air and supporting fiber. The increased temperature causes it to evaporate more quickly. Being a thin film, it has no bulk liquid to cool it by convective heat transfer. The capillary action of the porous wick quickly replaces the evaporated fuel to sustain the evaporation or combustion.

Flammability (Explosive) Limits

Mixtures of flammable gases or vapors with air will combust only when they are within particular ranges of concentration. When a gas is present at a concentration below its lower explosive limit (LEL, or lower flammability limit—LFL), it is considered too lean a mixture to burn and cannot be ignited. At concentrations above its upper explosive limit (UEL), the fuel/air mixture is too rich to burn and will not ignite. The explosive range between these two limits is illustrated in Figure 2-17 and Tables 2-3 and 2-4. Some materials, such as hydrogen, carbon monoxide, and carbon disulfide, have very wide ranges within which flame will propagate to create an explosion. However, most fuels, such as petroleum distillate hydrocarbons, have quite narrow explosive ranges. Fuel/air mixtures are often considered to be in either closed or open systems, as discussed next.

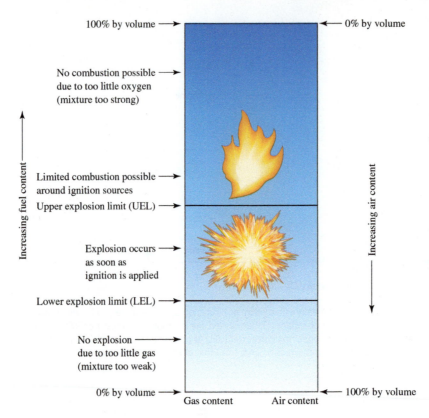

FIGURE 2-17 Schematic of flammable gas/air mixtures above and below explosion limits. *Based on Brannigan, F. L., R. G. Bright, and N. H. Jason, eds.* Fire Investigation Handbook. *NBS Handbook 134. Washington, DC: US Government Printing Office, 1980, p. 139.*

TABLE 2-3	Flammability (Explosive) Limits and Ignition Temperatures of Common Gases				
	EXPLOSIVE LIMITS (IN AIR)		**IGNITION TEMPERATURE (MINIMUM)**		**MINIMUM IGNITION ENERGY**
Fuel	**Lower**	**Upper**	**°C**	**°F**	**mJ**
Natural gas	4.5	15	482–632	900–1,170	0.25
Propane (commercial)	2.15	9.6	493–604	920–1,120	0.25
Butane (commercial)	1.9	8.5	482–538	900–1,000	0.25
Acetylene	2.5	81[a]	305	581	0.02
Hydrogen	4	75	500	932	0.01
Ammonia (NH_3)	16	25	651	1,204	—
Carbon monoxide	12.5	74	609	1,128	—
Ethylene	2.7	36	490	914	0.07
Ethylene oxide	3	100	429	8041	0.06

Sources: NFPA. 2003. *Fire Protection Handbook.* 19th ed. Quincy, MA: National Fire Protection Association, Table 8-9.2; and SFPE. 2008. *SFPE Handbook of Fire Protection Engineering.* 4th ed. Quincy, MA: Society of Fire Protection Engineers and the National Fire Protection Association, Table 3-18.1.
[a]Higher concentrations (up to 100) may detonate.

TABLE 2-4	Flash Points and Flame (Fire) Points of Some Ignitable Liquids					
	FLASH POINT (CLOSED CUP)*		**FLASH POINT (OPEN CUP)**		**FIRE POINT**	
FUEL	°C	°F	°C	°F	°C	°F
Gasoline (auto, low octane)	−43	−45	—	—	—	—
Gasoline (100 octane)	−38	−38				
Petroleum naphtha[a]	−29	−20				
JP-4 (jet aviation fuel)	−23 to −1	−10 to −30				
Acetone	−20	−4				
Petroleum ether	<−18	<0				
Benzene	−11	−12				
Toluene	4	40				
Methanol	11	52	1(13.5)[†]	34(56)	1(13.5)	34(56)
Ethanol	12	54				
n-Octane	13	56				
Turpentine (gum)	35	95				
Fuel oil (kerosene)	38[b]	100				
Mineral spirits	40	104				
n-Decane	46	115	52[†]	125	61.5[†]	143
Fuel oil #2 (diesel)	52 (min.)	126				
Fuel oil (unspecified)	—	—	133[a]	271	164[a]	327
Jet A	43–66	110–150				
p-Xylene	25[§]	77[§]	29[§]	84[§]	—	—
JP-5 (Jet aviation fuel)	66	151				

Sources: *NFPA. 2001. *Fire Protection Guide to Hazardous Materials.* Quincy, MA: National Fire Protection Association, except as noted.

[†]Calculated minimum limit for open-cup tests with flame igniter. Higher values in parentheses are for spark source ignition. *Source:* Glassman, I., and Dryer, F. L. 1980–1981. "Flame Spreading across Liquid Fuels." *Fire Safety Journal* 3: 123–38.

[‡]SFPE. 2008. *SFPE Handbook of Fire Protection Engineering.* 4th ed. Quincy, MA: NFPA, Table 2-8.5.

[§]www.ScienceLab.com, MSDS *p*-xylene, 2008.

[a]Generic name for miscellaneous light petroleum fractions used in such consumer products as cigarette lighter fuels and fuels for camping stoves and lanterns.

[b]The flash point of kerosene is set by law in many jurisdictions and may be higher in compliance with local laws.

Closed Systems

Within a closed system, if the mixture will not explode, it will not ignite. For this reason, the explosive range and flammability range of a gas or vapor may be thought of as one and the same. The explosive ranges and vapor pressures of possible fuels at a fire scene must be carefully considered, for they can play a significant part in determining accidental or incendiary origin and in ruling out some hypothetical situations. As can be seen from Figure 2-18, flammability limits are temperature dependent: the higher the initial temperature, the wider the range. Technically, the explosive limits and flammability limits are determined under different conditions—constant pressure versus constant volume—and are therefore very nearly the same.

Open Systems

In an open system, other variables control the ignitability of the fuel/air mixture. If a mixture of vapor and air is initially too lean for an explosion, efforts to ignite it may raise the

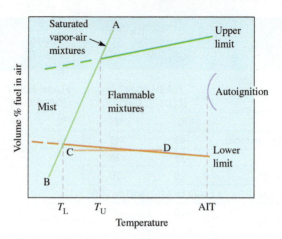

FIGURE 2-18 The flammability limits of a vapor/air mixture as a function of initial temperature at a constant pressure, showing the higher the temperature, the wider the explosion range. *From Zabetakis, M. G. 1965. "Flammability Characteristics of Combustible Gases and Vapors." US Bureau of Mines, US Government printing Office, 3.*

temperature and increase the amount of material volatilized sufficiently to cause ignition. More important, probably, is the too-rich mixture that will not ignite. The application of a brief arc will not be expected to cause a fire; however, prolonged application of a flame may add so much additional heat that the flammability limit is affected or may produce so much turbulence as to mix in additional air and thus start a fire. Because of the initial overly rich mixture, this resultant fire is expected to develop into what is known as a rolling fire of some intensity. It is important to understand that the reason fire is ignited in both cases is that the system was altered by introduction of heat from the ignition source.

Such an alteration is not possible in a closed system and will not be effective in producing a fire any more than in producing an explosion. Thus, on a warm day, when the gasoline/air mixture inside a tank of gasoline is richer in gasoline vapor than the upper explosive limit, an arc could safely be produced inside the tank with no ignition. At *very* low temperatures, when fewer vapors are produced and therefore may form a mixture with the air that is within the explosive range, an explosion may result (see Table 2-3).

Vapor pressure considerations play a critical role in evaluating incidents where the flame external to a partially full container of flammable liquid is thought to have caused the vapor inside the container to explode by combustion. As we saw in Figure 2-16, the vapor pressure of pentane (the major, most volatile liquid component in automotive gasoline) is, at saturation, well above its UEL (8 percent) for any reasonable temperature (above −20°C; −4°F) (Drysdale 1999). This means that if there is a significant quantity of liquid in the container and a reasonable time has elapsed, the concentration of vapors inside the container will be far too rich to support combustion. A flame can be sustained at the mouth of the vessel if there is enough vapor emanating to mix with the surrounding air, but no explosion will occur. Heating of a closed vessel containing liquid can cause a mechanical explosion if the heating is sufficient to create a vapor pressure that exceeds the mechanical strength of the vessel.

To test the theoretical (calculated) concept, Novak and DeHaan in cooperation with the New Zealand Police Service conducted empirical testing of plastic fuel containers filled with gasoline (DeHaan 2004). In each case, gasoline vapors emanating from the filler spout were ignited readily. There was no explosion, but there was a small clear flame about 12 cm (5 in.) high in each test, as shown in Figure 2-19A. As the plastic container melted, the opening increased in area (Figures 2-19A and B), and heat was absorbed by the gasoline (sometimes to boiling). The flame plume got larger, but there was no propagation into the can to cause an explosion. Eventually, the entire top of the can melted or burned away, exposing the entire horizontal surface of the gasoline, as seen in Figures 2-19D and E. Figure 2-19F shows where the underside of melted containers bear the molded information. When cutting the container open, it can show pockets that often trap residual liquid fuel, as shown in Figure 2-19G. Figure 2-19 illustrates an ignition test of 3.8 L (1 gal) plastic container filled with gasoline, with open filler spout.

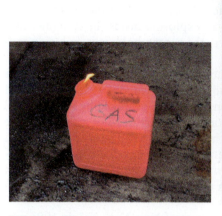

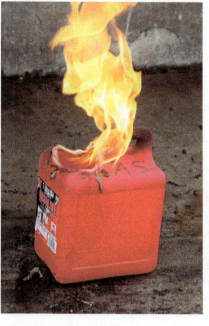

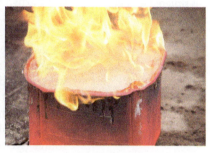

FIGURE 2-19A Vapors of one gallon of gasoline in a plastic container ignited at open spout. *Courtesy of Jamie Novak, Novak Investigations and St. Paul Fire Dept.*

FIGURE 2-19B Burning vapors at 10 minutes. *Courtesy of Jamie Novak, Novak Investigations and St. Paul Fire Dept.*

FIGURE 2-19C Gasoline boiling as vapors burn at 20 minutes. *Courtesy of Jamie Novak, Novak Investigations and St. Paul Fire Dept.*

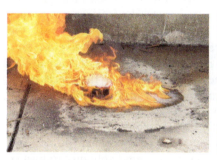

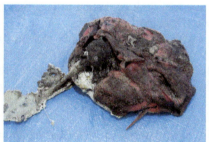

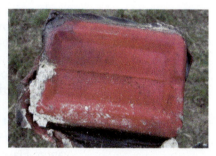

FIGURE 2-19D Melted remains of plastic can with burning gasoline. *Courtesy of Jamie Novak, Novak Investigations and St. Paul Fire Dept.*

FIGURE 2-19E Melted gasoline container after fire (top). *Courtesy of Jamie Novak, Novak Investigations and St. Paul Fire Dept.*

FIGURE 2-19F Underside of melted container bears molded information. *Courtesy of Jamie Novak, Novak Investigations and St. Paul Fire Dept.*

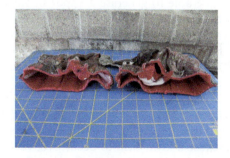

FIGURE 2-19G Container cut open showing pockets that often trap residual liquid fuel. *Courtesy of Jamie Novak, Novak Investigations and St. Paul Fire Dept.*

FIGURE 2-19 Ignition test of 3.8 L (1 gal) plastic container filled with gasoline, with open filler spout.

For liquid fuels with lower vapor pressures, propagation or ignition can occur within a fuel container. This is a problem with ethanol-based motor fuels, where ignition inside fuel storage tanks is possible at normal temperatures (Gardiner, Barden, and Pucher 2008). Guidry reported an incident in which denatured (ethyl) alcohol (whose vapor pressure curve is much lower than that of pentane and has a much broader explosive range) caused an explosion within a container (Guidry 2005). Under the **ambient temperature** and use conditions, an ignitable vapor concentration existed inside the container. When a flame ignited the stream of liquid pouring from the container, the flame propagated into the container. This caused an explosion inside the container that split the container and spewed burning alcohol over the person holding it, inducing serious burns.

In cases involving home storage of gasoline, burn injuries can occur when the canister is tipped or knocked over, spilling its contents and dispersing vapors within the area of the container. In a case study of 25 burned children less than 6 years old by Kennedy and Knapp, the research showed that in each case vapors from overturned or spilled gasoline were ignited by a pilot light from either a water heater or dryer. The study noted that children at this age are totally unaware of the hazards gasoline introduces into their environment. The study also showed that older children and adults who misuse gasoline as an inhalant, solvent, or fire starter expose themselves to the vapors to a competent ignition source (Kennedy and Knapp 1997).

The tragic explosion of flight TWA 800 off the coast of New York in July 1996 was caused by a very unusual set of conditions when a nearly empty jet fuel tank was heated by ambient summertime conditions and the operation of onboard air conditioners. The fuel was then exposed to a reduced atmospheric pressure as the aircraft gained altitude (increasing the fuel's partial vapor pressure). At 4,000 m (13,000 ft.), an accidental electrical ignition source within the tank ignited the vapors as they reached their LEL. The resulting internal fuel tank explosion caused massive damage to the fuselage and brought the plane down (Dorsheim 1997).

Automotive fuel tank explosions in movies are created by using high explosives. In real life, automotive fuel tanks very rarely explode, but when a tank does, it is usually as a result of a collision that ruptures it and allows all the liquid to drain out; the concentration of vapor in the tank can then fall below the UFL, and the vapor may explode if ignited.

Flash Point

The flash point of a material is the lowest temperature at which it produces a flammable vapor. Flash point can be used to assess the fire hazards of flammable or combustible ignitable liquids. At its flash point temperature, the vapor pressure of the fuel (as a percentage of 760 mmHg) is equal to that fuel's lower limit of flammability. For example, the flash point of *n*-decane is 46°C (115°F). Its vapor pressure at that temperature is 6 mmHg, which is 0.78 percent of 760 mmHg. This value is very close to the measured lower explosive limit of 0.75 percent.

A liquid fuel must be able to generate a vapor in sufficient quantity to reach that lower limit in air before it can burn. This does not mean that the vapor will ignite spontaneously at this temperature but only that it can be ignited by a flame, a small arc, or other local source of heat. For example, the flash point of low-octane automotive gasoline is about −43°C (−45°F). This flash point value means only that gasoline produces a vapor that can be ignited at any temperature above about −43°C, not that gasoline will spontaneously ignite at such an extremely low temperature.

The flash point is determined by placing a small sample of the fuel in the cup of a testing apparatus and heating or cooling it to the lowest temperature at which an arc or small pilot flame will cause a little flash to occur over the surface of the liquid. No fire results from such a test other than the little flash of flame, which immediately extinguishes itself.

Several recognized flash point testers are used today, including the Pensky-Martens, Cleveland, and Tagliabue (Tag) testers. Each device has a particular temperature range and fuel type for which it is most accurate. The Tag closed-cup tester, for example, is the accepted method (described in *ASTM D56-05*) for testing nonviscous liquids with a flash point below 93°C (200°F) (ASTM International 2005). The Pensky-Martens tester (closed-cup) is best suited for liquids with a flash point above 93°C (200°F) and is described in *ASTM D93* (ASTM International 2015a). The open-cup tests are used for evaluating hazards of ignitable liquids where they are encountered in open-air situations—during transportation or spills, for instance. The Tag open-cup method is described in *ASTM D1310-14* (ASTM International 2014), and the Cleveland open-cup method is described in *ASTM D92-12b* (ASTM International 2012). Most tables of flash point data for fire safety purposes list the closed-cup flash point of most materials. As a general rule, the open-cup flash points for the same materials would be a few degrees (<10 percent) higher than the closed-cup values.

The NFPA *Fire Protection Handbook* describes flash point tests used in the industry and contains extensive tables of flash point data for all types of flammable liquids. See Table 2-4 for representative flash points and Table 2-5 for minimum autoignition temperatures, flammable ranges, and specific gravities of some common ignitable liquids.

TABLE 2-5	Minimum Autoignition Temperatures, Flammable Ranges, and Specific Gravities of Some Common Ignitable Liquids				
FUEL	**IGNITION TEMPERATURE (°C)**	**(°F)**	**MINIMUM IGNITION ENERGY (MJ)**	**FLAMMABLE RANGE (% IN AIR @ 20°C)**	**SPECIFIC GRAVITY**
Acetone	465	869	1.15	2.6–12.8	0.8
Benzene	498	928	0.2	1.4–7.1	0.9
Diethyl ether	160	320	—	1.9–36.0	0.7
Ethanol (100 percent)	363	685	—	—	0.8
Ethylene glycol	398	748	—	—	1.1
Fuel oil #1 (kerosene)	210	410	—	—	
Fuel oil #2	257	495	—	—	
Gasoline (low octane)	280	536	—	1.4–7.6	0.8
Gasoline (100 octane)	456	853	—	1.5–7.6	0.8
Jet fuel (JP-6)	230	446	—	—	
Linseed oil (boiled)	206	403	—	—	
Methanol	464	867	0.14	6.7–36.0	0.8
n-Pentane	260	500	0.22	1.5–7.8	0.6
n-Hexane	225	437	0.24	1.2–7.5	0.7
n-Heptane	204	399	0.24	—	0.7
n-Octane	206	403	—	1.0–7.0	0.7
n-Decane	210	410	—	—	0.7
Petroleum ether	288	550	—	1.1–5.9	0.6
Pinene (alpha)	255	491	—	—	
Turpentine (spirits)	253	488	—	—	<1

Sources: Data taken from NFPA. 2001. *Fire Protection Guide to Hazardous Materials.* Quincy, MA: National Fire Protection Association; Turner, C. F., and J. W. McCreery. 1981. *The Chemistry of Fire and Hazardous Materials.* Boston: Allyn and Bacon.

The NFPA (Friedman 1998) classifies ignitable liquids according to their reported flash points:

- Class I: Flashpoint below 38°C (100°F) (**flammable liquids**)
- Class II: Flashpoint between 38°C and 60°C (100°F–140°F) (**combustible liquids**)
- Class III: Flashpoint above 60°C (140°F) (combustible liquids)

Flame Point/Fire Point

The **flame point** or **fire point** is the lowest temperature at which a liquid produces a vapor that can sustain a continuous flame (rather than the instantaneous flash of the flash point). It is usually just a few degrees above the rated flash point. Although it is not often reported, the flame point is probably a more realistic assessment of a fuel's contribution to a fire environment than the flash point. The fire points of a few common fuels are shown in Table 2-4. The exact values of flash point and flame point temperatures of tested fuels depend on the following factors (Friedman 1998):

- the size of the ignition source,
- how long it is held over the source each time,
- the rate of heating of the liquid, and
- the degree of air movement over the fuel.

Glassman and Dryer (1980–1981) (see Table 2-4) reported minimum fire points for alcohols to be equal to their minimum flash points and observed a significant difference between values obtained using flame igniters and those using electrical arc ignition, apparently as a result of the infrared absorption characteristics of alcohol fuels.

Ignition Temperature

The **ignition temperature**, sometimes called the **autoignition temperature** (AIT) or spontaneous ignition temperature (SIT), is the temperature at which a fuel will ignite on its own without any additional source of ignition. For purposes of comparing liquid and gaseous fuels, ignition temperature can be measured by injecting a small quantity of fuel into a hot-air environment (usually a closed container) at various temperatures. In the standard test, *ASTM E659,* the test chamber is an electrically heated 1 L glass flask (sometimes called a Setchkin apparatus) (ASTM International 2015b). When the container is at or above the fuel's ignition temperature, the fuel will burst into flame upon injection. For example, low-octane gasoline, with a flash point of −43°C (−45°F), requires a minimum temperature of about 280°C (536°F) to catch fire (100 octane gasoline has an AIT of 456°C). This is the minimum temperature that must be reached by the match, spark, lighter, or other igniting instrument in order for that material to burn.

With one or two exceptions, such as catalytic action, the temperature of at least a portion of the fuel must be raised to its ignition temperature before fire can result from any fuel. Ignition temperatures of common materials are generally so high as to rule out spontaneous combustion, except for a very small category of materials and only under very special conditions. Carbon disulfide (CS_2), used as an industrial cleaning solvent, is one exception. Carbon disulfide has various reported AITs of 90°C to 120°C (194° to 240°F). In general, for a given series of hydrocarbons, the longer the carbon backbone, the lower the AIT of the material. For example, *n*-pentane has an AIT of 260°C, while *n*-octane and higher alkanes have an AIT of around 208°C.

Catalytic oxidation of some fuels can occur at temperatures much lower than the AIT, but these reactions are very rare and occur under special conditions. For example, platinum in a finely divided state may serve to allow (catalyze) combustion of certain flammable gases in air at low initial temperatures. In a fuel cell or a hand warmer this may be important, but it is very rare in general fires. For solids, in which pyrolytic decomposition must precede ignition, there is another value, called the piloted ignition temperature.

flammable liquid ▪ A liquid that has a closed-cup flash point that is below 37.8°C (100°F) and a maximum vapor pressure of 2068 mm Hg (40 psia) at 37.8°C (100°F) (NFPA 2017d, pt. 3.3.85; *see also* pt. 3.3.34, Combustible Liquid).

combustible liquid ▪ CLASS II: Any liquid that has a flash point at or above 100°F (37.8°C) and below 140°F (60°C). CLASS IIIA: Any liquid that has a flash point at or above 140°F (60°C), but below 200°F (93°C). CLASS IIIB: Any liquid that has a flash point at or above 200°F (93°C) (NFPA 2016c).

fire point ▪ The lowest temperature at which a liquid ignites and achieves sustained burning when exposed to a test flame.

ignition temperature ▪ Minimum temperature a substance should attain in order to ignite under specific test conditions (NFPA 2017d, pt. 3.3.114).

autoignition temperature ▪ The lowest temperature at which a combustible material ignites in air without a spark or flame (NFPA 2017d, pt. 3.3.16).

Virtually all fires originate where there is a localized high temperature in a region in which an appropriate fuel/air mixture occurs. The local region may be very small, as in the case of an electrically induced arc, a mechanical spark, or a minute flame. The important concept is that at this very small point in space, a temperature in excess of the ignition temperature occurs in the presence of appropriate fuel and air (or oxygen), and this energy is transferred to an adequate volume of ignitable fuel. Such circumstances are not unusual, but from the investigative standpoint, it must always be accepted that these circumstances constitute a *minimum* requirement for *any* fire whatever to result. That tiny initial flame then propagates through adjoining mixtures in the **flammable range**.

Many times, no source of such relatively high temperatures appears to be present, and the origin of a fire seems very mysterious. In such instances, it is actually not difficult to produce a source of energy in a very small area. Fires can be kindled by rubbing two sticks together, by the flint-and-steel method (which strikes a very small but hot spark), and by other similar means. In the start of a fire, it is only the heat content of the source (as reflected in part by its temperature) that counts—not the area over which the temperature holds. A nail in a shoe heel striking a rock may ignite a fire, not because the shoe is hot but because a small spark reaches a very high temperature.

Except in industrial fires, where there are pressurized vessels and delivery lines, it is rare for any large amount of fuel to be heated past its ignition temperature. If even a small portion of fuel is heated so that the temperature is above the ignition point, a fire can result. This is why so many fires occur under conditions that do not seem to be hazardous. As long as the fuel gas or vapor concentration is within its flammability range in the vicinity of this small but intensely energetic source, there can be ignition. The fundamental consideration is not the temperature of an ignition source compared with the ignition temperature of the fuel, but the transfer of heat energy from the source to the fuel. An ignition source may be present that is at a temperature that is technically higher than the AIT listed for that fuel, but there still may not be ignition if enough energy is not transferred to the fuel.

AIT is a minimum environmental temperature measured by a particular laboratory technique (*ASTM E659* being the most common) and is dependent on the size, shape, and even surface material and texture of the confinement vessel used in the test apparatus. The real-world ignition sources that a fuel might encounter will usually have different size, shape, and confinement and so will almost always have to be at a temperature considerably higher than the listed AIT.

AIT data are more for reference and comparison than for a specific determination. Some minimum ignition temperatures of common fuels are listed in Tables 2-3 and 2-4. Because the minimum ignition temperature is dependent on the method used for its determination, that value should be used primarily for comparisons between fuels. Testing has revealed that hot surface ignition of gasoline in open air, for instance, requires that the temperature of the surface be at least 200°C (360°F) above the listed autoignition temperature [i.e., 500°C to 700°C (930°F to 1,300°F)]. It is thought that the hot surface produces rapid evaporation, which minimizes contact time (American Petroleum Institute 1991). The material and texture of the hot surface will also affect minimum ignition temperatures. The grade of gasoline is also critical: the higher the grade or octane rating, the higher the AIT.

Ignition Energy

Every fuel gas or vapor has a minimum **ignition energy**, or amount of energy that must be transferred to the fuel to trigger the first oxidation. For most fuels, this is a very small amount of energy; for hydrocarbon fuels, the minimum ignition energy is on the order of 0.25 millijoule (mJ) (see Table 2-3). This amount is dependent on the concentration of the vapor and is often at its minimum when the fuel vapor is at its stoichiometric or ideal concentration (as shown in Figure 2-20). For a vapor/air mixture to ignite, there are four required conditions.

flammable range ■ The range of concentrations between the lower and upper flammable limits (NFPA 2017d, pt. 3.3.86; *see also* NFPA 2013).

ignition energy ■ The quantity of heat energy that should be absorbed by a substance to ignite and burn (NFPA 2017d, pt. 3.3.113).

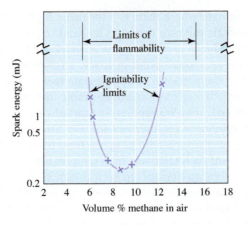

FIGURE 2-20 Ignitability curve and flammability limits for methane/air mixtures at atmospheric pressure and 20°C. *From Zabetakis, M. G. 1965. "Flammability Characteristics of Combustible Gases and Vapors." Washington, DC: US Bureau of Mines, US Government Printing Office: 2.*

First, an ignition source must have adequate energy (above the minimum ignition energy for that fuel); second, the fuel must be present at a concentration within its flammability range; third, there must be contact between the source and the fuel while it is in that range; and finally, the contact must be of sufficient duration for enough energy to be transferred from the source to the fuel. Unless all four of these conditions are met, there will not be an ignition.

Several flammability properties are interrelated. For instance, the minimum ignition energy of a fuel is dependent on fuel concentration, as can be seen in Figure 2-20. This means that a very energetic source can ignite mixtures closer to the flammability limits for that fuel, while a very weak source may be competent only when the mixture is near its stoichiometric mixture. In addition, the flammability limits are dependent on starting, or initial, temperature, as was shown in Figure 2-18: the warmer the starting (pre-fire) mixture, the wider the limits.

flame front ▪ The flaming leading edge of a propogating combustion reaction zone (NFPA 2017d, pt. 3.3.81).

In gaseous-phase explosions, the speed with which a **flame front** progresses through a fuel/air mixture is dependent on concentration. The flame speed reaches a maximum when the mixture is near its stoichiometric or ideal mixture. As a result, overpressures caused by rapidly expanding gases are at or near their maxima. A premixed hydrocarbon fuel/air mixture near its stoichiometric mixture theoretically can produce pressures up to 120 psi (8 bar) under ideal conditions (Harris 1983). A lean mixture propagates at a slower speed and produces less heat and, therefore, lower pressures. Because all the fuel is consumed in the reaction, there is no subsequent fire or flame. In contrast, a rich mixture results in a less vigorous explosion with less mechanical damage due to lower pressures and slower speeds. The excess fuel produces smoke or soot and a following flaming fire. Thus, the heat effects and blackening are often greater and the blast damage less when the mixture is rich than when it is lean.

boiling point ▪ The temperature at which the vapor pressure of a liquid equals the surrounding atmospheric pressure. For purposes of defining the boiling point, atmospheric pressure shall be considered to be 14.7 psia (760 mm Hg or 101.4 kPa). For mixtures that do not have a constant boiling point, the 20 percent evaporated point of a distillation performed in accordance with *ASTM D86, Standard Test Method for Distillation of Petroleum Products at Atmospheric Pressure*, shall be considered to be the boiling point (NFPA 2016b).

Boiling Points

Boiling points are sometimes important in fire investigations, but they are of secondary significance compared to other properties discussed in this chapter. Boiling point ranges are used to characterize many fuels encountered in fires. Most liquids may be expected to be heated to their **boiling point** in a fire. However, there is a very important distinction between a liquid fuel that is reasonably pure and will therefore have a reasonably definite boiling point and one that is a mixture of many components of variable boiling points.

A pure, single-component liquid fuel will have a definite boiling point at which an entire sample may be distilled without a change in temperature of the vapors. The general public can get relatively few pure liquid fuels compared with a much larger number of mixtures that have a boiling *range* rather than a boiling *point*. These mixtures range from gasoline, with more than 200 individual compounds, to mixtures manufactured for special purposes such as cleaning or industrial solvent action. When heated, these mixtures allow the distillation of their most volatile constituents first, followed by constituents of decreasing volatility (a process often called weathering). In general, the most volatile constituent of a mixture is the most significant as it relates to the fire hazard. When a liquid fuel such as gasoline that has a boiling point range burns, the more volatile species evaporate first and fastest from the surface layer. The bulk liquid beneath the surface will retain the lighter species for some time, since they will have to migrate by diffusion (aided by convective flows) through the bulk liquid to reach the surface before they can evaporate (DeHaan 1995). A consequence of fractional distillation is that the residue of a petroleum distillate may have a lower autoignition temperature than the bulk liquid, possibly posing a risk of delayed ignition (Kennedy and Armstrong 2007).

In initiating a fire, materials of high boiling point will rarely be above their flash point at ambient temperatures, and only the more volatile (low boiling point) will be expected to show special hazard. As a rule, the boiling point and the flash point tend to parallel each other, so the low-boiling material will usually have a low flash point as well. The presence of a mixture does not greatly diminish the fire hazard of the most volatile component in that mixture. A mixture of gasoline and diesel fuel, for instance, exhibits a flash point indistinguishable from that of gasoline alone until the gasoline represents less than about 5 percent of the mixture.

Vapor Density

The fundamental property of a vapor that predicts its behavior when released in air is its **vapor density**. The vapor density, that is, the density of a vapor relative to that of air, may be simply calculated by dividing the molecular weight of the vapor by the mean molecular weight of air, which is approximately 29. This relationship is represented by the equation

$$\text{Vapor density (gas or vapor)} = \text{Molecular wt of gas}/\text{Molecular wt of air} \quad (2.2)$$

For example, the lightest gas, hydrogen, has a molecular weight of only 2; therefore, its vapor density (V.D.) is

$$\text{V.D.} = 2/29 = 0.07 \quad (2.3)$$

Methane, the simplest hydrocarbon fuel gas found in swamp gas and natural gas, has a molecular weight of 16. Its vapor density, then, is roughly 16/29, or 0.55. Ethane, the other major component of natural gas, has a molecular weight of 30, making it almost exactly the same density as air, and giving it a vapor density of 1.03. The vapor densities of some common fuels are shown in Table 2-6.

Gases or vapors with a vapor density greater than 1.0 are heavier than air and tend to settle in the air into which they are released until they encounter an obstruction, such as a floor, after which they tend to spread outward at this level, much in the same manner as if they were liquids. In contrast, vapors lighter than air tend to rise through the air until an obstruction, such as a ceiling, is encountered, after which they spread at the high level. The tendency to spread is less absolute than with liquids because the difference in density as compared with air is much less than compared with any liquid, and air currents produce mixing. Some mixing with the air is inevitable, and the nearer the vapor density is to that of air, the greater the mixing of fuel and air. This effect of greater mixing is due to the process known as diffusion. All gases, regardless of their molecular weight or vapor density, tend to diffuse into each other when the opportunity exists.

Differences in diffusion rates of gases depend on their vapor density: when a fuel vapor is much heavier than air (V.D. >> 1.0), its diffusion rate will be much less than when its density is much closer to that of the air into which it is diffusing, that is, when its vapor density is close to 1.0. The diffusion of a vapor is a very slow process. In a closed container, diffusion of a vapor will eventually produce a uniform distribution after some hours. In an open system such as a room, diffusion of vapors from a volatile liquid does

vapor density ■ The relative weight of a gas or vapor compared to air, which has an arbitrary value of one. If a gas has a vapor density of less than one it will generally rise in air. If the vapor density is greater than one the gas will generally sink in air. [NFPA 2017d, pt. 3.3.197; *see also* pt 3.3.176, Specific Gravity (air) (vapor density)].

TABLE 2-6	Vapor Densities of Common Fuel Gases and Vapors

FUEL	VAPOR DENSITY (AT STANDARD TEMPERATURE AND PRESSURE)
Hydrogen	0.07
Methane	0.55
Acetylene	0.90
Carbon monoxide	0.97
Ethane	1.03
Propane	1.51
Butane	1.93
Acetone	2.00
Pentane[a]	2.50
Hexane[b]	3.00

[a]Lightest liquid component of gasoline.
[b]Lightest major component of camping fuels.

not produce a uniform distribution, but rather a gradient of concentration from very high (saturation vapor pressure) to very low, as represented in Figure 2-20.

Methane, as noted, is lighter than air and thus tends to rise in a room as long as its temperature is the same as that of the room air. Its rate of diffusion is greater than that for heavier molecules, and so it tends to mix with air and form a gradient of concentration, as illustrated in Figure 2-21(a). The same is true for natural gas, which is a mixture of methane and ethane and other light gases, so its vapor density will be between 0.55 and 1.0, depending on the relative proportions of the components. Ethane is rarely encountered by itself, but because its vapor density is close to 1, it will diffuse readily in air and neither rise nor settle in air, there being no gravitational separation. Diffusion acts to keep vapors diffused and mixed in air and, once mixed in air, vapors will not settle out to re-form layers of high concentration. The same is true for acetylene (C_2H_2) with a molecular weight of 26 and therefore a vapor density of 0.9, as well as ethene (C_2H_4) and carbon monoxide (CO), each with a molecular weight of 28 and therefore a vapor density of 28/29, or 0.97. All other commonly encountered fuel gases and vapors have a vapor density significantly greater than 1 and will tend to sink when released in air. For example, propane, the next heavier hydrocarbon, (V.D. = 1.51) will mix readily with air, but it will tend to sink as it does so.

A flammable propane/air mixture (2 to 9.6 percent) will have a vapor density very close to that of air. Butane (V.D. = 1.93) sinks more readily and tends not to diffuse as quickly. All higher hydrocarbons, characteristic of most petroleum products, will have slower diffusion rates (diffusivity) along with their greater vapor density. Gasoline vapors, for instance, contain a mixture of all the most volatile components of the liquid blend. This mixture, being considerably heavier than air, will sink rapidly to the floor or ground surface. Therefore, gasoline vapors will pour into low regions or down drains and will carry their intrinsic hazard to the lowest possible region (see Figures 2-21(b) and (c) for a graphic representation).

From a fire hazard standpoint, the vapor density and diffusion rate of the lightest, most volatile component of a mixture is what will determine the spread and ignitability of vapors, not the properties of the bulk liquid. For instance, gasoline has a range of components, some of which, like *n*-decane, have a very low vapor pressure at room temperature

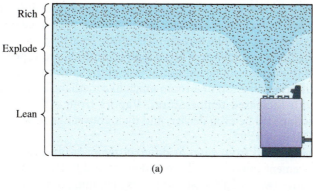

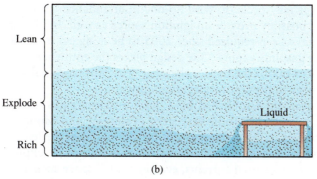

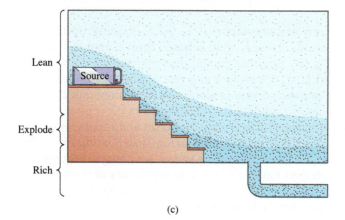

FIGURE 2-21 Typical mixtures of natural gas or flammable fluid vapors in closed rooms. (a) Natural gas (methane) in a room. (b) Gasoline in a room. (c) Gasoline (or butane) in a room with various elevations.

(a)

(b)

(c)

and a correspondingly high flash point. It is the isobutane and *n*-pentane content of automotive gasoline that generates the bulk of the vapors at ordinary room temperatures and produces the significant ignition risk. Gasoline's heavier components, such as the xylenes, do not contribute significantly to the vapors until the gasoline has been evaporating for many minutes, by which time the lighter components will have already been ignited (DeHaan 1995). In general, the vapors of fresh automotive gasoline will behave exactly like those of *n*-pentane in their movement.

It is apparent that various concentration layers will exist with a gradient of intermediate concentrations between the heaviest and lightest layers. Some of these vapor layers will be within their explosive flammable limits, while the mixture in other layers will be either too rich or too lean to be ignited. These distributions represent release into a sealed room with still air in which there is no physical activity and in which the vapors are at the same temperatures.

In an assessment of distribution of vapors, the effects of temperature and air currents must not be overlooked. A fan, furnace, operating machinery, or even someone walking will stir vapors into mixtures throughout a room. The draft created by a water heater burner, furnace burner, or open window may be enough to redistribute vapors and may draw them into contact with an open-flame ignition source at the same time. Even butane, if warmed sufficiently, will rise to the top of a room much like methane because the vapor density drops rapidly with increased temperatures. Vapors from a flammable liquid cooled by evaporative cooling will be even denser, and their convective flow will enhance their tendency to settle (DeHaan 1995).

When a gas mixture is formed from gases at different temperatures, the temperature alone may control its movement initially until the temperature differences are equalized. The alert investigator must be aware of all these influences (including timer- or thermostat-controlled equipment that may cycle on with no one in attendance) that can distribute and circulate vapors and possibly provide an ignition source as well. In the United States, gas-fired water heaters have been required since 2005 to be designed to make it difficult for their burners to ignite gasoline vapors. One design places the entire heater in an 18-in.-deep bucket to keep vapors out of the burner chamber. The other uses a flash suppressor on the combustion chamber to prevent propagation outward.

The concentration gradient established by a heavier-than-air gas (such as LP gas) leaking into still air has been shown to be very steep (Valentine and Moore 1974). This means that a person standing in the room may not be able to detect the leak by its odorant while a layer below knee height in the same room is within its explosive range. Experiments have shown that thermal currents, even in a small space such as a camper or RV, result in almost complete mixing of propane into air, with no detectable gradient (DeHaan 1995).

One interesting property of dense vapors (V.D. >2.5) is their propensity to flow horizontally, like a viscous liquid. Pentane vapor released from a pool at room temperature will diffuse upward only a few centimeters, and then the mass of vapor will slump sideways and spread outward along the surface at a rate of about 0.05 m/s in still air. This so-called advective flow can spread vapors along a surface more quickly than diffusion, but is easily overcome by even a modest draft (DeHaan 1995).

Careful consideration of the distribution of fuel gases and vapors must be made when assessing the likelihood of ignition by possible sources. If an ignition source like a candle flame is high up in a room, LP gases or gasoline vapors are going to require a long time to diffuse sufficiently to reach their flammable range in the vicinity of the candle flame unless there is some external means of circulation like a fan or strong draft, or the vapors are released under pressure (jet). Similarly, a kerosene heater burning normally at floor level in a room is unlikely to ignite natural gas leaking into the room until the gas can fill the room from the top down in the absence of mechanical circulation. The mere presence of an ignition source and a fuel source in the same room is not a guarantee that there will be ignition. The assessment of possible ignition sources for such vapor/air mixtures should take into account all of these contributing factors, including the heights of, and protective enclosures around, appliance burners.

It was once thought that the distribution of blast effects from a vapor/air deflagration was directly linked to the preignition distribution of vapors. However, experiments by one of the authors demonstrated that even when a highly localized (floor) layer of *n*-hexane vapors is ignited, the pressures are equalized throughout a moderate-sized compartment within 5 milliseconds (ms) (DeHaan et al. 2001). This means that the walls of the average compartment will be exposed to the same pressure at the same time from within and will therefore fail where it is weakest structurally.

It is frequently noted in explosions in wooden frame structures that it is the bottom of the wall that moves rather than the top, despite whether the deflagration was fueled by natural gas or LP gas. This result can mean that the bottoms of the walls were not as

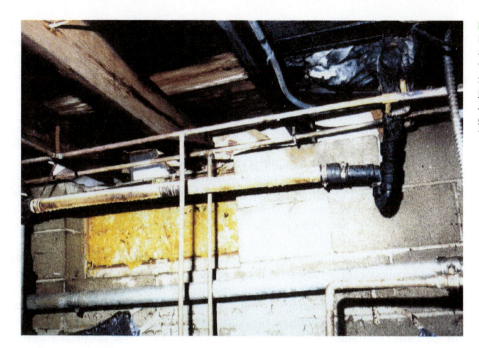

FIGURE 2-22 Pocketed burning of natural gas accumulated under this wooden floor produced significant charring of joists and floor. *Courtesy of Jamie Novak, Novak Investigations and St. Paul Fire Dept.*

well anchored to the foundation or slab as the tops of the walls were to the structure above. The bottoms of wood frame walls are also much more likely to be weakened by termites or dry rot.

When a fire follows an explosion, however, if the turbulence of the explosion has not completely dissipated the layer of fuel vapor, the fire will tend to burn at the interface between the richest layer of fuel and the air (as discussed previously). Thus, a fire following a hexane (or gasoline) vapor explosion will tend to burn atop or within a remaining layer of dense vapor (where the fuel-rich layers will burn longest). The distribution of fire damage low down in the room after a vapor ignition indicates that a heavier-than-air vapor has been involved. The reverse will occasionally occur on the underside of a natural gas layer trapped or pocketed on the underside of a floor or roof structure, as in Figure 2-22. In either case, the location and distribution of postexplosion fire damage may give important clues as to the vapor density of the fuel responsible.

The volume of vapor generated by the evaporation of a known volume of a volatile liquid may be important in evaluating the ignition potential of accidental or even intentional spills. If total evaporation can be assumed, the volume of vapor generated (at standard temperature and pressure) by 1 US gallon (3.8 L) of liquid can be calculated from the empirical relationship

Vapor (in cubic feet, ft^3) = 111 × Specific gravity of liquid* ÷ Vapor density of liquid

For example, 1 US gallon of diethyl ether, with a specific gravity of 0.7 and a vapor density of 2.55, will produce

$$111 \times 0.7/2.55 = 30.47 \text{ ft}^3 \text{ of diethyl ether vapor}$$

Because diethyl ether has a flammability or explosive range of 2 to 36 percent in air, 30.47 ft^3 of vapor, if uniformly distributed, will produce an explosive mixture in a room of 84 to 1,520 ft^3 in volume. In metric units the equivalent relationship for 1 L of liquid (0.001 m^3) is

Vapor (in cubic meters, m^3) = 0.85 × Specific gravity ÷ Vapor density

For commercial propane, the liquid/vapor expansion rate is approximately 272; that is, 1 L of liquid propane will produce about 272 L of vapor at standard temperature and pressure. Commercial butane has an expansion factor of approximately 234 (*NFPA 58*) (NFPA 2017a). The expansion rate for LP gas itself will vary with the composition of the LP gas, since the rates for each component are different.

Heat of Combustion

The heat of combustion of the fuels is another property of fuels often of great importance to the investigator. If the approximate amounts of fuels in a room can be estimated by weight, the intensity of burning observed can be compared with the possibilities of various combinations of fuels. The rate at which heat is released is more critical to reconstructing the events of a fire than the total amount of heat. Sometimes, it is useful to be able to recognize when the fire damage to a room simply does not tally with the amount of heat that should have been produced by the fuels known to be present. The causes for such differences can then be explored.

The scientific method raises the questions: Was there so much damage that it cannot be accounted for by assessment of fuel loads normally present? Was there reduced fuel because stock had been removed prior to the fire? Was there reduced ventilation available, or was there enhanced combustion due to oxygen enrichment? Was the lack of damage due to the incomplete or inefficient combustion of the available fuels? Some of the most common fuels, such as wood, have such variable properties as to give only approximations of the actual output in a specific instance. Table 2-7 summarizes the heat of combustion of a few of the most important fuels from the standpoint of the fire investigation.

The heat of combustion is used to calculate a theoretical adiabatic flame temperature for each fuel. These calculated values are sometimes erroneously used to estimate the potential effect the flames will have on surrounding materials. Work by Henderson and Lightsey (1984) indicates that the actual measured flame temperatures produced by these fuels when burned in air are much lower than previously thought. The measured temperatures they reported are included in Table 2-7. The roles of the flame temperatures and heat of combustion in fire investigation will be explored in later chapters. The real-world maximum open-flame temperatures of nearly all normal fuels burning in turbulent diffusion flames is about 900°C (1700°F), and this figure is used in most calculations. Some fuels like styrene, crude oil, and urethane foam that burn with very smoky flames, so that the heat produced cannot be readily lost (low emissivity), produce very high temperatures in the flames. Fuels that burn cleanly with no soot or pyrolysis products (alcohols) also have a low emissivity and high flame temperatures.

Pyrolysis and Decomposition of Liquids

Although some unstable liquids decompose at fairly low temperatures, most fuel liquids reach their boiling point and boil away before being subject to pyrolytic decomposition. Even when liquids are exposed to an intense general fire, convection within a deep pool as opposed to a thin film helps mix the cooler and warmer liquids. The liquid at the surface boils off into the flame, with the heat absorbed from the flames being lost by evaporative cooling. This process maintains the temperature of the entire pool at or just below the boiling point of the liquid; the liquid pool protects the surface on which the pool is sitting. When dealing with viscous liquids with impaired circulation such as asphalt, plastic resins, or some foods, portions of the liquid in contact with an intense heat source can reach and exceed their pyrolysis temperatures and begin to char and decompose like a solid. The pyrolysis products then enter the flame in the same way as those driven off a solid.

In tank or pool fires involving heavy crude oils, the residue formed on the burning surface by distillation of the lighter components may become denser than the surrounding liquid. The hot residue can then settle into the tank and contact water in the bottom, producing a steam explosion that propels the burning fuel above outward with disastrous

TABLE 2-7	Heats of Combustion and Flame Temperatures of Some Fuels

FUEL	HEAT OF COMBUSTION (MJ/kg) NET		FLAME TEMPERATURE (°C) ADIABATIC	ACTUAL
Acetylene	49.9[a] (55.8MJ/m^3)	48.2[b]	2,325	
Butane	49.5[b] (112.4 MJ/m^3)[c]	45.7	1,895	
Carbon monoxide	(11.7 MJ/m^3)[c]	10.1		
Charcoal	33.7	34.3	2,200[d]	1,390[d]
Coleman fuel				770[e]
Coal (anthracite)	30.9–34.8			
Cotton	16			
Ethane	47.5 (60.5 MJ/m^3)[c]	47.4	1,895	
Ethyl alcohol	29.7	26.8		840[e]
Fuel oil #1 (kerosene)	46.1			
Hexane	48.3 (164.4 MJ/m^3)[c]	43.8	1,948/2,200[e]	
Hydrogen	130.8 (12.1 MJ/m^3)[c]			
Gasoline	43.7			810[e]
Methane	55.5 (34 MJ/m^3)[c]	50	1,875[e]	
Propane	50.4 (86.4 MJ/m^3)[c]	46.4	1,925[e]	970[e]
Polyethylene	43.2			
Polypropylene	43.2			
Polystyrene	40			
Polyurethane	23			
Wood	20	16–20	1,590[f]	~600–1,000[f]

[a]NFPA. 2003. *Fire Protection Handbook.* 19th ed. Quincy, MA: National Fire Protection Association, Table A.1.
[b]SFPE. 2008. *SFPE Handbook of Fire Protection Engineering.* 4th ed. Quincy, MA: Society of Fire Protection Engineers and the National Fire Protection Association, Tables 1-5.3 and 1-5.6.
[c]Harris, R. J. 1983. *The Investigation and Control of Gas Explosions in Buildings and Heating Plant,* New York: E and FN Spon, 6–7.
[d]Henderson, R. W., and G. R Lightsey. 1985. "Theoretical Combustion Temperature of Wood Charcoal." *National Fire and Arson Report* 3: 7.
[e]Henderson, R. W., and G. R Lightsey. December 1984. "The Effective Flame Temperatures of Flammable Liquids." *Fire & Arson Investigator* 35: 8.
[f]Henderson, R. W., and G. R Lightsey. December 1985. "Theoretical vs. Observed Flame Temperatures during Combustion of Wood Products." *Fire & Arson Investigator* 36.

results. This situation can also occur with nonpetroleum liquids like cooking oils that can pyrolyze and form a true char.

Liquid fuels are categorized by their flash point (see Table 2-4.) Flammable liquids are all those that have a flash point below 100°F (37.8°C) (NFPA Classification: Class I), with Class IA and IB liquids having flash points below room temperature, 73°F (22.8°C). Combustible liquids are those with a flash point above 100°F (37.8°C) [NFPA Class II, flash point between 100°F and 140°F (37.8°C and 60°C), and Class III, flash point above 140°F (60°C)]. Class III combustible liquids are further divided into Class IIIA (flash point between 140°F and 200°F) and Class IIIB (flash point above 200°F (93°C)] (NFPA 2008). In the United Kingdom, highly flammable liquids are those that have a flash point below 32°C (90°F); flammable liquids are those with a flash point between 32°C and 60°C; and combustible liquids are those with a flash point above 60°C (140°F) (Drysdale 1999). Ignitable liquids are a category of liquid fuels that includes both flammable and combustible liquids.

2.10.2 HYDROCARBON FUELS

Hydrocarbons ranging from the light gas methane to heavier compounds, including oils and asphalts, are the most important fuels to be considered in a fire investigation.

Natural Gas

Natural gas, primarily methane, from different geological formations shows considerable variation in composition and may contain some noncombustible gases. Natural gas is typically 70 to 90 percent methane, 10 to 20 percent ethane, and 1 to 3 percent nitrogen, with traces of other gases (NFPA 2008). In most cases, the investigator may consider its properties to be the same as those of methane, without introducing serious error.

Liquefied Petroleum Gas

Liquefied petroleum gas (LPG), commonly used in rural areas where natural gas is not available, is a mixture of propane and *n*-butane, with small quantities of ethane, ethylene, propylene, isobutane, and butylene (NFPA 2008). Depending on its source and its intended use, it can be quite variable in its composition, ranging from almost pure propane to a heavier mixture largely composed of butane. For LPG sold in the United States, the investigator can consider LPG the same as propane in its physical and combustion properties without serious error. In some other countries, LPG can be primarily butane. If butane is known to have been involved (from lighters, torches, or aerosol containers), it is best to use its reference values for calculations.

Petroleum

Petroleum in its crude state is a thick oil varying in color from light brown to black. It contains a large number of compounds and different types of compounds, which are separated to a considerable extent in the manufacture of petroleum fuels. Products obtained from the distillation of petroleum include gases, petroleum ether, straight-run gasoline, kerosene, medium distillates including paint thinner–type mixtures and solvents, diesel fuels, heavy lubricating oils, petroleum jelly, paraffin, waxes, asphalt, and coke. The distillation curve of petroleum products is represented in Figure 2-23.

Gasoline

Gasoline, widely used in vehicles and appliances and perhaps the most important fuel of petroleum origin, is a mixture of volatile, low-boiling, and midrange hydrocarbons. It contains hydrocarbon compounds with boiling points between approximately 32°C (90°F) and 205°C (400°F). The average molecular weight of gasoline is sometimes taken to be close to that of *n*-octane, about 114. The petroleum distillate described as straight-run gasoline contains the raw hydrocarbons that distill off between 40°C and 200°C (100°F to 395°F) and is used as camping fuel and sometimes called white gas or naphtha. The range of compounds included is often measured by the carbon number or molecular length of *n*-alkanes included. In this case, this distillate cut includes C_4 (butane) to C_{12} (dodecane).

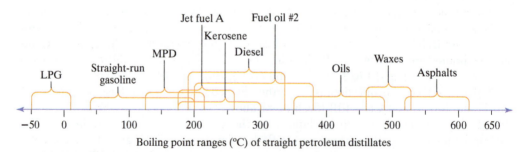

FIGURE 2-23 Boiling point ranges of straight petroleum distillates.

Modern automotive gasoline contains more than 200 hydrocarbons in a complex mixture that is not just the straight cut or fraction but a blend of many compounds, especially aromatics whose relative component concentrations vary little from refinery to refinery. This means that it is not generally possible to identify one oil company's product from another based on a comparison of the basic hydrocarbon profiles of the gasoline. Recently, forensic chemists have noticed that component ratios are changing and substitutions are being made, so laboratory identification of gasoline as an **accelerant** is no longer as straightforward as it once was. Before gasoline is sold as a motor fuel, a variety of additives are added by the refinery. These additives often include compounds to improve the burning characteristics of the fuel. Dyes were once added to distinguish leaded from unleaded motor fuels. Today, nearly all automotive gasoline is unleaded. Dyes are rarely seen except to identify lower-taxed fuels for agricultural use.

accelerant ▪ A fuel or oxidizer, often an ignitable liquid, intentionally used to initiate a fire or increase the rate of growth or spread of fire (NFPA 2017d, pt. 3.3.2.).

Oxygenates, especially ethanol and methanol, are very common in automotive gasoline. In many areas, they are completely replacing MTBE (methyl *t*-butyl ether), once commonly used as an oxygenate additive. The additive packages used by manufacturers differ and offer a means of distinguishing fresh, unburned, and uncontaminated gasoline. Unfortunately, due to the industry practice of exchanging raw petroleum feedstocks, additive packages, and even finished gasoline depending on market and supply conditions, it is not possible, in most cases, to identify a particular retail brand of gasoline from a sample of the fuel as it is delivered to the retail customer. However, recent advances in gas chromatography and data interpretation are making it possible to compare unburned fuels against suspected sources with considerable specificity.

Kerosene and Other Distillates

Kerosene as defined by *ASTM D3699* has a boiling point range from 175°C to 300°C (350°F to 572°F) with a minimum flash point of 38°C (100°F) (ASTM International 2013a). Kerosene and the distillate fuels of higher boiling ranges were considered useful only for illumination until the diesel motor became a common device. Although diesel fuel is similar to kerosene, it spans a wider range of less-volatile components.

The modern jet engine and other turbine-driven engines increased the use and economic significance of kerosene-like fuels. The classification scheme used for laboratory characterization of ignitable liquids (those liquids considered either flammable or combustible) includes an intermediate range called medium petroleum distillates [having a boiling point range between about 125°C and 215°C (250°F to 400°F)]. This range includes carbon numbers from C_9 to C_{17}. Many household and commercial products fall into this class—paint thinners, mineral spirits, some charcoal starters, and even some insect sprays.

Kerosene and similar petroleum distillates have long been a suspect in the setting of deliberate fires. Their lower volatility presents a lesser hazard to the user than does gasoline. The liquid evaporates more slowly, so that less haste is required in its ignition, and there is much less danger of explosion. Kerosene-class compounds have very low autoignition temperatures, on the order of 210°C (410°F) (see Table 2-5). Interestingly, despite their lower AITs, their high flash points make them less likely to aid the spread of fire (see Table 2-4). Their compositions involve several series of higher-molecular-weight hydrocarbons. Kerosene (fuel oil #1, Jet Fuel A) generally contains paraffinic and **olefinic** hydrocarbons in the C_{10} to C_{16} range. This range denotes hydrocarbons having 10 to 16 carbon atoms linked together. These have boiling points between 175°C and 260°C (350°F to 500°F) and therefore fall in the fraction that follows (with some overlap) gasoline in the simple distillation of crude oil.

olefinic ▪ Characteristic of, or containing, olefins.

Diesel Fuel

Diesel fuel contains predominantly paraffinic hydrocarbons with low sulfur content and additives to improve combustion. It covers the boiling point range from 190°C to 340°C

(375°F to 650°F), which includes carbon numbers from C_{10} to C_{23}. Fuel oil, or domestic heating oil, is the next-heavier product, representing a distillation range of approximately 200°C to 350°C (400°F to 675°F). Diesel fuel and domestic heating oil may both sometimes be described as fuel oil #2, depending on local usage. The product for home use is carefully controlled to minimize sulfur and water content, which could corrode heating units having minimal service.

Those fuels intended for industrial service have higher sulfur and ash content and cover a range of products and applications. Diesel fuels have a higher autoignition temperature (250°C or higher) and a low vapor pressure. In a fire, unless present on a porous wick or as an aerosol, diesel fuels only reluctantly support fire. Dyes may be added to denote diesel fuel intended for farm use, which is often taxed at a lower rate than that for road use.

Lubricating Oils

Lubricating oils include a variety of hydrocarbons with a wide range of viscosities and thermal and frictional characteristics to suit every lubrication need. Although lubricating oils are not readily combustible at ordinary temperatures, at elevated temperatures they can add to the fuel load of an established fire. Release of an oil under pressure creates an aerosol of fine droplets that are more easily ignited than the bulk liquid. Used motor oil, often stored in a casual fashion, contains a significant percentage of gasoline residues. Contaminated oil can have a much lower flash point than pure oil and can be the source of accidental fire.

Specialty Petroleum Products

Specialty petroleum products are not true petroleum distillates but are used in such a wide variety of consumer products that they will show up in fire debris even if they are not involved directly in the fire's ignition. These products are manufactured or blended for specific chemical and physical properties. Isoparaffinic blends are made in various boiling point ranges and may be found in copier toners, cigarette lighter fuels, charcoal starters, lamp oils, and even in some waterless hand cleaners (Exxon Corp 1990). Aromatic blends, sometimes called low-paraffinic aromatics (LPAs), are blends of aromatics and naphthenic hydrocarbons intended for use in adhesives and some insecticides. They can be found as background volatiles in household furnishings and are chemically similar to the aromatic fractions found in automotive gasoline (Gialamas 1994). There are also single-component products such as limonene (used as a cleaner) and *n*-tridecane (fuel for liquid candles). They are all combustible liquids, are rapidly replacing many traditional petroleum distillates in consumer products, and are being used as arson accelerants.

2.10.3 COMBUSTION OF LIQUID FUELS

When an ignitable liquid is poured or spilled on a surface, only its vapors, not the liquid itself, actually combust. The behavior of the liquid and its vapors is generally predictable. On a nonporous surface like linoleum, vinyl, or painted concrete, the viscosity and surface tension of the liquid will determine the depth of the freestanding pool that results. The depth determines how large an area the pool will cover for a given quantity of fuel. Viscous liquids like kerosene or diesel fuel form a deeper pool (~1 mm) that will not cover as large an area as a nonviscous fuel like methanol or gasoline, whose freestanding pool may be only 0.1 to 0.5 mm deep (DeHaan 1995).

On other surfaces, the depth of the pool will be determined by the nature of the surface, as shown in Figure 2-24. A semiporous surface like raw wood or concrete will allow some penetration, 2 or 3 mm or so, with a proportional reduction in the area of the pool. Carpets or other porous surfaces allow very deep penetration, so the resulting pools can be very small. The pre-fire evaporation rate from such porous surfaces is considerably

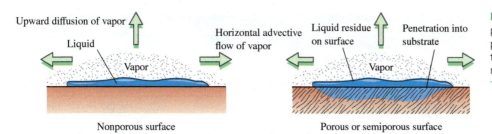

FIGURE 2-24 Liquid pools on nonporous and porous surfaces with vertical and horizontal movement of vapors.

Nonporous surface

Porous or semiporous surface

faster than the rate from a freestanding pool of the same diameter and the same liquid at the same temperature due to the capillary drive of the substrate (the wick effect) (DeHaan 1999).

As described previously, prior to ignition the vapors generated by a pool will rise by diffusion and spread sideways by advective flow, as in Figure 2-24. Upon ignition, the flames are established everywhere the vapors have diffused into the surrounding air in a flammable mixture. The radiant heat from flames near the center of the pool is in part absorbed by the liquid remaining in the pool, and the radiant heat from flames at the edges is absorbed in part by the adjoining floor surface that is not protected by the liquid. This radiant heat may be enough to damage or even ignite the floor exterior to the pool, as in Figure 2-25. Meanwhile, the heat being absorbed by the liquid is being distributed through the liquid by convective circulation, and the temperature of the entire pool begins to rise. The liquid does not really cool the surface beneath it, but it can protect it because the temperature, obviously, cannot exceed the boiling point of the liquid.

For a low-boiling-point fuel like methyl alcohol, the temperature of the floor under the pool will not exceed about 65°C (150°F), the boiling point of methyl alcohol. Therefore, the floor under the pool escapes all damage until the alcohol evaporates. With gasoline, there is progressive distillation and consumption of the components from light to heavy until only the heaviest remain controlled by the diffusion mechanism through the bulk liquid as described earlier. The bulk liquid temperature is limited only by the boiling point of the heaviest constituents, such as n-dodecane with a boiling point of 216°C (421°F). As the lighter components boil off, the liquid can reach temperatures such that some floor materials may be scorched.

When heavy petroleum products like diesel fuel are burning, the temperatures of the liquid can be as high as 340°C (650°F), which is above the ignition temperatures of solid fuels like some woods. (See boiling points in Table 2-8.) As discussed earlier, partial evaporation of petroleum distillates changes the ratio of components, since lighter ones evaporate faster than heavier ones. This process explains why some fuels produce halo-type burns, and others scorch and char the floor more extensively. Because they are so shallow, freestanding pools of most ignitable liquids burn away quite rapidly. The rate is dependent on the nature of the surface and the size of the pool, with very small pools (<0.1 m; 4 in. in diameter) burning away faster than larger pools. When there are cracks

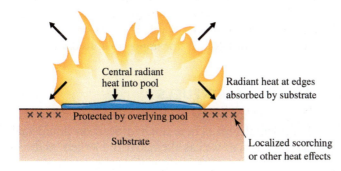

FIGURE 2-25 Distribution and effects of radiant heat from burning pool of ignitable liquid.

TABLE 2-8	Properties of Petroleum Products		

PETROLEUM DISTILLATE	BOILING POINT/RANGE	FLASH POINT	AUTOIGNITION TEMPERATURE
Ethanol	78.5°C (173°F)*	13°C (55°F)	363°C (685°F)
Toluene	110.6°C (231°F)*	4.4°C (40°F)	
Gasoline (low octane)	32°C–190°C (90°F–375°F)	−43°C (−45°F)	257°C (495°F)
Methanol	64.7°C (148.5°F)*		
Medium petroleum distillate	125°C–215°C (250°F2400°F)	13°C (55°F)	220°C (428°F)
Mineral spirits	Varies	40°C (104°F)	245°C (473°F)
VM & P Naphtha (regular)		−2°C (28°F)	232°C (450°F)
Kerosene (C_{10}–C_{16})	175°C –300°C (350°F –500°F)	38°C (100°F)	210°C (410°F)
n-Dodecane	216°C (421°F)*	74°C (165°F)	203°C (397°F)
Fuel oil #1	175°C–260°C (350°F–500°F)	43°C–72°C (110°F–162°F)	210°C (410°F)
Diesel fuel (fuel oil #2)	200°C–350°C (400°F–675°F)	52°C (125°F)	257°C (494°F)
n-Pentane	36°C (97°F)	−40°C (−40°F)	260°C (500°F)

Sources: NFPA. 2001. *Fire Protection Guide to Hazardous Materials.* Quincy, MA: National Fire Protection Association.
*Merck & Co. 1989. *The Merck Index.* 11th ed. Rahway, NJ: Merck.

(a)

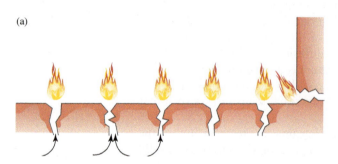

FIGURE 2-26A Pocketed burning from liquid in cracks or seams in a floor may be enhanced by any upward draft and radiant heat feedback within cracks.

(b)

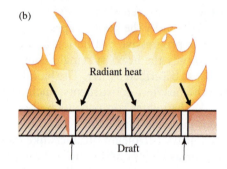

FIGURE 2-26B Radiant heat striking a wood plank floor can initiate charring of the exposed edges, causing a beveled appearance. Combustion between the planks can be enhanced by draft from below. This can be very difficult, if not impossible, to differentiate from (A).

or crevices, localized burning can take place for longer periods of time, inducing localized charring of the floor at the joints and seams, as illustrated in Figure 2-26A. If extra ventilation can then be drawn through these cracks, severe but localized floor damage can result. Downward radiant heating can produce "beveled" edges on floorboards, as pictured in Figure 2-26B. It can be very difficult, if not impossible, to differentiate between these effects.

2.10.4 NONHYDROCARBON LIQUID FUELS

Many materials other than hydrocarbons can be used as accelerants and can play a part in the ignition and spread of accidental fires. These nonhydrocarbon liquid fuels include alcohols, solvents, and similar materials, as well as alternative or biofuels, as discussed next.

Alcohols, Solvents, and Similar Nonhydrocarbons

Methyl alcohol was formerly widely used in spirit (mimeograph) duplicating machines, as an alternative motor fuel, and as a thinner for shellacs and finishes. Ethyl alcohol, especially in reagent (190 proof) or high-proof beverage form (85 or higher proof), can also be used to start fires even though its heat output is not very high. Isopropyl (rubbing) alcohol is flammable at the concentrations packaged for retail use.

All of the simpler alcohols can provide fuel for the incendiary fire and accidental fire and are difficult to detect in post-fire debris because of their extreme volatility and water solubility. Ketones such as acetone and methyl ethyl ketone are widely used as solvents for paints and finishes, as are ethyl acetate and related compounds. Although more and more paints are water-based, thus requiring no volatile solvents, many wood finishes employ turpentine as thinner or linseed oil (or related organic oil) as part of the finish.

A tremendous variety of proprietary mixtures used as mop cleaners, dust attractants, insecticide solvents, copier toners, glue solvents, and plastic resin solvents are encountered at fire scenes. They require mention because of a predisposition to think of liquid fuels only in terms of petroleum distillates. Such thinking can be totally erroneous in many fires. Industrial and commercial fires are often fed and intensified to extremes by special-purpose cleaning agents and solvents. The general properties of many of these compounds have already been discussed.

2.10.5 ALTERNATIVE FUELS OR BIOFUELS

Currently, there are motor fuels in wide use that are not petroleum derivatives. Alternative fuels or biofuels are based on vegetable materials—either processed food oil or ethanol produced by fermentation of corn or other vegetable materials. These fuels can be pure biofuels or, more commonly, a blend of biofuel and petroleum product (Kuk and Spagnola 2008).

Biodiesel

Biodiesel, sometimes denoted as Bl00, is produced by chemically treating vegetable oils (corn, peanut, safflower, canola, etc.) or, more rarely, animal fats to yield a mixture of four fatty acid methyl esters. The ratios of the few components depend on what oil or fat was the starting point. There are presently more than 770 commercial outlets for B100 biodiesel in the United States and countless informal producers.

Biodiesel can be used as a direct substitute for diesel fuel in vehicles with minor mechanical modifications. A 20/80 blend of biodiesel and petroleum diesel denoted as B20 is also in widespread use because it requires no mechanical modifications for use in most motor vehicles. Its performance as a fuel in a motor or in an open fire depends on its diesel fuel constituents. Biodiesel fuels may contain residues of methanol and water from the production process. Because the molecular weights of biodiesel components are similar to those of C_{18} to C_{23} alkanes, the flash points are going to be similar (>100°C). The presence of significant quantities of residual methanol will obviously greatly reduce the flashpoint.

Ethanol

Pure ethanol is not suitable as a motor fuel. The most common variety is E85, a mixture of 85 percent ethanol and 15 percent gasoline. This mixture is being sold across the United States for use in Flex Fuel vehicles. Motor gasoline in the United States has contained up to 10 percent ethanol as an oxygenated additive to reduce CO content. As a motor fuel, this product must meet the same flash point, vapor pressure, and ignition temperature standards as gasoline fuel. The effect on hazard, then, is expected to be minimal. However, its detection after a fire with water extinguishment presents a challenge to the fire investigator.

2.10.6 FUEL GAS SOURCES

Sources of fuel gases of particular interest to the fire investigator include gas lines, natural gas, liquefied petroleum gas, containers, and appliances.

Gas Lines

Although gas lines do not normally represent a source of ignition, they do represent a source of readily ignitable fuel. Because of the properties of gas, gas enclosed in a pipe does not normally pose any hazard. There isn't any danger unless the gas mixes with air to form a combustible or explosive mixture. Such an escape is possible when there is (1) leakage due to inadequately sealed joints or corroded pipes, (2) mechanical fracture of lines from external causes, and (3) failure of lines because of excessive heat, which may melt essential sealing components of the line, valves, regulator, or gas meter.

Natural Gas

Fuel gas in the form of natural gas or LP gas is delivered to appliances via a system of tanks, regulators, pressurized delivery pipes, and flexible connectors. Natural gas in the United States is piped underground via transmission pipelines that may be pressurized to as high as 1,200 pounds per square inch (psi). Distribution pipelines or mains operate at typical pressures of about 60 psi (but may be up to 150 psi). A line regulator at each service location then drops the pressure to 0.14 to 0.36 psi, or to a 4 to 10 in. water column (w.c.) for delivery to residential appliances (1 psi = 27.67 inches w.c.) (NFPA 2017d). Pressures in piping inside commercial buildings for industrial furnaces may be up to 5 psi (but may be higher under special circumstances) (NFPA 2015a). The delivery piping may be steel, wrought iron, copper tubing (if the gas is low sulfur), brass, coated aluminum alloy tubing, or stainless steel. Cast iron pipe is not to be used. Plastic pipe or tubing can be used only on outside underground installations. Natural gas has very little odor of its own, so an **odorant** mixture (usually *t*-butyl mercaptan, thiophane, or another mercaptan) is added during pumping into the delivery pipeline.

odorant ■ A chemical compound that has a smell or odor.

2.10.7 LP GAS

Although natural or manufactured gas is common in urban areas, many rural and isolated regions use liquefied petroleum (LP) gases.

Characteristics and Uses

LP gases are normally either propane, butane, or a mixture of the two, with small quantities of other hydrocarbons. Propane has a boiling point of −42°C (−44°F) at atmospheric pressure and is kept in liquid form by pressure, i.e., its vapor pressure at the ambient temperature. Commercial propane contains propylene and traces of other gases and ethyl mercaptan as an odorant. Butane (pure *n*-butane) has a boiling point of −0.5°C (33°F) at atmospheric pressure, so it can briefly exist as a free liquid at very low temperatures. It, too, contains butylenes and other trace gases and an odorant such as ethyl mercaptan (Lapina 2005). LP gas is supplied in fixed or portable containers of various sizes normally refilled by transferring liquid fuel under pressure from a delivery truck or facility.

Most installations are designed so that only gas, not the liquefied fuel, is vented to the appliance. The most common exceptions are LPG tanks for forklifts and similar equipment, in which the tank is designed to deliver liquid fuel to the motor. Only gas is vented by having the delivery tube above the maximum fill level of the tank or cylinder, as shown in Figure 2-27. When the cylinder is filled to its normal maximum, 80 percent of capacity, liquid propane spills out of the spill tube via the bleed valve, and the operator knows the tank is full. If the tank is improperly positioned or overfilled and then connected to an appliance, the liquid can overwhelm the delivery system and spill out via the main delivery valve.

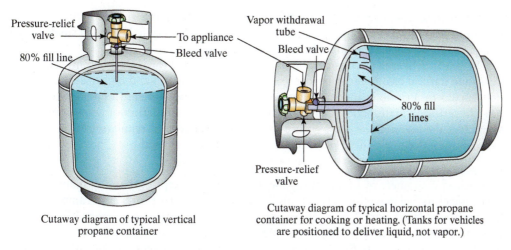

Pressure-relief valve

80% fill line

To appliance

Bleed valve

Cutaway diagram of typical vertical propane container

Vapor withdrawal tube

Bleed valve

80% fill lines

Pressure-relief valve

Cutaway diagram of typical horizontal propane container for cooking or heating. (Tanks for vehicles are positioned to deliver liquid, not vapor.)

FIGURE 2-27 Cross sections of typical horizontal and vertical propane containers.

The pressure within the vapor space of the tank is controlled by the temperature of the tank and its contents. This can range from 28 psi for propane at 0°F (−18°C) to 127 psi at 70°F (21°C) to 286 psi at 130°F (54°C). A pressure relief valve on the container is usually set to bleed off gas when pressures exceed 250 psi (Ettling 1999). A one- or two-stage regulator reduces the tank pressure to a working pressure of 11 to 14 in. w.c. (0.4 to 0.5 psi) for introduction into a typical nonindustrial appliance (NFPA 2017d). Operating pressures for undiluted LP gas systems in buildings shall not exceed 20 psi, according to *NFPA 54: National Fuel Gas Code* (NFPA 2015a).

The same observations with regard to leaks and failures that apply to LP gas delivery systems, with some additional conditions, apply to flexible rubber connectors (hoses) found on connections to portable cylinders for campers and barbecue grills. The portability of tanks exposes them to weather and mechanical damage from handling, especially as they are refilled. Tanks are labeled to reflect their capacities and the dates of their manufacture and pressure (hydrostatic) testing. The necessity to disconnect and reconnect them repeatedly for filling makes them susceptible to damaged connectors that can cause leaks. Flexible connections can crack with age or misuse.

Because both propane and especially butane are heavier than air, their escape into the air is somewhat different from that of methane, a major constituent of natural gas. Being heavy, propane and butane vapors behave more like the fumes of gasoline, which accumulate at low levels in enclosures, where they are less likely to be smelled but more likely to encounter ignition sources. When propane with a vapor density of 1.5 is involved, its density is sufficiently close to that of air to mix more readily with air than heavier fuel gases. In its flammable range, a propane/air mixture is almost the same density as air itself, so it may not settle at all. Modest mechanical stirring in a room, or even the thermal stirring caused by sunlight heating one side of an enclosure, has been shown to mix propane quite uniformly in an enclosed space (Thatcher 1999). Release of gas under pressure causes turbulent mixing.

LP gases give rise to fires (and asphyxiations) more frequently than natural gas due to the nature of the fuels themselves and also to the method of installation, the uses of the appliances, and the storage and distribution equipment. While natural gas is normally delivered from heavy iron pipe, permanently installed and under the specifications of local building ordinances, LP gases are more often delivered through semi-flexible copper tubing installed in an uncontrolled manner by amateur installers, and from removable tanks. In addition, the supply of gas has to be replenished from tank trucks or with portable tanks rather than from a permanent installation. Thus, there is considerably increased chance of poor connections, broken tubing, leaking valves, and similar deficiencies. LP gas water heaters have also been installed to replace costly electric heaters in small closets where ventilation is inadequate when the door is closed.

LP gas is delivered at considerably higher pressures and through differently sized orifices than natural gas. Because of its higher heat of combustion and higher density, it also delivers 2.5 to 3 times as much energy per unit volume. Equipment fitted for one type of gas can seriously malfunction if used with the other. If malfunction of a gas appliance is suspected, the investigator must ensure that the correct type of regulator, burner orifice, and control valve(s) are all in place to match the type of gas used.

Pressurized Containers

Pressurized containers of LP gas, propane, or butane are kept on hand in many types of occupancies to fuel everything from tools like handheld propane torches to camping stoves and barbecues (see Figure 2-27). These containers come in various sizes from 1 lb. to 28 lb. capacity (rated by weight of water equivalent) and are usually not hard to recognize even when fragmented by a **BLEVE** (a boiling liquid expanding vapor explosion). However, there is another source of LP gases that is not as readily identified. A variety of aerosol products, from lubricants, paints, and insecticides to air fresheners, hair sprays, and deodorants, are pressurized with dimethyl ether or mixtures of butane, isobutane, and propane instead of the inert fluorocarbons used for so many years (DeHaan and Howard 1995). These aerosol containers may hold as much as 120 ml of pressurized liquid fuel, which vaporizes immediately upon release. Such small quantities do not present an ignition risk when uniformly diluted throughout an average-size room. But, when enclosed in a cabinet or an appliance, they can form an explosive mixture on release within that space.

Failure of a single aerosol can inside a vehicle will produce explosive concentrations that can do considerable damage. Despite the manufacturer's advice, aerosol products are sometimes used to excess. Entire apartments and houses have been damaged by the release and subsequent ignition of multiple cans. The solvents used in these products, e.g., kerosene for insecticides, alcohols for cosmetics, pose an additional risk of fire if released in the vicinity of an open flame.

Natural gas is also shipped and stored as a cryogenic liquid (CNG) with a boiling point of −160°C (−260°F). When released, CNG causes the formation of a dense vapor cloud denser than air, which poses a significant ignition risk as it spreads (Raj 2006).

Leaks

A gas line may show leakage from inadequate sealing of the joints during installation, from deterioration of joints, or from corrosion severe enough to penetrate the walls of the line. Rigid metal lines can fracture if subjected to severe vibration, mechanical movement, or loading. Leaks may also occur from worn or defective valves, regulators, and fittings. In any of these events, it is expected that the odorant intentionally added to all natural gas will serve as a warning of escaping gas because natural and some manufactured gases are inherently odorless.

Leakage has also followed lightning strikes whose induced current caused perforations of stainless steel and copper gas lines. Goodson reported that corrugated stainless steel tubing (CSST) with a plastic covering intended for residential gas delivery systems has been shown to be perforated by the passage of induced current from lightning strikes, causing perforations 0.04 to 0.15 in. across. These perforations allowed gas leaks into attics and other enclosed spaces where ignitable concentrations could accumulate (Goodson and Hergenrether 2005). Sanderson (2005) has described multiple penetrations of polyethylene gas piping caused by discharge of static electricity built up on the interior of such piping by the passage of particulates (dust and rust) through the pipe. These very small diameter perforations would release gas at low rates that could accumulate in concealed spaces (such as the steel pipe riser near the meter). Chemical corrosion can also cause multiple leaks in any metallic tubing, as shown in Figure 2-28.

BLEVE ■ Boiling liquid expanding vapor explosion (NFPA 2017d, pt. 3.3.20).

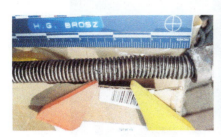

FIGURE 2-28A Corrosion of propane gas flex line caused sufficient leak to cause explosion. *Courtesy of Peter Brosz, Brosz & Associates Forensic Services Inc.; Professor Helmut Brosz, Institute of Forensic Electro-Pathology.*

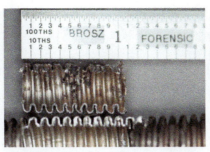

FIGURE 2-28B Internal close-up of chemical corrosion. *Courtesy of Peter Brosz, Brosz & Associates Forensic Services Inc.; Professor Helmut Brosz, Institute of Forensic Electro-Pathology.*

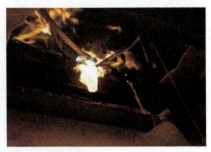

FIGURE 2-28C Electric arc–induced perforation of CSST and ignition of gas. *Courtesy of Jamie Novak, Novak Investigations and St. Paul Fire Dept.*

Assuming that such a leak exists and that it is not noted, the sequence of events is as follows. Initially, the gas is too low in concentration to be ignited from any source. When the gas reaches its lower combustible limit, it will have formed an explosive mixture throughout the area in which the gas concentration has reached this limit. This will normally occur only in a confined or partially confined space, but that space will be under great danger of an explosion—not a fire, initially at least.

If there is a source of ignition, such as a pilot flame, or if a match is ignited by a smoker at this time, an explosion will occur. It can be very forceful, which is characteristic of a stoichiometric mixture, and without continuing flame. If the mixture is not ignited until it accumulates to form a rich mixture, it will generate less mechanical force but will sustain a flame after the explosion. If ignited right at the leak, where there may be some gas/air mixture within the combustible limits locally, a continuing fire is expected. This fire can play, in a blowtorch effect, on other fuels in a direct line and ignite them. The distance the flame will project depends on the pressure of the gas being fed to the line. Typical residential delivery pressures of 0.5 psi or less produce a horizontal jet of flame only 1 or 2 ft. (0.3 to 0.6 m) in length. Industrial or service pressures are much higher, and the flame-jet length will be proportionately longer. Due to the odorants used in utility gas, most gas leaks are detected by residents long before combustible mixtures are produced.

Mechanical Fracture

Release of gas from a mechanically fractured line is rare. However, it is probably more common than is generally believed and occurs even in the absence of natural catastrophes such as earthquakes, landslides, and similar major causes of destruction. For example, a gas line was laid under a street over which there was heavy trucking. Failure to tamp the soil properly around the pipe allowed it to buckle under the recurrent loads until the line parted, filling the soil with gas, which eventually percolated through porous soil to accumulate inside a structure, which led to an explosion and fire.

In another instance, a small gas stove was attached to the gas line with a copper tube and with a soldered connection. The stove was moved around somewhat, with recurrent flexure on the connection. Finally, the joint parted and resulted in both a fire and multiple asphyxiations by the combustion products. As depicted in Figure 2-29, misuse can also lead to leaks. The corrugated flexible connector pipes used on many gas appliances are subject to corrosion by ammonia or sulfur-containing contaminants in the gases and can become dangerously leaky even when not moved. Many lines are now coated to minimize such corrosion.

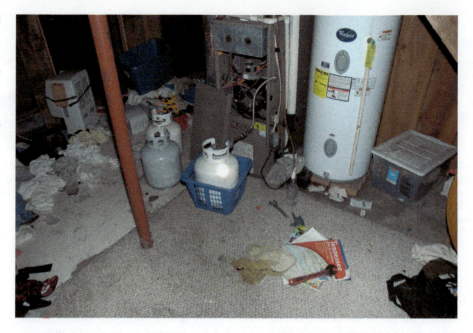

FIGURE 2-29 Improvised use of portable LP tanks for household furnace (note empty cylinders and wrenches). *Courtesy of Greg Lampkin, Knox County Sheriff's Office, Tennessee, Fire Investigation Unit.*

Gas, natural or LP, released from a buried pipe can migrate considerable distances along the loose earth or void space surrounding some gas lines or through porous soils. This migration can result in gas accumulations inside buildings some distance from the actual leak. This process is enhanced if the overlying soil is sealed by pavement, ice, or even frozen soil, which minimizes upward losses. Such percolation through soil can also scrub the gas of its odorant, which means that a leak can exist without witnesses reporting the usual gas odors. Both natural gas and LP gas can also lose their odorants by chemical adsorption onto the walls of new pipe, either steel or plastic, or new containers, or by oxidation by the red iron (oxide) rust inside old, disused, or newly installed steel pipe (NFPA 2017d).

Improperly plumbed gas appliances connected by rubber tubing or even garden hose have been found responsible for leaking fuel that resulted in a fire or explosion. These connections most often leak at joints or connections to metal fittings. The low delivery pressures in most residential structures rarely lead to failure by bursting, but rubber products can degrade from age, sunlight, or exposure to chemicals and can crack or split as they become brittle.

Another type of mechanical malfunction is failure of pressure regulators in gas delivery systems. A failure due to corrosion, mechanical damage, or freezing in any of these regulators can result in massive overpressures being delivered to the appliances. These overpressures, in turn, result in flames exiting the appliances as the burners and vents are unable to accommodate the extra flames and exhaust volume.

As with leakage, release of gas under those circumstances can lead to fire when the gas is ignited directly as it first emerges from the fractured line. If the leaking gas mixes with enough air before it is ignited, there will be an explosion in the accumulated mixture. This explosion is almost always followed by a continuous flame at the source of the fuel gas.

Failure from Heat

Usually, failure of a gas line from excessive heat will be limited to a fire in which the gas is not causally related. Lines are frequently joined by low-melting alloys such as solder. If such a joint is heated by exterior flames or even hot gases, the joint may fail. In very hot structure fires, it is not uncommon to have brass or bronze fittings partially melt (see Figure 2-30). Because brass or bronze fittings are regularly used in connection with gas lines, these failures will be found after the fire. Severe fire heating can cause differential

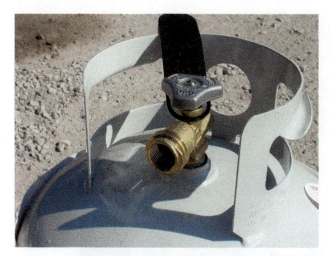

FIGURE 2-30A New LP tank fittings. *Courtesy of Greg Lampkin, Knox County Sheriff's Office, Tennessee, Fire Investigation Unit.*

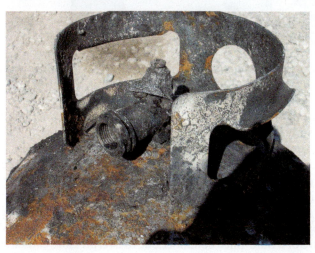

FIGURE 2-30B Post-fire. Partially melted valve and fittings from fire exposure may require X-ray examination to reveal whether they are open or closed. *Courtesy of Greg Lampkin, Knox County Sheriff's Office, Tennessee, Fire Investigation Unit.*

expansion of brass connectors and steel/iron pipe fittings, sometimes resulting in loose connections after cooling.

Because there must already be a fire to melt the attachment in these situations, it is clear that the escaping gas will merely feed additional fuel to the fire locally and will produce a characteristic blowtorch type of burning in front of the opening. A melted connection is not to be considered as a cause of the fire but only as a result of and a contributing factor to the intensity of the fire. The gas cannot spread under these conditions to augment the flames except ahead of the line opening. Under no conceivable circumstances will gas escaping into a burning fire avoid burning locally to be consumed at a distance from the opening. The large blowtorch type of flame will have the effect of causing a burned-out area immediately in front of the opening or charring to adjacent surfaces, as pictured in Figure 2-31. Its effect on the remainder of the fire will be negligible in virtually every circumstance. At worst, the blowtorch type of flame may alter the fire pattern because of local intensity, which tends to deflect air currents to the hottest part of the fire.

Despite the facts, it is quite common for claims to be made that escaping gas severely augmented the total fire throughout a building. This would necessitate that the unburned gas passed through, around, or over burning areas to reach distant portions of the fire. Unusual release conditions might provide mixtures that are too rich to ignite or gases that are moving too quickly to be ignited by a fire in the vicinity of the leak (until they are sufficiently diluted or slowed). This movement would normally be expected to mix

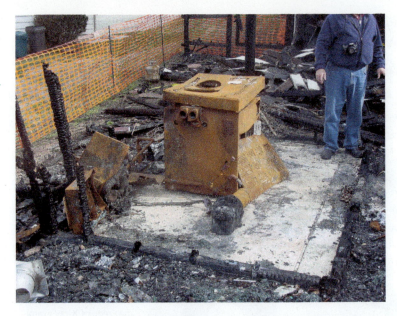

enough air and flames into the gas stream by turbulence that ignition would readily occur immediately.

Another dangerous situation occurs when ignitable liquids are packaged in sealed containers, such as solvents in metal cans or glass bottles. When these containers are exposed to a fire, pressure built up by the expanding liquid prevents the liquid from evaporating. Because evaporation allows a liquid to maintain its temperature at or below its boiling point, the temperatures inside the containers exceed the boiling point of the liquid and may trigger pyrolysis of the liquid. The containers are then filled with a mixture of pressurized liquid, vapor, and (sometimes) gaseous pyrolysis products, which can add greatly to the fuel load of the fire when the containers erupt. These eruptions can occur with explosive force and suddenly and dramatically affect the course and intensity of the general fire. Failure of a fluid-filled container due to overpressure caused by extreme heating is often called a BLEVE, even if the fluids and gases involved are not in themselves combustible.

PART 2: Basic Fire Dynamics

2.11 Basic Fire Dynamics

The body of fire dynamics knowledge as it applies to fire scene reconstruction and analysis is derived from the combined disciplines of physics, thermodynamics, chemistry, heat transfer, and fluid mechanics. Accurate determination of a fire's origin, intensity, growth, direction of travel, duration, and extinguishment requires that investigators rely on and correctly apply all principles of fire dynamics. Investigators must realize that variability in fire growth and development is influenced by a number of factors, such as available fuel load, ventilation, and physical configuration of the room.

Fire investigators can benefit from a working knowledge of published research involving the application of the expertise that exists in the area of fire dynamics. The published research includes several recent textbooks and expert treatises, traditional fire protection engineering references, US government research done primarily by the National Institute of Standards and Technology (NIST) and the US Nuclear Regulatory Commission (NRC), and fire research journals.

Many fire investigators do not routinely have access to all these resources. Bridging this knowledge gap is the primary purpose of this chapter. Many basic fire dynamics concepts are described in *NFPA 921* (NFPA 2017d, Chapter 5). These basic concepts and other, more advanced ones will be discussed later in this textbook. Existing real-world examples and training exercises illustrate their application and describe how basic fire dynamics principles apply to fuels commonly found at fire scenes. Case examples are offered in this chapter along with discussions on the application of accepted fire protection engineering calculations that can assist investigators in interpreting fire behavior and conducting forensic scene reconstruction.

2.11.1 BASIC UNITS OF MEASUREMENT

The common units of measurement and dimensions used in fire scene reconstruction come from two systems: United States (US) and metric. The United States is in the gradual process of converting to the international standard, which is known as the International System of Units (SI, from the French, Système International). It is customary to show all measurements and calculations using the SI system, and in most cases, we give the equivalent English units in parentheses for reference. Table 2-9 lists many commonly used fundamental dimensions from fire dynamics along with their typical symbol, unit, and conversion factor.

The most fundamental property of fire dynamics is heat. All objects above absolute zero (−273°C, −460°F, 0 K) contain heat owing to the motion of their molecules. Sufficient heat transfer by conduction, convection, and radiation to an object increases its temperature and may ignite it, which may spread fire to neighboring objects.

TABLE 2-9	Fundamental Dimensions Commonly Used in Fire Dynamics		
DIMENSION	**SYMBOL**	**SI UNIT**	**CONVERSION**
Length	L	m	1 m = 3.2808 ft.
Area	A	m^2	1 m^2 = 10.7639 ft^2
Volume	V	m^3	1 m^3 = 35.314 ft^3
Mass	M	kg	1 kg = 2.2046 lb.
Mass density	ρ	kg/m^3	1 kg/m^3 = 0.06243 lb./ft^3
Mass flow rate	$\dot{m}$	kg/s	1 kg/s = 2.2 lb./s
Mass flow rate per unit area	$\dot{m}''$	$kg/(s \cdot m^2)$	1 $kg/(s \cdot m^2)$ = 0.205 lb./$(s \cdot ft^2)$
Temperature	T	°C	$T\,(°C) = [T\,(°F) − 32]/1.8$ $T\,(°C) = T\,(K) − 273.15$ $T\,(°F) = [T\,(°C) \times 1.8] + 32$
Temperature	T	K	$T\,(K) = T\,(°C) + 273.15$ $T\,(K) = [T\,(F) + 459.7]0.56$
Energy, heat	Q, q	J	1 kJ = 0.94738 Btu
Heat release rate	$\dot{Q}, \dot{q}$	W	1 W = 3.4121 Btu/hr = 0.95 Btu/s, 1 kW = 1 kJ/s
Heat flux	$\dot{q}''$	W/m^2	1 W/cm^2 = 10 kW/m^2 = 0.317 Btu/$(hr \cdot ft^2)$

Sources: Derived from Drysdale 2011; Karlsson and Quintiere 2000; Quintiere 1998; and SFPE 2008.

2.11.2 THE SCIENCE OF FIRE

exothermic ■ a chemical reaction that releases heat energy.

Fire is simply a rapid oxidation reaction or combustion process involving the release of energy. Friedman (1998) refers to combustion as "an **exothermic** (heat producing) chemical reaction between some substance and oxygen." Although a fire's energy release may be visible in the form of flames or glowing combustion, nonvisible forms exist. Nonvisible forms of energy transfer may include heat transfer in the form of radiation or conduction (Quintiere 1998). Oxidation processes like rusting of iron or yellowing of newsprint generate heat, but so slowly that the temperatures of the objects do not increase perceptibly.

Fire Tetrahedron

fire tetrahedron ■ A geometric representation of the four factors necessary for fire: fuel, heat, an oxidizing agent, and an uninhibited chemical chain reaction.

For fires to exist, four conditions must coexist, which may be represented by what is commonly known as the **fire tetrahedron**, shown in Figure 2-32. The basic components of the tetrahedron are (1) the presence of fuel or combustible material, (2) sufficient heat to raise the material to its ignition temperature and release fuel vapors, (3) enough of an oxidizing agent to sustain combustion, and (4) conditions that allow uninhibited exothermic chemical chain reactions to occur. The science of fire prevention and extinguishment is based on the isolation or removal of one or more of these components.

The action of heat on a flammable liquid fuel causes simple evaporation (i.e., liquid transformed into a vapor). The action of heat on most solid fuels causes the chemical breakdown of the molecular structure, called pyrolysis, into vapors, gases, and residual solid (char). The pyrolysis also absorbs some heat from the reaction, i.e., it is an **endothermic** process.

endothermic ■ a chemical reaction that absorbs heat energy.

The flaming combustion of the gases from a liquid or solid generally takes place within an area above the fuel's surface. Heat and mass transfer processes create a situation in which the fuel generates a region of vapors that can be ignited and sustained with the proper conditions (Figure 2-33).

Types of Fires

There are four recognized categories of combustion or fire types: (1) diffusion flames, (2) premixed flames, (3) smoldering combustion, and (4) spontaneous combustion (Quintiere 1998). Diffusion flames make up the category of most natural-fuel–controlled flaming fires such as candles, campfires, and fireplaces. These occur as fuel gases or vapors diffuse from the fuel surface into the surrounding air. In the zone where appropriate concentrations of fuel and oxygen are present, flaming combustion will occur. Oxygen in the air will move (diffuse) to the flame reaction zone as it is consumed in the combustion process.

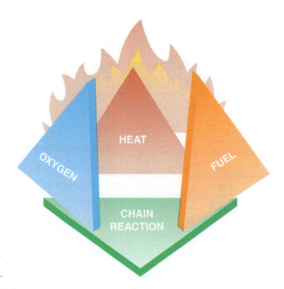

FIGURE 2-32 The fire tetrahedron.

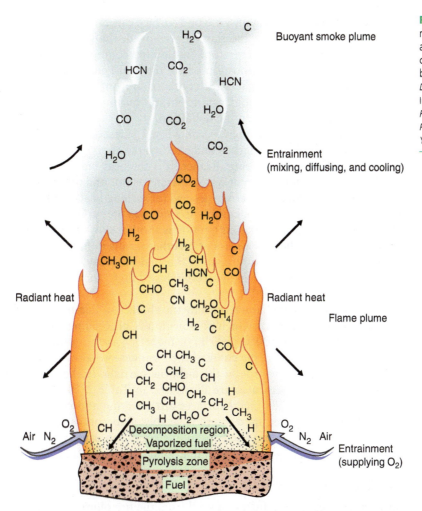

FIGURE 2-33 Schematic representation of the heat and mass transfer processes associated with a burning surface. *From DeHaan, J. D. 2012.* Kirk's Fire Investigation. *7th ed. Reprinted by permission of Pearson Education, Inc., New York Inc.*

If fuel and oxygen are combined prior to ignition, the resulting combustion process is known as premixed flames. These fuels generally consist of either vaporized liquid fuels or gases. Ignition of these gas or vapor mixtures is possible within regions bounded by upper and lower fuel/oxygen concentrations. In a jet engine, a special type of flame can occur when the fuel vapor is released under pressure into the air and mixes by mechanical action to produce an ignitable mixture.

Smoldering is typically a slow-propagating, self-sustained exothermic process in which oxygen combines directly with the fuel at its surface or within it, if it is porous. If enough heat is being produced, the surface may glow with incandescent reaction zones. Smoldering fires are characterized by visible charring and absence of flame. A discarded or dropped cigarette on the surface of a couch, mattress, or other upholstered furniture can cause a smoldering fire. Although smoldering combustion does not emit a visible glow, it does generate heat detectable by touch.

The terms **glowing combustion** and smoldering combustion are often used interchangeably, but there is a distinction between the two. Both terms refer to flameless oxidative exothermic combustion where oxygen is combining directly with the solid fuel surface and creating heat. Glowing combustion occurs where direct surface reactions become dominant on charring materials (Babrauskas 2003). If ventilation is aided by draft or extra oxygen, the glowing can be maintained (as observed when bellows are used on a smoldering wood fire). This type of combustion is dependent on external heating and may not be a self-sustaining reaction.

smoldering ■
Combustion without flame, usually with incandescence and smoke (NFPA 2017d, pt. 3.3.164).

glowing combustion ■
Luminous burning of solid material without a visible flame (NFPA 2017d, pt. 3.3.97).

A torch flame played against a wood surface can cause it to char and glow where the flame is applied, but when the flame is removed, the glow stops and the combustion diminishes, often to a complete stop. Smoldering combustion can best be described as a self-sustaining flameless combustion where the heat generated by the reaction heats surrounding fuel to the point where the combustion front advances and continues to grow. The layperson often uses smoldering to mean "burning with flames that are not large," but this is not the correct scientific definition.

A similar misperception may occur when a surface heated by radiant or convective heat transfer is observed to darken and emit white vapors. This process is sometimes erroneously described as smoldering. Rather, it is the heat-induced pyrolysis of the fuel surface that causes the formation of wisps of water vapor and other vapors, sometimes called off-gassing. This is an endothermic process (absorbing heat), and when the external heating is halted, the vapor or smoke emission stops as the surface temperature drops rapidly.

Like smoldering, spontaneous ignition is another slow chemical reaction. **Self-heating** can produce enough heat in a mass of fuel that results in flaming or sustained smoldering combustion at a critical point known as **thermal runaway**. Spontaneous combustion usually involves naturally occurring vegetable-based fuels, such as those found in peanut and linseed oils (Babrauskas 2003).

A smoldering fire is characterized by the absence of flame but the presence of very hot materials on the surface of which combustion is proceeding. If the temperature of that surface is high enough [500°C (900°F) or higher], a visible glow or incandescence can be seen. As we shall see later, the color of the incandescent glow on the surface is related to its temperature, as is also true of the airborne particles in the flame. Some visible colors and their related temperatures are illustrated in Table 2-10. These are not the temper colors visible on polished metal surfaces after heating and cooling. The words glowing and smoldering are often used interchangeably. Babrauskas (2003), however, describes glowing combustion as a non-self-sustaining condition usually as a result of forced ventilation, while smoldering is self-sustaining solid gas combustion.

2.11.3 HEAT TRANSFER

During a fire, heat is usually transferred from the fire plume to surrounding objects, compartment surfaces, and occupants by three fundamental methods: (1) conduction, (2) convection, and (3) radiation.

The relative importance of these three methods that dominate a fire depends on not only the intensity and size of the fire but also the physical environment. The heat

self-heating ■ The result of exothermic reactions, occurring spontaneously in some materials under certain conditions, whereby heat is generated at a rate sufficient to raise the temperature of the material (NFPA 2017d, pt. 3.3.153).

thermal runaway ■ An unstable condition when the heat generated exceeds the heat losses within the material to the environment. The temperature rise is so large that stable conditions no longer exist (NFPA 2017d, pt. 5.7.4.1.3).

TABLE 2-10	Visual Color Temperatures of Incandescent Hot Objects	
COLOR	APPROXIMATE TEMPERATURE (°C)	APPROXIMATE TEMPERATURE (°F)
Dark red (first visible glow)	500–600	930–1,100
Dull red	600–800	1,110–1,470
Bright cherry red	800–1,000	1,470–1,830
Orange	1,000–1,200	1,830–2,200
Bright yellow	1,200–1,400	2,200–2,550
White	1,400–1,600	2,550–2,910

Source: Data taken from Turner, C. F., and J. W. McCreery. 1981. *The Chemistry of Fire and Hazardous Materials.* Boston: Allyn and Bacon, 90. See also Drysdale, D. D. 1999. *An Introduction to Fire Dynamics.* 2nd ed. Chichester, UK: Wiley, 53.

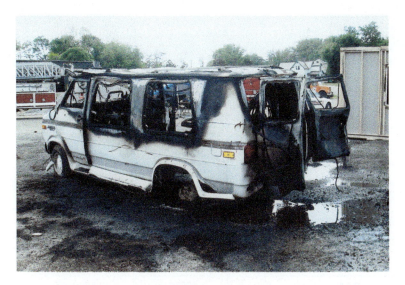

FIGURE 2-34 Example of internal conductive heat transfer through the rear doors from a fire inside the vehicle. *Courtesy of Capt. Sandra K. Wesson, Donan Fire Investigations.*

transferred increases the surface temperature of the target, which can cause observable and measurable effects.

Conduction

Through the process of **conduction**, thermal energy passes from a warmer to a cooler area of a solid material. Heat conducted through walls, ceilings, and other adjacent objects often leaves signs of fire damage based on the varying temperature gradients (Figure 2-34).

The general equations used in conductive heat transfer through a solid whose faces are at different temperatures, T_1 (cooler) and T_2 (warmer), are:

$$\dot{q} = \frac{kA(T_2 - T_1)}{l} = \frac{kA(\Delta T)}{l}, \tag{2.4}$$

$$\dot{q}'' = \frac{\dot{q}}{A} = \frac{kA(\Delta T)}{Al} = \frac{k(\Delta T)}{l}, \tag{2.5}$$

where

$\dot{q}$ = conduction heat transfer rate (J/s or W),
$\dot{q}''$ = conductive heat flux (W/m^2),
k = thermal conductivity of material [W/(m · K)],
A = area through which the heat is being conducted (m^2),
$\Delta T = (T_2 - T_1)$ wall face temperature difference between the warmer, T_2,
and cooler, T_1, (K or °C) surfaces, and
l = length of material through which heat is being conducted (m).

Conduction requires direct physical contact between the source and the target receiving the heat energy. For example, heat from a fire in a living room may be conducted through a poorly insulated common wall to an adjoining room, producing surface demarcation patterns. In an investigation, examine and record damage to both sides of interior and exterior walls and surface materials. Interior wall finishing materials such as wood paneling may also have to be removed to evaluate the effects of heat transfer. See Table 2-11 for the thermal characteristics of typical materials found at fire scenes.

conduction ■ Process of transferring heat through a material or between materials by direct physical contact. The transfer of energy in the form of heat by direct contact through the excitation of molecules and/or particles driven by a temperature difference (NFPA 2017d, pt. 3.3.38).

MATERIAL	THERMAL CONDUCTIVITY k [W/(m · K)]	DENSITY ρ (kg/m³)	SPECIFIC HEAT c_p [J/(kg · K)]	THERMAL INERTIA $k\rho c_p$ [W² · s/(m⁴ · K²)]
Copper	387	8940	380	1.30×10^9
Steel	45.8	7850	460	1.65×10^8
Brick	0.69	1600	840	9.27×10^5
Concrete	0.8–1.4	1900–2300	880	2×10^6
Glass	0.76	2700	840	1.72×10^6
Gypsum plaster	0.48	1440	840	5.81×10^5
PPMA	0.19	1190	1420	3.21×10^5
Oak	0.17	800	2380	3.24×10^5
Yellow pine	0.14	640	2850	2.55×10^5
Asbestos	0.15	577	1050	9.09×10^4
Fiberboard	0.041	229	2090	1.96×10^4
Polyurethane foam	0.034	20	1400	9.52×10^2
Air	0.026	1.1	1040	2.97×10^1

TABLE 2-11 Thermal Characteristics of Common Materials Found at Fire Scenes

Sources: Data derived from Drysdale 2011, 37.

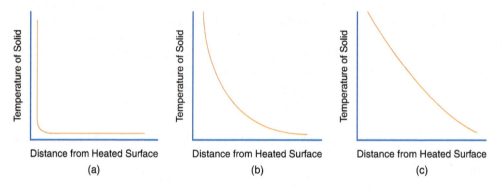

FIGURE 2-35 Temperature distribution through conduction for (a) short duration, (b) medium duration, and (c) steady state.

The graphs in Figure 2-35 illustrate the temperature during short- and medium-duration conductions and steady-state conduction through a solid material. During short-duration conduction, heat flux events produce high surface temperatures, with the inner core staying much cooler. Increasing the time duration of heat transfer increases the internal temperature of the solid and eventually produces a nearly linear temperature gradient from front (hot) to rear (cool).

Convection

The second process, **convection**, is the transfer of heat energy via movement of liquids or gases from a warmer to a cooler area, also known as Newton's law of cooling. An indicator of convective heat transfer damage may be found in the region where a fire plume contacts the ceiling directly above the plume.

convection ■ Heat transfer by circulation within a medium such as a gas or a liquid (NFPA 2017d, pt. 3.3.39).

The general equations used in convective heat transfer are

$$\dot{q} = hA(T_\infty - T_s) = hA(\Delta T), \qquad (2.6)$$

$$\dot{q}'' = \frac{\dot{q}}{A} = \frac{hA(\Delta T)}{A} = h\Delta T, \qquad (2.7)$$

where

$\dot{q}$ = convective heat transfer rate (J/s or W),
$\dot{q}''$ = convective heat flux (W/m^2),
h = convective heat transfer coefficient [W/(m^2 · K)],
A = area through which the heat is being convected (m^2), and
$\Delta T = (T_\infty - T_s)$ temperature difference between the fluid, T_∞, and the surface, T_S (K or °C).

The term h, the convective heat transfer coefficient [W/(m^2 · K)], is dependent on the nature of the surface and the velocity of the gas. Typical values for air are 5 to 25 W/(m^2 · K) for free convection and 10 to 500 W/(m^2 · K) for forced convection (Drysdale 2011).

Closer examination of surface features will usually indicate the direction and intensity of the fire plume and ceiling jet, which contain heated products of combustion such as hot gases, soot, ash, pyrolysates, and burning embers. During the early stages of fire development, the most extensive damage normally exists at the plume's impingement on the ceiling directly above the fire source. Generally, materials farther from the fire plume will exhibit less damage. In the later stages of fire development, the more extensive convection-related damage may be located remote from the fire origin. This damage can be associated with the flow of heated combustion products through vents and adjacent compartments and may include the intense burning of pyrolysates (fuel) where adequate mixing with oxygen occurs.

Radiation

The third process, **radiation**, is the emission of heat energy via electromagnetic waves from a surface at a temperature above absolute zero (0 K). Heat transfer by radiation often damages surfaces facing the fire plume, including immobile objects such as furniture. Convection and radiation are responsible for most victim burn injuries. Radiant heat travels in straight lines and can be reflected by some materials and transmitted by others. The total thermal effect on a material's target surface may be a combination of conductive, convective, and radiative heat transfer rates.

radiation ■ Heat transfer by way of electromagnetic energy (NFPA 2017d, pt. 3.3.153).

The equation for radiative heat flux received by a target surface is represented in general terms by

$$\dot{q}'' = \varepsilon \sigma T_2^4 F_{12}, \qquad (2.8)$$

where

$\dot{q}''$ = radiative heat transfer flux (kW/m^2),
ε = emissivity of the hot surface (dimensionless),
σ = Stefan-Boltzmann constant = 5.67×10^{-11} (kW/m^2)/K^4 *or* kW/(m^2 · K^4),
T_2 = temperature of the emitting body (K), and
F_{12} = configuration factor (depends on the surface characteristics, orientation, and distance).

On heated solid and liquid surfaces the emissivity is commonly 0.8 ± 0.2. The emissivities for gaseous flames depend on their fuel and thickness, and may be very low if the layer is thin. Most are approximately 0.5 to 0.7 (Quintiere 1998).

Guidelines for interpreting the damage due to radiation are simple—the investigator should generally start with the least damaged surfaces farthest from the apparent fire plume, systematically advancing toward the apparent area of most intense fire. Areas of more intense damage to these surfaces often are closer to the most severe radiant heat source. By comparing these damaged surfaces, an investigator can often determine the direction of the fire movement and intensity as it developed. After this evaluation, the investigator assesses the fire development and spread to assist in determining an area and potential point of fire origin.

Superposition

superposition ■ The combined effect of two or more fires or heat transfer effects, a phenomenon that may generate confusing fire damage indicators.

Superposition is the combined effect of two or more fires or heat transfer effects, a phenomenon that may generate confusing fire damage indicators. The predominant heat transfer mode through direct flame impingement (flame contact, for example) involves both radiant and convective heat transfer from the flaming gases to the surface, as well as some conduction through the surface. Direct flame impingement is a case of superposition in which the high radiant heat flux and high convective transfer of the flame quickly affect the exposed fuels. Such combined effects can quickly ignite fuels and raise others to very high surface temperatures.

Because the goal of an arsonist is often the rapid destruction of a building, multiple-set fires are often encountered. These fires, which initially consist of separate plumes, can confuse even the most experienced investigator, particularly when their sequence of ignition is unknown, and the effects of separate fires overlap. Additionally, separate multiple fires can occur when there is a collapse or fall down of burning materials, such as hanging draperies or window shades involved as fire spreads from a single origin. If multiple points of fire origin are suspected, the investigator should evaluate the combined heat transfer effects or superposition of these plumes.

EXAMPLE 2-1 ■ Heat Transfer Calculations

Problem. A fire in a storage room in an automobile repair garage raises the temperature of the interior surface of the brick walls and ceiling over a period of time to 500°C (932°F or 773 K). The ambient air temperature on the outside of the brick wall of the garage is 20°C (68°F or 293 K). The thickness of the brick wall is 200 mm (0.2 m), and its convective heat transfer coefficient is 12 W/(m² · K). Calculate the temperature to which the exterior of the wall will be raised.

Suggested Solution: Conductive-Convective Problem. In this solution, the configuration is considered a plane wall of uniform homogenous material (brick) having a constant thermal conductivity, a given interior surface temperature of $T_S = 500°C$ (932°F or 773 K), and exposed to an external garage ambient air temperature of $T_a = 20°C$ (68°F or 293 K). The external surface temperature, T_E, of the wall is unknown. This temperature might be important later if combustible materials come into contact with this wall surface.

Since the steady-state heat transfer rate of conduction through the brick wall is equal to the heat transfer rate of convection passing into the ambient air outside the garage,

$$\dot{q}'' = \frac{\dot{q}}{A} = \frac{T_S - T_E}{L/k} = \frac{T_E - T_a}{1/h}, \tag{2.9}$$

where

$\dot{q}$ = conduction heat transfer rate (J/s or W),
$\dot{q}''$ = conductive heat flux (W/m²),
h = convective heat transfer coefficient [W/(m² · K)] (brick to air),
k = thermal conductivity of material [W/(m · K)] (through brick),
L = path length through which heat is being conducted (m),
A = area through which the heat is being conducted (m²), and
$\Delta T = (T_S - T_E)$ wall face temperature difference between the warmer T_S and cooler T_E(K).

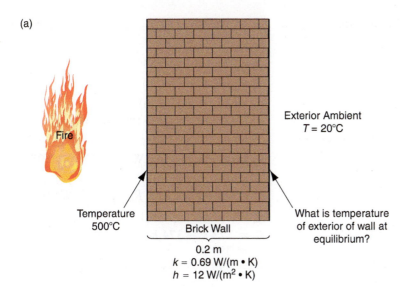

(a)

Fire

Exterior Ambient
T = 20°C

Temperature
500°C

Brick Wall

What is temperature
of exterior of wall at
equilibrium?

0.2 m
$k = 0.69 \text{ W/(m} \cdot \text{K)}$
$h = 12 \text{ W/(m}^2 \cdot \text{K)}$

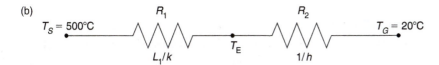

(b)

$T_S = 500°C$ R_1 R_2 $T_G = 20°C$

T_E

L_1/k $1/h$

FIGURE 2-36 (a) Heat transfer by conduction: surface temperature calculation. (b) Heat transfer by conduction: electrical analog.

$$\frac{773 \text{ K} - T_E}{0.2 \text{ m}/[0.69 \text{ W}/(\text{m} \cdot \text{K})]} = \frac{T_E - 293 \text{ K}}{1/[12 \text{ W}/(\text{m}^2 \cdot \text{K})]}$$

$$2665 - 2.448 T_E = 12.05 T_E - 3530$$

$$T_E = \frac{6195}{15.49} = 399 \text{ K} = 126°C \ (258°F)$$

Suggested Alternative Solution: Electrical Analog. Assuming that the brick maintains its integrity during the fire, determine the steady-state temperature of the wall's surface in the garage [example modified from Drysdale (2011)]. A one-dimensional electrical circuit analog, shown in Figure 2-36(a), is used in this solution because we can look at the way heat transfers through a material in the same way that current flows through resistors.

Solutions by electrical analogs are often used. The steady-state heat transfer solution is best illustrated by a direct-current electrical circuit analogy, where the temperatures are voltages ($V = T$) and the thermal resistances of heat convection and conduction are represented as electrical resistances ($R_1 = L_b/k_n$, and $R_2 = 1/h_h$, respectively). The heat flux, $\dot{q}''$, whose units are W/m^2, is analogous to the current, that is, $I = \dot{q}''$.

The problem can be represented as shown in Figure 2-36(b) as a steady-state electrical circuit analog, where R_1 and R_2 are the thermal resistances of the brick wall and inner air of the garage, respectively.

Temperature in storage room	$T_S = 500°C$ (773 K)
Temperature in garage	$T_G = 20°C$ (293 K)
Thermal conductivity	$k = 0.69$ W/(m·K)
Thickness of the brick	$L = 200$ mm (0.2 m)
Conductive thermal resistance	$R_1 = \Delta L/k = (0.2$ m$)/(0.69$ W/ (m·K)$) = 0.290$ (m²·K)/W
Convective heat transfer coefficient	$h = 12$ W/(m²·K)
Convective resistance	$R_2 = 1/h = (1)/[12$ W/(m²·K)$] = 0.083$ (m²·K)/W
Total heat flux	$\dot{q}'' = (T_S - T_G)/(R_1 + R_2) = 1287$ W/m²
	$T_E = 773$ K $- (\dot{q}'')(R_1)$
Exterior wall temperature	$T_E = 773$ K $- 374$ K
	$= 399$ K
	$T_E = 399$ K $- 273 = 126°C$ (258°F)

2.11.4 HEAT RELEASE RATE

heat release rate (HRR) ▪ The rate at which heat energy is generated by burning (NFPA 2017d, pt. 3.3.105).

watt (W) ▪ Unit of power, or rate of work, equal to one joule per second, or the rate of work represented by a current of one ampere under the potential of one volt (NFPA 2017d, pt. 3.3.203).

The **heat release rate (HRR)** of a fire is the amount of heat released per unit time by a heat source. The term is often expressed in **watts** (W), kilowatts (kW), megawatts (MW), kilojoules per second (kJ/s), or Btus per second (Btu/s) and is denoted in formulas as $\dot{Q}$ (the dot over the Q means per unit time). For general conversion purposes, 3412 Btu/hr = 0.95 Btu/s = 1 kJ/s = 1000 W = 1 kW.

Release Rates

The HRR is essentially the size or power of the fire. Three important effects of HRR make it the single most important variable in describing a fire and the hazards associated with its interaction with buildings and their occupants (Babrauskas and Peacock 1992; Bukowski 1995b):

- Heat release rate increase (increases the size of the developing fire)
- Correlation with other effects (smoke production, temperature)
- Occupant tenability

First, and most important, heat released by a fire is the driving force that subsequently produces more fuel by evaporation or pyrolysis. This increased fuel production can lead to a further increase in HRR (a growing fire). As long as adequate quantities of fuel and oxygen are available, the transfer of heat from the burning fuel causes pyrolysis or an exothermic condition, and more heat is released from it and surrounding fuels. It is not guaranteed that all the fuel will burn. As with burning characteristics of fuels, there are physical limits to theoretical and actual HRRs.

Second, another important role of the HRR in forensic fire scene reconstruction is that it directly correlates with other variables. These include the production of smoke and toxic by-products of combustion, room temperatures, heat flux, mass loss rates, and flame height.

Third, there is direct correlation between high HRRs and lethality of a fire. High HRRs produce high mass loss rates of burning materials, some of which may be very toxic. High heat fluxes, large volumes of high-temperature smoke, and toxic gases may overwhelm occupants, preventing their safe escape during fires (Babrauskas and Peacock 1992).

Drysdale (1985) introduced the concept of HRRs to fire investigators in 1985, when he introduced formulas for the calculation of estimated flame heights and onset time for flashover.

TABLE 2-12 Peak Heat Release Rates for Common Objects Found at Fire Scenes

MATERIAL	TOTAL MASS (kg)	PEAK HEAT RELEASE RATE (kW)	TIME (s)	TOTAL HEAT RELEASED (MJ)
Cigarette	—	0.005 (5 W)	—	—
Wooden kitchen match or cigarette lighter	—	0.050 (50 W)	—	—
Candle	—	0.05–0.08 (50–80 W)	—	—
Wastepaper basket	0.94	50	350	5.8
Office wastebasket with paper	—	50–150	—	—
Pillow, latex foam	1.24	117	350	27.5
Small chair (some padding)	—	150–250	—	—
Television set (T1)	39.8	290	670	150
Armchair (modern)	—	350–750 (typical)–1.2 MW	—	—
Recliner (synthetic padding and covering)	—	500–1000 (1 MW)	—	—
Christmas tree (T17)	7.0	650	350	41
Pool of gasoline (2 qt., on concrete)	—	1 MW	—	—
Christmas tree (dry, 6–7 ft.)	—	1–2 MW (typical)–5 MW	—	—
Sofa (synthetic padding and covering)	—	1–3 MW	—	—
Living room or bedroom (fully involved)	—	3–10 MW	—	—

Sources: Data derived from Gorbett, Pharr, and Rockwell 2016, 133; Karlsson and Quintiere 2000, 26; and SFPE 2008, Chapter 3-1.

The peak heat release rate is dependent on the fuel present, its surface area, and its physical configuration. The HRRs of many typical fuels are available on the NIST website, www.fire.nist.gov. Other fire dynamics factors that relate to the HRR include mass loss, mass flux, heat flux, and combustion efficiency.

These equations attempted to answer the following important questions:

- How intense was the fire, and could it ignite nearby combustibles or produce thermal injuries to humans?
- Was an ignitable liquid of sufficient quantity used in the fire, and how high did the flames reach?
- Were conditions right for flashover to occur?
- When did the smoke detectors and/or sprinklers activate?

An investigator's basic question centers on the peak HRR, which can range from several watts to thousands of megawatts. Table 2-12 lists peak HRRs for common burning items of potential interest to fire investigators.

Heat of Combustion

A material's heat of combustion is the amount of heat released per unit of mass during combustion, expressed in (MJ/kg) or kilojoules per gram (kJ/g). The term Δh_c denotes the complete heat of combustion and is used when all the material combusts, leaving no fuel behind. The effective heat of combustion, denoted by Δh_{eff}, is reserved for more realistic cases where combustion is not complete, and the heat lost to heating the fuel is considered.

Mass Loss

The mass loss rate or burning rate of a fuel typically depends on three factors: type of fuel, configuration, and area involved. For example, a campfire constructed with small sticks of dry wood arranged in a tent configuration will burn more quickly and yield a higher HRR over a shorter period of time than one using wet, large-dimensioned wood placed in a haphazard arrangement. This burning rate is expressed in kilograms per second (kg/s) or grams per second (g/s).

The HRR can be calculated from the mass loss rate and heat of combustion of an object. The HRR can be calculated using the general equation (2.6). Mass loss rates can be experimentally determined by simply weighing a fuel package while it burns.

The heat release rate, $\dot{Q}$, can be calculated from

$$\dot{Q} = \dot{m}\Delta h_c, \tag{2.10}$$

where

$\dot{Q}$ = heat release rate (kJ/s or kW),
$\dot{m}$ = burning rate or mass loss rate (g/s), and
Δh_c = heat of combustion (kJ/g).

Mass Flux

Another concept related to the HRR is a material's mass flux, or mass burning rate per unit area, expressed in $kg/(m^2 \cdot s)$ and denoted by $\dot{m}''$ in equations. It is measured in laboratory tests where the fuel surface area or pool diameter and orientation are controlled variables, because they can affect $\dot{m}''$ dramatically. When the horizontal burning area of a material is known along with the burning rate per unit area, the heat release rate equation is written

$$\dot{Q} = \dot{m}''\Delta h_c A, \tag{2.11}$$

where

$\dot{Q}$ = total heat release rate (kW),
$\dot{m}''$ = mass burning rate per unit area $[g/(m^2 \cdot s)]$,
Δh_c = heat of combustion (kJ/g), and
A = burning area (m^2).

The amount of heat needed to convert a solid or liquid fuel to a combustible form, gas or vapor, is called the latent heat of vaporization and represents heat that has to be created to initiate and sustain combustion. The energy needed to evaporate a mass unit of fuel, expressed in kilojoules per kilogram (kJ/kg), is denoted by H_L in equations. Solids, unlike liquids, have values of H_L that are grossly time dependent. It is very hard to obtain accurate H_L values for solids. Values for Δh_c, $\dot{m}''$, and H_L are listed in Table 2-13 and are available in the reference literature for various fuels.

heat flux ■ The measure of the rate of heat transfer to a surface, expressed in kW/m² or W/cm² (NFPA 2017d, pt. 3.3.103).

Heat Flux

Another fire dynamics concept vital to interpreting ignition, flame spread, and burn injuries is **heat flux**. Heat flux is the rate at which heat is falling on a surface or passing through an area, measured in kilowatts per square meter (kW/m²), and is represented by the symbol $\dot{q}''$.

TABLE 2-13 — Typical Mass Flux, Heat of Vaporization, and Effective Heat of Combustion for Common Materials

COMMON MATERIAL	MASS FLUX $\dot{m}''$ [g/(m² · s)]	HEAT OF VAPORIZATION H_L (kJ/g)	HEAT OF COMBUSTION (EFFECTIVE) ΔH_{eff} (kJ/g)
Gasoline	44–53	0.33	43.7
Kerosene	49	0.67	43.2
Paper	6.7	2.21–3.55	16.3–19.7
Wood	70–80	0.95–1.82	13–15

Sources: Derived from SFPE 2008; Quintiere 1998.

The radiant heat output (emissive power) of a surface at temperature T is expressed as

$$\dot{q}'' = \varepsilon\sigma T^4, \tag{2.12}$$

where

ε = emissivity of the source fire,
σ = Stefan-Boltzmann constant, and
T = Kelvin temperature of the surface,

so the higher the temperature of a source, the greater the heat flux from that source. Heat flux increases as a function of temperature, T (K), to the fourth power.

Two important pieces of information can be obtained if an investigator can estimate the heat flux and its duration: (1) whether ignition of a secondary or target surface can be achieved and (2) whether thermal injury to a victim exposed to a fire is possible. The minimum heat flux needed to produce thermal injuries and to ignite some common fuels is presented in Table 2-14.

TABLE 2-14 — Impact of a Range of Radiant Heat Flux Values

RADIANT HEAT FLUX (kW/m²)	OBSERVED EFFECT ON HUMANS AND WOODEN SURFACES
170	Maximum heat flux measured in post-flashover fires
80	Thermal protective performance (TPP) test
52	Fiberboard ignites after 5 seconds
20	Floor of residential family room at flashover
16	Pain, blisters, second-degree burns to skin at 5 seconds
7.5	Wood ignites after prolonged exposure (piloted or not)
6.4	Pain, blisters, second-degree burns to skin at 18 seconds
4.5	Blisters, second-degree burns to skin at 30 seconds
2.5	Exposure while firefighting, pain and burns after prolonged exposure
<1.0	Exposure to sun

Sources: Derived from *NFPA 921* (NFPA 2017d, Table 5.5.4.2) and Gratkowski, Dembsey, and Beyler 2006

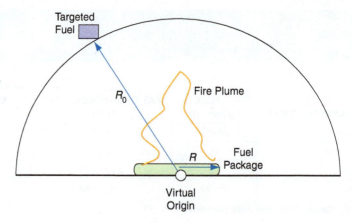

FIGURE 2-37 Schematic illustration of radiant heat transfer from a point source (virtual origin) of a fire plume to a target.

Heat fluxes from various flames and fires are listed in detail in the *Ignition Handbook* (Babrauskas 2003). Because, in most cases, these values are difficult to measure and even more difficult to accurately estimate, the investigator should consult these published experimental data.

In the simplest of cases, radiant heat flux from a fire plume can be approximated as emerging from a single point source known as the virtual origin. A schematic illustration of the concept of radiant heat transfer from a point source of a flame to a target is shown in Figure 2-37 (NFPA 2008).

The equation used to predict the incident heat flux falling on an object or victim from a point-source fire, as in Figure 2-37, is

$$\dot{q}_0'' = \frac{P}{4\pi R_0^2} = \frac{X_r \dot{Q}}{4\pi R_0^2},$$
(2.13)

where

$\dot{q}_0''$ = incident radiation flux on target (kW/m²),
P = total radiative power of the flame (kW),
R_0 = distance to the target surface (m),
X_r = radiative fraction (typically 0.20 to 0.60), representing the percentage of heat released from the source as radiant heat, and
$\dot{Q}$ = total heat release rate of source (kW),

or, by rearrangement,

$$R_0 = \left(\frac{X_r \dot{Q}}{4\pi \dot{q}''_0} \right)^{1/2}.$$
(2.14)

This equation is valid when the ratio of the distance to the targeted object to the radius (R) of the burning fuel package is

$$\frac{R_0}{R} > 4,$$
(2.15)

that is, when the radius of the burning surface of the fire, R, is small compared with the distance between the target and the fire, R_0, as shown in Figure 2-37.

For cases where

$$\frac{R_0}{R} \leq 4,$$
(2.16)

the source cannot be treated as a point, and the geometry of the target surface relative to the source becomes critical. For each geometry, a configuration factor will have

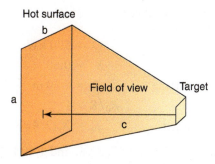

FIGURE 2-38 A small target facing a large radiant heat source (a by b in size) a distance c away is subject to heating from a wide angle of view.

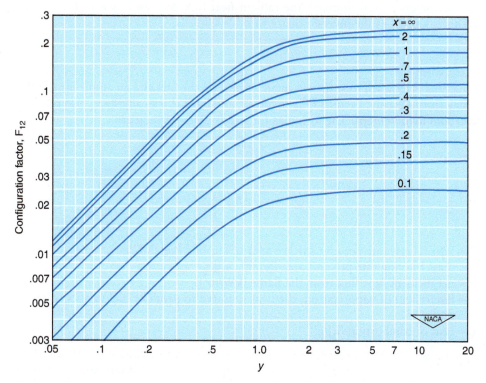

FIGURE 2-39 The configuration factor F_{12} for a geometry like that shown in Figure 2-38 is determined from this monograph, where $x = a/c$, and $y = b/c$. The curve with the closest value for x is selected. The intersection of that curve with the vertical line equal to the calculated value of y gives F_{12}. *From Hamilton and Morgan, NACA Tech. Note 2836, December 1952.*

to be calculated. The configuration factor (F_{12}) appears in the general radiant heat relation

$$\dot{q}'' = \varepsilon \sigma F_{12} T^4 \quad \text{or} \quad \dot{Q} F_{12}. \tag{2.17}$$

Because the calculations can be very complex, F_{12} for a geometry such as that in Figure 2-38 is usually determined from a nomograph such as that in Figure 2-39. Nomographs for various geometries are found in the *SFPE Handbook of Fire Protection Engineering* (SFPE 2008, Appendix D, A44-47).

EXAMPLE 2-2 ■ Heat Flux Calculation

Problem. A 500 kW fire represented as a point source as shown in Figure 2-37 has a surface radius of 0.2 m. Assume the radiative fraction to be 0.60. What is the heat flux falling on the target fuel at distances of R_0 equal to 1, 2, and 4 m?

Suggested Solution. The expected heat release rate can be calculated from equation (2.6).

Heat release rate $\qquad\qquad\qquad\qquad$ $\dot{Q} = 500 \text{ kW}$

Radiative fraction $\qquad\qquad\qquad\qquad$ $X_r = 0.60$

Radius of the burning fuel surface $\qquad$ $R = 0.20 \text{ m}$

Equation ratio test $\qquad\qquad\qquad\qquad$ $R_0/R > 4$

Incident radiation flux on target $\qquad$ $\dot{q}_0'' = X_r\dot{Q}/4\pi R_0^2$

At R_0 equal to 1, 2, and 4 m $\dot{q}_0'' = 23.87, 5.96,$ and 1.49 kW/m^2, respectively.

Note that as the distance is doubled, the radiant heat flux decreases by a factor of one-fourth. This is known as the inverse square rule.

Steady Burning

Once a material is exposed to sufficient incident heat on the fuel and an ample air supply, the fire may spread evenly, become fully involved, and burn at a steady state, also referred to as **full room involvement**. The formulas for steady-state burning are

> **full room involvement** ■ Condition in a compartment fire in which the entire volume is involved in combustion of varying intensities (NFPA 2017d, pt. 3.3.95).

$$\dot{m}'' = \dot{q}''/H_L \qquad (2.18)$$

and

$$\dot{Q}'' = \frac{\dot{q}''}{L_V}\Delta h_c, \qquad (2.19)$$

where

$\dot{Q}''$ = heat release rate per unit surface area of burning fuel (kW/m²),
$\dot{m}''$ = mass burning rate per unit area [g/(m² · s)],
$\dot{q}''$ = net incident heat flux from the flame (kW/m²),
L_V = latent heat of vaporization, the heat required to produce fuel vapors (kJ/g), and
Δh_c = heat of combustion (kJ/g).

These equations are useful because they allow investigators to estimate the steady-state burning rate. For many solid fuels, latent heat of vaporization (L_V) is not constant due to char formation and complex heat and mass transfer processes. L_V can vary with time and is not easily measured.

Combustion Efficiency

The **combustion efficiency** of a substance is the ratio of its effective heat of combustion to the complete heat of combustion and is expressed by the term X, where

> **combustion efficiency** ■ The ratio of a substance's effective heat of combustion to the complete heat of combustion.

$$X = \Delta h_{\text{eff}}/\Delta h_c. \qquad (2.20)$$

Thus, for fuels with more complete combustion, values of X approach 1. Fuels with lower combustion efficiencies—characterized by flames containing products of incomplete combustion, which produce sootier and more luminous fires—have values of X between 0.6 and 0.8 (Karlsson and Quintiere 2000). For example, gasoline typically has a Δh_c of 46, but its Δh_{eff} is 43.8 owing to incomplete combustion ($X = 0.95$). Examples of soot-producing substances include many flammable liquids and thermoplastics.

To account for incomplete combustion for fuels such as plastics and ignitable liquids, the combustion efficiency can be inserted into the equation for the convective heat release rate, $\dot{Q}_c$, where X_r is the energy loss attributable to radiation (typically 0.20 to 0.40):

$$\dot{Q}_c = X\dot{m}''\Delta h_c A(1 - X_r). \qquad (2.21)$$

In calculations of mean flame heights and virtual origins, $\dot{Q}$, is used. When other properties of fire plumes, such as plume radius, centerline temperatures, and velocity are calculated, the convective heat release rate, $\dot{Q}_c$, is used (Karlsson and Quintiere 2000).

EXAMPLE 2-3 ■ Ignitable Liquid Fire

Problem. An arsonist pours a quantity of gasoline onto a concrete floor, creating a 0.46 m (1.5 ft.)-diameter pool. The arsonist ignites the gasoline, creating a fire very similar to a classic burning pool. Estimate the heat release rate from the burning pool using historical fire testing results.

Suggested Solution. Assuming an unconstrained pool fire, the expected heat release rate can be calculated from equation (2.8).

Heat release rate	$\dot{Q} = \dot{m}\Delta h_{eff}A$
Mass flux rate for gasoline	$\dot{m}'' = 0.036\ \text{kg}/(\text{m}^2 \cdot \text{s})$ (reduced by incomplete combustion)
Heat of combustion for gasoline	$\Delta h_{eff} = 43.7\ \text{MJ/kg}$
Area of the burning pool	$A = (\pi/4)(D^2) = (3.1415/4)(0.46^2) = 0.166\ \text{m}^2$
Heat release rate	$\dot{Q} = (0.036)(43,700)(0.166) = 261\ \text{kW}$

The heat release rate of a real fire under these conditions would be expected to be in the range 200 to 300 kW; but in actuality, a thin layer of gasoline will show a heat release rate of only approximately 25 percent of the value computed by the preceding equations, which were developed for pools of substantial depth. For a detailed discussion, see the work by Putorti, McElroy, and Madrzykowski (2001) of NIST.

2.11.5 FIRE DEVELOPMENT

Fires, particularly those within enclosed structures, burn in a predictable manner over time. For the purpose of fire scene reconstruction, development can be divided into four separate fire phases, each containing unique characteristics and its own time frame. These phases are applicable to both single fuel packages and well-ventilated compartment fires. These fire development curves are often referred to as the **fire signature**. The phases and associated physical signs are as follows:

> **fire signature** ■ A fire development curve of time versus heat release rate typically having four phases of incipient ignition, growth, fully developed, and decay.

- *Phase 1:* Incipient ignition—Low heat, some smoke, no detectable flame
- *Phase 2:* Growth—More heat, lots of smoke, flame spread
- *Phase 3:* Fully developed fire—Massive heat and smoke output, extensive flame
- *Phase 4:* Decay—Decreased flame and heat, considerable smoke, with increased smoldering

As shown in Figure 2-40, these phases form a characteristic fire signature or design curve fire, which is often studied for items identified as the source of the first fuel burned in typical structural fires. These phases are important to understanding a fire's growth and its physical effects on the compartment and its contents; calculating the activation of smoke, heat, and automated sprinkler systems; estimating evacuation times; and determining the risk of heat exposure to occupants.

At the transition from phase 2 to phase 3, flashover may occur, depending on the total amount of heat released, the amount of ventilation, the amount of fuel available, and the size and configuration of the compartment. In the absence of flashover, the fire may not become fully developed and instead may reach a maximum size because of limited available fuels, flame spread, or a ventilation limit.

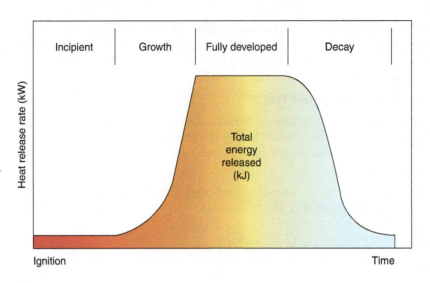

FIGURE 2-40 Fire development phases that often form a fire signature, consisting of (1) ignition, (2) growth, (3) fully developed fire, and (4) decay. *From the* SFPE *Handbook of Fire Protection Engineering, 4th ed., 2008, by permission of Society of Fire Protection Engineers.*

Phase 1: Incipient Ignition

The fundamental properties that influence an object's ignitability are its density, ρ, heat capacity, c_p, and thermal conductivity, k. The calculated product of these three characteristics ($k\rho c_p$) is often referred to as an object's **thermal inertia** and the calculated value $k/\rho c_p$ is called the thermal diffusivity. As with mechanical inertia—where the higher the inertia of an object, the harder it is to move—the higher the thermal inertia, $k\rho c_p$, of a material, the harder it is to ignite—that is, more heat has to be applied or longer exposure is required for ignition to occur.

Table 2-15 lists the ignition properties of some common fuels, where T_{ig} is the approximate surface temperature observed at ignition, and $\dot{q}''_{critical}$ is the minimum heat flux needed to bring about ignition (Drysdale 2011). These results are applicable to short-term exposures (10 to 30 minutes) of fresh, whole products. If heating is prolonged (hours), much lower $\dot{q}''_{critical}$ values may be found. For example, wood products may ignite at approximately 7.5 kW/m² under such conditions. These values do not include long-term heating (i.e., months to years) for the self-heating properties of wood and some other materials.

The temperature of an object is a measure of the relative amount of heat (energy) contained within it. This heat is determined by the mass of the object and its heat capacity, or specific heat. The heat capacity, c_p, of an object is a property that determines how much heat must be added to the object to increase its temperature.

The ignition of an object can be calculated when it is exposed to radiant or convective heat flux, $\dot{q}''$, with no initial contact with flames (autoignition). The calculation assumes that a first burning object (ignition source) provides sufficient radiant heat flux to ignite a second, nonburning fuel object nearby. Experimental fire testing by Babrauskas has established three levels of ignitability: easy, normally resistant, and difficult (SFPE 2002). To establish these relationships, this fire testing included paper, wood, polyurethane, and polyethylene fuels.

Thin materials such as paper and curtains will easily be ignited when exposed to a threshold radiant flux of 10 kW/m² or greater. Thicker or more massive items with low thermal inertia values such as upholstered furniture will ignite when exposed to a radiant flux of 20 kW/m² or greater. Solid materials with thicknesses greater than 13 mm (0.5 in.), such as plastics or dense woods having large thermal inertia values, will ignite when exposed to a radiant flux of 40 kW/m² or greater (SFPE 2008). However, there are exceptions.

thermal inertia ■ The properties of a material that characterize its rate of surface temperature rise when exposed to heat. Thermal inertia is related to the product of the material's thermal conductivity (k), its density (ρ), and its heat capacity (c_p) (NFPA 2017d, pt. 3.3.186).

TABLE 2-15	Ignition Properties		
MATERIAL	**THERMAL INERTIA $k\rho c_p$ KW/$(m^2 \cdot K)s^2$**	**IGNITION TEMPERATURE T_{ig} (°C)**	**CRITICAL HEAT FLUX $\dot{q}''_{critical}$ (kW/m^2)**
Plywood, plain (0.635 cm)	0.46	390	16
Plywood, plain (1.27 cm)	0.54	390	16
Plywood, FR (1.27 cm)	0.76	620	44
Hardboard (6.35 mm)	1.87	298	10
Hardboard (3.175 mm)	0.88	365	14
Hardboard, gloss paint (3.4 mm)	1.22	400	17
Hardboard, nitrocellulose paint	0.79	400	17
Particleboard (1.27 cm stock)	0.93	412	18
Douglas fir particleboard (1.27 cm)	0.94	382	16
Fiber insulation board	0.46	355	14
Polyisocyanurate (5.08 cm)	0.020	445	21
Foam, rigid (2.54 cm)	0.030	435	20
Foam, flexible (2.54 cm)	0.32	390	16
Polystyrene (5.08 cm)	0.38	630	46
Polycarbonate (1.52 mm)	1.16	528	30
PMMA, type G (1.27 cm)	1.02	378	15
PMMA, polycast (1.59 mm)	0.73	278	9
Carpet #1 (wool, stock)	0.11	465	23
Carpet #2 (wool, untreated)	0.25	435	20
Carpet #2 (wool, treated)	0.24	455	22
Carpet (nylon/wool blend)	0.68	412	18
Carpet (acrylic)	0.42	300	10
Gypsum board, common (1.27 mm)	0.45	565	35
Gypsum board, FR (1.27 cm)	0.40	510	28
Gypsum board, wallpaper	0.57	412	18
Asphalt shingle	0.70	378	15
Fiberglass shingle	0.50	445	21
Glass-reinforced polyester (2.24 mm)	0.32	390	16
Glass-reinforced polyester (1.14 mm)	0.72	400	17
Aircraft panel, epoxy fiberite	0.24	505	28

Source: Derived from Quintiere and Harkleroad 1984.

The following equations (2.22), (2.23), and (2.24) are derived from data plots from Babrauskas (1982) published in *SFPE Engineering Guide to Piloted Ignition of Solid Materials under Radiant Exposure* (SFPE 2002). These equations represent piloted ignitions where a burning piece of furniture ignites a second item. They should not be applied to heat release rates from sources that can burn indefinitely e.g., gas jets.

The heat release rates, $\dot{Q}$, needed for a fire source to ignite another fuel package a distance D (measured in meters) away, can be calculated for fuels classified as easy $(\dot{q}''_{\text{crit}} \geq 10 \text{ kW/m}^2)$, normally resistant $(\dot{q}''_{\text{crit}} \geq 20 \text{ kW/m}^2)$, and difficult $(\dot{q}''_{\text{crit}} \geq 40 \text{ kW/m}^2)$, as shown, respectively, in the following equations:

$$\dot{Q} = 30 \times 10^{\left(\frac{D+0.8}{0.89}\right)}, \qquad \dot{q}'' \geq 10 \text{ kW/m}^2, \tag{2.22}$$

$$\dot{Q} = 30\left(\frac{D + 0.05}{0.019}\right), \qquad \dot{q}'' \geq 20 \text{ kW/m}^2, \tag{2.23}$$

$$\dot{Q} = 30\left(\frac{D + 0.02}{0.0092}\right), \qquad \dot{q}'' \geq 40 \text{ kW/m}^2, \tag{2.24}$$

where

$\dot{Q}$ = heat release rate of the source fire (kW), and
D = distance from the radiation source to the second object (m).

The time to ignition for thermally thin and thermally thick materials can be estimated by several equations contained in engineering practice guides developed by the SFPE (2002, 2008). The generally accepted equations for ignition time of thermally thin and thermally thick materials are (2.25) and (2.26), respectively. Under thermally thin conditions, $l_p \leq 1$ mm, (l = thickness of the material),

$$t_{\text{ig}} = \rho c_p l_p \left(\frac{T_{\text{ig}} - T_\infty}{\dot{q}''}\right). \tag{2.25}$$

In thermally thick conditions, $l_p \geq 1$ mm, the thickness term disappears:

$$t_{\text{ig}} = \frac{\pi}{4} k \rho c_p \left(\frac{T_{\text{ig}} - T_\infty}{\dot{q}''}\right), \tag{2.26}$$

where

t_{ig} = time to ignition (s),
k = thermal conductivity [W/(m · K)],
ρ = density (kg/m^3),
c_p = specific heat capacity (kJ/kg · K),
l_p = thickness of material (m),
T_{ig} = piloted fuel ignition temperature (K),
T_∞ = initial temperature (K), and
$\dot{q}''$ = radiant heat flux (kW/m^2).

The ignition behavior of liquids is different, and the preceding equations for solids should not be used.

Phase 2: Fire Growth

Fire growth rates, as shown in Figure 2-42, can sometimes be modeled using mathematical relationships that show the flame spread and fire growth estimations using heat release rates. The growth of the flame front across a horizontal fuel surface of a solid fuel is known as the lateral flame spread and can be expressed by the equation (Quintiere and Harkelroad 1984)

$$V = \frac{\dot{q}''}{\rho c_p A (T_{\text{ig}} - T_S)^2} \tag{2.27}$$

or as

$$V = \frac{\phi}{k \rho c_p (T_{\text{ig}} - T_S)^2} \tag{2.28}$$

TABLE 2-16	Example Lateral Flame Spread Data		
MATERIAL	**PILOTED IGNITION TEMPERATURE** T_{ig} (°C)	**AMBIENT SURFACE TEMPERATURE** T_S(°C)	**IGNITION FACTOR ϕ** (kW²/m³)
Wool carpet			
Treated	435	335	7.3
Untreated	455	365	0.89
Plywood	390	120	13.0
Foam plastic	390	120	11.7
PMMA	378	<90	14.4
Asphalt shingle	356	140	5.4
Acrylic carpet	300	165	9.9

Source: Derived from *ASTM E1321* (ASTM International 2009).

where

V = lateral velocity of flame spread (m/s),
$\dot{q}''$ = radiant heat flux (kW/m²),
ρ = density (kg/m³),
c_p = specific heat capacity [kJ/(kg · K)],
A = cross-sectional area affected by the heating of $\dot{q}''$,
ϕ = ignition factor from flame spread data (kW²/m³) (experimentally derived),
k = thermal conductivity [W/(m · K)],
T_{ig} = piloted fuel ignition temperature (°C), and
T_S = unignited, ambient surface temperature (°C).

ASTM E1321-13: Standard Test Method for Determining Material Ignition and Flame Spread Properties defines the values for ϕ and other variables needed for calculating lateral flame spread (ASTM International 2013b). Table 2-16 lists the horizontal flame spread data for several common materials. An external draft pushes the flame down against the downwind side and increases its radiant heat effect on the fuel in front of its path; the flame front will grow faster if wind aided.

Lateral or downward flame spread on thick solids such as wood is typically slow, on the order of 1×10^{-3} m/s (1 mm/s). In contrast, upward spread on solid fuels is typically 1×10^{-2} to 1 m/s (10 to 1000 mm/s). Lateral flame spread rates across liquid pools are typically 0.01 to 1 m/s, depending on the ambient temperature and the flash point of the liquid (Figure 2-41). Premixed vapor/air mixtures can have flame spread rates of 0.1 to 0.5 m/s for laminar flames. Turbulent flames cause higher flame spreads (1 to 2 m/s over pools of gasoline are typical). Some fuel/air mixtures can produce pressure-driven flames that accelerate to **detonation** velocities (over 1000 m/s) (Drysdale 2011).

Another example of lateral surface flame spread over a solid fuel is a grass, or wildland, fire. Lateral flame spread in this type of fire depends on several key variables: the type of fuel and its configuration, wind velocity and direction, humidity, and terrain. The brush or duff along the forest floor is usually involved in the initial phases of the fire. The terrain, radiant heat transfer, and wind-induced convective heat transfer can contribute significantly to the flame spread along the forest floor. Flame spread through the canopy of trees or brush is a different process and is part of the complexity being studied in ongoing research relating to wildland–urban interface fires.

detonation ■
Propagation of a combustion zone at a velocity greater than the speed of sound in the unreacted medium (NFPA 2013).

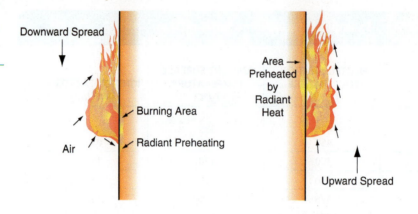

FIGURE 2-41 Radiant heat ahead of an existing flame determines its rate of spread.

Downward Spread

Burning Area

Radiant Preheating

Air

Area Preheated by Radiant Heat

Upward Spread

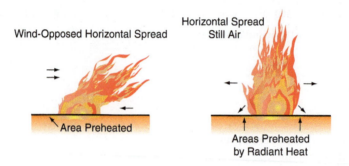

Wind-Opposed Horizontal Spread

Area Preheated

Horizontal Spread Still Air

Areas Preheated by Radiant Heat

The Thomas formula (1971), which can be used to approximate wind-aided horizontal flame spread in grass fires on flat ground, is

$$V = \frac{k(1 + V_\infty)}{\rho b},$$ (2.29)

where

V = velocity of flame spread (m/s),
k = 0.07 wildland fire, 0.05 wood crib (kg/m^3),
V_∞ = wind speed (concurrent) (m/s), and
ρb = bulk density of the fuel (kg/m^3).

EXAMPLE 2-4 ■ Estimating Lateral Flame Travel Velocity

Problem. An investigator determines that a fire ignited at the edge of an untreated wool carpet. What was the estimated velocity of the lateral flame spread, assuming a high radiant heat impact that produced an initial ambient surface temperature of 365°C?

Suggested Solution. Use the Quintiere and Harkelroad equation (2.28) and *ASTM E1321-13* data from Table 2-16.

Ignition factor	ϕ	$= 0.89 \, kW^2/m^3$
Fuel thermal inertia	$k\rho c_p$	$= 0.25 [kW^2 \cdot s/(m^4 \cdot k^2)]$
Piloted fuel ignition temperature	T_{ig}	$= 455°C$
Ambient surface temperature	T_S	$= 365°C$
Velocity of flame spread	V	$= \phi/k\rho c_p (T_{ig} - T_s)^2 = 0.89/0.25(455 - 365)^2$
		$= 0.33 \times 10^{-3}$ m/s $= 26$ mm/min

Notice that the lower the initial temperature (T_S) is, the larger the denominator of equation (2.23) is, and the slower V will be. If the fuel surface is not preheated, the ambient surface temperature becomes $T_S = T_a = 25°C$, where $T_a =$ ambient air temperature, and the velocity of the flame spread V is calculated as follows:

$$V = \phi/kpc_p(T_{ig} - T_s)^2 = 0.89/0.25(455 - 25)^2$$
$$= 0.019 \times 10^{-3} \text{ m/s} = 1.14 \text{ mm/min.}$$

EXAMPLE 2-5 ■ Wildland Flame-Spread Velocity

Problem. Children playing with matches set a fire during a dry season of the year in a flat-terrain wildland area. The wind is blowing at a velocity of 2 m/s, and the bulk density of the low brush along the forest floor is 0.04 g/cm^3. Determine the velocity of the flame spread from this fire with and without considering the effect of the wind.

Suggested Solution. Use the Thomas equation (2.29).

Velocity of flame spread	$V = k(1 + V_\infty)/\rho_b$
Wind speed	$V_\infty = 2$ m/s
Bulk density	$\rho_b = 0.04$ g/cm$^3 = 40$ kg/m^3
Equation constant	$k = 0.07$ kg/m^3
Flame spread velocity (with $V_\infty = 0$ m/s)	$= (0.07)(1 + 0)/(40)$ $= 0.00175$ m/s $= 1.75$ mm/s $= 0.1$ m/min
Flame spread velocity (with $V_\infty = 2$ m/s)	$= (0.07)(1 + 2)/(40)$ $= 0.00525$ m/s $= 5.25$ mm/s $= 0.315$ m/min

Fire growth rates during the initial phases of development can sometimes be modeled using mathematical relationships. One common relationship assumes that the initial growth rate geometrically approximates the square of the time that a fire has burned (also called a t^2 fire), as shown in Figure 2-42. A perfect fire, unlimited by fuel or ventilation

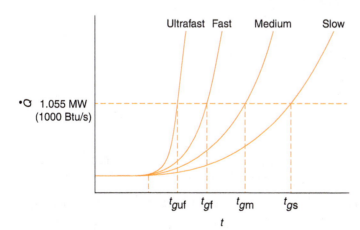

FIGURE 2-42 The fire growth factor α is derived from the graph of Q versus time, where $\alpha = (1055/t_g^2)$, and t_g is the time required for the heat release rate to grow from its baseline (incipient fire) value to 1.055 MW (1000 Btu/s).

factors, would have an exponential growth rate. This behavior applies only to the growth phase.

This accepted growth rate formula is

$$\dot{Q} = (1055/t_g^2)t^2 = \alpha t^2, \qquad (2.30)$$

where

t = time (s),
t_g = time required for fire to grow from ignition to 1.055 MW (1000 Btu/s),
$\dot{Q}$ = heat release rate (MW) at time t, and
α = fire growth factor (kW/s²) for the material being burned.

According to an accepted principle used by *NFPA 72* (detectors) (NFPA 2016a) and *NFPA 92* (NFPA 2015b) (smoke control systems), Table 2-17 and Figure 2-43 illustrate four types of growth times used to define fires by the time required to reach 1.055 MW (1000 Btu/s). The time t_g is obtained from repeated calorimetry tests of specific fuel packages.

TABLE 2-17	Four Growth Rates in t^2 Fires		
TYPE OF FIRE	**EXAMPLE OBJECTS**	**TIME** t_g **(s)**	**FIRE GROWTH FACTOR** α **(kW/s²)**
Slow	Thick wooden objects (tables, cabinets, dressers)	600	0.003
Medium	Lower-density objects (furniture)	300	0.012
Fast	Combustible objects (paper, cardboard boxes, drapes)	150	0.047
Ultrafast	Volatile fuels (flammable liquids, synthetic mattresses)	75	0.190

Sources: Derived from *NFPA 92* (NFPA 2015b) and *NFPA 72* (NFPA 2016a).

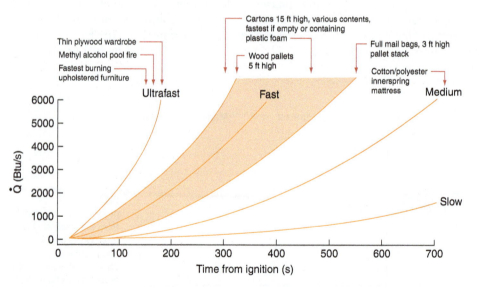

FIGURE 2-43 Relation of t^2 fires to several individual fire tests. The heat release rate is (1000 Btu/s = 1.055 MW). *Courtesy of NIST, from Nelson and Tu, 1991.*

TABLE 2-18	Typical Ranges for Fire Behavior of Materials Stored in Warehouses	

MATERIAL	TYPICAL HEAT RELEASE RATE PER FLOOR AREA COVERED (MW/m²)	CHARACTERISTIC TIME FOR t^2 FIRES TO REACH 1 MW (s)
Wood pallets		
Stacked 0.46 m (1.5 ft.) high	1.3	155–310
Stacked 1.5 m (5 ft.) high	3.7	92–187
Stacked 3.1 m (10 ft.) high	6.6	77–115
Stacked 4.6 m (15 ft.) high	9.9	72–115
Polyethylene bottles in cartons, stacked 4.6 m (15 ft.) high	1.9	72
Polyethylene letter trays, stacked 1.5 m (5 ft.) high	8.2	189
Mail bags, filled, stored 4.6 m (15 ft.) high	0.39	187
Polystyrene jars in cartons, 4.6 m (15 ft.) high	14	53

Source: Based on data from Heskestad, G. 1991. "Venting Practices" Sec. 6, Chap. 10 in Fire Protection Handbook, National Fire Protection Association Quincy, MA: 6.101-6.116.

Table 2-18 shows typical ranges for the heat release rates per unit area and characteristic times for a fire to reach 1.055 MW (1000 Btu/s) in size. These data were obtained from actual fire testing of common materials stored in warehouses.

The slow growth curve ($t_g = 600$ s) usually applies to thick solid objects such as solid wood tables, cabinets, and dressers. The medium growth curve ($t_g = 300$ s) applies to lower-density solid fuels such as upholstered and lightweight furniture. The fast growth curve ($t_g = 150$ s) applies to thin combustible items such as paper, cardboard boxes, and drapes. The ultrafast growth curve ($t_g = 75$ s) is for some flammable liquids, some older types of upholstered furniture and mattresses, or materials containing other volatile fuels (NFPA 2008). The geometry of the objects also has an impact on growth rates.

The t^2 growth rate applies after the initial incipient fire phase, during which the growth rate is nearly zero. In some cases involving polyurethane upholstered furniture, the steady-state phase does not exist, and the approximation for the heat release rate resembles a triangular shape. The approach of fitting a triangular shape to model the heat release rate signatures of furniture can represent up to 91 percent of the total heat released (Babrauskas and Walton 1986).

EXAMPLE 2-6 ■ Loading Dock Fire

Problem. A fire, which was extinguished by an automatic sprinkler system, occurred on the back loading dock of a supply distribution center. A nearby security camera captured the silhouette of a young male running from the loading dock prior to the activation of the sprinkler system.

On examination of the fire scene, the investigator determines that the fire was intentionally set in a cart of polyethylene letter trays on two pallets stacked 1.56 m (5 ft.) high on the loading dock. Determine for the investigator the heat release rate 30 s and 120 s after the arsonist set the fire.

Suggested Solution. Use equation (2.30) for t^2 fire growth and data from Table 2-18 on typical ranges for fire behavior of polyethylene letter trays.

Time to reach 1 MW	$t_g = 189$ s
Growth time of fire	$t = 30$ s
Heat release rate	$\dot{Q} = (1055/t_g^2)t^2$
	$= (1055/189^2)(30^2) \cong 25$ kW
and for	$t = 120$ s
	$\dot{Q} = (1055/189^2)(120^2) = 425$ kW

Phase 3: Fully Developed Fire

The fully developed phase is also referred to as the steady-state phase, either when the fire reaches its maximum burning rate based on the amount of fuel available or when there is insufficient oxygen to continue the growth process (Karlsson and Quintiere 2000). Fuel-controlled fires are associated with steady-state fires, particularly when sufficient oxygen is supplied. The term *fully developed* does not distinguish post-flashover fires from those that die out due to a lack of oxygen.

When there is insufficient oxygen, the fire becomes ventilation-controlled. In this case, the fire is usually in an enclosed room, and temperatures may become higher than in fuel-controlled fires. Fully developed fires in compartments are often postflashover fires in which all the fuel is involved, and the size of the fire becomes ventilation-controlled.

Phase 4: Decay

The fire decay during phase 4 usually occurs when approximately 20 percent of the original fuel remains (Bukowski 1995a). Although most fire service and fire protection specialists are interested in the first three phases of a fire, there are significant problems associated with the decay phase.

In high-rise buildings, for example, even after the fire is extinguished, trapped occupants may need to be rescued. Furthermore, fire investigators entering the building may also be exposed to residual amounts of toxic by-products of combustion, since high concentrations of CO and other toxic gases are produced during the decay phase often dominated by smoldering.

EXAMPLE 2-7 ■ Reliable Test Data

Problem. A fire investigator is trying to develop reliable test data on the length of time a fire may have burned and an estimate of the corresponding heat release rate. The fire was reportedly started by a child playing with a cigarette lighter while sitting at the center of a mattress. The mattress was the only piece of furniture involved in the fire in the room, and a smoke detector in the hallway reportedly activated shortly after the fire began.

Suggested Solution. The information needed by the investigator is found at the "Fire on the Web" Internet site of NIST (www.fire.nist.gov). Collections of actual test data for commonly found items in residential and commercial settings can be found in the Fire Tests/Data section. The data files include still photos, video, graphs, miscellaneous data, and setup data for NIST fire modeling software programs.

Figure 2-44 shows the information needed to compare this case with a similar fire under laboratory testing conditions. The fire test data revealed that the peak heat release rate occurred at approximately 150 seconds (2.5 minutes) after ignition, resulting in a 750 kW fire. When forming the hypothesis for the fire, the investigator could evaluate whether the fire's timeline is reasonably consistent with witness accounts, damage indicators, and heat release data. The investigator needs to remember that the test mattress may not be the same construction as the one involved in the fire and that even the same mattress will

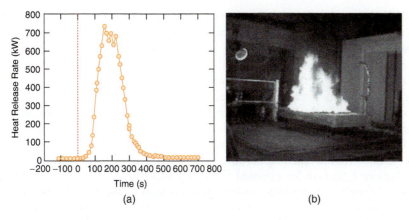

FIGURE 2-44 Reliable fire test data on (a) the heat release rate and (b) the fire after 120 seconds to support an investigation of a mattress fire. *Courtesy of NIST, "Fire on the Web," www.fire.nist.gov.*

behave differently if ignited at a corner or from underneath. The test was conducted in a large enclosure so as to minimize heat radiation effects (which would increase the rate of burning) and ventilation effects (which could limit the maximum rate). The investigator needs to consider these variables when testing the relevant hypothesis. Good documentation of the fire scene will be the key to success.

2.11.6 ENCLOSURE FIRES

The growth of a fire confined to a room is usually constrained by the ventilation-limited flow of air, smoke, and hot gases into and out of the enclosure. Confining variables may include the ceiling height, ventilation openings formed by windows and doors, room volume, and location of the fire in the room or compartment. While the fire gases are constrained, flashover may occur as a consequence of the heat release rate of the combustible materials contained within the room.

Minimum Heat Release Rate for Flashover

In the growth of a compartment (room) fire, flashover is defined by *NFPA 921* (2017d) as the transition phase in the development of a compartment fire in which surfaces exposed to thermal radiation reach ignition temperature more or less simultaneously, and fire spreads rapidly throughout the space, resulting in full room involvement, or total involvement, of the compartment or enclosed space. This transition may occur in just a few seconds in small, heavily fueled rooms, or over a period of minutes in large rooms, or may not take place at all due to an insufficient heat release rate of the fire. A useful reference on this subject is *NFPA 555: Guide on Methods for Evaluating Potential for Room Flashover* (NFPA 2017b).

Fire researchers have documented other observations during this transition phase. Defining observations often include one or more of the following criteria that address the effects of flashover: ignition of floor targets, high heat flux (>20 kW/m^2) to the floor, and flame extension out of the compartment's vents (Babrauskas, Peacock, and Reneke 2003; Milke and Mowrer 2001; Peacock et al. 1999).

The investigator may observe the following during flashover:

- Flames are emitted from openings in the compartment.
- Upper-layer gas temperature rises to $\geq 600°C$.
- Heat flux at floor level reaches ≥ 20 kW/m^2.
- Oxygen level in upper portions of the room decreases to approximately 0 to 5 percent.
- There is a small, short-term pressure rise of approximately 25 Pa (0.0036 psi).

There are two fundamental definitions for the occurrence of flashover. The first looks at flashover as a thermal balance in which critical conditions are produced when the compartment exceeds its ability to lose heat. The second definition views the compartment as being in a mechanical fluid-filling process. In this approach, the point at which the compartment's cool air layer is replaced with hot fire gases is flashover.

Because flashover represents a transition phase, defining the exact moment of occurrence is often a problem. Prior to flashover, the highest average temperatures are found in the upper, or hot gas, layer. If the average temperature of the hot gas layer exceeds 600°C, with or without the flaming ignition of the hot smoke called **flameover** or rollover, the radiant heat from the layer that is reaching all other exposed fuel in the room exceeds the minimum ignition radiant heat flux for exposed fuels, and those fuels ignite. If flashover occurs, temperatures throughout the room reach their maximum (1000°C is not uncommon) as the two-layer environment of the room breaks down and the entire room becomes a turbulently mixed combustion zone—from floor to ceiling.

The active mixing promotes very effective combustion with oxygen concentrations dropping below 3 percent and producing very high temperatures. This environment produces radiant heat fluxes of 120 kW/m^2 or higher, ensuring rapid ignition and burning of all exposed fuel surfaces, including walls, carpets, flooring, and low-lying fuels like baseboards. Also, combustion near ventilation points is enhanced.

Ignition of carpets can produce floor-level flames that sweep under chairs, tables, and other surfaces that were initially protected from the downward radiant heat from the hot gas layer alone. Burning proceeds throughout the room until the fuel supply is exhausted or some attempt is made at extinguishment.

Several variables can influence the minimum heat release rates necessary for flashover to occur. First, the size of the compartment may influence the impact of radiation from the fire to the surfaces of the walls, floor, and ceiling. For small compartments, radiation from the fire enhances rapid temperature increase of exposed surfaces. Also, small compartments may negate the two-zone model.

Vent openings have an impact on flashover because large vent openings make it necessary to have a very large fire in a room to produce flashover and may produce inaccurate calculations for vent flows. The surface materials on the walls can influence the minimum flashover energy, and some calculations take the heat transfer characteristics of the materials into account (Peacock et al. 1999).

Recent work on flashover calculations along with comparison with experimental data demonstrates that the wall surfaces play a role in heat transfer. Researchers report a trend that shorter exposure times increase the needed minimum heat release rate for flashover (Babrauskas, Peacock, and Reneke 2003).

An approximation for the minimum heat release rate required for flashover in a room, $\dot{Q}_{fo}$, can be found using the following equation, called the Thomas correlation (1981):

$$\dot{Q}_{fo} = 378A_o\sqrt{h_o} + 7.8A_w,\qquad(2.31)$$

where

$\dot{Q}_{fo}$ = heat release rate for flashover (kW),
A_o = area of the opening to the compartment (m^2),
h_o = height of the compartment opening (m), and
A_w = area of the walls, ceiling, and floor minus the opening (m^2).

flameover ■ The flaming ignition of the hot gas layer in a developing compartment fire. The condition in which unburned fuel (pyrolysate) from the originating fire has accumulated in the ceiling layer to a sufficient concentration, i.e., at or above the lower flammable limit, that it ignites and burns. Flameover can occur without ignition of, or prior to the ignition of, other fuels separate from the origin. Also known as rollover (NFPA 2017d, pt. 3.3.82).

EXAMPLE 2-8 ■ Calculating Flashover

Problem. Given a 10 m × 10 m room, with a 3 m-high ceiling and a 2.5 m × 1 m opening (see Figure 2-45), determine the minimum heat release rate needed to cause flashover.

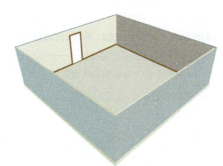

Suggested Solution. Use equation (2.31).

Area of compartment opening	A_o	$= (2.5 \text{ m})(1 \text{ m}) = 2.5 \text{ m}^2$
Height of compartment opening	h_o	$= 2.5 \text{ m}$
Area calculations	A_w	$= \text{floor} + \text{walls} + \text{ceiling} - \text{compartment opening}$

$$\text{One floor} = (10 \text{ m})(10 \text{ m}) = 100 \text{ m}^2$$
$$\text{Four walls} = (4)(10 \text{ m})(3 \text{ m}) = 120 \text{ m}^2$$
$$\text{One ceiling} = (10 \text{ m})(10 \text{ m}) = 100 \text{ m}^2$$
$$= 320 \text{ m}^2 - 2.5 \text{ m}^2 = 317.5 \text{ m}^2$$

Flashover heat release rate
$$\dot{Q}_{fo} = 378 A_o \sqrt{h_o} + 7.8 A_w$$
$$= (378)(2.5)\sqrt{2.5} + (7.8)(317.5)$$
$$= 1494 + 2477 = 3971 \text{ kW} = 3.97 \text{ MW}$$

A realistic answer would be about 4 MW.

Alternative Methods for Estimating Flashover

When applying the scientific method, the investigator needs to consider alternative methods for estimating the minimum heat release rate necessary for flashover, evaluate the results of fire models, and compare them with eyewitness accounts of the fire.

The first alternative approach assumes a flashover criterion temperature of a suitable increase in temperature, $\Delta T = 575°C$ (Babrauskas 1980), where

$$\Delta T = T_{fo} - T_{ambient} = 600 - 25 = 575°C. \tag{2.32}$$

$$\dot{Q}_{fo} = 0.6 A_v \sqrt{H_v}, \tag{2.33}$$

where

$\dot{Q}_{fo}$ = heat release rate for flashover (MW),
A_v = area of the door (m^2), and
H_v = door height (m).

The term $A_v \sqrt{H_v}$ is often referred to as the ventilation factor and frequently appears in similar equations. In actual experiments, two-thirds of the cases agree and are bounded by the following equations (Babrauskas 1984):

$$\dot{Q}_{fo} = 0.45 A_v \sqrt{H_v}, \tag{2.34}$$

$$\dot{Q}_{fo} = 1.05 A_v \sqrt{H_v}. \tag{2.35}$$

EXAMPLE 2-9 ■ Calculating Flashover: Alternative Method 1

Problem. Repeat the calculation for minimum heat release rate needed to cause flashover as previously presented in Example 2-8 using an alternative method.

Suggested Solution. Use equations (2.28), (2.29), and (2.30), also known as the Babrauskas correlation formulas.

Area of the door opening	$A_v = (2.5 \text{ m})(1 \text{ m}) = 2.5 \text{ m}^2$
Height of door opening	$H_v = 2.5 \text{ m}$
Flashover heat release rate	$\dot{Q}_{fo} = 0.6 A_v \sqrt{H_v}$
	$= (0.6)(2.5)\sqrt{2.5} = 2.37 \text{ MW}$
Minimum heat release rate	$\dot{Q}_{fo} = 0.45 A_v \sqrt{H_v} = 1.78 \text{ MW}$
Maximum heat release rate	$\dot{Q}_{fo} = 1.05 A_v \sqrt{H_v} = 4.15 \text{ MW}$

The second alternative approach is based on test data and a flashover criterion temperature difference of $\Delta T = 500°C$ (Lawson and Quintiere 1985; McCaffrey, Quintiere, and Harkleroad 1981):

$$\dot{Q}_{fo} = 610\sqrt{h_k A_s A_v \sqrt{H_v}}, \tag{2.36}$$

where

> h_k = enclosure conductance to ceiling and walls $[\text{kW}/(\text{m}^2 \cdot \text{k}) \text{ or } (\text{kW}/\text{m}^2)/K]$,
> A_s = thermal enclosure surface area, excluding vent or door area (m^2),
> A_v = total area of vent or door opening (m^2), and
> H_v = height of vent or door opening (m).

The McCaffrey, Quintiere, and Harkleroad (MQH) approach requires an estimate for the effective heat transfer enclosure conductance coefficient, h_k, of the enclosure. Assuming uniform heating of the enclosure with adequate thermal penetration, the conductance coefficient h_k can be estimated as

$$h_k = \frac{k}{\delta}, \tag{2.37}$$

where

> h_k = enclosure conductance to ceiling and walls $[(\text{kW}/\text{m}^2)/K]$,
> k = thermal conductivity of enclosure material $[(\text{kW}/\text{m})/K]$, and
> δ = enclosure material thickness (m).

EXAMPLE 2-10 ■ Calculating Flashover: Alternative Method 2

Problem. Repeat the calculation for the minimum heat release rate needed to cause flashover given an enclosure lined with 16 mm $\left(\frac{5}{8}\text{-in.}\right)$-thick gypsum board. Also calculate the estimated enclosure conductance.

Suggested Solution. Assuming uniform heating of the enclosure with adequate thermal penetration of the enclosure material, the typical values are as follows:

Heat release rate	$\dot{Q}_{fo} = 610\sqrt{h_k A_s A_v \sqrt{h_v}}$
Thermal conductivity	$k = 0.00017 \text{ (kW/m)}/K$
Enclosure thickness	$\delta = $ enclosure

Enclosure conductance	h_k	$= k/\delta$
		$= 0.00017/0.016 = (1.062 \times 10^{-2})[(kW/m^2)/K]$
Total surface area	A_s	$= 317.5\ m^2$
Total vent area	A_v	$= 2.5\ m^2$
Height of vent	H_v	$= 2.5\ m$
Flashover heat release rate	$\dot{Q}_{fo}$	$= 610\sqrt{(0.01062)(317.5)(2.5)\sqrt{2.5}}$
		$= 2226.9\ kW = 2.23\ MW$

A realistic answer would be about 2.2 MW.

The results 4.0 MW (Example 2-8) and 2.23 MW (Example 2-10) fall within the minimum and maximum calculated range of 1.78 to 4.15 MW, from equations (2.29) and (2.30). Taking a numerical average of the three $\dot{Q}_{fo}$ predictions is an inappropriate calculation.

Importance of Recognizing Flashover in Room Fires

Those who examine a fire scene after extinguishment or burnout should be aware of the importance of recognizing whether flashover did actually occur and the impact it may have had on the burning of a room's contents.

Post-flashover burning in a room produces numerous effects that were once thought to be produced only by accelerated arson fires involving flammable liquids such as gasoline. A fireball of burning gasoline vapors can sometimes produce floor-to-ceiling damage. The brief duration of such fires will result in shallow penetration. No matter how the fire began, walls scorched or charred from floor to ceiling can be due to post-flashover burning as well as from a fireball of burning gasoline vapors.

The combustion of carpets and underlying pads, once considered by fire investigators to be fairly unusual in accidental fires, is quite common in rooms filled with today's high-heat-release materials such as polyurethane foam and synthetic (thermoplastic) fabrics in upholstery, draperies, and carpets. Less expensive carpets and the backings of nearly all wall-to-wall carpets are made of highly combustible fibers like polypropylene. These carpets can melt, shrink, and ignite under moderate radiant heat flux, exposing the combustible urethane foam pad underneath to the radiant heat and flames. This combustion produces intense fires at floor level that can create deep irregular burn patterns on the floor beneath. The involvement of common carpet in corridor fires was the reason that the flooring radiant panel test was developed. Due to the extremely turbulent combustion, the intense radiant heat effects in post-flashover fires are not uniform; therefore, the effects on floors are not uniform (DeHaan 2001).

Other published experiments report the presence and absence of burn-throughs with gasoline poured and ignited on flooring along with various tile and carpet arrangements (Sanderson 1995). The experiments reported that without the presence of carpet padding, burn-throughs did not occur. However, burn-throughs sometimes were reported with carpet padding, but not at the location where the gasoline was poured. Babrauskas (2005) concurs with the authors that the most common reason for burn-throughs of flooring is radiant heat from above, and not the burning of combustible liquid on the floor. Extended slow combustion of collapsed furniture and bedding can also produce localized burn-throughs of flooring.

Fire damage under tables and chairs, once thought to be the result of the burning of flammable liquids at floor level, can be produced by the flaming combustion of the carpet and pad as they ignite during flashover. High temperatures and total room involvement, at one time thought to be linked to flammable liquid accelerants, are produced during post-flashover burning without accelerants. The extremely high heat fluxes produced in post-flashover fires can char wood or burn away other material at rates up to 10 times the rate at lower heat fluxes (Babrauskas 2005; Butler 1971).

Prolonged post-flashover burning can make the reconstruction of the fire very difficult as post-flashover or full room involvement fires typically ignite all exposed fuel surfaces from floor to ceiling. Localized patterns of smoke and fire damage that can help locate fuel packages, characterize their flame heights, and reveal the direction of flame spread can be destroyed. Some larger rooms sometimes exhibit progressive flashover, with floor-to-ceiling ignition at one end and undamaged floor covering at the other. Brief exposure (less than five minutes) to post-flashover fires does not necessarily compromise fire patterns on walls (see Hopkins, Gorbett, and Kennedy 2007).

In pre-flashover burning, the most intense thermal damage will be in areas immediately around or above burning fuel packages. The higher temperatures of the hot gas layer will produce more thermal damage in the upper half or upper third of the room. In post-flashover fires, all fuels are involved, the fires may become ventilation limited, and the most efficient (highest temperature) combustion occurs in turbulent mixing around the ventilation openings, where the oxygen supply is greatest. Oxygen-depleted burning occurs in many post-flashover rooms where the available fuel exceeds the air supply. See the work by Carman (2008) on improving the understanding of post-flashover fire behavior. He has done extensive testing on the production of clean burn patterns by ventilation effects in ventilation-controlled fires (Carman 2010).

Interviews of first-in firefighters may reveal whether a room was fully involved, floor to ceiling, when entry was first made. Investigators must be aware of the conditions that can lead to flashover and how to recognize whether it has occurred. A thorough understanding of heat release rates and fire spread characteristics of modern furniture and the dynamics of flashover will be of great assistance (Babrauskas and Peacock 1992).

Post-flashover Conditions

As previously stated, the average hot gas temperature in a room or compartment at flashover rises to $\geq 600°C$. At post-flashover conditions, the entire compartment is treated as a single homogenous, turbulent, and well-mixed volume sharing a common temperature and fuel/oxygen concentrations of oxygen and other by-products of combustion.

For ventilation-controlled fires during post-flashover, the heat release rate of the fuel within the compartment is regulated by the available ventilation. Specifically, the rate of inflow of fresh air and the outflow of gases is determined by a combination of the temperature differential across the vent and the ventilation factor ($A_v\sqrt{H_v}$).

Understanding this, we can use the relationship of mass flow into an opening to estimate the maximum heat release rate of fuels burning within a compartment. The mass flow rate of air through an opening is approximately (Karlsson and Quintiere 2000)

$$\dot{m}_{\text{air}} = 0.5A_v\sqrt{H_v}. \tag{2.38}$$

Because the heat release rate is regulated by the amount of available air, the following relationship can be used to estimate this rate:

$$\dot{Q} = \dot{m}_{\text{air}}\frac{\Delta h_c}{r}, \tag{2.39}$$

$$\dot{Q} = 0.5A_v\sqrt{H_v}\frac{\Delta h_c}{r}, \tag{2.40}$$

where

    Δh_c = heat of combustion of the fuel (kJ/kg),
    $\dot{m}_{\text{air}}$ = mass of air required to burn a mass of fuel [kg (air)/kg (fuel)],
    $\dot{Q}$ = heat release rate (kJ/s or kW), and
    r = air-to-fuel ratio 5.7 kg (air)/kg (wood).

The term is approximately constant for most fuels. For example, for wood,

$$\Delta h_c = 15{,}000 \text{ kJ/kg}$$

$$r = 5.7 \text{ kg (air)/kg (wood)}$$

$$\frac{\Delta h_c}{r} = 2630 \text{ kJ/kg (air)}$$

For a wood-fueled fire in a room, the maximum-sized fire can be estimated by assuming 100 percent efficiency. Substituting this value into equation (2.35), we obtain

$$\dot{Q} = 1370 A_v \sqrt{H_v} \text{(kJ/s = kW)}. \tag{2.41}$$

In post-flashover fires, the temperature of the compartment, which may reach 1100°C (2012°F), can also be estimated. The combined work of Thomas (1974) and Law (1978) produced the following correlation for predicting the maximum post-flashover temperature, assuming natural ventilation:

$$T_{fo(max)} = 6000 \frac{\left(1 - e^{-0.1\Omega}\right)}{\sqrt{\Omega}} \tag{2.42}$$

$$\Omega = \frac{A_T - A_v}{A_v \sqrt{H_v}} \tag{2.43}$$

where

$T_{fo(max)}$ = maximum compartment temperature at flashover,
Ω = ventilation factor
A_T = total area of the compartment-enclosing surfaces, excluding the area of vent openings (m^2),
A_V = total area of the vent openings (m^2), and
H_V = height of the vent openings (m).

EXAMPLE 2-11 ■ Calculating Maximum Heat Release Rate and Temperature in a Ventilation-Controlled Compartment Fire

Problem. Given a ventilation-controlled fire consisting of burning wooden furniture in a 10 m × 10 m room, with a 3 m-high ceiling and a 2.5 m × 1 m opening (see Figure 2-47), determine the minimum heat release rate and maximum compartment temperature, assuming natural ventilation.

Suggested Solution. The minimum heat release rate for a fire to progress in this room with the given opening can be calculated from equation (2.36).

Minimum heat release rate	$\dot{Q}$	$= 1370 A_v \sqrt{H_v}$
Height of opening	H_v	$= 2.5$ m
Area of opening	A_v	$= (1)(2.5) = 2.5 \text{ m}^2$
Minimum heat release rate	$\dot{Q}$	$= 1370 A_v \sqrt{H_v}$
		$= 1370(2.5)\sqrt{2.5} = 5415 \text{ kW} = 5.415 \text{ MW}$
Maximum compartment temp. at flashover	$T_{fo(max)}$	$= 6000 \dfrac{(1 - e^{-0.1\Omega})}{\sqrt{\Omega}}$
Ventilation factor	Ω	$= \dfrac{A_T - A_v}{A_v \sqrt{H_v}}$
Total area of the vent opening	A_v	$= (1)(2.5) = 2.5 \text{ m}^2$

Total area of the compartment-enclosing surfaces, excluding area of vent opening

$$\text{One floor} = (10 \text{ m})(10 \text{ m}) = 100 \text{ m}^2$$

$$A_T = \text{Four walls} = (4)(10 \text{ m})(3 \text{ m}) = 120 \text{ m}^2$$

$$\text{One ceiling} = (10 \text{ m})(10 \text{ m}) = 100 \text{ m}^2$$

$$= 320 \text{ m}^2 - 2.5 \text{ m}^2 = 317.5 \text{ m}^2$$

Height of the vent opening $H_v = 2.5 \text{ m}$

Ventilation factor $\quad \Omega \quad = \dfrac{A_T - A_v}{A_v \sqrt{H_v}} = \dfrac{317.5 - 2.5}{2.5\sqrt{2.5}} = \dfrac{315}{3.95} = 79.75$

Maximum compartment temperature at flashover

$$T_{fo(\max)} = 6000\dfrac{(1 - e^{-0.1\Omega})}{\sqrt{\Omega}}$$

$$= 6000\dfrac{(1 - e^{-7.975})}{\sqrt{79.75}}$$

$$= 6000\dfrac{0.999}{8.93} = 671.6°C$$

Discussion. Since we earlier predicted that a fire of 3 to 4 MW would be at the verge of triggering flashover in this large room, and the ventilation opening will support a fire of 5 MW or better, there is agreement that the maximum predicted temperature 671°C will exceed the threshold for flashover (i.e., 600°C).

2.11.7 OTHER ENCLOSURE FIRE EVENTS

Duration

As part of forensic fire scene reconstruction and analysis, other features of fire behavior in enclosures also become important to investigators. The following are commonly cited features: (1) smoke detector activation, (2) heat and sprinkler system operation, and (3) limited-ventilation fires.

Enclosure fire features can be helpful in answering several questions that arise during an investigation. For example: How long did the fire effectively burn? and, When during this time period did the smoke detector or sprinkler head activate? Answers to these questions can be placed on a timeline of information needed to fill the voids, particularly when fire deaths occur.

In tightly closed rooms, a fire consumes available oxygen and pumps oxygen-depleted air into the hot smoke layer. This layer descends until it reaches the level of the fire. The fire then experiences reduced burning, existing on what oxygen is available to it in the smoke layer, and reducing, accordingly, its heat release rate. If there is a leak or vent high in the room, the smoke layer may rise to where the fire is back in normal room air, and the fire resumes its full heat release rate, until the layer descends again. This sequence may produce a cyclical behavior of open flame/smolder/open flame/smolder until the fuel is depleted.

NFPA 555 specifies two methods for estimating the duration of burning in a tightly closed compartment—one for fires with a steady heat release rate of $\dot{Q}$, the second for unsteady t^2 fires (NFPA 2017b).

For steady fires:

$$t = \dfrac{V_{O_2}}{\dot{Q}(\Delta h_c \rho o_2)}. \qquad (2.44)$$

For growing fires:

$$t = \left[\frac{3V_{O_2}}{\alpha(\Delta h_c \rho o_2)} \right]^{1/3}$$

(2.45)

where

t = time (s),
V_{O_2} = volume of oxygen available to be consumed in the combustion process (m³),
$\dot{Q}$ = heat release rate from steady fire (kW),
$\Delta h_c \rho o_2$ = heat release rate per unit volume of oxygen consumed (kJ/m³), and
α = constant governing the speed of fire growth (kJ/s³) (slow 2.93×10^{23}, medium 11.72×10^{-3}, fast 46.88×10^{-3})

The quantity Vo_2 is generally considered to be half the total available oxygen in the room [so $Vo_2 = 0.5(0.21\ V_{room})$], since flaming combustion will generally not be sustained once O_2 levels are in the range of 8 to 12 percent, as cited in *NFPA 555* (NFPA 2017b). This relationship also assumes that the fire is at floor level in the room; if the fire is elevated and not so large that it will induce a great deal of localized turbulent mixing, Vo_2 will be controlled by the volume of the room at and above the level of the fire.

Smoke Alarm Activation

Fire investigators often have a problem determining when on a timeline of events a thermal fire detector, smoke alarm, or sprinkler system was activated. Historically, fire protection engineers have done much work on this area, specifically the DETACT-QS program (Evans and Stroup 1986). These significant events are usually noticed by a witness or electronically reported by alarm systems and often serve as critical markers in an investigation.

Figure 2-46 shows the measurements needed to calculate these activations. The dimension H is the distance to the ceiling above the fuel surface, and r is the radial distance

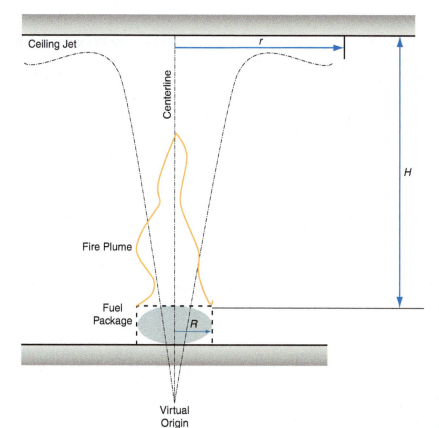

FIGURE 2-46 Fire plume measurements needed in fire detector, smoke detector, or sprinkler system calculations, consisting of fuel surface to ceiling along centerline (*H*), radius of burning fuel surface (*R*), and radial distance of ceiling jet from centerline (*r*).

from the plume centerline to the heat detector or sprinkler head. The centerline is the imaginary vertical line emerging from the center of the fuel source to the ceiling. R is the equivalent radius of the burning fuel package.

Three common methods are used in estimating smoke detector response time, namely, Alpert (1972), Milke (1990), and Mowrer (1990). The Alpert and Milke methods use the convective portion of the heat release rate, $\dot{Q}_c$, in calculations. The convective heat release rate fraction, X_c (typically 0.70), is used, where $\dot{Q}_c = X_c\dot{Q}$.

In the Mowrer method, two calculations are necessary to estimate smoke detector activations for steady-state fires. The first calculates the time for the fire gases to reach the ceiling at the plume centerline, or the plume lag time. The second calculates the time for the gases to reach the detector from the plume centerline, or the ceiling jet lag.

For a steady-state fire of heat release rate $\dot{Q}$, these equations are expressed as

$$t_{pl} = C_{pl}\frac{H^{4/3}}{\dot{Q}^{1/3}} \tag{2.46}$$

$$t_{cj} = \frac{1}{C_{cj}}\frac{r^{11/6}}{\dot{Q}^{1/3}H^{1/2}} \tag{2.47}$$

where

t_{pl} = transport lag time of plume (s),
t_{cj} = transport lag time of ceiling jet (s),
C_{pl} = plume lag time constant = 0.67 (experimentally determined),
C_{cj} = ceiling jet lag time constant = 1.2 (experimentally determined),
r = radius of distance from plume centerline to the detector (m),
H = height of ceiling above top of fuel (m), and
$\dot{Q}$ = heat release rate of the fire (kW).

EXAMPLE 2-12 ■ Smoke Detector Activation by Wastepaper Basket Fire

Problem. A business owner closed his shop and later claimed that he may have caused a fire by carelessly discarding a lit match into a wastepaper basket before leaving. The fire ignited a small 0.3 m (0.98 ft.)-diameter basket filled with ordinary papers. The fire developed quickly to reach a steady-state heat release rate of 100 kW.

The initial temperature of the room was 20°C (293 K, 68°F). The distance from the top of the wastepaper basket to the ceiling is 4 m (13.12 ft.). A smoke detector attached to the ceiling is located radially 2 m (6.56 ft.) from the fire plume's centerline. Assuming that there are negligible radiation losses in a smooth, level ceiling, determine the time of the smoke detector's activation by the heated ceiling jet gases.

Suggested Solution. Assume that steady-state conditions exist, along with immediate activation.

Height of ceiling above fuel	H	= 4 m
Radius from plume centerline	r	= 2 m
Plume lag time constant	C_{pl}	= 0.67
Ceiling jet lag time constant	C_{cj}	= 1.2
Heat release rate	$\dot{Q}$	= 100 kW
Plume transport time lag	t_{pl}	$= C_{pl}\dfrac{H^{3/4}}{\dot{Q}^{1/3}} = 0.92$ s
Ceiling jet transport lag time	t_{cj}	$= \dfrac{1}{C_{cj}}\dfrac{r^{11/6}}{\dot{Q}^{1/3}H^{1/2}} = 0.32$ s
Detector activation time	t	$= t_{pl} + t_{cj} = 0.92 + 0.32 = 1.24$ s

Discussion. Owing to variables such as fire size, room geometry, the type of detector (photoelectric or ionization), and environmental interactions, the time to activate a smoke detector may vary, especially with ceiling-mounted units. Therefore, the preceding solution may not be accurate because it does not account for the lag time for the smoke to enter the detector's sensing chamber. The solution assumes that an instantaneous fire of 100 kW occurs, something that takes a real-world fire 30 or more seconds to develop. A suggested practice for determining the activation time for ceiling-mounted smoke detectors is to consider the temperature of the smoke layer (Heskestad and Delichatsios 1977).

Testing by Collier (1996) showed that, approximately, a 4°C rise at the detector location is sufficient for an activation. In several approaches to predicting the time for smoke, heat, and sprinkler systems to activate, the engineering calculations typically use only the convective heating of the sensing elements by the hot fire gases and do not account for any direct heating by radiation from the flames. In heated rooms, the smoke layer from low-energy fires may not be buoyant enough to reach the detector through the fire's static hot layer.

For comparison, the methods of Alpert and Milke provide estimates of 5.89 and 12.48 seconds, respectively, for this problem. Experimental reenactment of a fire condition may reveal critical variables (e.g., placement/location on a wall, ceiling vent location, or time required for development of the fire to steady state).

Sprinkler Head and Heat Detector Activation

In estimating the time to activate a sprinkler head or heat detector, both the ceiling jet temperature and its velocity must be calculated along with the ratio r/H. The equations for these estimates are based on data from a series of actual tests for 670 kW to 100 MW fires (Alpert 1972; NFPA 2008).

The first calculation necessary is the centerline temperature directly above the plume produced by the burning fuel source:

$$T_m = 16.9\frac{\dot{Q}^{2/3}}{H^{5/3}} + T_\infty \quad \text{for} \quad r/H \leq 0.18. \tag{2.48}$$

For r/H ratios greater than 0.18, the detector or sprinkler falls within the ceiling jet portion of the plume.

$$T_{m_{jet}} = 5.38\frac{(\dot{Q}/r)}{H} + T_\infty \quad \text{for} \quad r/H > 0.18, \tag{2.49}$$

where

T_m = plume gas temperature above fire (K),
$T_{m_{jet}}$ = temperature of ceiling jet (K),
T_∞ = ambient room temperature (K),
$\dot{Q}$ = heat release rate from fire (kW),
$\dot{Q}_c$ = convective heat release rate (kW), where $\dot{Q}_c = X_c\dot{Q}$
r = radial distance from plume centerline to device (m), and
H = distance above fuel surface (m).

For calculating the time to activation of a sprinkler head, the generally accepted engineering practice is to consider only the convective heating of the sensing elements by the hot fire gases (Iqbal and Salley 2004). This practice does not account for direct heating by radiation and assumes that conduction of heat from the sprinkler to the piping is negligible. Therefore, the value for the convective heat release rate for the fire is often used in place of the total heat release rate, $\dot{Q}$.

To study detector and sprinkler activation problems in a more depth, the maximum velocity of the ceiling jet, U_m, needs to be calculated. The following correlations depend on the value of the r/H ratio.

For maximum jet velocity close to the centerline,

$$U_m = 0.96\left(\frac{\dot{Q}}{H}\right)^{1/3} \quad \text{for} \quad r/H > 0.15. \tag{2.50}$$

For jet velocities farther away from the centerline,

$$U_m = 0.195\left(\frac{\dot{Q}^{1/3}H^{1/2}}{r^{5/6}}\right)^{1/3} \quad \text{for} \quad r/H > 0.15, \tag{2.51}$$

where

U_m = gas velocity (m/s),
$\dot{Q}$ = heat release rate (kW),
H = distance above fuel surface (m), and
r = radial distance from plume centerline to device (m).

Determination of the time to activation of the heat detector or sprinkler during steady-state fires relies on the response time index (RTI). This index assesses the ability of a heat detector to activate from an initial condition of ambient room temperature. Because the detector of a sprinkler has a finite mass, the RTI takes into account the time lag before the temperature of the detector rises.

$$t_{operation} = \frac{RTI}{\sqrt{U_m}}\log_e\left(\frac{T_m - T_\infty}{T_m - T_{operation}}\right), \tag{2.52}$$

where

RTI = response time index $(m^{1/2} \cdot s^{1/2})$,
U_m = gas velocity (m/s),
T_m = plume gas temperature above fire (K),
T_∞ = ambient room temperature (K), and
$T_{operation}$ = operation temperature (K).

RTI values are specified by the manufacturer for each style or model of sprinkler.

EXAMPLE 2-13 ■ Sprinkler Head Activation to Wastepaper Basket Fire

Problem. A closer examination of the debris in Example 2-12 shows that the wastebasket actually contains both paper and plastic, producing a steady-state fire of 500 kW. A standard-response bulb sprinkler head, whose operation temperature is 74°C (165°F, 347 K) and RTI is 235 $m^{1/2} \cdot s^{1/2}$, is located directly above the basket. The ambient temperature of the room is 20°C (68°F, 293 K). Estimate the time to activation of the sprinkler head. When calculating the ceiling jet temperature, use the convective heat release rate, $\dot{Q}_c$.

Suggested Solution. Since the area of interest is directly above the fire plume, the radius from the centerline is zero, which gives a ratio $r/H < 0.18$. Also, the conservative assumption is that the convective heat release rate fraction (X_c) of the fire is 0.70. Therefore, use the appropriate equations to calculate the temperature and velocity.

Heat release rate	$\dot{Q}_c$	= 500 kW
Convective heat release rate	$\dot{Q}_c$	= 350 kW
Distance above fuel surface	H	= 4 m
Ambient room temperature	T_∞	= 20°C + 273 = 293 K
Response time index	RTI	= 235 $m^{1/2} \cdot s^{1/2}$
Temperature of operation	$T_{operation}$	= 74°C + 273 = 347 K
Temperature of ceiling jet	T_m	= $16.9(\dot{Q}^{2/3}/H^{5/3}) + T_\infty$
		= $(16.9)(350^{2/3}/4^{5/3}) + 293$
		= $83 + 293 = 376$ K = 103°C

| Ceiling jet velocity | U_m | $= 0.96\left(\dfrac{\dot{Q}}{H}\right)^{1/3}$ |

$$= (0.96)(500/4)^{1/3} = 4.8 \text{ m/s}$$

| Time to operation | $t_{\text{operation}}$ | $= (\text{RTI}/\sqrt{U_m})\log_e[(T_m - T_\infty)/(T_m - T_{\text{operation}})]$ |

$$= (235/\sqrt{4.45})\log_e[(376 - 293)/(376 - 347)]$$

$$= 61.8 \text{ s} \approx 1 \text{ min}$$

The calculations for ceiling jet behaviors are valid only for smooth, level ceilings. Open joists, ceiling ducts, or pitched surfaces will dramatically affect the movement of gases.

CHAPTER REVIEW

Summary

Fire is a chemical reaction that produces physical effects. Consequently, the fire investigator should have some familiarity with the simpler chemical and physical properties and processes involved. Because fire consists of a number of chemical reactions occurring simultaneously, it is important to understand first what a chemical reaction is and how it is involved in a fire.

Furthermore, the body of fire dynamics knowledge as it applies to fire scene reconstruction and analysis is derived from the combined disciplines of physics, thermodynamics, chemistry, heat transfer, and fluid mechanics. Accurate determination of a fire's origin, intensity, growth, direction of travel, duration, and extinguishment requires that investigators rely on and correctly apply all principles of fire dynamics. Investigators must realize that variability in fire growth and development is influenced by a number of factors such as available fuel load, ventilation, and physical configuration of the room.

Review Questions

1. The smallest unit of an element that takes part in a chemical reaction is a/an _____.
2. What natural element is necessary for normal combustion?
3. What three compounds are produced by the combustion of hydrocarbon fuels?
4. What is the difference between hydrocarbons and carbohydrates?
5. What is the difference between glucose and cellulose?
6. What is the heat of combustion of a fuel?
7. Name four classes of petroleum products.
8. What chemical structure is characterized by the designation alkane?
9. What chemical structure is characterized by the designation aromatic?
10. Define an organic compound.
11. According to the ideal gas law, if the temperature of a fixed amount of gas rises from 300 K (27°C) to 600 K (327°C), what will be its change in volume?
12. Describe the phenomenon of pyrolysis.
13. Describe four of the routes by which a solid can be converted to a vapor.
14. Describe what happens when wood burns.
15. What conditions usually accompany low-temperature ignition of wood?
16. Describe the difference between thermoplastic and thermosetting synthetic materials.
17. Why is latex foam different from synthetic foams in its combustion properties?
18. What behavior affects the combustion of thermoplastics like polypropylene, nylon, or polystyrene?
19. What metals burn readily in air?
20. What factors control the phenomenon of a dust explosion?
21. Describe the difference between cellulosic and synthetic materials. Which is more easily ignited by a glowing cigarette?
22. What is saturation vapor pressure and how is it measured?
23. What is meant by the lower explosive limit?
24. What happens at the flash point of a liquid fuel?
25. What is the difference between flash point and autoignition temperature?
26. What is the equation used to determine the vapor density of a gas or vapor?
27. Which compounds have the widest flammability ranges?
28. Name five common petroleum-based fuels and describe each.
29. What are three differences between natural gas and LP gas?
30. At what pressures is natural gas delivered in distribution lines? Regulator to residential line? To appliance burner?
31. What is the difference between flammable, combustible, and ignitable liquids?

References

Albers, J. 1999. "It's Time to Reduce Upholstered Furniture-Driven Flashover." *American Fire Journal* July: 6–8.

Alpert, R. L. 1972. "Calculation of Response Time of Ceiling-Mounted Fire Detectors." *Fire Technology* 9: 181–95.

———. July 2008. "Cover Story." *California Fire/Arson Investigator*: 25.

American Petroleum Institute. January 1991. "Ignition Risk of Hydrocarbon Vapors by Hot Surfaces in the Open Air." API Publication 2216.

Angell, H. W. 1949. *Ignition Temperature of Fireproofed Wood, Untreated Sound Wood, and Untreated Decayed Wood*. Forest Products Research Society.

ASTM International. 2005. *D56-05, Standard Test Method for Flash Point by Tag Closed Tester*. West Conshohocken, PA: ASTM International.

———. 2012. *D92-12b, Standard Test Method for Flash and Fire Points by Cleveland Open-Cup Tester*. West Conshohocken, PA: ASTM International.

———. 2013a. *D3699-13be1, Specification for Kerosene*. West Conshohocken, PA: ASTM International.

———. 2013b. *E1321-13, Standard Test Method for Determining Material Ignition and Flame Spread Properties*. West Conshohocken, PA: ASTM International.

———. 2014. *D1310-14, Standard Test Method for Flash Point and Fire Point of Liquids by Tag Open-Cup Apparatus*. West Conshohocken, PA: ASTM International.

———. 2015a. *D93-15b, Standard Test Methods for Flash Point by Pensky-Martens Closed-Cup Tester*. West Conshohocken, PA: ASTM International.

———. 2015b. *E659-15, Standard Test Method for Autoignition Temperature of Liquid Chemicals*. West Conshohocken, PA: ASTM International.

Babrauskas, V. 1980. "Estimating Room Flashover Potential." *Fire Technology* 16: 94–103, 112.

———. 1982. *Development of The Cone Calorimeter, A Bench Scale Heat Release Rate Apparatus Based on Oxygen Consumption*. NASA STI/Recon Technical Report N, 83.

———. 1984. "Upholstered Furniture Room Fires—Measurements, Comparison with Furniture Calorimeter Data, and Flashover Predictions." *Journal of Fire Sciences* 2(1): 5–19.

———. 2001. "Ignition of Wood: A Review of the State of the Art." In *Interflam 2001*, 71–88. London: Interscience Communications.

———. 2003. *Ignition Handbook*. Issaquah, WA: Fire Science Publishers.

———. 2004. "Charring Rate of Wood as a Tool for Fire Investigations." In *Interflam 2004*, 1155–76. London: Interscience Communications.

———. 2005. "Charring Rate of Wood as a Tool for Fire Investigators." *Fire Safety Journal* 40: 528–54

Babrauskas, V., B. F. Gray, and M. L. Janssens. 2007. "Prudent Practices for the Design and Installation of Heat-Producing Devices near Wood Materials." *Fire and Materials* 31: 125–35.

Babrauskas, V. and R. D. Peacock. 1992. "Heat Release Rate: The Single Most Important Variable in Fire Hazard." *Fire Safety Journal* 18(3), pp. 255–272.

Babrauskas, V., R. D. Peacock, and P. A. Reneke. 2003. "Defining Flashover for Fire Hazard Calculations. Part II." *Fire Safety Journal* 38: 613–22.

Babrauskas, V. and W. D. Walton. 1986. "A Simplified Characterization of Upholstered Furniture Heat Release Rates." *Fire Safety Journal* 11: 181–92.

Bowes, P. C. 1984. *Self-Heating: Evaluating and Controlling the Hazards*. Amsterdam: Elsevier.

Brown, C. R. October 1934. "The Ignition Temperatures of Solid Materials." *NFPA Quarterly* 28, no. 2: 134–35.

Browning, B. L., ed. 1951. *The Chemistry of Wood*. New York: Wiley-Interscience.

Bukowski, R. W. 1995a. "How to Evaluate Alternative Designs Based on Fire Modeling." *Fire Journal* 89 (2):68-70, 72-74.

———. 1995b. "Predicting the Fire Performance of Buildings: Establishing Appropriate Calculation Methods for Regulatory Applications." ASIAFLAM '95. International Conference on Fire Science and Engineering, Kowloon, Hong Kong, March 15-16, 1995.

Butler, C. P. 1971. "Notes on Charring Rates in Wood." *Fire Research Note No FR 896*. Borehamwood, UK: Fire Research Station.

Carman, S. W. 2008. "Improving the Understanding of Post-flashover Fire Behavior." Proceedings of the International Symposium on Fire Investigation Science and Technology, Sarasota, FL.

———. 2010. "Clean Burn Fire Patterns—A New Perspective for Interpretation." Interflam, Nottingham, UK, July 2010.

Collier, P. C. R. 1996. "Fire in a Residential Building: Comparisons Between Experimental Data and a Fire Zone Model." *Fire Technology* 32(3): 195–217.

Conkling, J. A. 1985. *The Chemistry of Pyrotechnics and Explosives*. New York: Marcel Dekker.

Cooke, G. 1998a. "When Are Sandwich Panels Safe in a Fire? Part 1." *Fire Engineers Journal* 58, no. 195.

———. 1998b. "When Are Sandwich Panels Safe in a Fire? Part 2." *Fire Engineers Journal* 58, no. 196.

CPSC. March 2006. *16 CFR 1633: Standard for the Flammability (Open Flame) of Mattress Sets*. Federal Register 70, no. 50.

Cuzzillo, B. R., and P. J. Pagni. Spring 1999. "Low Temperature Wood Ignition." *Fire Findings* 7, no. 2.

———. 2000. "The Myth of Pyrophoric Carbon." In *Fire Safety Science—Proceedings of the Sixth International Symposium*, 301–12. Bethesda, MD: IAFSS.

Damant, G. 1988. California Department of Consumer Affairs, Bureau of Home Furnishings. Personal communication.

DeHaan, J. D. 1995. "The Reconstruction of Fires Involving Highly Flammable Hydrocarbon Liquids." PhD dissertation, Department of Pure and Applied Chemistry, University of Strathclyde.

———. 1999. "The Influence of Temperature, Pool Size, and Substrate on the Evaporation Rates of Flammable Liquids." Paper presented at Interflam, Edinburgh, Scotland.

———. 2001. "Compartment Fires 1996–98." *CAC News,* Spring.

———. 2004. "Exploding Gas Cans and Other Fire Myths." *CAC News*: 20–26.

DeHaan, J. D., and K. Bonarius. 1988. "Pyrolysis Products of Structure Fires." *Journal of Forensic Sciences* 28: 299–309.

DeHaan, J. D., D. Brien, and R. Large. October–December 2004. "Volatile Organic Compounds from the Combustion of Human and Animal Tissue." *Science and Justice* 11, no. 4: 223–36.

DeHaan, J. D., D. Crowhurst, D. Hoare, M. Bensilum, and M. P. Shipp. 2001. "Deflagrations Involving Heavier-than-Air Vapor/Air Mixtures." *Fire Safety Journal* 36, no. 7: 693–710.

DeHaan, J. D., and W. Howard. 1995. "Combustion Explosions Involving Household Aerosol Products." In *Proceedings of the Fourth International Symposium of the Detection and Identification of Explosives*, Chantilly, Virginia.

DeHaan, J. D., and S. Nurbakhsh. 1999. "The Combustion of Animal Carcasses and Its Implications for the Consumption of Human Bodies in Fires." *Science and Justice,* January.

Dorsheim, M. A. 1997. "Fuel Ignites Differently in Aircraft, Lab Environments." *Aviation Week and Space Technology* July, 61–63.

Drysdale, D. 1985. *An Introduction to Fire Dynamics*. New York: John Wiley & Sons.

———. 1999. *An Introduction to Fire Dynamics*. 2nd ed. Chichester, UK: Wiley.

———. 2011. *An Introduction to Fire Dynamics*. 3rd ed. John Wiley & Sons.

Ettling, B. V. 1999. "Venting of Propane from Overfilled Portable Containers." *Fire & Arson Investigator* April: 54–56.

Evans, D. D., and D. W. Stroup. 1986. "Methods to Calculate the Response Time of Heat and Smoke Detectors Installed Below Large Unobstructed Ceilings." *Fire Technology* 22(1): 54–65.

Exxon Corp. 1990. *Isopars*. Houston, TX.

Fire, F. L. 1985. "Plastics and Fire Investigations." *Fire & Arson Investigator* December: 36.

———. 2005. "Panel Perspectives." *Fire Engineering Journal and Fire Prevention* September: 44–46.

Fleischer, H. O. 1960. *The Performance of Wood in Fire*. Report No. 2202. Madison, WI: Forest Products Laboratory.

Forest Products Laboratory. 1945. "Report No. 1464." *Wood Products* 50, no. 2: 21–22.

Friedman, R. 1998. *Principles of Fire Protection Chemistry and Physics*. 3rd ed. Quincy, MA: National Fire Protection Association.

Gardiner, D., M. Barden, and G. Pucher. 2008. "An Experimental and Modeling Study of the Flammability of Fuel Tank Vapors from High Ethanol Fuels." Washington, DC: National Renewable Energy Laboratory, Subcontract Report NREL/SR-540-44040. Golden, CO: US Department of Energy.

Gardiner, W. C. 1982. "The Chemistry of Flames." *Scientific American* 246, no. 2: 110–25.

Gialamas, D. M. Spring 1994. "Is It Gasoline or Insecticide?" *CAC News*.

Glassman, I., and F. L. Dryer. 1980–1981. "Flame Spreading across Liquid Fuels." *Fire Safety Journal* 3: 123–38.

Goodson, M., and M. Hergenrether. 2005. "Investigating the Causal Link between Lightning Strikes, CSST, and Fire." *Fire & Arson Investigator* October: 28–31.

Gorbett, G. E., J. L. Pharr, and S. Rockwell. 2016. *Fire Dynamics*. Upper Saddle River, NJ: Pearson.

Graf, S. H. 1949. "Ignition Temperatures of Various Papers, Woods, and Fabrics." *Oregon State College Bulletin* March, 26.

Guidry, D. May 2005. Personal communication.

Harris, R. J. 1983. *The Investigation and Control of Gas Explosions*. New York: E & FN Spon.

Henderson, R. W., and G. R. Lightsey. 1984. "The Effective Flame Temperatures of Flammable Liquids." *Fire & Arson Investigator* December, 35.

Heskestad, G. H., and M. A. Delichatsios. 1977. *Environments of Fire Detectors—Phase 1: Effects of Fire Size, Ceiling Height, and Material*. NBS-GCR-77-86 and NBS-GCR-77-95. Gaithersburg, MD: National Bureau of Standards.

Hodges, D. J. 1963. *Colliery Guardian* 207, no. 678.

Holleyhead, R. H. 1999. "Ignition of Solid Materials and Furniture by Lighted Cigarettes." *Science and Justice* 39, no. 2: 75–102.

Hopkins, R. L., G. Gorbett, and P. M. Kennedy. 2007. *Fire Pattern Persistence and Predictability on Interior Finish and Construction Materials During Pre- And Post-Flashover Compartment Fires*. Fire and Materials 2007, San Francisco, January 29–31.

Iqbal, N., and M. H. Salley. 2004. *Fire Dynamics Tools (FDTs)*. Quantitative fire hazard analysis methods for the U.S. Nuclear Regulatory Commission Fire Protection Inspection Program. Washington, DC.

Jackson, P. E. 1998. "Intumescent Materials." *Fire Engineers Journal* 58: 194.

Karlsson, B. and J. G. Quintiere. 2000. *Enclosure Fire Dynamics*, Boca Raton, FL: CRC Press.

Kennedy, C. S., and J. F. Knapp. 1997. "Childhood Burn Injuries Related to Gasoline Can Home Storage." *Pediatrics* 99: e3.

Kennedy, P., and A. Armstrong. 2007. "Fraction Vaporization of Ignitable Liquids: Flash Point and Ignitability

Issues." Paper presented at Fire and Materials 2007, 10th International Conference and Exhibition, Interscience Communications, San Francisco, January 29–31.

Kirk, P. L. 1969. *Fire Investigation*. New York: Wiley.

Krasny, J. F., W. J. Parker, and V. Babrauskas. 2001. *Fire Behavior of Upholstered Furniture and Mattresses*. Norwich, NY: Noyes/William Andrew.

Kuk, R. J., and M. V. Spagnola. September 2008. "Extraction of Alternative Fuels from Fire Debris Samples." *Journal of Forensic Sciences* 53, no. 5: 1123–29.

Lapina, R. 2005. "Propane Fire & Explosion Investigation." *Fire & Arson Investigator* April: 46–49.

Law, M. 1978. *Fire Safety of External Building Elements— The Design Approach*. AISC Engineering Journal (Second Quarter)

Lawson, J. R., and J. G. Quintiere. 1985. *Slide-Rule Estimates of Fire Growth*. NBSIR 85-3196. Gaithersburg, MD: National Bureau of Standards

Lightsey, G. R., and R. W. Henderson. 1985. "Theoretical vs. Observed Flame Temperatures during Combustion of Wood Products." *Fire & Arson Investigator* December: 36.

Madrzykowski, D., N. Bryner, W. Grosshandler, and D. Stroup. 2004. "Fire Spread through a Room with Polyurethane Foam Covered Walls." In *Interflam 2004*, 1127–38. London: Interscience Communications.

McCaffrey, B. J., J. G. Quintiere, and M. F. Harkleroad. 1981. "Estimating Room Fire Temperatures and the Likelihood of Flashover Using Fire Test Data Correlations." *Fire Technology* 17(2): 98–119

McGraw, J. M., and F. W. Mowrer. 1999. "Flammability of Painted Gypsum Wallboard Subjected to Fire Heat Fluxes." In *Interflam 1999*, 1320–30. London: Interscience Communications.

McNaughton, G. C. 1944. *Ignition and Charring Temperatures of Wood*. US Department of Agriculture, Forest Service.

Milke, J. A. 1990. "Smoke Management for Covered Malls and Atria." *Fire Technology* 26(3): 223–43

Milke, J. A., and F. W. Mowrer. 2001. *Application of Fire Behavior and Compartment Fire Models Seminar*. Tennessee Valley Society of Fire Protection Engineers (TVSFPE), Oak Ridge, September 27–28.

Mowrer, F. W. 1990. "Lag Time Associated with Fire Detection and Suppression." *Fire Technology* 26, no. 3 (August): 244–65.

———. 2003. "Ignition Characteristics of Various Fire Indicators Subjected to Radiant Heat Fluxes." In *Fire and Materials 2003*, 81–92. London: Interscience Communications.

NFPA. 2008. *Fire Protection Handbook*. 20th ed. Quincy, MA: National Fire Protection Association.

———. 2013. *NFPA 705: Recommended Practice for a Field Flame Test for Textiles and Films*. Quincy, MA: National Fire Protection Association.

———. 2014. *NFPA 1033: Standard for Professional Qualifications for Fire Investigator*. Quincy, MA: National Fire Protection Association.

———. 2015a. *NFPA 54: National Fuel Gas Code*. Quincy, MA: National Fire Protection Association.

———. 2015b. *NFPA 92: Standard for Smoke Control Systems*. Quincy, MA: National Fire Protection Association.

———. 2015c. *NFPA 99: Health Care Facilities Code*. Quincy, MA: National Fire Protection Association.

———. 2016a. *NFPA 72: National Fire Alarm and Signaling Code*. Quincy, MA: National Fire Protection Association.

———. 2016b. *NFPA 35: Standard for the Manufacture of Organic Coatings*. Quincy, MA: National Fire Protection Association.

———. 2016c. *NFPA 115: Standard for Laser Fire Protection*. Quincy, MA: National Fire Protection Association.

———. 2016d. *NFPA 53: Recommended Practice on Materials, Equipment, and Systems Used in Oxygen-Enriched Atmospheres*. Quincy, MA: National Fire Protection Association.

———. 2017a. *NFPA 58: Standard for Storage and Handling of LP Gases*. Quincy, MA: National Fire Protection Association.

———. 2017b. *NFPA 555: Guide on Methods for Evaluating Potential for Room Flashover*. Quincy, MA: National Fire Protection Association.

———. 2017c. *NFPA 414: Standard for Aircraft Rescue and Fire-Fighting Vehicles*. Quincy, MA: National Fire Protection Association.

———. 2017d. *NFPA 921: Guide for Fire and Explosion Investigations*. Quincy, MA: National Fire Protection Association.

Nurbakhsh, S. 2006. California Bureau of Home Furnishings. Personal communication.

Peacock, R. D., P. A. Reneke, R. W. Bukowski, and V. Babrauskas. 1999. "Defining Flashover for Fire Hazard Calculations." *Fire Safety Journal* 32(4): 331–45.

Perry, R. H., and D. Green. 1997. *Perry's Chemical Engineers' Handbook*. 7th ed. New York: McGraw-Hill.

Putorti, A. D., McElroy, J. A., and Madrzykowski, D. 2001. *Flammable and Combustible Liquid Spill/Burn Patterns*. US Department of Justice, Office of Justice Programs, National Institute of Justice.

Quarles, L., L. G. Cool, and F. C. Beall. 2005. "Performance of Deck Board Materials under Simulated Wildfire Exposures." Paper presented at Seventh International Conference on Woodfiber-Plastic Composites, Madison, Wisconsin, May 19–20, Retrieved April 10, 2005. www.cnr.berkeley.edu.

Quintiere, J. G. 1998. *Principles of Fire Behavior*. Albany, NY: Delmar.

Quintiere, J. G., and M. Harkleroad. 1984. New Concepts for Measuring for Flame Spread Properties, NBSIR 84-2943. Gaithersburg, MD: National Bureau of Standards, November 1984.

Raj, P. K. 2006. "Where in a LNG Vapor Cloud Is the Flammable Concentration Relative to the Visible Cloud Boundary?" *NFPA Journal* March–June: 68–70.

Sanderson, J. L. 1995. "Tests Add Further Doubt to Concrete Spalling Theories." *Fire Findings* 3(4): 1–3.

Sanderson, J. 2005. "Electrostatic Pinholing." *Fire Findings* 13, no. 4: 1–3.

SFPE. 2002. *SFPE Engineering Guide to Piloted Ignition of Solid Materials under Radiant Exposure.* Edited by SFPE Task Group on Engineering Practices. Bethesda, MD: Society of Fire Protection Engineers.

———. 2008. *SFPE Handbook of Fire Protection Engineering.* 4th ed. Quincy, MA: Society of Fire Protection Engineers and the National Fire Protection Association.

Shaffer, E. L. 1980. "Smoldering Initiation in Cellulosics under Prolonged Low-Level Heating." *Fire Technology* 23 (February).

Shipp, M., K. Shaw, and P. Morgan. 1999. "Fire Behavior of Sandwich Panels Constructions." In *Interflam 1999,* 98. London: Interscience Communications.

Stark, N. M., R. H. White, and C. M. Clemons. 1997. "Heat Release Rate of Wood-Plastic Composites." *SAMPE Journal* 33, no. 5: 26–31.

Stauffer, E. 2004. "Sources of Interference in Fire Debris Analysis." In *Fire Investigation,* edited by N. Nic Daeid. Boca Raton, FL: CRC Press.

Stauffer, E., J. A. Dolan, and R. Newman. 2008. *Fire Debris Analysis.* Boston, MA: Academic Press.

Thatcher, L. March 1999. RVFOG Results. Personal communication.

Thomas, P. H. 1971. "Rates of Spread of Some Wind-Driven Fires." *Forestry* 44: 155–75

———. 1974. *Fire in Model Rooms.* Conseil Internationale du Batiment (CIB) Research Program, Building Research Establishment, Borehamwood, Hertfordshire, England.

———. 1981. "Testing Products and Materials for Their Contribution to Flashover in Rooms." *Fire and Materials* 5 (3):103-111. doi: 10.1002/fam.810050305.

Valentine, R. H., and R. D. Moore. 1974. "The Transient Mixing of Propane in a Column of Stable Air to Produce a Flammable but Undetected Mixture." New York: American Society of Mechanical Engineers.

White, R. H., and E. V. Nordheim. 1992. "Charring Rate of Wood for ASTM E 119 Exposure." *Fire Technology* 28: 5–30.

Xiang, X. Z., and J. J. Cheng. 2003. "A Model for the Prediction of the Thermal Degradation and Ignition of Wood under Constant Variable Heat Flux." In *Fire and Materials 2003,* 71–79. London: Interscience Communications.

Yudong, L., and D. D. Drysdale. 1992. "Measurement of the Ignition Temperature of Wood." Paper presented at First Asian Fire Safety Science Symposium, Hefei, Anhui Province, People's Republic of China.

Legal Reference

Truck Insurance Exchange v. MagneTek, Inc., 360 F.3d 1206 (10th Cir. 2004).

3

Chemical Fires and Explosions

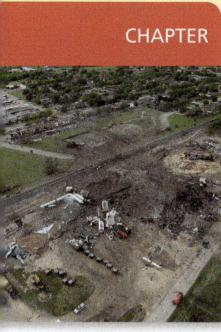

Devastation after ammonium nitrate detonation
in West Texas on April 17, 2013.
The seed room and fertilizer storage facility were decimated.
Source: Chip Somodevilla/Staff/Getty Images News/Getty Images

KEY TERMS

backdraft, *p. 182*

BLEVE, *p. 195*

brisance, *p. 189*

consumer fireworks, *p. 183*

deflagration, *p. 181*

detonation, *p. 174*

explosion, *p. 174*

explosive, *p. 176*

fragmentation, *p. 183*

high explosive, *p. 188*

high-order damage, *p. 192*

low explosive, *p. 186*

low-order damage, *p. 192*

mechanical explosion, *p. 192*

nonflammable, *p. 231*

physical hazard material, *p. 209*

seat of explosion, *p. 197*

stoichiometric, *p. 177*

unconfined vapor cloud explosion (UCVE), *p. 181*

vapor, *p. 178*

vapor density, *p. 178*

OBJECTIVES

After reading this chapter, you should be able to:

- Understand the scientific methodology used to identify and conduct investigations of chemical fires and explosions.
- Describe techniques used during scene examination, evidence recovery, and laboratory analysis.
- Explain the multiple potential causes of and contributing factors to chemical fires and explosions.
- Identify key reference materials on chemical hazards.
- List flammable gases, solid fuels, and hazardous liquids typically found in chemical fires and explosions.
- Identify the common causes of diffuse-phase explosions by gases, vapors, and suspended combustible dust.

- Identify common types of dense-phase explosives, their uses, and whether they are high or low explosives.
- Describe the chemical compounds associated with the production of improvised high explosives.
- Recognize, explain, and know the limitations of DOT hazard warning systems for the transport of hazardous materials.
- Recognize, explain, and know the limitations of NFPA hazard classes for the storage, use, and handling of hazardous materials.
- Interpret potential fire hazards from product labels and safety data sheets.

Fire is a chemical reaction. Fuels are decomposed (burned) in air to produce heat and products of combustion (CO, CO_2, H_2O, unburned hydrocarbons). Although most fires in buildings and passenger road vehicles involve typical combustible fuel contents like wood, paper, textiles, and petroleum products, many fires and explosions may involve or be the result of reacting or hazardous materials. Examples include thermite reactions between a susceptible metal and an oxide (i.e., titanium and iron oxide); reactions between a solid oxidizer and a contaminant (high-concentration calcium hypochlorite and brake fluid); release of heat from a exothermic decomposition reaction; and evolution of flammable gases from chemical processes (e.g., during pickling of steel).

Fires involving reacting or hazardous materials may be more intense or have higher heat release rates and burning temperatures, exhibit lower ignition propensities, dramatically increase the rate of fire spread, and make suppression a challenge or more dangerous by producing toxic gases, flammable gases, or explosive compounds. For example, water applied to a fire involving trichloroisocyanurate (pool chemicals) may produce nitrogen trichloride—a known explosive compound. Water applied to burning metal can be split to produce oxygen that intensifies a fire and hydrogen gas that, if confined, further fuels a fire, creating a potential explosion hazard.

explosion ■ The sudden conversion of potential energy (chemical or mechanical) into kinetic energy with the production and release of gases under pressure, or the release of gas under pressure. These high-pressure gases then do mechanical work such as moving, changing, or shattering nearby materials (NFPA 2017, pt. 3.3.56).

An **explosion** is defined by *NFPA 921* as "the sudden conversion of potential energy (chemical or mechanical) into kinetic energy with the production and release of gases under pressure, or the release of gas under pressure. These high-pressure gases then do mechanical work such as moving, changing, or shattering nearby materials" (NFPA 2017, pt. 3.3.56). Fire investigators should be able to discriminate the effects of explosions, per NFPA 1033, (NFPA 2014, pt. 4.2.9).

detonation ■ Propagation of a combustion zone at a velocity greater than the speed of sound in the unreacted medium (NFPA 2017 , pt. 3.3.46; see also NFPA, 2013a).

Fires and explosions frequently accompany each other. Explosions range in violence from the diffuse type of rolling, progressive flame resulting from combustion of a rich mixture of flammable gases or vapors in air, to the violent, almost instantaneous **detonation** of condensed-phase chemicals or an explosive mixture. The destructive effects of explosions from high-explosive detonations vary widely and range from broken windows and dislodged bricks to the complete destruction of buildings or vessels. *NFPA 921* specifically defines detonation as "the propagation of a combustion zone at a velocity greater than the speed of sound in the unreacted medium" (NFPA 2017, pt. 3.3.46; see also NFPA 2013a and 2013b).

The four basic types of explosions that the fire investigator may encounter are the following:

1. chemical, including explosible dusts,
2. mechanical,
3. electrical, and
4. nuclear.

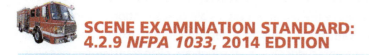

SCENE EXAMINATION STANDARD:
4.2.9 *NFPA 1033*, 2014 EDITION

TASK:

Discriminate the effects of explosions from other types of damage, given standard equipment and tools, so that an explosion is identified and its evidence is preserved.

PERFORMANCE OUTCOME:

The investigator will identify explosive effects on glass, walls, foundations, and other building materials, distinguish between low and high order explosion effects, and analyze damage to document the blast zone and origin.

CONDITIONS:

Given standard equipment and tools and a mock scenario of an explosion.

TASK STEPS:

1. Identify the type of explosion
2. Identify the possible cause of the explosion
3. Identify any explosive effects on glass, walls, foundations, and other building materials
4. Distinguish between low and high order explosion effects
5. Analyze damage to document the blast zone and origin

Source: Derived and updated from Washington State Patrol, Form No. 3000-420-081 (Sept. 2014) Fire Protection Bureau, Standards and Accreditation, Olympia, Washington http://www.wsp.wa.gov/fire/docs/cert/fire_invest.pdf

Explosions may be intentional or unintentional. Explosions may result from solid fuels—ranging from fine particulate solids like dust, to massive piles, to incompatible liquids and confined flammable or combustible gases. Chemical and mechanical explosions are more common than electrical and nuclear and may be related. For instance, incompatible reactive chemicals can evolve heat and gaseous compounds that result in a mechanical failure of a vessel. Purely mechanical explosions typically involve some form of containment and a subsequent failure and sudden release of a gas or liquid under conditions of pressure exceeding the rated pressure of a a container, vessel, or pipe.

The fire investigator is tasked with determining the conditions that caused mechanical explosions and whether the failure is a cause or consequence of the environment. For example, aluminum tanks for liquid propane gas are acceptable for ambient temperatures, whereas an aluminum propane tank exposed to an external fire can expand faster than the tank's relief valve can function, causing the tank to swell—ultimately exceeding the rated strength of the tank—and explode. The aluminum tank will fracture open with a clean edge; shrapnel from straps may be found at a distance from the event. The aluminum propane tank was a victim of an existing exposure fire. In a similar fashion, the release and ignition of natural gas inside a structure, once ignited, will expand with a flaming front and overpressures. Ammonium nitrate in the prill form, while stable at ambient temperatures and pressure, can detonate under conditions of exposure to fire, confinement, shock, and/or contamination, causing high overpressures and extensive damage.

A runaway reaction between one or more chemicals in a vessel can overcome the relief vent, causing the vessel to rupture. Furthermore, some mechanical explosions can initiate a secondary chemical explosion.

A pressure vessel, compressed air tank, or line failure, can disturb and suspend a combustible dust in air, which, if above the minimum explosible concentration and in the presence of an ignition source, can ignite, causing a secondary dust explosion. Electrical explosions occur when large currents suddenly flow through air, oil in transformers or switch gears, or undersized conductors. The extremely rapid heating causes the expansion of surrounding gases, the boiling and expansion of the oil, or evaporation of the conductor. This expansion occurs so quickly, as in a lightning strike, that explosive effects can be created, especially if the event is confined. Nuclear explosions cause massive blast effects by extremely rapid heating of surrounding gases and evaporating solids. All explosions involve the sudden release or production of gases that exert force and inflict damage on nearby materials.

Like other fire investigation scenarios, there is a methodology for performing an investigation of chemical fires and explosions. The first step is to assess the form of material first ignited and the fire cause as chemical.

3.1 Chemical Explosions

The conversion of chemical energy to kinetic energy can take on a variety of forms, and the energy released can exhibit a range of effects. The reaction paths and processes involved and the speed with which the reaction progresses depend not only on the chemistry of the starting materials involved but also, in some cases, on their physical form and environment (i.e., contamination with and without confinement, exposure to heat and fire). Explosive materials can be thought of as falling into two general categories—diffuse explosive mixtures and condensed-phase, or concentrated, explosives.

explosive ■ Any chemical compound, mixture, or device that functions by explosion (NFPA 2017 ed., pt. 3.3.58).

While diffuse explosive mixtures are most often combinations of a combustible gas with air, the condensed-phase explosion is not dependent on oxygen from the air but results from a combustive oxidation of the explosive. An **explosive** is any chemical compound, mixture, or device that functions by explosion NFPA 2017, pt. 3.3.58). An explosive can be a material that contains a mixture of both a fuel for the combustion and an internal oxidizer, or one that is unstable and capable of rearranging its chemical structure when stimulated, with highly exothermic effects. Black powder is an example of the first mixture type, while dynamites, TNT, nitroglycerine, PETN, and lead azide are examples of the second (single compound). All contain in themselves all the essential components for almost instantaneous conversion to gases with great kinetic energy (heat).

3.1.1 DIFFUSE-PHASE EXPLOSIONS

A diffuse-phase explosion is the rapid combustion of a fuel (gas, vapor, mist, or dust) premixed with air or oxygen and then ignited. The reaction proceeds as a flame front extends from the ignition source into the premixed fuel/air mixture and then grows larger in volume and surface area with time. Its effects are dependent on its type of fuel, concentration, ignition mechanism, and degree of confinement.

3.1.2 GASES

Perhaps the most common example of an accidental diffuse-phase explosion in the build environment is that the release of natural or liquid propane (LP) gas is able to mix with air and then be ignited. Depending on the amount of gas escaping, the amount of air in the space, and the leak rate and mixing that takes place, the reaction mixture can reach the explosive range. When a volume of natural gas is uniformly mixed with about 10 volumes of air, a mixture close to its ideal explosive ratio, ~9 percent, results. If this mixture fills a room and is ignited, the combustion is a deflagration, a propagation of a combustion zone at a velocity that is less than the speed of sound in the unreacted medium (NFPA 2017, pt. 3.3.43). The rate is pressure and temperature dependent and will increase as the ignition proceeds and the flame front expands, so it can become considerably higher.

The combustion produces a great amount of heat very suddenly, and the combustion gases (and remaining atmospheric gases—nitrogen, etc.) are quickly heated and expand violently. This expansion is restricted by the walls, floor, and ceiling of the room. The resulting overpressure, which is typically a few pounds per square inch (psi), several kilopascals (kPa), or a fraction of a bar (1 atmosphere = 14.7 psi = 1.013 bar = 101.32 kPa, so 1 psi = 6.89 kPa = 0.07 bar = 70 mbar = 27.67 in. w.c.), pushes the walls, floor, and ceiling, or breakable portions like windows and doors, outward. If enough gas is premixed with room air, the destruction can be extensive, as shown in Figures 3-1A–M.

Typically, early in the investigation, it is determined that utility gas contributed to the explosion. Processing a fire scene where a natural or LP gas explosion has occurred requires attention to gas piping and utilizing devices and appliances. Data regarding recent repair work or appliance installations, if any, should be gathered to establish a source for the fugitive gas.

This explosion process meets the definition of a deflagration because of the speed of propagation and moderate pressure that develop. With the heat generated in such a short time, items that are most readily ignited, charred, or damaged will be affected. Eyebrows and scalp hair may be singed, but flesh will not be deeply burned, because a longer time is needed for heat to penetrate and damage skin than hair. Clothing and thin draperies may be scorched or set on fire, but furnishings will be little affected because finer, less massive fabrics ignite more readily than upholstery and wood.

The pressures produced may move walls outward, break doors and windows, and even lift the roof or floors. However, a person in the room, especially one close to the source of ignition, may not be seriously injured by the blast itself. The compressive pressure wave near the origin is usually slight enough not to cause permanent injury and is moving away from the ignition source, and the flash fire may be transitory enough that an occupant may not be seriously burned, and combustibles may not be ignited. The pressures are not such that a localized seat of shattered or pulverized material is produced.

The combustion rate grows as the surface area of the flame front expands. As a result, anything that increases the surface area by turbulent mixing can increase the combustion rate. This mixing can be caused by furniture or by passage of the flame front through doorways or across barriers. Expansion of gases in the room of origin may also pressurize and heat the mixture in adjoining rooms. Because higher pressures and temperatures increase the intensity of the combustion and its propagation rate, the reaction accelerates. While a gas/air explosion originates at its ignition source, the greatest destruction will occur at distances from the ignition source while still within the premixed volume.

Ideal Mixture

Every fuel has a ratio with its oxidizer at which its production of heat and reaction velocity are at their maximum and combustion will be most efficient. This is called the ideal or **stoichiometric** ratio or mixture, and it is often close to the midpoint between the lean limit (LEL) and rich limit (UEL). The total damage done by a gas or vapor/air mixture will be maximized, because the amount of gaseous products and heat produced and the rates will all be at their respective maxima (NFPA 2017, pt. 5.1.5.2.2).

NFPA 921 advises (NFPA 2017, pt. 23.8.2.1) that explosions that occur in mixtures at or near the LEL or UEL of a gas or vapor can produce less violent explosions than those near the optimum concentration, which is just slightly rich of stoichiometric. Generally, investigators find and document that these explosions tend to produce low-order damage, particularly. This effect is related to the fact that the less-than-optimum ratio of fuel and air results in lower flame speeds, lower rates of pressure rise, and lower maximum pressure.

stoichiometric ■ Every fuel–air mixture has an optimum ratio at which point the combustion will be most efficient. This ratio occurs at or near the mixture known by chemists as the stoichiometric ratio. When the amount of air is in balance with the amount of fuel (i.e., after burning there is neither unused fuel nor unused air), the burning is referred to as stoichiometric. This condition rarely occurs in fires except in certain types of gas fires (NFPA 2017, pt. 5.1.5.2.2; see also pt. 23.8.2.1).

Rich Mixture

Consider now the "rich" mixture, where the escaping natural gas has mixed with the room air to form a mixture of 15 percent gas in air, or consider that the mixture of gas and room air is not uniform and there are pockets in which the gas concentration is much higher than in other parts of the room. When the mixture is ignited, there is an explosive thump, but there is insufficient air (oxygen) available for immediate and total combustion. Much of the natural gas is not burned, and the speed and force of the reaction are diminished. There is leftover and heated fuel in the area. The combustion products and remaining fuel expand when heated but cool immediately afterward, and air is drawn into the partial vacuum that results. This mixing provides more oxygen to combine with the remaining hot gas, and a rolling fire results as the turbulence caused by the initial combustion mixes the remaining fuel and air.

Because the reaction takes place over a longer period of time than in the case of an ideal mixture, a significant pressure wave may not develop, and the reaction may more accurately be classified as a combustion than as a deflagration. A victim may generally describe the event as "I heard a 'whoosh' and was on fire." Interestingly, a concussive thump will be more apparent to a listener outside the room than to someone within. Destruction by rich-mixture ignitions may far exceed that caused by theoretically perfect mixtures of gas and air, because such explosions are followed by fire, and the fire may consume a building that otherwise would have been subjected only to a sudden expansion that might move its walls but not destroy its contents. In some cases, stratified levels of fuel-rich mixtures create flammable mixtures and potentially strong explosions, which are pushed out a vent opening and mix with the ambient air.

The preceding discussion applies to natural gas (methane/ethane) or LP gas. Other gases behave differently. Hydrogen and acetylene, for instance, burn at much higher speeds than methane and exert much higher pressures. Acetylene can also detonate under some conditions. The chemical properties of any potential fuel gas must be carefully considered when assessing a blast scene.

Lean Mixture

The lean mixture combusts differently than the others in an explosion. Because the propagation rate for a gas/air mixture is greatest when the mixture is near its ideal or stoichiometric ratio, the lean-mixture explosion may be heard or felt as sharper than in the rich-mixture case. The force of a lean-mixture deflagration may be considerable, and its noise is very startling. However, with insufficient fuel to develop maximum speed, heat, and pressure during the blast or lingering, rolling post-blast fire, the damage from a lean-mixture deflagration may be minor compared with that of the other mixtures. No following fire is expected from a lean-mixture deflagration except for filmy materials like sheer curtains that may be ignited and then go on to set other fuels alight. Generally, although not in every instance, an explosion of this type produces purely physical forces and not an established fire.

3.1.3 VAPORS AND VAPOR DENSITY

Not all explosions involve fuel gases. Many involve the combustion of **vapors** generated by the evaporation of flammable liquids.

Vapor Density

Explosions that result from the ignition of vapors from liquid fuels are more likely to produce post-explosion fires than are those that result from the ignition of gases. The explosion itself produces heat to volatilize remaining liquid fuel, and provides an ignition source for the new vapors being generated. Gaseous fuels will be largely consumed or physically displaced, leaving little for continuous flaming fire afterward unless there is a continuous source of new gaseous fuel, such as a broken supply pipe.

The **vapor density** of organic liquid vapors must be considered in connection with special circumstances of the environment. For example, machines are sometimes degreased with hydrocarbon solvents. Not only is there possibly a high concentration of flammable

vapor ▪ The gas phase of a substance, particularly of substances that are normally liquids or solids at ordinary temperatures (NFPA 2017, pt. 3.3.196; see also pt. 3.3.96, Gas).

vapor density ▪ See *NFPA* 3.3.176, Specific Gravity (air) (vapor density) (NFPA 2017, pt. 3.3.197). The ratio of the average molecular weight of a gas or vapor to the average molecular weight of air (NFPA 2017, pt. 3.3.176).

vapors in the area, but also drains and service pits provide lower regions into which the vapors can sink. If vapors accumulate in a depression, it is there that the hazardous condition is first established. Any arc or flame in this vicinity can cause an explosion, even though it may be separated from the working area by some distance. Drains, sewers, heating ducts, elevator shafts, tunnels, and utility shafts are all possible areas for remote ignition. The density of flammable liquid vapors can produce rapid flame spread through the layer where the premixed fuel/air mixture is in the flammable range.

Because natural gas is lighter than air and mixes freely with it, natural gas deflagrations are good examples of the effects of various concentrations of fuel/air mixtures. Natural gas, however, is one of a few gases (hydrogen, methane, carbon monoxide) that are lighter than air. All vapors generated by evaporation of ignitable liquids at ordinary temperatures are *heavier* than air at the same temperature. Pentane vapors, for example, are about 2.5 times as heavy as air. Most petroleum distillates are less volatile than pentane, and their vapors are even heavier. Fresh automotive gasoline contains up to 8 percent *n*-butane and its related isomers, as well as pentane, so its initial evaporation and ignition properties are dominated by those of butane and pentane (DeHaan 1995).

Solvents

Most solvents like lacquer thinners, petroleum ether, and acetone have vapors, like those of gasoline, that are heavier than air. The fire investigator must understand their mixing properties in air. Dense vapors like these can be visualized as having fluid properties like maple syrup. When released, the vapors form a pool a few centimeters deep and then spread in a thick layer, seeping under doors, flowing down stairs, and collecting in pools in low spots of the room or structure. These vapors are heavy enough to concentrate at the bottom of low spots and form a very rich mixture. The vapors then mix slowly into overlying still air by diffusion, creating a gradient of concentration from the too rich to the too lean.

The combustion of a gradient concentration will usually progress quickly, but a rolling fire may be sustained as the rich layers are mixed by the turbulent combustion of the overlying layers. Ignition of gasoline vapors in the house shown in Figures 3-1A–E produced enough force to blow window assemblies from the building, but the following fire was limited to one room due to an excess of fuel vapors and insufficient ventilation elsewhere, producing too rich a mixture.

Mechanical Mixing

If sufficient mixing of gases or vapors with air occurs before ignition, there can be a massive deflagration. A layer-cake condition will exist only in a space where there is no mechanical mixing of the vapor/air layers. This mixing can be caused by open windows, doors, chimneys, machinery, or even by people walking through the area. Mechanical mixing will complicate the interpretation of the resulting fire. Propane releases are very sensitive to thermal mixing. Solar heating onto or into a compartment can cause enough circulation in the room to mix a propane/air mixture throughout. This may dilute small amounts to concentrations below the LEL or create ignitable mixtures throughout a room, despite the vapor density of pure propane.

Draft Conditions and Pilot Lights

When considering remote points of ignition of flammable vapors, draft conditions should be considered. The propagation of a layer of vapor along a horizontal surface from a container or spill of flammable liquid can be predicted to occur at a particular rate on the order of 2 to 5 cm/s (0.8 to 2 in./s) for pentane at 20°C (68°F) in still air depending on the volatility of the liquid and the temperature of the surroundings (Ellern 1961). Even small drafts caused by fans, mechanical equipment, or the pilot light of a stove or heater can cause a positive flow of vapors toward an ignition source at a much faster rate than expected.

A pilot light creates small volumes of hot gas that rise because of the reduced density of hot gases; cool air then flows into the base of the flame, giving rise to a slow but definite flow of air toward the flame. If heavy vapors are being released, even at some distance, this

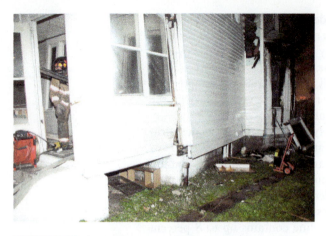

FIGURE 3-1A A gasoline vapor explosion severely damaged this abandoned house. *Courtesy of Jamie Novak, Novak Investigations and St. Paul Fire Dept.*

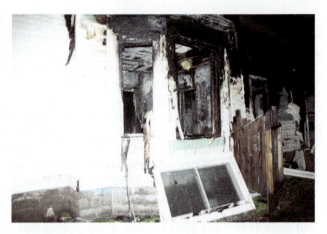

FIGURE 3-1B Only the room where windows had blown out suffered fire damage. *Courtesy of Jamie Novak, Novak Investigations and St. Paul Fire Dept.*

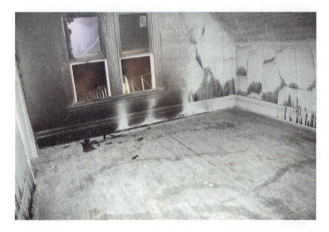

FIGURE 3-1C Gasoline had been poured throughout the house, but there was inadequate oxygen to allow full propagation. *Courtesy of Jamie Novak, Novak Investigations and St. Paul Fire Dept.*

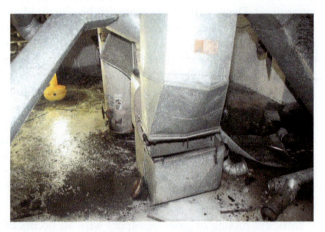

FIGURE 3-1D Furnace ductwork was badly damaged by overpressure within. *Courtesy of Jamie Novak, Novak Investigations and St. Paul Fire Dept.*

FIGURE 3-1E In the basement, the mixture was so rich that raw gasoline was still detected. Gasoline had pooled around the furnace and water heater (possibly ignited by the furnace). *Courtesy of Jamie Novak, Novak Investigations and St. Paul Fire Dept.*

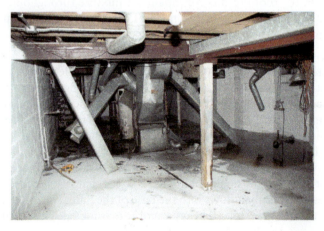
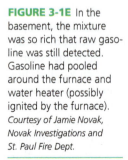

slow air flow will move the vapors toward the pilot and may result in ignition. The layer of vapors lies close to the floor, and if the combustion chamber is elevated, the vapors will not accumulate to an ignitable concentration. Pilot lights not only provide the arsonist with an open-flame ignition source but also draw the explosive vapors toward it. Ignition of the main burner or start-up of the fan causes the flow to occur much more quickly.

NFPA 921 (NFPA 2017, pt. 10.9.4.2) cautions that investigators should be aware that modern pilot light systems are designed to prevent gas flow to pilot lights on appliance burners by using a thermocouple to sense the presence of a lit pilot flame. However, if the cutoff system fails to close the gas supply to the pilot, the quantity of escaping gas is not large enough to fuel significant fires or explosions. The exception to this assumption is in spaces where little or no ventilation exists (NFPA 2017, pt. 10.9.4.3).

3.1.4 DEFLAGRATIONS

Although fires involving the vapors of flammable liquids can fall into the general descriptive class of combustion—with rolling flame fronts and minimal pressures produced—depending on circumstances of fuel, mixing, concentration, and confinement, they can readily achieve the next, more violent class of oxidation, **deflagration**. For a pressure effect to be produced, however, the deflagrating gas or vapor/air mixture must be confined to some extent. This confinement normally takes the form of a rigid container or even a room or structure.

If very large quantities of gaseous materials are involved, sufficient confinement may be produced by the inertia of the gas cloud. Although small quantities of a vapor/air mixture may deflagrate when confined in a rigid container, very large masses of the mixture must be present to provide a confinement effect in open air to produce what is sometimes called an **unconfined vapor cloud explosion** (UVCE) (see NFPA 2017, pt. 23.11.4). This open-air confinement effect is noticeable only in large clouds of airborne vapor above very large spills of volatile liquids.

An unconfined vapor cloud explosion is a more common occurrence at refineries or industrial premises where a large quantity of volatile liquid fuel is released quickly, often at high temperature and pressure. This quickly produces a very large vapor cloud that can then be ignited by any appropriate source in contact with it. This was the mechanism, for instance, for the huge UVCE at Flixborough, UK in 1974, when a large quantity of cyclohexane was released from a failed pipe joint. The explosion destroyed the large plant and killed 28 employees (USFA 1988).

The time required for a deflagration to occur differentiates deflagrations from other violent forms of combustion. A deflagration may take from several milliseconds to as much as a second to develop (Zalosh 2008a, 2008b). The time scales for detonations are much shorter. Similarly, the peak pressures developed by deflagrations are many times lower than those developed by detonations. Lower pressures and slower rates of pressure rise have a different effect on their surroundings than those from detonations.

Gaseous fuels are susceptible to transitioning from combustion to deflagration to detonation. This is especially true if they are heated and pressurized in contact with enough oxygen to support combustion. Heat and pressurization extend the explosive range, so what is not an explosive mixture at room temperature may be explosive under the conditions of actual use. As gases expand during combustion there is often a pressure-piling action that raises pressures and temperatures ahead of the actual reaction front.

The geometry of the confining vessel is also critical to deflagration/detonation transitions. If the mixture is confined in a pipe (or even long corridor) whose length (l) is significantly greater than its width or diameter (D) (typically $l/D > 100$; for some gases, it is as low as $l/D > 10$), the flame front stretches out due to frictional drag at its sides. This increases the surface area of the flame front and increases the combustion rate. When this acceleration reaches a certain point, the reaction transitions to a detonation (Lewis and Von Elbe 1961).

Interestingly, the detonation limits of such mixtures are not the same as the flammability/explosive limits discussed earlier, and the maximum velocities are not necessarily achieved at

deflagration ■ Propagation of a combustion zone at a velocity that is less than the speed of sound in the unreacted medium (NFPA 2017, pt. 3.3.43; see also NFPA 2013a).

unconfined vapor cloud explosion (UCVE) ■ When a flammable vapor is released, its mixture with air will form a flammable vapor cloud. If ignited, the flame speed may accelerate to high velocities and produce significant blast overpressure [American Institute of Chemical Engineers (AIChE), Glossary of Terms, 2017].

a central or ideal concentration. Detonation velocities ranging from 1,500 m/s to 2,000 m/s (between 4.2 and 50 percent) (4,920 to 6,560 ft/s) for acetylene in air were measured by Breton, depending on concentration (Lewis and Von Elbe 1961). Pure (98 percent) acetylene under pressure (5 kg/cm^2) detonates at 1,050 m/s (3,445 ft/s). Hydrogen detonation limits in air are reported to be 18.3 to 59 percent; carbon monoxide and hydrogen in air: 19 to 59 percent; and acetylene/air: 4.2 to 50 percent (Lewis and Von Elbe 1961).

The strength of the initiating source also can play a role in determining whether the reaction will be a deflagration or detonation. The stronger the source, the more likely a detonation will take place in a susceptible explosive or mixture.

Backdraft

backdraft ■ A deflagration resulting from the sudden introduction of air into a confined space containing oxygen-deficient products of incomplete combustion (NFPA 2017, pt. 3.3.17).

One special case of deflagrations that many investigators do not always consider is that of **backdraft**, or smoke, explosions. The gases, vapors, and solids produced by a smoky fire constitute a vapor-state fuel. If supplied with enough oxygen and a source of ignition, accumulations of smoke can deflagrate with sufficient energy to break windows, move light walls, and injure firefighters, producing pressures of 0.03 to 0.1 bar (0.5 to 1.5 psi) (Harris 1983, 126). See Figures 3-2 and 3-3 for an illustration of the explosive potential of a backdraft. Depending on the combustion rate of the accumulated smoke, there may not be sufficient overpressure to inflict physical damage. The expansion of the burning smoke layer, however, may fill portions of the building that were clear moments before and force smoke out door and window openings.

Dust Suspensions

Coal dust in mines, flour dust in granaries, metallic dust in machine shops, sawdust in lumber mills, or any fuel in powdered form can be dispersed in a cloud to form an explosive fuel/air mixture. Although we do not normally think of a solid fuel deflagrating in a diffuse-phase mixture, it can happen. As in gas- or vapor-based mixtures, there are ranges of concentration (typically measured in grams of fuel per cubic meter of air) for each fuel that will support combustion.

The behavior of the ignited solid/air mixture parallels the behavior of rich, lean, and ideal mixtures of gases and vapors. Unlike gases, however, there are restrictions on the particle size for each fuel that will sustain combustion. Generally, the finer the dust, the more likely it is to both remain airborne in suitable concentrations in air and to combust readily to contribute to a self-sustaining reaction. Organic dusts such as cornstarch, soy flour, sugar, and wheat starch are capable of creating maximum pressures of 8.5 to 9.9 bar

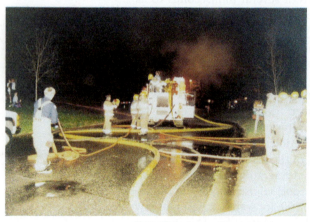

Figure 3-2

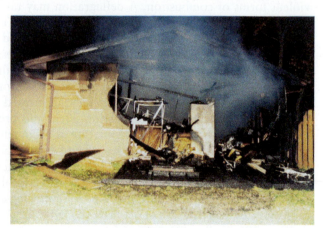

Figure 3-3

FIGURES 3-2 AND 3-3 Front windows and side wall of a garage blown out by a smoke explosion observed by arriving firefighters. Fire ignited against wood siding outside the front door. *Courtesy of Jamie Novak, Novak Investigations and St. Paul Fire Dept.*

(850 to 990 kPa or 123 to 144 psi) under ideal conditions (fine particles, suitable concentrations, strong ignition source) (Zalosh 2008a; Zalosh 2008b). One major difference between gas/air deflagrations and dust explosions is that accumulations of dust on surfaces are agitated by the initial deflagration, and this additional fuel will propagate the deflagration much longer, often gaining considerable energy in later stages (Spencer 2008, 57–61). More energetic ignition sources are frequently required for dust suspensions than for gas/air mixtures.

Turbulence caused by the initial combustion of fireworks can aerate such mixtures, allowing almost instantaneous combustion throughout (because flame will then come into contact with the fuel/oxidizer particles throughout the dust cloud). Unstable materials like acetylene and ethylene oxide are capable of transition to a detonation even when not airborne dusts.

3.1.5 IGNITION

In addition to open flames, other sources of heat can initiate ignition. No matter what other concentrations of vapors are present in the area, the fuel mixture *must* be present at combustible concentrations in the immediate area of the heat source to be ignited. With a fire, continued heating of a pyrolyzable fuel will create the conditions for the fire, but not for the explosion. Any hot spot or region, regardless of its size, can initiate an explosion of vapors if it meets the following criteria:

- There has to be contact between the ignition source and the fuel.
- At some point, the temperature of the source is well above the autoignition temperature of the flammable material involved.
- At the ignition point, the fuel/air mixture is within its explosive range.
- These conditions of contact last long enough for enough heat to be transferred to the fuel to trigger a self-sustaining combustion.

These criteria apply to all flames; electric arcs, including those created by static electric discharge; and hot solids, such as heated metal and incandescent sparks. Interestingly, smoldering combustion, as on the tip of a lighted cigarette, is generally incapable of initiating an explosion in a fuel vapor/air mixture.

Unlike an open flame that produces a continuous source of high temperature, an electric arc may be only of short duration. Either the vapors in contact with the arc are in their

CHEMICAL SAFETY BOARD (CSB)

The US Chemical Safety and Hazard Investigation Board (CSB; http://www.chemsafety.gov) is a nonregulatory, independent federal agency charged with investigating industrial chemical accidents. Headquartered in Washington, DC, the agency's board members are appointed by the president and confirmed by the Senate.

The CSB conducts origin and cause investigations of chemical accidents, such as dust, flammable vapor, gas, fire, and chemical explosions at fixed industrial facilities. The CSB does not issue fines or citations, but makes recommendations as to prevention measures to plants, regulatory agencies such as the Occupational Safety and Health Administration (OSHA), the Environmental Protection Agency (EPA), industry organizations, and labor groups.

ILLICIT EXPLOSIVE DEVICES

The term **consumer fireworks** is a misnomer when referring to "M-80" type devices. With their explosive filler—1 to 20 g of highly reactive flash powder—and cardboard containers, this class of explosives constitutes a significant risk from thermal and blast effects. The solid end plugs produce missile and **fragmentation** effects capable of causing injury and even death. These devices are dangerous and are controlled as illicit explosive devices under federal law in the United States.

consumer fireworks ■ Small fireworks devices containing restricted amounts of pyrotechnic composition, designed primarily to produce visible or audible effects by combustion, that comply with the construction, chemical composition, and labelling regulations of the US Consumer Product Safety Commission (CPSC), as set forth in CPSC 16 CFR 1500 and 1507, 49 CFR 172, and APA Standard 87-1, Standard for the Construction and Approval for Transportation of Fireworks, Novelties, and Theatrical Pyrotechnics (NFPA 2014).

fragmentation ■ The process by which the casing of an artillery shell, bomb, or grenade is shattered by the detonation of the *explosive* filler.

explosive range and explode, or they are not, in which case nothing happens as a result of the arc. A similar effect is produced when a small charge of high explosive is used to disperse gasoline from a plastic or glass container. The high explosive generates gases at very high temperatures (thousands of degrees), but they are of short duration, and the explosion pushes the gasoline (fuel) and oxygen mixture away from the ignition source. More often than not, no ignition occurs. If a metal container is used for the gasoline, however, the metal fragments (shrapnel) are superheated by the initiating blast and frictional tearing and will often act as point sources of ignition, as they retain their heat longer than do the gases of the reaction.

3.2 Condensed-Phase Explosions

Condensed-phase explosions involve solid or sometimes liquid or gel explosives in which either the fuel and oxidizer are mechanically mixed or the monomolecular material itself is capable of undergoing extremely rapid conversion. Explosions of higher energy than the deflagrations described previously usually involve a condensed-phase or dense-phase chemical, because detonation of a diffuse-phase system is very rare. These detonations may occur in high-pressure or high-temperature gas systems or in systems involving sensitive compounds such as acetylene or ethylene oxide.

Oxidation reactions that fall into the detonation category differ greatly from combustion and deflagration reactions in a number of ways, as graphically represented in Figure 3-4. There are major differences in the reaction time and in the reaction volume of the explosive reaction.

Compared with the milliseconds or seconds required for a deflagration, detonations occur throughout the charge within microseconds. The forces generated and their effects on the surroundings will be different more because of this time relation than because of the total force generated. The pre-blast reaction volume of a stick of dynamite in a room is the small volume occupied by that stick, virtually a point source from which all the explosive forces are generated as the post-blast gases occupy some 1,500 times the pre-blast volume. If the same room is filled with an explosive mixture of vapors and air, the explosive volume is that of the entire room, which, upon combustion, tries to occupy up to 8 times its original volume. In physical terms, this is the chief distinction between diffuse- and condensed-phase explosions. In chemical terms, of course, there are many differences.

Even though the total forces produced (i.e., total work done) may be similar, the specific effects of the two types of explosions will be quite different. While the energy released

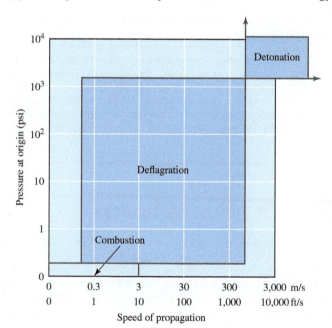

FIGURE 3-4 Phase diagram showing ranges of pressure and speed of propagation for general states of explosive combustion, deflagration, and detonation.

by the complete deflagration of a quantity of gasoline can be compared to that released by a detonation quantity of high explosives, the damage potential of the two events is vastly different due to the time frames and dynamics involved. The energy released by TNT detonating is on the order of 4.56 MJ/kg, while the heat of combustion of methane is 55 MJ/kg and that of gasoline is 46 MJ/kg (Kirk-Othmer, ed. 1998).

Most condensed-phase high explosives require an initiating mechanical shock that triggers a cascade effect of reactions throughout the reaction volume. Materials that detonate have chemical bonds sensitive to energy applied in the form of pressure and are disrupted by the transmittal of pressure or shock throughout the mass of the explosive charge.

The characteristic feature of detonation is the shock wave that propagates the reaction moving through the explosive at a speed greater than the speed of sound in that matrix. Unlike the high-speed oxidations of gaseous explosive mixtures, detonations of a condensed-phase explosive do not require confinement except when small quantities of material are involved. Many sensitive materials will still detonate when unconfined, but not very efficiently. The pressures produced will be low, and a considerable amount of the material will remain undetonated in what is called a *low-yield* or *nonideal* explosion. Some materials will detonate when heated to a critical temperature that is often pressure dependent.

All explosives have a critical diameter. If a mass of explosive is too thin or too small in cross section there will be no propagation. Such critical diameters are taken into account when commercial preparations such as dynamite cartridges, grenades, or high-explosive boosters are being designed but are ignored in many improvised criminal devices.

3.2.1 CHEMICAL AND PHYSICAL PROPERTIES

Materials that explode or detonate have a different chemistry from those that require the addition of an external source of oxygen to enable the reaction. The molecules of materials that can detonate have the capability of shattering into fragments when properly stimulated. As those molecular fragments recombine, they release large quantities of heat in a fraction of the time it takes for combustion to take place.

Because many nitrogen compounds are basically unstable from the standpoint of their compositional (potential) chemical energy, nitrogen compounds are probably the most common types of chemicals used in the formulation of explosive materials. Nitrogen is an element that resists chemical combination with other elements. This means that the compounds of nitrogen tend suddenly to rearrange themselves to yield elemental nitrogen. In doing so, they release their potential chemical energy as heat and light in an explosively sudden manner. Oxygen is often combined with nitrogen in various carbon-containing organic compounds in common explosives. In the explosion, nitrogen is released from its chemical structure along with a great deal of energy, and the oxygen combines with carbon compounds during the reaction to produce even more energy.

Materials that undergo explosive decomposition almost always contain one or more characteristic chemical structures that are responsible for the sudden release of great energy. These structures include the following groups:

- —NO_2 and —NO_3 in organic and inorganic nitrates
- —N_3 in inorganic and organic azides
- —NX_2, where X is a halogen
- —ON≡C in fulminates
- —$OClO_2$ and —$OClO_3$ in inorganic and organic chlorates and perchlorates, respectively
- —O—O— and —O—O—O— in inorganic and organic peroxides and ozonides, respectively
- —C≡C— in acetylene and metal acetylides
- [M—C], a metal atom bonded with carbon in some organometallic compounds (Urbanski 1964)

There are many mixtures containing both fuel and oxidizer that are subject to deflagration. These produce generally low-energy deflagrating explosions, but can produce severe damage when encountered in improvised explosive devices. For instance, black powder is a mixture of carbon, sulfur, and potassium nitrate (as the oxidizer), and flash powder is commonly a mixture of aluminum powder and sulfur (as fuels) and a perchlorate (as the oxidizer).

In addition to their similar chemistries, materials that explode or detonate have several performance properties in common—they all produce large amounts of heat and, when properly initiated, convert nearly completely to gaseous products (with the rare exception of the metal acetylides that produce carbon and metal and no gaseous products). These gases and atmospheric gases nearby in turn expand rapidly due to the heat generated. Most explosive materials are sensitive to heat in some degree. Raising the temperature will cause explosion or detonation, but unlike combustible vapors, explosive materials, due to their chemistry, do not have precise ignition temperatures (Henkin and McHill 1952, 1391). The ignition temperature measured depends on the rate of rise of the temperature. The faster the temperature rises, the lower the autoignition temperature appears to be.

3.3 Types and Characteristics of Explosives

In addition to being sensitive to heat, most explosives are also sensitive, to a greater or lesser degree, to initiation by mechanical shock. Thus, the sensitivity of an explosive material to both such effects is of interest to the fire and safety investigator. Based on the sensitivities and oxidation processes of these materials, explosives are often classified as propellants, low explosives, or high explosives. Explosions may also be characterized as high order or low order.

Common explosives and their compositions are summarized in Table 3-1.

3.3.1 PROPELLANTS OR LOW EXPLOSIVES

low explosive ■ Low explosives are characterized by deflagration (subsonic blast pressure wave) or a relatively slow rate of reaction and the development of low pressure when initiated. Common low explosives are smokeless gunpowder, flash powders, solid rocket fuels, and black powder. Low explosives are designed to work by the pushing or heaving effects of the rapidly produced hot reaction gases (NFPA 2017, pt. 23.12.1.1).

Propellants or **low explosives** are combustible materials that carry both fuel and the necessary oxygen for their combustion. Low explosives are designed to work by the pushing or heaving effects of the rapidly produced hot reaction gases. *NFPA 921* characterizes low explosives as those that produce deflagration (subsonic blast pressure wave) or a relatively slow rate of reaction and the development of low pressure when initiated (NFPA 2017, pt. 23.12.1.1).

Nitrocellulose propellants ignite at approximately 190°C (374°F) and combust when burned in small quantities at normal atmospheric pressures (Davis 1943). This oxidation rate is pressure (confinement) dependent. Modest confining pressures elevate it to a deflagration, which becomes extremely fast at the pressure developed inside a cartridge when confined by a bullet. For example, the burning rate of Bullseye smokeless powder at normal atmospheric pressure is 0.23 mm/s (0.009 in./s); at 34.5 bar [3.45 MPa (500 psi)] its burning rate is 6 mm/s (0.24 in./s); while at 2,410 bar [241 MPa (35,000 psi)] (a typical breech pressure inside a weapon) its burning rate is 300 mm/s (11.8 in./s) (Cooper and Kurowski 1996, 43). Double-base smokeless powders contain nitroglycerin in addition to nitrocellulose and can be sensitive to sympathetic (pressure) initiation and detonation if nitroglycerin is present in high enough concentration. They do not detonate under most conditions.

Black powder, on the other hand, deflagrates even when burned in small quantities at atmospheric pressure and can produce high-intensity blast effects when confined by only a moderate pressure (such as the inertia of the surrounding charge itself). Black powder has a burning rate of 17 mm/s (0.67 in./s) at atmospheric pressure, 30 mm/s (1.2 in./s) at 34.5 bar [3.45 MPa (500 psi)], and only 62 mm/s (2.44 in./s) at 2,410 bar [241 MPa (35,000 psi)] (Cooper and Kurowski 1996, 43). It is not subject to sympathetic (pressure) initiation and does not detonate at any time.

TABLE 3-1 Common Explosives

TYPE	COMPOSITION	CHARACTERISTICS
High Explosives *Primary/Main* Charge Straight dynamite	Nitroglycerin (NG) Ethylene glycol dinitrate (EGDN) Sodium nitrate Wood pulp	Water resistant High strength
Gelatin dynamite	NG/EGDN Nitrocellulose (gelling agent) Wood pulp Sulfur (in some cases)	Water resistant High strength
Ammonia dynamite	NG/EGDN Ammonium nitrate (NH_4NO_3) Sodium nitrate ($NaNO_3$) Wood pulp Sulfur	Less expensive Reduced water resistance
Nitrostarch dynamite	Nitrostarch Aluminum flakes	Similar to nitrocellulose No NG headaches Does not separate or decompose
Military dynamite	RDX Trinitrotoluene (TNT) Cornstarch Oil	Insensitive to shock, friction Stable in storage
TNT	Trinitrotoluene	Military uses High brisance
Initiators PETN	Pentaerythritol tetranitrate	High brisance Also used in detonating cord and Semtex
RDX	Cyclotrimethylenetrinitramine	High brisance Also used in detonating cord and Semtex
Blasting Agents Slurries	Ammonium nitrate or sodium nitrate, often with fuels such as carbon or aluminum	Used in bulk or prepackaged form Main charge only Require booster Can detonate
Water gels	Ammonium nitrate Sodium nitrate Sensitized with organic nitrates (e.g., monomethylamine nitrate) In emulsion form	Require booster Can detonate
Low Explosives	Commonly used in improvised explosive devices Also used in explosive hardware and tool applications	Deflagrate, but can produce detonation-like effects if adequately confined
Black powder	Potassium nitrate Sulfur Charcoal	Easily ignitable Filler in safety fuse Firearm propellant
Single-base smokeless powder	Nitrocellulose	Firearm propellant
Double-base smokeless powder	Nitrocellulose Nitroglycerin	Firearm propellant

Both smokeless powder and black powder function as small-arms propellants when they are ignited as thin flakes or small granules as illustrated in Figure 3-5. The finer the size, the faster they will burn to completion. Deflagrations can produce pressures of up to 2,760 bar [276 MPa (40,000 psi)] (solid explosives) with reaction velocities of up to

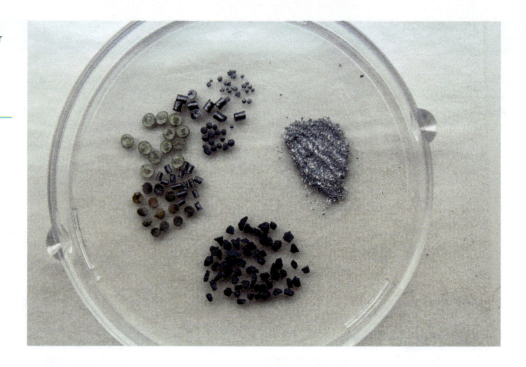

FIGURE 3-5 Common pipe bomb fillers. Upper left: various smokeless powders. Upper right: flash powder. Bottom: black powder. *Courtesy of Wayne Moorehead.*

1,000 m/s (3,280 ft/s) (depending on chemistry, confinement, and manner of initiation). Depending on their means of ignition, geometry, and confinement, some materials, like double-base smokeless powder and potassium perchlorate/aluminum ($KClO_4/Al$) flash powders, can detonate. Under some conditions, they can be considered to be high explosives.

3.3.2 HIGH EXPLOSIVES

high explosive ■ A material that is capable of sustaining a reaction front that moves through the unreacted material at a speed equal to or greater than that of sound in that medium [typically 1000 m/sec (3000 ft/sec)]; a material capable of sustaining a detonation (NFPA 2017, pt. 3.3.107; see also pt. *3.3.46, Detonation*).

High explosive materials are intended to detonate and will detonate when properly initiated by heat or shock. Localized heating produced by mechanical shock is sufficient to rupture some of their chemical bonds and initiate a chain reaction in which heat from one bond disruption is quickly transmitted to surrounding bonds in a cascade, which results in the explosion of the entire mass within a few microseconds.

High explosive detonations have velocities of 1,000 to 9,000 m/s (3,280 to 29,500 ft/s) with maximum pressures (at the surface of the explosive charge) of more than 68.9 bar [6,890 MPa (1,000,000 psi)]. Such localized high pressures result in a seat of most intense damage—often shattering or pulverizing nearby surfaces.

Properties of Straight Dynamite

At one time, probably the most common high explosive was ordinary nitroglycerin or *straight* dynamite. Straight dynamite is compounded with nitroglycerin (NG) and ethylene glycol dinitrate (EGDN) soaked into a solid absorbent or filler such as sawdust. This type of dynamite is very sensitive to shock, friction, degradation, separation (weeping), and thermal ignition and is very rarely used today except for ditching applications, where water resistance and sympathetic initiation are desirable features. The strength of a straight dynamite is based on the actual percentage of NG present by weight.

Properties of Gelatin Dynamite

Gelatin dynamite, which uses a combination of NG dissolved in nitrocellulose, is a formulation that is water resistant and very energetic but is expensive to make and prone to separation, "weeping" liquid nitroglycerin. These expensive components (NG and nitrocellulose) are sometimes replaced (all or in part) with ammonium nitrate or sodium nitrate. These combinations are still effective high explosives but are sensitive to water, which can render them unusable. When ammonium nitrate is used, the product is called an *ammonia* or *semigelatin* dynamite. These ammonia dynamites are rated in strength *equivalent* to a particular percentage of NG (i.e., 40 percent ammonia dynamite does not contain 40 percent NG but contains the energy equal to 40 percent–strength straight dynamite).

Alternative High Explosives
Due to the expense and danger of making and storing nitroglycerin dynamites, they have been largely replaced by water-gel dynamites that use organic nitrates as sensitizing agents and ammonium nitrate as the main explosive ingredient. Today, nitroglycerin dynamites are made only in small quantities for special applications. Some dynamites are made with nitrostarch as the explosive agent. This dynamite contains no nitroglycerin, and the attendant risks are absent. The water-gel explosives are based on formulations of ammonium nitrate and organic nitrates such as monomethylamine nitrate or monoethanolamine in a water-based gel or guar gum or similar agent.

There are also slurry-type blasting agents that contain ammonium or sodium nitrates and aluminum or coal tar powders as fuel. Such materials are more stable than nitroglycerin but less sensitive, requiring a substantial detonation to trigger them. These explosives degrade to inert compounds rather than to more dangerous forms (e.g., straight dynamite "weeping" nitroglycerin). Due to their physical form as an emulsion, suspension, or slurry containing water, they are less sensitive at cold temperatures, are rendered unusable by freezing, and cannot be used in wet applications.

3.3.3 HIGH EXPLOSIVE CATEGORIES
High explosives may be further categorized as *primary*, or *initiating*, explosives and *main charge* explosives. Initiators like mercury fulminate, lead azide, picric acid salts, and others are highly sensitive to mechanical shock, friction, heat, and electricity and are commonly used in blasting caps and primers to initiate a larger explosion. Main charge explosives include dynamite, TNT, PETN, RDX, and the like. When dispersed, main charge explosives often simply burn, but in any mass at all (more than a few grams) these materials can detonate. Their actual performance may depend on the size and shape of the charge and the manner of initiation.

High explosives are rated by factors related to their intended application. Generally, commercial explosives are used in pushing or heaving applications, while military explosives are usually needed for their shattering power or **brisance**. Commercial high explosives are formulated in dilutions or mixtures of components to control not only the energy released but also the brisance, because different applications require different explosive properties.

brisance ■ The shattering effect or power of an explosion or explosive.

Blasting Agents
Blasting agents are explosive materials that generally require a high-explosive booster to initiate a detonation. Ammonium nitrate/fuel oil (ANFO) and its variants are the most common blasting agents. They are often sold in bulk rather than as individual units.

Binaries
There are a small number of high explosives called *binaries* which are made up of two components that by themselves are not explosives. When the components are mixed together, binaries form a cap-sensitive high explosive. Mixtures of nitromethane and ammonium nitrate or nitromethane and organic amines have been marketed as binary explosives (Cooper and Kurowski 1996, 43). Tannerite, a filler for exploding firearms targets, is sold as a binary today. It consists of an ammonium nitrate and ammonium perchlorate mixture as one component and fine aluminum powder as the second. Mixed together, they constitute a powerful, impact-sensitive high explosive.

Improvised Explosives
A number of high explosives can be synthesized by fairly simple chemical processes to be used in improvised explosive devices (IEDs). These include nitrogen triiodide (NI_3),

triacetone triperoxide (TATP), hexamethylene triperoxide diamine (HMTD), hydroxyl ammonium nitrate (HAN), ammonium dinitro amide (ADN), and metallic azides, fulminates, and acetylides. These are powerful and sensitive primary explosives (initiated by heat, friction, shock, or even static electricity) that would leave minimal detectable residues in post-blast debris if properly made and functioned (high order) (Muller et al. 2004).

Other high explosive blasting agents that have been easily synthesized and used in criminal bombings include ammonium nitrate/sugar and urea nitrate. These mixtures were estimated to have detonation velocities of 3,730 m/s for urea nitrate and 3,560 m/s for ammonium nitrate/sugar (Phillips et al. 2000). Silver acetylide [Ag—C≡C—Ag] is an example of a rare category of explosive that produces only solid residues (carbon and metallic silver) and no gas during its detonation. The enormous heat produced, however, heats the surrounding air to several thousand degrees, and the resulting expansion of gases exerts explosive force. Despite its unstable and sensitive nature, TATP has become the most widely used improvised explosive. It can be formulated using acetone, hydrogen peroxide, and acid from easily obtainable consumer products (e.g., nail polish remover, hair bleach, and batteries). The processes are simple and can be carried out with a few jars, filters, and ice.

3.3.4 COMPONENTS
High explosives usually require the use of initiators, time fuses, and boosters.

Blasting Caps
High-explosive main charges often require a detonation to initiate them. As shown in Figure 3-6, a small detonation source can be contained in a blasting cap consisting of an igniter compound, time delay, primary explosive, and, typically, a high explosive. An electric blasting cap has two leg wires and a bridge wire embedded in the ignitor. Applying electric current causes the bridge wire to overheat quickly, igniting the deflagrating material. A delay is often built in to increase the time between application of current and initiation of the primary explosive (typically from 10 to 200 milliseconds). The primary charge detonates, triggering the high explosive filler, which, in turn, provides the shock needed to cause the main charge to detonate. All this is contained within a metal (often aluminum) sleeve or tube, about 5 mm (3/16 in.) in diameter and 40 to 65 mm (1-1/2 to 3 in.) in length.

Nonelectric blasting caps have a hollow end that is crimped over the open end of a traditional safety fuse. Shock tube caps can be triggered only by the detonation of a fine coating of high explosive on the inside of a small-diameter plastic tube. These caps are safer to use than traditional caps, since they cannot be triggered by stray electric currents or flame. The propagation of the detonating coating is confined to the interior of the plastic tube.

Boosters
Boosters are small, specially formed high explosive charges made of TNT, PETN, or RDX that may be shaped like ice cubes, finger-sized sleeves, or cylinders. They are used as

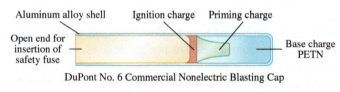

DuPont No. 6 Commercial Nonelectric Blasting Cap

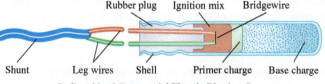

FIGURE 3-6 Typical blasting caps. Top: non-electric. Bottom: electric.

DuPont No. 6 Commercial Electric Blasting Cap

intermediates between blasting caps and main charge explosives. High explosive detonating cord is sometimes threaded through boosters or even used as a substitute booster by knotting it around or threading it through a main charge high explosive. Detonating cord is filled with PETN or RDX high explosive and itself requires a blasting cap to initiate it.

Time Fuse

Fire and explosion investigators will see different types of fuses. A common type is pyrotechnic or hobby fuse, in which a core of pyrotechnic powder is wrapped with windings of fine string and coated with nitrocellulose lacquer. When ignited, it burns with a visible exposed flame. Although intended to burn at rates of 12 to 25 mm/s (1/2 to 1 in./s), it can burn faster when crimped or crushed.

A safety fuse consists of a core of finely ground black powder protected by wrappings of string, tar, and plastic. When this fuse is ignited at one end, a small spurt of flame is emitted at the other end. There is no exposed flame anywhere along its length. It burns at 80 to 100 cm/min (30 to 40 in./min) and, due to its waterproofing layers, it can burn underwater.

Igniter cord consists of a perchlorate-based incendiary filler with a multiple spiral wrap of fine nickel-chrome-iron wire. It burns very quickly and is rarely seen in improvised devices.

Improvised fuses can include string or paper impregnated with black powder or pyrotechnic powders. Fuse materials removed from commercial fireworks such as quick match (black powder core wrapped in layers of paper) are also encountered.

Firing Trains

The combination of initial heat source, fuse, blasting cap, booster, and main charge is often called the firing train, or fuzing system. High explosives generally require a small detonation to initiate them but will not be initiated by a simple flame or electric arc. Time delays, blasting caps, and boosters may not be present, depending on the explosive involved and the intended use.

The accidental explosion of a munitions ship in December 1917 in the harbor of Halifax (Nova Scotia) is a good example of an accident with a complete firing train. Collision with another ship caused the release and ignition of drums of benzene (as deck cargo). The fire triggered the detonation of picric acid explosive, which in turn caused the detonation of the main cargo of TNT. A total of 2,925 tons of high explosive disintegrated the ship and flattened the center of Halifax, causing some 2,000 deaths and injuring 9,000 (Flemming 2004).

3.3.5 HIGH-ORDER EXPLOSIONS

Explosives are often categorized as *high order* or *low order*. Only high explosives can achieve *detonation*, the term referring to the propagation of a supersonic reaction wave within the explosive charge. This shock wave actually causes the rupture of the chemical bonds holding the explosive together. The entire mass of explosive converts to gas and heat at supersonic speeds, causing extremely high temperatures and pressures as well as shock, all of which bring about the shattering effect commonly associated with such explosives. All other explosive mechanisms are deflagrations (by our definition), because they propagate at subsonic speeds. The energy and heat produced in the initial charge are transferred within the charge at lower speeds (often by particle-to-particle transfer of thermal energy), and combustion of the individual fuel elements then proceeds at the surface of each particle. Heat and gases are produced at a slower rate, and lower pressures are produced. The external effects are less shattering than with a detonation, but they can be substantial in terms of the total kinetic energy produced.

High explosives are materials that are capable of sustaining a reaction front that moves through the unreacted material at a speed equal to or greater than that of sound in that medium [typically 1000 m/sec (3000 ft/sec)], a material capable of sustaining a detonation (NFPA 2017, pt. 3.3.107). High explosives need not initiate and propagate perfectly each time. This is particularly true with improvised explosive devices. Commercial explosive charges and military munitions are carefully designed to convert as completely to kinetic energy as possible so that the explosive effects are predictable. These complete conversions are referred to as *ideal*, *high-yield*, or *high-order detonations*. Improvised devices contain shapes and sizes of charges that cannot detonate completely, even when high explosives are used.

NFPA 921 characterizes **high-order damage** by a rapid pressure rise or high-force explosion producing a shattering effect on the confining structure or container and long missile distances (NFPA 2017, pt. 3.3.108).

Explosives have characteristic minimum diameters below which detonation is incomplete. If the initiating charge or device is inadequate in size (energy) or poorly placed in the main charge, detonation may not take place at all. For this reason, even when traditional high explosives (TNT, nitroglycerine, PETN, dynamite, RDX) are used, they may not detonate completely or at all. This is referred to as *low-yield*, *nonideal*, or *low-order detonation*. Premixed gas or vapor fuel/air mixtures at their ideal or stoichiometric mixture can be said to sometimes propagate high order because they function at maximum efficiency with no residual starting material.

3.3.6 LOW-ORDER EXPLOSIONS

Low-order explosives like black powder and nitrocellulose do not detonate even when confined and initiated under ideal circumstances and, because of the inefficiency or ineffectiveness of the thermal processes involved, do not explode high order. Double-base smokeless powder, because it contains both a low explosive (nitrocellulose) and a high explosive (nitroglycerin), can act as either a low or high explosive, depending on its initiation and confinement.

NFPA 921 characterizes the **low-order damage** by a slow rate of pressure rise or low-force explosion characterized by a pushing or dislodging effect on the confining structure or container and by short missile distances (NFPA 2017, pt. 3.3.127).

When a powder, such as Alliant Red Dot or Bullseye, with a high nitroglycerin content is used and is initiated with a suitable blasting cap, it can detonate, especially if an improvised container of high bursting strength such as a gas cylinder is used, but will rarely reach ideal or high-order conditions. In most improvised devices, the containment is weak or the initiation is inadequate, and the resulting blast, while terribly destructive, is not ideal (high order) and there will be intact, unreacted explosive scattered about. So when asked, "Did such-and-such a material explode high order?" the correct answer is usually, "It depends." That determination often depends on careful assessment of thermal and mechanical effects (indicators) at both macro and microscopic scale.

3.4 Mechanical Explosions

In a **mechanical explosion**, a container, vessel, or pipe bursts when internal gas or liquid pressures exceed the tensile strength of the container. The resulting release of high-pressure gas can produce blast effects (pressure, shock, and fragmentation), which can damage or destroy vehicles and buildings. Because an exothermic chemical reaction is not involved, heat is not released except in the tearing or shattering of metals. If liquid is released at temperatures or pressures far above ambient conditions, it vaporizes nearly instantaneously, and the rapidly expanding vapors exert their destructive forces on nearby surfaces.

Mechanical explosions may occur by themselves or before, during, or after fires. When associated with a fire, they may be the cause of the fire, or simply add to its destruction. Once the general nature of the explosion has been deduced, the search for pieces of the explosive device or the accidental mechanism responsible, or for residues of the chemicals involved (if any), can be undertaken more efficiently.

Mechanical explosions can produce blast effects that may be difficult to distinguish from those of chemical explosions. In either case, fluids or gases at very high pressures strike surfaces, distorting and sometimes shattering them to produce energetic secondary

high-order damage ■ A rapid pressure rise or high-force explosion characterized by a shattering effect on the confining structure or container and long missile distances (NFPA 2017, pt. 3.3.108).

low-order damage ■ A slow rate of pressure rise or low-force explosion characterized by a pushing or dislodging effect on the confining structure or container and by short missile distances (NFPA 2017, pt. 3.3.127).

mechanical explosion ■ An explosion where a container, vessel, or pipe bursts when internal gas or liquid pressures exceed the tensile strength of the container.

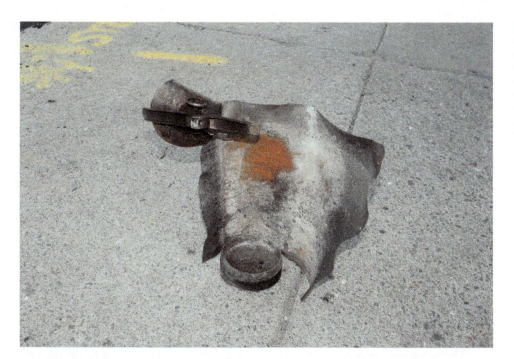

FIGURE 3-7 Fire extinguisher casing after mechanical explosion caused by exposure to sustained fire. *Courtesy of Vic Massenkoff, Contra Costa County Fire Protection District.*

missiles, or shrapnel. Cylinders of compressed gases, aerosol cans, storage tanks, hydraulic lines, pipelines, and similar systems can be overpressurized due to mechanical failures of compressors, relief valves, or regulators. Such containers may also be exposed to heat with a resulting increase in internal pressure. When the pressures developed within the line or vessel exceed its bursting strength, it will fail, and the pressurized fluid will be released, potentially with catastrophic results. The escaping gases inflict shock or pressure effects on nearby surfaces and may propel resulting fragments at high velocities.

Mechanical explosions can sometimes produce a localized seat of damage, similar to that produced by condensed-phase explosives. They are usually gaseous phenomena, except that changes in chemical or physical state are not involved, and that heat is not produced (other than heat created by the rapid tearing of a metal container). The absence of fire or other thermal damage is often a reliable indicator that a mechanical explosion occurred. When external heating has been involved, it will be seen that heated metals have lower tensile strengths than do those same metals at ordinary temperatures. An externally heated vessel is most likely to fail where it is heated.

See Figure 3-7 for an exploded fire extinguisher. Propane cylinders often fail with a typical "fish-mouth" hole where exposed to fire that produces little explosive effect. The location and orientation of that failure will direct the flow of released gases, sometimes causing the container itself to become a projectile.

3.4.1 ACID, GAS, OR BOTTLE BOMBS

A variety of improvised explosive devices function by creating a gas, usually non-flammable, by chemical reaction that causes the mechanical explosion of a confining vessel, most commonly a plastic soft-drink bottle. The reactions may produce CO_2 with little evolution of heat or may be strongly exothermic and produce steam as well as gas. These devices usually involve common household products, and they are easily accessible. They can produce high pressures and toxic or caustic gases capable of inflicting serious injuries as well as mechanical destruction (McDonald and Shaw 2009). Table 3-2 lists some of the more common combinations of ingredients.

Mixtures that produce flammable gas (hydrogen or acetylene) can have a double explosive effect—the mechanical failure of the confining container followed by the

| TABLE 3-2 | Common Ingredients Found in Acid, Gas, and Bottle Bombs |

COMBINATION	PRODUCT OF REACTION
Dry ice and water	Carbon dioxide
Alka-Seltzer and vinegar	Carbon dioxide
Calcium carbide and water	Acetylene gas
Sugar, dry bleach, and water	Steam, bleach
Aluminum foil and Drano	Hydrogen
Metal foil and hydrochloric acid	Hydrogen
Toilet, pool, or spa treatment and alcohol/ammonia or hydrogen peroxide (Newest products contain chlorinated or brominated hydantoins or chlorinated isocyanuric acids)	Chlorine gas or bromine gas[a] [a]Also nitrogen trichloride or nitrogen tribromide explosives

deflagration of the turbulently mixed fuel/air mixture. This deflagration may be nearly instantaneous if an open-flame ignition source (such as a lighted candle) is placed nearby, or delayed if the mixture has to spread to find an ignition source.

The pressures produced by the failure of a soft-drink bottle can be on the order of 200 psi. Chemical hazards from residual acid, base, or bleach can cause injuries to persons nearby. Due to the hazards of explosive, incendiary, and chemical injuries, states now consider these devices to be explosive devices in prosecutions.

The post-blast solid residues may be very limited in amount and subject to degradation from exposure to water. As seen in Figure 3-8, the aluminum (or other metal used) and unreacted acid or base are often found. The bottle used will have characteristic deformation due to the heat produced and internal pressure. Dry-ice devices fail with extreme cold fractures and no visible residues. Due to the unpredictable time intervals between mixing and explosion, the maker of the device is sometimes among the injured.

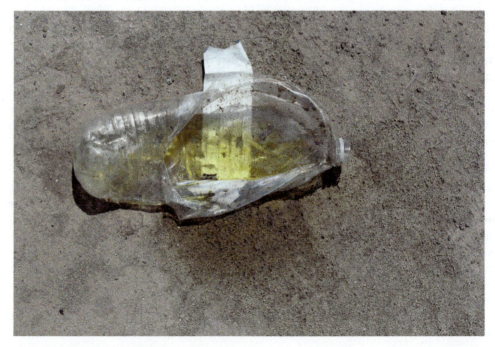

FIGURE 3-8 Melted and heat-distorted 2-L soda bottle is the remains of an acid–metal bottle bomb. Residues of unreacted hydrochloric acid and metal are present. *Courtesy of Wayne Moorehead.*

3.4.2 BLEVEs

If the original contents are liquid rather than gas, heating causes the liquid to reach a temperature far above its normal boiling point, since the liquid would ordinarily shed its excess heat as vapors to maintain its boiling point temperature. A failure of the vessel results in a **BLEVE** (boiling liquid expanding vapor explosion). The gases initially involved are supplemented by the superheated liquid that turns to vapor immediately on contact with normal atmospheric pressure. These explosions can be extremely destructive because of the energy contained in the liquid, even when the liquid and its vapor are noncombustible. BLEVEs involving 40-gallon water heaters have been known to demolish houses. BLEVEs involving superheated water or steam explosions are notable for their absence of fire/thermal effects.

BLEVE ■ Boiling liquid expanding vapor explosion (NFPA 2017 ed., pt. 3.3.20).

When the contents are flammable, the ensuing fires can be overwhelming. Remnants of gas cylinders, boilers, containers, or pipelines in mechanical explosions can reveal clues to cause and origin. When a liquid storage vessel is exposed to an external fire, the liquid inside in contact with the heated vessel wall absorbs the heat by conduction, while the wall in contact with only gas or vapor is not cooled. This may result in a tide mark on the exterior of the vessel that can tell the investigator what the level of liquid was in the vessel during the fire or the position of the vessel during fire exposure. This also means a vessel engulfed in fire will usually fail first where it is not in contact with liquid contents, because that portion will reach its tensile failure temperature before the portion that is in contact with liquid (Raj 2005, 37–49).

3.5 Electrical Explosions

The passage of high currents through air, insulating oil, or undersized conductors can cause very rapid heating, which, in turn, causes extremely rapid expansion of surrounding gases or liquids. The ultimate example of the explosive effects of arc-heated air is the lightning bolt, which can involve current flows of over 100,000 A. In the case of oil, as in oil-filled transformers or switchgear, the oil boils and turns to a vapor upon failure of the vessel. This vapor may be ignited by the continuing electric arc to produce an extensive fireball. Conductors can vaporize, producing a gaseous vapor moving at high speeds. Such failures can cause flash burns as well as blast and pressure damage, as illustrated in Figures 3-9A–B and 3-10.

3.6 Investigation of Explosions

Explosions can occur as the result of accidental mechanisms in materials in industrial applications or processes, household mishaps, or the deliberate criminal act of setting off a bomb. In rare instances, a bomb may be military ordnance that is being misused, but much more often, a bombing involves an improvised explosive device (IED). The ATF reported that there were an average of 576 bombings and attempted bombings reported in the United States in 2004 through 2007 (US Bomb Data Center 2009), with some 59 percent being pipe, tubing, or gas cylinder containers (pipe bombs).

Smokeless powder, black powder, and flash powder were the dominant explosive fillers used (US Department of Justice 2016). During 2014, some 37 percent of the total 642 bombing incidents contained explosives, while 24 percent were improvised explosive devices (IEDs).

It is the responsibility of the investigator *not* to presume that every event is caused by an accident or a bomb, but to treat each scene as a *potential* crime scene from the standpoint of scene security, preservation, and documentation. Evidence that an explosion is the result of a particular accidental cause can be just as important as evidence that proves it was a criminal act, and requires the same standard of care.

The examination of an explosion scene is generally carried out using the same scientific methodology as a fire investigation and, in fact, is most often carried out as part of the examination of the fire of which the explosion was a part. However, unlike at a

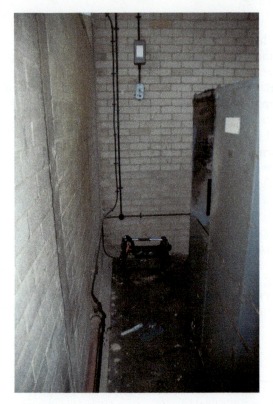

FIGURE 3-9A Electrical explosion caused when service person shorted out 10 kV at switch gear. Blast pattern on wall. *Courtesy of Paul Spencer, London Fire Brigade (Retired).*

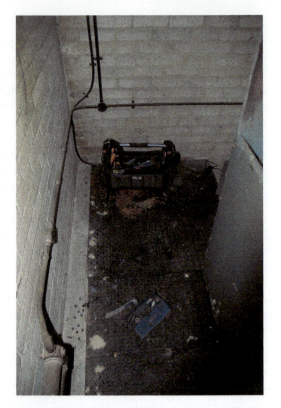

FIGURE 3-9B Fire-damaged tools; door of cabinet on floor around corner. *Courtesy of Paul Spencer, London Fire Brigade (Retired).*

FIGURE 3-10 Flash pattern on insulators. Serviceman fatally injured by arc blast. *Courtesy of Paul Spencer, London Fire Brigade (Retired).*

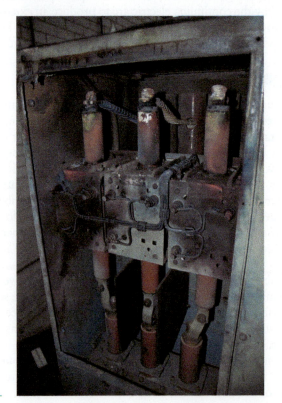

fire scene, it is most important that evidence or structural members not be moved prior to careful examination, because the relationship between the various pieces may be critical to reconstructing the cause of the explosion, much more so than in fire evidence.

Witness interviews are especially important in explosion investigations to reveal what someone was doing or where they were when the event occurred and what was observed. Surveillance cameras are becoming more commonplace, and they have captured critical events just before and during explosions.

3.6.1 THE SCENE SEARCH

A preliminary search of the scene will reveal the extent and direction of the spread of fragments (blast pattern) of the building, vehicle, device, or victim, as well as an apparent **seat of explosion**. Scene overview and photographic documentation can best be accomplished from a fire department aerial platform. Figures 3-11A–D show how much more information can be gained from an aerial view of a structure explosion compared with a ground-level view of the same scene. The distance from the apparent seat to the farthest discovered fragment should be multiplied by at least 1.5 (150 percent) to establish a preliminary

seat of explosion ■ A craterlike indentation created at the point of origin of some explosions (NFPA 2017, pt. 3.3.161).

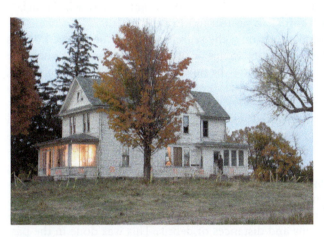

FIGURE 3-11A A view of initial propagation of a structural propane explosion from ground level. *Courtesy of Jamie Novak, Novak Investigations and St. Paul Fire Dept.*

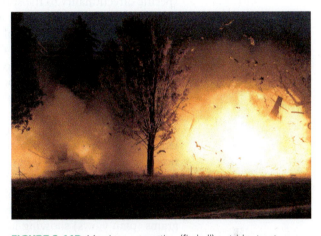

FIGURE 3-11B Massive propagation (fireball) outside structure. *Courtesy of Jamie Novak, Novak Investigations and St. Paul Fire Dept.*

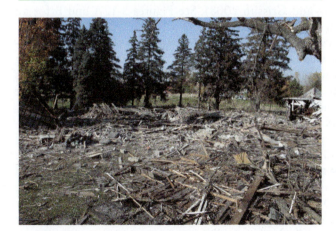

FIGURE 3-11C High-energy shattering of a large structure illustrates the power of a deflagration at near-ideal concentration. *Courtesy of Jamie Novak, Novak Investigations and St. Paul Fire Dept.*

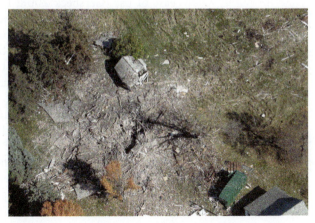

FIGURE 3-11D Aerial view of the same scene records the distribution of fragments (note cruciform distribution perpendicular to the four main walls). *Courtesy of Jamie Novak, Novak Investigations and St. Paul Fire Dept.*

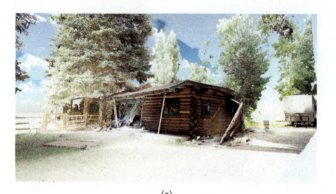
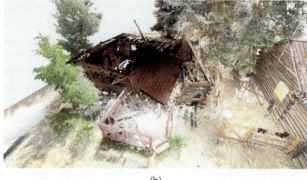

(a)

(b)

FIGURES 3-12A AND B Documentation of a fire scene using a Faro(tm) laser scanner allows production of aerial and eye-level views. *Compliments of Robert K. Toth, IAAI-CFI (R) - IRIS Fire Investigations Inc.*

perimeter. This perimeter may have to be expanded as the search progresses and reveals a specific directionality to the spread (as with pipe bombs, whose end caps may be launched hundreds of meters away), but will suffice to protect most of the evidence.

In order to secure the explosion scene, only the searchers should be allowed access during the early stages. Unlike evidence at fire scenes or ordinary crime scenes, where the evidence is readily visible, explosion evidence may be tiny fragments of paper, wire, metal, or wood that are easily overlooked and may stick, unnoticed, to the shoes of anyone in the scene and thus be carried off and lost forever.

The perimeter should be clearly marked with banner tape, rope, or barricades and closely monitored to ensure that only authorized personnel essential to the search are admitted. The perimeter can be expanded if searching and evaluation indicates there is some directionality to the distribution of fragments. Deflagrations, especially of diffuse-phase mixtures, tend to produce omnidirectional distribution, but devices like pipe bombs can produce directional effects, as pipe caps are often expelled great distances along the axis of the device.

Documentation includes thorough photographic coverage of the scene as well as diagrams (plan views) showing locations and distances of debris. This was done in the past with tape measures and protractors, and more recently with Total Station surveying systems. The advent of laser scanning systems that can accurately document locations up to 500 m (1,600 ft) in day or night conditions is likely to set new standards of accuracy and ease of use (Gersbeck 2008; Haag and Grissim 2008). See Figures 3-12A and B for an example of the usefulness of such scanning technology.

The size of the search sectors will be determined by the size of the scene and the number of searchers. They should be small [less than 0.4 m² (4 ft²)] near the seat, becoming larger [up to 10 m² (100 ft²)] toward the margins of the search area where the debris is lightly scattered. The sectors can be marked with chalk, string, or rope with stakes; or with tape stuck on the ground, and must be numbered for later reference.

Once the scene is secured and the sectors marked, the search can begin, with a perimeter search and photographic documentation, just as in a fire scene. The size, shape, and conditions of the scene and the number of qualified searchers available will determine the organization of the search. Using a grid, sector, or spiral search pattern, the search should start from the outside perimeter and work inward. This allows better preservation of the critical explosion seat and improved protection against souvenir hunters. The primary goal of the scene search and documentation is the identification of displaced debris or fragments and measurement of their displacement (distance from starting position).

The Four Rs

The scene search can be thought of as the first step in the investigative process, which may be remembered as the "Four Rs": Recognition, Recovery, Reassembly, and Reconstruction.

Recognition at the scene includes assessment of the blast damage (location, intensity, direction) as well as recognition of pieces of physical evidence to be used in the later stages. Physical evidence of an accidental situation or mechanism that brought about an explosion can be just as important as the evidence of a deliberate act of bombing. The training and experience of examiners or searchers is critical to the investigation, because important evidence can be small and appear inconsequential. Such evidence is easily overlooked by untrained searchers.

Recovery involves not only the physical process of picking up evidence, but its documentation and preservation as well. This process must take into account the fact that explosions produce blast, pressure, and thermal effects.

Reassembly of the device or mechanism may take place within the laboratory or at the scene, but is a necessary test to see whether the entire chain of circumstances is accounted for.

Reconstruction of the scenario. What was present? What was the initiator? How did it happen? Who was present?

The Four Cs

Just establishing that there was an explosion of a particular kind of material (gas, liquid, or solid) is usually not adequate. One way to remember all the necessary elements is the "Four Cs": Container, Concealment, Content, and Connections. While these are most applicable to criminal bombings, they are useful even for assessing accidental explosions.

Container   What evidence is there for the means of containment of gases, vapors, or low explosives sufficient for the blast effects we see? This may be fragments of pipe, furnace, wall, or vehicle. Fragments of the device are called primary fragmentation; fragments of everything else shattered by the blast are called secondary fragmentation. High explosives require no container to develop their maximum explosive effect. The absence of any container, then, may be construed to imply that a high explosive was used. Blast effects must corroborate this hypothesis.

Concealment   Bombs are often concealed in some manner to prevent premature discovery. Are there fragments of wrapping, container, or other mode of concealment? Is the location of the blast seat such that an explosive device could have been concealed there? Is there an intended target from whom the device had to be concealed? The concealing container does not form the actual containment of the explosive charge and can be anything from a paper bag or suitcase to a vehicle. The question is: Did this item belong at the scene naturally or was it brought here?

Content   What was the actual explosive material? In improvised devices or accidental explosions, the explosive is never totally consumed. Residues may be visible to the naked eye and be easily found or they may require sophisticated laboratory analysis, but they can be found if the investigator thinks to recover debris that was close to the initiating explosive charge. In accidental explosions, gases, vapors, or solids can accumulate from manufacturing processes or poor housekeeping, or inadequate safety measures may bring about destruction of normal stock. Interviews and review of fire inspections or previous accidents may reveal the content of potential explosive products.

Connections   Finally, connections must be examined—not just electrical wires, but any physical arrangement or sequence of events that could initiate an explosion. How did it start? In bombings, such considerations include where the device was placed (vehicle, dwelling, business), how it was triggered (movement, timer, on-command, etc.), and what the sequence was from power source to initiator to main charge (sometimes called the firing train).

The answers to these questions help reconstruct the entire event, including the intent of the bomber—to destroy, to intimidate, or to kill? In accidental situations, the same questions help establish cause and effect so that proper liability can be determined, and, more important, similar accidents can be avoided in the future. In accidental electrical explosions, an appropriate source of very high amperage electrical power must be identified, along with a conductive path. It must be remembered that some portions of the path may be obliterated by movement, fire damage, or the passage of current itself.

3.6.2 SPEED AND FORCE OF REACTION

When interpreting explosion damage at a fire scene, it is important to remember the differences between deflagrations and detonations. The differences in speed of reaction and in the forces and temperatures generated are responsible for characteristic effects on a structure or vehicle. In determining whether a combustion, deflagration, or a detonation took place, one guideline to keep in mind is *the smaller the pieces and the farther they are thrown, the higher the energy of explosion—combustion, deflagration, detonation.* The time required for a deflagrative explosion is on the order of hundredths of a second as compared with that of a detonation, which is on the order of thousandths or millionths of a second.

The relative slowness of a deflagration is important in distinguishing its effects on targets at close range, because they will be subjected to a more or less progressive pressure pulse that is subsonic with respect to the target material. This gives the material a chance to spread the pressure out, resulting in less shattering and more pushing of larger pieces. The abrupt pressure or shock wave from a detonation is supersonic at close range; the material cannot respond and is shattered rather than pushed. This intense shattering effect gives rise to the localized damage called the seat. As energy dissipates, the damage becomes less severe. The shock wave from a detonation compresses air into a very thin layer that does a great deal of the shattering. It is followed by a high-pressure front that does a great deal of the physical movement. The effects of an explosion may be categorized as blast wave, overpressure, missile, and thermal.

There is a difference in effect between, for example, a deflagration of gasoline vapor and the detonation of military dynamite in a wood-frame structure. The pressures produced by a deflagration are very low in the vicinity of the ignition source and grow as the flame front expands through the premixed fuel/air mixture. The lower, more uniform pressures of a deflagration usually do not produce a localized seat of more intense damage. Published tests by DeHaan (DeHaan et al. 2001, 693-710) have shown that pressures produced by a deflagration of a shallow hexane vapor layer [0.1 to 0.2 m deep (4 to 8 in.)] on the floor of a compartment [3.6 × 2.4 × 2.4 m in size (10 × 8 × 8 ft)] equilibrate at all surfaces of the compartment within a few milliseconds of one another. This pressure was seen to grow over a period of about 100 milliseconds until the failure pressure of the vent panel [5 to 6 kPa (0.75 psi)] was reached. This equalized pressure would cause the failure of the weakest part of the compartment (in this case, the vent panel).

In a real-world building this weakest part may be the roof, the windows, the bottoms of walls weakened by decay, or other components. The stronger the structure, the greater the confinement, and the higher the pressures that can be developed by a deflagration, from less than 7 kPa (1 psi) to 700 kPa (100 psi) or more, depending on the chemistry and quantity of fuel gas/air mixture present (Harris 1983).

In a detonation, the confinement of the structure plays no significant role in the pressures developed. Any pressure pulses can be reflected from large flat surfaces and bounce back to induce damage around corners or over or under barriers. The more energetic the explosion, the more pronounced such effects can be. Reflected pressure pulses can add to the originating pulse and create even more damage in the room of origin.

When the pressure or shock wave is transmitted through air, it drops off in a predictably rapid fashion. Finally, the temperatures produced in a deflagration would not be expected to exceed 1,500°C (2,700°F) but can reach several thousand degrees in a detonation. As one would expect, these differences in speed, pressure, and temperature produce different effects on the target materials. As we saw in Figure 3-11, a near-stoichiometric mixture of propane ignited below grade vented upward, completely shattering the building above. An analyst familiar with the differences can accurately estimate the type of explosion, and often the location of the ignition, that took place by examining fragments of the target and their distribution. Beveridge and others have published excellent descriptions of the characteristic features (Beveridge 1998, 2004; Yallop 1980).

Explosion Damage

The pressures produced by a deflagration are usually fairly low and do not *generally* shatter or pulverize, but they can cause serious structural damage to a building. Exceptions are shown in Figure 3-13. The pressure wave moved at subsonic speed and retained its destructive force longer as it moved away from the source, where an ideal mixture of LP gas and air was achieved. Because the rate of reaction of a deflagrating fuel/air mixture increases with the expanding surface area of the expanding flame front, the force exerted increases as the distance from the ignition source increases. For this reason, the area of most destruction of a fuel/air deflagration will usually not be in the vicinity of the ignition source but rather some distance away from it.

This pattern makes establishing the actual ignition source very difficult. Once the limit of the premixed volume is reached, the energy falls off with distance. The mixing and turbulence caused by the passage of the flame front around furniture and through doorways can dramatically increase the surface area of the flame front. Pre-ignition heating and pressurization of the fuel/air mixture in adjoining rooms can also result in more energetic deflagration than in the room of ignition (Pape, Mniszewski, and Longinow 2009). This in turn increases the damage done by the extensions of the blast into areas away from the ignition source. The deflagration pressure wave can be vented by the loss of doors or windows in a structure, minimizing damage to the walls. The normal appearance of such a scene, then, is substantial destruction over a wide area with large fragments and projectiles.

In contrast, a detonation, with its peak pressures in the tens of thousands of pounds per square inch, shatters and pulverizes materials in its immediate vicinity and creates a shock wave with a massive positive-pressure front with a negative-pressure wave or zone right behind it. The negative-pressure wave creates a partial vacuum that is filled by air rushing back in toward the explosion seat. This current can be strong enough to move light debris or even topple weakened masonry walls in a direction opposite the original blast. Windows can be sucked out of a wall as a blast wave moves parallel to it. The negative-pressure pulse that follows the positive-pressure wave from a confined deflagration is low in energy. The hexane vapor tests described earlier revealed a negative-pressure pulse about one-third as strong as the positive-pressure peak (DeHaan et al. 2001). This may be enough to move draperies back through broken windows, pull pictures off walls, pull unsupported doors into a room, or cause further collapse of structural members weakened by the positive pressure.

The detonation pressure wave initially moves at supersonic speeds but very quickly dissipates, making its damage highly localized. Because of its supersonic speed, the pressure wave is not subject to venting and can destroy a nearby wall whether it has windows and doors or not. The normal appearance of a detonation scene, then, is highly localized destruction with pulverization, shattering, and a large number of very small pieces, some of which will be projected large distances away. Keep in mind that all explosive detonations produce what becomes a low-energy pressure wave at large distances from the source.

The distance that window glass fragments are thrown from their origin is directly proportional to the pressure on the glass pane at the time of failure. Plain glass is thrown 50 to 60 m (180 to 200 ft) by a pressure of 27.6 to 34.5 kPa (4 to 5 psi), 30 to 35 m (100 to 120 ft) by pressures on the order of 13.8 kPa (2 psi), and 12–15 m (40 to 50 ft) by overpressures of 4.83 to 6.89 kPa (0.7 to 1 psi) (Harris 1983). Wire-reinforced or plastic-film-laminated glass, which has higher failure pressures, will be thrown shorter distances by the same pressures.

High explosives have been used to vaporize flammable liquids in combination devices used as anti-personnel weapons. These scenes bear post-fire evidence of both types of explosions. In the immediate vicinity of the device, the shattering effects of the high explosive predominate, as shown in Figure 3-13. Elsewhere in the structure the effects of the deflagrating gasoline vapor are the most apparent. The pressures produced by detonations often pulverize nearby surfaces, creating a crater, or seat, whose depth and dimensions reflect the size and sometimes the shape of the explosive charge. Such seats are not produced by diffuse-phase explosions (Kinney and Grahm 1985).

Pre-fire and Trans-fire Explosions

Because explosions can occur before a fire (as the means of ignition) or during a fire, the presence or absence of pyrolysis products on debris ejected from a building can reveal whether the fire was underway before the explosion. Smoke explosions or BLEVEs involving ignitable liquids occurring *during* a fire will often produce ejected debris that show thermal effects or combustion residues, while debris from deflagrations or detonations that initiate a fire usually have little or no such residues. If it is energetic enough to disrupt the ceiling or roof of the confining structure, a natural gas explosion will cause the combustion and release of the accumulated gas. This results in minimal post-blast burning except in the vicinity of the source of the gas.

Although the pressures of a deflagration inside a structure equilibrate at the speed of sound and, as a result, usually produce no localized blast effects, the pre-explosion distribution of fuel gas or vapor may produce localized *thermal* effects as the overrich layers or pockets of fuel burn off. Scorching or "flame-washed" effects may be caused by fuel/air

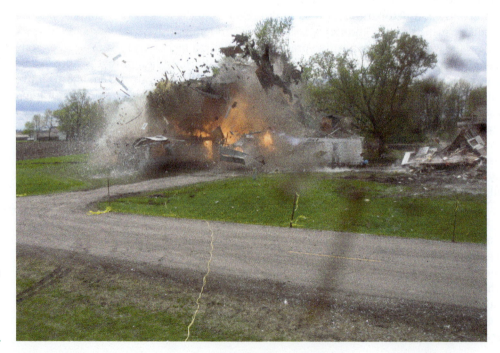

FIGURE 3-13 Massive deflagration of a near-ideal mixture of LP gas and air produced extensive fragmentation and high velocities. *Courtesy of Denise DeMars, Streich DeMars Inc., and Jamie Novak, Novak Investigations and St. Paul Fire Dept.*

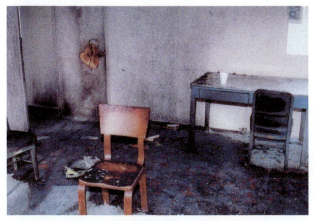

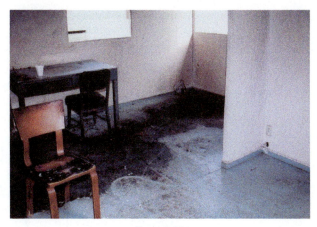

Figure 3-14

Figure 3-15

FIGURES 3-14 AND 3-15 Ignition of commercial LP gas released into this structure produced floor-level charring of vinyl tile and walls. Notice pronounced irregular charred areas and limited extension to baseboards and some walls. *Courtesy of Senior Special Agent Steven Bauer, ATF (retired).*

deflagrations in wood structures. The distribution of melting or scorching of materials (particularly thin, low-mass materials like paper or plastic) may reveal whether the pre-blast accumulation layer of gas or vapor was lighter or heavier than air. As debris is documented and collected, its appearance should be noted.

When flammable liquid vapors in a closed room are ignited, the flame propagates only through the vapor layer near floor level. Ide demonstrated extension of flames out the lower portion of a door opening when gasoline vapors were ignited in the adjoining room. These flames charred the lower legs of trousers worn by a mannequin placed in the doorway (Ide 1999). Observation and documentation of the distribution of thermal effects are critical to evaluation of the pre-blast distribution of vapors or gases. See Figures 3-14 and 3-15 for an example of thermal effects from a vapor explosion where LP gas was released into a room.

3.6.3 SCENE EVALUATION AND HYPOTHESIS FORMATION

Once the preliminary evaluation of the explosion debris and thermal patterns is completed, the investigator will be able to direct the search in certain areas with specific types of evidence in mind. The search of an explosion scene can be inward spiral, sector search, strip search, or grid search. Searches of larger scenes will be aided by laying out grid lines with string or rope and processing grid sectors in sequence. This is especially useful if search personnel are limited in number.

A detailed sketch of the scene is useful at this stage of the investigation. Because items of evidence can be described on the sketch, along with measurements of their distance from a reference point and a reconstruction of their line of flight, a sketch can clarify the relationships between those items. If properly done, the sketch will show how the paths tend to intersect at one area. This indicates that the seat of the explosion (or the point of ignition of a deflagrating fuel/air mixture) was probably in that area and allows the investigator to focus the search for pieces of the device (or ignition source) itself in that room or area. The distribution, distance, and trajectory of window glass fragments are especially important, because windows are usually broken in an explosion (see Figure 3-16). A sample of the glass should be preserved, or at least documented as to thickness and type (safety, plate, plain, wired, etc.). If the distance, thickness, and type are known, the pressure produced inside the structure can be estimated.

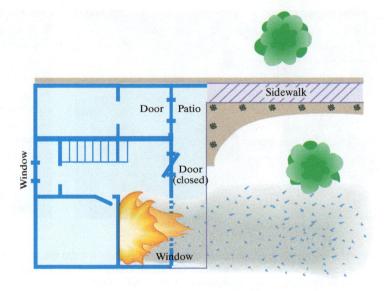

FIGURE 3-16 Distribution of glass fragments indicates the gasoline vapor deflagration was initiated in the room in the lower right corner of the structure.

3.6.4 EVIDENCE RECOVERY

In spite of the ultrahigh temperatures and pressures developed in a high-order detonation, some pieces of the device, however small, will remain in an identifiable form. Safety fuse is particularly resistant to blast effects and will survive, sometimes even with a remainder of the blasting cap still attached. Due to the frequent use of pipe bombs, the examination of a scene should include an examination of any broken bottles, pressure cylinders, or fragments of pipe or pipe cap found in the debris. The fragmentation of pipe, when used as a pipe bomb, follows a very predictable pattern. The larger the total number of fragments and the smaller the fragments, the higher the energy of the explosive filler (Oxley et al. 2001; Whitaker et al. 2009). This information can be useful in quickly establishing the nature of the device and explosive filler and alerting the investigator to other types of evidentiary materials that might be at the scene.

Small fragments of metal or plastic pipe, wire, or cardboard may easily be overlooked by inexperienced searchers or compromised by being stepped on. Explosion scenes should be searched grid-by-grid (preferably by two different searchers). Any item or debris that looks out of place needs to be photographed and recovered for later evaluation. Some examiners prefer to have each grid swept up after the visual search and all materials bagged for later examination under controlled conditions.

Sifting screens can be used to sift for fragments, but unlike fire scene evidence, the debris must be sifted dry, because many of the post-blast residues of low explosives are water soluble and will be lost if the debris is wet sifted. The clothing and the bodies of any victims (living or deceased) must be carefully examined for the presence of fragments (either primary or secondary). The patterns of thermal or impact injury to the clothing and skin may also be critical in reconstructing the event (whether the explosion was an accident or a bombing) and must be documented by photograph and diagram (DeHaan and Dietz 1987). Medical treatment can quickly alter the damage patterns of injuries, so documentation and recovery of evidence from victims must take place as soon as possible. X-rays are irreplaceable in assisting the search for fragments, but it should be remembered that PVC and other plastics have the same physical texture and x-ray density as cartilage or bone in the body and can very easily be overlooked during x-ray or visual examination of the wounds. Whitaker et al. (2009) reported velocities of PVC pipe nipple fragments to be as high as 290 km/h (465 mi/h; 80 m/s) and capable of inducing injuries despite their low mass.

There exist several engineering equations for predicting the effects of explosives published by the International Ammunition Technical Guidelines (IATG 2015), United Nations Office for Disarmament Affairs (See: https://www.un.org/disarmament). These equations can be used to estimate the size of explosives based upon their quantity, and the distance from the explosive. These rules are known as *Quantity-Distance (Q-D) criteria*, and are based on the approach derived from the *Hopkinson-Cranz Scaling Law* (Hopkinson 1915; Cranz 1916). The UN Guidelines also use the *Rankine-Hugoniot equations* (Rankine 1979) for assessing shock wave and particle velocities. The *Gurney Equations* (Gurney 1943) are a range of formulas used to predict how fast an explosive will accelerate a surrounding layer of metal or other material when the explosive detonates. This is useful in determining how fast fragments are released on detonation.

Low explosives like black powder or smokeless powder are not completely consumed when used in improvised devices (unless there has been a significant post-blast fire), and traces will often adhere to larger pieces of the containers (such as the nipple of a pipe bomb) or to large, cool surfaces near the exploding device or be buried into nearby wood surfaces. Organic explosives can be absorbed into plastic surfaces such as wire insulation, vinyl upholstery or luggage, or plastic bottles. It is much better to recover any item suspected of bearing explosive residues for laboratory examination and extraction than to attempt to swab the contaminated surface and submit just the swabs. For this reason, all loose debris from the seat, or crater, should always be collected and preserved in clean new cans or jars.

Polyethylene plastic bags and paper envelopes will allow volatile organic explosives to migrate into and through the container with the possibility of generating cross-contamination concerns and should be avoided for the blast seat debris or bulk organic explosives, if possible. Polyethylene (Ziploc) bags are suitable for small components and small items where high concentrations of organic explosive residues are not expected. Special plastic bags such as nylon or Kapak (by Ampac) are suitable for explosive evidence, but ragged, sharp-edged debris can puncture them, so careful handling is required.

Large immobile objects such as buildings will require swabbing with clean cotton gauze or cotton swabs wetted with methyl or isopropyl alcohol, distilled water, or acetone (Phillips et al. 2000). The swabs then need to be sealed in a clean glass or plastic vial. The hands and fingernails of persons suspected of handling explosives can be sampled with swabs, and fingernail scrapings recovered with clean flat wooden toothpicks. As with fire debris evidence, maintaining the collected evidence in cool, dark surroundings until submitted to the lab will minimize degradation or evaporation. Any comparison materials or reference specimens (bulk explosives) should, of course, be kept isolated from scene debris.

3.6.5 LABORATORY ANALYSIS

Although high explosives like nitroglycerin or TNT can detonate with nearly 100 percent efficiency, traces of the unexploded material can usually be detected on portions of the device, its container, or nearby surfaces, especially with the sensitivity of today's laboratory tests. These tests require solvent extraction of selected fragments of debris and analysis of the solution by very sensitive laboratory methods including thin-layer chromatography, capillary electrophoresis, gas chromatography, high-pressure liquid chromatography (HPLC), ion chromatography, and mass spectrometry. Forensic scientists who have extensive experience in explosives casework [such as those at the US Department of Justice—Bureau of Alcohol, Tobacco, Firearms and Explosives, and the Defense Explosives Research Agency (DERA) in the United Kingdom] have developed effective analytical schemes for the detection and identification of traces of high explosives and the more commonly used low explosives.

Military high explosives in their original packaging and many slurry- and water-gel blasting agents often leave virtually no detectable chemical residues if properly initiated. Highly sensitive analytical methods such as ion mobility spectrometry and liquid chromatography/mass spectrometry have been shown to be useful in identifying such traces (Cochran 2009). Even residues of peroxide-based explosives have been identified post-blast (Bottegal McCord, and Adams 2007; Sigman and Clark 2007). Portions of the packaging, such as the plastic wrappers, the heavy metal wire staples crimped on the ends of some cartridges, and even the metal end panels from TNT charges, have survived. Metallurgical tests on fragments may reveal the speed of reactions to which a container was subjected, even when the explosive itself cannot be identified (Chumbley and Lacks 2005, 104-110). These tests are especially valuable when examining debris from aircraft incidents, in which the mechanical impact can shatter metal components, but not at the velocities created by detonating high explosives.

Portions of the timing or triggering mechanisms of IEDs will survive if they are not in immediate contact with the explosive charge. In many instances, fragments of clockwork or electronic timers and the batteries used to power timers and electric blasting caps are identifiable by experienced laboratory analysts. Much of the laboratory reconstruction and identification of bomb components is visual, so the more complete the photographic documentation of the scene (with close-ups of the evidence in place before recovery) and the more thorough the search and recovery process, the higher the chances of success will be.

Recently, more techniques have been developed for examining melted components such as electrical or duct tape, and characterizing unburned smokeless powder (Briley and Goodpaster 2007). DNA has been identified on post-blast bomb fragments. New analytical methods are being introduced that make it possible to identify batches or sources of explosives on the basis of ion ratios (Ehleringer and Lott 2007).

Not all forensic labs are equipped with the personnel and specialized equipment required to identify explosive residues and reconstruct explosive devices (Corbin and McCord 2009). The investigator is encouraged to contact nearby laboratories to determine what services are available before submitting evidence to them.

Gas chromatography/mass spectrometry using vapor concentration recovery methods has been successfully applied to identify gaseous fuels (propane, butane, pentane) trapped in clothing of victims and in lung tissue and skin of decedents (Kimura et al. 1988; Schuberth 1994). Clothing, including shoes of explosion victims (living or deceased), should be collected as soon as possible and stored separately in airtight metal cans or glass jars for analysis. Porous materials such as upholstery, *if* exposed to high concentrations of gases or vapors and not exposed to extensive fire afterward, may contain identifiable residue.

3.6.6 INCIDENT ANALYSIS

The analysis of explosion incidents follows the scientific method requiring gathering data, formulating and testing hypotheses, and reaching a testable, defensible conclusion. Recent studies have focused on the damage and deformation of road signs, power poles, and adjacent vehicles as a means of reconstructing the amounts of blasting agent in large car bombs (Phillips et al. 2000). Some of the analytical tools (such as computer models) useful in fire reconstruction do not work on diffuse combustion explosion events due to the very different dynamics of gas movement, pressure, and heat production.

See Figure 3-14 for an example of a very destructive LP gas deflagration. It is easier to analyze a condensed-phase explosion because it is a more predictable single-pressure event. Combustion explosions can be very complex, with multiple propagations dependent on the geometry of the building, distribution of fuel, failure mechanisms, and the location of the ignition. In tests, ignition of a uniform natural gas/air mixture produced minimal flame extension out the vent/window and modest pressures when the mixture was ignited from the center of the room. When a similar mixture was ignited from the rear wall, a mass of unburned fuel was pushed through the window to create a very large, energetic fireball outside the compartment. The pressure from this *external* deflagration stripped drywall lining off the walls of the test compartment (DeHaan 1995). Mniszewski and Campbell (1998) have offered some examples of analytical tools that can be of use, including some CFD computer models of explosions. Models of fuel concentration and distribution are two ways of testing hypotheses about fuel sources and ignition mechanisms. Recently, the CFD software FLACS has been shown to be a powerful analytical tool for modeling gas or vapor dispersion and deflagration dynamics (Davis et al. 2010).

3.6.7 BOMB ARSON TRACKING SYSTEM (BATS)

In 2003 the US Bomb Data Center (USBDC) and the ATF developed a web-based data system for tracking fire, explosion, and explosives-related incidents occurring in the United States. The Bomb Arson Tracking System (BATS), provided free of charge, allows police and fire agencies to enter incident information, including location, description, area of origin, scene details, names of victims, witnesses, or suspects. The BATS database can be searched by all law enforcement and fire investigation agencies. Each agency is responsible for administering its own BATS account.

BATS is part of the USBDC's mission to collect, analyze, and disseminate timely and relevant information for use by US federal, state, local, and tribal agencies. BATS has been designated by the US Attorney General as the sole repository for information pertaining to explosives- and arson-related incidents. It combines data on IEDs and suspected bomb events, stolen and recovered explosives, and fire investigations (structural, vehicle, and wildland) so that trends and possible links can be identified. The system automatically encodes all locations into GIS coordinates and offers mapping options.

BATS is capable of generating and printing out standardized reports for consistency throughout the fire and explosion investigation community. Printed BATS reports are customized with each participating agency's header and seals. It can function as a case management tool as well. BATS has drop-down menus for fire descriptors and scene details, as well as provisions for narratives and paste-ins of photos, diagrams, log sheets, and supplemental reports. It has provisions for read-only or read/write access designated by the user to allow collaboration with other agencies on joint investigations. BATS can also function as a bomb/arson unit management system, because time spent on cases, court, training, travel, and maintenance can be tracked individually and as a unit.

Information can be designated as Restricted or Unrestricted. If a case is designated as Restricted, only contact information for the investigator logging in the case is provided. The USBDC provides two options to public safety agencies for access to BATS: Law Enforcement and Non-Law Enforcement. Users from an agency with an NCIC-issued ORI number have full access from any computer with Internet access. (Fire department investigators gain full access through cooperative agreements with local police agencies or after receiving an ORI from their state CJIS coordinator.) As of summer 2009, they can also choose the "Non-Law Enforcement" role, which limits their access to their own and other non-LE agency information. Data are released only to agencies authorized specifically by the user.

Because BATS has been designated as the sole reporting system by Congress and the attorney general, regular reporting provides investigators with a powerful tool for access to critical incident information. Arson investigators can compare local case specifics in real time against a jurisdictional database without the limitations that NFIRS reporting includes. (NFIRS is intended for documenting fire department responses to fire incidents, not for documenting investigations. Its information is subject to unrestricted access by all fire department personnel. According to the US Fire Administration, NFIRS is not intended as a case management system.)

In September 2009 the House passed a bill (H.R. 1727: Managing Arson Through Criminal History; the MATCH Act) establishing a *National Arsonist & Bomber Registry*. The legislation would authorize the attorney general to establish and maintain a database within ATF that would be built into BATS. The registry would require convicted arsonists and bombers to report where they live, work, and go to school and would include descriptions of vehicles they own, an up-to-date photograph, and a photocopied I.D. In addition to that information, the database would include finger and palm prints. This legislation will provide an important tool to law enforcement by enabling investigators to track arsonists and bombers, regardless of where they live, across jurisdictions. By querying a zip code to locate convicted arsonists living or working in the vicinity of a fire, or by querying the components database for previous incendiary or bomb components that match those used in an unsolved arson or bombing investigation, the process of narrowing down suspects would be expedited. H.R. 1727 passed the House on September 30, 2009, and on October 2009 was read in the Senate and referred to the Committee on the Judiciary. The bill was allowed to die without action.

BATS is being used by police and fire agencies across the United States, and it promises to dramatically improve the quality of information sharing and comparisons for the fire and explosion investigation community. For more information, public investigators are encouraged to contact the US Bomb Data Center (usbdc@atf.gov) or BATS (www. BATS.gov).

3.7 Chemical Fires and Hazardous Materials

3.7.1 INTRODUCTION

A chemical fire is here defined as one resulting from the reaction of one or more chemicals with the release of a flammable gas and/or sufficient heat to cause ignition of a reaction product or nearby combustible fuel. Most fire investigators are likely familiar with examples of fire resulting from the contamination of solid pool chemicals with brake fluid, fires from self-heating animal- or vegetable-type oils under the right conditions; and perhaps, thermite-type reactions. Fire investigators typically have or will encounter chemical fires in their careers ranging from simple to complex. Fire investigators may have various roles and degrees of involvement in chemical fire investigations. This chapter will address chemical fires with the objective of providing the fire investigator with some basic skills and knowledge to supplement their investigation methodology.

Three of the 16 topics in *NFPA 1033* that fire investigators shall have and maintain up-to-date basic knowledge on and apply to *all* fire investigations are fire chemistry, thermodynamics, and hazardous materials (NFPA 2014). What requisite knowledge and requisite skills should a fire investigator have to identify a fire as resulting from an adverse chemical reaction? After a fire, how would a fire investigator know what appears to be soot on a light fixture is conductive paint particles or the expelled products from a lithium ion polymer battery or calcium hypochlorite? Should the fire investigator have as much familiarity with basic chemistry including adverse chemical reactions as with electricity, electrical faults, and damage to electrical appliances and devices from fire scenes? What references should the fire investigator add to their library for basic chemical-related hazards? *NFPA 921: Guide for Fire and Explosion Investigations* (NFPA 2017) has topical or subject chapters on electricity, fire and building fuel gas systems, appliances, motor vehicles, and marine craft.

Chemical reaction hazards are likely to occur where chemicals are produced, used, handled, stored, and disposed of. There are numerous codes and standards for, and literature and guidance on, the safe production, use, handling, storage, and disposal of hazardous chemicals. Quantity, confinement, temperature, presence or absence of process controls, contamination, and concentration are all recognized factors contributing to the severity of a loss event involving chemicals. Some chemicals may have multiple inherent hazards; others exhibit hazards as a result of external input such as shock, contamination, or exposure to fire. Fire investigators are comfortable with understanding exposure to fire resulting in over-pressurization; however, over-pressurization may also result from chemical reactions. Overpressure through chemical reactions evolving gaseous products (Carson and Mumford 1996) can occur from:

1. reaction with water;
2. reaction due to contaminants;
3. corrosion;
4. reaction with construction materials;
5. decomposition; and,
6. self-initiated reactions

This section provides a description of chemical fires, chemical fire site investigation requirements, sampling plan and kits, analysis plan, chemical reaction hazards, and related codes, standards, and literature. Fundamental physical hazard properties of commonly encountered gases, liquids including solvents, and solids that can be involved in fires and explosions, are described.

3.7.2 REGULATIONS, CODES, AND STANDARDS

Hazardous materials are defined in *NFPA 400: Hazardous Materials Code* (NFPA 2016a) and by the IFC as "a chemical or substance that is classified as a physical hazard material or a health hazard material, whether the chemical or substance is in usable or waste condition." Health and physical hazard materials are further defined in *NFPA 400* as follows: "Health Hazard Material. A chemical or substance classified as a toxic, highly toxic, or corrosive material in accordance with definitions set forth in this code."

A **physical hazard material** is a chemical or substance classified as a combustible liquid, explosive, flammable cryogen, flammable gas, flammable liquid, flammable solid, organic peroxide, oxidizer, oxidizing cryogen, pyrophoric, unstable (reactive), or water-reactive material.

Because of their physical and health hazards, hazardous materials including waste are the subject of numerous regulatory agencies (EPA, OSHA, DOT) and the IFC and NFPA Codes and Standards. The IFC's Chapter 50 on Hazardous Materials also applies to treatment, storage, and disposal facilities (TSDFs), as well as the applicable Chapters 51–67, depending on the range of hazardous materials at each TSDF. Chapter 1 of the IFC describes how the operational permits should be issued for these facilities, which would include annual inspections by the AHJ for continued compliance. The IFC also includes waste in the definition of hazardous material. Applicable NFPA and IFC code language regarding waste are reviewed below. *NFPA 1: Fire Code* (NFPA 2015a) and *NFPA 400: Hazardous Materials Code* (NFPA 2016a) are the principal applicable codes and pointer documents to other NFPA standards. For example, some waste is or contains combustible metals, explosives, and flammable and combustible liquids; therefore, *NFPA 484: Standard for Combustible Metals* (NFPA 2015c), *NFPA 495: Explosives Code* (NFPA 2013b), and *NFPA 30: Flammable and Combustible Liquid Code* (NFPA 2015b), respectively, and possibly other codes are applicable.

The regulations are not unified. Not all EPA hazard characteristics are covered by NFPA. For example, EPA's hazard characteristic "spontaneously combustible" is not an

physical hazard material ■ A chemical or substance classified as a combustible liquid, explosive, flammable cryogen, flammable gas, flammable liquid, flammable solid, organic peroxide, oxidizer, oxidizing cryogen, pyrophoric, unstable (reactive), or water-reactive material.

NFPA 400 physical hazard. Combustible dusts are not included in *NFPA 400*; they are the subject of *NFPA 652: Standard on the Fundamentals of Combustible Dust* (NFPA 2016b). The EPA ignitability hazard characteristic has some test methods: flash point, ignition and propagation of flaming combustion by solids and oxidizers, and propensity to self-heat. The EPA's test method for waste containing oxidizers is different from the DOT's test method (Tests O.1 and O.3) and *NFPA 400*, Annex G. With respect to the DOT, the DOT packing group assignments are the inverse of the NFPA oxidizer Class. There are no EPA test methods for reactivity.

Most but not all chemical-related fire investigations will require refreshed 40-hour Hazardous Waste Operations and Emergency Response (Hazwoper) training and a current respirator fit test. Site personnel and the lead investigator will establish the level of personal protective equipment, respirator cartridges required, decontamination procedures, and other safety requirements to access and investigate the loss site. Yellow chemical Tyvek, chemical boots, chemical gloves, and safety glasses are typical minimum required personal protective equipment. Unknown mixtures especially present numerous potential physical and health hazards and should be respected as such.

Basic data, information, and documentation as collected from any fire scene (e.g., witness accounts, timeline, photographs, video recordings, drawings) during chemical fire and explosion investigations should comply with pertinent sections of *NFPA 921*. Other specific data required are any and all chemical and process information such as safety data sheets, starting materials, waste streams, lots numbers, certificates of analyses, inventory, process information, piping and instrumentation diagrams, standard operating procedures, housekeeping procedures, and so on. Pertinent process conditions include at a minimum temperature, pressure, and other environmental influences. Any identified physical, chemical, or process deviations are particularly important.

Two fundamental principles for sampling at chemical fire scenes are "earlier and more." Active mitigation of a hazardous or unidentified chemical hazard release is likely to occur very early after a loss event; therefore, samples must be identified with an abundance of forethought as well as caution. Samples identified and collected may not be analyzed first or at all.

After a chemical fire, the following information regarding chemicals is required: the class of material(s) present, and its (their) composition, concentration, form, and mass or quantity. Part of a chemical fire investigation is to identify and collect relative and related solid, liquid, and possibly gaseous samples and controls for laboratory characterization and testing. A sampling objective and sampling plan should be developed in conjunction with on-site personnel. If a reaction occurred inside a vessel, samples should be identified and collected from the inside of the vessel (top, bottom, lid, walls, and center) as well as any equipment associated with the tank (e.g., drums, secondary containment, tray, hoppers, conveyors, piping, semi-trailers). If a reaction involved super-sacks of solids, samples should be collected from a reasonable number of other super-sacks to provide a cross section of the material(s) present or potential variations. Should sampling have to comply with standards, there are numerous ASTM and DEQ standards and monographs the investigator can apply or modify accordingly. Split samples are typically requested. A split sample is one collected from the same location at the same time; it has the same appearance but is split into two or more containers for two or more parties.

In addition to typical fire investigation tools and basic sampling, a chemical fire scene sampling kit should contain pre-cleaned, wide-mouth glass jars and vials with Teflon-lined lids (see www.scispec.com); zip-lock bags of various sizes for over-packaging sample jars and vials and some solid samples; sterile scoops; sterile wipes; filter papers; anti-static plastic scoops; Coliwasa for sampling 55-gallon drums and some tanks; pH or litmus paper; and bonding and grounding straps and clamps. Samples collected are recorded on a sample log to the level of detail specified in the sampling plan. Typical information on the sample log includes form (solid, liquid, gas, mixture), a detailed description of the sample's location including GPS coordinates, and its potential hazard (e.g., acidic). A sketch of the loss site with the sample locations identified is a good practice, as are photographs showing the sample location when collected. It is often expected that samples from chemical fire scenes be stored in coolers while on site and similarly stored in a refrigerator at the laboratory.

An analysis plan should be developed based on the site and process specific data, and samples collected. The goal of the analysis plan, like that of other fire investigations, is to identify the ignition source and first fuel ignited resulting in the release of energy responsible for an over-pressurization, runaway reaction, flash fire, fire, or explosion. Post loss event, samples collected will likely represent products of one or more reactions or may be used to identify constituents. For example, chemical analysis can distinguish between calcium hypochlorite and dichlor isocyanurate–based pool chemicals or reactants that may be a thermite pair.

Basic chemical analyses for solids and semi-solids include Fourier transform infrared (FTIR) spectroscopy, energy dispersive x-ray spectroscopy (EDS), moisture content, particle morphology, and size distribution. For liquids, FTIR, pH, and conductivity may be important parameters. Other analyses may include simple or fractional distillation and x-ray diffraction. Thermal analyses include cone calorimetry, differential thermal analysis, or thermal gravimetric analysis. Additional laboratory tests may be performed to further understand or establish a reaction path. Tests may include ad hoc, standard, or modified standard test methods. An example is use of UN Test N.1 to establish the combustibility of metal fines, flake, powder, and so on. Testing is likely required to establish the reaction leading to a fire. Factors contributing to increased chemical hazards include a change in form (i.e., combustible dusts) and contamination, including moisture.

Based on information from the loss site, the results of characterizing samples from the area of origin, and literature, possible reactions to account for the release of energy are developed. One or more chemicals can react under certain conditions to produce other chemicals and, in some cases, heat. Equation 3.1 is the standard form of a simple reaction where A and B are reactants, the arrow indicates a forward reaction path with heat, and C and D are reaction products. Fire investigators have some awareness and basic knowledge of chemistry. They know that typical hydrocarbon-based fuels, when heated, evolve gases, which burn to release gaseous carbon monoxide (CO), carbon dioxide (CO_2), water (H_2O), and in some cases hydrogen cyanide (HCN), hydrogen chloride (HCl), and solid particulate.

$$A + B \xrightarrow{\Delta} C + D \qquad (3.1)$$

Chemical reactions range from simple to complex. Thermite reactions, which are a class of reactions that involve a metal reacting with a metallic (M) or a non-metallic oxide (AO) to form a more stable oxide (MO) and the corresponding metal or non-metal (A) of the reactant oxide, are a well-known class of adverse exothermic chemical reactions that evolve significant heat (ΔH) (Mei, Halldearn, and Xiao 1999):

$$M + AO \rightarrow MO + A + \Delta H \qquad (3.2)$$

Heats of reaction can be estimated from the above equation, or the specific chemicals can be combined and the heat evolved measured. Examples include iron oxide (Fe_2O_3) and aluminum (Al):

$$Al + \tfrac{1}{2}Fe_2O_3 \rightarrow \tfrac{1}{2}Al_2O_3 + Fe \ (T \ up \ to \ 3100K) \qquad (3.3)$$

The calculated iron oxide-aluminum thermite reaction enthalpy (at 298K) is −426.2 kJ/mol. Other common thermite pairs are iron oxide with titanium and magnesium with similarly high reaction enthalpies −395.8 kJ/mol and −326.7 kJ/mol, respectively (Weiser et al. 2010).

3.7.3 CAUSES OF REACTIVE CHEMICAL HAZARDS

Causes and chemicals or materials involved in the various emergency incidents are summarized in Tables 3-3 through 3-6. Tables 3-3 and 3-4 list the causes of the fires/explosions and releases, respectively. Tables 3-5 and 3-6 list the chemical(s) or materials identified as involved in fires and explosions, respectively. The chemicals include oxidizer solids, flammable solids, flammable solvents, explosive precursors, and reactive chemicals. Seventeen events were attributed to improper identification of chemicals and lack of chemical hazard awareness.

Cozzani, Smeder, and Zanelli identified that the process operations during which "unwanted reaction" accidents took place were predominantly fluid/solid handling/transfer followed by storage, "unknown," chemical reaction, transport, and mixing (Cozzani,

TABLE 3-3	Causes Identified in TSDF Fires and Explosions (Number of Incidents)
Equipment failure (13)	
Incorrect combination of chemicals (7)	
Operator error (5)	
Processing failure (5)	
Incorrect identification of chemical (4)	
Mixed incompatible reactive and/or ignitable waste (3)	
Incorrect identification of chemical properties (3)	
Welding sparks ignited vapors (3)	
Electrical outage (1)	
Pressure transient (1)	
Welding on out-of-service tank (1)	
Faulty equipment (1)	

TABLE 3-4	Causes Identified in TSDF Emergency Incidents Resulting in Releases (Number of Incidents)
Equipment failure (15)	
Lack of control of vapor emission (2)	
Spill from bulk container (2)	
Cooling water system rupture	
Failure to attach screw auger	
Incorrect storage	
Poor maintenance of tank trucks	
Aluminum waste not identified on manifest	
Fugitive emissions from process	
Rail car transfer	
Disgruntled employee(s)	
Improper release of contaminated water	
Incorrect identification of chemical	
Incorrect identification of chemical properties	
Improper identification of chemical combinations	
Inadequate system	

TABLE 3-5   Chemicals Resulting in Fires at TSDFs (1977–1998)

Unburned propane	Non-RCRA aerosol containers
Acid residue	Elemental phosphorus, combustible packaging
Molybdenum paste mixed with wood flour	Natural gas
Lithium manganese batteries	Hot gases
Alkaline batteries	Corrective sulfonation acid sludge, sulfuric acid mixture
Oil, grease, caustic manure with aluminum turnings	Wood debris, heat-generating waste streams
Oil dry, epichlorohydrin	Farm waste oil
Landfill	Combustible gases, air
Reagent sulfur, waste	Dirt, debris, and oxidizer mixture
D004/D018 Hazardous waste–portland cement mixture	Bromine, chlorine, air
Nitrocellulose	

Smeder, and Zanelli 1998). Certain handling and processes can and have resulted in ignition sources; some process equipment were not adequately sized. Cozzani and colleagues identified "unwanted reaction" accidents that usually involved "substances of quite simple structure and of low molecular weight." A table of substances involved in 300 unwanted reactions were mostly corrosives and toxics but listed seven oxidizers, seven flammables, and two metals (aluminum and zinc). Three oxidizers (nitric acid, sodium hypochlorite, and calcium hypochlorite) made the top five most unwanted reaction-involved substances; the other two were hydrochloric acid and sulfuric acid. After a review of numerous hazardous materials databases, Cozzani and colleagues identified 50 chemicals frequently involved in unwanted reactions and further reduced known unwanted reactions into specific GHS Hazard and Risk Phrase combinations. Sixty out of

TABLE 3-6   Chemicals Resulting in Explosion Incidents at TSDF (1977–1998)

CHEMICALS	PROCESS-RELATED
10% Nitroglycerine, 90% lactose	Molten slag, ash
Nitrocellulose	Hot slag, ash quench water
Acetone	Molten metal, ash quench
Nitrobidi	Natural gas (3 incidents)
Tetrazole	
Acid sludge, water-based coating, paper	**Ammunitions**
Spent oxygen breathing apparatus	Ammonium nitrate in ammunition
PCB-Contaminated paint waste	Detonator components
Solvent (not specified)	Live rounds of ammunition
Sodium azide	

78 accidents were the consequence of contact of acids with substances classified as R31 (contact with acid liberates toxic gas) and R32 (contact with acid liberates very toxic gas) and contact of flammable/oxidant, acid/base substances or by substances classified R14 (reacts violently with water) or R15 (contact with water liberates extremely flammable gas) (Cozzani, Smeder, and Zanelli 1998). Compounds that react exothermally and violently with water, particularly with restricted amounts of the latter, are acid anhydrides, acyl halides, alkali metals, alkyl aluminum derivative, alkyl non-metal halides, complex hydrides, metal halides, metal hydrides, metal oxides, non-metal halides and their oxides, and non-metal oxides (Bretherick and Urben 1999). Other literature on reactive chemicals includes AIChE's *Guidelines for Safe Storage and Handling of Reactive Materials*. Additional references are provided at the end of this chapter.

Other literature calls attention to losses involving the handling of hazardous waste where there is inadvertent heating (Cox, Carpenter, and Ogle 2014). In other cases, operations result in ignition (e.g., hot work, equipment failure, and process upsets). Clearly, hazardous waste is subject to mischaracterization and to other unrealized hazards such as incompatibility and reactivity.

3.7.4 GASES

Compressed hazardous gases are common in automotive shops, where fabrication (e.g., cutting, welding) occurs, hospitals, laboratories, and various chemical plants. The cylinders may release a toxic gas, contribute to a fire, or overpressurize if exposed to an external fire.

Compressed gases are usually packaged in metal bottles at pressures up to 20,000 kPa (3,000 psi) for shipment and storage. The containers are normally manufactured and inspected periodically to pressures at several times the recommended working pressure. According to the ideal gas law for a constant volume system, increasing temperature results in an increase in pressure. When heated, the contents can exceed the rated pressure for the container and the container fails. The resulting mechanical explosion can cause damage to nearby structures similar to that produced by a low-order explosion. The damage may often be unidirectional because the container will generally fail in only one direction—along a longitudinal seam or at a welded top or valve, for instance.

Even if the gas is inert, the rapidly increasing pressure can do serious mechanical damage. If the gas is flammable, the fuel made available to the fire may have a dramatic effect on the extent of the fire and its rate of spread. A somewhat different problem is encountered when the gas is subject to explosive or detonating decomposition when heated under pressure. Under those conditions, the result is equivalent to the detonation of a large quantity of a high explosive. When such a detonation occurs, massive destruction of the structure surrounding the exploding tank is usually the result along with the creation of an explosion seat.

Hydrocarbon Gases

Typical hydrocarbon gases include methane, ethane, propane, butane, ethylene, and acetylene. Propane and butane are widely used as fuel gases. The gases have similar flammability ranges. Fire investigators are being involved in more oil-field related fires including fracking fires.

Methane (CH$_4$)

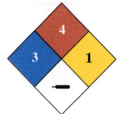

Methane is a colorless, odorless gas also known as swamp gas, marsh gas, or sewer gas because it is produced by the decomposition of organic materials in swamps, marshes, sewers, and landfill dumps. Methane is the major constituent of natural gas for heating and power generation. It burns readily in air and can explode if pressurized when heated. It is much lighter than air, having a vapor density of 0.55. Methane has a fairly narrow explosive range, from 5 to 14 percent by volume in air. Methane, once made by heating coal or coke to make town gas or producer gas for illumination and cooking, resulted in high concentrations of carbon monoxide (CO) along with the methane. Today it is most often recovered during oil drilling, but methane is also being made as a commercial fuel by the controlled fermentation of agricultural waste products in biogas conversion facilities. The product is odorized with sulfur or mercaptan compounds to ensure leaks are detected; however, under some circumstances, the odorant may be scrubbed out of the gas, resulting in an undetected or odorless leak. Methane from sewers or swamps has a strong odor due to the sulfur compounds (chiefly hydrogen sulfide) that accompany it.

A well sample, consisting of a gas and liquid, was analyzed and the data combined to arrive at the well stream composition. The well gas was predominantly methane (77 mole%) with 13% ethane, 5% propane, and 2% carbon dioxide, 1% *n*-butane, and less than 1% iso-butane and higher alkanes. The liquid fraction had heavier hydrocarbons with 63% by volume heptanes and higher alkanes. Well gases rich in propane and butane released in the area of diesel engines, automotive or on generators, can cause the diesel engine to overspeed. One article reports that 3.5 to 15 volume percent methane can result in diesel engine runaway (Mejia and Waytulonis 1984). Gas and well blowouts have been identified as causes of releases and leaks that can contribute to a diesel engine overspeed condition (Bhalla 2010). One paper reports physical indicators of overspeed within the engine (Ferrone Sinkovits 2005).

Ethane (C_2H_6)
This colorless, odorless gas is the other major constituent of natural gas fuel. It has a vapor density of 1.03, so it mixes readily with air, whose vapor density is 1, to form an explosive mixture at concentrations of 3 to 12.5 percent by volume.

Propane (C_3H_8)
Propane is one of the most common hydrocarbon fuels. LP or liquefied propane gas is used, handled, and stored in a variety of containers for torch gases, recreational vehicles, forklift fuel, heating, cooking, and industrial applications. Propane has a boiling point of −42°C (−44°F) and is heavier than air, with a vapor density of 1.52. Its flammable mixture range is between 2.2 and 9.6 percent by volume in air. Propane gas is considered to pose a severe explosive hazard when exposed to flame in suitable concentration. The properties of propane and natural gas are different; orifices unique for each gas are required for gas utilizing appliances.

Butane (C_4H_{10})
Butane is a colorless gas that is most often encountered as a component of liquefied petroleum gas used as fuel for torches, heating, cooking, and industrial uses. It is very flammable and will ignite at concentrations between 1.9 and 8.5 percent in air. The gas itself has a negligible odor but is usually (not always) odorized with methyl mercaptan or sulfur compounds to allow detection of leakage. The gas has a vapor density of about 2.0 and tends to disperse as a cloud along the ground. Under some circumstances it may be encountered as a liquid, because it has a boiling point of −0.5°C (30°F). The temperature of a butane torch flame is ~1100°C. Butane from hand-torch cylinders or lighter-refill containers is often used as an extraction solvent in clandestine drug labs or in the production of marijuana "oil" or "hash oil."

Acetylene (C_2H_2)
Acetylene is a flammable gas used extensively in welding operations. It is particularly hazardous in an enveloping fire because it has a very wide explosive range and a vapor density of 0.9, allowing it to mix readily with air. Acetylene forms an explosive mixture in concentrations between 2.5 percent and 81 percent by volume, but pure acetylene can detonate under certain conditions of heat and pressure. Even when simply burning in air,

acetylene can cause considerable damage because of the extremely high temperatures developed. In most commercial applications, the acetylene is dissolved in acetone in a cylinder containing a porous cement-like filler. If the contents are released while the cylinder is on its side, liquid acetone will be released along with the gas. Heating of acetylene cylinders can trigger decomposition that can cause explosions some time later, even after the cylinders are cooled.

Ethylene (C_2H_4)

Ethylene is a colorless, pleasant-smelling gas that burns or explodes very readily. It has a vapor density of 0.96, so it mixes readily with air. Ethylene forms an explosive mixture in air at concentrations between 3 percent and 30 percent. It can readily react with oxidizing materials and has been known to explode its compressed gas cylinder when exposed to heat and mechanical shock. Ethylene is likely to be encountered at process industries.

Other Gases

Non-hydrocarbon gases of particular interest to the fire investigator are hydrogen, oxygen, ammonia, and ethylene oxide.

Hydrogen (H_2)

Hydrogen is a colorless, odorless gas that is used in a variety of chemical, medical, and industrial processes. Ammonia absorption refrigerator cooling units are pressurized with hydrogen gas. Hydrogen gas can be released as a by-product of many processes including lead-acid battery charging, pickling of steel, electroplating, and some chemical reactions. Hydrogen is the lightest gas, with a vapor density of 0.07, and dissipates very quickly in open air. It has a wide range of explosive concentrations—from 4 to 74 percent by volume in air. Because of its flammability and explosive limits, hydrogen is considered by some to be the most hazardous of the compressed gases.

Hydrogen can be evolved from chemical reactions. Safety Data Sheets should be consulted. For example, Portland cement reacts with aluminum to evolve hydrogen. When pickling steel in an acid bath, hydrogen from the acid reacts with the surface of the metal. In one operation, two coils of steel rod were submerged in a fresh pickling bath at the same time. The amount of hydrogen gas evolved exceeded the local ventilation and the gas was ignited. Once ignited, the fire spread through the ventilation system. Hydrogen gas may also be liberated by the dissociation of water in contact with combustible metal (magnesium, titanium) fires. The temperature required to split water into hydrogen and oxygen is on the order of 1500°C. For this reason, firefighters should exercise extreme caution when considering the application of water to burning metal fires.

NFPA 2 is the Hydrogen Technologies Code (NFPA 2016c) and has requirements for hazard management of hydrogen processes.

Oxygen (O_2)

Oxygen exists as a pure material (oxidizing gas), 21 percent in air, and a product of chemical reactions (e.g., solid oxidizer decomposition). Oxygen promotes or accelerates the burning of typical combustible fuels. While oxygen is not a flammable fuel or toxic gas, oxygen in solid and liquid oxidizers and from pressurized tanks and process piping can have a considerable effect on intensifying a fire. Oxygen may be present in industrial applications as a compressed gas or as a supercold liquid [boiling point −183°C (−297°F)]. Small oxygen bottles for use with propane-oxygen torch kits are readily available in hardware stores. Liquid oxygen and chemical oxygen generators are used to assist breathing.

When present, oxygen can dramatically increase the ignitability of ordinary combustibles, increase the temperatures developed by burning materials, and increase the rates of combustion and the peak heat release rate. Solid oxidizers are a source of oxygen gas.

(See also the section on solid oxidizers later in this chapter.) Organic greases in compressed oxygen atmospheres become so readily ignitable (by friction or electrical discharge) that they are forbidden. Many ordinary combustibles when exposed to liquid oxygen become so readily oxidizable that they become virtually explosive. Even materials such as synthetic fabrics and polymers, which are not considered flammable, become hazardous when exposed to liquid oxygen or saturated with gaseous oxygen. Sacks of carbon black saturated with liquid oxygen were used as a cap-sensitive blasting agent for many years.

Solid and liquid oxidizers are covered in *NFPA 400*, Chapter 15 and Annex G (NFPA 2016a).

Ammonia (NH₃)

Ammonia is a colorless, sharp-smelling gas that is used in very large quantities as a fertilizer in agriculture and as a refrigerant in industrial plants and food cold storage and distribution centers. Anhydrous ammonia is the liquefied form of the gas. While not often thought of as an explosive gas, ammonia can explode when mixed with air. It has a vapor density of 0.6, so it behaves like natural gas (methane) when released, typically creating a dense, white cloud. Its explosive range is 16 to 25 percent by volume in air. Ammonia can be corrosive to metal valves, especially brass valves. It is also extremely toxic. Ammonia readily dissolves in water, forming the caustic ammonium hydroxide, which attacks the mucous membranes of the eyes, mouth, and respiratory tract.

Ethylene Oxide (CH₂OCH₂)

Technically a flammable liquid, but with a boiling point of 11°C (51°F), ethylene oxide is usually encountered in gaseous form. It is water soluble, and even dilute (5 percent) solutions in water may be flammable. Like acetylene, ethylene oxide is ignitable over a wide flammability range (3.6 to 100 percent) and can detonate in pure form. It has a vapor density (1.52) similar to that of propane. Ethylene oxide can ignite spontaneously on contact with pure oxides of iron or aluminum, or with alkali metal hydroxides (sodium, calcium, potassium).

3.8 Hazardous Liquids

Hazardous liquids include flammable and combustible liquids, oxidizing liquids, corrosives, and incompatible or reactive mixtures. Liquids may be pure, at near 100%, or exist as mixtures with water or other hazardous liquids. Safety data sheets, labels, and technical data sheets contain important information on the physical hazards of products, including solvents, strippers, sealers, and organic coatings. Vapors from flammable liquids and mixtures can result in flash fires and pool fires; vapors can travel to remote ignition sources.

While not a combustible liquid at room temperature, asphalt binder when heated is a combustible liquid and if ignited will support combustion and burn and spread as a pool fire. Consult Safety Data Sheets (SDS) for hazard information. For mixtures, the chemical in the highest concentration is typically the chemical of interest. SDS may be used to determine incompatible mixtures. Hazardous liquids are covered by various NFPA Codes and Standards including *NFPA 30: Flammable and Combustible Liquids Code* (NFPA 2015b) and *NFPA 400: Hazardous Materials Code* (NFPA 2016a).

Many hydrocarbon-based flammable and combustible liquids volatilize to form explosive or combustible vapors at room temperature and at temperatures developed in structure fires. Because of their flammability, most petroleum distillates are considered hazardous liquids. Liquids with flashpoints below 100°F are flammable liquids and those with flashpoints above 100°F are combustible liquids. Flashpoint is the lowest temperature of the liquid required for the liquid to evolve vapors that can be ignited. The fire point is sustained combustion. The form of the liquid further contributes to its physical hazard(s). Combustible liquids dispersed as a mist can have increased ignition propensity like flammable vapors, including hot surface ignition. Products and chemicals that have flashpoints at or below room ambient temperature can evolve flammable vapors. The lower flammable limits of hydrocarbon solvents and mixtures are low: 0.8 to 7 percent by volume in air. Often open flame ignition sources, including burners and pilot lights, are responsible for fires; other known ignition sources are sparks and hot surfaces such as 500 W halogen lamp bulbs.

More detailed chemical background, molecular structure, and properties information is contained in *Fire Debris Analysis* by Stauffer, Dolan, and Newman (2007). Useful source calculations of evaporating or spilled solvents are found in *Chemical Process Safety*, 2nd Edition by Crowl and Louvar (2001).

3.8.1 SOLVENTS

Flammable and combustible liquid solvents of particular interest to the fire investigator are household, commercial, and industrial chemicals for uses ranging from strippers, mastic removers, coatings, sealers, and the like. These products are typically formulated with volatile carrier solvents for the coating or pigment that evaporate when the material is applied to floors and other surfaces. Solvent vapors can be ignited by 500 W halogen lamp bulbs, open flames, and parting arcs. Some examples are provided below.

Alcohols

Methyl Alcohol (CH$_3$OH)   Methyl alcohol, or methanol, is a clear, colorless liquid used in many chemical manufacturing processes including drug, plastic, paint, varnish, and glue production. Methanol is available as a solvent from hardware stores. Higher-purity methanol is a typical laboratory solvent. It is also used as a fuel for high-performance automobile and boat engines. Methyl alcohol is a flammable liquid with a low flash point (11°C).

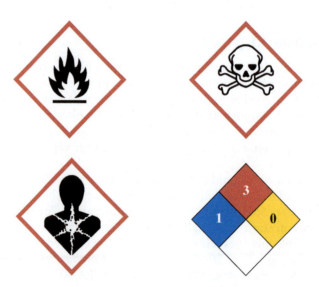

Because methyl alcohol burns completely leaving no residue, its flame is nearly transparent and blue in color. It can burn fiercely and yet not be visible until the flames impinge on another combustible that produces normal luminous flames. Methyl alcohol's flames have a very high average temperature. It burns to form carbon dioxide and water vapor, but if combustion is incomplete, it produces formaldehyde, a highly toxic material.

Ethyl Alcohol (CH₃CH₂OH) Ethyl alcohol, or ethanol, is a flammable liquid typically encountered more recently in the form of biofuel blends (gasoline-ethanol) and laboratory solvents. Ethyl alcohol is also the form of alcohol found in alcoholic beverages (grain alcohol); it is not encountered in its pure form except as a laboratory reagent. Ethanol may be used in a variety of concentrations in mixtures with water. Its flammability properties depend on its concentration, sometimes referred to (especially in beverages) as "proof" (50 proof = 25 percent alcohol, 100 proof = 50 percent alcohol, and so on). Grain alcohol intended for industrial purposes is usually at 95 percent concentration (190 proof) and is denatured by the addition of a small quantity of a poisonous substance to make it undrinkable. This denaturant may be methyl alcohol, sulfuric acid, benzene, gasoline, or some other toxic material.

Although ethyl alcohol will burn at higher concentrations, it does not produce as much heat per unit mass as do similar volatile petroleum products. It, like methyl alcohol, burns with a clear blue flame with little smoke. Because of the relatively low emissivity of burning ethyl alcohol, it is not a very good radiator of heat, and fires ignited with it grow more slowly than those involving petroleum distillates.

Acetone (CH₃O₂)

A very common solvent in the manufacture of plastics, fabric dyes, lacquers, paints, oils, waxes, and other products, acetone may be encountered in clandestine drug and explosive laboratories. It is a colorless, watery liquid with a mintlike odor, and burns with a yellow flame.

Ethyl Ether

Also known as diethyl ether or ether, ethyl ether is used as a solvent in pharmaceutical formulations and is very common in clandestine drug laboratories. It has been used for many years as an inhalant anesthetic in medicine, but ethyl ether also has wide use as a solvent for fats, greases, and resins. Because of its extreme volatility, wide range of flammable concentrations, and low ignition temperature, ethyl ether is extremely dangerous as a fresh liquid. Upon aging, it can form unstable peroxides, especially when exposed to air. These peroxides are sensitive to initiation by heat or shock and can cause a detonation. Burning vapors of ethyl ether may be difficult to detect, as the flame produced is nearly transparent.

Methyl Ethyl Ketone (MEK)

Also called butanone, MEK is used in paints, varnishes, lacquers, glues, and general solvents. It may be found as an intermediate solvent in clandestine drug laboratories. It is similar in its physical and combustion properties to acetone.

Cyclohexanone

Cyclohexanone is another ketone like acetone and MEK, with similar physical and chemical properties. Cyclohexanone is a moderate fire hazard that is used in clandestine drug laboratories in conjunction with other flammable solvents.

Rubbing Alcohol (Isopropyl Alcohol)

Usually sold in water solutions (70 percent), isopropyl alcohol is a flammable liquid readily available to consumers. It burns with a yellow, sootless flame.

Carbon Disulfide

A very common solvent in industrial processes, carbon disulfide is highly dangerous in the presence of heat, flame, sparks, or even friction. At normal temperatures it is a toxic material that affects the central nervous system like a narcotic or anesthetic. When heated, carbon disulfide gives off highly toxic sulfur oxides as it decomposes. Because of its volatility and extremely low autoignition temperature [100°C (212°F)], carbon disulfide is considered one of the most hazardous materials known. It can explode readily at vapor concentrations of around 5 percent but has a wide flammability range of 1.3 to 50 percent.

Aromatics

The aromatics—benzene, toluene, and the xylenes—are often found in combinations of one another because of their similar chemical properties. All of them produce toxic vapors, and all have been linked to some extent with causing cancer in animals chronically exposed to them. Benzene has the lowest flash point and greatest volatility; the properties of an aromatic mixture will largely be determined by the benzene concentration. Benzene is common in the plastic-, resin-, wax-, and rubber-manufacturing industries. Toluene and the xylenes may also be found as solvents for paints, lacquers, dyes, and petroleum products. They are used in making explosives and high-performance aviation fuel. All aromatics burn with a yellow, very sooty flame.

Bromobenzene

Bromobenzene is a low fire and explosion hazard because of its relatively high boiling point [156.2°C (313°F)] and low vapor pressure. It is common in clandestine drug laboratories and can generate toxic bromine-compound fumes when heated to decomposition.

Nitroethane and Nitromethane

Like other nitrated materials, these colorless, slightly oily liquids pose a potential fire and, particularly, explosion hazard. Both have relatively low flash points and ignition temperatures and will generate poisonous nitrogen oxides when heated. When they are contaminated with virtually any organic compound, particularly organic amines, they become potent shock- and heat-sensitive explosives.

Nitroethane and nitromethane pose a potential fire and, particularly, explosion hazard. Although nitromethane is used in large quantities as a lacquer and varnish solvent, when sensitized it becomes an explosive with 95 percent the strength of TNT. Nitromethane is often found in smaller quantities as a fuel for model cars and airplanes and as a fuel additive for gasoline engines. A nitroparaffin plant explosion occurred on May 1, 1991, in Sterlington, Louisiana, when a compressor failed and caught fire under a pipe rack with process pipe containing nitromethane. Confined heating of the nitromethane resulted in adiatic compression and detonation of the liquid explosive in two directions. Eight people perished, 120 were injured, and the small town was evacuated.

3.8.2 PETROLEUM PRODUCTS

Because virtually all petroleum products of significance in accidental or incendiary fires are a mixture of many separate chemical compounds that constitute a boiling point range or "cut," it should be kept in mind that the flammability hazard of a simple mixture of chemicals is largely determined by the properties of the lightest, most volatile component.

For example, although automotive gasoline contains more than 100 compounds, many of which have flash points above 50°C (122°F), the flash point (FP) of gasoline is close to that of its most volatile major component, n-pentane [FP −49°C (−56°F)]. Petroleum ether constitutes a narrow range of hydrocarbons that distill from petroleum at temperatures between 70°C and 90°C (158°F and 194°F).

Petroleum ether contains n-pentane, n-hexane, and n-heptane, and hydrocarbons of similar properties. It may be called benzine, benzin, or even naphtha depending on its components and its intended use. It may be considered to have the same hazardous properties as gasoline. Because of its excellent solvent properties, high volatility, and negligible residue, petroleum ether is widely used in pharmaceuticals and is often encountered in clandestine drug operations.

3.8.3 MISCELLANEOUS LIQUIDS

Other liquids of particular interest to fire investigators include organic amines, turpentine, and glycerin.

Organic Amines

Diethylamine and dimethylamine, like most organic amines, have a characteristic fishy odor. While dimethylamine is a gas at room temperature [boiling point: 7°C (44°F)], it is most commonly encountered as a water solution that is considered to be a flammable liquid. Dimethylamine has an ignition temperature of 400°C (725°F). Diethylamine is a liquid at room temperature [boiling point 57°C (134°F)] but has a very low flash point [−23°C (−9°F)] and an ignition temperature of only 312°C (594°F). Both diethylamine and dimethylamine are extremely toxic and are important precursors in the illicit manufacturing of LSD and methadone and may be encountered in fires involving clandestine laboratories.

Turpentine

Gum turpentine, not to be confused with mineral spirits or mineral turps, is an oil obtained by steam distillation of the resins of various pine and fir woods. It consists largely of the terpenes and other oleoresins found in the wood of those trees (Trimpe 1993, 53–55). Because it is a natural product, turpentine will vary depending on the wood from which it is made and on the gums or oils added to it for particular properties. Turpentine is considered a flammable liquid, although its high flash point [35°C (95°F)] makes it difficult to ignite at room temperature in the absence of a wick. Turpentines of various types are widely used in the paint, rubber, and plastics industries.

Glycerin

Glycerin (also glycerine and glycol) is a combustible liquid with a very high flash point that is completely soluble in water. Because it is safe for foods, it is widely used in food wrappings and in cosmetics as a plasticizer. It is also used in paints, cigarettes, and the manufacture of nitroglycerin explosives. It is becoming widely used as an antifreeze additive in domestic fire sprinkler systems. Unlike ethylene glycol, glycerin is compatible with plastic sprinkler piping and cements.

3.9 Solids

Most fuels in a structure fire are solids—wood, cloth, carpet, paper, and the like—converted to combustible vapors by pyrolytic action of the flames. There are some solids that, by virtue of their chemical properties, pose special hazards in terms of their flammability or speed of combustion. These solids will most often be encountered as part of the fuel load of commercial or manufacturing structures when they burn. As such, they can contribute significantly to the speed of and intensity of the fire.

Fire investigators who are not aware of the potential damage that can be caused by these compounds are liable to misinterpret the diagnostic signs left by their combustion. In addition, it is precisely because of their ease of ignition or intensity of reaction that certain materials are used to initiate incendiary fires in all types of targets. It is because of their unusual fire properties that certain hazardous solids will be examined here.

3.9.1 INCENDIARY MIXTURES

The most common incendiary solids are simple mechanical mixtures of various components—usually a fuel and an oxidizer, sometimes with initiators, catalysts, and the like, added to increase the efficiency of the reaction. Some of these mixtures include black powder, flash powder, matches, safety flares or fusees, thermite, Cadweld, and aluminum powder/plaster.

Black Powder

An explosive used in blasting, early firearms, and fireworks, black powder, or gunpowder, is a mixture of potassium nitrate, charcoal, and sulfur, usually in ratios of about 75:15:10. (The ratio can be changed to affect the rate of burning.) When dry, black powder can be ignited by a small spark, flame, or friction. It has an approximate AIT of

350°C (662°F). It can be rendered inert by absorbing water from the atmosphere. Temperatures on the order of 2,000°C (3,600°F) are produced during its combustion. When unconfined, black powder deflagrates and can be used as a trailer to transmit flame from one point to another. It forms the central flammable core in safety fuse. Black powder is now made in the United States at only one plant in Pennsylvania for military, antique firearms, and fireworks users (Conkling 1981).

Flash Powder

Flash powder, a mixture of a readily oxidizable metal such as powdered aluminum or magnesium with a strong oxidizer such as potassium perchlorate or barium nitrate, will produce an intensely hot flame in an almost instantaneous deflagration. Sulfur is usually present to promote uniform burning. These mixtures require minimal energy in the form of spark, heat, or friction to ignite and can produce temperatures in excess of 3,000°C (5,400°F). They are most often encountered in small explosive devices (including those sold as cherry bombs or M-80s) and in their larger, more destructive variants—military artillery simulators. Because of their sensitivity and destructive potential, devices using flash powder should be opened or dismantled only by qualified EOD personnel, even for evidentiary analysis.

The factories that make devices using these fillers pose serious explosion hazards because of airborne dusts, thin films on working surfaces, and product stored in bulk. Some powders include a sulfur and potassium chlorate mixture. The self-ignition propensity of this mixture has been well known since the 1890s. It has been banned from commercial fireworks by most Western countries but is occasionally found in devices made in China or Mexico (Tanner 1959).

Matches

Although innocuous enough in single use, the ignitable heads of common matches can be combined into substantial incendiary devices. Safety matches normally require frictional contact with a striker containing red phosphorus and powdered glass in a binder. These matches contain sulfur (fuel), potassium chlorate (oxidizer), and a variety of glues, binders, and inorganic fillers. When ignited by flame or spark, this mixture produces considerable heat and evolves sufficient gases to permit match heads to be used as propellants in improvised firearms.

By contrast, "strike-anywhere" matches usually consist of two layers of material with different flammability characteristics. Both contain potassium chlorate, phosphorus sesquisulfide (P_4S_3), rosin, and powdered glass, but the upper igniter button contains a higher percentage of P_4S_3 and glass, while the lower contains paraffin and sulphur (Ellern 1961). This combination allows the tip to ignite when struck against any hard surface, while the lower part has good flame characteristics but poor frictional sensitivity. Match strikers in bulk are extracted with a volatile solvent to provide phosphorus for methamphetamine production.

Safety Flares or Fusees

Safety flares and fuses contain a fuel of sulfur, wax, and sawdust and an oxidizer of strontium nitrate (for burning with a red flame) and potassium perchlorate. These devices burn with a very hot flame [in excess of 2,000°C (3,600°F)] and leave a white or gray lumpy residue consisting almost entirely of oxides of strontium. The mixture requires a high-heat source for ignition, and an igniter button is built into the end of each flare to provide it.

Thermite (or Thermit)

A mixture of powdered aluminum and iron oxide (Fe_2O_3), thermite, when ignited, will burn with extreme violence, spattering molten metal and producing temperatures in excess of 2,500°C (4,500°F)—sufficient heat to melt iron, steel, and even concrete. Fortunately, the reaction requires considerable heat input to begin. Usually, a magnesium strip is ignited as an initiator. Once ignited, a thermite fire is very difficult to extinguish because it supplies its own oxygen.

Cadweld

A mixture of powdered aluminum–copper alloy and iron powder that functions in the same way as thermite, Cadweld (see www.erico.com) produces a pool of molten copper as a residue and is used to weld large copper buss bars in heavy-duty electrical equipment. The temperature produced is on the order of 2,000°C (3,600°F). The mixture requires a high-temperature igniter, but the commercially prepackaged containers include a small quantity of magnesium powder so that the whole sample can be ignited with a match.

Aluminum Powder/Plaster

A fine aluminum powder, mixed with plaster of Paris and cast into ice cube–size blocks with a magnesium ribbon igniter, has recently been suspected as an ignition source in an arson case. It burns similarly to thermite, with a very hot, intense flame. This mixture was used as an improvised incendiary device in World War II.

3.9.2 OXIDIZERS

Solid sodium chlorate (NaOCl) oxygen generators onboard passenger aircraft evolve oxygen gas when the sodium chlorate decomposes into salt, heat, and oxygen. The decomposition reaction is accompanied by high temperatures. If combustible materials were present, a fire would occur. Other solid oxidizers and peroxides similarly liberate oxygen, intensifying combustible fuel fires.

Oxidizers, by definition, are not combustible in and of themselves but promote the burning of combustible fuels. The degree by which an oxidizer promotes combustion is related to the number of oxidizing gas molecules it can release. Consult the safety data sheet and other chemical hazard information. Typical strong oxidizer safety data sheet warnings include: "Fire: Not combustible, but substance is a strong oxidizer and its heat of reaction with reducing agents or combustibles may cause ignition. Explosion: Can cause explosions in contact with combustible dusts or vapors, occasionally explosive by shock or friction. Sensitive to mechanical impact."

All compounds containing chlorate or perchlorate salts are considered potentially hazardous materials because of their potency as oxidizing agents. In combination with virtually any oxidizable substance, these salts as well as nitrate salts of inorganics, or nitrate esters of organics can produce deflagrations with potential for serious structural damage. Virtually all nitrogen-containing compounds are unstable to some extent, and nitrates are generally even more unstable, as they are very active oxidizers. Some inorganic nitrates such as sodium nitrate are used as a substitute for more expensive explosives in dynamites and blasting agents. Although ammonium nitrate in its pure form will explode when heated, when it is contaminated with any organic material (such as charred paper or oil) to act as a fuel, it explodes with less stimulation and considerably more force (USFA 1988).

This phenomenon is responsible for the frequent use of ammonium nitrate–fuel oil (ANFO) as a blasting agent for both legitimate and criminal purposes. For many years ammonium nitrate fertilizer was thought to be so stable that dynamite was used to break up masses of it in damp warehouses. But when these same piles of fertilizer were contaminated with oil, they detonated in sympathy with the smaller dynamite charges. Exposure to fire also can cause detonation. This mechanism was the cause of the Texas City, Texas, explosion of 1947 (Stephens 1997). Sodium chlorate recovered from home-hobbyist welding torches or from weed killers has been used as an oxidizer in improvised explosive and incendiary devices.

3.9.3 REACTIVE METALS

Reactive metals include sodium metal, potassium, phosphorus, and magnesium.

Sodium Metal

Sodium metal is used in drug synthesis and related organic chemistry reactions. It is a soft metal that looks like silvery white putty. It is normally stored in a kerosene or oil bath because it reacts strongly with any water available, even that in the air or on human skin. When exposed to dry heat, sodium metal gives off very toxic oxides and in a general fire will flame spontaneously in air. It has an ignition temperature of about 115°C (240°F). In water, it generates large quantities of explosive hydrogen gas and caustic sodium hydroxide (lye) in a violently exothermic reaction, which spews flame and spatters hot lye and molten sodium.

Potassium

Potassium is used less frequently in chemical synthesis than sodium metal but presents the same serious hazards as sodium. In its pure form it is a silvery metallic crystal. Potassium generates hydrogen gas, potassium hydroxide, and a great deal of heat on contact with water. In addition, potassium can react with atmospheric oxygen to form a yellowish layer of explosive peroxides and a superoxide on the metal. These oxides can detonate when initiated by friction. In moist air, potassium can develop sufficient heat to ignite spontaneously.

Phosphorus

Phosphorus occurs in two forms of waxlike metal: one white (or yellow) and the other red. The two forms have quite different properties. White phosphorus is one of the few known materials that will burst into flames when exposed to air, so it is stored under water or a petroleum distillate. It has an ignition temperature of 30°C (86°F) and will react with most oxidizers, producing very toxic phosphorus oxides. In spite of its flammability, white phosphorus is not often encountered in accidental or incendiary fires (Meyer 2009) but has been used in the form of "Fenian fire"—a dispersion of a fine powder in a volatile solvent. When this substance is thrown onto a target, the solvent quickly evaporates, and the phosphorus bursts into flame.

If exposed to sunlight, white phosphorus can crystallize into the more stable red phosphorus, which does not burn when exposed to air and has an ignition temperature of 360°C (500°F). It will burn, however, and react violently, even explode, on contact with strong oxidizers. It is used as an igniter in frictional ignition devices, including those on matches and safety flares. It has found increasing favor in illicit methamphetamine manufacturing, where a mixture of red phosphorus and other precursors is often allowed to react unmonitored.

Magnesium

When people imagine the hottest flame possible, they often think of burning magnesium. Although not readily ignitable in large masses with small surface areas, magnesium shavings, powder, or ribbon can readily be lit with a common match. Magnesium fires can reach temperatures of 3,000°C (5,400°F) and produce toxic oxides, most often a dense, white, fluffy powder. When heated, magnesium can react with water or steam and produce flammable hydrogen gas as well as heat.

3.10 Clandestine Laboratories

As used here, the term *clandestine laboratories* refers to clandestine drug labs, marijuana cultivation, and clandestine explosives laboratories.

3.10.1 CLANDESTINE DRUG LABORATORIES

A significant number of structure fires are caused every year by accidental ignition of the highly flammable solvents or vapors used in the illicit manufacturing of drugs. According to the Drug Enforcement Administration DEA, in 2014 there was a total of 9,338 meth lab incidents, including labs, dumpsites, and chemical and glassware seizures.

The DEA also reports that seizures of clandestine drug labs and dumpsites have decreased dramatically since 2005, when 12,619 were seized, down to 5,910 in 2007, and 6,783 in 2008. The highest numbers are no longer recorded in California (286 to 470 in that same period); they are now reported in larger numbers in Missouri, Indiana, Illinois, and Tennessee (DOJ). Some 97 percent of the labs seized were reportedly producing methamphetamine, but amphetamine, phencyclidine (PCP), methadone, methaqualone (very rare), hallucinogens such as lysergic acid diethylamide (LSD), and methylene dioxyamphetamine (MDA) or methylene dioxymethamphetamine (MDMA) are also found.

The most common method of large-scale (10 lb or more) illicit manufacture of methamphetamine uses hydriodic acid (HI) and red phosphorus. Hydriodic acid is extremely corrosive, and red phosphorus can be converted to the more reactive white (or yellow) forms by the application of heat. Large glass flasks containing these reactants readily overheat and boil over, starting fires in all manner of buildings. Small batches of methamphetamine can be made in a bathroom sink with just a few glass jars. The reaction uses anhydrous ammonia, metallic (elemental) lithium (or sodium), and iodine. The lithium may be purchased or extracted from lithium batteries; the iodine may be purchased in solid form or extracted from medical iodine solutions (tinctures), and the phosphorus extracted from the striker strips of matchbooks. The starting materials themselves are often extracted from large quantities of over-the-counter cold tablets. Anhydrous ammonia, used extensively as an agricultural fertilizer, has been stolen in quantities from gallons to tractor-trailer loads. Sometimes the anhydrous ammonia is transferred to empty propane tanks. It is corrosive to the tank fittings and will cause them to leak badly, as shown in Figure 3-17.

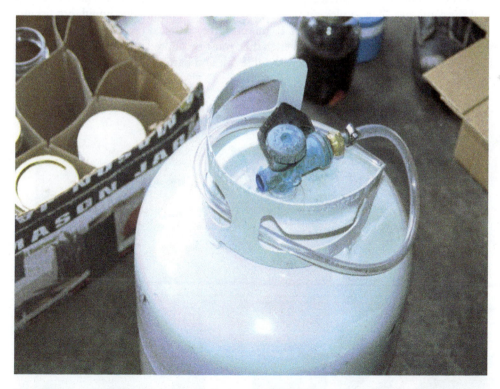

FIGURE 3-17 LP bottle used to transport anhydrous ammonia with cross-threaded "adapter." Green/blue corrosion on brass valve will eventually cause leakage of the valve. Note red phosphorus reaction in the glass jar behind the bottle. *Courtesy of the US Department of Justice, Drug Enforcement Administration.*

Until recently, Freon was used as the extraction solvent, but with the increasing scarcity of fluorocarbons, flammable solvents are used. If bulk anhydrous ammonia is not available, ammonium nitrate fertilizer can be converted to anhydrous ammonia using household lye. Empty lye containers or fertilizer bags would be significant evidence of the use of this process.

All these extraction and manufacturing processes involve the use of large quantities of flammable liquids—methyl alcohol, butane, acetone, lacquer thinner, ethyl ether, toluene, petroleum ether, camping fuel, and even gasoline—as solvents (which are then often evaporated by heating on hotplates or cookstoves). Many of the intermediate reactions take place in such solutions, and almost invariably the final product is "salted out" of a solution using hydrogen chloride (HCl) gas or even table salt. The resulting mixture must then be allowed to dry, and the room or building then fills with the vapors of evaporating solvent—often to explosive concentrations.

The explosions are initiated by the electric arc of a switch or motor, the overheating of reactant materials, the flames of a cookstove, or the match of an anxious observer. The ensuing fire is fueled by the large volumes of available flammable liquids on hand. Because of the potential profits, the large-scale laboratories can be surprisingly sophisticated, well equipped, and capable of turning out large quantities of fairly pure dangerous drugs. (See Figure 3-18, for example. An example of a typical backyard meth lab is shown in Figure 3-19.)

The newest twist in clandestine methamphetamine manufacture is called the "one pot" method. Here, Pseudoephedrine from cold medications is mixed with ammonium nitrate, lithium metal (from lithium batteries), lye (sodium hydroxide), water, and a flammable solvent such as ethyl ether or white gas in a single container such as a 2 L soft drink bottle, or similar jar or metal can. The reaction produces heat and a great deal of hydrogen gas. If the container is not vented repeatedly, the pressure can cause a mechanical explosion of the container. This explosion releases hydrogen, hot flammable liquid, hot lithium metal, and caustic hydroxides. In about 20 minutes, the chemical reaction produces methamphetamine base (oil) in the solvent, which then must be "salted out" with HCl gas. This gas is often generated in a separate jar with table salt and battery acid, or metal strips with

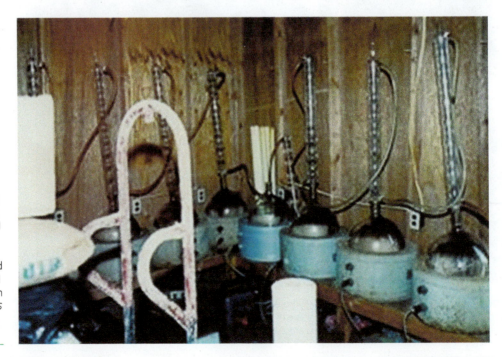

FIGURE 3-18 Clandestine drug laboratories can include reactive and toxic materials in elaborate and expensive glassware and other preparation equipment. Investigators should be cautious so as to avoid disturbing any reactions in progress. *Courtesy of the US Department of Justice, Drug Enforcement Administration.*

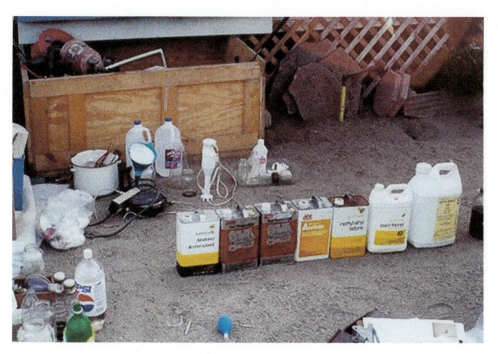

FIGURE 3-19 Typical "backyard" meth lab with hot plate, mixers, extraction solvents, and extraction/reaction vessels (soda bottles). *Courtesy of the US Department of Justice, Drug Enforcement Administration.*

hydrochloric acid. The final result, once filtered and washed, is a relatively pure meth with no telltale odors of bulk chemicals (Hunt, Kuck, and Truitt 2006).

To avoid detection, these laboratories are usually located in remote houses, garages, shacks, barns, or even trailers—anywhere electric power can be made available. More frequently, clandestine labs are appearing in motorhomes and camping trailers as isolated, self-contained plants with their own power generators or batteries and closed water-cooling systems. Clandestine drug labs have also been found in motels, rented houses, or apartments in urban areas, sometimes close to police and fire facilities.

The presence of one or more of the following at a fire scene should be a warning of a potential clandestine drug lab:

- Large numbers of empty containers:
    - Cold/allergy medicines or diet aids with Pseudoephedrine (see Figure 3-20)
    - Lithium batteries (e.g., for cameras, watches, or calculators)
    - Butane (lighter refills)
    - Lye (drain cleaner)
    - Camping fuel or automotive fuel additive
    - Muriatic acid (hydrochloric acid)
    - Iodine solution
    - Dimethyl sulfone (MSM) (used as a diluent or cutting agent)
- Cylinders or tanks of the following:
    - Anhydrous ammonia
    - HCl (hydrogen chloride)
    - H_2 (hydrogen)
    - LP gases (modified or corroded)
- Matchbooks without striker strips (in very large quantities)
- Multiple hotplates, electric skillets, or camp stoves
- Large quantities of alcohol (methyl, ethyl, or isopropyl), acetone, or MEK
- Ice-water baths in sinks, pans, or beer coolers with miscellaneous jars or tubing
- Residues that look like oatmeal dumped outside

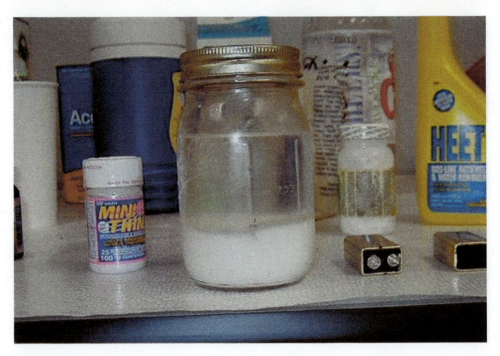

FIGURE 3-20 Pseudoephedrine extraction of powdered diet tablets using automotive fuel additive. Lithium will be extracted from the batteries. *Courtesy of the US Department of Justice, Drug Enforcement Administration.*

These scenes are very hazardous to investigate. Flammable, caustic, and highly toxic chemicals in gaseous, liquid, and solid forms may be encountered in such labs. Proper personal protective equipment (PPE) is essential. This is due to the complexity of the chemistries involved and hazardous materials present—flammable solvents; organic amines; methylamine; strong acids [sulfuric (H_2SO_4), hydrochloric (HCl), and especially hydriodic (HI)]; caustic bases; dangerous gases such as H_2, HI, and HCl; and extremely reactive materials such as anhydrides, phosphorus, and metallic lithium, sodium, and potassium (not to mention the toxic intermediate products including iodine vapors and phosphine gas).

At the first appearance of stored chemicals, glassware, laboratory equipment, pumps, ovens, and related apparatus, the assistance of a qualified forensic drug chemist is essential. The agency should seal off the scene and notify the appropriate narcotics enforcement team or DEA. In the interim, personnel should not turn on equipment that is off, should not turn off equipment that is on, and should not remove bottles, jars, or flasks from ice-water baths, if present. Many of the synthesis reactions are strongly exothermic and are being cooled by immersion or circulation to prevent a runaway buildup of heat that can cause the reactant mass to explode. These scenes should be approached with extreme caution because of the hazards of the solids, liquids, and even gaseous materials present.

3.10.2 MARIJUANA CULTIVATION

"Grow-ops" for the concealed cultivation of marijuana have been found in every type of structure in nearly every locale in North America—private residences, commercial premises, apartments, storage rental units, underground mines, even motorhomes and trailers. Except for the flammable solvents used for extraction of "hashish" oils, their main fire risk is the massive power needs of the high-intensity lamps used to promote rapid growth. Power connections (often illicit bypasses) can be haphazard or very sophisticated (see Figure 3-21). Electrical fires caused by these connections are the most common means by

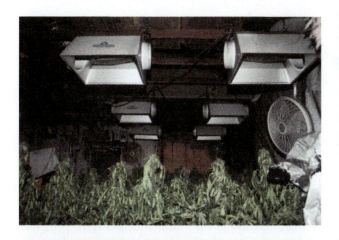

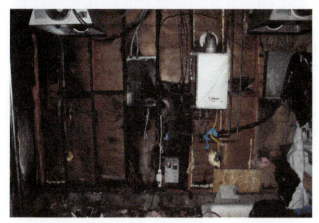

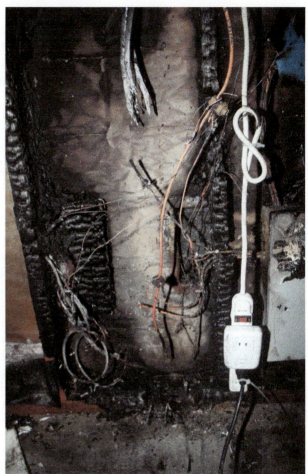

FIGURE 3-21 Marijuana "grow operations" are often detected when illicit power connections (meter bypasses) fail. *Courtesy of Vic Massenkoff, Contra Costa County Fire Dept.*

which these "grow-ops" are discovered. Fans, pumps (for water or hydroponic solutions), timers, and the lamps all provide ignition sources (Reed and Reed 2005). The high-intensity lamps used (often metal halide) can also ignite structural materials or growing plants by direct contact, or ignite nearby wood by radiant or conducted heat.

3.10.3 CLANDESTINE EXPLOSIVES LABORATORIES

Improvised explosive mixtures, typically involving hydrogen peroxide solutions and acetone (from consumer products), are becoming more common. The intermediate and final products are all hazards due to their extreme sensitivity and explosive power. The volatile solvents pose the usual fire risks. EOD units should handle all suspected explosive evidence and decontamination. Even innocuous-looking solids and liquids can be highly sensitive explosives at such scenes. If in doubt, call for EOD assistance.

3.11 Warning Systems

There are two different warning systems in common use in the United States to warn those handling or transporting hazardous materials of the types and severities of dangers posed if a material is exposed to heat or fire. These systems are the *NFPA 704* system and the Department of Transportation Hazardous Materials Transportation System.

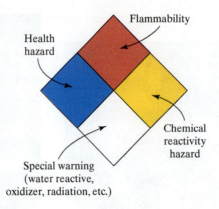

FIGURE 3-22 *NFPA 704* system for labeling hazardous material containers. *Based on NFPA 704 Standard System for the Identification of the Hazards of Materials for Emergency Response, 2012.*

3.11.1 *NFPA 704* SYSTEM

NFPA 704: Standard System for the Identification of the Hazards of Materials for Emergency Response, is used on storage tanks, exteriors of buildings, entry doors, pipelines, and the like (NFPA 2012). This system warns of the hazards relative to health, flammability, and chemical reactivity with a numbering system in which 0 represents no significant hazard, and 4 represents the highest degree of that hazard. The NFPA label is in the form of a diamond-shaped sign, as shown in Figure 3-22.

The topmost quadrant (often color-coded red) is the fire hazard. The left-hand quadrant is the health hazard (often color-coded blue), and the right-hand quadrant is the chemical reactivity hazard (susceptible to release of energy) and is usually color-coded yellow. The bottom quadrant is for special warnings when appropriate: the three-bladed propeller for radiation hazard; the letter W with a horizontal line through it to designate materials that are reactive to water (and therefore water should not be applied during fire emergencies). The letters OXY in the lower quadrant signify that the material is an oxidizer, while the letter P designates materials that can undergo polymerization (an exothermic reaction). The numeric designations are graded as follows:

A. Health Hazard

   4: Materials that can cause death or major injury upon very short exposure even if medical aid is given immediately
   3: Materials that can cause serious temporary or residual injury on short exposure
   2: Materials that could cause temporary incapacitation upon intense or repeated exposure unless medical aid is offered immediately
   1: Materials that can cause irritation only if no medical aid is given
   0: Materials that offer no hazard beyond that of any combustible material

B. Flammability

   4: Materials that will evaporate or vaporize completely on exposure to air at normal temperature and pressure, will mix with air, and will burn readily
   3: Liquids and solids that can be ignited under almost all ambient conditions
   2: Materials that will ignite if heated moderately or exposed to high ambient temperatures
   1: Materials that must be preheated before they will ignite
   0: Materials that will not burn

C. Reactivity

   4: Materials capable of detonation or explosive decomposition at normal temperatures
   3: Materials that are capable of detonation or explosive reaction but require a strong initiator, heating under confinement, or water reactivity

2: Materials that become unstable at elevated temperatures and pressures, may react violently with water, or form potentially explosive mixtures with water

1: Materials that can become unstable at elevated temperatures or pressures or react with water

0: Materials that are stable even under fire exposure conditions, and are not reactive with water

3.11.2 FEDERAL HAZARDOUS MATERIALS TRANSPORTATION SYSTEM

There are also designations for hazardous materials under the US Dept. of Transportation under the Federal Hazardous Materials Transportation Law (49 C.F.R. Parts 171–179). Under this system, each material classified as hazardous has a three- or four-digit number preceded by the prefix UN for United Nations (international shipping) or NA for North America (United States, Canada, and Mexico).

DOT labels are diamond-shaped and color-coded to a specific hazard class and usually include a warning pictograph. They are affixed to the outside of shipping containers (boxes, drums, etc.) and in some cases on placards on a vehicle transporting them. The classifications are as follows:

Class 1: Explosives, with subdivisions reflecting sensitivity: 1.1 for detonating explosives to 1.6 for materials with a negligible probability of accidental initiation

Class 2: Gases (flammable, **nonflammable**, poisonous)

Class 3: Flammable liquids [materials with a flash point of less than 60.5°C (141°F)]

Class 4: Flammable solids, spontaneously combustible materials, or materials that are dangerous when wet

Class 5: Oxidizers and organic peroxides

Class 6: Poisonous materials and infectious materials

Class 7: Radioactive materials

Class 8: Corrosive materials

Class 9: Miscellaneous hazardous materials

The reader is encouraged to review the emergency response literature for more specific information. Note that under this classification system, liquids with a flash point of less than 60°C (141°F) are classified as flammable liquids [as opposed to the 38°C (100°F) classification used by NFPA].

Many contributions and updates to this chapter courtesy of Elizabeth C. Buc, PhD, PE, CFI, Fire And Materials Research Lab, LLCl, Livonia, Michigan.

nonflammable ■
(1) Not readily capable of burning with a flame. (2) Not liable to ignite and burn when exposed to flame. Its antonym is *flammable* (NFPA 2017, pt. 3.3.131).

CHAPTER REVIEW

Summary

Explosions may occur as part of the progress of a normal fire, as the manner of initiation of a fire, or by themselves with no accompanying fire. Hazardous materials can be the cause of a chemical fire or explosion (as the first fuel ignited or source of heat) or involved in the fire as an additional fuel. Because of the reactivity or intensity of reaction of hazardous materials, their presence can significantly change the behavior of a fire.

Although the destructive power of an explosion is released in a much shorter time than that of a fire, many similarities exist between explosions and fires. As in all fire investigations, the investigator should pinpoint (1) the cause and origin of the fire or explosion, (2) the competent source of ignition for that explosion or fire, and (3) the sequence of events that led to the initiation.

Review Questions

1. Name the four categories of "explosion" and describe the features of each.
2. What is a mechanical explosion?
3. Name three major differences between a condensed- or solid-phase explosion and a diffuse-(gas/vapor) phase explosion.
4. What is a blast propagation diagram and how is it useful in an explosion investigation?
5. Name five examples of high explosives.
6. What are primary high explosives?
7. How do low explosives function?
8. What are the four Rs of an explosion scene investigation?
9. Why is it important to map the distance and direction of travel of debris at an explosion scene?
10. What are the four Cs of an explosion device reconstruction?
11. Name three of the most hazardous flammable hydrocarbon gases.
12. Name three flammable nonhydrocarbon gases.
13. Why are ethyl ether and carbon disulfide so dangerous from a flammability standpoint?
14. What is thermite (or thermit) and what residues does it leave behind?
15. Name three metal–oxidizer mixtures that can be used as incendiary materials.
16. Name four of the chemicals used in illicitly manufacturing methamphetamine.
17. What solvents have been found in clandestine drug labs?
18. List five of the waste materials or discards that indicate a clandestine meth lab is (or was) present.
19. Why are reactive metals so dangerous?
20. Why do nitromethane and nitroethane pose a special safety risk?

References

American Institute of Chemical Engineers. 2017. "Glossary of Terms." New York, NY.

Beveridge, A., ed. 1998. *Forensic Investigation of Explosions*. London: Taylor & Francis.

———. 2004. *Forensic Investigation of Explosions*. The Working Group on Fires and Explosions, Guidelines for Explosives Analysis. University of Central Florida, Orlando, FL: TWGFEX, November.

Bhalla, J. 2010. *Diesel Engine Runaway Safety Risk in Hazardous Environments*. Manama, Bahrain: Society of Petroleum Engineers.

Bottegal, M. N., B. R. McCord, and L. Adams. 2007. "Analysis of Trace Hydrogen Peroxides by HPLC-ED and HPLC-FD." Paper presented at AAFS, San Antonio, TX, February.

Bretherick, L., and P. Urben. 1999. *Bretherick's Handbook of Reactive Chemical Hazards*. San Diego: Butterworth-Heinemann.

Briley, E. M., and J. V. Goodpaster. 2007. "Practical Applications of Pattern Recognition to the Post-Blast Analysis of Black Electrical Tape." Paper presented at AAFS San Antonio, TX, February.

Carson, P.A., and C. J. Mumford. 1996. *The Safe Handling of Chemicals in Industry, Vol 3.* John Wiley & Sons.

Chumbley, L. S., and F. C. Lacks. 2005. "Analysis of Explosive Damage in Metals Using Orientation Imaging Microscopy." *Journal of Forensic Sciences* 50, no. 1 (January): 104–10.

Cochran, J. 2009. "Optimization of Explosives Analysis by Gas Chromatography and Liquid Chromatography." Paper presented at AAFS, Denver, CO, February.

Conkling, J. A. 1981. "Chemistry of Fireworks." *Chemical and Engineering News,* June 29, 24–32.

Cooper, P. W., and S. R. Kurowski. 1996. *Introduction to the Technology of Explosives.* New York: Wiley-VCH.

Corbin, M. B., and B. R. McCord. 2009. "Analysis of Smokeless Powder Components by Capillary Chromatography–TOF Mass Spectrometry." Paper presented at AAFS, Denver, CO, February.

Cox, B. L., A. R. Carpenter, and R. A. Ogle. 2014. *Process Safety Progress,* March.

Cozzani, V., M. Smeder, and S. Zanelli. 1998. *Journal of Hazardous Materials* A: 63, 131–42.

Cranz, C. 1916. *Lehrbuch der Ballistik.* Berlin: Springer-Verlag.

Crowl, D. A., and J. F. Louvar. 2001. *Chemical Process Safety: Fundamentals with Applications.* 2nd ed. Upper Saddle River, NJ: Pearson Education.

Davis, S. G., D. Engel, F. Gavelli, P. Hinze, and O. R. Hansen. 2010. "Advanced Methods for Determining the Origin of Vapor Cloud Explosions. Case Study: 2006 Danvers Explosion Investigation." Pp. 197–207 in *Proceedings ISFI 2010.* Sarasota, FL: International Symposium on Fire Investigation Science and Technology.

Davis, T. L. 1943. *The Chemistry of Powder and Explosives.* Hollywood, CA: Angriff Press.

DeHaan, J. D. 1995. "The Reconstruction of Fires Involving Highly Flammable Hydrocarbon Fuels." Ph.D. dissertation, Strathclyde University. (Also, University Microfilms, Ann Arbor, Michigan, 1996.)

DeHaan, J. D., D. Crowhurst, D. Hoare, M. Bensilum, and M. P. Shipp. 2001. "Deflagrations Involving Stratified Heavier-than-Air Vapor/Air Mixtures." *Fire Safety Journal,* 36: 693–710.

DeHaan, J. D., and W. R. Dietz. 1987. "Bomb and Explosion Investigations." *National Association of Medical Examiners*, September.

Ehleringer, J., and M. Lott. 2007. "Stable Isotopes of Explosives Provide Useful Forensic Information." Paper presented at AAFS, San Antonio, TX, February.

Ellern, H. 1961. *Modern Pyrotechnics.* New York: Chemical Publishing.

Ferrone, C. W., and C. Sinkovits. 2005. "The Runaway Diesel—A Side by Side Mechanical Analysis." *Proceedings of ASME International Mechanical Engineering Congress and Exposition.* Orlando, FL.

Flemming, D. B. 2004. "Explosion in Halifax Harbor." Halifax, NS: Formac.

Gersbeck, T. G. 2008. "Advancing the Process of Post-Blast Investigation." Paper presented at AAFS, Washington DC, February.

Gurney, R. W. 1943. *The Initial Velocities of Fragments from Bombs, Shells, and Grenades, BRL-405.* Aberdeen, MD: Ballistic Research Laboratory.

Haag, M. G., and T. Grissim. 2008. "Technical Overview and Application of 3-D Laser Scanning for Shooting Reconstruction and Crime Scene Reconstruction." Paper presented at AAFS, Washington DC, February.

Harris, R. J. 1983. *The Investigation and Control of Gas Explosions in Buildings and Heating Plant.* New York: E & FN Spon.

Henkin, H., and R. McHill. 1952. "Rates of Explosive Decomposition of Explosives." *Industrial Engineering Chemistry,* 44: 1391.

Hopkinson, B. 1915. UK Ordnance Board Minutes 13565.

Hunt, D., S. Kuck, and L. Truitt. 2006. *Methamphetamine Use: Lessons Learned.* Final report to the National Institute of Justice (NCJ 209730). Cambridge, MA: Abt Associates. Retrieved January 31, 2006 from www.ncjrs.gov/pdffiles1/nij/grants/209730.pdf.

IATG. 2015. International Ammunition Technical Guidelines, IATG 01.80:2015[E]. United Nations Office for Disarmament Affairs. Retrieved January 7, 2017, from https://www.un.org/disarmament.

Ide, R. H. 1999. "Petrol Vapour Explosion: A Reconstruction." Pp. 757–63 in *Proceedings Interflam 1999.* London: Interscience Communications.

Kimura, K., T. Nagata, K. Hara, and M. Kageura. 1988. "Gasoline and Kerosene Components in Blood: A Forensic Analysis." *Human Toxicology* 7.

Kinney, G., and K. Grahm. 1985. *Explosive Shocks in Air.* New York: Springer-Verlag.

Kirk-Othmer, ed. 1998. *Encyclopedia of Chemical Technology.* 4th ed. Vols. 1–27. New York: Wiley.

Lewis, B., and G. Von Elbe. 1961. *Combustion, Flames and Explosions of Gases.* 2nd ed. New York: Academic Press.

McDonald, K., and M. Shaw. 2009. "Identification of Household Chemicals Used in Small Bombs via Analysis of Residual Materials." Paper presented at American Academy of Forensic Sciences, February.

Mei, J., R. D. Halldearn, and P. Xiao. 1999. *Scripta Materialia* 41 (5), 541–548.

Mejia, L. C., and R. W. Waytulonis. 1984. *Overspeed Protection for Mine Diesels—A Literature Review.* US Department of Interior, Bureau of Mines, Information Circular 9000.

Meyer, E. 2009. *Chemistry of Hazardous Materials.* 5th ed. Upper Saddle River, NJ: Pearson/Brady.

Mniszewski, K. R., and J. A. Campbell. 1998. "Analytical Tools for Gas Explosion Investigation." In *Proceedings Interflam 1998.* London: Interscience Communications.

Muller, D., A. Levy, R. Shelef, S. Abramovich-Bar, D. Sonenfeld, and T. Tamiri. 2004. "Improved Method for the Detection of TATP after Explosion." *Journal of Forensic Sciences* 49, no. 5 (September): 935–40.

NFPA. 2001. *Fire Protection Guide to Hazardous Materials.* Quincy, MA: National Fire Protection Association.

———. 2012. *NFPA 704: Standard System for the Identification of the Hazards of Materials for Emergency Response.* Quincy, MA: National Fire Protection Association (next edition 2017).

———. 2013a. *NFPA 68: Standard on Explosion Protection by Deflagration Venting.* Quincy, MA: National Fire Protection Association.

———. 2013b. *NFPA 495: Explosives Code.* Quincy, MA: National Fire Protection Association.

———. 2014. *NFPA 1033: Standard for Professional Qualifications for Fire Investigator.* Quincy, MA: National Fire Protection Association.

———. 2015a. *NFPA 1: Fire Code.* Quincy, MA: National Fire Protection Association.

———. 2015b. *NFPA 30: Flammable and Combustible Liquid Code.* Quincy, MA: National Fire Protection Association.

———. 2015c. *NFPA 484: Standard for Combustible Metals.* Quincy, MA: National Fire Protection Association.

———. 2016a. *NFPA 400: Hazardous Materials Code.* Quincy, MA: National Fire Protection Association.

———. 2016b. *NFPA 652: Standard on the Fundamentals of Combustible Dust.* Quincy, MA: National Fire Protection Association.

———. 2016c. *NFPA 2: Hydrogen Technologies Code.* Quincy, MA: National Fire Protection Association.

———. 2017. *NFPA 921: Guide for Fire and Explosion Investigations.* Quincy, MA: National Fire Protection Association.

Oxley, J. C., J. Smith, E. Resende, E. Rogers, R. Strobel, and E. Bender. 2001. "Improvised Explosive Devices: Pipe Bombs." *Journal of Forensic Sciences,* 46, no. 3: 510–34.

Pape, R., K. R. Mniszewski, and A. Longinow. 2009. "Explosion Phenomena and Effects of Explosions on Structures." *Practice Periodical on Structural Design and Construction.* American Society of Civil Engineers.

Phillips, S. A., A. Lowe, M. Marshall, P. Hubbard, S. Burmeister, and D. Williams. 2000. "Physical and Chemical Evidence Remaining after the Explosion of Large Improvised Bombs." *Journal of Forensic Science* 45, no. 2: 324–32.

Raj, P. K. 2005. "Exposure of a Liquefied Gas Container to an External Fire." *Journal of Hazardous Materials* A122: 37–49.

Rankine, W. J. H. 1979. *The Dynamics of Explosion and Its Use.* Amsterdam: Elsevier.

Reed, C., and A. Reed. 2005. "Fire Investigation of Clandestine Marijuana Grow Operations." Pp. 365–78 in *Proceedings Fire and Materials 2005.* London: Interscience Communications.

Schuberth, J. 1994. "Post-Mortem Test for Low Boiling Arson Residues of Gasoline by GC/MS." *Journal of Chromatography* 662.

Sigman, M. E., and D. Clark. 2007. "Optimized Analysis of Triperoxide by GC-MS." Paper presented at AAFS, San Antonio, TX, February.

Spencer, A. B. 2008. "Dust: When a Nuisance Becomes Deadly." *NFPA Journal* November–December: 57–61.

Stauffer, E., J. A. Dolan, and R. Newman. 2007. *Fire Debris Analysis.* Academic Press.

Stephens, H. W. 1997. *The Texas City Disaster—1947.* Austin, TX: University of Texas Press.

Tanner, H. G. 1959. "Instability of Sulfur–Potassium Chlorate Mixtures." *Journal of Chemical Education* 36, no. 2: 58.

Trimpe, M. A. 1993. "What the Arson Investigator Should Know about Turpentine." *Fire and Arson Investigator* 44, no. 1: 53–55.

Urbanski, T. 1964. *Chemistry and Technology of Explosives.* Vol. 1. New York: Pergamon.

US Bomb Data Center. 2009. Washington, DC: Bureau of Alcohol, Tobacco, Firearms and Explosives.

US Department of Justice. 2016. *2014 Annual Explosives Incident Report.* Washington, DC: US Bomb Data Center, Bureau of Alcohol, Tobacco, Firearms and Explosives, April 6, 2016.

USFA. 1988. "Six Firefighter Fatalities in Construction Site Explosion, Kansas City, Missouri (November 29, 1988)." FEMA, USFA National Fire Data Center.

Weiser, V., E. Roth, A. Raab, M. Juez-Lorenzo, S. Kelzenberg, and N. Eisenreich. 2010. *Propellants, Explosives, Pyrotechnics* 35, 240–47.

Whitaker, K. M., et al. 2009. "Coming Apart at the Seams: The Anatomy of a Pipe Bomb Explosion." Paper presented at AAFS, Denver, CO, February.

Yallop, H. J. 1980. *Explosion Investigation.* Harrogate, UK: Forensic Science Society Press.

Zalosh, R. G. 2008a. "Explosion Protection." Chaps. 3–15 in *SFPE Handbook of Fire Protection Engineering.* 4th ed. Quincy, MA: National Fire Protection Association.

———. 2008b. "Explosions." Chap. 8, sec. 2 in *Fire Protection Handbook.* 20th ed. Quincy, MA: National Fire Protection Association.

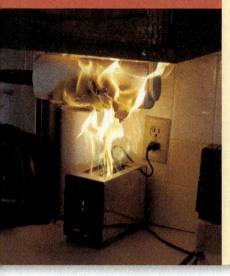

Courtesy of Jamie Novak, Novak Investigations and St. Paul Fire Dept

OBJECTIVES

After reading this chapter, you should be able to:

- Describe common ignition sources and their typical heat release rates.
- Recognize secondary sources of ignition.
- Identify the role of appliances in starting fires.
- Explain the role of smoking as a fire origin.

4.1 Introduction to Ignition Sources

Ignition can be defined as the initiation of self-sustaining combustion in a fuel. The fundamental properties that influence an object to ignitability are its density, thermal capacity, and thermal conductivity. Taken together, these properties constitute the material's *thermal inertia.* Ignition requires transfer of enough energy quickly enough to overcome the thermal inertia and trigger sufficient combustion to become self-sufficient. If that occurs, the ignition source is said to be *competent* (for that fuel under those conditions). Ignition involves bringing at least a part of the fuel to a characteristic temperature by means of conducted, convected, or radiant heat transfer until it can sustain combustion.

In gaseous fuels, this process involves raising the temperature of only a small volume to ignition. In solids, it usually involves the surface of the fuel (the exception being self-heating, in which the heat is being generated within the bulk of the fuel). No matter what the nature of the fuel, without some source of ignition, that is, without some source of energy, there won't be a fire. Without exception, the source is some type of hot object or mass, chemical reaction, flame, or electric current.

Except for the self-heating case, the temperature of the source must exceed the ignition temperature of the fuel, and it must be able to transfer enough heat into a suitable mass of fuel before there can be ignition. In the case of self-heating, ignition will cause self-sustaining smoldering combustion, in which oxygen from the surrounding air diffuses into the surface of the charring fuel to create enough heat to advance the reaction, but smoldering combustion can be started equally well by an external heat source. Although ignition of smoldering combustion is sometimes of interest to the fire investigator, for the most part the onset of flaming combustion is the event of most concern. Flaming combustion of a solid material occurs when sufficient gases or vapors are generated from the pyrolyzing fuel to support flames.

As a general rule, the lower the energy of the ignition source, the closer the source and first fuel have to be for ignition to take place. The ignition source may be small and inconspicuous compared with the destructive fire that follows. There may be intermediate stages from initial ignition to full involvement of the first fuel package, and then the fire may spread as other fuel packages in the room ignite. This item-to-item growth must obey the same physical laws. Material that is intentionally heated by electricity, friction, chemical reaction, or a controlled flame may be dropped or blown into fuel that then ignites. These intermediate occurrences must always be taken into consideration in dealing with the source of ignition. The challenge to the fire investigator is to identify the fuel first ignited and then determine how the ignition source managed to transfer enough heat to that fuel for it to kindle into flame.

In this chapter we examine a wide variety of heat sources and their thermal properties. The fundamental processes of heat transfer, heat release rate, and fire propagation must be applied to each scenario. In applying the scientific method to ignition processes, the investigator must evaluate likely sources.

4.2 Primary Ignition Sources

The primary source of ignition of virtually every fire is heat. The heat can originate from a hot surface, a hot particle, a chemical reaction, or a distant radiant heat source; however, the small open flame of a common match or lighter is among the most effective primary ignition sources for fires. These sources are responsible for a large percentage of both accidental as well as deliberate fires. Other sources include mechanical sparks (incandescently hot or burning particles) or electric arcs ranging from very small to lightning bolt size. All these sources generate enough localized heat to ignite many fuels, although not all sources will ignite all fuels. Heat may also be generated by the passage of current through wires (particularly in an overload condition) through a high-resistance connection or through an unintended conductive path. Heat is also generated by numerous chemical reactions of the exothermic type, some very slow, some very fast.

4.2.1 MATCHES

The match is specifically and exclusively designed to initiate combustion and is the most basic source of flame. Whether it directly initiates the destructive fire or merely sets a controlled fire that is later responsible for the larger fire is immaterial to the investigation of the source of ignition, but may be very material to the investigation of the larger fire.

The match is a stick treated to be readily combustible combined with a head that includes both fuel and oxidizer in a form that can be ignited by localized heat produced by friction. Matches are found in two general categories: the *strike-anywhere* match and the *safety* match. The strike-anywhere, or kitchen, match contains an oxidant such as potassium chlorate mixed with an oxidizable material such as sulfur or paraffin, a binder of glue or rosin, and an inert filler like silica.

The tip, which is more easily ignitable by friction, contains a high percentage of both phosphorus sesquisulfide (P_4S_3) and ground glass. The head of the safety match contains an oxidizer and a fuel such as sulfur. It will ignite only when struck against the strip containing red phosphorus, glue, and an abrasive like ground glass. The stick of the match is often treated with a chemical to suppress afterglow. Paper matches are generally impregnated with paraffin to improve both water resistance and the burning characteristics of the head.

The heat output of a large kitchen match is between 50 to 80 W (see Table 4-1), and the *average* flame temperature (once the incendiary tip has burned away) is between 700°C to 900°C (1300°F to 1650°F). Because the match flame is laminar and involves wood (or cardboard) and wax, temperatures within the thin combustion zone near the outside of the plume are similar to those of a laminar candle flame and can be as high as 1200°C to 1400°C (2200°F to 2500°F) (Karlsson and Quintiere 2000).

This energy and temperature are adequate for ignition of many fuels as long as that energy can be transferred into the fuel. A low heat flux output is not sufficient to ignite most fuels by radiant heat, so there is usually direct contact between the flame and fuel before ignition. This is true of ordinary combustible solids, but combustible gases or vapors can be drawn into the flame by entrainment flow, so there may appear to be ignition without direct contact.

US and Foreign-Manufactured Matches

Minor variations in match formulation and manufacturing detail exist among US manufacturers, although some matches are custom-made with special head or shaft designs for promotional purposes. Large differences in appearance (and sometimes in action) are expected only with matches of foreign origin. For instance, some foreign-made matches have been known to ignite by frictional contact between their heads.

Considerations for Fire Investigators

It is common to attempt to compare matches from a scene with suspected sources such as partial matchbooks on the basis of their length, width, color, and the paper content of the cardboard stems. On some occasions, the torn bases of the paper matches can be physically compared, jigsaw fashion, to the stubs in the matchbook. Most US book matches today, however, are pre-perforated, which makes them tear uniformly and thus reduces the chances for accurate comparisons. It is sometimes possible to trace the origin of partially consumed matches at a fire scene by conducting an elemental analysis on the unburned match heads (Andrasko 1978).

4.2.2 LIGHTERS

There are two general types of lighters: the electric-element type usually found in vehicles, and liquid-fuel lighters. In most fires, the electric lighter may be disregarded as a source of

TABLE 4-1	Heat Release Rates and Burn Times of Common Ignition Sources			
	TYPICAL OUTPUT (kW)	TYPICAL BURN TIME (s)[a]	MAXIMUM FLAME HEIGHT FLAME (mm)	MAXIMUM HEAT FLUX (kW/m²)
Cigarette 1.1 g (not puffed, laid on solid surface) bone dry	0.005	1,200	—	42
Cigarette 1.1 g (not puffed, laid on solid surface) conditioned to 50% R.H.	0.005	1,200	—	35
Methenamine pill, 0.15 g	0.045	90		4
Candle (21 mm, wax)*	0.075	—	42	70[b]
Wood cribs, BS 5852 Part 2				
No. 4 crib, 8.5 g	1	190		15[c]
No. 5 crib, 17 g	1.9	200		17[c]
No. 6 crib, 60 g	2.6	190		20[c]
No. 7 crib, 126 g	6.4	350		25[c]
(Crumpled) brown lunch bag, 6 g	1.2	80		
(Crumpled) wax paper, 4.5 g (tight)	1.8	25		
Newspaper—folded double sheet, 22 g (bottom ignition)	4	100		
(Crumpled) wax paper, 4.5 g (loose)	5.3	20		
Newspaper—crumpled double sheet, 22 g (top ignition)	7.4	40		
Newspaper double sheet newspaper, 22 g (bottom ignition)	17	20		
Polyethylene wastebasket, 285 g, filled with 12 milk cartons (390 g)	50	200[d]	550	35[e]
Plastic trash bags, filled with cellulosic trash (1.2–14 kg)[f]	120–350	200[d]		
Small upholstered chair	150–250	—	—	—
Upholstered (modern foam) easy chair	350–750	—	—	—
Recliner (PU foam, synthetic upholstery)	500–1000	—	—	—
Gasoline pool on concrete (2 L) (1/m² area)	1000	30–60	—	—
Sofa	1000–3000	—	—	—

Sources: V. Babrauskas and J. Krasny, *Fire Behavior of Upholstered Furniture*, NBS Monograph 173 (Gaithersburg, MD: US Department of Commerce, National Bureau of Standards, 1985).

*From S. E. Dillon and A. Hamins, "Ignition Propensity and Heat Flux Profiles of Candle Flames for Fire Investigation" in *Proceedings: Fire and Materials 2003* (London: Interscience Communications), 363–76.

[a]Time duration of significant flaming.

[b]Centerline—immediately above flame; <4 kW/m² outside.

[c]Measured from 25 mm away.

[d]Total burn time in excess of 1800 s.

[e]As measured on simulation burner.

[f]Results vary greatly with packing density.

ignition because it depends on the battery of a vehicle to heat the wire heating element. The electric lighter is not operative except with its electrical connections to a battery; therefore, its use is restricted.

The liquid-fuel lighter ignites the flammable vapors from a fuel-soaked wick or liquid reservoir by means of a spark produced when a steel strikes the surface of a flint. Cigarette lighter flints are made of misch metal, an alloy of rare earths like cesium, lanthanum, or neodymium whose sparking potential is very high (Babrauskas 2003, 509). Thus, a spark or hot particle ignites a fuel vapor under controlled conditions, leading to a small, predictable flame. These lighters are a convenient substitute for a match and are, no doubt, responsible for many incendiary fires. They are rarely left behind and are therefore unlikely to be recovered as evidence.

When lighters are recovered, there may be latent fingerprints (especially on a removable fuel reservoir inside the case) and trace evidence. Some lighters ignite the vapors by catalytic oxidation or piezoelectric effect on a crystal, but since the flame produced is the same as that from a regular flint lighter, their use as an ignition source remains functionally the same. The heat release from a wick-type lighter is similar to that of a large kitchen match (50 to 80 W), and maximum temperatures are similar to those reported for pool fires of hydrocarbon fuels, $\approx 1000°C$ ($1830°F$) (Drysdale 2011).

Disposable lighters filled with butane have replaced traditional lighters in which the user refueled with a light liquid petroleum product. In the latter, the butane fuel compartment is under pressure, and the fuel is delivered through a metering valve to be ignited (in the manner described earlier) as a small, laminar jet flame. The adiabatic temperatures of these flames have been reported as $1895°C$ ($3440°F$), so real-world maximum temperatures might be expected on the order of $1400°C$ ($2500°F$). Research at the University of Maryland on cigarette lighters with port-type and Bunsen-type burner designs (adjusted to produce 75-W flames) reported temperatures reaching 2022 K ($1749°C$; $3180°F$) and peak heat fluxes as high as $169 kW/m^2$ (25 mm from tip axially) (Williamson and Marshall 2005).

Tests of disposable butane lighters indicated a fuel release rate of 0.001 to 0.002 g/s and a flame less than 20 mm (0.8 in.) in height. Based on a delta change ("Δ") of ΔH_c 46 kJ/g, this fuel consumption would produce an estimated 40 to 90 W. These lighters can explode if exposed to high temperatures and are subject to leakage when dropped or exposed to reduced atmospheric pressure, as in airplane cabins. The metering valve can sometimes be adjusted to release a fairly voluminous stream of flammable gas, and the resulting flame can be several inches high (with corresponding increase in heat release rate). These non-refillable lighters are intended to be disposable and are likely to be left at the point of ignition of a fire.

4.2.3 TORCHES

A variety of torches used in industrial and residential applications include traditional blowtorches using manually pressurized white gas delivery and drip torches using kerosene or diesel fuel for setting controlled back fires in wildlands. Handheld or long-wand roofing torches use propane, butane, or MAPP [methyl acetylene ($H_3C—C≡CH$) and propadiene ($H_2C≡C≡CH_2$)] as fuels. Acetylene/oxygen and acetylene/air handheld torches are very well known. Certain paint-stripping devices (heat guns) that are either propane-fueled or electrically powered can produce very high gas temperatures and high heat fluxes.

Fire Findings reported that flame temperatures in a propane hand torch ranged from $332°C$ ($629°F$) at the tip to $1333°C$ ($2071°F$) at the flame center to $1200°C$ to $1350°C$ ($2190°F$ to $2460°F$) at the tip of the "inner flame" cone (Sanderson 2005b). Any of these propane torches can cause accidental and intentional fires if applied to suitable fuels. Cellulosic materials are most susceptible to ignition by torch application, especially if finely divided, because brief application of a flame to a solid wood surface will cause only surface scorching and (possibly) brief glowing combustion that ceases as soon as the flame is withdrawn.

Finely divided materials (dried leaves, needles, sawdusts) are very susceptible to ignition, usually in two stages: smoldering followed by flame. More massive materials are susceptible when the torch flame is played into narrow crevices or spaces, where radiant losses from surface ignition are minimized. In these cases, ignition can be caused within the cavity that may not be readily detectable or extinguishable from the outside. Crevices can retain sawdust and detritus from termite attack, making ignition even more likely. In hot torch work on roofs, torches are used to cause tar to adhere to roof structures or liquefy the asphaltic adhesive on the flexible membrane as it is laid. Under either condition, smoldering ignition triggered in crevices or in debris is then concealed under the hot tar or membrane. Roof fires following several hours of concealed smoldering have occurred.

Microtorches are advertised as intended for welding and brazing operations but are primarily being sold in smoke shops. These use butane as a fuel and premix it in a special torch tip that can produce extremely hot flames. (See Figure 4-1.) These microtorches are small enough to be concealed in the hand and can be ignited and left burning. Due to their application as welding devices, these microtorches normally lack any child-resistant features. The maximum temperatures measured in the combustion zones of a microtorch should be the same as for a full-size one [1200°C to 1350°C (2200°F to 2470°F)]. These torches are often used in the inhalation of drugs like crack cocaine.

4.2.4 CANDLES

Once candles were only a consideration of fire causation during power failures. Now with increased use, candles are a consideration in many residential fires. The National Candle Association estimates that candles are used in 7 of 10 American homes and that candle sales increase by 15 percent each year. The USFA estimates that candles are responsible for more than 9,400 residential fires each year. The CPSC estimated an even higher number—12,800 fires causing 170 deaths and 1,200 injuries (Dillon and Hamins 2003, Ahrens 2002). The NFPA estimated that in 2002, candles started 18,000 reported home fires, causing 130 deaths, 1,350 injuries, and property losses of $333 million in the United States alone (Nicholson 2005).

A traditional paraffin or beeswax candle produces about 50 to 80 W of heat with a laminar flame and an *average* flame temperature of 800°C to 900°C (1470F to 1650°F), but like a match flame, a candle flame has an outer combustion zone that can have temperatures as high as 1200°C to 1400°C (2200°F to 2550°F). Because of the candle's steady, prolonged flame and high temperature zone, it is possible to melt thin copper or even iron wire in a candle flame if it is held steadily in the very hot combustion zone. However, the thermal conductivity of metal wire conducts the heat away too quickly to permit the melting of larger-diameter wire.

Dillon and Hamins reported that a 21-mm (0.8-in.)-diameter candle had a mass loss rate of 0.09 to 0.11 g/min. With a net ΔH_c of 43 kJ/g, this produced a flame 40 mm (1.6 in.) high, with an HRR of ~65 to 75 kW. They measured the total heat flux along the vertical centerline and showed a maximum of about 70 kW/m^2 at the tip of the flame, dropping to ~40 kW/m^2 at 50 mm (2 in.) above the tip and ~20 kW/m^2 at 170 mm (6.7 in.) above the tip (Dillon and Hamins 2003). Just 13 mm (0.6 in.) from the centerline, the total heat flux at the level of the flame tip was about 27 kW/m^2, showing the significant amount of heat in the buoyant plume. These results confirm direct observations of the propensity for a candle flame to ignite fuels at some distance immediately above the flame but not target fuels at the side of the flame.

A well-designed candle melts at just the right rate to maintain a steady supply of wax for the wick to deliver to the flame: too little wax and the candle extinguishes for lack of fuel; too much wax and the wick gutters and drowns (Faraday 1993). Ideally, the wax burns completely to carbon dioxide (CO_2) and water. The combustion of carbon soot occurring in the outer high temperature zone is essentially complete; virtually no soot escapes the laminar flame. If the wick is too long and the flame becomes turbulent, soot can escape. If the wax is contaminated with oils or other organic materials, these may not burn completely, and a large quantity of soot can be released. If the wick is not symmetrically placed in the candle, the candle can fail and slump, exposing large lengths of wick.

The heat release rate (and therefore the flame length) of a candle is determined by the amount of exposed wick. If charred matchsticks are dropped into a candle, they can act as supplemental wicks, dramatically increasing the size of the flame. The larger flame can impinge on adjacent fuels or heat the container in which the candle is placed, creating increased risk of accidental fires (Townsend 2000, 10).

Candles cause fires when combustibles come into contact with the flame (e.g., loose material can move into the flame), the candle can tip over while lighted (especially with taper or column-style candles as opposed to pillar or votive styles), or the candle fails as the wick comes loose or otherwise becomes more exposed. This last situation causes a larger flame. Ignition can also occur when combustibles are included in the candle as decorations.

Candles with aromatic oils are used for aromatherapy and then left to burn while the occupant goes to sleep. Large decorative candles with multiple wicks and burning times of several days create prolonged risks of ignition of draperies, furniture, and clothing (Sanderson 1998a; Singh 1998).

4.3 Secondary Ignition Sources

For purposes of this chapter, *secondary ignition sources* include sparks and arcs, hot objects and surfaces, friction, radiant heat, and chemical reaction.

4.3.1 SPARKS/ARCS

The **spark** per *NFPA 921* (NFPA 2017b, pt. 3.3.175; see also *NFPA 654*, 2017c) is defined as "a moving particle of solid material that emits radiant energy due either to its temperature or the process of combustion on its surface." The true definition of spark is ambiguous because the term can refer to one of two situations:

- an electric arc of brief duration where electric current is discharging through air or another insulator, or
- a tiny fragment of burning or glowing solid material moving through the air

The electric spark is not readily distinguished from the electric **arc**, except for duration. Babrauskas (2003, 70) has suggested that an arc represents a stable electrical flow, whereas an electric spark represents an initial flow of electric current across a gap between conductors. The arc, "a high-temperature luminous electric discharge across a gap or through a medium such as charred insulation" (NFPA 2017b, pt. 3.3.7), persists as a discharge for a considerable time interval, while an electric spark is virtually instantaneous. Therefore, it is simpler to regard all such electrical phenomena as arcs of various durations and leave the term *spark* to represent a solid particle or molten droplet heated by some process to incandescence. The longer an arc persists, the more time it has to heat its immediate surroundings and transfer heat to surrounding fuel. The energy that can be released from an electric arc can range from millijoules to millions of joules. Because the arc can persist from microseconds to hundreds of seconds, the total heat released can be within a very broad range—from a tiny, brief arc of static electricity on a household doorknob to a massive lightning strike.

The capacity of arcs to ignite fuels, then, depends greatly on their duration, current flow, and the susceptibility (physical and chemical properties) of nearby fuels. The latter

spark ■ A moving particle of solid material that emits radiant energy due either to its temperature or the process of combustion on its surface (NFPA 2017b, pt. 3.3.175).

arc ■ A high-temperature luminous electric discharge across a gap or through a medium such as charred insulation (NFPA 2017b, pt. 3.3.7).

conception of a spark, that is, a tiny fragment of burning or glowing material moving through the air, has become the standard usage and will be used here. Sparks, then, can be produced by a sharp blow between two dissimilar materials like steel and flint, by extreme frictional contact between two moving materials, by extreme heating and melting of conductors in electrical failures, or by the airborne debris of a solid-fuel fire. These incandescently hot particles are capable of igniting fires in vapors and some solids that will be addressed later in this chapter.

Mechanical sparks include burning brands or very hot embers, fragments of debris from an existing fire, droplets of metal from extremely hot combustion or electric arcing events, incandescent or burning metal from impact or mechanical friction, or soot/particulates from engines of many types. These will be considered as a special case of hot objects in the following section.

4.3.2 OBJECTS/HOT SURFACES

Most hot objects are heated either by being in or close to a flame, by frictional heating, or by the flow of electric current through them. In electric appliances, ceramic or wire heating elements carry current and generate heat as a result. If combustible materials come into contact with these heating elements, they can cause fires by igniting and then spreading the fire to other fuels nearby. These appliances are not primary sources of ignition but lead to loss of control of a designed heat source. Malfunctions can also lead to the production of hot surfaces when electricity flows through conductive paths for which they were not intended or at rates that exceed the design of intended conductors. Hot objects play an important role in transmitting the heat of various chemical and physical processes to fuels, thereby spreading a fire. As seen in Table 4-1, the visible light emitted by the surface of a hot object can give an indication of its temperature. The capacity of this object to ignite a fire depends not only on its initial temperature but also on its mass and thermal capacity, which together determine how much heat this mass contains.

The evaluation of a possible ignition of a fuel by hot object or surface is not a simple matter of noting the temperature of the surface or mass or comparing it with the listed AIT (**autoignition temperature**) of the fuel. Ignition of any fuel will not occur unless enough heat is transferred into a sufficient mass of fuel to establish a persistent flame. The transfer of that heat from a surface depends on the nature and contour of the surface (even its roughness and cleanliness), the nature of contact, and whether the fuel can maintain the contact long enough. The AIT of a liquid or gaseous fuel varies with the test method used, the volume and shape of the test cell, and the material used for the test cell (Holleyhead 1996).

For example, clean, polished metal hot surfaces produce ignitions at lower temperatures than do similar metals that have an oxide layer. Very short contact or *residence times* do not allow enough heat to be transferred. A volatile liquid fuel dripped onto a flat, hot metal surface is likely to cool the immediate contact area by evaporation; the resulting vapors rise by convection away from the hot surface, thus reducing the residence time. The temperature of the surface, then, would have to be hundreds of degrees hotter than the AIT for that fuel for there to be ignition, and even then it would not be a guaranteed result.

The lower the flash point of the liquid fuel, the higher the temperature of the hot surface necessary to achieve ignition (Babrauskas 2003). Hot-surface ignition of liquid or gaseous fuels is achieved at lower temperatures if they are confined (in a tube or other enclosure). Other variables include surface type, droplet size, and airflows near the surface. When hot particles can penetrate or burrow into a solid fuel, residence time is no longer a factor, but the total amount of heat that the mass can carry is critical. If the thermal energy of the particle is too low (insufficient mass or density, inadequate thermal capacity), there may not be ignition even if the object is buried in the fuel and transfers all

autoignition temperature ■ The lowest temperature at which a combustible material ignites in air without a spark or flame (NFPA 2017b, pt. 3.3.15).

its heat. Hot objects that land on a rigid surface are even less likely to ignite a solid fuel due to the extra convective and radiative losses to the surrounding air.

It is tempting to measure the temperatures of hot surfaces as they occur in open air and then compare those temperatures against ignition temperatures of potential fuels (as has been reported in *Fire Findings*), but temperatures are only a guide to the processes taking place. If the temperature on the surface of a glass light bulb in the open is measured at 200°C (400°F), that value reflects only the steady-state temperature of that surface achieved by the balance between the heat flux (input) striking the inside of that bulb from the hot filament and the heat losses from convective, radiative, and even conductive processes on the outside of the bulb. If the rate at which the heat is lost is changed by placing the bulb in contact with a surface or by burying it in an insulating material, the temperature of that surface will rise, often dramatically. The new temperature then poses a very different source for transfer of heat to a potential fuel. To summarize, burying even a low-wattage heat source in a deep layer of cellulose insulation poses an ignition risk even when the open-air temperature of that heat source would make it seem safe.

As a reference point, however, knowledge of open-air temperatures of some hot surfaces is useful. The surface temperatures of halogen work-light lamps (bulbs) have been reported to be 593°C to 685°C (1100°F to 1266°F; i.e., sufficient to ignite flammable vapor/air mixtures as well as solids), and the glass face of a 300-W halogen work light to range from 180°C to 215°C (357°F to 418°F) (Corwin 2001). The open-air surface temperatures of heating elements of electric range tops ranged from 370°C (700°F) for small burners to 590°C (1100°F) for large burners in older appliances, and 500°C to 730°C (925°F to 1350°F) for equivalent burners in new ranges (Sanderson 2000, 5). Most modern electric ranges have a great deal of power in each cooking element, as well as high temperature. Goodson and Hardin reported wattage ratings for various electric range heating elements ranges from 1,200 to 2,500 W (Goodson and Hardin 2003).

As we have seen, with complex fuels like cellulosics, the increase in temperature may bring about physical and chemical changes in the fuel that make it more susceptible to ignition than the original fuel. The heat transfer rate to the fuel surface is probably more useful than temperature as an indicator of ignitability. The chemical and physical nature of the fuel has to be considered, and the effects of radiant heat have to be tested as part of the hypothesis testing phase of the scientific method. The higher the radiant flux applied to a fuel, the lower the observed ignition temperature will usually be, dramatically decreasing the time to ignition.

If the fuel is a thermoplastic, it may melt, sag away from the ignition source, or form a nonporous mass and become less likely to be ignited. Materials that char upon initial heating may become more susceptible with initial heating if the charring produces a porous residue that will support a smoldering combustion. Charring may also produce a pyrolyzed fuel that requires more energy to ignite.

4.3.3 FRICTION

Friction between two moving surfaces generates heat (as in the disc brakes of an automobile, which can become extremely hot). Although traditionally, rubbing sticks together to start a fire has been taught as a survival technique, friction in other contexts is more important in igniting fires, especially in machinery. Wood is a poor conductor of heat.

Any bearing that does not have adequate lubrication can become hot through friction, and contact of the hot object with a readily ignited fuel can lead to a fire. Lack of lubrication is one of the relatively common sources of fire where machinery is in use. Conveyor or power transmission belts can jam or be forced to run against frozen rollers and cause extreme frictional heating. Once ignited, the moving belt can spread fire very rapidly.

If frictional heat becomes extreme, one or both of the surfaces may disintegrate, producing a shower of incandescent particles. This disintegration may be the end result of massive overheating or very localized surface heating where the temperature of the mass itself may not rise appreciably. The temperatures of hot particles generated by this process are limited by the melting temperatures of the material involved. For instance, a mechanical spark generated from a copper-nickel alloy surface may have a maximum temperature of 300°C (570°F) (and not be incandescent at all), while a fragment of tool steel may be at 1400°C (2550°F) and be bright sparkling white (NFPA 2017b, Table 5.7.1.1). This situation can occur with any moving machinery. Bearings in conveyor systems, for instance, can clog with abrasive dust or seize from lack of lubrication and create large numbers of incandescent sparks for long periods of time. Bearings in automotive turbochargers can fail in seconds if lubrication is interrupted, due to their very high rotational speeds (up to 25,000 rpm).

Not only bearings give rise to dangerous temperatures from excessive friction. High-speed rotors like those found in airplane motors that come into contact with the housing have been known to produce enough heat to melt the housing and ignite related hardware. Fragments of overheated brake shoes in malfunctioning train or truck brakes can be thrown from the moving vehicle for miles before being detected. Mufflers, tailpipes, tailgates, chains, and other equipment dragging on the road surface can generate substantial showers of incandescent metal particles with enough heat to ignite roadside fuel (dried grass, leaves, or litter). Machining operations (milling machines, lathes) can generate showers of hot particles that can ignite waste in or under the tool.

4.3.4 RADIANT HEAT

Although the heat radiated from a fire may ignite other fires at a distance, ignition is not primary but is secondary to an already large, established fire. Radiant heat plays a great role in spreading most fires. As a primary ignition source, radiant heat alone is less frequently encountered. Radiant heat from fireplaces, stoves, and heaters has been seen to bring *nearby* cellulosics to their ignition temperatures and thus start fires. When devices are permanent fixtures, their remains will usually still be detectable after the fire.

Other sources may not be so easily identifiable. The investigator must remember that direct physical contact between the heat source and the first fuel is not always necessary when sufficient radiant heat is brought to bear on the fuel surface. Here the reflective and absorptive qualities of the fuel are critical, as are its density and thermal conductivity. All that is required is for the target fuel to absorb more heat than it can dissipate and for that heat to raise the local (surface) temperature above the fuel's spontaneous ignition temperature.

Rays from direct sunlight (at a typical heat flux of 1 kW/m^2) are not intense enough to ignite common fuels, but if they are concentrated or focused by a transparent object that is round in cross section, either spherical or cylindrical, or by a concave reflective surface such as a shaving mirror or the polished metal bottom of some aerosol cans, they can reach 10 to 20 kW/m^2 at the focal point of the light path. If a cellulosic fuel is located at or near that focal point, the fuel can be heated to its ignition temperature and catch fire. Figures 4-1 and 4-2 illustrate two examples of ignition by sunlight focused by shaving mirrors. This mechanism is often blamed for starting wildland fires, but the conditions have to be just right: the object has to produce a sharply focused area of sunlight, and the dry fuel has to be located precisely at the focal point of that lens or mirror before ignition will take place. Empty glass bottles, broken glass, or flat reflectors do not have a measurable focal length and will *not* cause ignition by this means.

Table 4-1 shows the maximum heat fluxes of some common small flaming ignition sources [at a distance of 25 mm (1 in.)]. Some tools and appliances, even when operating as designed, can act as nonflaming ignition sources. Radiant heat from floodlights (particularly quartz halogen), projection lamps, heat lamps, and flameless torches can be

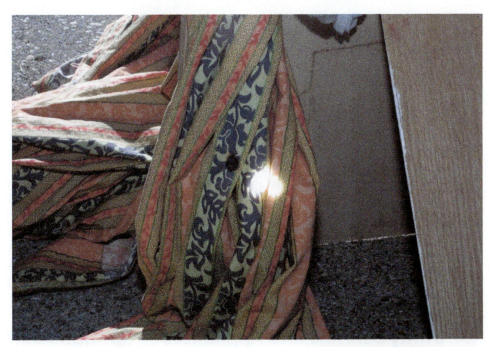

FIGURE 4-1 Sunlight focused on cloth target by a shaving mirror can reach heat flux sufficient to ignite fabrics. *Courtesy of Jamie Novak, Novak Investigations and St. Paul Fire Dept.*

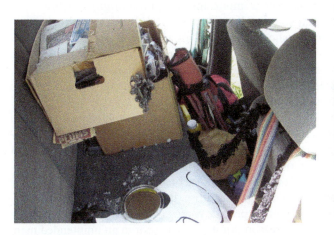

FIGURE 4-2A Shaving mirror (foreground) focused sunlight onto a corner of a box above it in a parked car. *Courtesy of Scott R. Schuett, Lebanon, CT.*

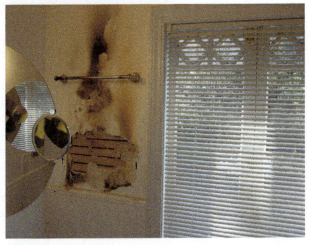

FIGURE 4-2B Shaving mirror (on left) focused sunlight from a window onto towels, which ignited on the rack. *Courtesy of Kyle Binkowski, Fire Cause Analysis.*

enough to ignite cellulosic fuels at close range (Sanderson 2000; Lowe and Lowe 2001). A noncombustible covering (e.g., sheet metal, tile, asbestos, or plasterboard) can allow heat to be transferred to a fuel surface beneath while impeding the loss of heat by convection, thus making it susceptible to ignition even when concealed. Hot surfaces in vehicles, such as brake rotors, exhaust manifolds, and catalytic converters, have the potential to ignite fuels by both radiant and conducted heat.

Radiant heat is also linked to the ignition of wood even when the heat flux is not enough to create ignition temperatures directly. In installations of heaters, furnaces, boilers, and even chimneys and vent flues, radiant heat at low levels may induce degradation of the wood to charcoal. Charring of wood can occur when temperatures on the order of 105°C (230°F) or greater are maintained for very long periods of time.

4.3.5 CHEMICAL REACTION

A number of chemical mixtures are capable of great heat generation and even formation of flame. They are only of occasional consequence in ordinary investigation of fires. Some accidental fires in warehouse-style home-supply stores have been linked to leaks or spills of corrosives (acids or bases) that came into contact with metals, or strong oxidizers (swimming pool chlorines) that came into contact with fuels such as automobile brake fluids and underwent an exothermic reaction. They play a role in a limited number of incendiary fires because of the lack of knowledge about them on the part of the arsonists. These reactions are more likely to be encountered in industrial or clandestine drug lab fires than elsewhere, and they require the attention of the chemical specialist.

Drying oils, decomposing cellulosic and organic materials causing biochemical reactions can generate as well as heat and can contribute to ignition. Salvage and recycling operations may produce mixtures of chemicals that spontaneously combust on contact, producing dangerous, large fires (Hall, Wanko, and Nikityn 2008, 68–73). Many chemical fires are due to ignition or decomposition of hazardous chemicals, some of which may be related to hypergolic reactions. In these cases, a highly exothermic redox reaction between two substances can occur spontaneously at ambient temperatures. In sealed containers, these hypergolic reactions can cause combustion, deflagration, or explosions (Buccola 2011).

4.4 Utility Services and Appliances as Ignition Sources

As many fires are either started by or attributed to utility **services** or appliances, consideration of these as possible ignition sources is important. When the origin of a fire is not determined, it is easy to conclude that some malfunction of an appliance or a **short circuit** in electrical wiring caused the fire. A short circuit is "an abnormal connection of low resistance between normal circuit conductors where the resistance is normally much greater; this is an overcurrent situation but it is not an overload" (NFPA 2014b, pt. 3.3.167). This conclusion is especially convenient because, in many fires, there is so much damage to wiring, or melting of appliances.

In modern building construction, electrical wiring is widely distributed as an integral part of nearly all parts of the structure, and gas lines and appliances are also very common. In structures, it is the rare fire that does not engulf such items to some extent at least, thus possibly focusing attention on them.

The investigator must remember that the mere presence of an electrical wire or a gas line does not constitute proof of responsibility for igniting a fire. If an electrical wire is not energized (that is, no voltage applied to it), it cannot provide energy to ignite any fuel. Even if it is energized, there has to be a mechanism, a reason, for it to create heat in an unintended manner. It is the investigator's responsibility to establish this mechanism and demonstrate how it can create enough heat to ignite the first fuel. Gas lines, even when charged or pressurized with gas, do not constitute an ignition source (except under the most exceptional circumstances when they can conduct misdirected electrical energy) but are merely a source of fuel.

4.4.1 GAS APPLIANCES AS IGNITION SOURCES

Gas appliances used for nonindustrial purposes include stoves, ranges, room heaters, furnaces, clothes dryers, and water heaters. All of these appliances have open flame burners that create heat. Thus, regardless of the exact type of heating device, the investigations, as well as all the possible hazards that attend the use of the device, are similar. The investigator needs to consider the heat output rating of the appliance, whether the flame was correctly adjusted, how the flame could come into contact with combustibles, and whether the automatic control mechanisms were functioning.

One of the few ways in which the gas furnace or dryer in normal operation is likely to initiate a fire is the simultaneous failure of the thermostat and the high-level or "high limit" control. The high-level device is a second thermostat or **thermal cutoff** (TCO) located in the circulating-air ducting of a furnace. It is usually coupled in series with the regular thermostat and is adjusted to break the circuit (and close a valve on the gas delivery line) at a maximum temperature above which the furnace cannot be safely operated. This temperature varies but is usually above 90°C (200°F). A simultaneous failure of both thermostats allows the furnace to continue operating indefinitely with the production of heat and possibly a resulting fire.

The failure of pressure regulators can cause an appliance to become an ignition source. Although these regulators may or may not be part of the appliance, their failure can cause masses of flame to escape from the burner compartment of the stove, furnace, or water heater affected. These flames can then ignite nearby combustibles by radiant heat or by direct flame impingement. Even under normal operation, the burners create considerable heat. Some appliances may not have adequate standoff or may be installed improperly, thereby exposing combustible walls or floors to radiant or conducted heat, as illustrated in Figures 4-3A–B and 4-4. Inadequate air supplies can result in excessive soot formation in the combustion chamber that can then induce smoldering ignition of nearby combustible surfaces.

thermal cutoff ■ An electrical safety device that interrupts electric current when exposed to heat at a specific temperature.

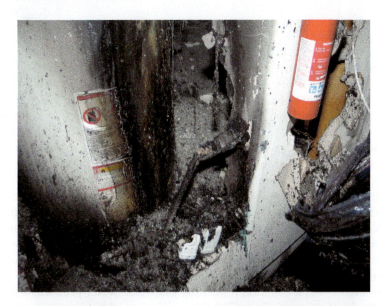

FIGURE 4-3A Fire in water heater closet as found (unit less than 1 year old). *Courtesy of Battalion Chief Kurt Hubele, Richland, (WA) FD.*

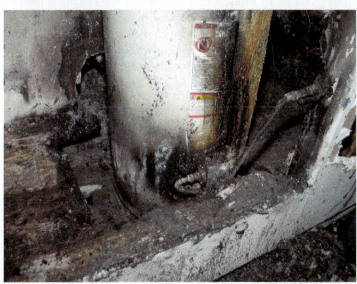

FIGURE 4-3B After cleanup—no floor left in closet. *Courtesy of Battalion Chief Kurt Hubele, Richland, (WA) FD.*

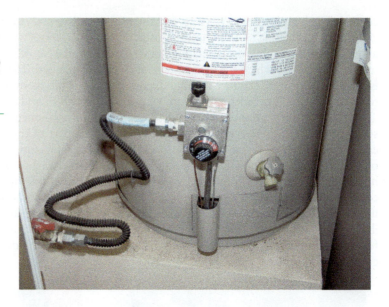

FIGURE 4-4 Exemplar heater in next apartment showed heater installed on plywood floor with no stand-off legs. *Courtesy of Battalion Chief Kurt Hubele, Richland (WA) FD.*

The standing pilot flame once standard on gas water heaters, furnaces, ranges, and ovens that offered a small but continuous and potentially competent ignition source, has largely been replaced by electric igniters. These igniters may be in the form of a high-voltage arc, an electric spark created by capacitive discharge or piezoelectric effect, or a glow bar (electrically heated hot surface). The investigator should examine all gas appliances carefully before concluding their status as an ignition source (Sanderson 2005a, 6).

Although gas appliances do start fires, they are probably less often the cause of a fire than generally assumed. Gas is the chief fuel in many places, and its intrinsic hazards tend to encourage an abnormal fear of it as a source of fire. Gas can serve as a convenient probable cause when the inexperienced investigator finds no other provable cause. Occasionally, gas is released as a result of a failure within the electrical system of the appliance and then ignited as it is released (Goodson, Sneed, and Keller 1999). The investigation of any fire involving fuel gases should include examination and documentation of the condition of the fuel supply, the ventilation available to the flame, electrical control system(s), and the system for removal of products of combustion (vents, flues, and chimneys).

As diagrammed in Figure 4-5, a common residential gas water heater produces a fire of 24,000 to 36,000 Btu/hr (6.66 to 10 Btu/s, 7 to 10.5 kW). A steel baffle is inserted in the central flue to slow the exhaust gases and give them more time to transfer heat to the water. There is typically a draft hood at the top of the heater to entrain room air into the exhaust gases and cool them. The vent is usually single-walled metal except where it passes through walls or ceilings, where it is at least double-walled. The flue-gas temperature at the top of the tank for steady-state operation of a 30,000 Btu/hr residential water heater is on the order of 300°C to 315°C (569°F to 601°F) with the baffle in place. If the baffle is left out, the gas temperature rises to 565°C (1050°F). The draft hood allows entrainment of room air, reducing the gas temperature in the flue (with baffle) to around 200°C to 250°C (400°F to 450°F) (Dwyer 2000).

On-Demand Heaters

Energy conservation issues are prompting the installation of on-demand, or tankless, water heaters instead of traditional 30- to 50-gal reservoir units. These units can be gas or electrically fueled. They are typically wall-mounted metal boxes approximately 0.9 m (36 in.) high, 0.5 m (20 in.) wide, and 0.3 m (12 in.) deep that may be concealed in closets or service areas. They provide hot water only when they sense water flow. A gas-fueled burner provides 120,000 to 200,000 Btu/hr (31 to 57 kW) of heat to heat 4 to 8 gal of water per minute. Due to their very high heat outputs, on-demand units have to be properly installed

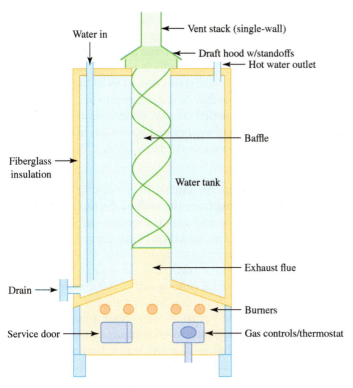

Water in

Vent stack (single-wall)

Draft hood w/standoffs

Hot water outlet

Baffle

Fiberglass insulation

Water tank

Exhaust flue

Drain

Burners

Service door

Gas controls/thermostat

Typical Temperatures during Normal (Steady-State) Operation

Center of flue (top of tank)
    With baffle 300°C–315°C (569°F–600°F)
    Without baffle 565°C (1,050°F)
Exterior of vent connector 73°C (164°F)
Top of 4-ft vent stack (gas temp.) 183°C–205°C
    (362°F–400°F)
    Without baffle 400°C (750°F)
Water 60°C–80°C (140°F–175°F)
Top exterior of tank 36°C (96°F)
Underside of front 63°C (145°F)

FIGURE 4-5 Cross section of typical residential gas water heater and some typical temperatures developed. *Some data courtesy* Fire Findings. *Additional data from tests by author (unpublished).*

and vented. Most gas units have external electrical connections for their ignition and control devices (Sanderson and Schudel 1998).

Fire Cause Considerations

The fire pattern will usually indicate if a gas appliance started the fire. The pattern reveals the origin to be behind, around, or over the gas appliance. Only a combination of factors including malfunction, improper installation, or other detectable fault or defect can be considered as proof of origin from a gas appliance. The arsonist often will set the fire under or close to a gas appliance to make it appear that the appliance was responsible for the fire. Liquid flammables may have been poured around the appliance so that the origin of the fire seems to be associated with the appliance. An incorrect assessment can result without careful scene examination. Ignitable liquids may have penetrated below the appliance, and possibly below the floor, and produced the characteristic charring and damage in regions a gas fire could not reach. Natural gas fires are unlikely to burn much below their point of release, because the fuel is significantly lighter than the surrounding air. Fuel oil and the vapors from flammable liquids will settle downward. Propane released under pressure (i.e., from a delivery line or as a jet) mixes with air sufficiently that it will neither rise nor settle.

People often store flammable liquids in furnace or water heater closets. Leaks or spills from stored containers create vapors that are quickly drawn into the combustion chamber of the appliance by the convection of either the pilot flame or the main burner. If there is sufficient vapor mixed with the air, an explosion, usually followed by sustained fire of the liquid, will result.

Recent changes in water heater design have been aimed at reducing the chances of ignition of flammable liquid vapors (called FVIR—flammable vapor ignition resistant—designs). For many years, building codes have required gas water heaters to be at least 18 in. (45.7 cm) above floor level if they are placed in a garage where accidental releases of flammable liquids are likely. Testing has revealed that unless flammable liquid is poured near the heater and the room tightly sealed (to prevent losses by advective flow under doors), this elevation precaution will prevent ignition. One design places a standard water heater into a steel bucket (or "weir") with sides 18 inches high in order to prevent the ignition of spilled flammable liquids. Testing has revealed this design to be highly efficient in preventing ignitions (Hoffman et al. 2003). Another new design employs a flash suppressor screen on the combustion chamber and sealed service, electrical, and plumbing entry ports. This design will prevent any ignition of vapors or fugitive gas starting in the combustion chamber from propagating into the room (Sanderson 2004, 1–4).

Insulation

Some type of insulation surrounds all approved gas appliances. In circulating heaters, this insulation consists merely of an outer wall separated from the wall of the firebox, through which circulates the cool air that is to be heated. The wall will not become significantly hotter than the ambient air that circulates behind it if air circulation is maintained both within the heat exchanger and outside the appliance. Presence of combustible trash against an appliance wall will not normally lead to ignition of the trash. But the wall of the combustion chamber may still be hot enough to ignite material coming into direct contact with it.

Shifting or even partial collapse of air-space insulation may create hot spots on the exterior, as will settling of packed insulation. These hot spots then create a higher ignition risk. Improper clearances between vent stacks (flues) and wood framing can result in ignition. The absence of the draft hood or central baffle in a gas water heater will cause higher-than-design (normal) gas temperatures on the outside of the vent, which can trigger degradation and ignition of nearby wood.

Backfire or Rollout

The claim that there has been a backfire from a furnace or other heating appliance carries more credibility than an ignition of combustibles against the heater. Nevertheless, a backfire is an extremely rare happening that can result only from improper use of or malfunction within the appliance. For a backfire to occur, a quantity of gas needs to accumulate in the combustion chamber before it is ignited. Accumulation can occur as a result of overpressure in the delivery system, use of the wrong fuel delivery orifice, or blockage of the heat exchanger or exhaust vent (Bertoni 1996). On ignition, a small explosion occurs and flames may blow out of the open front of the appliance. If there is a suitable combustible fuel in the path of this small amount of flame, a fire could result. The combination of factors is so unlikely, however, that this type of claim must be very carefully scrutinized before being accepted.

With a pilot light, accumulation of sufficient gas for a significant backfire is unlikely. In the absence of a pilot light, the gas will not ignite until it diffuses or spreads to some other source of ignition, which in all probability will require enough gas to produce an explosion. In addition, escaped natural gas will often pass harmlessly up the vent pipe into a chimney.

Electric ignition systems on gas furnaces, stoves, and water heaters are replacing continuous ignition sources—the pilot light—with an intermittent source that does not function until demanded. This system could allow for the buildup of a volume of gas/air mixture with explosive potential instead of providing a continuous ignition source to burn off small quantities as they reach their lower flammable limit.

With a fuel oil–fired furnace, the motor-driven pump can produce a sustained fire outside the furnace housing if the exhaust or heat exchanger is blocked. The failure of a fuel gas pressure regulator (either in the appliance or external in the delivery system) can cause continuous massive overfueling that results in the exit of burner flames via appliance service doors or vent openings (**rollout**).

rollout ▪ Exiting of burner flames in an appliance due to massive overfueling.

Direct Contact

Another manner in which a gas appliance can start a fire involves direct contact of a normal gas flame with flammable or combustible material. In general, this will occur only with open flames (e.g., gas range tops or broilers), although flammable materials can sometimes be drawn into a protected flame. The electric elements of stoves or broilers can also ignite solid fuels that come into direct contact with them, or the contents of skillets or pans.

Plugged Vent

Dwyer (2006) reported that if the vent of a gas water heater or furnace is plugged, the lack of a chimney can induce sufficient back pressure that the flames are forced out of the burner enclosure, possibly into contact with nearby combustibles. Examination of these devices should include careful examination of the exhaust duct for the remains of bird nests, dead leaves, construction debris, and the like. Blockage of the vent stack alone should cause the hot gases to vent from the draft hood if it is properly installed. The investigator should also check to see that the lower flame shield under the burner has not been removed and that the service doors are in their proper locations. Careless owners often neglect to replace the service doors after igniting the pilot light and should be interviewed to determine the last time the equipment was serviced or lighted.

Open Flames

Open flames—most common on kitchen ranges, laboratory and industrial burners, and special types of heating appliances—are hazardous as sources of fire. A common example is the ignition of cooking oils and greases in the kitchen, as well as towels, clothing, curtains, or paper, near open flames. Fires started by stoves and ovens are the leading cause of residential fires (Nicholson 2006). Autoignition temperatures of lard or vegetable cooking oils are quite high [over 350°C (662°F)], but enough boiling and splattering oils can splash onto the burner below to cause **piloted ignition** at lower temperatures.

Skillet fires can be very large. Grease ignitions are especially common as a cause of fires in restaurants, where there is a lot of cooking, but not enough time is spent cleaning stove hoods. These fires may spread upward in grease-coated exhaust ducts, where fans and vents carry the fire up with increasing magnitude. Most building codes require automatic fire protection of the cooking area and lower hood. This configuration can do little if the flame is established in the exhaust ducting above the hood. The ignition temperatures and flash points of cooking oils are listed in Table 4-2. The fire points are well above the normal cooking oil maximum temperature of 205°C (400°F) (Babrauskas 2003). Note in Table 4-2 that the fire point, AIT, and hot-surface ignition temperatures of all cooking oils decrease with use.

piloted ignition temperature ■ Minimum temperature that a substance should attain in order to ignite under specific test conditions (NFPA 2017b, pt. 3.3.139. See also pt. 3.3.114, Ignition Temperature).

TABLE 4-2	Properties of Cooking Fats Measured at Fire Research Station							

FAT	FLASH POINT (°C)		FIRE POINT (°C)		AIT (°C)		HOT-SURFACE IGNITION TEMP. (°C)	
	VIRGIN	AFTER 8 HEATING CYCLES	VIRGIN	AFTER 8 HEATING CYCLES	VIRGIN	AFTER 8 HEATING CYCLES	VIRGIN	AFTER 8 HEATING CYCLES
Corn oil	254	227	NA	321	309	283	526	542
Drippings (bacon)	254	241	NA	331	348	276	553	537
Hydrogenated cooking fat	260	210	NA	331	355	273	568	554
Lard	249	218	NA	326	355	282	541	568
Olive oil	234	218	NA	316	340	280	562	543
Peanut oil	260	243	347	335	342	280	552	535

From *Ignition Handbook* by V. Babrauskas, © 2003, p. 886, Fire Science Publishers. Used by permission.

Small gas appliances that are not part of a permanent installation can be displaced or upset, with occasional drastic results. Laboratory burners are especially subject to being tipped over. They can start fires by playing the flame on top of a wooden table or against some other combustible material. Similar considerations may be true for small portable gas heaters sometimes used in homes and similar areas. These heaters may be permanently installed or temporary and may not meet any standard of safety or building codes.

The investigator is referred to *NFPA 54: National Fuel Gas Code* (NFPA 2015) or *NFPA 58: Liquefied Petroleum Gas Code* (NFPA 2017a), which give detailed instructions for the proper installation and operation of all types of gas-burning appliances. *Fire Findings* reported the air venting from a 60,000 Btu/hr (17 kW) kerosene-fueled salamander portable heater had a temperature of 639°C (1182°F). Due to turbulent mixing, the temperature of the maximum hot-air stream dropped to 238°C (460°F) at 0.3 m (1 ft) and 148°C (298°F) at 0.6 m (2 ft) from the heater (Sanderson 2005b).

Altered Gas Nozzle

An unlikely, but possible, type of fire causation from a gas appliance involves tampering with or altering the gas nozzle in the venturi, possibly by partial or total unscrewing of the nozzle or installation of the incorrect fuel nozzle. If this happens, much larger than normal quantities of gas would reach the flame, which, in turn, might grow and spill from the top or front of the appliance. These fires would occur at the first use of the appliance after the opening was enlarged, which should again make their detection and proof of cause relatively simple. The service and repair history of the appliance may reveal recent problems or repairs. The venturi used must match the fuel gas and pressure regulator being used. Often, X-rays will reveal internal failures, blockages, or the open/closed position of fire-damaged valves and regulators.

4.4.2 PORTABLE ELECTRIC APPLIANCES

Electricity represents a source of ignition in the form of arcs, electrically heated wires, and heating elements, and even lightning. Heat-producing electric appliances can cause ignition of susceptible fuels even when operating normally. Electric heaters, toasters, or toaster ovens with exposed Nichrome (resistance) heater wires offer an ignition source with surface temperatures on the order of 600°C (1150°F) or greater. These hot surfaces are not able to ignite most flammable gases or vapors but can ignite most cellulosics (including foods) if they come into contact or near contact with them (see Figure 4-6).

Heater elements in clothes dryers are especially susceptible to such contact. Dryer lint, usually a mixture of fine cellulosic, synthetic, and natural fibers (wool and hair), is one of the most readily ignitable solids. Accumulations of lint on heater grids or on adjacent surfaces of venting both inside the dryer and out are one of the most common first fuels in dryer fires.

The radiant heat produced by most portable electric heaters is approximately 10 kW/m² or less at the wire guard. This may be enough to ignite cellulosics or char elastomeric and thermosetting materials if contact is prolonged. Cellulosic fuels that are brought into contact with the heater element itself are likely to be ignited quickly. Today, most consumer-type portable electric heaters have tilt switches to shut power off if the unit is knocked over, in addition to thermostats and TCOs. Investigators must carefully examine heaters to determine what, if any, safety devices are present and if they have failed or been tampered with.

4.4.3 KEROSENE HEATERS

The fuel in kerosene heaters may be delivered to a constant flame by vertical transport up a wick that is partially inserted in a fuel reservoir, in the same way as in a kerosene lamp. A more effective means of fuel delivery is a barometric delivery system in which the fuel is delivered to a shallow horizontal reservoir from a vertically oriented removable tank. The

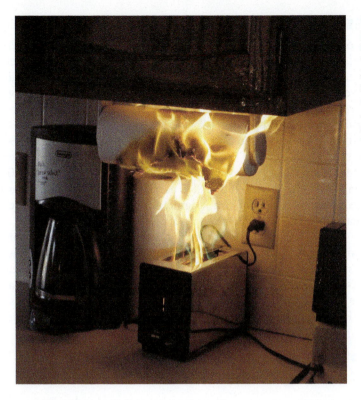

FIGURE 4-6 Toaster pastries ignited by repeated operation of a toaster cause flames 30 cm (~12 in.) high, sufficient to ignite nearby combustibles. *Courtesy of Jamie Novak, Novak Investigations and St. Paul Fire Dept.*

flow of fuel is controlled by a barometric valve in the tank. A partial vacuum above the fuel in the tank prevents the fuel from flowing into the reservoir until the level drops below that preset by the valve.

Modern heaters have a shutoff mechanism that extinguishes the wick if the heater is tipped over or subjected to excessive vibration. The main safety problem with kerosene heaters is that the capacity of the tank exceeds that of the reservoir, so that if there is a loss of the vacuum in the tank, the excess fuel can flood the reservoir and create a spill external to the heater, which then ignites with catastrophic results (Lentini 1990). This loss of vacuum can occur as the result of a leak in the tank or its associated parts, or as the result of fueling the heater with a fuel like gasoline or camping fuel with a higher vapor pressure than that of kerosene. In these cases, the vapor then replaces the partial vacuum that holds back the flow of fuel, resulting in a flood of fuel that overwhelms the reservoir.

Although a newer anti-flare-up device is available, most older heaters encountered pose a serious fire risk from this type of failure (Henderson and Lightsey 1994). Accidental spills during refilling can cause significant fires, especially if the burner is not extinguished. Any residual fuel left in a heater should be collected and preserved for testing to establish its actual content.

4.4.4 STOVES AND HEATERS

A variety of liquid fuel portable heaters are made for camping and boating use. These range from pressurized fuel delivery systems (Primus stoves) to denatured alcohol fuel burning on the surface of a noncombustible wick element. These heaters are subject to spillage of burning fuel if tilted or overturned. Although these heaters are not intended for use in enclosed spaces, they are often found in tents and campers. Because these heaters may consist of a small circular burner pan and a perforated metal shield over it, the investigator may not identify them as ignition sources.

4.4.5 OIL STORAGE

External heating (fuel) oil storage tanks are common in both residential and commercial premises. Traditionally, these are welded steel tanks with rigid metal pipe connections. Those features, combined with the low vapor pressure (high flash point) of typical heating fuels, mean they do not constitute a high risk of ignition (either accidental or intentional). However, when fuels are absorbed on porous materials that can act as a wick, their low ignition temperatures [~205°C (400°F)] pose a risk.

If plumbing connections are exposed to an external fire, they can fail quickly. Some jurisdictions allow fuel storage tanks to be made of high-density polyethylene (owing to their corrosion resistance and lower costs). Testing has shown that tanks in 300- to 400-gal sizes can be caused to fail by external fires. If 5 L (1.5 gal) of gasoline is poured over the outside, or a modest cardboard/newspaper fire is ignited underneath the tank, a catastrophic failure and release of the tank contents can result.

Placement of a cloth wick into the mouth of the tank also causes failure, since it continues to burn within the tank (due to the low vapor pressure) until the tank melts. The melted plastic of the tank can support a large pool fire of molten polyethylene, so that even an empty tank poses a fire risk (McAuley 2003). Oil-fueled furnaces can cause fires by creating heavy soot if burners are maladjusted, or more commonly, leaks from fuel connections can support flames outside the combustion chamber, which then ignite nearby combustibles.

4.5 The Role of Hot and Burning Fragments in Igniting Fires

Hot or burning particles, or sparks, are a special category with regard to kindling of fires. As pointed out earlier in the chapter, the designation spark is an ambiguous one, because it can refer to incandescently hot metal from a mechanical or electrical source or to hot bits of debris from an established fire. Most fragments from an established fire are glowing, although at times they may be flaming. Bits of wood, paper, and other light organic fuels are susceptible to the formation of glowing fragments, and larger pieces of paper may travel while still flaming. Bits of paper or tobacco may become detached during lighting of a cigarette or pipe. These particles can ignite other fuels with which they come in contact if they retain enough heat. Most fragments will be carried upward by the draft from the fire that generates them, and air currents may carry them for significant distances to ignite other fuel.

4.5.1 WINDBLOWN SPARKS

The question frequently arises: How far can windblown sparks travel and still cause a secondary fire? Although no precise answer is possible, several factors can be identified. The ambient wind is important as sparks tend only to rise with the buoyant flow over the fire, drift a short distance, and fall nearby, unless propelled by wind.

Another factor is the type and weight of material that is burning. Very small fragments and thin materials like paper will normally be totally consumed before they return to some combustible surface. Fragments of wood, excelsior, or corrugated cardboard will burn considerably longer and travel farther before igniting something else. Tests by DeHaan demonstrated that burning wood chips and straw could be carried up to 15 m (50 ft) from their source in a 32-km/hr (20-mph) wind to ignite cloth, straw, and wood shavings targets (DeHaan et al. 2001). Light items will rarely travel as much as 6 m (20 ft), except under significant wind conditions.

Another factor is the height that fragments reach before being blown to one side. The higher they go, the more time they have to burn up totally or to cool off, and the longer their exposure to any air movement. Documentation of the intensity and direction of wind at the time of the fire is critical to the evaluation of mechanisms. Distances in excess of 9 to 12 m (30 to 40 ft) are to be accepted only with the greatest caution.

Throughout this discussion of spark travel, the role of wind has repeatedly been referred to as modifying the fire spread. No investigation involving the distance or effectiveness of spark ignition is complete without ascertaining from meteorological records, or at least from eyewitnesses, the wind conditions at the time in question. It is evident that violent winds will produce very different effects from mild ones.

A strong wind will blow a spark farther than a weak wind but will also speed the rate of combustion. With a given size of burning fragment, the wind effect does not vary greatly with different wind velocities. The most significant effect of the strong wind is its ability to blow large fragments of material, which will naturally burn longer than small ones.

A wad of burning newspaper on the ground will not ordinarily travel along the ground for any significant distance if propelled only by a breeze. In a strong wind, however, it may roll for a considerable distance before it is consumed. The relation of importance is the time necessary for it to burn as compared with the speed with which it is moving laterally with the wind.

The consideration should be given to materials at ground level than to those that emerge from chimneys, because very large burning objects are rarely carried up a chimney to any significant height. In very large fires, however, the updraft can loft large pieces of burning debris, boards, branches, cardboard, and rags high enough that they can be carried hundreds of yards by the prevailing wind, igniting remote fires. This has been observed to be a major means of fire spread in large fires in both urban and wildland settings, as depicted in Figures 4-7A and B.

In one recent major conflagration, burning wood fire brands (some as large as 2 × 4s) were lofted some 60 m (200 ft) above a multistory condo/retail complex under construction and were blown more than 680 m (0.4 mi) to ignite wooden shake-shingle roofs of two apartment complexes (see Figure 4-7A). At the time, the winds were 2 to 27 km/hr (13 to 17 mph) (USFA 2004). See Figure 4-7B for an illustrative map.

There are several common origins for hot fragments, and because these are the primary source of the fire that may result, they will be considered individually.

4.5.2 FIREPLACES AND CHIMNEYS

Fireplaces are blamed for igniting many fires. Nevertheless, the mere fact that a possible fire origin is close to a fireplace is not a definitive indication that the fire was initiated by the fireplace. The condition of any chimney spark arrestor should also be documented.

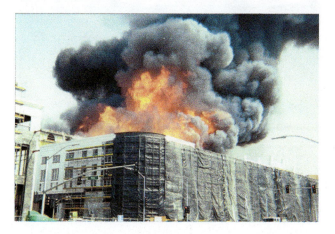

FIGURE 4-7A Massive fire engulfing six-story residential/commercial complex (wood framed). *Courtesy of Kyle Binkowski, Fire Cause Analysis.*

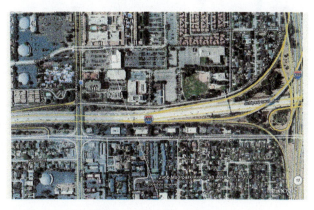

FIGURE 4-7B Map showing trajectory of burning brands 0.7 km (0.4 mi) from a fire scene to ignite the roof of an apartment complex 0.8 km (0.4 mi) away. © 2009 Google—Map data—© Tele Atlas

Emission of Sparks or Blazing Materials from the Front or Open Portion

Sparks or blazing materials may ignite nearby combustible floor coverings or furnishings, but these fires are rare because the top of a wooden floor is very difficult to ignite to a sustained combustion. Scorch marks are not uncommon and are annoying, but wood floors do not usually represent the first fuel ignited. Light fuels like paper may readily be ignited, so pre-fire actions and conditions may be critical. Some rugs or carpets are sufficiently flammable to be ignited under these circumstances, and furniture may occasionally be ignited. Most building codes require a noncombustible hearth extending well to the front and sides of a fireplace opening. Burning fragments of Christmas wrappings apparently ignited a large pile of crumpled wrappings in front of the fireplace in the fire shown in Figures 4-8 and 4-9. Thus, there is a hazard from this source, but it is readily interpreted when encountered (when pre-fire activities are described).

Intense Radiant Heat from a Fireplace Stove Filled with Inappropriate Fuels or Overfueled

Sufficient radiant heat can be generated by intense fires in the firebox to create heat fluxes of 10 to 20 kW/m^2 through the front opening. These can ignite ordinary combustibles in line of sight of the opening if they are within 1 m (3 ft). Inappropriate fuels include crumpled masses of paper, Christmas tree branches, plastics, foams, cardboard boxes, and similar commodities. Some fuels are intended for fireplace use (e.g., compressed-sawdust artificial logs), but may cause overheating if overfueled. The manufacturer of artificial logs typically includes package instructions requiring that not more than one log be put on the fire at a time. Overheating of the firebox is also liable to cause ignition of wood materials located behind the fireplace or inside the wall.

Emission of Sparks or Blazing Materials from a Chimney

Chimney fires occur because soot, bird or rodent nests, creosote, dust, cobwebs, and a variety of combustible materials accumulate in the chimney, where they may be ignited by a spark or flame from the fire below and lead to a large blaze within the chimney itself. When this happens, large quantities of burning fragments will be expelled from the chimney top and increase the danger of igniting a roof or other adjacent combustible structure. The blazing residues (firebrands) or large glowing sparks (embers) of roof fires may travel and ignite larger fires elsewhere.

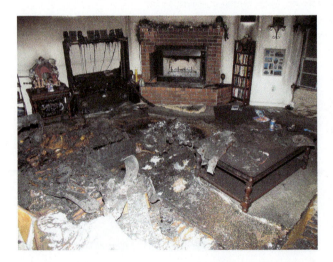

FIGURE 4-8 Living room furniture burned when fragments of burning Christmas wrappings escaped from a fireplace to ignite a pile of wrappings on the floor. *Courtesy of Derrick Fire Investigations.*

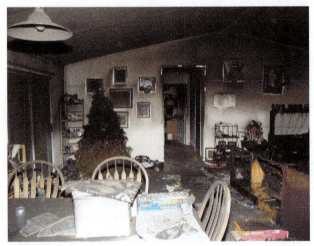

FIGURE 4-9 Heat and smoke layer enveloped the top of this Christmas tree but only scorched it (oxygen-deprived smoke layer). *Courtesy of Derrick Fire Investigations.*

The effect of wind on chimney action is also relevant. Wind blowing across a chimney opening exerts what is known as the *Bernoulli effect*, that is, a lowering of the pressure at the chimney mouth. The result is a stronger draft up the chimney, which can increase the size of fragment that can move upward and be ejected into the stronger wind stream. This is an additional reason for the investigator to consider wind velocity when there is a possibility that spark movement started a fire.

Emission of Sparks or Blazing Materials Resulting from Defects or Holes in a Chimney

Although rare, possibly serious fires can be caused by sparks igniting timber or other construction material adjacent to the chimney. Few chimneys become so defective by use or abuse as to pose any real danger of leaking sparks or burning materials through their walls. However, defects can result from anything that causes serious deterioration of the house, as the earth settling or slippage, earthquakes, or extreme age and decrepitude. Some manufactured chimneys can separate at their joints due to corrosion or mechanical failure. A chimney fire may damage the chimney lining, so that gaps develop that allow hot gases to escape the flue and begin to char wooden structures. If there is another chimney fire, gaps may permit flames and sparks to contact combustible framing directly. Because of the characteristic pattern and behavior of a roof fire, the cause of the fire will not be difficult to determine. The recent history of use should be established by interviews with the occupants.

Overheating of Combustible Materials near or in Contact with a Fireplace or Chimney

Overheating of combustible materials by radiant heat from or direct contact with the hot surfaces of fireplaces or chimneys is probably less important in fires involving stone or masonry fireplaces than in those with metal ones. Fires in the immediate vicinity of chimneys are not uncommon, and many people attribute them automatically to overheating of wood structural elements.

The insulative capacity of intact stone or brick is such that these chimneys rarely transmit enough heat to damage the structure. Metal chimneys and fireboxes are more common today. Loose insulation between the double walls of metal fireplaces can settle, allowing spaces with minimal insulation capacity. The outer walls can then reach temperatures in excess of what they should, and these may be dangerously close to combustibles.

Chimney enclosures today are often of wood construction. They are supposed to be lined with drywall, but this lining is not always installed. Manufacturers of metal fireplaces provide detailed installation instructions, and if violated by the installer, a fire may occur. Violations include disregarding required clearance from combustibles, using the wrong fluepipes, blocking of required air-circulation openings, or altering the manufactured unit.

The often-specified triple-wall flue pipes depend on proper flow of cooling air through the annular segments. Improper installation can block the flow of cooling air. Occasionally a tradesperson may simplify the installation of a fireplace by removing protuberant standoffs designed to enforce a certain distance of clearance. The term *zero clearance* is an inappropriate marketing catchphrase and should not be taken to mean that a unit can be installed in any relationship to combustibles that the installer might wish. Fireplaces lacking an Underwriters Laboratories (UL) (or equivalent) listing obviously may be presumed to be intrinsically defective and unsafe.

Circumstances of recent use may be valuable in establishing the actual cause of chimney-related fires. Unusually large or hot fires from burning a dry Christmas tree or sustained fireplace use may trigger ignition previously avoided by normal use.

Similar considerations apply to furnace and water heater flue pipes where they pass through openings in wooden structures. In these instances, there is usually a chimneylike insulator structure surrounding the actual chimney or vent. Any fire that starts from any

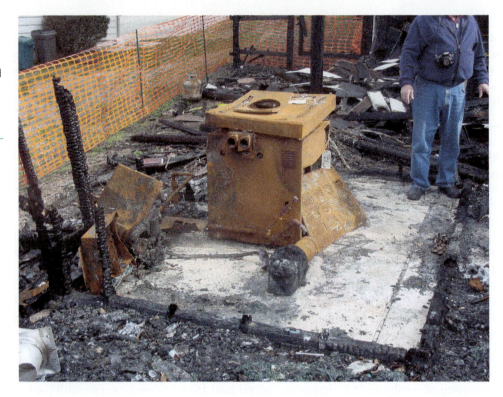

cause in the vicinity of a penetration will be drawn up it, often localizing the fire in the region around the suspected chimney or vent. Insulators or thimbles may be required around exhausts for heaters, stoves, and emergency generators. For this reason and others, a postulated origin of fire should be scrutinized carefully before it is accepted. Considerations of the properties of purported first fuels are relevant.

Changes in equipment such as the installation of high-efficiency heaters or fireboxes (fireplace inserts) can change the airflow of an old chimney or dramatically increase the surface temperatures of fireboxes and flues, thus creating problems where none existed before. These increases may be enough to overwhelm the designed insulation or induce more heating by conduction through brick or stone, resulting in degradation of wood structural members in contact.

Gaps can develop between the top front of the firebox and the facing brick or stone. Because the chimney and fireplace are not likely to be destroyed by the fire, evidence of gaps in its structure, added to the fire pattern, should reveal its contribution to starting the fire. Some units require that firebox side edges be tightly sealed with noncombustible material. A gap there can allow hot air emanating from the front of the unit to get sucked into the chase behind the fireplace, causing overheating of wood materials there. This is another possible source of fire.

Embers and "Hot Ashes" Removed from Fireplaces and Barbecues

Embers from fireplaces, campfires, and barbecues can cause delayed ignition fires remote from the fireplace, campfire, or grill. Due to low heat release rate (HRR) and slow combustion and the insulative properties of ashes and the charred wood, the embers are undetected when removed. Usually, the homeowner cleans out the ashes and places them in a combustible box, bag, or trash can, assuming they are out. Wood or charcoal embers, insulated by ashes, can continue to smolder for 3 to 4 days under the right conditions and can result in ignition after being removed (Bohn 2003).

4.5.3 LONG-TERM HEATING (LOW-TEMPERATURE IGNITION)

Wood, especially in massive form, requires a considerable amount of heat to cause its ignition. For flaming combustion, there must be enough heat flux to pyrolyze volatiles from the wood and ignite those vapors. Temperatures around proper flues and chimneys in good repair are not expected to reach the 250°C (482°F) minimum ignition temperatures for fresh wood. However, it has been reported that exposure to much lower temperatures (below 105°C or 221°F) causes degradation of wood to charcoal (Schwartz 1996; Cuzzillo and Pagni 1999b). This charcoal, also erroneously called pyrophoric carbon, is sometimes found in wood around heat sources like furnaces and chimneys. Although the term **pyrophoric** is technically misapplied here because it refers to materials that ignite spontaneously in air at moderate temperatures 54°C (130°F) or below, it is widely used in fire investigation in discussing wood that appears to ignite at temperatures far below its usual ignition temperatures.

pyrophoric material ■ Any substance that spontaneously ignites upon exposure to atmospheric oxygen (NFPA 2017b, pt. 3.3.151).

It is apparent to experienced fire investigators that fires have begun in confined spaces in wooden structural components where exposure to a source of some heat for long periods of time has caused far more charcoal to form than would be expected from the duration of the reported (or observed) fire.

Our review of fire cases that present the strongest argument for the formation of self-heating charcoal shows that the circumstances are often as Bowes predicted: a heat source near wood that is protected by a barrier of metal or tile or in a very confined area like a pipe or flue snugly fitted through a wooden beam for a long period of time, followed by structural collapse or other change that allows a sudden inrush of fresh air, can precipitate a flaming fire (Bowes 1984). Production of this charcoal is clearly a long-term phenomenon, often requiring many months, and more typically years, to reach combustible form and critical mass. Martin and Margot reported that temperatures as low as 105°C (221°F) were capable of degrading wood but that the lower the temperature, the longer the time required (Martin and Margot 1994).

The mechanism for this process is complex and has been the subject of some debate, especially concerning the applicability of a predictive thermodynamic technique called Frank-Kamenetskii after its creator (Drysdale 2011, 12–14). There are several important features of these processes that have to be recognized:

■ The conversion of fresh wood to a charred or cooked state can occur at low temperatures [well below 250°C (482°F) and possibly as low as 77°C (170°F)] over a long period of time.

■ Fresh wood when heated produces gases and vapors that will support flaming combustion but requires that significant heat be applied to effect this pyrolysis and then ignition, whereas charcoal has many fewer volatile components and supports only very limited flaming combustion but will readily support glowing combustion.

■ Fresh whole wood (i.e., sawed lumber) will not self-heat unless very hot, but charcoal will.

■ Fresh wood has a much higher permeability to air along its growth axis than across it.

■ Smoldering combustion can result from runaway self-heating.

■ A mass of fuel undergoing smoldering combustion can transition to open flame if ventilation causes a high enough heat release rate (either external, as from a draft of wind, or enhanced buoyant flow around or through the mass).

When all these factors are taken into consideration within the context of the previously described scenarios, we can see that there is a supportable hypothesis for these fires. First, heat is applied to a mass of wood that has, by its mass or covering, limited exposure to air (Cuzzillo and Pagni 1999a). The wood degrades to a cooked form with the gradual release of the volatile fuel vapors insufficient to support flames (with the characteristic flat, shrunken surfaces with sharp-edged segments). The charred, cooked wood has a high permeability to air enhanced by the multiple cracks into the wood produced by the cooking, a low thermal inertia, and an ability to self-heat, all very different from fresh wood. Continued application of heat to such a material can induce runaway self-heating, especially if air is admitted as the result of shrinkage or separation from sealing materials. This runaway self-heating is the critical step in the process.

At this point, there is ignition (self-sustained smoldering combustion), but it may not be recognized from outside the cavity or concealed space where it is taking place. If enough air is admitted and the enhanced ventilation causes a high enough heat release rate, the smoldering combustion can transition to flaming combustion (with the rapid involvement of adjacent intact wood structural members). The flaming stage is often detected as the "fire."

The conditions have to be nearly perfect—temperatures typically between about 100°C and 200°C (212°F and 392°F) with limited ventilation so that heat is not readily dispersed and oxygen is generally excluded, and there is an adequate mass of wood. There are extensive data on the relationship between fuel mass, environmental temperature, and time to develop runaway self-heating. These conditions are sometimes found in accidental fires investigated, but the investigator must be careful of blaming "pyrophoric carbon" for any fire in the vicinity of a flue or hot water pipe merely because no other cause can be identified. As Bowes pointed out:

- The temperatures of heating surfaces have to be at high temperatures [although nowhere as high (200°C; 400°F) as his calculations indicated];
- The wood has to have substantial mass (plywood floors are more likely to simply char through than to ignite);
- The temperature of the hot surface has to be high enough to maintain heat flux on the wood to overcome losses due to conduction or convection;
- The time has to be long enough (weeks, months, or years, depending on the intensity of the applied heat); and
- There has to be exclusion (or limited circulation) of air in the vicinity until just prior to detection of the fire (Bowes 1984).

One case involving all five of these elements was the result of a water heater that sat on a wooden platform protected by a steel sheet and an asbestos barrier. Some weeks after a new water heater was installed, the platform began to burn and the fire was detected. Figure 4-3 illustrates a similar case.

It should be remembered that smoldering combustion (in charcoal) requires very low oxygen concentrations and that fresh air, with its richer oxygen supply, is required to sustain open flames. Because of the time required for the production of charcoal, low-temperature ignition of wood can generally be eliminated as a cause of fires in very new buildings. Interestingly, Babrauskas, Gray, and Janssens reported that wood in contact with a surface with a temperature in excess of 77°C (170°F), even if periodic, should be considered a potential ignition scenario (Babrauskas, Gray, and Janssens 2007). Both Underwriters Laboratories (UL) and the Building Code of the City of New York (Section C26-1400.6) cite 170°F as the upper safe temperature for wood surfaces.

As with most other accidental ignition sources, careful investigation and evaluation must be carried out before concluding that low-temperature ignition or an overheated chimney is a cause. In addition to there being much more char than expected, if the wood timber is cross sectioned, the char should also gradually change from complete char, to partially pyrolyzed, to undamaged as one moves away from the purported heat source. Unfortunately, the processes involved and their interaction are complex, and currently there are no data showing an exact relationship between temperature of exposure and time to ignition.

4.5.4 TRASH BURNERS AND INCINERATORS

Fires started by trash burners will rarely require much investigation because of the obvious nature of the origin and the fact that the pattern will trace directly to the burner in most instances. The types of material normally destroyed by burning in trash burners are those most likely to form airborne burning fragments, and the openings in the incinerator to allow ventilation of the fire also allow escape of burning fragments.

Accidental fires, particularly of dry grass or brush in the area, are commonly associated with trash burners and incinerators. The strength and direction of the wind and the ignitability of possible first fuels including fuel moisture and nature of materials being burned are all important considerations.

4.5.5 BONFIRES

The bonfire poses a different problem than the trash burner, despite also being an exterior fire. To maintain a satisfactory bonfire, it is customary to use relatively massive wood instead of paper, packing, cardboard, and similar items of trash. The wood poses less hazard from rising fragments of burning material than does trash. However, unlike trash burners, there is no restraint or protection of the fire from winds. In a high wind, a bonfire becomes very dangerous and can start larger, uncontrolled fires.

If adjacent to dry grass or leaves, a bonfire is always hazardous. Here also, the investigation is likely to be rather simple. Sometimes, it is difficult to distinguish the remains of a small bonfire from those of a general fire that involved a concentration of fuel at a point that may leave excessive ash and charcoal, which appear similar to the remains of a bonfire. Careful examination will usually distinguish the two. In many instances the remains of bonfires contain, in addition to wood ash, the remains of food containers or other indications of human activity.

The direction of the prevailing wind and the contour of the land are critical to correctly determining fire origins. The considerations of ignition by airborne brands include type of fuel being burned, size of fragments that can escape, and size of the fire (creating the upward buoyancy). The larger the fragments and the more massive they are, the longer they can burn. Flat brands, such as fragments of cardboard or wood shingles, have better aerodynamics than needle or spherical shapes and can remain airborne much longer and travel farther.

4.5.6 HOT METALS

Metals occasionally can be a direct source of fires, but more often are a source of burning metal sparks from grinding or cutting operations or droplets of molten metals. Molten metal may carry enough heat to ignite susceptible fuels with which it comes in contact and is therefore capable of starting fires, as are burning fragments. Because a considerable amount of heat is required to melt the metal, dangers are usually associated only with special operations in metal fabrication. However, the dangers are often exaggerated, because many alloys, including types of solder, will not carry enough heat to ignite the fuel material on which they fall.

Molten ferrous alloys like steel are more dangerous than solders due to their higher melting temperatures and often higher thermal capacities. Thus, welding and cutting of steel with an arc or a torch in the presence of susceptible organic fuels is a very dangerous practice. See *NFPA 51B: Standard for Fire Prevention during Welding, Cutting, and Other Hot Work* (NFPA 2014a) for safety during those operations.

The state of subdivision of a solid fuel is critical in determining its susceptibility. It is, for example, almost impossible to ignite a large timber accidentally by the short, direct application of a torch flame or by the molten metal from it. In contrast, finely divided fuels (e.g., shredded packing materials, sawdust, shavings, or loose paper) may be ignited under the same conditions. Directing a flame into a narrow crack or split in a piece of wood, however, may cause ignition of both surfaces. The close spacing causes reduced losses and enhanced feedback, resulting in ignition.

Molten metal can also be produced by the fusion caused by the heat of a short circuit or failure of a component in electrical equipment. Although ejection of molten material from the equipment presents a hazard, the greatest danger may be from direct ignition by the short circuit itself, but only if a current protection device does not interrupt the current. Thus, the metal may be considered a secondary and less probable source of ignition.

In considering hot or molten metal fragments as sources of ignition, the investigator must keep in mind that most metals have a high density, and the hot fragment will fall rapidly, in contrast to bits of paper or wood, which tend to rise in the convective plume of the fire itself. Aluminum is of relatively low density. In flat form, such as a roof section, aluminum sheet may rise in a buoyant fire plume rather than fall, but this will not be true of solder, molten brass, iron, or copper. Aluminum, because of its low density, ease of oxidation, and low melting point, is very unlikely to play a role in spreading fire as airborne debris and is not a likely source of ignition. But, in the case of high-voltage power lines made from aluminum, globs of molten aluminum may land on dry vegetation and ignite wildland fires. Molten masses are generated when two power lines unexpectedly make contact, resulting in conductor clashing, because of extreme winds, failed insulators, failed supports, or excessively stretched conductors, for example.

Despite their higher melting temperature, copper particles are a less effective ignition source than are aluminum particles. Although metals can burn, most metals are extremely difficult to ignite except when very finely divided. Magnesium is the chief exception. Either alone or alloyed with aluminum, magnesium is more easily ignited.

Occasionally, massive metal pieces heated by torch cutting or welding operations can ignite ordinary combustibles they contact. This is more likely if the fuel is a char-forming material rather than a thermoplastic. This mechanism is extremely unlikely, however, if more than a few minutes have elapsed between the hot work and observed ignition (due to the high thermal conductivity of the metal). Investigation and thorough interviews will be needed to test hypotheses. Fire watches after hot-work operations are typically only 30 minutes long, but some smoldering ignitions from hot-work operations have been known to take hours, instead of minutes, to manifest in a flaming fire.

4.5.7 MECHANICAL SPARKS

Iron, steel, and some other metals will spark when a frictional contact rips a fragment of the ferrous alloy out with sufficient energy to heat it beyond its ignition temperature [on the order of 700°C to 800°C (1300°F to 1475°F)]. The particle ignites in the air and burns (at >1600°C; 2900°F), leaving a sometimes incandescent flake of carbon and iron oxide as an ash (Babrauskas 2003). These sparks are small but finite heat sources that can ignite some flammable vapors. If the ash flakes are hot enough and large enough to transfer sufficient heat to their surroundings, they can ignite readily combustible (finely divided) solid materials on which they fall. These fires happen along railroad tracks where mechanical sparks from overheated brake shoes can be dropped for many hundreds of yards.

Many grass and brush fires along railroads are ignited by particles emitted from diesel locomotive exhaust or eductor tubes. These particles, consisting of carbon, calcium oxide, and the oily residues of fuel and lubricant, are emitted along with the exhaust. Under some conditions of engine operation they are emitted while still burning and can ignite dry grass along the track or even several feet from it (Maxwell and Mohler 1973). Many states require spark arrestors on all engines operating in high fire-hazard areas, but they are sometimes overlooked or even intentionally eliminated during maintenance.

The cutting or grinding of iron or steel using a carborundum blade grinder can create sparks. Incandescent particles have been observed up to 5 m (15 ft) from a handheld grinder being used on a steel reinforcing bar. Such sparks reportedly have a starting temperature of 1600°C to 2130°C (2900°F to 3866°F) and an energy of 1 kJ. Impact of a steel tool on concrete (particularly quartz) or aluminum-coated or contaminated rusty steel can also create mechanical sparks capable of igniting flammable gases (Babrauskas 2003).

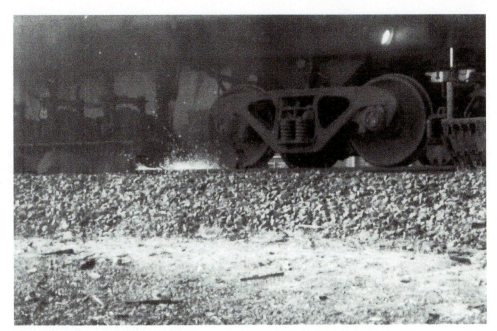

FIGURE 4-11 Sparks from this rail grinder were thought to be responsible for igniting a sawdust bin in a lumberyard. Typical water spraying would extinguish fires on the railroad right-of-way but would not necessarily affect hot sparks buried in sawdust adjacent to the track. *Courtesy of Joe and Chris Bloom, Bloom Fire Investigation, Grants Pass, OR.*

The rail-grinding equipment used on railroads creates large quantities of hot sparks that can be projected some distance from the track. Because this equipment, as shown in Figure 4-11, is not stationary, its operation is not controlled and may escape scrutiny.

The exhaust systems of off-road motorcycles and trucks are also liable to emit hot carbon particles occasionally. Some vehicles may be required to have spark arrestors before being permitted to operate in forest areas. Catalytic converters on vehicles have been known to decompose and to spew chunks of their ceramic matrix at very high temperatures into grass and brush.

4.5.8 FIREARMS RESIDUES

The burning residues of firearms ammunition occasionally ignite forest and grass fires, as well as structure fires. Although modern smokeless powder is almost completely consumed during the discharge of rifles and shotguns, some flakes escape while still burning from the muzzle of a short-barreled handgun. Although they are low in mass and thermal content, these flakes can ignite finely divided cotton and similar combustibles at very close range [less than 0.3 m (1 ft)].

Black powder, in contrast, produces large quantities of burning particles of powder and incandescent ash from both short- and long-barreled guns. Although generally limited to antique handguns, rifles, and cannons, the use of black powder for sporting purposes is undergoing a strong resurgence in popularity (Babrauskas 2005). Because residues from these weapons can ignite dry fuels like paper, cloth, wood shavings, and leaves, even at distances of up to 1.3 m (4 ft), the investigator must consider the possibility of accidental ignition in identifying the cause of exterior, and even some interior, fires.

4.5.9 EXPLODING AMMUNITION

Exploding ammunition, the projectile of which contains a percussion cap and a small powder charge, has been sold to the public and represents an occasional fire danger. Foreign armor-piercing rifle ammunition with a steel insert has been thought to be the cause of some wildland fires behind target ranges, because the steel is capable of striking mechanical sparks as it ricochets off bare rock.

Exploding paper targets employing a shock-sensitive explosive such as Tannerite, which is the brand name of a patented invention (Tanner 2005), have also been implicated in accidental wildland fires. Tannerite is an exploding firearms practice target that contains a binary explosive of ammonium nitrate and/or ammonium perchlorate (oxidizers) and aluminum powder, both combined together before use.

4.5.10 MILITARY AMMUNITION

Tracer and incendiary bullets, normally used only in military weapons, are more dangerous sources of ammunition fires. Tracer ammunition contains a mixture of strontium nitrate, magnesium powder, and an active oxidizer like calcium peroxide. Incendiary ammunition usually contains white phosphorus or a similar material with a low ignition temperature. Either type of ammunition is a fire hazard because of the high-temperature flames produced in the fired projectile. Both will initiate destructive fires in dry leaves, brush, or needles (duff). Ammunition has, on rare occasions, been used by arsonists to set remote fires that are inaccessible to fire crews.

Virtually all military ammunition is marked by characteristic color bands on each projectile, but some foreign military surplus ammunition brought into the United States has been cleaned and repackaged, precluding ready identification (Few 1978). Hunters buying recycled ammunition have inadvertently discharged these missiles during hunting and target practice, sometimes with serious consequences. With the characteristic paint removed, identification of incendiary projectiles requires x-ray or visual laboratory examination. Signaling or rescue flares, which are available for even small-caliber handguns, present the same sort of risk because they, too, contain pyrotechnic or incendiary mixtures that burn for up to 40 seconds. Some have a parachute to slow their descent, thereby prolonging burning time and making them subject to winds, while others are simply ballistic meteors (Powerboat Reports 1994).

4.6 Smoking as a Fire Origin

There is no question that the carelessness of smokers is the primary reason for the high incidence of both indoor and outdoor fires. However, theories about how smoking caused a fire can be totally inappropriate, and the alleged ignition would not have been successful under the circumstances.

Smoking involves both burning tobacco and the matches and lighters used to ignite it. Whether the flame is from a match or a lighter, this flame will inevitably start a fire if it comes in contact with suitable fuel. Thus, the discarding of a match into dry grass, before the match is extinguished, has been the cause of many exterior fires. Both match flames and lighters will cause explosions and fires with volatile flammables in the vicinity. Many persons have attempted to commit suicide by turning on the gas, but then they wish a last cigarette. Sometimes, the explosion that follows kills them, but more often puts them in the hospital with serious burns.

4.6.1 CIGARETTES

The burning characteristics of cigarettes vary from brand to brand. Modern tobacco cigarettes contain a complex chemistry of additives to control the moisture content and burning rates of both the tobacco and the paper. US cigarettes sometimes used to include a chemical additive to keep them burning even when not being puffed. Now, cigarettes designed to self-extinguish have become common.

The temperature distribution within the burning tobacco and its ash is complex and difficult to measure. Baker reported that surface (solid) temperatures reached 850°C to 900°C (1560°F to 1650°F) at the edge of the glowing mass during the puff or draw using x-ray measurement techniques (Holleyhead 1996). After the draw stopped, the hottest part of the mass shifted to the center, with temperatures of 775°C (1427°F), and the

Puffing

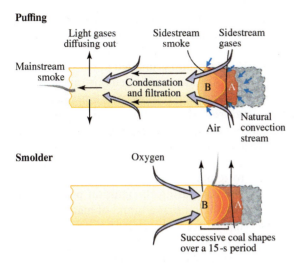

FIGURE 4-12A Airflow in a cigarette at rest and while being puffed. *Data from Mitler and Walton 1993*

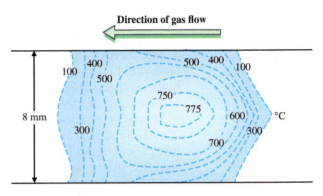

FIGURE 4-12B Temperature distribution in a burning cigarette at very start of puff. *Data from Gann, Harris, Krasny, Levine, Mitler and Ohlemiller 1998*

temperature of the ash at the edge dropped to approximately 300°C (572°F), as illustrated in Figure 4-12A. These temperatures are in general agreement with test results reported by Béland (1994) and by *NFPA 921* (NFPA 2017b).

Variations in the types and cut of the tobacco used will affect the temperatures developed as well as the burning rates (Gann 2007). This is especially true of hand-rolled cigarettes, whether of tobacco or other vegetable material, whose properties have not been studied in detail. Research by Baker et al. (2016) confirms that a static smoldering cigarette emits about half the heat of complete combustion of an equivalent amount of tobacco.

Tests conducted by the California Bureau of Home Furnishings measured the temperature characteristics of many common tobacco cigarette brands. Maximum temperatures produced ranged from 400°C (760°F) for one variety to 780°C (1440°F) for another. Temperatures rose by as much as 100°C as the burning reached the end of each cigarette. Some brands of cigarettes consistently self-extinguished when not smoked; others always burned to completion (Damant 1979). Although the rate at which a cigarette will burn depends on its orientation and the direction and intensity of any draft, the rate was also found to vary from brand to brand. Tests by the California Department of Forestry measured rates from 6 to 8 mm (1/4 to 1/3 in.) per minute and total burn times of 13 to 15 minutes for unaided horizontal burning (Eichman 1980).

The heat release rate for an average tobacco cigarette has been reported as approximately 5 W. Such a low level emphasizes the necessity for a fuel to be in direct contact with the smoldering tip of the cigarette before ignition can be ensured. A lit cigarette will occasionally set fire to dry fuel, such as upholstery or dry grass, on which it rests uncovered. A linear scorch will result, but it will rarely cause ignition. If the fuel is loose enough that the burning cigarette can burrow into it as it burns, ignition is more likely. When a single layer of light cloth covers the same cigarette, the insulation prevents the radiation of the heat, and temperatures up to 100°C (212°F) higher can result. This temperature difference may be sufficient to allow ignition of the fuel.

If the cigarette burrows down into loose cellulosic fuels or is pushed partially between two upholstered cushions, enough heat may build up to cause ignition if the arrangement conserves the heat without restricting the air supply. On exposed polyurethane foam, which is often very susceptible to flame, heat from the cigarette melts the rubber away from it so that, as the cigarette burns, it forms a trough in the foam. In combination with some fabric coverings, however, polyurethane can support a smoldering fire (Sanderson 2007). Although most modern upholstery foam rubbers are made to resist ignition, a cigarette can ignite latex rubber foams.

Sanderson (1998b) showed that cigarettes discarded into crumpled paper trash transitioned to flames in only about 1 percent of tests. An uncommon demonstration is the ignition of toilet paper rolls by placing a cigarette inside the roll (as sometimes occurs in public toilets). These often transition to a flaming fire within 20 minutes. As discussed in Holleyhead's extensive review of cigarette ignition, many cellulosic products, including toilet tissue, cardboard, paper towels, and office carbon paper, are all susceptible if the contact and geometry are suitable (Holleyhead 1999).

Not all cigarettes have the same potential to ignite cellulosic fuels. *ASTM E2187-2016* (ASTM 2016) is a standard test method for comparing the ignition potential of tobacco cigarettes. The general test protocol consists of lighting a brand of manufactured cigarette, placing it on filter paper, and observing whether the cigarette burns the full length of the tobacco column. The test is repeated 40 times per brand of cigarette, recording the proportion of cigarettes that burn their entire length. If 25 percent or fewer burn their entire length, that brand of cigarettes is deemed "fire-safe" (Gann et al. 2001).

Recent efforts to reduce accidental fires caused by cigarettes have focused on redesigning cigarettes to make them self-extinguish (as do cigars) when not being actively smoked by changing the paper or the tobacco. A common approach to produce a Fire Safe Cigarette (FSC), also referred to as Reduced Ignition Propensity (RIP) cigarette, is to add material onto the wrapping paper in the form of bands. The process used to place these bands onto the paper is through printing, using a water or solvent mixture, onto one side of the paper. The process works by blocking portions of the fine pores on the paper surface responsible for gas diffusion while burning (Eitzinger, Gleinser, and Bachmann 2015).

All 50 US states and the District of Columbia have passed laws and regulations mandating FSC cigarettes. These new cigarettes are required to self-extinguish when not being smoked (Shannon 2009; Gann et al. 2001; Yau and Marshall 2014). In addition, Canada, Australia, and the European Union (EU) have enacted similar legislation. This legislation was expected to have a significant impact on the frequency of cigarette-induced fires.

Recent research by Yau and Marshall (2014) concluded that implementation of the FSC is associated with reductions in US residential fire mortality rates. Using data during 2000 to 2010 obtained from the National Center for Health Statistics (NCHS), their study examined the statistical association between state-level implementation of fire-safe cigarette legislation and the rate of residential fire deaths in 32 states after implementation of fire-safe cigarette legislation. In 12 states there was either less than a 5 percent decrease or an increase, and seven states had insufficient deaths to evaluate state-level changes.

Yau and Marshall's study used Poisson regression and defined a decrease as a drop of at least 5 percent in residential fire mortality death rates. For purposes of their study, a death was considered unintentional and fire-related if one of the causes of death was exposure to smoke, fire, and flames as defined in the International Statistical Classification of Diseases and Related Health Problems-10 (ICD-10) codes X00–X09.

4.6.2 BEDDING AND FURNISHINGS

While changes in the construction materials of modern furnishings have made them less susceptible to ignition by cigarette, fires still occur. Cigarettes and cigars, being sources of sustained smoldering combustion, are more likely to ignite finely divided cellulosic fuels like cotton padding than thermoplastics and foams that melt rather than char. Years ago, mattresses and upholstered furniture were made of cushions of cotton batting, kapok, or sisal (or latex foam rubber, which will also smolder), covered with natural fiber fabrics of linen or cotton. Thus, a dropped cigarette could burrow into fuel, which would in turn support a smoldering fire for an extended period of time.

Newer furniture is made with polyurethane foam cushions covered in thermoplastic fabric. Neither of these materials is likely to be ignited by a smoldering source such as a cigarette. But the cushions are sometimes wrapped in cotton batting instead of a polyester fiber blanket, so the risk of cigarette ignition is not entirely absent. The synthetics are much more susceptible to ignition by an open flame and, once ignited, will support a much larger, more energetic fire than will the older furnishings.

Cotton sheets and blankets may similarly be ignited by cigarettes, but only when they are presented as a wadded mass of fuel. Single flat layers of fabrics will be penetrated by a smoldering cigarette but not ignited, due to the heat lost to convection. Kapok, sometimes used as a pillow stuffing, is very susceptible to glowing ignition sources, but feathers are not (although both will support smoldering once established). Decorative pillows may be filled with anything and should not be overlooked as an intermediate fuel that is ignited by a cigarette and then grows into a flaming fire that involves a urethane mattress. The investigator must be aware of complex interactions, must search the debris as well as interview the owner or tenant, and must obtain samples of all the likely first fuels, if possible.

Despite significant advances in improving the fire resistance of furnishings, smoking in bed remains a threat to life safety. The reasons are simple. Bedding often contains cotton, which is readily ignited by smoldering sources and is capable of sustaining a smoldering fire for an extended period. If the smoker falls asleep, so that a lighted cigarette drops into wadded sheets, pillowcases, or onto a cotton-stuffed mattress or pad, a fire can result. Statistics indicate that this type of fire is common (DeHaan, Nurbakhsh, and Campbell 1999). A special hazard of fire that involves upholstered furniture or bedding occurs when the drowsing smoker is awakened by the heat but, being confused, adopts incorrect measures to control the situation. People have attempted to throw the burning bedding out the window or carry it to the exterior and, in the process, have extended the fire over large areas of the building.

The time between ignition from a smoldering cigarette to open flaming combustion of upholstered furniture varies. One test, depicted in Figure 4-13, shows a delay of 42 minutes between placement and flame ignition. The time depends on the combination of cellulosic and synthetic materials and the extent and location of contact with the cigarette.

The National Bureau of Standards [now the National Institute of Standards and Technology (NIST)] reported that of six upholstered chairs in one test, three went to flaming ignition in 22 to 65 minutes, while the remaining three simply smoldered (Braun et al. 1982). The California Bureau of Home Furnishings reported that of fifteen upholstered chairs, nine went to flaming combustion in times ranging from 60 to 306 minutes, five self-extinguished, and one was still smoldering when extinguished at 330 minutes (McCormack et al. 1986). Krasny, Parker, and Babrauskas (2001) have published an extensive study of the variability of cigarette and flaming ignition of furniture, and the reader is referred there for more information.

In experiments observed by DeHaan, flaming combustion was achieved in older, cellulosic-filled upholstered furniture and bedding in times ranging from 22 minutes to over 2 hours from the placement of the burning cigarette. (If the fabric covering is torn, and the cigarette is placed against the cotton stuffing, the time to flame can be as little as 18 minutes.) The correct combination of fabric and padding (stuffing) can reduce the ignitability of furnishings. Even cotton-padded furniture can be cigarette-ignition resistant if covered with a heavy fabric made of thermoplastic (synthetic) fiber (Damant 1994; Holleyhead 1999). If a piece of furniture appears to have been ignited by a cigarette, samples of covering and padding should be recovered for later examination.

Even in the absence of flaming combustion, bed and furniture fires increase the danger of death by burns or smoke inhalation. The combination of smoking in bed and excessive alcohol consumption increases the hazard.

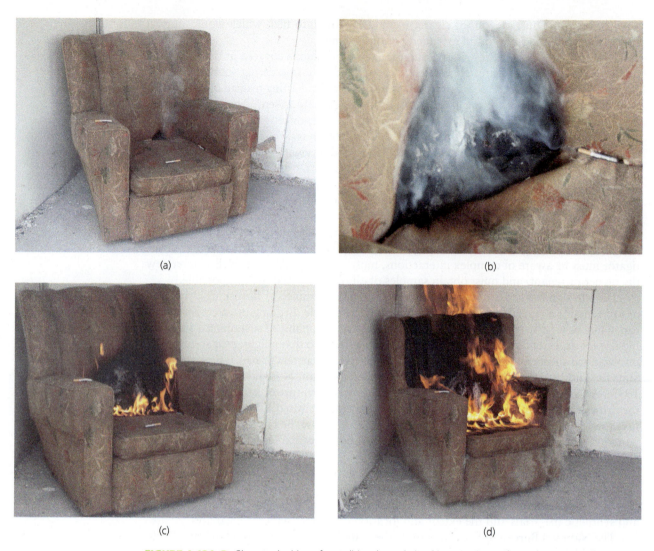

(a)

(b)

(c)

(d)

FIGURE 4-13A–D Cigarette ignition of a traditional armchair taking 42 minutes from placement to flames. Note location of ignition and failure of other cigarettes on other surfaces. *Courtesy of Jamie Novak, Novak Investigations, and St. Paul Fire Dept.*

4.6.3 CIGARETTES AND FLAMMABLE LIQUIDS AND GASES

Another fallacy about cigarettes is that they will readily ignite flammable liquids or gases. Repeated attempts to cause explosions by inserting a lighted cigarette into an explosive gasoline vapor–air mixture have resulted in failure, even with the ash knocked off and the cigarette being puffed strongly. Tests involving throwing or dropping lighted cigarettes into gasoline vapors above or alongside a spill on pavement have not resulted in an ignition until a lighted match was dropped into the same vapor. This is not proof that an explosion cannot happen, but any claim that it has occurred should be viewed with the greatest skepticism.

In his extensive review of the dynamics of tobacco cigarettes and flammable vapors, Holleyhead (1999) describes several factors revealed by the tests of Baker (2016) and others that make ignition of gasoline vapors by a glowing cigarette most unlikely. Tests have shown the oxygen levels in the cigarette in the vicinity of the combustion zone to be very low and carbon dioxide levels to be very high, both factors that significantly reduce the

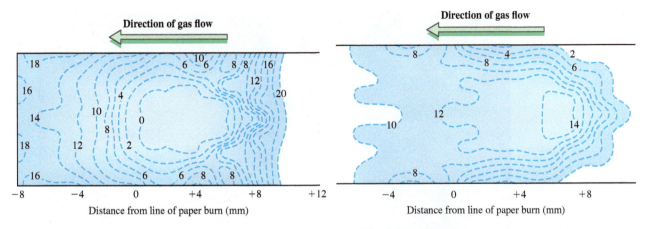

FIGURE 4-14A Oxygen concentrations in a cigarette—at the start of a concentration in a cigarette at the start of a "puff." Note the extremely low O_2 concentration throughout the high-temperature zone preventing ignition of gases/vapors.

FIGURE 4-14B Carbon dioxide levels are very high whether the cigarette is being actively smoked or not. This will inhibit ignition of all but the most sensitive gases.

chances of vapor ignition, as illustrated in Figure 4-14. Furthermore, the residence time of airborne vapors in the cigarette being puffed is so short that there is not enough time for any but the most reactive species to ignite.

In a commercially made cigarette, the suppressing of any sustained ignition is minimized by the spacing between the fuel elements such that the quenching distance of most of the reactive gases is not exceeded. Kirk suggested that the ash surrounding the burning tobacco may act in the same manner as the screen around a miner's safety lamp, acting to suppress any flame by quenching it between closely spaced elements. Finally, while the surface temperatures of the burning tobacco inside the cigarette tip are high, the presence of incombustible ash may reduce the efficiency of heat transfer to the fuel vapor (Damant 1994; Holleyhead 1999). These heat transfer considerations are validated by the published test data, which showed that only hydrogen, hydrogen sulfide, carbon disulfide, acetylene, ethylene oxide, phosphine, and diethyl ether are susceptible to cigarette ignition, while gasoline vapors and methane are not (Babrauskas 2003).

Tests by the ATF Fire Research Laboratory involved contact of burning tobacco cigarettes of different brands with gasoline vapors from a pool at room temperature. In 137 attempts using both smoldering (passive) and actively drawn (puffing) cigarettes no ignitions were observed. Further testing involved multiple applications of 157 burning cigarettes to or near a gasoline-saturated cotton blouse with no ignitions observed (Malooly and Steckler 2005; Tontarski et al. 2007). Contaminants or irregularities in the filling or in the paper may occasionally promote a very brief, tiny flame that would be capable of igniting a suitable fuel/air mixture.

Peer-reviewed published research by Marcus and Geiman (2014) examined the propensity of lit cigarettes to ignite gasoline vapors. In over 4,500 instances of exposure of a lit cigarette to ignitable concentrations of gasoline vapor in air, they reported no instances of the ignition of gasoline vapors. The 70 distinct tests used 723 cigarettes and five major brands of commercially-manufactured tobacco cigarettes. Their experiments exposed lit cigarettes, both at idle and under draw, to gasoline vapors in various configurations including pools/pans of gasoline, gasoline on textile substrates (clothing), and gasoline sprays.

The damage to clothing or upholstery when scorched or burned by a cigarette will very rarely ignite the fire that burns the house. In any instance where smoking is claimed to be the source of a fire, careful attention must be given to determine that the claimed

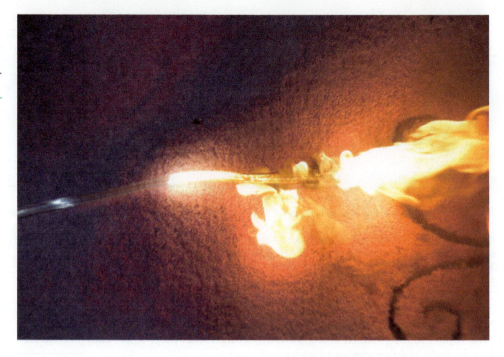

FIGURE 4-15 Oxygen mask readily ignited by match flame burns with great intensity. *Courtesy of Jamie Novak, Novak Investigations, and St. Paul Fire Dept.*

fuel is one that could be lighted by burning tobacco or, alternatively, the flame from a discarded burning match, which is actually a much more likely source. Consideration must also be given to time factors. Due to their low HRR, cigarettes require contact time to transfer enough heat to cause ignition of another fuel. This generally means at least 15 minutes have to elapse. A slight draft, however, has been observed to shorten this time by 2 to 3 minutes (Sanderson 2007).

In his own tests, DeHaan has confirmed those ignition times and that only incendiary materials (like gun cotton, gunpowder, or flash powder) can be ignited immediately on contact with a glowing cigarette. The use of medical oxygen by a smoker makes all materials saturated with oxygen more ignitable. This includes clothing, bedding, facial hair, and the plastic mask and cannula, as seen in Figure 4-15.

4.6.4 PIPES AND CIGARS

Pipe and cigar smoking is not basically different in its fire potential from cigarettes. Cigars tend to go out when not puffed, but this does not prevent some fires from being ignited when cigars fall onto a suitable target. Discarded pipe embers, like lighted cigarette embers, can burn their way through crumpled papers in a wastebasket until the embers lodge where there is thicker fuel (and ventilation) and then ignite it. Pipe ashes will also scorch upholstery or clothing, actually burning holes in cloth in many instances. They rarely cause flaming fire except with sawdust, cotton packing, or similar readily ignitable materials. Hot pipe and cigar ashes are often physically larger than cigarette ashes and have more heat to transfer to fuels they contact but do not sustain combustion on their own for very long.

4.6.5 PLANTINGS

Finely divided cellulosic materials can be encountered in gardens and decorative plantings of both real and artificial plants. Dry potting soils, peat moss, and Spanish moss have been shown to be readily ignitable by contact with a smoldering cigarette. Smokers often assume plantings are in regular (mineral or garden) soil and are therefore non-combustible (Schuh and Sanderson 2009, 1–3).

4.7 Spontaneous Combustion (Self-Heating)

Spontaneous ignition is the "initiation of combustion of a material by an internal chemical or biological reaction that has produced sufficient heat to ignite the material" (NFPA 2017b, pt. 3.3.180). **Spontaneous combustion** "due to self-heating is a special form of smoldering ignition that does not involve an external heating process. An exothermic reaction within the material is the source of the energy that leads to ignition and burning" (NFPA 2017b, pt. 5.7.4.1.1.5).

A frequent claim is that a fire started from spontaneous combustion (DeHaan 1996b). At first, this suggestion seems to violate the basic premise that there must be fuel, oxygen, and heat before there can be combustion and implies that in some mysterious manner fires simply set themselves on occasion. The term *spontaneous chemical causation* would be more accurate, for in such cases the mass of fuel, rather than igniting from one point or even one surface, ignites throughout its mass at very nearly the same time; and the heat has been accumulating, not from some exterior source, but from chemical processes occurring within the fuel mass. When such combustion occurs, it is an example of the balance of physical and chemical processes that occur in all fires but on a time scale that allows their individual roles to be better appreciated. Taken as a whole, however, their interactions make them hard for the fire investigator to understand.

The single driving force is an exothermic reaction generating heat. If that heat is not dissipated by normal mechanisms as fast as it is made, it can build up in a fuel mass and raise the temperature of the mass. Because reaction rate generally doubles with every increase in temperature of about 10°C (18°F), the reaction, by generating heat, tends to make itself go faster and faster with a constantly increasing heat production rate. When there is insufficient dissipation of the heat, the temperature may rise to the point of ignition of the entire reacting mass. The process is treated in more detail in the fire investigation literature (DeHaan 1996a). Not all chemical reactions are sufficiently exothermic (self-heating) to cause ignition, and not all exothermic reactions are sensitive enough to temperature rises to drive them to ignition. The NFPA *Fire Protection Handbook* (NFPA 2008) lists commonly encountered materials, rated according to their susceptibility to self-heat.

4.7.1 CHARACTERISTICS OF SELF-HEATING

Self-heating is "the result of exothermic reactions, occurring spontaneously in some materials under certain conditions, whereby heat is generated at a rate sufficient to raise the temperature of the material" (NFPA 2017b, pt. 3.3.164). The general rule that applies to self-heating is that the mass of material needed to accomplish ignition is inversely related to the reactivity of the material, and the time needed is directly related to the mass required (i.e., the lower the reactivity, the larger the necessary mass and the greater the time needed). Catalytic reactions (such as the setting of fiberglass resin) require only a very small mass because the reaction is highly exothermic and can take place in a few seconds.

Self-ignition is "the initiation of combustion by heat but without a spark or flame" (NFPA 2017b, pt. 3.3.165). Drying oils can trigger self-ignition in a few hours and require as little as 25 to 50 ml (1 to 2 fl. oz.). Activated charcoal can self-heat in masses of a few pounds and requires several hours to a few days.

Laboratory studies have demonstrated that charcoal barbecue briquettes are unlikely to self-heat to ignition unless presented in large masses [more than 50 lb (20 kg)] or at high ambient temperatures over 100°C (Wolters et al. 1987). However, these data must be understood as applying to pure and uncontaminated charcoal briquettes. Credible reports exist of fires that originated from small bags of charcoal briquettes where external ignition sources like cigarettes were successfully excluded. These fires appear to have been due to briquettes contaminated by chemical substances that promoted combustion. Some charcoal briquette bag ignitions have taken place, however, after unwise individuals returned hardly burned briquettes to the bag.

spontaneous ignition ▪ Initiation of combustion of a material by an internal chemical or biological reaction that has produced sufficient heat to ignite the material (NFPA 2017b, pt. 3.3.180).

spontaneous combustion ▪ Due to self-heating; a special form of smoldering ignition that does not involve an external heating process. An exothermic reaction within the material is the source of the energy that leads to ignition and burning (NFPA 2017b, pt. 5.7.4.1.1.5).

self-heating ▪ The result of exothermic reactions, occurring spontaneously in some materials under certain conditions, whereby heat is generated at a rate sufficient to raise the temperature of the material (NFPA 2017b, pt. 3.3.164).

self-ignition ▪ See autoignition. Initiation of combustion by heat but without a spark or flame (NFPA 2017b, pt. 3.3.165).

Hays and grasses require significant masses (100 kg/220 lb or more) and days to weeks before ignition, even at moderate temperatures. Coal and bulk materials will not self-heat to ignition unless they are present in very large masses (many tons) and given weeks or even months. The higher the starting temperature, the faster the process can progress. Cotton laundry that has not been allowed to cool down properly from drying has been known to ignite after just a few hours. The presence of cooking oils that have not been removed by laundering may contribute to self-heating of laundry, as may residues of bleaches (oxidizers). The self-heating of residues of cooking oils in clothes dryer lint may lead to some fires in clothes dryers (Reese, Kloock, and Brien 1998; Sanderson and Schudel 1998). Tests have revealed that triglyceride oils like corn, cotton, or linseed oils are not very soluble in water and will be retained in clothes after laundering [and may be detectable in the residual water in the washing machine pump if the clothes in the dryer have been fire damaged (Mann and Fitz 1999)].

Some suspected sources of spontaneous heating can be tested by subjecting them to the Mackey test, which was developed to assess the hazards of oils used to improve the weaving qualities of cotton and linen fiber, or, preferably, by establishing their critical temperature for various mass sizes and shapes (Mackey 1895; Frank-Kamenetski 1969). Some processes can be tested by differential scanning calorimetry (DSC) to determine the rate at which they yield heat. The likelihood that a process can be an ignition source can then be evaluated. Because the environment has so much to do with self-heating (porosity, oxygen supply, thermal conductivity, heat transfer coefficient, etc.), simple chemical or thermal tests of materials may not reveal all their tendencies to self-heat.

Although time consuming, the most accurate analysis is to place various masses of the suspect material into ovens and expose them to slowly increasing environmental temperature. Internal temperature monitoring of the mass will reveal when runaway self-heating occurs. Brian Gray (2001) warned about simple reliance on small-scale tests in predicting self-heating in industrial situations where products have relatively high critical temperatures when tested in small, single packages but whose critical temperatures as stored assemblies are considerably lower. He cited two cases in which hot storage conditions of bulk product changed the thermodynamics in critical fashion. In one case, drums of calcium hypochlorate (whose generation of oxygen is an exothermic reaction) were stored in an exterior storage container and produced a runaway self-heating reaction. In the other case, small packages of instant noodles were originally packed at a packing temperature of 81°C (177°F), below the estimated critical temperature for the shipping assembly (in cartons on pallets) of 106°C (222.8°F). A change in manufacturing process caused the product to be packed at 113°C to 120°C (235°F to 248°F), a change that caused a massive fire loss (Babrauskas 2003).

In one case in New York, a large warehouse fire was traced to a storage area where cases of latex rubber surgical gloves had been stored for several years. Because the gloves were packaged in separate boxes in each case as shown in Figure 4-16A, investigators could not believe that the latex had self-heated until they found cases on the periphery of the main fire whose contents displayed the entire range of self-heating damage from mildly discolored to deeply charred as shown in Figures 4-16B and C. The gloves had been stored in an unventilated area, and the high summer temperatures finally tipped the balance toward runaway self-heating (Hevesi 1995).

Powders (dusts) or dried aerosols (from catalytic-setting paints) have been seen to accumulate on ventilation filters or hot surfaces like lamps and develop into self-heating masses, causing fires. These processes are often aided by airflow and elevated temperature of the substrate (Kong 2003).

4.7.2 SELF-HEATING OILS

The most commonly encountered consumer product that can self-heat to spontaneously ignite is drying oil such as linseed (extracted from flax seeds), tung nut, fish, or soybean oil. As the name implies, drying oils harden by oxidation of the double bonds of the fatty

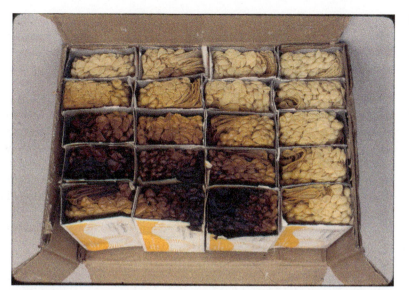

FIGURE 4-16A Self-heating of latex surgical gloves stored for years in a warehouse. *Courtesy of US Department of Justice, Bureau of Alcohol, Tobacco and Firearms and Explosives.*

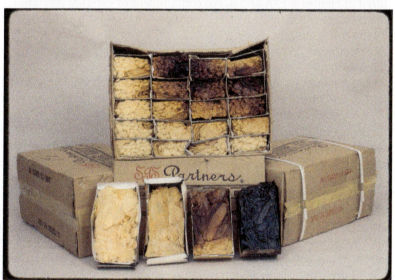

FIGURE 4-16B Showing gradations of damage in cartons. *Courtesy of US Department of Justice, Bureau of Alcohol, Tobacco and Firearms and Explosives.*

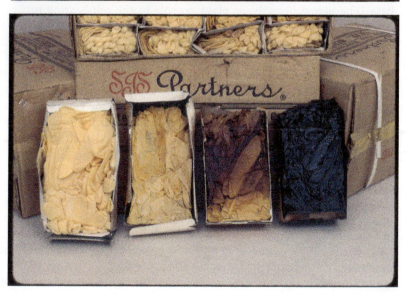

FIGURE 4-16C Note limited damage to individual boxes. *Courtesy of US Department of Justice, Bureau of Alcohol, Tobacco, Firearms and Explosives.*

acids in the oils, particularly the linolenic acid component (Howitt, Zhang, and Sanders 1995). As they oxidize they polymerize to form a tough, natural plastic coating. This coating property is why these oils have been used in paints and finishes for centuries. The oxidation process relies on oxygen in the air and generates heat. The reaction rate depends on the amount of drying oil that is presented to the air.

A quantity of oil in a can will not self-heat to a detectable degree, but if the oil is spread as a thin layer on a porous substrate like cotton cloth, there can be enough surface area to promote rapid oxidation and heating. If this heat is trapped by insulation in a manner that oxygen can still diffuse into the mass, the reaction rate will rise.

Raw linseed oil will demonstrate this effect but often will not spontaneously ignite, because bulk raw linseed oil contains oleic and linoleic acids, which are not as reactive as linolenic acid. Raw linseed oil does not dry as fast and hard as boiled linseed oil, which is made by boiling the product to concentrate the amount of the less saturated, more reactive fatty acids or, more commonly, by adding a drying agent, most often a metallic oxide. The drying agent triggers rapid setting and thereby more rapid heat generation. The effect is that a quantity of cotton rags smeared with boiled linseed oil can self-heat to the point of autoignition when kept at room temperature for a period of just a few hours, as pictured in Figures 4-17A and B. No containment or external insulation is necessary, because the reaction is enhanced by the availability of oxygen, and enough insulation is provided by the overlying rags.

As little as 25 to 50 ml (1 to 2 fl. oz.) is adequate if other factors are optimum. Reactions monitored in one series of tests revealed temperatures in excess of 400°C (750°F) within the mass of rags (Howitt, Zhang, and Sanders 1995). Once the mass of rags bursts into open flame, there will be enough heat to ignite other ordinary fuels in the vicinity. This is the mechanism thought to be responsible for the fire in the Meridian Plaza high-rise office building, and has been identified as the heat source in numerous fires in furniture shops and home workshops where wood-finishing products containing boiled linseed oil were used and residues wiped up with cloth rags (Dixon 1992; Ziegler 1993).

The key elements that must be present are presence of a drying oil (most commonly of vegetable or animal origin), a porous support medium that allows free access of oxygen to diffuse into the mass and that does not melt when the temperature rises, provision of an adequate oxygen supply, and time for the reaction to occur. The higher the ambient or starting temperature, the faster the reaction will proceed. If the ambient temperature is below about 10°C (50°F), linseed oil is unlikely to self-heat to flaming ignition.

Many wood stains and varnishes contain both a petroleum solvent and a linseed oil base. The petroleum solvent plays no role in the self-heating process except to slow it down by evaporative cooling. If the product is sprayed and then wiped up, the solvent will largely have evaporated and will not serve as a delay mechanism.

Self-heating does not occur with hydrocarbon (lubricating) oils or animal lard except at unusually high ambient temperatures and does not usually occur with the cooking oils commonly found in household kitchens [e.g., peanut, corn, olive, safflower, rapeseed (canola)] at relatively low ambient temperatures. One exception occurs when these oils are absorbed into porous foods like flour or onto cotton towels and are then exposed to high starting temperatures. This mechanism is likely when the oil has been used to deep fry fish. Then, the effluent will contain fish oils that can self-heat, and porous bread or batter crumbs, all at high temperatures (Dixon 1995). Rags used to wipe down hot cooking griddles with various oils and then thrown into waste or laundry bins while still hot can also self-heat to ignition. Self-heating fires have occurred when hydrocarbon oils leaked into porous insulation lagging covering pipes running at an elevated temperature, but such fires will occur only in an industrial environment (Babrauskas 2003).

Gaw (2005) reported that stacks of cotton towels oiled with linseed oil, then laundered and washed and stored at 93°C (200°F) self-heated to 575°C (1067°F) and then ignited into flaming combustion. He noted that significant oil remained in the towels after

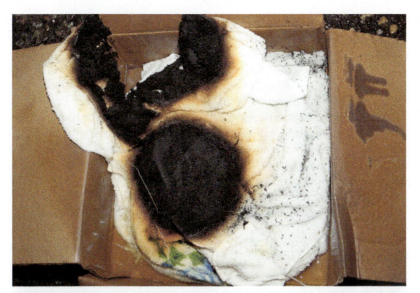

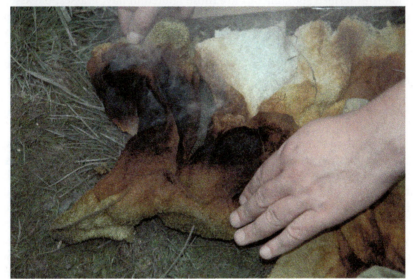

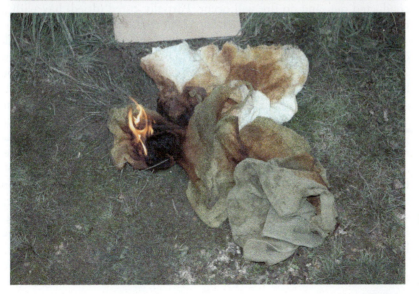

laundering, that bleach had no effect on the amount of oil removed, and that residual oil was recovered from the clothes washer pump even after laundering oiled towels and then a full load of non-oiled towels.

The reactivity of oils is measured by its **iodine number**, which is "a measure of the unsaturation of a substance (as an oil or fat) expressed as the number of grams of iodine or equivalent halogen absorbed by 100 grams of the substance" (Merriam-Webster 2017). While there are exceptions, generally, the higher the iodine number, the more susceptible the oil is to self-heating. For example, linseed oil has an iodine value of 173 to 201, tung oil: 150 to 176, soybean oil: 137 to 143, cottonseed oil: 108 to 110, corn oil: 111 to 130, and peanut oil: 85 to 105 (Vlachos and Vlachos 1921). The NFPA has rated many common products (both natural and synthetic) with respect to their susceptibility to self-heating (NFPA 2008). Stauffer has carried out extensive work in the chemistry and forensic identification of these products and the reader is referred there for more detail (Stauffer 2005).

4.7.3 SELF-HEATING OF VEGETATION

Aside from occasional serious fires that occur in the storage of chemicals, the most common fires termed spontaneous are those ignited in hay, grasses, bagasse, or other vegetation residues. The phenomenon has been known since ancient times, and considerable experimental work has been performed in attempting to explain its mechanism (Hoffman 1941; Firth and Stuckey 1945).

In 1873, Ranke Viljer, a Danish scientist, observed and recorded a case of spontaneous fire in a pile of hay. He performed further experiments in support of his theory of strong adsorption of oxygen by pyrophoric carbon. This was apparently the first detailed and well-documented description and served as the starting point for nearly all later work on the subject (Ranke 1873).

Several sources of heat can contribute to self-heating of hays and grasses. First, there is the heat of respiration of microbial populations and living materials such as freshly cut grass. This can raise the temperature of a fuel mass to over 70°C (160°F), at which temperatures the cells and microorganisms die. In order for most vegetable materials to undergo self-heating, there must be favorable moisture content to allow a fermentative process to proceed.

Unlike the fuels already described, which undergo chemical changes, self-heating of vegetable materials is often a biological process dependent on oxygen and living microorganisms, at least at first. If the hay is well cured (dried), it will not allow destructive fermentation; if it is too wet, not enough oxygen can diffuse into the mass, too much heat is conducted out, and no fire will occur. Partially cured (dried) hay with moisture content between 12 and 21 percent is best for self-heating.

The activity of the microorganisms will heat the hay to the thermal death point of the organisms as a limiting temperature. This temperature, too, is in the neighborhood of 70°C (160°F) and is lower for many organisms. Regardless of insulation that exists in a large mass of the vegetable material, temperatures in this range fall far short of the necessary ignition point of the hay, which is on the order of 280°C (540°F) and above.

The biological temperature limit makes clear that microorganisms can raise the temperature only to a point at which some exothermic chemical process(es) can be initiated to raise the temperature much higher. This phase of the process has been the subject of much attention and has produced various theories, including the production of pyrophoric carbon, pyrophoric iron, heat from enzyme action, and even auto-oxidation of the oils contained in seeds. Firth and Stuckey (1945) reported that much acid is generated in the early stages of the process and that this is accompanied by marked browning of the hay. This high acidity has been used as a means of determining whether spontaneous combustion has occurred as contrasted with external ignition.

Perhaps the most widely accepted theory is that of Browne, who postulated the formation of unsaturated compounds by the action of microorganisms (Browne 1935).

These could form peroxides with oxygen of the air, and later form hydroxy compounds along with heat. Others do not agree that acidic degradation products are formed (Bowes 1984). Rathbaum's work explored the complex role of temperature, ventilation, and moisture content for hay and other grasses (Rathbaum 1963). There are several possible chemical routes that do not rely on biological mechanisms. Gray has demonstrated that bagasse (the waste material from sugar cane extraction) can self-heat in the hot, dry climate of inland Australia even in the absence of any microorganisms (Gray 1990). Apparently, between 70°C and 170°C (160°F and 340°F), chemical decomposition reactions supported by moisture dominate, and above 170°C (340°F) oxidation reactions dominate as long as oxygen is available.

Whatever the actual mechanism may be, it is certain that it consists of a number of steps, the most important being chemical in nature. The packing density of the hay or grass, the size of the stack or bale, and its moisture content when left are critical factors. Other facts that are of importance to the investigator concern the environment—rainfall prior to ignition and ambient temperature of storage.

Spontaneous fires in stacked hay do not usually occur in less than 10 to 14 days after stacking and generally require 5 to 10 weeks. Under ideal conditions of moisture and very high ambient temperature (35°C to 40°C; 95°F to 105°F), ignition could be observed in 6 to 7 days (Lowenseent 1981). The fire that occurs is in the center of the stack and burns to the exterior, usually forming some type of chimney or flue to the exterior. A fire from an outside source (accidental or intentional) burns toward the inside (Firth and Stuckey 1945). Unburned hay in a stack in which spontaneous combustion has occurred will often be very dark in color with a color gradation ranging from gold-brown, to chocolate colored, to blackened, to char and may have a higher acidity than normal hay.

Odors described as caramel-like or tobacco-like have been described. If a burning stack is spread apart, hay that is not on fire may suddenly burst into flame when fresh oxygen is introduced if spontaneous combustion is the cause of the fire, which has preheated the fuel mass. Depending on the geometry of the stack, some exterior fires may preheat the interior. This is not expected to occur when the hay has been fired exteriorly, but small interior fires have been found after deliberately ignited test fires.

An interesting indicator of spontaneously ignited hay fires is the formation of hay clinkers. These glassy, irregular masses, gray to green in color, can be found throughout the pile wherever temperatures were the highest and most prolonged, but are likely to be concentrated near the center. The clinkers are composed of the inorganic residues of silicon, sodium, and calcium from the plant stems as well as impurities baled with the hay (soil, dust) fused into a glassy mass by the heat developed in the fire. Hicks has done an in-depth study of hay clinkers that strongly indicates that the inorganic constituents of various grasses may be linked to their propensity to form such glasses (Hicks 1998). Recently, Tinsley, Whaley, and Icove performed a series of live fire experiments examining the formation of hay clinkers in externally ignited fires. The result of that study indicated that the formation of hay clinkers is dependent on a variety of factors, none of which reliably indicate the origin or cause of the fire (Tinsley, Whaley, and Icove 2010).

Hay fires in pole barns with metal roofs may cause the formation of numerous large masses as opposed to a few smaller clinkers. Clinkers do not occur in all self-heating hay fires, so their absence cannot be taken as proof of incendiary cause, and their presence should not be taken as proof of spontaneous origin. A hay clinker may be mistaken for the residue of an incendiary device. Elemental analysis is essential. Spontaneous combustion is an easy decision to reach when the cause of the fire is not known. Many fires that have been attributed to spontaneous causes were actually deliberately set.

When other materials of vegetable origin such as fiberboard are involved, some input of external heat is necessary to trigger enough oxidation. Fiberboard, pressboard, and plywood are made by subjecting a wood product and a resin to high pressures at high temperatures. When these products are manufactured, if they are not stacked so as to allow excess heat to escape, residual heat remaining in the stacked mass may trigger self-heating.

Sawdust piles and other materials of wood have also been thought to ignite spontaneously, but they are unlikely to do so unless a drying oil or similar external contaminant is present. Sanding waste from freshly varnished wood has been linked to self-heating, triggered by residual heat from the sanding process. This tendency is aggravated if the wood has been recently coated with a catalytic polymer finish whose setting involves an exothermic reaction, not just simple evaporation of a solvent.

4.7.4 OTHER MATERIALS SUBJECT TO SELF-HEATING

In addition to the two best-known examples of systems subject to spontaneous ignition, oily rags and hay, a number of other fuel systems may ignite spontaneously. One of the more troublesome and common ones is coal, lying unmined in the ground or at times in large piles or storage bins above ground, since the wetting of coal can cause generation of heat (Hodges 1973). As with hay, exposure to water and the accumulated moisture content has been found to be critical to self-heating (Smirnova and Shubnikov 1951). Without doubt, the process itself is a slow exothermic chemical one in which heat is generated faster than it can escape in an environment that is well insulated. Other factors of importance are the type of coal (some grades of which ignite far more readily than others) and the coal size (finer dusts being more susceptible). Massive quantities are needed, and days or weeks are required before flaming ignition can be achieved.

4.7.5 IMPLICATIONS FOR THE FIRE INVESTIGATOR

There is a temptation to label many accidental fires as spontaneous because there is no identifiable ignition source or obvious human intervention. If the materials and processes cannot be specifically characterized as susceptible to self-heating under the prevailing conditions, then the cause must be considered to be unknown. Spontaneous ignition (with very rare exceptions) does not occur instantaneously, and the time frame for development is linked to the chemistry and mass of the reactant. Flaming ignition is always preceded by smoke and odors that should be detectable by anyone in the vicinity for some time prior to flaming ignition.

4.8 Other Sources of Ignition

Although accidental fires can be ignited by a small flame, electric arc, burning fragments, or other hot objects, there are some sources of ignition that do not fall into those categories. Lightning, spontaneous combustion, electric lighting, discarded batteries, and animal interaction are also sources of ignition.

4.8.1 LIGHTNING

Long before humans learned to start a fire, it is likely that their knowledge of fire came from fires ignited by bolts of lightning. Lightning is an electrical discharge of natural origin that is not fundamentally different from the electric arc, except in intensity. It is a massive discharge of the static electric charges built up in clouds of moisture or dust. The clouds and the earth act as the plates of a condenser or capacitor; the potential across them can reach up to 100 million volts. The discharge usually consists of several strokes back and forth, each lasting a few millionths of a second and 40 to 80 thousandths of a second apart. The currents involved are typically around 20,000 amperes, although much higher values are occasionally reached (Fuchs 1977).

Lightning strikes are usually accompanied by the physical destruction of any poor electrical conductor in their path. Windows can be blown out, wood can be splintered and shattered, and electric appliances can be exploded (see Figures 4-18A–B and 4-19). The

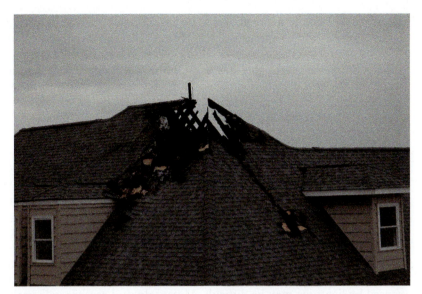

FIGURE 4-18A Light-
ning strike on house roof.
Fire damage to roof
where struck. *Courtesy of
Greg Lampkin, Knox County
Sheriff's Office, Tennessee,
Fire Investigation Unit.*

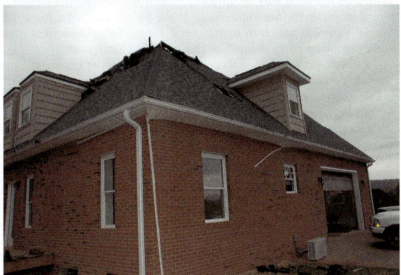

FIGURE 4-18B Limited
fire damage, down pipe
dislodged. *Courtesy of Greg
Lampkin, Knox County
Sheriff's Office, Tennessee,
Fire Investigation Unit.*

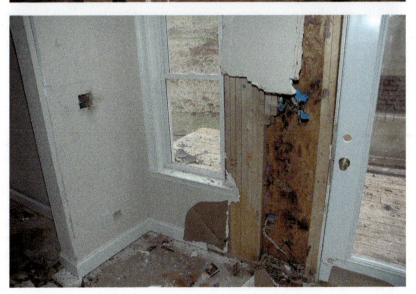

FIGURE 4-19 Interior
wall damage as lightning
followed electrical cables.
*Courtesy of Greg Lampkin,
Knox County Sheriff's
Office, Tennessee, Fire
Investigation Unit.*

air in the path of the main strike can be heated to a temperature of 30,000°C (54,032°F) and is expanded at a supersonic speed as a result. The resulting pressure shock wave can damage nearby structures with explosive force. In a lightning flash, the heat generated by the flow of current through a struck solid object will often ignite it. This is especially true when the object is dry. Although protective devices now available have markedly reduced loss, lightning-induced fires continue to damage structures.

4.8.2 LIGHTNING AND TREES

Lightning only occasionally strikes trees which depend upon their susceptibility to combustion. An old, dead, dry trunk is more likely to catch fire than a living tree, which is both a better conductor and less flammable. In general, many bolts of lightning will strike for every fire that is initiated. In regions where thunderstorms are common, the risk is great. The probability of ignition of ground fuels is controlled by their fuel moisture and the depth of the accumulated ground layer (Fuchs 1977, 62–63).

In most instances, lightning fires are easily traced. When a fire of undetermined origin occurs in a remote area of mountain or forest, the investigation as to whether it was caused by lightning may be difficult. Meteorological records will establish whether there was a storm in the questioned area at the right time. Some forestry services maintain a special lightning watch to monitor and record lightning strikes in wildland areas, and there are meteorological satellites that record lightning activity.

Lightning detection services can help to confirm or eliminate lightning as an ignition source. Vaisala Inc. maintains a lightning strike service called StrikeNet (thunderstorm .vaisala.com), which uses a network of electronic detectors. Its reports claim accuracy of 500 m as to location and can be requested online for particular time frames and various distances from a street address or GPS location. A typical StrikeNet report may uncover a tree or other object that was split or damaged by means other than the fire itself. If this finding corresponds to the origin of the fire as indicated by study of the pattern, it is probable that lightning was the origin.

The investigator needs to be familiar with the effects of lightning when it strikes objects. The most common effects are splitting of wood and mechanical disruption of structures. Most of these effects arise from sudden volatilization of water inside the tree or structure by heat from the electric current, so that the effect is that of an internal explosion. The effects are extremely variable, being determined by both the intensity of the electrical discharge and the localized condition of the object that is struck. Lightning strikes can induce power surges in nearby power or phone lines (causing failure and sometimes ignition of appliances connected to them). Examination of appliances (including computers and telephones) throughout a structure or even in adjacent buildings is important in verifying the role of lightning (or lone power surges) in igniting a fire, as all appliances plugged in at the time are likely to be damaged.

4.8.3 IGNITION BY ELECTRIC LIGHTING

Incandescent light bulbs can generate temperatures in open air at the surface of the glass bulb or envelope ranging from 74°C (165°F) to 267°C (513°F) depending on the wattage of the lamp and its position, as seen in Figure 4-20 (General Electric 1984). These temperatures can scorch cellulosics or melt synthetics but would probably not result in flaming ignition. However, higher temperatures can be produced if the bulb is enclosed in a housing or wrapped or buried in insulating material. Low-wattage bulbs normally produce a surface temperature inadequate to ignite common combustibles. As wattage is increased, especially with bulbs in housing types that restrict ventilation, temperatures can increase. Thus, potentially, a large incandescent light bulb (>50 W) can start a fire if in prolonged contact with suitable fuel.

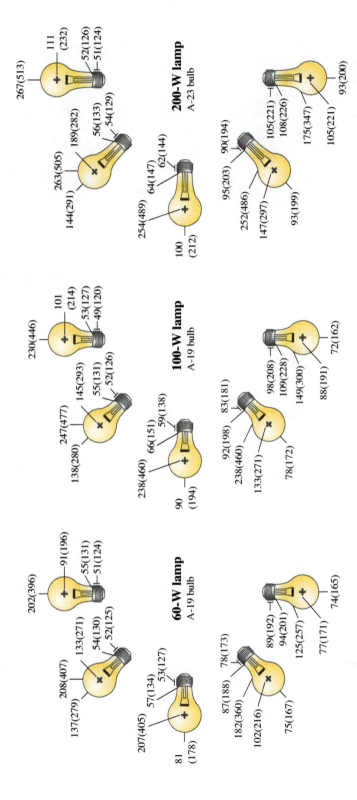

FIGURE 4-20 Surface temperatures of bulb and socket for typical incandescent lamps in open air (unlimited circulation) as a function of position. (Numbers in parentheses are temperatures in degrees Fahrenheit.)

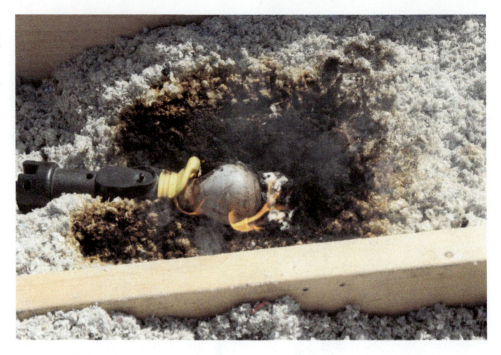

FIGURE 4-21 A 75-W lamp igniting cellulose insulation. *Courtesy of Jamie Novak, Novak Investigations and St. Paul Fire Dept.*

As pointed out earlier in this chapter, the circumstances of contact between a heat source and a fuel determine whether there is ignition. If a hot surface is placed in contact with a fuel long enough, the surface may provide insulation and reduce the heat losses from that surface, thereby increasing its temperature and its potential for ignition. (See Figure 4-21.) Gruehn recorded smoldering ignition of a wood floor by prolonged contact with a 75-W light bulb (Gruehn 1988). Even low-wattage lamps (<15 W), if buried or wrapped in an insulating material, can generate sufficient temperatures to ignite paper, cloth, sawdust, and grain. These occurrences are uncommon, not because of the lack of a high enough temperature, but rather, because something easily ignitable (such as a cellulosic material) must be in contact with the bulb, and this rarely occurs. The most likely areas for such ignitions are basements, storage rooms, and shops where packing material is allowed to be in contact with an operating bulb.

In tests conducted by DeHaan and Albers, a 60-W incandescent bulb buried in crumpled newspapers ignited them to flames in just 10 minutes 5 seconds. A 75-W bulb buried in sawdust (uncontrolled fuel moisture) caused smoke in 6 minutes 13 seconds, but no flames were observed prior to suspension of the test at 28 minutes. There was melting and smoke generation of polyester fiberfill burying a 100-W bulb, but no ignition for 32 minutes. A 150-W decorative lamp had no effect on polyurethane foam resting atop it for 30 minutes due to the large surface area and limited contact area, but a 100-W lamp buried under polyurethane foam caused ignition after two hours (see Figures 4-22A–B and 4-23) (DeHaan and Albers 2007).

The breakage of any lit incandescent lamp, even low-voltage and low-wattage ones, introduces two additional sources of possible ignition: the filament and an arc. The operating temperature of a tungsten filament is approximately 1500°C (2700°F). The filament begins to burn up as soon as air contacts it. The filament begins to cool as soon as the circuit is interrupted by failure of the filament, but it may retain enough heat to ignite flammable vapors or solids that come into contact with it shortly after failure. In addition, the brief arc produced when the filament fails produces the same risk of ignition as any other electric arc if flammable gases or vapors are in the vicinity.

Fluorescent lights operate at much lower temperatures than incandescent lamps, with the exterior of the tube rarely exceeding 60°C to 80°C (140°F to 180°F) (Cooke and

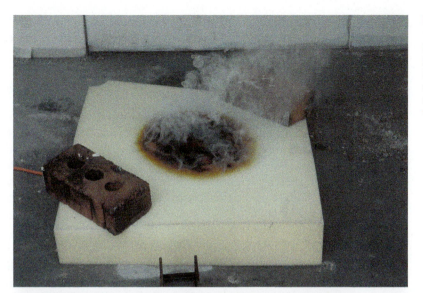

FIGURE 4-22A A 100-W lamp buried in polyurethane foam forces pyrolytic decomposition and char formation. *Courtesy of John Galvin, London Fire Brigade (Retired).*

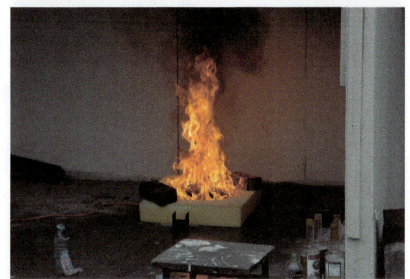

FIGURE 4-22B Leading occasionally to flames. *Courtesy of John Galvin, London Fire Brigade (Retired).*

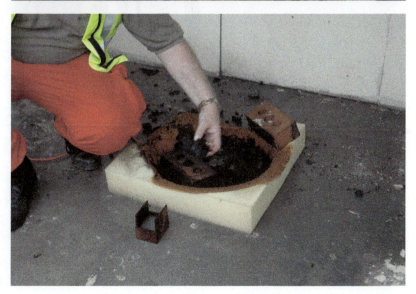

FIGURE 4-23 After flaming combustion, a rigid, porous, but very fragile char is formed around the heat source. *Courtesy of John Galvin, London Fire Brigade (Retired).*

Ide 1985). Quartz halogen lamps contain a quantity of iodine or bromine vapor and a tungsten filament operating at very high temperatures. The surface temperature of the fused quartz envelope can be as high as 600°C to 900°C (1100°F to 1650°F), and the temperature of a nearby reflector can be proportionately high (Lowe and Lowe 2001). Even brief contact between a fuel and the lamp (or even the reflector) could result in flaming ignition (see Figure 4-24).

Halogen lamps can also ignite fuels by radiant heat and melt diffusers, shades, and fixtures. They have also been known to shatter while lit, scattering hot fragments of glass and metal onto combustibles (Lowe and Lowe 2001). An example of a high-wattage metal halide lamp whose element shattered, with the fragments penetrating both the inner and outer enclosures, is shown in Figure 4-25. The hot metal and quartz fragments were believed to have ignited cellulosic materials directly beneath. Lamps with an extra-shatter-resistant glass shroud are available but are rarely used because of their significant extra cost.

4.8.4 IGNITION FROM DISCARDED BATTERIES

Most batteries for consumer devices (1.5 to 9 V) can support current discharges of up to 1 A when fresh. If metal can form a conductive path between the terminals, sufficient electric current heating can occur to ignite cellulosic materials in direct contact. Nine-volt batteries have both terminals at one end, so a coin or a piece of aluminum foil can act as a heating element if contact is made with both terminals. Lithium-ion battery failures can also cause fires.

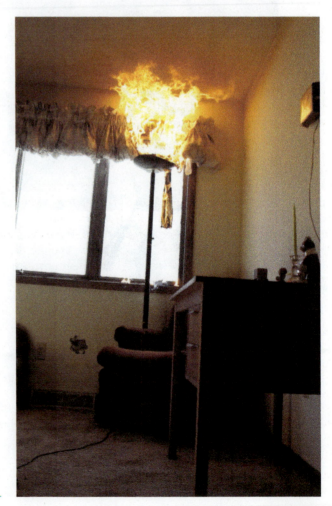

FIGURE 4-24 A halogen lamp ignites a curtain valance after less than one minute of contact. *Courtesy of Jamie Novak, Novak Investigations and St. Paul Fire Dept.*

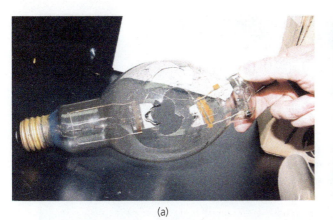

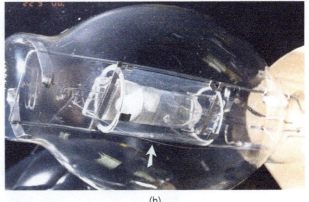

(a)   (b)

FIGURE 4-25 Metal halide lamp failure caused ignition. *Courtesy of Peter Brosz, Brosz & Associates Forensic Services Inc.; Professor Helmut Brosz, Institute of Forensic Electro-Pathology.*

4.8.5 ANIMAL INTERACTION WITH SOURCES OF IGNITION

Sometimes, animals cause fires. Both rodents and birds may carry lighted cigarettes or other burning objects, which then ignite combustibles, possibly even rooftops. Many rodents and birds store a variety of materials for nest building or other reasons. Birds may carry sticks, nest materials, and other objects and drop them down the roof vents of heating appliances. If the object were a lit cigarette and dropped onto flammable material, a fire could result. As previously mentioned, bird nests and rodent nests in chimneys and flues present fire hazards. Birds have also built nests on top of or adjacent to high-wattage flood lamps or other intermittent heat sources. When the lamp or appliance is turned on, a delayed ignition can occur.

A rat may chew a strike match head anywhere and thereby ignite it. Some evidence has been found that a rat or mouse carrying a strike-anywhere match in its mouth could strike it accidentally against a rough surface such as brick or concrete, lighting it in passing. The final effect will be the same as with any other match-ignited fire, but the combination of factors makes it most unlikely to occur.

Mice and rats have also been known to chew the insulation off wires, either short-circuiting them directly or leaving the exposed conductors awaiting some other contact. A simple short across the exposed conductors will be unlikely to ignite a fire but may simply trip the circuit protection. If foreign materials (from saltwater to portions of the animal's anatomy) can sustain current flow, the heat generated can degrade the insulation and lead to ignition of the insulation and other fuels in the immediate vicinity. This mechanism probably represents the single most significant contribution to fire causation by animals. Post-fire signs may be minimal once the surrounding insulation has been destroyed, but unburned insulation has a gnawed appearance, as seen in Figure 4-26. (See also Figure 4-27.)

Snails, slugs, birds, and other animals have been known to short out electrical equipment, thereby starting fires both inside and outside structures. Dogs and cats have been known to knock over containers of flammable liquids, which are then ignited by remote ignition sources. They have also been known to knock candles, Christmas trees, and lamps (such as the heat lamps used to keep pets, poultry, and livestock warm) into contact with combustibles. Moths have been proposed as a mechanism for starting spot fires by catching fire in a candle flame and then flying some distance to ignite remote fuels. Cooke and Ide (1985) dispelled this myth by saying, "A moth on fire would be aerodynamically unstable and unable to fly very far even if the chitin from which the wings are made supported combustion."

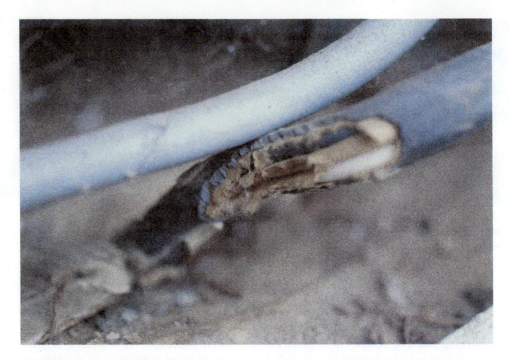

FIGURE 4-26 Rodent-gnawed wires in this RV refrigerator came close to being a fire cause. Fortunately, only the bare ground and neutral conductors had been exposed at this point. *Courtesy Joe Bloom, Bloom Fire Investigation.*

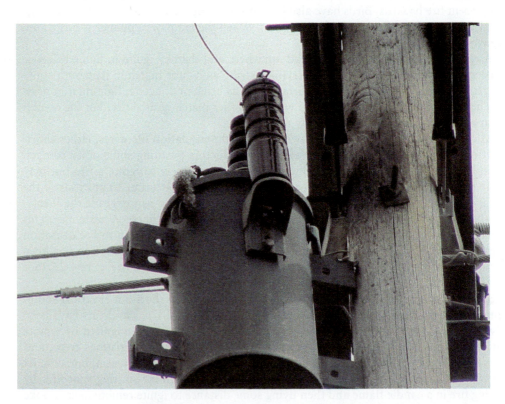

FIGURE 4-27 A grass fire started at the base of this power pole. The remains of the perpetrator can be seen as the tail and the foot on the left side of the transformer. Note "flash burn" on the adjacent pole. *Courtesy David J. Icove, University of Tennessee.*

There appears to have been little or no study, at this time, made of the habits of animal species in relation to fire hazard. Even without scientific study, it is apparent that animals have started fires; thus, a thorough investigation needs to consider the possibility of the role of animals.

4.9 Assessing Ignition Sources at the Fire Scene: The Ignition Matrix™

Nearly every room (or vehicle) offers multiple possible ignition sources—not only from inherent energy sources such as fixed wiring, fixtures, outlets, heaters (gas or electric), or other appliances—but also from the variety of human activities that may bring more ignition sources into action. These additional ignition sources include smoking materials, use or misuse of electric tools or appliances and devices, extension cords and power strips, candles, and countless more items.

Fire investigators face the challenge of identifying all potential ignition sources in the area of origin and then eliminating them until they are down to one (based on reasonable data or methods). The scientific method of fire investigation requires the investigator to reach a defensible conclusion by demonstrating not only how this source could have started the fire but also how all other reasonably possible sources have been excluded. If two or more ignition sources are deemed possible at the end of the investigation, the cause has to be declared to be undetermined. Demonstrating these conclusions can be difficult, especially in a concise, yet comprehensive, manner.

Electrical engineer Lou Bilancia developed the Ignition Matrix™, a grid, to evaluate ignition sources and also document competency to ignite a particular first fuel. Based on physical examination of the scene, interviews with occupants, or pre-fire photos or videos, the investigator identifies and lists all potential first fuels in the room in a vertical column, as shown in Figure 4-28. The investigator then lists all the possible ignition sources in a row across the top of the page. Each square, then, represents the interaction between an energy source and a first fuel (Bilancia 2007). Each combination is then evaluated on four primary values:

1. Is this ignition source competent to ignite this fuel? Yes or no.
2. Is this ignition source close enough to this fuel to be capable of igniting it? Yes or no.
3. Is there evidence of ignition? Yes or no.
4. Is there a pathway for a fire ignited in this first fuel to ignite the main fuel? Yes or no.

There are often comments or notes concerning each evaluation, such as the following:

- This source was not energized (appliance or power cord) or not in use (candle).
- "Too far away" or "Depends on duration being adequate," or "Unknown—must test exemplar."
- Physical or visual evidence of burning or ignition was witnessed or recorded in video.
- Plume developed from first fuel sufficient, or flashover produced ignition.

The matrix can then be color-coded to indicate which combinations are capable, which are excluded, and which need further data.

A typical bedroom may have 15 or more potential first fuels: bed (mattress, box spring, frame), bedding (blankets, pillows, sheets, comforters), carpet and pad, dresser, TV cabinet, clothes, posters, chairs, draperies, books, bookshelves, and so on. Wall and ceiling coverings must also be included if they are combustible. Based on physical examination of the scene, pre-fire photos or videos, and interviews with recent occupants, the investigator may identify additional potential ignition sources like fixed wiring, outlets, switches, and fixtures; table lamps, clock, radio, TV, electric blanket, extension and power cords, cigarettes, candles, and matches. Although there may be many competent

FIGURE 4-28 Ignition Matrix™ —identified fuels along vertical axis; ignition sources along horizontal. *Courtesy of Lou Bilancia, Synnovation Engineering Inc. Copyright 2008–17. All rights reserved. Used with permission.*

Heat sources / Fuels	Clock radio	Cell phone charger	Cigarette	Candle	Compact fluorescent lamp	Plug-in room refresher
Lace night table cover	1. yes (a) 2. yes close 3. no (d) 4. yes path	1. yes (a, c) 2. not close 3. 4. yes	1. 2. yes close 3. no evid. 4.	**1. yes comp** **2. yes** **3. yes** **4. yes**	1. yes (a, c) 2. yes 3. no (d) 4. yes gravity	1. yes (a) 2. not close 3. no (d) 4.
Sheets or bed covers	1. no (c) 2. not close 3. no (d) 4. yes gravity	1. yes (a, c) 2. yes close 3. no (d) 4. yes	1. 2. not close 3. no evid. 4.	1. yes comp 2. not close 3. 4.	1. yes (a, c) 2. no 3. no (d) 4. no	1. yes (a) 2. yes close 3. 4.
Curtains	1. no (c) 2. not close 3. no (d) 4. yes path	1. yes (a, c) 2. yes close 3. no (d) 4. yes	1. 2. not close 3. no evid. 4.	1. yes comp 2. not close 3. 4.	1. yes (a, c) 2. no 3. no (d) 4. yes shade	1. yes (a) 2. yes close 3. no (d) 4.
Plastic decorative flowers	1. no (c) 2. not close 3. no (d) 4.	1. yes (a, c) 2. not close 3. no (d) 4. no	1. not comp. 2. 3. no evid. 4.	**1. yes comp** **2. yes close** **3. yes** **4. yes**	1. no (a, c) 2. no 3. no (d) 4. yes shade	1. no (a, c) 2. not close 3. no (d) 4. no
Lamp shade	1. yes comp 2. not close 3. no (d) 4. yes path	1. yes (a, c) 2. not close 3. no (d) 4. no	1. 2. not close 3. no evid. 4.	1. yes comp 2. not close 3. indirect 4. yes path	1. no (a, c) 2. yes close 3. no (d) 4. yes	1. no (c) 2. not close 3. no (d) 4. no

1. Competent ignition source Y/N?
2. Proximity, ignition close to fuel Y/N?
3. Evidence of ignition Y/N?
4. Initial fuel path to fuel load Y/N?

Color legend
Red = Competent and close
Blue = Not competent
Yellow = Competent but ruled out
White = Uninvestigated

Codes
P = plume or flashover
W = witnessed
F = open flame
N = not energized

Notes
a. *if the device failed*
b. *if fuel was cellulosic with a breeze*
c. *only with open flame*
d. *device was intact*

ignition-fuel combinations, many will be excluded based on physical separation. A candle on the dresser will not be capable, for instance, of directly igniting first fuels more than an inch or two away. Movement of these ignition sources must always be considered. If the definable and defensible area of origin is small, then the lists of first fuels and ignition sources will be considerably shorter than if the whole room is being considered. The investigator must be careful, however, of excluding fuels or sources merely because they are outside the area of origin by a few inches.

This approach forces the investigator to consider a range of alternative hypotheses and consider each one on the basis of factors such as heat release rate, heat flux, separation distances, thermal inertia, and routes of fire spread. A completed matrix offers a concise demonstration that all potential ignition sources have been considered and all (but one, presumably) eliminated. The Ignition Matrix™ is also more easily verified than the traditional item-by-item list, improving the investigator's own review process.

Summary

An ignition source must be of sufficient energy and in contact with (or at least capable of transferring heat to) appropriate fuel long enough to raise the fuel to its ignition temperature to trigger the combustion of that fuel under the ambient conditions present. That combustion may be in the form of a self-sustaining smolder or open flames, and each requires particular conditions. Flames, arcs, sparks, self-heating, and heated objects can all initiate fires under the right conditions, and all must be considered whenever a fire scene is being examined. It is not enough simply to have an ignition source with a given temperature. The cause of a fire is the source of energy, the first fuel ignited, and the circumstances under which those were brought together that resulted in ignition.

The circumstances of ignition and the contact that precedes it may change the temperature of the source, the chemical properties of the fuel, or the physical state of the fuel in complex ways. All materials and reactions must follow certain physical and chemical laws, and fuels and oxidizers are no exceptions. The analytical fire investigator must ensure that a postulated sequence of events in a fire not only fits observed conditions, but also follows these laws. Reliance on published data to confirm some ignition hypotheses may be enough if the conditions of the published tests are a reasonable match to the fire conditions. If they are not, properly designed and executed tests may be necessary to prove or disprove a particular hypothesis.

Review Questions

1. List five different open-flame fires (ignition sources) and list their heat release rates.
2. Why are candles a more common accidental ignition source today?
3. What effect does "insulation" have on the temperature of an ignition source like a light bulb?
4. Name three ways in which gas appliances can start accidental fires.
5. How can kerosene room heaters cause fires?
6. What fuel surface temperature is required to ignite fresh whole wood? What temperature is considered a potential ignition risk for wood exposed on a long-term basis?
7. Name three sources of frictional mechanical sparks.
8. Why will cigarettes not ignite gasoline vapors but will ignite acetylene or hydrogen?
9. Name three ways in which animals can cause fires.
10. List five conditions required for spontaneous combustion to occur.

References

Ahrens, M. 2002. *Home Candle Fires*. Quincy, MA: National Fire Protection Association.

Andrasko, J. 1978. "Identification of Burnt Matches by Scanning Electron Microscopy." *Journal of Forensic Sciences* 24: 627–42.

ASTM. 2016. *E2187-2016: Standard Test Method for Measuring the Ignition Strength of Cigarettes*. West Conshohocken, PA: ASTM International.

Babrauskas, V. 2003. *Ignition Handbook*. Issaquah, WA: Fire Science Publishers.

———. 2005. "Risk of Ignition of Forest Fires from Black Powder or Muzzle-Loading Firearms." Report for US Forest Service. San Dimas: T & D Center.

Babrauskas, V., B. F. Gray, and M. L. Janssens. 2007. "Prudent Practices for the Design and Installation of Heat-Producing Devices near Wood Materials." *Fire and Materials* 31: 125–35.

Baker, R. R., et al. 2016. "The Science Behind The Development and Performance of Reduced Ignition Propensity Cigarettes." *Fire Science Reviews* 5(1): 2.

Béland, B. 1994. "On the Measurement of Temperature." *Fire and Arson Investigator* September.

Bertoni, J. 1996. "The Essentials of Gas and Oil Fired Forced Warm Air Furnaces." *Fire and Arson Investigator* (December): 15–18.

Bilancia, L. 2007. "The Ignition Matrix." November. CCAI.

Bohn, J. A. 2003. "Woodstove Ashes Staying Hot for 110 Hours." Personal communication, Longmont Fire Department, February.

Bowes, P. C. 1984. *Self-Heating: Evaluating and Controlling the Hazards*. Amsterdam: Elsevier.

Braun, E., et al. 1982. "Cigarette Ignition of Upholstered Chairs." *Journal of Consumer Product Flammability* 9.

Browne, C. A. 1935. "The Ignition Temperature of Solid Materials." *NFPA Quarterly* 28, no. 2.

Buccola, K. 2011. *A Survey of the Use of Homemade Overpressure Chemical Devices in Several Cities in the United States: Determining the Impact on the United States*. Doctoral dissertation, Arizona State University.

Building Code of the City of New York, Sec. [C26-1400.6] 27-792 and Sec. [C26-1409.1] 27-809. See also *UL127: Factory Built Fireplaces* (Northbrook, IL: Underwriters Laboratories).

Cooke, R. A., and R. H. Ide. 1985. *Principles of Fire Investigation*. Leicester, UK: Institution of Fire Engineers.

Corwin, S. 2001. "Halogen Work Light Testing." *Fire Findings* 9, no. 2: 12–13.

Cuzzillo, B. R., and P. J. Pagni. 1999a. "Low Temperature Wood Ignition." *Fire Findings* 7, no. 2: 7–10.

———. 1999b. "The Myth of Pyrophoric Carbon." Pp. 301–12 in *Proceedings Sixth International Symposium on Fire Safety Science*. Poitiers, France.

Damant, G. H. 1979. Lecture, California Conference of Arson Investigators. Sacramento, CA: California Department of Consumer Affairs, Bureau of Home Furnishings, June.

———. 1994. "Cigarette Ignition of Upholstered Furniture." Sacramento, CA: Inter-City Testing and Consulting.

DeHaan, J. D. 1996a. "Spontaneous Combustion: What Really Happens." *Fire and Arson Investigator* 46 (January and April).

———. 1996b. "Spontaneous Ignition: What Really Happens, Part I." *Fire and Arson Investigator* 46 (March); "Part II." *Fire and Arson Investigator,* 46 (June).

DeHaan, J. D., and J. C. Albers. 2007. *Low-Energy Ignition Tests*. CCAI, November 7, 2007 (unpublished data).

DeHaan, J. D., D. Crowhurst, D. Hoare, M. Bensilum, and M. P. Shipp. 2001. "Deflagrations Involving Stratified Heavier-Than-Air Vapor/Air Mixtures." *Fire Safety Journal* 36(7): 693–710.

DeHaan, J. D., S. Nurbakhsh, and S. J. Campbell. 1999. "The Combustion of Animal Remains and Its Implications for the Consumption of Human Bodies in Fire." *Science and Justice* 39, no. 1 (January): 27–38.

Dillon, S. E., and A. Hamins. 2003. "Ignition Propensity and Heat Flux Profiles of Candle Flames for Fire Investigation." Pp. 363–76 in *Proceedings Fire and Materials 2003*. London: Interscience Communications.

Dixon, B. 1992. "Spontaneous Combustion." *Journal of the Canadian Association of Fire Investigators* March.

———. 1995. "The Potential for Self-Heating of Deep-Fried Food Products." In *Proceedings FBI International Symposium on the Forensic Aspects of Arson Investigators*. Fairfax, VA.

Drysdale, D. D. 2011. *An Introduction to Fire Dynamics*. 2nd ed. Chichester, UK: Wiley.

Dwyer, N. 2000. "How Hot Does It Get?" *Fire Findings* 8, no. 2 (Spring): 5.

———. 2006. "Flame Rollout." *Fire Findings* 14, no. 1 (Winter): 12–13.

Eichman, D. A. 1980. "Cigarette Burning Rates." *Fire and Arson Investigator* June.

Eitzinger, B., M. Gleinser, and S. Bachmann. 2015. "The Pore Size Distribution of Naturally Porous Cigarette Paper and Its Relation to Permeability and Diffusion Capacity." *Beiträge zur Tabakforschung/Contributions to Tobacco Research* 26 (7): 312–19.

Faraday, M. 1993. *The Chemical History of a Candle*. Atlanta: Cherokee.

Few, E. W. 1978. "Ammunition Identification Guide." *Arson Investigator*. California Conference of Arson Investigators, Spring, 24–29.

Firth, J. B., and R. E. Stuckey. 1945. *Society of the Chemical Industry* 64, no. 13; and 65, no. 275. Proceedings International Symposium: Self-Heating of Organic Materials. Delft, Netherlands, February 1971.

Frank-Kamenetski, D. A. 1969. *Diffusion and Heat Transfer in Chemical Kinetics*. New York: Plenum.

Fuchs, V. 1977. *Forces of Nature*. London: Thames and Hudson.

Gann, R. G. 2007. *Measuring the Ignition Propensity of Cigarettes*. Gaithersburg, MD: NIST, January 2001. http://fire.nist.gov/ bfrlpubs/fire07/PDF/f07068.pdf.

Gann, R.G., R.H. Harris, J.F. Krasny, R.S. Levine, H. Mitler and T.J. Ohlemiller, 1998. "The Effect of Cigarette Characteristics on the Ignition of Soft Furnishings." Gaithersburg, MD: NIST, January 1988.

Gann, R. G., K. D. Steckler, S. Ruitberg, W. F. Guthrie, and M. S. Levenson. 2001. *Relative Ignition Propensity of Test Market Cigarettes*. NIST Technical Note 1436. Gaithersburg, MD: NIST.

Gaw, K. 2005. "Autoignition Behavior of Oiled and Washed Cotton Towels." In *Proceedings Fire and Materials,* San Francisco, CA.

General Electric Co. 1984. *Incandescent Lamps*. General Electric Publication TP-110R2.

Goodson, M., and G. Hardin. 2003. "Electric Cooktop Fires." *Fire and Arson Investigator* October: 31–34.

Goodson, M., D. Sneed, and M. Keller. 1999. "Electrically Induced Fuel Gas Fires." *Fire and Arson Investigator* July: 10–12.

Gray, B. F. 1990. "Spontaneous Combustion and Its Relevance to Arson Investigation." Paper presented at IAAI-NSW Annual Conference, Sydney, Australia, September.

———. 2001. "Interpretation of Small Scale Test Data for Industrial Spontaneous Ignition Hazards." Pp. 719–29 in *Proceedings Interflam 2001*. London: Interscience Communications.

Gruehn, R. L. 1988. "To Be Prepared Is Everything." *Fire and Arson Investigator* 39, no. 1 (September): 54.

Hall, R. J., J. J. Wanko, and M. E. Nikityn. 2008. "Special Hazards Fire Investigation." *NFPA Journal* November–December: 68–73.

Henderson, R. W., and G. R. Lightsey. 1994. "An Anti-Flareup Device for Barometric Kerosene Heaters." *Fire and Arson Investigator* 45, no. 2 (December): 8.

Hevesi, D. 1995. "Warehouse Caught Fire When Gloves Combusted." *New York Times,* August 10, 1995.

Hicks, A. J. 1998. "Hay Clinkers as Evidence of Spontaneous Combustion." *Fire and Arson Investigator* July, 10–13.

Hodges, D. J. 1973. "Spontaneous Combustion: The Influence of Moisture in the Spontaneous Ignition of Coal." *Colliery Guardian* 207, no. 678.

Hoffman, E. J. 1941. "Thermal Decomposition of Undercured Alfalfa Hay in Its Relation to Spontaneous Ignition." *Journal of Agricultural Research* 61: 241.

Hoffman, J. M., et al. 2003. "Effectiveness of Gas-Fired Water Heater Elevation in the Reduction of Ignition of Vapors from Flammable Liquid Spills." *Fire Technology* 39: 119–32.

Holleyhead, R. 1996. "Ignition of Flammable Gases and Liquids by Cigarettes: A Review." *Science & Justice* 36, no. 4: 262–66.

———. 1999. "Ignition of Solid Materials and Furniture by Lighted Cigarettes: A Review." *Science and Justice* 39, no. 2: 75–102.

Howitt, D. G., E. Zhang, and B. R. Sanders. 1995. "The Spontaneous Combustion of Linseed Oil." In *Proceedings International Conference of Fire Safety*. San Francisco, CA, January.

Karlsson, B., and J. G. Quintiere. 2000. *Enclosure Fire Dynamics*. Boca Raton, FL: CRC Press.

Kong, D. 2003. "How to Prevent Self-Heating (Self-Ignition) in Drying Operations." *Fire and Arson Investigator* October: 45–48.

Krasny, J. F., W. J. Parker, and V. Babrauskas. 2001. *Fire Behavior of Upholstered Furniture and Mattresses*. Norwich, NY: William Andrew.

Lentini, J. J. 1990. "Vapor Pressures, Flash Points, and the Case against Kerosene Heaters." *Fire and Arson Investigator* 40, no. 3 (March).

Lowe, R. E., and J. A. Lowe. 2001. "Halogen Lamps II." *Fire and Arson Investigator,* April: 39–42.

Lowenweent, L. 1981. "Fire Investigation." *International Criminal Police Review* no. 344 (January): 2–3.

Mackey, W. M. 1895. *Journal of the Society of Chemical Industries* 14, no. 940.

Malooly, J. E., and K. Steckler. 2005. "Ignition of Gasoline by Cigarette." ATF (May 2005).

Mann, D. C., and M. Fitz. 1999. "Washing Machine Effluent May Provide Clues in Dryer Fire Investigations." *Fire Findings* 7, no. 4 (Fall): 4.

Marcus, H. A., and J. A. Geiman. 2014. "The Propensity of Lit Cigarettes to Ignite Gasoline Vapors." *Fire Technology* 50 (6): 1391–1412.

Martin, J. C., and P. Margot. 1994. "Approche Thermodynamique de la Recherche des Causes des Incendies. Inflammation du Bois I." *Kriminalistik und Forensische Wissenschaften* 82 (1994): 33–50.

Maxwell, F. D., and C. L. Mohler. 1973. *Exhaust Particle Ignition Characteristics*. Riverside, CA: Department of Statistics, University of California Riverside.

McAuley, D. 2003. "The Combustion Hazard of Plastic Domestic Heating Oil Tanks and Their Contents." *Science and Justice* 43, no. 3 (July–September): 145–58.

McCormack, J. A., et al. 1986. "Flaming Combustion of Upholstered Furniture Ignited by Smoldering Cigarettes." North Highlands, CA: California Department of Consumer Affairs, Bureau of Home Furnishings.

Merriam-Webster. 2017. "Iodine Number." Merriam-Webster.com. Accessed January 10, 2017 from https://www.merriam-webster.com/dictionary/iodine number.

Mitler, H.E. and G.N. Walton. 1993. "Modeling the Ignition of Soft Furnishings by a Cigarette." Gaithersburg, MD: National Institute of Standards and Technology.

NFPA. 2008. *Fire Protection Handbook,* 20th ed. National Fire Protection Association, Quincy, MA.

———. 2014a. *NFPA 51B: Standard for Fire Prevention during Welding, Cutting, and Other Hot Work*. Quincy, MA: National Fire Protection Association.

———. 2014b. *NFPA 1033: Standard for Professional Qualifications for Fire Investigator*. Quincy, MA: National Fire Protection Association.

———. 2015. *NFPA 54: National Fuel Gas Code*. Quincy, MA: National Fire Protection Association.

———. 2017a. *NFPA 58: Liquefied Petroleum Gas Code*. Quincy, MA: National Fire Protection Association.

———. 2017b. *NFPA 921: Guide for Fire and Explosion Investigations*. Quincy, MA: National Fire Protection Association.

———. 2017c. NFPA 654: Standard for the Prevention of Fire and Dust Explosions from the Manufacturing, Processing and Handling of Combustible Particle Solids. Quincy, MA: National Fire Protection Association.

Nicholson, J. 2005. "When You Go Out—Blow Out." *NFPA Journal* September–October: 68–73.

———. 2006. "Watch What You Heat." *NFPA Journal* September–October, 67–73.

Powerboat Reports. 1994. "Skyblazer Best in Low-Cost Aerial Pyrotechnics." September.

Ranke, H. 1873. *Liebig's Annals of Chemistry* 167: 361–68.

Rathbaum, H. P. 1963. "Spontaneous Combustion of Hay." *Journal of Applied Chemistry* 13 (July): 291–302.

Reese, N. D., G. J. Kloock, and D. J. Brien. 1998. "Clothes Dryer Fires." *Fire and Arson Investigator* July: 17–19

Sanderson, J. L. 1998a. "Candle Fires," *Fire Findings* 5, no. 4 (Fall).

———. 1998b. "Cigarette Fires in Paper Trash." *Fire Findings* 6, no. 1 (Winter).

———. 2000. "Heat-Bulb Testing: Wood, Straw and Towels Respond Differently at Close Distances to Lamps." *Fire Findings* 8, no. 4 (Fall).

———. 2004. "Manufacturers Vary Methods to Incorporate FVIR Technology." *Fire Findings* (Fall): 1–4.

———. 2005a. "Hot Surface Ignition." *Fire Findings* 13, no. 2 (Spring): 6.

———. 2005b. "Propane Torch Flame Exceeds 2400°F." *Fire Findings* 13, no. 2 (Spring): 5.

———. 2007. "Cigarette Fires in Fabrics." *Fire Findings* 15, no. 3 (Summer): 1–3.

Sanderson, J. L., and D. Schudel. 1998. "Clothes Dryer Lint: Spontaneous Heating Doesn't Occur in Any of 16 Tests." *Fire Findings* 6, no. 4 (Fall): 1–3.

Schuh, D. A., and J. L. Sanderson. 2009. "Cigarette Testing Reveals Dry Potting Soil, Peat Moss Can Be Viable Fuel Sources." *Fire Findings* 17, no. 2 (Spring): 1–3.

Schwartz, B. A. 1996. "Pyrophoric Carbon Fires." *Fire and Arson Investigator* December: 7–9.

Shannon, J. M. 2009. "Fire-Safe Cigarettes; Keep Fighting." *NFPA Journal* March–April: 6.

Singh, H. 1998. *Hazard Report on Candle-Related Incidents*. Washington, DC: US CPSC.

Smirnova, A. V., and A. K. Shubnikov. 1951. "Effect of Moisture on the Oxidative Processes of Coals." *Chemical Abstracts* 51, no. 18548 (November 25, 1951).

Stauffer, E. 2005. "A Review of the Analysis of Vegetable Oil Residues from Fire Debris Samples." *Journal of Forensic Science* 50, no. 5 (September): 1091–1100.

Tanner, D. J. 2005. US Patent 6848366, "Binary Exploding Target, Package Process and Product." Issued February 1, 2005.

Tinsley, A. T., M. Whaley, and D. J. Icove. 2010. "Analysis of Hay Clinker as an Indicator of Fire Cause." Paper presented at *ISFI 2010,* Adelphi, MD, September 27–29.

Tontarski, R. E., et al. 2007. "Who Knew? Cigarettes and Gasoline Do Mix." Presentation B84 at American Academy of Forensic Sciences 59th Annual Meeting, San Antonio, TX, February 19–24.

Townsend, D. 2000. "Fires and Tea Light Candles." *Fire Engineers Journal* January: 10.

USFA. 2004. *Santana Row Development Fire*. USFA-TR-153. Emmitsburg, MD: FEMA.

Vlachos, W., and C. A. Vlachos. 1921. *The Fire and Explosion Hazards of Commercial Oils*. Philadelphia, PA: Vlachos & Co.

Williamson, J. W., and A. W. Marshall. 2005. "Characterizing the Ignition Hazard from Cigarette Lighter Flames." *Fire Safety Journal* 40, no. 5 (July 2005): 491–92.

Wolters, F. C., P. J. Pagni, T. R. Frost, and D. W. Vanderhoot. 1987. *Size Constraints on Self-Ignition of Charcoal Briquets*. Pleasanton, CA: Clorox Technical Center.

Yau, R. K., and S. W. Marshall. 2014. "Association between Fire-safe Cigarette Legislation and Residential Fire Deaths in the United States." *Injury Epidemiology* 1.

Ziegler, D. L. 1993. "The One Meridian Plaza Fire: A Team Response." *Fire and Arson Investigator* September.

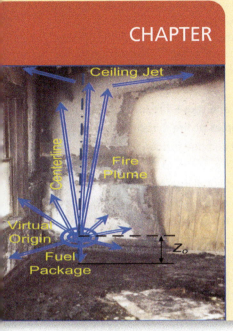

Courtesy of David J. Icove, University of Tennessee.

annealing, *p. 335*

backdraft, *p. 332*

calcination of gypsum, *p. 326*

ceiling jet, *p. 315*

char, *p. 326*

clean burn, *p. 333*

conduction, *p. 325*

convection, *p. 302*

craze, *p. 333*

diffusion flame, *p. 351*

entrainment, *p. 305*

eutectic melting, *p. 334*

fire effects, *p. 320*

fire patterns, *p. 294*

fire spread, *p. 297*

flammable, *p. 303*

ghost marks, *p. 329*

heat transfer, *p. 294*

isochar, *p. 327*

overhaul, *p. 297*

oxidation, *p. 325*

plume, *p. 302*

radiant heat, *p. 303*

radiation, *p. 342*

rekindle, *p. 341*

soot, *p. 303*

spalling, *p. 328*

spoliation, *p. 293*

thermal inertia, *p. 350*

trench effect, *p. 316*

vent, *p. 296*

ventilation, *p. 294*

venting, *p. 324*

OBJECTIVES

After reading this chapter, you should be able to:

- Understand and correctly apply the professional standards of care during the examination of fire scenes.
- Identify, comprehend, and apply the concepts of fire dynamics when examining fire scenes for their origin and cause.
- Determine dynamics in the fire's growth and development.
- Recognize fire patterns and their causes.
- Translate the pattern's relation to fire dynamics.
- Correlate fire plume calculations to assist in explaining fire patterns.
- Recognize and minimize the possibility of **spoliation** when processing a fire scene.

spoliation ■ Loss, destruction, or material alteration of an object or document that is evidence or potential evidence in a legal proceeding by one who has the responsibility for its preservation (NFPA 2017, pt. 3.3.178).

- Calculate the visible flame height given the heat release rate and effective diameter of a fire.
- Explain the effects of environmental conditions on fire.
- Distinguish between Type III (ordinary) construction and Type V (wood frame) construction as seen in single-family residences in the United States.

In order to accurately examine fire scenes for the origin and cause, fire investigators need to have a basic understanding of the underlying principles of fire dynamics that directly relate to the damage caused by the fire, particularly the damage formed by **fire patterns**. To determine the onset, growth, and development of a fire, scene examinations are best approached from a three-dimensional viewpoint. Two-dimensional interpretations of damage to the exposed contents, such as with V-patterns on walls and burn patterns on floors and carpets, may lead the investigator to a wrong hypothesis as to the fire's origin and cause.

The body of fire dynamics knowledge as it applies to fire scene reconstruction and analysis is derived from the combined disciplines of physics, thermodynamics, chemistry, **heat transfer**, and fluid mechanics. Accurate determination of a fire's origin, intensity, growth, direction of travel, duration, and extinguishment requires that investigators rely on and correctly apply all principles of fire dynamics. Investigators must realize that variability in fire growth and development is influenced by a number of factors such as available fuel load, **ventilation**, and physical configuration of the room.

Fire investigators can benefit from published research involving the application of the expertise that exists in the area of fire dynamics. The published research includes recent textbooks and expert treatises (DeHaan and Icove 2012; Drysdale 2011; Karlsson and Quintiere 2000; Quintiere 1998, 2006), traditional fire protection engineering references (SFPE 2008), US government research done primarily by the National Institute of Standards and Technology (NIST) and the US Nuclear Regulatory Commission (NRC) (Iqbal and Salley 2004), and fire research journals. These journals include peer-reviewed fire-related ones such as *Fire Technology*, the *Journal of Fire Protection Engineering*, and *Fire Safety Journal*. Fire-related research also appears in peer-reviewed forensic journals such as the *Journal of Forensic Science* and *Science and Justice*. Many basic fire dynamics concepts are described in *NFPA 921*, 2014 ed., pt. 6 (NFPA 2017).

Many fire investigators do not have access to all these resources. The primary purpose of this chapter is to bridge this knowledge gap. Existing real-world examples and training exercises illustrate their application and describe how basic fire dynamics principles apply to fuels commonly found at fire scenes. Case examples are offered in this chapter along with discussions on the application of accepted fire protection engineering calculations that can assist investigators in interpreting fire behavior and conducting forensic scene reconstruction.

As a result of the *Daubert*, *Daubert II*, *Kumho Tire*, and *Benfield* decisions as well as others regarding admissibility of expert witnesses and their opinions, following an investigative protocol is an expectation of courts. Before attempting to investigate a fire, the investigator should be familiar with the principles of fuels, ignition, and fire behavior. He or she must have a clear understanding of the purposes and goals of the investigation and a rational, orderly plan for carrying it out to meet those purposes.

Reconstructing the pre-fire scene as completely as possible using a step-by-step plan is critical to evaluating fire patterns accurately. This includes not only physically relocating fuel packages in their original locations but also identifying wall, floor, and ceiling coverings;

TABLE 5-1	Professional Levels of Job Performance for Fire Investigators as Cited in *NFPA 1033*, 2014 Edition

CATEGORY	JOB PERFORMANCE REQUIREMENT
4.1 General Requirements for a Fire Investigator	**4.1.1** Shall meet the job performance requirements defined in Sections 4.2 through 4.7.
	4.1.2 Shall employ all elements of the scientific method as the operating analytical process throughout the investigation and for the drawing of conclusions.
	4.1.3 Site safety assessments shall be completed on all scenes and regional and national safety standards shall be followed and included in organizational policies and procedures.
	4.1.4 Shall maintain necessary liaison with other interested professionals and entities.
	4.1.5 Shall adhere to all applicable legal and regulatory requirements.
	4.1.6 Shall understand the organization and operation of the investigative team within an incident management system.
4.2 Scene Examination	**4.2.1** Secure the fire ground
	4.2.2 Conduct an exterior survey
	4.2.3 Conduct an interior survey
	4.2.4 Interpret effects of burning characteristics on materials
	4.2.5 Interpret and analyze fire patterns
	4.2.6 Examine and remove fire debris
	4.2.7 Reconstruct the area of origin
	4.2.8 Inspect the performance of building systems
	4.2.9 Discriminate the effects of explosions from other types of damage
4.3 Documenting the Scene	**4.3.1** Diagram the scene
	4.3.2 Photographically document the scene
	4.3.3 Construct investigative notes
4.4 Evidence Collection and Preservation	**4.4.1** Utilize proper procedures for managing victims and fatalities
	4.4.2 Locate, collect, and package evidence
	4.4.3 Select evidence for analysis
	4.4.4 Maintain a chain of custody
	4.4.5 Dispose of evidence
4.5 Interview	**4.5.1** Develop an interview plan
	4.5.2 Conduct interviews
	4.5.3 Evaluate interview information

Source: NFPA 1033: Standard for Professional Qualifications for Fire Investigator. Published by National Fire Protection Association (NFPA), © 2014.

determining window and door openings; and conducting a fire engineering analysis for a reconstruction of fire spread. No two fire scenes are ever alike, and no routine can be applied in the same way to each fire.

Table 5-1 summarizes a step-by-step plan in compliance with *NFPA 1033* (NFPA 2014).

5.1 Investigative Information During Suppression

One of the major difficulties of fire investigation is that the fire scene may be accidental, natural, undetermined, or intentional. The ideal crime scene has no personnel present besides the investigator and any co-workers. Fire scenes almost always involve a number of firefighters and their supervisors, onlookers, and the press. Fire is usually detected by an outsider who may compromise what would be considered to be ideal crime scene security right at the outset. A great deal of damage and disorder is caused by the fire and its suppression.

Unlike other crime scenes where a body, a broken window, or a gunshot indicates that a crime has been committed, suspicions of criminal fire activity are often not raised until long after the efforts of suppression. Arson is unique because the crime destroys rather than creates evidence as it progresses. The firefighter's prime responsibility is to protect life and property. Protecting public safety by the detection of criminal activity is secondary to other functions and does not fall within the official purview of the fire service at all in some countries.

5.1.1 RESPONSIBILITY OF THE FIREFIGHTERS

The first person on the scene is the most valuable witness to the nature of the undisturbed scene and the circumstances surrounding it. Line firefighters are often the first independent witnesses at the scene. Investigators can familiarize line firefighters with some aspects of fire investigations and physical evidence. In some progressive jurisdictions, firefighters are instructed that in the event of any suspicious nature of a fire, they are to use extra caution in the suppression, overhaul, and salvage of that fire scene because, if the process is not implemented properly, the fire scene can be compromised.

With the proper precautions, unnecessary damage or disruption may be prevented. For instance, the use of excessive quantities of water at high pressures can flush important evidence away from the scene or can complicate the investigation by causing collapse of plaster and sheetrock, forcing investigators to spend many hours removing pounds of waterlogged plasterboard and fiberglass insulation from the scene. In smaller structures, the use of straight streams of water should be avoided. Fog streams are not only less destructive but usually more effective as a firefighting technique.

Unnecessary structural damage, such as removal or destruction of windows, walls, and doors, should be avoided. The use of straight hose streams to break windows or strip siding off frame buildings may be necessary for suppression, but excessive use is to be strongly discouraged. The use of high-pressure streams inside small buildings can strip interior walls and ceilings of their gypsum board or plaster coverings and destroy invaluable burn patterns on those surfaces. High-pressure streams can also disturb badly burned bodies and destroy the fragile remains of incendiary devices.

Fog or modified fog streams are more effective in most interior attacks and are less destructive. Fire crews have been known to push the walls of buildings into a burning pile to minimize post-fire cleanup, a practice detrimental to the preservation of a fire scene. On many occasions, rapid entry to a fire scene may be gained only by forcible entry; and subsequent requirements to **vent** the scene may result in breakage of windows. Firefighters should mentally note which doors or windows were broken or open as well as those that were locked upon arrival. The recognition of signs of forced entry, such as broken door frames or torn window screens, is also valuable to the investigation. These observations should be related to the investigator.

During the early stages of suppression, firefighters are in the best position to detect possible multiple points of fire origin. The realization that several fires simultaneously established themselves in *separate* areas of a building is an important step in the detection

vent ■ An opening for the passage of, or dissipation of, fluids, such as gases, fumes, smoke, and the like (NFPA 2017, pt. 3.3.198).

of multiple arson sets, a common technique used by fire setters. The fire investigator will be interested in not only the location and extent of the fire but also the direction of suppression efforts, the points at which the fire was attacked, and the manner in which the structure was vented, because all these can affect the fire patterns within. The firefighters should note any unusual flames or smoke colors, odors, and weather conditions (wind direction and intensity, temperature, etc.), and condition (operability) of fire detection and suppression systems in the building.

Smith (1997) has published an excellent in-depth review of firefighters' responsibilities and their important role in successful fire investigation. It is the ultimate responsibility of the fire department to maintain custody and control of the scene until the investigation is complete, even if that entails hiring a private guard.

5.1.2 MINIMIZING POST-FIRE DAMAGE

The primary sources of post-fire damage to the scene are firefighting, overhaul, and salvage operations.

Overhaul

Overhaul of the fire scene includes the removal and destruction of possible pockets of smoldering fire in walls, floors, and upholstered furniture. These overhaul activities should be limited to those necessary to prevent a recurrence of the fire Wallace and DeHaan (2000). The investigator should note the following items:

■ Were walls or floors torn up? If so, what was their condition?
■ Were the rugs in place?
■ Or were the rugs folded up and thrown in a corner?
■ Was the furniture in place?
■ Were the walls and floors intact or had someone removed their covering materials previously?

> **overhaul** ■ A firefighting term involving the process of final extinguishment after the main body of the fire has been knocked down. All traces of fire must be extinguished at this time (NFPA 2017, pt. 3.3.135).

Sometimes, an arsonist will intentionally open ceilings, remove attic access panels, or open holes in fire-resistant plaster or gypsum board walls to expose the internal studding and improve the rate of **fire spread** from room to room. Large items of fire-damaged upholstered furniture, such as sofas and beds, may be removed to the outside of the building during overhaul. The dumping of furniture and contents from a house into a single pile can make the subsequent investigation impossible. When furniture is removed, someone should remember or note the locations from which pieces were removed. When conditions permit, all contents from all the rooms should not be dumped into a single pile, but placed in separate piles with locations established for the contents of each room. Only the minimum amount of overhaul necessary for safety should be allowed until the origin of the fire has been determined.

> **fire spread** ■ The movement of fire from one place to another (NFPA 2017, pt. 3.3.78).

Gasoline-powered fans, pumps, and saws are often used during overhaul. Use of these possible sources of contamination should be restricted to exterior placement and then carefully documented. All fueling of tools should be carried out in an area remote from the fire. Electric or hydraulic tools are preferable if they are available.

Salvage and Security Concerns

During the salvage portion of the fire scene cleanup, owners, tenants, and employees are sometimes allowed to enter the fire scene to remove items of value. The fire official responsible for the scene should not allow any unauthorized persons to enter a fire scene and especially should not allow materials to be removed from the scene until the investigator has had a chance to evaluate those items.

Cases have been reported in which victims returned to the fire scene to pick up some valuables and then proceeded to destroy the evidence of one or more arson sets for which they were responsible. Therefore, fire crews have the best opportunity to detect suspicious circumstances because, on entry, they can be aware of unusual conditions, contents, or fire behavior.

5.2 The Investigation

A fire investigation can begin while the fire is still burning or may not begin until long after suppression due to circumstances of the fire or the resulting criminal or civil litigation. Every fire should be investigated to detect the crime of arson, or to seek out dangerous products or practices to preserve the safety of the community. If feasible, every good fire scene investigation begins with an initial "non-invasive" survey of the scene and its immediate surroundings.

It is vital to the success of the inquiry to remember that the most productive investigation will be done right at the fire scene, regardless of the time sequence of the investigation as related to the fire itself. However useful interviews may be for suggesting lines of inquiry or corroborating conclusions, the irrefutable physical evidence of the fire's origin and cause will be found only by careful examination of the fire scene.

5.2.1 DURING THE FIRE

Whenever possible, it is helpful for the investigator to be present during the fire and its suppression. The region of the structure in which the fire started may be apparent or may be obscured by flames and smoke that prevent close inspection. The investigator can benefit from observing the suppression activities of the firefighters, because these can alter the course and intensity of a fire as well as cause unusual burn patterns. The investigator can also photograph or videotape the sequence of the fire and begin the search for witnesses. Preliminary interviews with witnesses to establish what they saw or heard, and where and when, are an important part of most fire investigations.

The responsibilities of the firefighters to fire investigations go beyond merely extinguishing the fire. Firefighters are often the first witnesses on the scene and have enormous control over the fate of all types of evidence at the scene—from burn patterns, to human remains, to residues of the ignition source. The observations of responding firefighters are often crucial in detecting the origin and causes of fires, particularly when arson is suspected. The National Fire Protection Association (NFPA) booklet, "The Firemen's Responsibility in Arson Detection," summarizes the responsibilities of firefighters (NFPA 1949). See Table 5-2.

5.2.2 IMMEDIATELY AFTER THE FIRE IS EXTINGUISHED

So that access to the scene remains secure, it is important for the investigator to be on the scene of the fire as soon as possible after extinguishment. Although the condition of the hot remains is often not suitable for anything approaching a complete investigation, some exterior surveys may be carried out to identify hazardous areas such as the potential for structural collapse, or chemical or electrical hazards. Fire investigators should follow *NFPA 1033* (NFPA 2014, pt. 4.2.1) in securing the fire scene and pt. 4.2.2 in conducting an exterior survey of the damaged fire scene, whether it is a structure, vehicle, forest, or grassland.

The general consequences of the fire may be more apparent at this time than later when the rubble is cleared out. Because of the large amount of collapsed rubble in some fires, it is virtually impossible to make an examination until some clearing has occurred. In small fires, however, much can be accomplished at this stage, because when the fire is localized, so is the damage, and reasonable access is available. In larger fires, it may be days or months before the completion of the investigation.

TABLE 5-2	Summary Guidance on "The Fireman's Responsibility in Arson Detection" as provided by the National Fire Protection Association (NFPA)
Observing general conditions at the fire in the vicinity of the fire	In the vicinity of the fire ■ Observe the elements ■ Observe persons and automobiles ■ Observe color of smoke and flame, odors prevalent ■ Observe size of fire and speed at which it is traveling Upon arrival ■ Observe the number of separate fires, intensity, and rapidity of spread ■ Observe odors ■ Observe products of combustion
Observing condition of building openings at the time of a fire	■ Find out whether doors and windows are locked ■ Look for evidence of burglary ■ Remember sequence of events
Observing owners, occupants, and bystanders at the time of fire	■ Observe manner of persons at the fire ■ Look for familiar faces
Locating evidence of fire causes	■ Look for indicators of arson intent ■ Look for arson materials and arson equipment
Protecting and preserving evidence of fire causes	■ Protect and guard evidence ■ Identify, preserve, remove, and safeguard evidence
Observing condition of contents of a building involved in a fire	■ Watch for indications of removal of personal property ■ Watch for indications of removal of valuable merchandise
Guard buildings and property involved in a fire	■ Control entrance ■ Accompany persons allowed to enter
Recording and reporting observations made at a fire	■ Provide a suitable notebook ■ Make brief entries
Appearing in court	■ Familiarize yourself with circumstances and conditions ■ Make a creditable appearance ■ Taking the oath and qualifying ■ Show respect, confidence, and a business-like attitude ■ Tell the story as you know it ■ Refer to notes ■ Identify evidence and exhibits

Source: NFPA. 1949. The Firemen's Responsibility in Arson Detection. Quincy, MA: National Fire Protection Association.

SCENE EXAMINATION STANDARD: 4.2.1 *NFPA 1033*, 2014 EDITION

TASK:

Secure the fire ground—given marking devices, sufficient personnel, and special tools and equipment—so that unauthorized persons can recognize the perimeters of the investigative scene and are kept from restricted areas, and all evidence or potential evidence is protected from damage or destruction.

PERFORMANCE OUTCOME:

The investigator will secure the general origin area to protect evidence and restrict access.

CONDITIONS:

Given a fire scene, ribbon or rope, information signs, tape, stapler, and an assistant.

TASK STEPS:

1. Upon arrival, document and record request for investigation, scene arrival information, agencies present, and present and predicted weather conditions
2. Obtain legal authority to inspection and entry
3. Conduct hazard and risk safety assessment of scene
4. Secure and document utilities (electric, gas, alarm systems)
5. Locate general origin area and items of potential evidence
6. Place ribbon or rope around the origin area and/or potential evidence items
7. Post signs and/or a guard outside the ribboned or roped area
8. Prevent unauthorized entry

Source: Derived and updated from Washington State Patrol, Form No. 3000-420-081 (Sept. 2014) Fire Protection Bureau, Standards and Accreditation, Olympia, Washington http://www.wsp.wa.gov/fire/docs/cert/fire_invest.pdf

SCENE EXAMINATION STANDARD: 4.2.2 *NFPA 1033*, 2014 EDITION

TASK:

Conduct an exterior survey, given standard equipment and tools, so that evidence is preserved, fire damage is interpreted, hazards are identified to avoid injuries, accessibility to the property is determined, and all potential means of ingress/egress are discovered.

PERFORMANCE OUTCOME:

Remaining alert for safety hazards, the investigator will conduct a 360-degree exterior survey of the scene. The investigator will identify entry/exit points, items of potential evidence, and post-fire indicators. The investigator will also indicate on a photo log where exterior photos are taken, if any, using the following task steps.

CONDITIONS:

Given a fire scene, a note pad, and a photo log.

TASK STEPS:

1. Locate fire scene
2. Proceed 360 degrees around the scene
3. Enter on the photo log where photos would be taken
4. Ribbon potential evidence items
5. Ribbon or mark entry/exit points
6. Document observations

Source: Derived and updated from Washington State Patrol, Form No. 3000-420-081 (Sept. 2014) Fire Protection Bureau, Standards and Accreditation, Olympia, Washington http://www.wsp.wa.gov/fire/docs/cert/fire_invest.pdf

5.2.3 DURING THE CLEARING OF THE SCENE

It is critical that *overhaul,* the removal of potential seats of smoldering fire for the prevention of rekindles, is kept to an absolute minimum until the investigator arrives and examines the scene. In scenes where there has been a death, overhaul in the vicinity of the body should be strictly limited to dousing of smoldering furnishings with a hand line to prevent reignition.

It is most important for the investigator to be present during cleanup and overhaul to conduct an interior survey in accordance with *NFPA 1033* (NFPA 2014, pt. 4.2.3). During this phase, if not supervised, significant evidence can be destroyed or disturbed, thereby reducing its interpretive value. Problems can be avoided if the investigator is present and able to take the necessary steps to preserve the evidence.

Many fire service personnel are trained to recognize evidence so that they can call the investigator's attention to relevant items as they are found. This interdependence is especially valuable when the investigator cannot supervise all areas of a large fire scene and must rely on capable and trained assistants. When it is necessary to remove furnishings during cleanup, it is critical to document the location of major fuel packages. It was once thought that the only fire patterns of value were on the floors, so all "debris could be shoveled or flushed out leaving a clean scene for the investigator." Wallace and DeHaan (2000) emphasize that it is essential that no debris be removed by fire crews prior to the arrival of fire investigators.

5.2.4 AFTER CLEANUP

After cleanup, the investigator has a chance to examine burn patterns, if they have not been destroyed by the demolition of unsafe portions of the building during cleanup. Dismantling

SCENE EXAMINATION STANDARD: 4.2.3 *NFPA 1033*, 2014 EDITION

TASK:

Conduct an interior survey, given standard equipment and tools, so that areas of potential evidentiary value requiring further examination are identified and preserved, the evidentiary value of contents is determined, and hazards are identified to avoid injuries.

PERFORMANCE OUTCOME:

Remaining alert for safety hazards, the investigator will conduct a 360-degree interior survey of the scene. The investigator will identify entry/exit points, items of potential evidence, and post-fire indicators. The investigator will also indicate on a photo log where interior photos are taken, if any, using the following task steps.

CONDITIONS:

Given a fire scene, a note pad, and a photo log.

TASK STEPS:

1. Locate fire scene
2. Proceed 360 degrees around the scene; observe and document effects of fire
3. Enter on the photo log where photos would be taken
4. Ribbon potential evidence items
5. Ribbon or mark entry/exit points
6. Document observations, including presence or absence of normal building contents

Source: Derived and updated from Washington State Patrol, Form No. 3000-420-081 (Sept. 2014) Fire Protection Bureau, Standards and Accreditation, Olympia, Washington http://www.wsp.wa.gov/fire/docs/cert/fire_invest.pdf

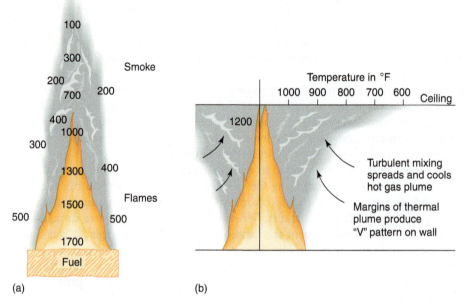

FIGURE 5-1 The fire plume includes both flames and buoyant smoke. The temperature (°F) distribution of gases in the buoyant plume: (a) unrestricted, (b) under ceiling.

and removal of the building (and its contents) should be prohibited, or kept to the minimum required for public safety, until the investigation is completed. The investigator must be thorough even if much of the building has been removed. Rubble or items removed from the structure should not be overlooked because it is possible to recover highly significant evidence from debris. The documentation of the debris' original location will be more difficult.

After extensive demolition or repair, investigation is handicapped to a considerable degree. Often, available photographs or videos can assist in evaluating the limited remains of the fire scene, but they are no substitute for original investigation at the scene. If photographic, diagrammatic, and interview documentation is sufficiently comprehensive, some fires can be reconstructed and accurately investigated long after the fact. But in some cases, if the scene has been extensively cleared, it is not possible to arrive at firm conclusions as to the cause of the fire.

If fire destruction is nearly complete, very little can be done in the way of fire pattern analysis, as depicted in Figure 5-1. Rarely can the investigator hope to prove the use of liquid flammables from the pattern of the fire, and then only when extensive post-flashover burning has not occurred and when the pattern is so distinctive as to leave no doubt as to whether flammables were used. Many investigators are tempted to limit their activities to the questioning of witnesses, almost to the exclusion of examining any physical evidence still remaining. Table 5-1 summarizes guidelines for the systematic examination of a typical structure fire scene.

5.3 Fire Plumes

The single most important factor in fire scene reconstruction is the fire **plume**, the buoyant column of hot gases produced by the combustion of a fuel source emitting a vertical column of flames, hot products of combustion, and smoke rising above a fire (Cox and Chitty 1982; McCaffrey 1979; Beyler 1986; Drysdale 2011). The plume can also be called convection column, thermal updraft, or thermal column (NFPA 2017, pt. 3.3.141), and heat transfer by **convection** plays a large part of the heat transfer by the plume.

plume ■ The column of hot gases, flames, and smoke rising above a fire; also called *convection column, thermal updraft,* or *thermal column* (NFPA 2017, pt. 3.3.141).

convection ■ Heat transfer by circulation within a medium such as a gas or a liquid (NFPA 2017, pt. 3.3.39).

Fire plumes can originate from any fuel combusting that has a sufficient heat release rate to generate a buoyant column of flames and smoke. They can be produced by floor-level pools of ignitable liquids. Many combustible solids, including certain types of foam mattresses and plastics, melt and collapse while burning and behave like liquid fuels. Fire plumes can also result from fuel geometries having multiple vertical and horizontal fuel surfaces, complex internal structures, and varying fuel types. We will treat the effects of fire plumes from a simple flat fuel array as behaving analogously to a pool fire.

The shape of burning pools that produce fire plumes depends on several variables including the geometry of the containment of the pool, the type of substrate on which the pool is resting, and, in some cases, the external winds. Because fire plumes are three-dimensional, their location can often be determined and documented by evaluating the patterns of heat transfer, flame spread, and smoke damage they cause to adjacent flooring, wall, and ceiling surfaces. A fire investigator can gain additional insight through a fundamental understanding of the nature, physics, and heat transfer characteristics of fire plumes, including **radiant heat**. The buoyancy of hot gases is the driving force behind the vertical movement and horizontal spread of fire plumes as they encounter obstacles.

Research with simulated pool fires in compartments shows that plumes lean with dominant air flow from their vertical position when influenced by air movement (Steckler, Quintiere, and Rinkinen 1982). With 55 full-scale steady-state experiments, except for the smallest openings in the compartment, disturbances caused by the incoming air flow behave much like a fire plume exposed to a cross wind.

5.3.1 FIRE PLUME DAMAGE CORRELATIONS

Testing by the FM Global (formerly the Factory Mutual Research Corporation) provided additional insight into the formation of V-patterns. In FM Global's testing, a closer examination of a fire plume's lines of demarcation reveals distinct areas of damage to the wall surfaces, also known as the *fire propagation boundary*. This boundary is a visually distinguishable line where the heavy pyrolysis of the surface ends.

Fire testing by FM Global has documented the close correlation of the fire propagation boundary with the *critical heat flux boundary*, which is where the minimum heat flux is at or below the point at which a **flammable** vapor/air mixture is produced by pyrolysis at the surface of the solid fuel (Tewarson 2008). Critical heat fluxes have also been experimentally determined by successive exposures of material samples to progressively decreasing incident heat fluxes until ignition no longer takes place (Spearpoint and Quintiere 2001).

Figure 5-2 illustrates the close correlation in FM Global's 8-m (25-ft) corner tests of a growing fire peaking at a 3 MW heat release rate (Newman 1993). This test is designed for evaluating fires involving low-density, high–char forming wall and ceiling insulation materials. In this figure, the dashed line and the visual damage evaluation as measured by radiometers attached to the surface indicate the critical heat flux boundary. Note how closely these observations correlate. The position and impact of the fire plume on the walls, ceilings, and surface areas are important to interpreting these correlations correctly when evaluating the various types of fire patterns.

At first, the **soot** and pyrolysis products of the smoke condense on the cooler surfaces, with no chemical or thermal effect. As hot gases from a plume come into contact with the surface, heat is transferred by convective and radiative processes. As the heat is transferred, the temperature of the surface increases. The heat may be conducted into the surface. At some point, the temperature increases to the point at which the surface coating begins to scorch, melt, or pyrolyze. At higher temperatures it may actually ignite. These temperatures are reached when the critical heat flux is reached for that material and sustained for a sufficient time. These observations allow us to characterize patterns as surface deposit only, thermal effect to surface only, charring and ignition, penetration, and consumption.

radiant heat ■ Heat energy carried by electromagnetic waves that are longer than visible light waves and shorter than radio waves; radiant heat (electromagnetic radiation) increases the sensible temperature of any substance capable of absorbing the radiation, especially solid and opaque objects (NFPA 2017, pt. 3.3.152).

flammable ■ Capable of burning with a flame (NFPA 2017, pt. 3.3.83).

soot ■ Black particles of carbon produced in a flame (NFPA 2017, pt. 3.3.173).

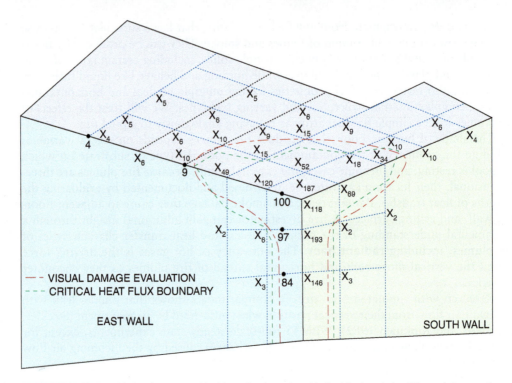

FIGURE 5-2 The correlation between critical heat flux boundary (dashed line) and visual lines of demarcation (dashed-dotted line) in an FM Global 25-ft corner fire test provides a scientific explanation for the formation of V patterns on walls.

Source: SFPE Handbook of Fire Protection Engineering, *3rd ed., 2002, by permission of Society of Fire Protection Engineers.*

When a fire scene is examined, often the only evidence remaining is the fire burn pattern indicators reflecting their thermal impact. In cases where a fire was extinguished quickly by fire suppression or self-extinguished, clearly defined burn patterns from the plume are left on the walls, floors, ceilings, and exterior surfaces of the structure. Many of these patterns are formed by the intersection of fire plumes with structure and other target surfaces.

There are four major types of plumes of interest in fire investigation and reconstruction (Milke and Mowrer 2001):

- axisymmetric
- window
- balcony
- line

Understanding these plume types provide a keener insight into the dynamics of more complex fires. The investigator examining the damage of these plumes must have a working knowledge of their origin, type of fuel package, and ventilation. Furthermore, empirical testing has established mathematical relationships describing the behavior, shape, and impact of these classes of fire plumes.

For a summary of physical-scale fire testing and computer modeling of thermal spill plumes, see the work by Harrison (2004) and later Harrison and Spearpoint (2007) at the University of Canterbury, Christchurch, New Zealand. These reports expand the earlier research by Morgan and Marshall (1975) regarding experimentally based theories on thermal spill plumes used to interpret conditions of smoke production and hazards in covered multilevel shopping malls.

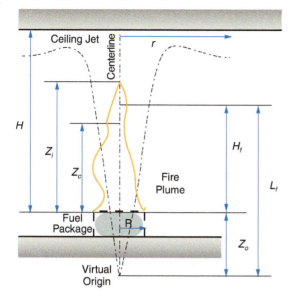

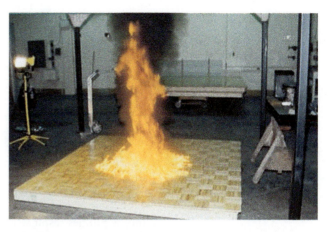

FIGURE 5-3 Schematic diagram of the typical axisymmetric fire plume and its interaction with a ceiling, where Z_0 is the distance from the fuel surface to the virtual origin, H_f is the mean flame height above the fuel surface, Z_c is the continuous flame height above the fuel surface, Z_i is the intermittent flame height above the fuel surface, H is the distance to the ceiling from the fuel surface, R is the radius of the fuel package, and r is the distance of the ceiling jet from the plume centerline. The statistical mean flame height is the portion of luminous flame that is visible during 50 percent of its total exposure time.

FIGURE 5-4 An axisymmetric fire plume under a NIST furniture calorimetry hood during research on flammable and combustible liquid spill and burn patterns. *Courtesy of Putorti, McElroy, and Madrzykowski (2001,15).*

5.3.2 AXISYMMETRIC PLUMES

Axisymmetric plumes have uniform radial distribution from a common vertical plume centerline. Generally, they occur in open areas or near centers of rooms where there is no nearby wall. Much research has been conducted on the correlations of the plume height, temperatures generated, gas velocities, and **entrainment**. Figure 5-3 shows the typical descriptions and measurements used for flame and plume characteristics describing the plume centerline, mean flame height, and virtual origin (Heskestad 2008). These measurements are used in calculations that show relationships of the fire plume with heat release rates, flame height, temperatures, and smoke production.

Figure 5-4 is an example of an axisymmetric fire plume under the NIST furniture calorimetry hood during research on flammable and combustible liquid spill and burn patterns (Putorti, McElroy, and Madrzykowski 2001, 15). These tests provide valuable data on heat release rates as well as on burn patterns on various flooring surfaces.

Plumes occurring near walls and corners do not behave as axisymmetric plumes. Their behavior will be discussed in a later section of this chapter.

5.3.3 WINDOW PLUMES

Plumes that emerge from doors and windows into large open spaces are known as window plumes. See *NFPA 92 NFPA 2015*, pt. 5.5.3, for a more complete description. These plumes emerge from openings during the fire and are commonly ventilation controlled. In Figure 5-5, the plume is emerging from the opening and measures Z_w above the soffit.

entrainment ■ The process of air or gases being drawn into a fire, plume, or jet (NFPA 2017, pt. 3.3.55).

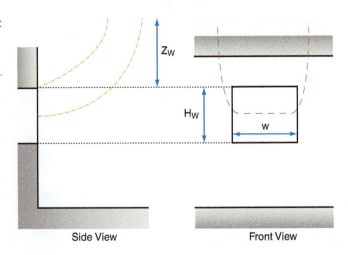

FIGURE 5-5 A schematic diagram of a window plume showing side and front orientations.

Side View

Front View

Window plumes result when the rate at which combustible vapors and gases are produced by pyrolysis inside the room exceeds the rate at which those products can be burned by combining with air entering the room and flow out through openings to burn outside the compartment. Window plumes are often, but not exclusively, associated with post-flashover burning in that room. As such, they may be a visible indicator of a fire's development.

Window plumes can be a major factor in vertical fire spread in multistory buildings, because entrainment can push the plume against combustible siding or spandrel panels or windows of stories above. The building facades above the window sometimes experience very high heat fluxes under such conditions, resulting in rapid failure (DeHaan and Icove 2012).

The area and height of the ventilation openings of window plumes can be used to estimate the maximum heat release rate of the fire in a compartment that is being ventilated by that opening. When a smoke plume is viewed as a window plume, a mathematical relationship based on actual experimental data for wood and polyurethane can be used to predict the maximum heat release rate, assuming that the single opening is ventilating the fire (Orloff, Modale, and Alpert 1977; Tewarson 2008).

Similarly, in the case of window plumes, the mass loss rate can also be determined. *NFPA 92* (NFPA 2015, pt. 5.5.3), uses the following equation for making this determination:

$$\dot{m} = \left[0.68 \left(A_w \sqrt{H_w} \right)^{1/3} (Z_w + a)^{5/3} \right] + 1.59 A_w \sqrt{H_w}, \tag{5.1}$$

where

$\dot{m}$ = mass flow rate at height Z_w (kg/s),
A_w = area of ventilation opening (m^2),
H_w = height of ventilation opening (m),
Z_w = height above the top of the window (m), and
a = $\left(2.40 A_w^{2/5} H_w^{1/5} \right) - 2.1 H_w$(m).

This formula is not valid if the temperature rise above ambient temperature is less than 2.2°C (4°F). But this method for estimating the mass flow rate may be relevant when considering the observations of on-scene eyewitnesses and responding firefighters. For example, the description of the window plume may be sufficient to estimate the extent of the involvement of the fire based on the observed area and height of the ventilation opening.

5.3.4 BALCONY PLUMES

Plumes that emerge under overhangs and from doors are known as balcony spill plumes as described in *NFPA 92* (NFPA 2015, pt. 5.5.3). Balcony spill plumes (Figure 5-6) are characteristic of fires occurring in enclosed rooms and spreading through patio doors or windows to covered porches, patios, or balconies. The buoyancy of product of combustion causes them to flow along the underside of horizontal surfaces until they can rise vertically.

The pattern of thermal damage or smoke damage to the underside of horizontal surfaces may be used to estimate the dimensions of the plume. The plume spreads laterally as it flows. The width of the plume is estimated by recreating the horizontal and vertical dimensions of its contact area such that

$$W = w + b, \tag{5.2}$$

where

  W = maximum width of the plume (m),
  w = width of the opening from the area of origin to the balcony (m), and
  b = distance from the opening to the balcony edge (m).

This calculation has been used in estimating the width and height of the fire plume to assess its smoke production. Locations of balcony plumes include exterior doors leading to garden apartments, internal hotel rooms in atrium-style buildings, multistory shopping malls, and multiple-level prison cells that face catwalks.

The characteristic of a balcony plume is that flames are deflected from the upper floor by the external overhang, or by an open porch or deck in an apartment or condominium. The overhang is an example of the use of passive fire engineering in building construction to reduce the chance that external plumes will spread fires to floors above the floor of fire origin by preventing re-entrainment against the building.

Figure 5-7 shows an example of a window plume coming into exterior contact with a porch overhang, creating a situation similar to a balcony spill. As the plume exits the window, it travels along the ceiling of the porch overhang, and flames are projected from the edge of the overhang by their buoyant momentum. This scenario is common in residential fires, particularly when the dwelling has a porch or a deck.

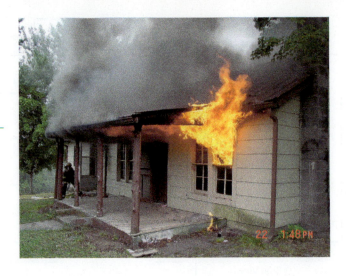

5.3.5 LINE PLUMES

Line plumes (Figure 5-8) have elongated geometric shapes that produce narrow, thin, shallow plumes. The relationship of the heat release rate to the flame height is described in a later section. A line plume can be used to describe a flame plume whose length is many times greater than its width.

Possible scenarios for line plumes include exterior fires in ditches where spilled ignitable liquids collect and ignite, a row of townhouses, a long sofa, the advancing front of a forest fire, flame spread over flammable wall linings, and even a balcony spill plume (Quintiere and Grove 1998). Line plumes can also be used to approximate elongated fires in open areas of atria or warehouses.

The relationship of the heat release rate to the flame height for line plumes (Figure 5-8), where $B > 3A$, is described next. For flame plume heights greater than five

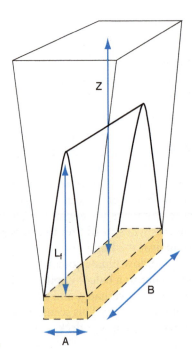

FIGURE 5-8 Illustration of a line source plume.

times the B measurement in Figure 5-8, the line plume more closely resembles an axisymmetric plume (Hasemi and Nishihata 1989):

$$L_f = 0.035\left(\frac{\dot{Q}}{B}\right)^{2/3} \quad \text{for} \quad B > 3A;$$

(5.3)

$$\dot{m} = 0.21z\left(\frac{\dot{Q}}{B}\right)^{2/3} \quad \text{for} \quad B < 3A \quad \text{and} \quad L < z < 5B,$$

(5.4)

where

L_f = flame height (m),
$\dot{Q}$ = heat release rate (kW),
A = shorter side of line plume base (m),
B = longer side of line plume base (m),
$\dot{z}$ = mass flow rate (kg/s), and
z = ceiling height above fuel (m).

The entrainment of air around a long line plume can be envisioned as air coming from two opposite sides of an axisymmetric plume. It has been modeled in a theoretical study by Quintiere and Grove (1998). For a wall fire where the flame is against a vertical, noncombustible wall, the entrainment is from one side only. If the $\dot{Q}$ for an equivalent fuel surface can be calculated, the $\dot{Q}$ (heat release rate per unit length of line) can be calculated from the ratio $\dot{Q}/B$.

The *Fire Protection Handbook* (SFPE 2008) gives the relationships

$$L_f = 0.017\dot{Q}^{2/3} \quad \text{for line fire plumes;}$$

$$L_f = 0.034\dot{Q}^{3/4} \quad \text{for wall fire plumes.}$$

5.3.6 AXISYMMETRIC FIRE PLUME CALCULATIONS

Investigators can benefit from information on fire plumes, which are merely the physical manifestations of the combustion process. Sound scientific and engineering principles, based on a combination of theoretical and actual fire testing data, describe fire plume behavior.

Information on fire plume behavior is expressed in terms of five basic calculated measurements often used in hazard and risk analysis (SFPE 2008). They model the following fire plume characteristics:

- Equivalent fire diameter
- Virtual origin
- Flame height
- Plume centerline temperatures and velocities
- Plume air entrainment

These basic characteristics constitute the bare minimum information needed for fire scene reconstruction. Several common equations for performing a fire engineering analysis of fire plumes rely on the energy or heat release rate and provide answers to the questions: How tall was the fire plume? What was the placement of the virtual source in relation to the floor? What was the depth of the burning flammable liquid pool?

A fire investigator must be able to use these calculations in applying basic fire science and engineering concepts. These calculations are essential in evaluating the various working hypotheses, such as the amount of fuel burned, the fire's time duration, and the impact of ventilation of the room of origin.

Many of these calculations are found in the various fire modeling software tools, such as FPETool and CFAST. The calculations are briefly explained here to demonstrate their underlying concepts and potential applications.

Equivalent Fire Diameter

In calculations of the flame height for fire plumes, the base of the fire is assumed to be circular. This is normally not the case when ignitable liquids are spilled onto a floor or when the fuel package is rectangular in shape. In these cases, the equivalent diameter must be calculated. For circular areas ($A = \pi r^2$, where $r = D/2$), the basic relationship is

$$D = \sqrt{\frac{4A}{\pi}}, \tag{5.5}$$

where

D = equivalent diameter (m),
A = total area of burning fuel package (m^2), and
π = 3.1416.

Areas of irregular pools can be calculated by recreating the shape and size of pools from fire scene photos and obtaining dimensions from fire scene notes and duplicating the shapes on paper cutouts. The cutouts can then be weighed using a postal scale and the area determined from the weight of a reference paper sample of known area. Areas can also be recreated from photogrammetry of the fire scene photos.

Investigators should be aware that the heat release rate of a smoke spill plume is much less than that of the plume emitted by a burning liquid pool of significant depth. This aspect will affect both the heat release rate and flame heights. For a detailed discussion on the fire forensics aspects and analysis of liquid fuel fires, see research by Putorti, McElroy, and Madrzykowski (2001) and Mealy, Benfer, and Gottuk (2011).

Rectangular contained spills include those produced when an oil-filled electric transformer or storage tank is compromised and spills its contents into a rectangular diked area and ignites. It is then necessary to determine the diameter of a circle containing the same area as the rectangular spill, using the aspect ratio of the spill (Figure 5-9).

The *aspect ratio* is the width-to-length ratio of the spill area. The equivalent diameter relationship generally holds true for pools with an aspect ratio ≤2.5. Aspect ratios >2.5, such as would be seen with trench or line fires, utilize other models (Beyler 2008).

In cases of short-duration fires, the area of a liquid fuel spill can be measured directly from the burned areas of the floor or covering. In post-flashover or prolonged fires where the floor covering is readily combustible, the fire-damaged areas may extend well beyond the margins of the original pool and are therefore not a reliable guideline.

Putorti, McElroy, and Madrzykowski (2001) addressed the relationship among surface area, volume of liquid, and type of surface that controls the equivalent depth of the pool. Mealy, Benfer, and Gottuk (2011) explored the forensic aspects through tests that provided insight into the differences in fire dynamics between pool and spill fires

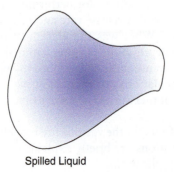
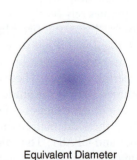

FIGURE 5-9 The equivalent-diameter concept used in estimating the diameter of a circle that represents the same area as a noncircular spill pattern.

Spilled Liquid   Equivalent Diameter

(i.e., thick and thin fuel depths). They provided a methodology by which liquid fuel fire events can be assessed and identified forensic indicators that can be used in the analysis of liquid fuel fire events.

Mealy, Benfer, and Gottuk (2011) confirmed that for spills on nonporous surfaces such as sealed concrete, the depth of a freestanding pool of gasoline is about 1 mm (1×10^{-3} m). The area (m^2) is then calculated by dividing the volume of the spilled liquid (m^3) by the depth (m), where

$$\text{Area (m}^2) = \frac{\text{Volume (m}^3)}{\text{Depth (m)}}. \tag{5.6}$$

For conversion of units, 1 liter (L) = 10^{-3} m^3.

On semi-porous surfaces such as wood, the equivalent depth is 2 to 3 mm (2–3 $\times 10^{-3}$ m). On porous surfaces such as carpet, the maximum depth will be the thickness of the carpet, assuming full saturation of the carpet.

EXAMPLE 5-1 ■ Equivalent Fire Diameter

Problem. A container filled with 3.8 L (1 gal or 3800 cm^3) of gasoline is accidentally tipped over onto an enclosed patio of sealed concrete. The depth of the spilled pool is 1 mm. Calculate the (1) coverage area and (2) equivalent diameter of a circle of the same area.

Suggested Solution.

$$\text{Area of spill} = \frac{\text{Volume of liquid}}{\text{Depth of pool}} = \frac{3800 \text{ cm}^3}{0.1 \text{ cm}} = 38{,}000 \text{ cm}^2 = 3.8 \text{ m}^2$$

The equivalent diameter D then is

Equivalent diameter	$D = \sqrt{4A/\pi}$
Total surface area	$A = 3.8 \text{ m}^2$
Constant	$\pi = 3.1416$
Equivalent diameter	$D = \sqrt{(4)(3.8)/3.1416} = 2.2 \text{ m}$

Virtual Origin

As shown in Figure 5-3, the *virtual origin* represents the actual fire as a point source. Its location is a point along the fire plume centerline where flames appear to originate, measured from the top burning surface of the fuel package. Identifying the virtual origin is helpful when evaluating the exposure of other targets fuels in the room to the fire. The investigator may need to make several assumptions depending on the distance to the target and the size of the burning fuel surface.

The virtual origin can be mathematically calculated, and its location can be helpful in reconstructing and documenting the fire's virtual source, point of origin, area, and direction of travel. The virtual origin is also used in some calculations for the measurement of the fire plume flame height.

The virtual origin, Z_0, is calculated from the *Heskestad equation* (1982, 1983):

$$Z_0 = 0.083\dot{Q}^{2/5} - 1.02D, \tag{5.7}$$

where

Z_0 = virtual origin (m),
$\dot{Q}$ = total heat release rate (kW), and
D = equivalent diameter,

for the conditions

$$T_{amb} = 293 \ K, \ (20°C, 68°F),$$
$$P_{atm} = 101.325 \ kPa \text{ (standard temperature and pressure), and}$$
$$D \ \leq 100 \text{ m (328 ft).}$$

The virtual origin, depending on the equivalent diameter and the total heat release rate, may fall above or below the fuel's surface. This placement depends primarily on the heat release rate and effective diameter of the fuel. The resulting value can then be used in equations and models of other fire plume relationships.

Small-diameter ignitable liquid spills are more likely to exhibit virtual origins above the fuel surface. Inspection of equation (5.7) reveals that the smaller the value of the fire's equivalent diameter, D, and/or the larger the value of the heat release rate, $\dot{Q}$, the greater the chance for a positive virtual origin, Z_0, that is, above the fire surface. Because not all fires burn at floor level, the concept of Z_0 is useful in estimating the effective origin of the fire plume in relation to the fuel surface and the compartment.

EXAMPLE 5-2 ■ Virtual Origin

Problem. A fire starts in a wastepaper basket filled with papers and quickly reaches a steady-state heat release rate of 100 kW. The basket measures 0.305 m (1 ft) in diameter. Determine the virtual origin of this plume using the Heskestad equation.

Suggested Solution. Use the equation for the virtual origin.

Virtual origin	$Z_0 = 0.083\dot{Q}^{2/5} - 1.02D$
Equivalent diameter	$D = 0.305$ m
Total heat release rate	$\dot{Q} = 100$ kW
Virtual origin	$Z_0 = (0.083)(100)^{2/5} - (1.02)(0.305)$
	$= 0.524 - 0.311 = 0.213$ m (0.698 ft, or 8.9 in.)

In this case the virtual origin is a positive number, indicating that it is above the surface of the fuel. If the same fuel were spread out over the floor such that its equivalent diameter was 1.0 m while its $\dot{Q}$ remained 100 kW, its virtual origin would be $Z_0 = -0.5$ m (1.64 ft, or 19.7 in., below the floor). This means that the impact of the fire on the room would be as if the fire were burning farther away from the ceiling.

Discussion. If the trash can were filled with gasoline and $\dot{Q} = 500$ kW, recalculate the virtual origin. What can you assume about the virtual origin when the heat release rate is raised?

Flame Height

Flames from plumes represent the visible portion of a fire's combustion process. They are visible owing to the luminosity of heated soot particles and pyrolysis products. The buoyancy of these fire gases allows a fire plume to rise vertically. The height of the flames is described by several terms, including continuous, intermittent, and average.

Knowing the flame height and the approximate duration of the fire allows the investigator to examine and confirm what potential damage can be expected based on heat transfer to the ceiling, walls, flooring, and nearby objects. Several equations, based on fitting regression formulas to actual fire testing, are used to estimate the flame height. As with all these equations, users are cautioned that the equations are bounded by the limitations of the testing.

Flames from burning fuels, especially pool fires, fluctuate in height. Researchers typically define flame height as the distance above the burning fuel surface at which the flame tip is observed at least 50 percent of the time. Zukoski, Cetegen, and Kubota (1985), in defining the mean flame height, examined the intermittent flame, the fraction of the time the flame is 0.5 times above a certain height. Audouin et al. (1995) defined in an analysis similar to Zukoski's that the continuous and intermittent flame heights were greater than 0.95 and less than 0.05 times, respectively. Stratton (2005) described a method to measure these heights, as well as the flame's pulsation frequency, from a three-dimensional cloud captured on video.

Within the flaming region, the two McCaffrey flame height measurements (McCaffrey 1979) along the centerline are depicted as continuous, Z_c, and intermittent, Z_i:

$$Z_c = 0.08\dot{Q}^{2/5}, \tag{5.8}$$

$$Z_i = 0.20\dot{Q}^{2/5}, \tag{5.9}$$

where

Z_c = continuous flame height (m),
Z_i = intermittent flame height (m), and
$\dot{Q}$ = heat release rate (kW).

Crude estimates of heat release rates based upon estimates of the flame heights made by witnesses and responding firefighters can be drawn by algebraically rearranging the McCaffrey flame height equation for intermittent flame heights:

$$\dot{Q} = 56.0Z_i^{5/2}. \tag{5.10}$$

EXAMPLE 5-3 ■ Flame Height: McCaffrey Method

Problem. For Example 5-2 involving the 100 kW wastepaper basket fire, determine the continuous and intermittent flame heights using the McCaffrey method.

Suggested Solution. Use the equation for the McCaffrey method.

Heat release rate $\qquad\qquad \dot{Q} = 100\,\text{kW}$

Continuous flame height $\quad Z_c = 0.08\,\dot{Q}^{2/5} = (0.08)(100)^{2/5}$
$$= 0.505\,\text{m (1.66ft)}$$

Intermittent flame height $\quad Z_i = 0.20\,\dot{Q}^{2/5} = (0.20)(100)^{2/5}$
$$= 1.26\,\text{m(4.1ft) above the fuel surface}$$

EXAMPLE 5-4 ■ Heat Release Rate from Flame Height: McCaffrey Method

Problem. A witness to an accident involving an overturned lawn mower sees the gasoline ignite and burn, forming an axisymmetric fire plume. He observes intermittent flames reaching 3 m (9.84 ft) into the air from the ground. Estimate the heat release rate, $\dot{Q}$, given off by the burning fuel spill.

Suggested Solution. Use the equation for the McCaffrey method.

General equation $\qquad\qquad Z_i = 0.20\,\dot{Q}^{2/5}$

Intermittent flame height $\qquad Z_i = 3.0\,\text{m}$

Estimated heat release rate $\quad \dot{Q} = 56.0\,Z_i^{2/5}$
$$= (56.0)(3.0)^{2/5} = 873\,\text{kW}$$

A practical estimate would be 800 to 900 kW.

EXAMPLE 5-5 ■ Calculating the Area of a Pool Fire

Problem. Calculate the area of the pool fire at 873 kW from Example 5-4.

Suggested Solution. Use the equation for the heat release rate.

General equation $\qquad\qquad\qquad\qquad \dot{Q} = \dot{m}'' \Delta h_c A$

Heat release rate $\qquad\qquad\qquad\qquad \dot{Q} = 873 \text{ kW}$

Mass burning rate per unit area $\qquad \dot{m}'' = 53 g/(m^2 \cdot s)$

Heat combustion $\qquad\qquad\qquad \Delta h_{eff} = 43.7 \text{ kJ/g}$

Area of pool fire $\qquad\qquad\qquad A = \dot{Q}/(\dot{m}'' \Delta h_c) = 873/[(53)(43.7)]$

$\qquad\qquad\qquad\qquad\qquad\qquad = 0.38 \text{ m}^2 (4.1 \text{ ft}^2)$

One assessment of the flame height is its statistical mean flame height, which is the portion of luminous flame that is visible during 50 percent of its total exposure time. When the human eye observes a pulsating flame, it tends to interpolate the variations into a rough approximation of the mean flame height.

A good estimate of the mean or average flame height, L_f, uses the *Heskestad equation*:

$$L_f = 0.235 \, \dot{Q}^{2/5} - 1.02D, \qquad\qquad (5.11)$$

where

D = effective diameter (m),
$\dot{Q}$ = total heat release rate (kW), and
$L_f = Z + Z_0$ = mean flame height above the virtual origin (m).

This equation includes a diameter term, accounting for the effects of large-diameter fuels on the visible flame. The larger the size of the burning fuel area, the lower the flames will be for the same heat release rate.

EXAMPLE 5-6 ■ Flame Height: Heskestad Method

Problem. From Example 5-2 involving the 100 kW wastepaper basket fire, determine the mean flame height, L_f, above the virtual origin, Z_0.

Suggested Solution. Use equation (5.11) for calculating the mean or average flame height.

Mean flame height $\qquad L_f = 0.235 \, \dot{Q}^{2/5} - 1.02D$

Diameter of basket $\qquad D = 0.305 \text{ m}$

Total heat release rate $\quad \dot{Q} = 100 \text{ kW}$

Mean flame height $\qquad L_f = 0.235 \, \dot{Q}^{2/5} - 1.02D$

$\qquad\qquad\qquad\qquad = (0.235)(100)^{2/5} - (1.0)(0.305)$

$\qquad\qquad\qquad\qquad = 1.17 \text{ m } (3.84 \text{ ft}) \text{ above the virtual origin } (3 \text{ to } 4 \text{ ft})$

The virtual origin from Example 5-2 was about 0.2 m above the fuel surface.

Entrainment Effects

When a fire is burning in the center of a room, the buoyant upward flow of the fire gases drags fresh room air into contact with it. This process, called entrainment because surrounding cooler air is mixed or entrained into the upward plume flow, changes the plume's temperature, velocity, and diameter above the fuel source. Entrainment reduces the plume temperature and increases its width.

If there is a horizontal ceiling and the fire plume reaches this height, the plume hits the ceiling and flows horizontally, forming what is called a **ceiling jet**. In this case ceiling entrainment also takes place (Babrauskas 1980).

When some of the heat is transferred to the air and is removed by convective processes, there usually is turbulent mixing that dilutes the rising column of hot gases and cools it further. Looking down on the fire plume from above, as in Figure 5-10a, we can see that the inward air currents are roughly equal around the entire perimeter, so the plume remains symmetrical and upright.

If the fire is against a wall, it cannot draw room air into itself equally from all sides, so the air being drawn from the free side acts like a draft to force the plume sideways against the wall as shown in Figures 5-10b and c. The entrainment reduced by 50 percent means that less cooling air is brought in, slowing the cooling process. Thus, the gases have more time to rise farther, stretching out the flame. This process can occur on nearby wall surfaces even if they are not vertical. This mechanism is responsible for external flame spread between floors of modern high-rise buildings.

When the windows of the room first involved fail, the plume exits the building and then entrains itself against the side of the building, as shown in Figure 5-10d. The windows and spandrel panels of the floors above are then exposed to the radiant and convective heat transfer ($>50 \text{ kW/m}^2$) of the plume and quickly fail, allowing the flames to enter the floor above and ignite the contents of that floor. If there is not sufficient fire protection to suppress this newly ignited fire, then fire can leapfrog up the building. In buildings with a ledge or balcony at each floor level, the plume is directed away from the side of the building, so it never gets a chance to attach to the facade. The chances of ignition by window failure of the floors above are much reduced by a ledge flame-guard effect, compared with a (sheer) curtain wall design.

If the fire occurs in a corner, the perimeter through which cooling air can be drawn is reduced to one-fourth its original size (there is still plenty of air reaching the combustion

ceiling jet ■ A relatively thin layer of flowing hot gases that develops under a horizontal surface (e.g., ceiling) as a result of plume impingement and the flowing gas being forced to move horizontally (NFPA 2017, pt. 3.3.26).

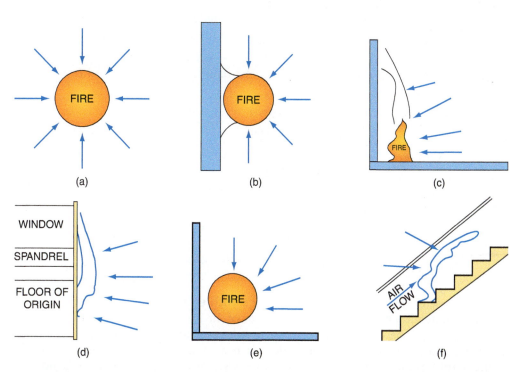

FIGURE 5-10 (a) Entrained air flow for an axisymmetric plume, from above; (b) entrainment in wall configuration; (c) side view; (d) typical high-rise fire plume; (e) entrainment in corner fire; (f) trench effect, side view.

zone, so the fire continues to burn at the same rate as represented in Figure 5-10e). In a corner, the gases cool even more slowly and have even more time to rise before cooling to the point at which they are no longer incandescent (500°C), and the visible flame becomes even taller. This effect is enhanced by the increased radiant heat that reaches the fuel surface after being reflected off the nearby wall or corner surfaces, thus increasing the heat release rate.

Because a nearby wall or corner reduces the cooling entrainment of room air into the rising plume and increases radiant heat feedback to the burning fuel, the height of the visible flame can be affected. In its 2004 edition, *NFPA 921* (NFPA 2004) listed relationships that are very useful to investigators and have been subjected to numerous studies and tests for determining the mean flame height near walls (Alpert and Ward 1984). These relationships are as follows:

$$H_f = 0.174 \, (k\dot{Q})^{2/5}, \tag{5.12}$$

$$\dot{Q} = \frac{79.18 H_f^{5/2}}{k}, \tag{5.13}$$

where

H_f = flame height (m),

$\dot{Q}$ = heat release rate (kW), and

k = wall effect factor, with

k = 1: no nearby walls,

k = 2: fuel package at wall, and

k = 4: fuel package in corner.

EXAMPLE 5-7 ■ Flame Height: NFPA 921 Method

Problem. Using Example 5-2 involving the 100 kW wastepaper basket fire, estimate the height of the flame in three configurations—in the middle of the room, near a wall, and near a corner. Assume that this is an unconstrained fire burning in a large room with no ventilation constraints.

Suggested Solution. From equation (5.12), the flame height H_f measured from the top of the fuel surface is as follows:

Total heat release rate	$\dot{Q} = 100 \text{ kW}$
Flame height	$H_f = 0.174(k\dot{Q})^{2/5}$
No nearby walls ($k = 1$)	$H_f = (0.174)(1 \times 100)^{2/5}$
	$\quad = (0.174)(100)^{0.4} = 1.10 \text{ m (3.61 ft)}$
Near a wall ($k = 2$)	$H_f = (0.174)(2 \times 100)^{2/5}$
	$\quad = 1.45 \text{ m (4.376 ft)}$
In a corner ($k = 4$)	$H_f = (0.174)(4 \times 100)^{2/5}$
	$\quad = 1.91 \text{ m (6.27 ft)}$

---

trench effect ■ A phenomenon, also known as the Coanda effect, in which there is the tendency of a fast-moving stream of air to deflect itself toward and along nearby surfaces.

A special case of this phenomenon called the **trench effect**, also known as the *Coanda effect*, is the tendency of a fast-moving stream of air to deflect itself toward and along nearby surfaces. The trench effect can occur wherever a fire starts on the floor of an inclined surface with walls on both sides, such as a stairway or escalator (shown in Figure 5-10f). In this case, the flow of the air drawn into the fire from below is aided by the confinement of the buoyant flow. When the fire reaches a critical size (i.e., a critical airflow), the plume lies down in the trench and is stretched out by the directional entrainment. If the floor and/or walls of the trench are combustible, they ignite, and the fire can spread the length of the stairway very quickly.

The trench effect was the mechanism that drove a small fire on the floor of an all-wood escalator in London's King's Cross underground station in 1987 to develop quickly into a massive fireball that engulfed the large ticket hall at the top of the escalator (Moodie and Jagger 1992). Further research by Edinburgh University identified four factors relating to the conditions that produce the trench effect: (1) the slope of the trench, (2) its geometric profile, (3) the combustible construction material, and (4) the fire ignition source (Wu and Drysdale 1996). Researchers determined that the critical angle above horizontal is 21° for a large trench and 26° for a small trench.

Plume Centerline Temperatures and Velocities

The temperature distribution along the centerline of a typical plume is represented in Figure 5-11a, and the temperature distribution along a horizontal cross section through the flames is represented in Figure 5-11b. Estimates of the centerline maximum temperature rise, velocity, and mass flow rate of a plume are useful in determining the impact of the fire plume in compartment fires. This impact includes the maximum effect of the plume as it is rising to the ceiling and may come into contact with other fuel packages. There are several formulas for estimating these values.

The *Heskestad method* (Heskestad 1982, 1983) used for estimating the centerline maximum temperature rise, velocity, and mass flow rate of a plume is

$$T_0 - T_\infty = 25 \left[\frac{\dot{Q}_c^{2/5}}{(Z - Z_0)} \right]^{5/3}, \tag{5.14}$$

$$U_0 = 1.0 \left[\frac{\dot{Q}_c}{(Z - Z_0)} \right]^{1/3}, \tag{5.15}$$

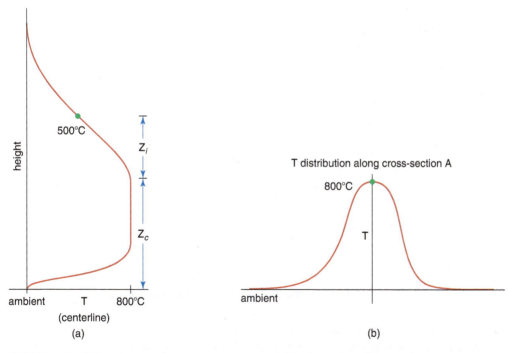

FIGURE 5-11 (a) Plot of average flame temperature versus height shows the uniform maximum temperature in the center of the continuous flame zone and the decreasing average flame temperature in the intermittent region. (b) Plot of average flame temperature versus horizontal position shows the maximum temperature at the axis of the flame plume.

$$\dot{m} = 0.0056\dot{Q}_c\frac{Z}{L_f} \quad \text{for} \quad Z < L_f \tag{5.16}$$

(i.e., for points within the flame plume),
where

$$\dot{Q}_c = 0.6\dot{Q} \quad \text{to} \quad \dot{Q}_c = 0.8\dot{Q}. \tag{5.17}$$

The *McCaffrey method* (McCaffrey 1979) for estimating the centerline maximum temperature rise, velocity, and mass flow rate of a plume is

$$T_0 - T_\infty = 21.6\,\dot{Q}^{2/3}Z^{-5/2}, \tag{5.18}$$

$$U_0 = 1.17\,\dot{Q}Z^{-1/3}, \tag{5.19}$$

$$\dot{m}_p = 0.076\,\dot{Q}^{0.24}Z^{1.895}. \tag{5.20}$$

An alternative method for estimating the maximum temperature rise and velocity of a plume is *Alpert* (Alpert 1972)

$$T_0 - T_\infty = \frac{16.9\,\dot{Q}^{2/3}}{H^{5/3}} \quad \text{for} \quad \frac{r}{H} \leq 0.18, \tag{5.21}$$

$$T_0 - T_\infty = \frac{5.38\,(\dot{Q}/r)^{2/3}}{H^{5/3}} \quad \text{for} \quad \frac{r}{H} > 0.18, \tag{5.22}$$

$$U = 0.96\frac{\dot{Q}^{1/3}}{H} \quad \text{for} \quad \frac{r}{H} \leq 0.15, \tag{5.23}$$

$$U = \frac{0.195\,\dot{Q}^{1/3}H^{1/2}}{r^{5/6}} \quad \text{for} \quad \frac{r}{H} > 0.15, \tag{5.24}$$

where

T_0 = maximum ceiling temperature (°C),
T_∞ = ambient air temperature (°C),
$\dot{Q}$ = total heat release rate (kW),
$\dot{Q}_c$ = convective heat release rate (kW),
Z = flame height along the centerline (m),
Z_0 = distance to the virtual origin (m),
$L_f = Z + Z_0$,
$\dot{m}_p$ = total plume mass flow rate (kg/s),
r = radial distance from the plume centerline (m),
H = ceiling height (m),
U = maximum ceiling jet velocity (m/s), and
U_0 = centerline plume velocity (m/s).

EXAMPLE 5-8 ■ Plume Temperature, Velocity, and Mass Flow Rate at Ceiling Level: McCaffrey Method

Problem. A fire is discovered in a wastepaper basket in a room that has a ceiling height of 2.44 m (8 ft). The heat release rate estimate is 100 kW. Assume that the ambient air temperature is 20°C (68°F). Estimate the plume temperature, velocity, and mass flow rate at the ceiling using the McCaffrey method. (The proper approach is to measure the distance from the top of the fuel source or the lowest point where the fuel can entrain air. You may want to consider subtracting the height of the wastepaper basket from the ceiling height.)

Suggested Solution. Use the McCaffrey equation.

Maximum plume ceiling temperature
$$T_0 = 21.6\,\dot{Q}^{2/3}Z^{-5/2} + T_\infty$$
$$= (21.6)(100)^{2/3}(2.44)^{-5/2} + 20 = 68.5°C$$

Centerline plume velocity
$$U_0 = 1.17\,\dot{Q}^{1/3}Z^{-1/3}$$
$$= (1.17)(100)^{1/3}(2.44)^{-1/3} = 4.033 \text{ m/s}$$

Plume mass flow rate
$$\dot{m}_p = 0.076\dot{Q}^{0.24}Z^{1.895}$$
$$= (0.076)(100)^{0.24}(2.44)^{1.895} = 1.244 \text{ kg/s}$$

Discussion. In Example 5-2, the calculated virtual origin, Z_0, was 0.213 m (0.698 ft) above the burning fuel surface. Solve this same problem using the methods of Heskestad and Alpert.

Smoke Production Rates

During a fire, the smoke production within a building can expose people and property to smoke, toxic gases, and flames. The spread of fire and smoke can also cause a significant amount of property damage, including the disruption of electronic equipment by deposits of soot on circuitry (Tanaka, Nowlen, and Anderson 1996). The smoke production rate is estimated to be close to twice that of the mass flow rate of gas produced by a fire plume. This assumption is based on the theory that the amount of air entrained into the rising plume equals the amount of smoke-filled gas (NFPA 2008, sec. 11, chap. 10).

In the *Zukoski method* (Zukoski 1978) for determining smoke production rates, the equation for estimating the rate of the plume mass flow above the flame at 20°C (68°F) is

$$\dot{m}_s = 0.065\,\dot{Q}^{1/3}\,Y^{5/3}, \tag{5.25}$$

where

$\dot{m}_s$ = plume mass flow rate (kg/s),

$\dot{Q}$ = total heat release rate (kW), and

Y = distance from virtual point source to bottom of smoke layer (m).

The best correlations to this theory are found in cases involving simple circular equivalent pool fires and in which the enclosure has ventilation in the lower layer.

Enclosure Smoke Filling

When smoke from a fire accumulates within an enclosure or compartment, it tends to rise to the ceiling. This accumulation or enclosure smoke-filling rate depends on the amount of smoke being produced by the fire and its ability to escape through vents within the compartment. As the smoke accumulates, a layer forms and descends toward the floor of the compartment.

The enclosure smoke-filling rate is important when estimating how much smoke accumulated below the ceiling. Factors contributing to how fast smoke stratifies and descends from the ceiling relate primarily to the amount of smoke produced and the size and location of smoke vents. Fire investigators finding a room with smoke stratification deposits evenly distributed in an enclosed room may find this evidence important when later determining the fire duration or the smoke exposure a victim might have encountered at a particular time. This research supports that at the time of the fire the level of the smoke in the room corresponds to smoke stratification deposits. It would not be unusual for smoke to fill the room, but the stratification deposits might be limited to 1.22 m (4 ft) down from the ceiling.

The relationship for the descent of this upper layer in a closed room is expressed as:

$$U_t = \frac{\dot{m}_s}{\rho_l A_r}, \tag{5.26}$$

where

U_t = rate of layer descent (m/s),

$\dot{m}_s$ = plume mass flow rate (kg/s),

ρ_l = density of the upper gas layer (kg/m^3), and

A_r = enclosure floor area (m^2).

The density of smoke varies inversely with temperature but is conservatively estimated to be the same as air at standard temperature and pressure (STP; 1.22 kg/m^3).

EXAMPLE 5-9 ■ Smoke Filling

Problem. The 100 kW fire discovered in a wastepaper basket in the previous example is in a closed room that has a ceiling height of 2.44 m (8 ft). The room measures 2.44 m (8 ft) square. Estimate the enclosure smoke-filling rate for this fire.

Suggested Solution. Use the data previously calculated using the McCaffrey method. Assume the lower limit of the velocity of descent by using the ambient density of air as 1.22 kg/m^3, and 17°C.

Rate of layer descent	$U_t = \dfrac{\dot{m}_s}{\rho_l A_p}$
Mass rate of smoke production	$\dot{m}_s = 1.244$ kg/s
Density of upper gas layer	$\rho_l = 1.22$ kg/m^3
Enclosure floor area	$A = (2.44)(2.44) = 5.95$ m^2
Rate of layer descent	$U_t = (1.244)/(1.22)(5.95) = 0.171$ m/s

---

5.4 Fire Patterns and Analysis

The ability to interpret and document fire patterns accurately is essential to investigators reconstructing fire scenes, per *NFPA 1033* (NFPA 2014, pt. 4.2.4). Fire patterns are often the only visible evidence remaining after a fire is extinguished. Smoke deposits, heat transfer, and flame spread are the major causes of change to the exposed surfaces and appearance of materials during a fire. Fire patterns are formed by the heating effects of fire plumes on exposed solid surfaces such as floors, ceilings, and walls. These burn patterns are influenced by a number of variables including the available fuel load, ventilation, and the physical configurations of the room. Many common combustible materials and ignitable liquids can produce these fire plumes and the resulting fire patterns.

5.4.1 TYPOLOGY

When reconstructing fire scenes, skilled fire investigators use numerous indicators to estimate the areas and points of origin, distribution, and behavior of a fire such as direction of spread. As seen in Table 5-3 these indicators, called fire patterns, are characteristically broken down into five major groupings: (1) demarcations, (2) surface effects, (3) penetrations, (4) loss of material, and (5) victim injuries. Some specific patterns are illustrated in Figure 5-12.

fire effects ■ The observable or measurable changes in or on a material as a result of a fire (NFPA 2017, pt. 3.3.71).

The first four of these patterns correlate to the categories of the **fire effects** discussed previously. Victim injuries can be considered a special case of applying those categories to human skin and tissue. Fire investigators should be trained in understanding how fire patterns are formed and be able to interpret and analyze fire patterns, per *NFPA 1033* (NFPA 2014, pt. 4.2.5).

TASK:

Interpret fire patterns, given standard equipment and tools and some structural/content remains, so that each individual pattern is evaluated with respect to the burning characteristics of the material involved and in context and relationship with all patterns observed and the mechanisms of heat transfer that led to the formation of the pattern.

PERFORMANCE OUTCOME:

The investigator will observe a fire scene and document burn patterns and characteristics of two different materials.

CONDITIONS:

Given a fire scene, necessary portable lighting, measuring device, a note pad, and a briefing of fire suppression activity.

TASK STEPS:

1. Locate fire scene
2. Locate equipment needed
3. Obtain fire suppression briefing
4. Observe and document burn patterns
5. Observe and document burn characteristics of two burned materials

Source: Derived and updated from Washington State Patrol, Form No. 3000-420-081 (Sept. 2014) Fire Protection Bureau, Standards and Accreditation, Olympia, Washington http://www.wsp.wa.gov/fire/docs/cert/fire_invest.pdf

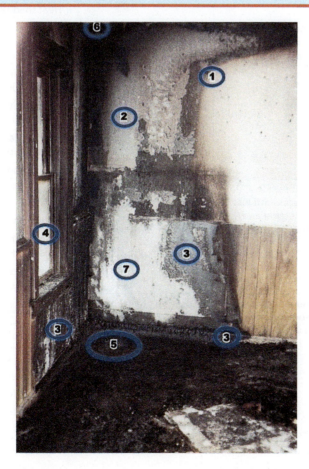

FIGURE 5-12 Fire pattern indicators found at fire scenes consisting of (1) demarcation, (2) calcination, (3) loss of material from wooden wainscoting and baseboard, (4) fractured glass, (5) ignitable liquid burn pattern on carpet, (6) penetration into the ceiling, and (7) area of clean burn where paper and pyrolysis products burned completely off the wall. *Courtesy of David J. Icove, University of Tennessee.*

TABLE 5-3	Typology of Common Fire Patterns		
TYPE OF PATTERN	**DESCRIPTION**	**VARIABLES**	**EXAMPLES**
Demarcations	The intersection of affected and unaffected areas on materials where smoke and heat impinge	■ Type of material ■ Fire temperature, duration, and rate of heat release ■ Fire suppression ■ Ventilation ■ Heat flux reaching surface	■ V patterns on walls ■ Discoloration patterns ■ Smoke stains
Surface effects	Determined by the boundary shape, areas of demarcation, and nature of heat application to various surface types	■ Surface texture (rougher surfaces sustain more damage) ■ Surface-to-mass ratio ■ Surface coverings ■ Combustible and noncombustible surfaces ■ Thermal conductivity ■ Temperature of surface	■ Spalling of floor surfaces ■ Combustible surfaces scorched or charred by pyrolysis and oxidation ■ Dehydration ■ Noncombustible surfaces changing color, oxidizing, melting, or burning cleanly ■ Smoke stains ■ Heat shadowing
Penetrations	Penetration of horizontal and vertical surfaces	■ Preexisting openings in floors, ceilings, and walls ■ Direct flame impingement ■ Heat flux ■ Duration of fire ■ Suppression	■ Downward penetrations under furniture ■ Saddle burns on exposed floor joists ■ Failure of walls, ceilings, and floors ■ Internal damage to walls and ceilings ■ Calcination
Loss of material	Combustible surfaces with loss of material and mass	■ Type of materials ■ Construction methods ■ Room contents and fuel loads ■ Duration of fire	■ Tops of wooden wall studs ■ Fall-down of debris ■ Isolated areas of consumed carpet ■ Beveling of corners and edges
Victim injuries	Areas, depths, and degrees of burns on victim's clothing and body	■ Location of victim in relation to other objects or victims ■ Actions taken prior to, during, and after the fire	■ Burns to face and hands ■ Absence of burn injuries where protected by clothing or furniture ■ Burns on lower torso ■ Heat shadowing

Source: Expanded from Icove 1995.

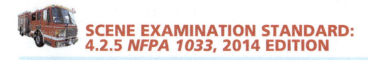

SCENE EXAMINATION STANDARD:
4.2.5 *NFPA 1033*, 2014 EDITION

TASK:

Interpret and analyze fire patterns, given standard equipment and tools and some structural or content remains, so that fire development is determined, methods and effects of suppression are evaluated, false origin area patterns are recognized, and all areas of origin are correctly identified.

PERFORMANCE OUTCOME:

The investigator will observe a fire scene and indicate on a rough sketch the area of origin and fire development.

CONDITIONS:

Given a fire scene, necessary portable lighting, and a sketch pad.

TASK STEPS:

1. Locate and observe the fire scene
2. Using burn patterns and fire development indicators, sketch the fire scene
3. Indicate area(s) of origin on the sketch
4. Indicate fire development patterns on the sketch
5. Observe and document effects of suppression activities

Source: Derived and updated from Washington State Patrol, Form No. 3000-420-081 (Sept. 2014) Fire Protection Bureau, Standards and Accreditation, Olympia, Washington http://www.wsp.wa.gov/fire/docs/cert/fire_invest.pdf

5.4.2 V PATTERNS

The impingement, intensity, and direction of the fire plume's travel form lines or areas of demarcation on walls, ceilings, floors, and other materials. As the hot gases and smoke rise from a fire, they mix with surrounding air, and the mixing zone becomes wider as hot gases rise above the fuel. Entrainment mixes and spreads the rising column, so it forms a V approximately 30° in width (i.e., half-angle of 15°) if unconfined in still air from a turbulent diffusion fire (You 1984). Therefore, the total width of the unconfined plume in still air is approximately half its height above the fuel surface.

As the fire gases mix, they are diluted and cooled. As a result, the diameter of the hottest part of the plume along the centerline becomes smaller with increasing height. The rapid cooling of fire gases by mixing with the air limits their thermal damage on noncombustible walls, so the thermal pattern on adjacent walls will not reflect the entire 30° angle width described for the plume.

Analyzing the shape of fire patterns caused by plumes can provide valuable information. For example, assuming that fuel is directly beneath the fire pattern, the most pronounced ceiling damage is often in the plume impingement area directly above the fuel source (as in Figure 5-3), a point from which a gas-movement vector points directly back to the fire's origin. The temperature of the gases determines the extent of thermal effects on surfaces they encounter. If their temperature is too low, the heat transfer will be insufficient and there may be no thermal effect; but combustion products will still condense on cooler surfaces.

Damage patterns forming lines of demarcation frequently appear in simple two-dimensional (cross-sectional) views of the location where the fire plume comes into contact with and damages wall surfaces. These lines are often referred to as *V-shaped fire patterns,* based on their characteristic upward-sweeping curves.

NFPA 921 (NFPA 2017) and *Kirk's Fire Investigation* (DeHaan and Icove 2012) dispel past misconceptions regarding the shape and geometry of V patterns, once thought to relate to the rapidity of fire growth. The shape of a V pattern is actually related to the heat release rate, geometry of the fuel, ventilation effects, ignitability and combustibility of affected surfaces, and intersection with vertical and horizontal surfaces.

If the V-shaped fire pattern's angle of demarcation is followed downward to its base, the area closest to the virtual origin of the plume can be located. Several mathematical relationships aid in documenting and analyzing the features of fire plume height, temperature, velocity, vortex shedding frequency, and virtual origin (Heskestad 2008; Quintiere 1998).

5.4.3 HOURGLASS PATTERNS

In certain cases, when a fuel package burns in a room adjacent to a wall or corner, the damage appears in the shape of an hourglass burn pattern instead of a V, as shown in Figure 5-12 (Icove and DeHaan 2006). Through both fire testing and mathematical analysis, the authors have shown that the formation of hourglass burn patterns is a direct function of the fire plume's virtual origin, which is mathematically tied to the heat release rate and surface area of the fuel package. A later section in this chapter will illustrate in full the formation of these hourglass patterns.

5.4.4 DEMARCATIONS

Demarcations occur in locations where smoke, heat, and flames impinge on materials, forming intersections between affected and unaffected areas. Examples include smoke layers deposited on walls and plume patterns on walls. See item 1 (demarcation) in Figure 5-12. Demarcations can vary depending on the type of exposed material, gas temperature, rate of heat release, and ventilation. Demarcations can identify deposits on the surface where temperatures have not been hot enough to thermally change the surface's covering. Areas of material loss are sometimes helpful in determining demarcations.

Heat and smoke levels, also referred to as horizons, refer to the height at which smoke or heat has stained or marked the walls and windows of a room. In fire modeling programs, these levels can be predicted throughout the structure being modeled and correlated with the duration and size of the fire. Heat and smoke levels are also important when evaluating victim accounts of whether they could see an exit if standing in a room or whether they would be affected by smoke or heat as they navigated through the building. In cases involving victims injured or killed in fires, the smoke and heat levels become important when evaluating whether victims stood up in a smoke-filled room and sustained their injuries from the cloud of heated toxic gases and smoky by-products of combustion.

As the ceiling jet plume extends throughout the room, demarcations are formed by stratified heat and smoke damage. In Figure 5-12, the ceiling plume extends to the right along the wall, forming the start of a stratified line. Notice the sharp demarcation in the degree of damage between the affected and the unaffected areas on the wall surface. Note also the acute angle between the demarcation line and the ceiling. This angle is the result of buoyancy-driven flow along the ceiling and is a very reliable indicator of direction of spread.

Fire suppression efforts such as the application of hose spray to the walls, ceilings, and floors can also affect demarcations. Ventilation efforts during fire suppression, such as the **venting** of the roof and the opening of doors and windows, also can affect the demarcations formed by heat and smoke throughout the structure. Figure 5-13 illustrates the formation of an upward pattern on the wall surface by the impact of a hose spray, which scoured the heat-affected paper and peeled it off the wall. The cooler the surface, the faster soot and pyrolysates will condense. Airflow will also control depositions. Figure 5-14 (a and b) shows the effects of airflow on soot deposition and how it can reveal the direction of hot gas spread.

venting ■ The escape of smoke and heat through openings in a building (NFPA 2017, pt. 3.3.201).

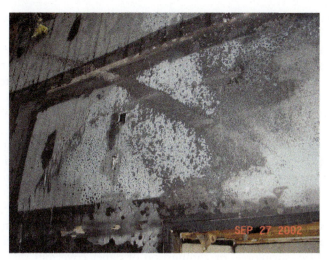

FIGURE 5-13 The impact of a hose spray on a wall during fire suppression efforts formed an upward pattern on the wall surface demarcations previously formed by heat and smoke. *Courtesy of David J. Icove, University of Tennessee.*

5.4.5 SURFACE EFFECTS

Surface effects occur when heat transfer is sufficient to cause discoloration of masonry surfaces, scorching or charring of combustible surfaces, melting or changes in color, or oxidizing of noncombustible surfaces. Areas not damaged by the heat and flames are called *protected areas* and are significant in cases where objects or bodies have been found or have been removed prior to inspection. Surface effects can also include nonthermal deposits of soot or pyrolysis products that condense on the cooler surfaces. The cooler the surface, the faster these deposits occur. Variables influencing surface effects include the type and smoothness of the surface, the thickness and nature of the coverings, and even the object's surface-to-mass ratio.

Extended post-flashover burning in a room exposes surfaces to high temperatures and heat fluxes. This "erases" the demarcations and surface effects (DeHaan and Icove 2012). Research at Eastern Kentucky University on burn patterns showed that brief (2 to 9 min) exposure to post-flashover fires did not always totally obliterate the fire patterns needed by investigators (Hopkins, Gorbett, and Kennedy 2007).

An example of a surface effect is the discoloration of paint on the external metallic surfaces of a burned automobile. Heat transfer through **conduction** often produces discernible fire patterns on the exterior and interior surfaces of the vehicles. Discoloration of metallic surfaces can also be caused by **oxidation**, which is a chemical process associated with combustion. Particularly with metal surfaces, the boundaries between higher and

conduction ■ Heat transfer to another body or within a body by direct contact (NFPA 2017, pt. 3.3.38).

oxidation ■ Reaction with oxygen either in the form of the element or in the form of one of its compounds (NFPA 2016).

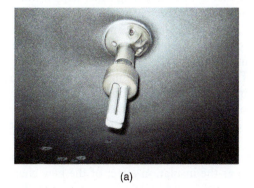

(a)

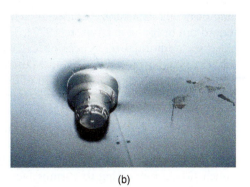

(b)

FIGURE 5-14 Deposits of soot (a) around light fixtures and (b) around a heat detector indicate direction of air movement. *Courtesy of Ross Brogan, NSW Fire Brigades, Greenacre, NSW, Australia*

lower temperatures can be observed and often can be documented through photographs and/or drawings.

Gypsum plasterboard or gypsum board is a material used in residential and commercial construction primarily for interior walls, in a process sometimes referred to as drywall construction. The drywall board contains gypsum (calcium sulfate dihydrate) bonded between two layers of paper. Fire-rated or X-type drywall is reinforced with glass fibers. The *ASTM C1396/C1396M-11* standard is the international standard for its manufacture (ASTM 2014).

Gypsum is a rock mineral that can be mixed with water and then dried into a hardened paste, resulting in a product that is 21 percent water by weight. The **calcination of gypsum** wallboard is a process by which heat transfer causes the calcium sulfate to dehydrate in two discrete steps at characteristic temperatures, typically around 100°C (212°F) and 180°C (356°F).

As gypsum dehydrates, it shrinks and loses the water of hydration, and its mechanical strength degrades. It can fail, exposing combustible wall structure, when it loses so much strength from dehydration, shrinkage, or combustion of paper coverings that it can no longer support its own weight. Eventually, the fully dehydrated gypsum turns powdery and loses all its mechanical strength, causing the wall to collapse. This process of calcination can also form lines of demarcation on the wall surface (DeHaan and Icove 2012). The effect of calcination on a gypsum board wall is shown as items 2 and 7 in Figure 5-12.

A change in color from white to gray to white is seen in a cross section of affected gypsum. Dehydration alone probably does not cause the gray-to-white change, because this is a colorless transition. During fire exposure other carbonaceous pyrolysis products accumulate that turn the absorbent gypsum gray. Subsequent heating burns away or evaporates these deposits, causing whitening to progress through the thickness of the gypsum.

During fire exposure, the exposed paper and painted surfaces of the gypsum wallboard burn away. This reduces the overall mechanical strength of the gypsum wallboard. The process in which dehydrated gypsum falls or flakes off the surface during heat exposure is called ablation, which occurs at 600°C (1112°F) for ceilings and 800°C (1472°F) for walls (König and Walleij 2000). Ablation reduces the thickness of the board (Buchanan 2001, 341). There are several techniques for documenting the measured post-fire loss of gypsum from the wall surface and estimating the radiant heat flux exposure time (Kennedy 2004; Schroeder and Williamson 2003). The measurements of depth of calcination of gypsum surfaces are often recorded on a plot of the room.

Research by Schroeder and Williamson (2001) indicates that gypsum wallboard is a useful source for documenting a fire's intensity, spread, and direction. In a series of experiments using an *ASTM E1354* cone calorimeter, they concluded that thermally induced changes in gypsum wallboard, along with x-ray diffraction analysis to document the crystalline structure change, provided a quantifiable method for assessing time, temperature, and heat flux exposure. Additional cited references on the thermal properties of gypsum board can be found in Lawson (1977), Thomas (2002), and McGraw and Mowrer (1999). Also see additional references on calcination of gypsum board during fire in Mowrer (2001), Chu Nguong (2004), and Mann and Putaansuu (2006).

Charring is the pyrolytic action of heat that converts the organic material, most often paper or wood, into its volatile fractions, leaving behind carbonaceous **char**. Depending on the type of wood, this char layer may burn off or flake off as the fire exposure continues. The linear depth of the pyrolyzed material affected, including the char layer and lost material, is referred to as the *char depth*.

The rate at which wood chars is not linear. Wood chars quickly at first and then at a much slower rate owing to various factors such as the insulation effect of the new char, reduced air–fuel interactions, ventilation, heat transfer, and physical arrangement. The reported charring behavior of large-section structural lumber has been modeled. A review of 55 specimens of 2 in. × 4 in. spruce-pine-fir lumber subjected to a constant-temperature

calcination of gypsum ■ A fire effect realized in gypsum products, including wallboard, as a result of exposure to heat that drives off free and chemically bound water (NFPA 2017, pt. 3.3.24).

char ■ Carbonaceous material that has been burned or pyrolyzed and has a blackened appearance (NFPA 2017, pt. 3.3.29).

exposure of 500°C (932°F) produced a linear model. The model showed a constant rate of charring of 1.628 mm²/s and 0.45 mm/min (Lau, White, and Van Zeeland 1999). Real-world fire exposures do not produce constant temperature or heat flux conditions.

Research to numerically simulate pyrolysis modeled the movement of the char/virgin front with good agreement of mass loss with experimental testing (Jia, Galea, and Patel 1999). Babrauskas offers a comprehensive analysis of charring rate of wood as a tool for fire investigators (DeHaan and Icove 2012, chap. 7). Babrauskas (2005) and Butler (1971) cite data illustrating the variability of char rates with type of wood and nature of fire exposure. The char rate is highly dependent on applied heat flux. During a fire, heat fluxes on a surface may vary from near zero to 50 kW/m² for contact by small flames, to 120 to 150 kW/m² under post-flashover conditions, resulting in a char rate varying from zero to several millimeters per minute.

To identify conductive heat transfer through walls, investigators often document the charring of wood studs within walls covered by materials such as wooden paneling or gypsum board. Figure 5-15 shows varying degrees of damage to a gypsum board–covered wall and previously protected wood studs within the wall after exposure to a test fire. The test results agreed with the varying degrees of charring damage predicted by a fire model known as WALL2D (Figure 5-16), which predicts heat transfer and char damage to wood studs protected by gypsum board and exposed to fire. The WALL2D developers reported good agreement of their heat transfer model with the results of both small- and full-scale fire tests (Takeda and Mehaffey 1998). An engineering study focused on WALL2D identified it as a viable fire model for users in both the regulatory and fire investigation communities (Richardson et al. 2000).

Char depth is usually documented using a penetrating tool and survey grid diagrams (NFPA 2017, pt. 18.4.3). In these diagrams, the data from the measurements are converted to lines of equal depth, called **isochar** lines. Each line connects depths of the same value. Investigators should consider recording elevation (height above the floor) measurements for greater precision (Sanderson 2002). Because variations in char rate can be caused by the differences in affected woods, coatings, and flame-retardant treatments, investigators are cautioned to recognize that char depths should be compared on similar types of wood (baseboards, door frames, etc.).

isochar ■ A line on a diagram connecting points of equal char depth (NFPA 2017, pt. 3.3.121).

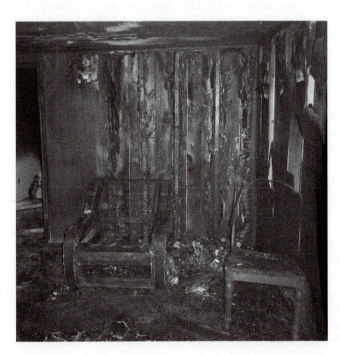

FIGURE 5-15 Varying degrees of damage to a paneled wall and previously protected wood studs within the wall after being exposed to a test fire. *Courtesy of David J. Icove, University of Tennessee.*

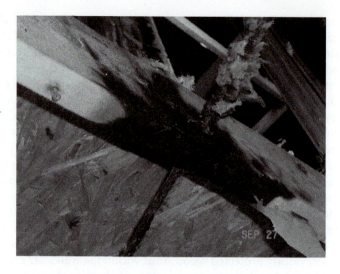

FIGURE 5-16 The progression of a char front upward through a wood ceiling joist after exposure to a test fire. *Courtesy of David J. Icove, University of Tennessee.*

Owing to the nonlinear nature of charring, the measurement of char depth cannot establish precise times of fire exposure, but deeper relative depths of char may indicate areas of more intense or prolonged burning. Also, the appearance of the char surface often depends on the individual characteristics of the wood and ventilation conditions (DeHaan and Icove 2012). However, char depth relationships assuming a constant 50 kW/m^2 incident flux have been suggested for fire protection engineering applications (Silcock and Shields 2001).

spalling ■ Chipping or pitting of concrete or masonry surfaces (NFPA 2017, pt. 3.3.174).

Spalling occurs during rapidly rising temperatures, typically 20°C to 30°C/min (70°F to 86°F/min) (Khoury 2000). Several factors influence spalling, but the moisture content and nature of the aggregate used (limestone versus granite) are the leading variables. Spalling can also be caused by suddenly cooling a very hot concrete surface with a hose stream. High-strength concrete tends to spall more than normal concrete owing to its higher density. The pores of the high-density concrete become filled more quickly with the high-pressure water vapor (Buchanan 2001, 228). Spalling can be reduced if the concrete is made with fine plastic fibers mixed into the slurry. As the fibers melt at low temperatures they provide pores to vent the internally produced steam.

Steel reinforcements expand more rapidly when heated than does concrete. Thus, if reinforcements are not protected deeply in the concrete, they expand and cause tensile failure of the concrete. Lightweight concrete spalls more readily because of the vermiculite used as an aggregate.

Testing by the SP Swedish National Testing and Research Institute on spalling reinforced the two classic explanations for concrete spalling. The most common cause is thermal stress, which forces water vapor out of the hotter side of the concrete. Experiments by Jansson (2006) documented that water vapor is also forced out of the cold side of the concrete during fire tests. During these fire tests, the internal pressures also started to fluctuate severely after 15 minutes. New material test methods have been proposed for determining whether an actual exposed concrete may suffer from explosive spalling at a specified moisture level. A specimen cylinder is used, which is a cost-effective alternative to full-scale testing (Hertz and Sorensen 2005).

Studies by the UK Building Research Establishment (BRE) about fire damage on natural stone masonry in buildings showed that natural stone can be seriously affected in building fires, with damage concentrated around window openings and doorways (Chakrabarti, Yates, and Lewry 1996). Color changes at 200°C to 300°C (392°F to 572°F) were followed by localized disintegration at 600°C to 800°C (1112°F to 1472°F). Color changes included the reddening of stones containing iron, which is irreversible and causes significant damage to historical buildings. Other damage noted by BRE included costly smoke staining and salt efflorescence resulting from fire hose streams.

BRE also reported that brown or light-colored limestone containing hydrated iron oxide changes to reddish brown at 250°C to 300°C (482°F to 572°F), more reddish at 400°C (752°F), and a gray-white powder at 800°C to 1000°C (1472°F to 1832°F). The depth of calcination of limestone is seldom less than 20 mm, which begins at 600°C (1112°F), reducing the stone's strength. Magnesium limestone is white or buff colored and changes to pale pink at 250°C (482°F) and pink at 300°C (572°F).

Sandstone changes to a brown color due to the dehydration of iron compounds starting at 250°C to 300°C (482°F to 572°F) and to reddish brown above 400°C (752°F). Structural weakening of sandstone starts at 573°C (1063°F), when the quartz grains internally rupture. Loss of strength of such stone is particularly critical when solid stone lintels are used above windows, doors, and gateways, as massive structural collapse can occur without warning.

Further research by BRE indicated that granite will show no color changes but will crack or shatter at temperatures above 573°C (1063°F) through quartz expansion, and marble's internal calcite crystals will undergo thermal hysteresis, causing a reduction in flexural strength. Marble has been known to crumble into a powder when exposed to extreme heat (>600°C, 1150°F). This is particularly dangerous for marble staircases in fires.

The UK Building Research Station published a historical review of the visible changes in concrete or mortar when exposed to high temperatures (Bessey 1950). The study examined aggregates, concrete, and mortar, and the reproducibility and interpretation of observed changes in terms of temperature. Research by Short, Guise, and Purkiss (1996) at the Department of Civil Engineering, Aston University, UK, using optical microscopy documents their use of color analysis in the assessment of fire-damaged concrete.

Flammable liquids very rarely produce significant spalling on bare concrete because a typical flammable liquid pool fire on bare concrete lasts only 1 to 2 min, and sometimes much less (DeHaan 1995). This leaves little time for heat to penetrate into the concrete, which has poor conductivity. Additionally, the radiant heat from the flame is, in part, absorbed by the liquid fuel during combustion, and the maximum temperature of the surface cannot significantly exceed the boiling point of the liquid in contact with it. Because the boiling point range of gasoline is 40°C to 150°C (104°F to 302°F), the concrete will not usually be heated to the point at which it will be affected (DeHaan and Icove 2012, chap. 7). Extensive experiments by Novak (unpublished data) have demonstrated the lack of spalling beneath flammable liquid pool fires on a variety of concrete surfaces that are readily spalled by a wood fire (see Figure 5-17).

If tile or carpet is present on the concrete, the gasoline flames can trigger localized charring, melting, and combustion of the floor covering. Because this combustion is more prolonged than the gasoline flame itself, the molten mass has a very high boiling point, and there is no freestanding liquid to protect the concrete; therefore, there is more opportunity for heat to affect the concrete and cause it to spall if it is susceptible. Figure 5-18 shows an example of localized burning due to a flammable liquid pour pattern on floor tiles. The collapse of molten burning plastic or roofing tar onto a concrete surface will produce significant and prolonged heat transfer that will induce spalling. Prolonged burning of structural wood collapsed onto a concrete floor surface is especially likely to cause spalling. Additional cited references on spalling of concrete include Canfield (1984), Smith (1991), Sanderson (1995), and Bostrom (2005).

Localized combustion of flammable liquids on vinyl- or asphalt-tiled concrete surfaces can produce a type of floor damage called **ghost marks**. Ghost marks are subsurface staining of the concrete beneath the joints of tile floors that appears to be caused by combustion of the cement/mastik dissolved by the applied flammable liquid. Radiant heat in post-flashover fires and long-term heating by fall down of burning materials can produce spalling but do not apparently produce ghost marks (DeHaan and Icove 2012, chap. 7). Charring of wood floors along tile seams is not the same.

ghost marks ■ Stained outlines of floor tiles produced on non-combustible floors by the dissolution and combustion of tile adhesive.

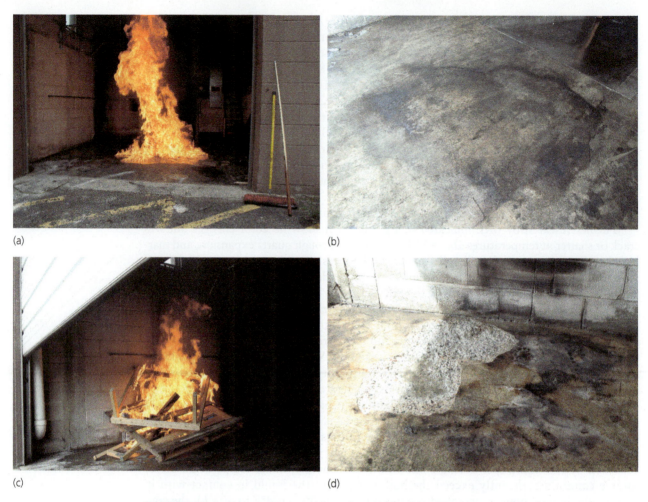

(a)

(b)

(c)

(d)

FIGURE 5-17 Spalling concrete tests: (a) gasoline pool fire, (b) staining but no spalling of concrete after gasoline fire self-extinguished, (c) wood pallet fire on same type concrete, (d) extensive spalling under wood fire. *Courtesy of Jamie Novak, Novak Investigations and St. Paul Fire Dept.*

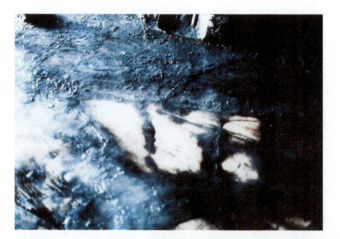

FIGURE 5-18 Surface effects due to a flammable liquid pour pattern (center of the photograph) that charred the floor tiles. Two parallel pour patterns are documented, characteristic of a back-and-forth spilling of flammable liquids as the arsonist backed out of the building. *Courtesy of David J. Icove, University of Tennessee.*

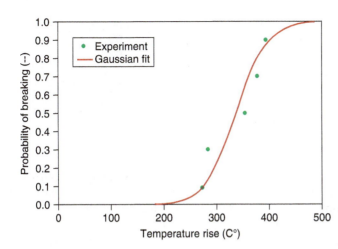

FIGURE 5-19 The probability of breakage of 3-mm-thick window glass fits a Gaussian statistical correlation with a mean temperature of 340°C (644°F) and a standard deviation of 50°C (122°F). *Courtesy of Babrauskas (2004); www.doctorfire .com.*

Fractured glass is another surface effect that usually occurs when glass is stressed by non-uniform heating. Common variables that affect glass breakage include its thickness, the presence of any defects, the rate at which it was heated or cooled, and the method used to secure the glass to the window frame (Shields, Silcock, and Flood 2001).

The potential for glass to fracture and break out has been the topic of several research initiatives. The prediction of the probability of breakage fits a Gaussian statistical correlation, as shown in Figure 5-19 (Babrauskas 2004). This relationship shows that the mean temperature for the breakage of 3-mm-thick (0.12 in.) window glass is 340°C (644°F), with a standard deviation of 50°C (122°F).

The fire modeling program BREAK1 (Berkeley Algorithm for Breaking Window Glass in a Compartment Fire) can calculate the temperature history of a glass window given several fire parameters combined with a physical composition of the glass (NIST 1991). The model also predicts the temperature gradients of the glass normal to the glass surface and the window breakage time. Large-scale glass fracturing by heat is often observed as a room approaches flashover and the temperatures and heat fluxes dramatically increase. This program computes only the cracking of glass, whereas the investigator is often interested in knowing when the glass failed enough so that pieces fell out, rather than the time when cracks first appeared. It is the physical loss of glass from windows that can affect the development of the fire in the room, sometimes dramatically.

Hietaniemi (2005) at the VTT Building and Transport, Finland, has produced a probabilistic simulation model for glass fracture and fallout in a fire. This approach uses two steps: The model first predicts the simulation time for the initial occurrence of a crack using the BREAK1 program, followed by a thermal response model of the glass.

Heat-induced failure of dual-glazed windows is considerably less predictable. Often, the inside pane fails, but its fragments protect the exterior glass pane. Dual-glazed windows have been observed to survive post-flashover room fires only to break when struck by hose streams. Dual glazing with heat-absorbing film is even more resistant to heat-induced failure.

One common mechanism for thermal fracturing of common window glass is the stress induced by non-uniform heating as a result of thermal shadow cast by framing or trim. When a window is exposed to radiant or convected heat, the exposed portions increase in temperature and begin to expand, but the areas shaded by the framing or window putty are not heated. Because glass is a relatively poor conductor of heat, shaded areas remain cool and do not expand, as shown in Figure 5-20a. This differentiation induces stress in the glass that can cause the glass to fracture, often in patterns roughly

FIGURE 5-20 Heat fractures of a window pane caused by shadowing of radiant heat. Fractures radiating out from a point on the right often are caused by a preexisting nick in the edge of the glass or by stress induced by a glazier point or frame nail.

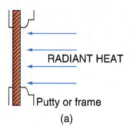

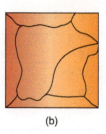

RADIANT HEAT

Putty or frame

(a)

(b)

FIGURE 5-20 Heat fractures of a window pane caused by shadowing of radiant heat. Fractures radiating out from a point on the right often are caused by a preexisting nick in the edge of the glass or by stress induced by a glazier point or frame nail.

parallel to the edges, as shown in Figure 5-20b. The fractures radiating from a single point on the right often are caused by a preexisting nick in the edge of the glass or by stress induced by a glazier point or frame nail (DeHaan and Icove 2012, chap. 7).

The observation that the windows blew out during a fire is rarely associated with an overpressure event but, rather, with thermally induced massive fracturing. The pressures produced by a flashover transition in a room are very rarely adequate to cause mechanical breakage (Fang and Breese 1980; Mitler and Rockett 1987; Mowrer 1998). However, the development of a **backdraft** condition, in which the fire becomes severely underventilated and is then given additional air, can produce overpressures sufficient to cause windows to break.

The edges of ordinary glass fractured by mechanical stress are characterized by curved, conchoidal ridge lines caused by the propagation of the fracture, as in Figure 5-21a. The fracture pattern on the face of glass when broken by mechanical shock or pressure is typically a spiderweb pattern of mostly straight fractures, as in Figure 5-21b. The pattern usually consists of a number of radial fractures from the point of contact and concentric fractures connecting them.

Mechanical impacts of very brief duration cause minimal radial fractures, because the glass does not have time to flex and may produce a domed plug of glass to be ejected from the side opposite a localized impact. Thermal stress usually results in more random patterns with wavy fractures. These fractures usually have mirror-smooth edges with minimal conchoidal ridges, because they are usually produced at lower speeds than mechanical fractures.

If enough glass can be recovered to jigsaw-fit pieces together for at least part of the pattern, and the inside or outside face can be identified by soil, paint, decals, or lettering, the direction of force can be established by the 3R rule: The conchoidal lines on radial fractures start at right angles on the reverse (side away from the force). The direction is reversed on concentric fractures. Toughened safety glass used in the side and rear windows

backdraft ■ A deflagration resulting from the sudden introduction of air into a confined space containing oxygen-deficient products of incomplete combustion (NFPA 2017, pt. 3.3.17).

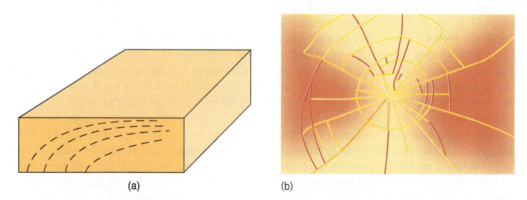

(a)

(b)

FIGURE 5-21 (a) Edge of glass fragment showing conchoidal fracture lines. (b) Face of glass sheet broken by mechanical impact near the center, with radial fractures and concentric fractures.

of vehicles and in structural doors and shower doors fractures into small, rectangular blocks. As a general rule, the cause and direction of failure of safety glass cannot be established, but under some conditions fragments trapped in the frame may reveal the approximate location of a mechanical impact point.

The sequence of impacts can be established from intersecting and ending fractures. Sequence of failure versus time of exposure to fire can be established by the presence or absence of soot on the broken edges. Direct contact with flame can heat glass to the point at which all accumulated soot and smoke deposits are oxidized off, a so-called **clean burn**. Glass breakage patterns can also reveal a great deal of information about an explosion (DeHaan and Icove 2012, chap. 12). The distance to which the glass is blown is related to the thickness of the glass, the size of the window, and the pressures developed (Harris, Marshall, and Moppett 1977; Harris 1983). As a general rule, the thinner the glass or the larger the surface area of the pane, the lower the failure pressure will be.

A distinctive form of glass fracturing called **crazing** is usually produced when fire suppression water spray strikes a heated glass surface. Crazing is characterized by a complex (road map–like) pattern of partial-thickness fractures and concave pitting (Lentini 1992). Field experiments during test fires confirmed that when a water spray was applied to the hot glass panes on one side of a heated window, crazing occurred. Common window glass softens when its temperature reaches 700°C to 760°C (1300°F to 1400°F).

Another descriptive form of surface burn pattern is called a clean burn (Kennedy and Kennedy 1985, 451; NFPA 2017, pt. 6.2.11; DeHaan 2007, 275). Clean burns leave a distinct and visible fire on noncombustible surfaces after combustible layer or layers containing soot, paint, and paper are burned away. When a solid surface is exposed to a fire environment, products of combustion—water vapor, soot, and pyrolysis products—will condense on it. The cooler the surface, the faster products will condense, giving rise to the shadowy outlines of studs, nail heads, and other hidden features of a wall structure that cause a temperature differential.

When a sooted surface is exposed to direct flame, it can reach high enough temperatures that the accumulated products can burn away, leaving behind a clean surface. This pattern can be used to identify areas of direct contact between a surface and the flaming portion of the plume. Surfaces not in contact with the flame will rarely reach sufficiently high temperatures to allow the complete combustion of condensed soot or pyrolysates.

An unpublished study by Ingolf Kotthoff indicates that for a clean burn to occur, the material must reach approximately 700°C (1300°F). A clean burn can also result where charred organic materials are burned away, leaving a bare noncombustible substrate exposed. *NFPA 921* cautions that the investigator should be careful not to confuse clean burn areas with spalling (NFPA 2017, pt. 6.2.11.2).

In ATF Fire Research Laboratory test burns in 2008 involving single-room compartments in ventilation-controlled conditions, each fire was started in the same manner and location (Carman 2010). The main variable in each of the tests was the length of time the fires burned. The results showed both similarities and differences in the ensuing burn patterns, particularly in clean-burn indicators. One hypothesis is that the mechanism for clean-burn pattern development may be different from the popular notion of combustion of previously deposited soot on that surface. The patterns may be due in part to high thermal gradients on surfaces that prevent localized deposition. Accordingly, further study of such mechanisms may improve the interpretation of such patterns and the timing of their creation.

Melted materials can also reveal information about the temperatures to which surfaces were exposed during the fire. Studies by the UK Building Research Station provided an estimation of the maximum temperatures attained in building fires from an examination of the debris. Researchers examined lead and zinc plumbing fixtures, aluminum and alloys used in small machinery, molded glass from windows and jars, sheet glass in window panes, silver jewelry and eating utensils, brass doorknobs and locks, bronze window

clean burn ■ A distinct and visible fire effect generally apparent on noncombustible surfaces after combustible layer(s) (such as soot, paint, and paper) have been burned away. The effect may also appear where soot has failed to be deposited because of high surface temperatures (NFPA 2017, pt. 3.3.31).

craze ■ The appearance of fine cracks in the surface of a helmet shell or other smooth surface of an ensemble element.

frames and bells, copper electric wiring, and cast iron pipes and machinery (Parker and Nurse 1950). The findings of this study demonstrated that the analysis of melted materials in a fire could identify and document areas of varying temperature exposure.

Plastics, glass, copper, aluminum, and tin are the most common melted materials found at fire scenes that can document the wide range of temperatures produced by the fire (DeHaan and Icove 2012). Melting points of thermoplastics can vary depending on the nature of their internal molecular structure. Glass melts, softens, or becomes molten over a range of temperatures. Table 5-4 lists approximate melting temperatures of common materials. It must be remembered that interactions between melting materials can cause unusual effects. Zinc or aluminum melting onto steel can produce alloying through **eutectic melting**, causing the steel to melt at ordinary fire temperatures. Zinc can come from pot-metal fittings or galvanized coatings. Aluminum is well-known for creating a eutectic alloy with copper with a very low melting point. Calcium sulfate (gypsum or plaster) can cause localized melting of black iron under fire conditions.

eutectic melting ■
Eutectic melting (alloying) involves damage that occurs when a metal of different composition contacts the subject metal. The original melting may or may not be electrically related, but the damage to the subject metal caused by deposition of the second does not involve an electrical current and is not a form of electrical damage (NFPA 2017, pt. 9.11.3).

TABLE 5-4	Approximate Melting-Point Temperatures of Common Materials	
MATERIAL	°C	°F
Aluminum alloys[a]	570–660	1060–1220
Aluminum (pure)[c]	660	1220
Copper[c]	1083	1981
Cast iron (gray)[a]	1150–1200	2100–2200
50/50 solder[a]	183–216	360–420
Carbon steel[a]	1520	2770
Tin[c]	232	450
Zinc[c]	420	787
Magnesium alloy[a]	589–651	1092–1204
Stainless steel[a]	1400–1530	2550–2790
Iron (pure)[c]	1535	2795
Lead (pure)[c]	327	621
Gold (pure)[c]	1065	1950
Paraffin (wax)[d]	50–57	122–135
Human fat[e]	30–50	86–122
Polystyrene[b]	240	465
Polypropylene[d]	165	330
Polyester (Dacron)[d]	dec 250	480
Polyethylene[b,c]	130* (85–110)	185–230
PMMA (acrylic plastic)[b]	160*	320
PVC[b]	dec 250*	480
Nylon 66[b]	250–260	480–500
Polyurethane foam[c]	dec 200	390

Sources: [a]Perry and Green 1984, Table 23-6, 23–40; [b]Drysdale 2011; [c]DeHaan 2007, 274–86; [d]*The Merck Index* (Merck Co. 1989); [e]DeHaan, Campbell, and Nurbakhsh 1999.
Note: dec = decomposes.
*Varies with cross-linking.

As we have seen, localized temperatures in any flame can readily reach 1200°C (2200°F), but the actual values recorded depend greatly on the measuring technique. Temperatures in a growing room fire can vary from ambient room temperature to over 800°C (1470°F). Post-flashover fires can produce temperatures of over 1000°C (1800°F) throughout a room. Burning plastics can produce localized flame temperatures of 1100°C to 1200°C (1980°F to 2200°F). Most other materials, whether ignitable liquids or ordinary combustibles, produce maximum flame temperatures in air of 800°C (1470°F). Evidence of high temperatures [800°C (1470°F) or higher] is not proof of the use of accelerants. Plastics can indicate the intensity and distribution of heat exposure as they soften and distort.

Annealed furniture springs result when their temperature exceeds the typical or **annealing** point (538°C, 1000°F), and the coiled steel springs lose their temper (Tobin and Monson 1989). Collapsed springs are indicators of this phenomenon, and an investigator should compare the relative degree of collapse to try to ascertain the direction and intensity of the fire (DeHaan and Icove 2012). This collapse is not an indicator that accelerants were used, because smoldering fires of accidental cause can readily produce these effects. The investigator should also examine the framework (usually metal or wood) for other signs of localized thermal damage, (NFPA 2017, pt. 6.2.14). Modern urethane foam furniture often burns so quickly that even the high-temperature flames cannot bring the steel springs to their annealing temperatures. Steel springs can also corrode to the point of failure from fire exposure due to stress-corrosion cracking, which occurs when normally ductile metals are subjected to a tensile stress at elevated temperature (NPL 2000).

annealing ■ Loss of temper in metal caused by heating.

5.4.6 PENETRATIONS

Another common fire pattern is the occurrence of penetrations through horizontal and vertical surfaces as direct flame impingement or intense radiant heat on walls, ceilings, and floors is sustained long enough to affect deeper layers of the material. Ceiling areas directly overhead of fire plumes may burn through or collapse, allowing flames to extend into confined spaces. In some cases, fall-down of combustible debris followed by extended smoldering can lead to localized penetration of wooden floors, sills, and toe plates in wood-framed structures.

Variables influencing penetrations include preexisting openings in floors, ceilings, and walls. Also, direct flame impingement coupled with high heat fluxes plays an important role in creating the conditions necessary for penetrations. The area where a fire plume intersects a ceiling is an example of a penetration into the ceiling directly above the fire plume due to the high heat flux and temperatures that caused the failure of the ceiling materials.

Penetrations are not always above the fire plume. During flashover conditions, downward penetrations are sometimes found. As discussed previously, the most common reason for penetrations through wooden flooring is radiant heat from above, not the combustion of ignitable liquids (DeHaan 1987; Babrauskas 2005). Sustained burning of collapsed furniture, bedding, or clothing also can result in localized penetrations. Fire testing involving no ignitable liquids in furnished rooms has demonstrated that the resulting post-flashover conditions can produce penetrations through carpet, pad, and plywood floors.

In post-flashover fires where ignitable liquids were poured onto carpeted floors, burning penetrations can char supporting joists from post-flashover fire, not the liquid fuel fire. In fire tests conducted by the US Fire Administration, 1.75 L (0.46 gal) of gasoline was poured onto carpeted floor (FEMA 1997). Flashover occurred at 40 seconds, with extinguishment at 10.3 minutes. An examination of the scene after extinguishment showed the fire to have burned through the carpet, carpet underpadding, and 9.5-mm (0.37-in.) plywood floor. As shown in Figure 5-22, there was widespread

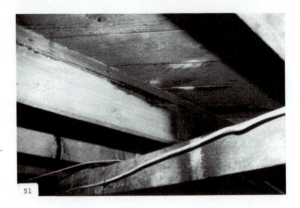

FIGURE 5-22 The burn-through of carpet, underpadding, and 12-mm (0.5-in.) plywood floor in a room fire test involving 1.75 L (0.5 gal) of gasoline and approximately 10 minutes of post-flashover burning. *Courtesy of the US Fire Administration.*

charring on the 2 in. × 8 in. supporting joists. The test involved nearly 10 minutes of post-flashover burning, which caused most of the observed damage long after the gasoline burned away.

Sometimes, burning foam mattresses drop enough burning molten liquid from pyrolysis onto the floor directly under the bed to cause burns through the floor. Burning thermoplastics such as polyethylene trash containers or thermoplastic appliance liners can do the same. Traditional cotton-stuffed upholstered furniture such as sofas, chairs, and mattresses can support combustion long enough to burn through wooden floors beneath them after they collapse.

Failure of walls, floors, and ceilings during a fire may also contribute to formation of penetrations through which the fire extends throughout a structure. These failures have been known to transport heat, flames, and smoke to other areas of the structure, leading inexperienced investigators to conclude improperly that two or more fires were set within the structure. Such penetrations can occur as gypsum wallboard fails, lath chars, plaster collapses, and metal ceilings or other noncombustible ceiling coverings peel away. Ventilation drafts up stairwells can cause very intense fires with rapid failure of doors and ceilings.

5.4.7 LOSS OF MATERIAL

Loss of material occurs in any combustible material located in the path of a fire's development and spread. This loss of material is helpful in determining the fire's intensity and direction of travel. *Heat shadowing* can affect the loss of materials by shielding the heat transfer and masking the potential lines of demarcation of other fire patterns (Kennedy and Kennedy 1985, 450; NFPA 2017, pt. 6.2.3.) Loss of material can be driven by direct flame impingement or radiant heat alone. Rapid charring caused by post-flashover radiant heat can be enhanced by ventilation from doors or windows to produce penetrations through floors near doors or windows, in the center of rooms, or across the room from vents where air flows, where post-flashover mixing is most efficient (DeHaan and Icove 2012). Extensive destruction around heater vents has been observed in rooms where there was prolonged post-flashover burning because of the extra oxygen the vents provided to fuels already burning. The results of full-scale fire tests reported by Carman (2008, 2009, and 2010) and supplemented by post-fire computer modeling further demonstrated the impact of open doorways on fire patterns.

In Figure 5-12, items 3 (loss of material from wooden wainscoting and baseboard) and 7 (areas of clean burn where paper and pyrolysis products burned completely off the wall) are two examples of loss of materials due to direct impingement of the fire plume. The most significant is the relative loss of the wooden wainscoting material. The closer the material is to the plume centerline, the deeper the charring. Localized damage to the wooden baseboard documents the radiant heat from above.

Loss of material may occur on the tops of wooden studs, on corners and edges of furniture and moldings, and floors and carpeted surfaces. This gives rise to beveling of solid fuels or extended V patterns that can reliably indicate direction of fire spread. Other forms of loss of material come from fall-down of debris from above. Typical examples include burning drapery or curtains, which ignite other objects in the room and sometimes mislead novice investigators into thinking that multiple fires may have been set.

NFPA 921 cautions that although mass loss of material can be used as an indication of the duration and intensity of the fire, it may not be valid is all cases (NFPA 2017, pt. 6.2.3.3). This is because mass loss rate involves a complex combination of factors involving both varying material properties and fire conditions.

Loss of material may clarify the nature and extent of fire damage to upholstered furniture exposed to smoldering versus flaming combustion. Tests by Ogle and Schumacher (1998) demonstrated that smoldering fire patterns often tended to consist of char zones with a thickness equal to that of the fuel element (i.e., the entire thickness). If the source of the smoldering fire was, for example, a cigarette, they found that the smoldering patterns persisted as long as the cigarette continued to smolder. Fire patterns created by smoldering fires were destroyed if a transition to flaming combustion occurred. In the case of cigarette-initiated fires, the cigarette itself was consumed in the flaming phase.

Flaming fire patterns had thin char zones with thicknesses smaller than the thickness of the fuel element. Ogle and Schumacher (1998) observed that the flaming fire consumed the cover fabric and underlying padding. When examining flame spread rates with polyurethane foam (PUF) seat cushions, they observed that horizontal burning was faster than vertical downward burning. Also, because the cushions were thermally thick, the depth of char into the foam tended to be thin when compared with the overall cushion thickness.

Figures 5-23, 5-24, and 5-25 show graphic representations of the burn patterns observed by Ogle and Schumacher in fires involving upholstered PUF

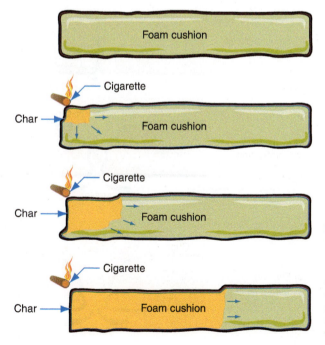

FIGURE 5-23 Cross-sectional view of the development of smoldering fire patterns in a cotton-upholstered foam cushion exposed to a smoldering cigarette at its corner.

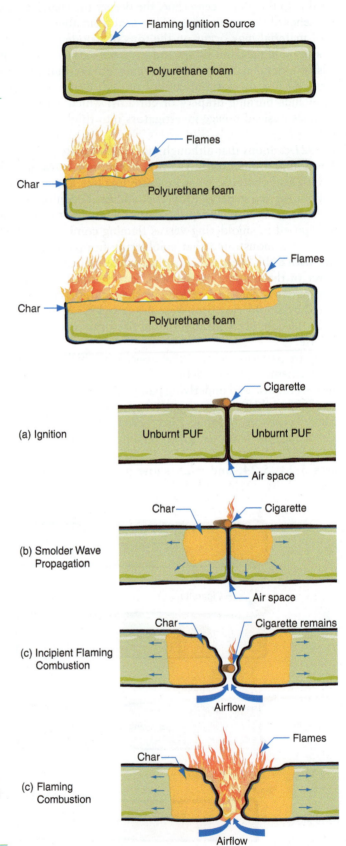

FIGURE 5-24 Cross-sectional view of the development of flaming fire patterns in a foam cushion exposed to a flaming ignition source at its surface.

Flaming Ignition Source

Polyurethane foam

Flames

Char

Polyurethane foam

Flames

Char

Polyurethane foam

Cigarette

(a) Ignition

Unburnt PUF

Unburnt PUF

Air space

Char

Cigarette

(b) Smolder Wave Propagation

Air space

Char

Cigarette remains

(c) Incipient Flaming Combustion

Airflow

FIGURE 5-25 Cross-sectional view of the development of a burn-through and the transition from smoldering to flaming combustion in a pair of upholstered foam cushions exposed to a smoldering cigarette at their junction.

Char

Flames

(c) Flaming Combustion

Airflow

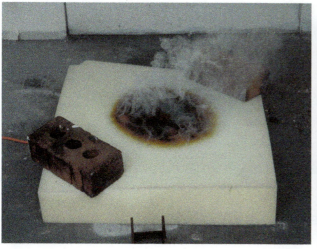 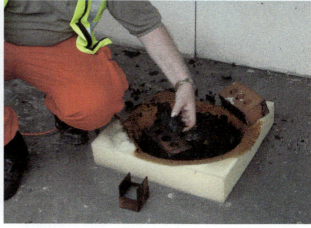

(a)   (b)

FIGURE 5-26 (a) A polyurethane foam cushion placed over a high-wattage lamp. (b) The foam around the lamp formed a dry, rigid, crusty char. When the cushion was ignited by open flame, the residue was the typical sticky liquid and semimolten combustion product. *Test courtesy of Jack Malooly. Photos (a) and (b) courtesy of John Galvin, London Fire Brigade (Retired).*

cushions. These figures show the cross-sectional views for smoldering, flaming, and transition, respectively. Although polyurethane foam by itself is not usually ignitable by a smoldering cigarette, PUF cushions are more likely to be ignited in combination with cellulosic fabrics and paddings (Holleyhead 1999; Babrauskas and Krasny 1985).

Hot surfaces or a sustained heat source such as a lighted incandescent bulb in contact with polyurethane foam can cause the formation of a cakelike, rigid char, whereas the flaming combustion of the same foam causes the production of viscous yellow polyol. Post-fire examination may reveal the different residues, as seen in Figure 5-26.

5.4.8 VICTIM INJURIES

Victim injuries may occur during discovery of, interaction with, or escape from a fire and may reveal actions taken during critical time periods. This is especially true in fire deaths where the only remaining fire pattern indicators are the areas and degrees of burns on the victim's body and clothing. Human tissues exhibit a variety of behaviors, much like the layers of a tree trunk. Body fat can also contribute to the combustion process in prolonged-exposure fires (DeHaan, Campbell, and Nurbakhsh 1999; DeHaan and Pope 2007; DeHaan 2012).

Radiant heat (infrared radiation) travels in straight lines and is absorbed to some extent by most materials. Some thin synthetic fabrics are sufficiently transparent to infrared that first- and second-degree burns can be induced through the fabric. Most materials to some degree absorb or reflect radiant heat, but its energy can be reflected from metallic surfaces with sufficient energy to induce thermal damage to secondary target surfaces. The bodies of victims incapacitated during fires may block radiant heat from reaching the surfaces on which they are lying, resulting in a heat or smoke shadowing pattern. In these instances, a silhouette of the victim is left on the bed, carpet, or chair, as illustrated in Figure 5-27.

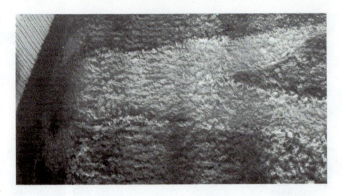

FIGURE 5-27 The bodies of incapacitated victims during fires may block heat from reaching the surfaces on which they are lying, resulting in a heat or smoke shadowing fire pattern. In these instances, a silhouette of the victim is left on the bed, carpet, or chair. *Courtesy of David J. Icove, University of Tennessee.*

5.5 Interpreting Fire Plume Behavior

5.5.1 FIRE VECTORING

A vector is a mathematical pointer that has a direction and a magnitude. An applied technique known as fire vectoring provides the investigator with a tool for understanding and interpreting the combined movement and intensity of plumes that create fire pattern damage. Fire investigators have used fire pattern indicators of various types since the earliest investigations.

Kennedy and Kennedy (1985) introduced the concept of heat and flame vector analysis. However, few investigators fully understood the application of the concept nor did they systematically apply it. Scientific research into fire scene investigations has addressed the topic only in the last decade.

Heat and flame vectoring, to which we refer simply as fire vectoring, is becoming a standard technique for using fire patterns to help determine a fire's area and point of origin (Kennedy 2004; NFPA 2017, pt. 18.4.2). Several examples throughout this text use this simple yet effective principle for tracing a fire's development, which was fully explained and used to document the 1997 USFA Burn Pattern Study (FEMA 1997).

Although the underlying concept of fire vectors has two components—direction of movement and relative intensity—some investigators successfully use only the vector's directional component. However, in post-flashover burning, heat fluxes due to turbulent fuel/air mixing may be high enough to result in the most severe burn damage to a room, irrespective of the fire's actual area or point of origin.

Movement patterns are caused by flame, heat, and by-products of combustion produced when the fire spreads away from its initial source. Evaluating areas of relative damage from the least to the most damaged areas can reveal the fire's movement, a technique for tracking a fire back to its possible room, area, and point of origin. Beveled edges to burned materials, smoke levels in a series of connected rooms, or protected areas on one side of an object are all examples of movement patterns. As long as the target material's thermal properties are considered, a trained investigator may make some interpretation of approximate duration.

Intensity patterns are the result of the fire's sustained impingement on exposed surfaces, such as walls, ceilings, furnishings, wall coverings, and floors. Various intensities of heat transfer result in thermal gradients along these surfaces and sometimes form lines of demarcation dividing burned and unburned areas.

The fire vector's position and length quantitatively indicate the intensity of the particular burn pattern, and its direction typically indicates the apparent flow from hottest to coolest. Once the vectors are documented and reviewed, their cumulative effect assists in determining the source of the fire. Each vector is assigned a number that is used for notations in the report. A fire vector diagram used in USFA Test 5 is shown in Figure 5-28 (FEMA 1997, 47). This technique is more acceptable and accurate in assessing pre-flashover fires.

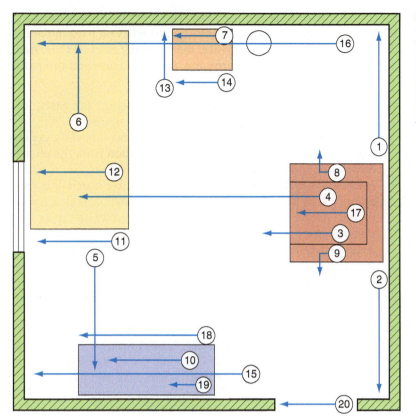

FIGURE 5-28 The fire vectoring technique uses the length of a drawn vector to indicate quantitatively the direction and intensity of the particular burn pattern. *Courtesy of FEMA (1997, 47).*

5.5.2 VIRTUAL ORIGIN

When a majority of the vectors point to the fire plume's base, it is often appropriate to consider this to be the location of the initial fuel package. Vectoring is helpful in estimating the location of the virtual origin or source of thermal energy of the fire. As discussed previously, the virtual origin is a point located along the plume's centerline that would give the same radiative output as the actual fire. This location is sometimes lower than the floor level. If the physical and thermal properties of the fuel package can be determined from the scene investigation, the virtual origin can be mathematically calculated, and its location can be helpful in reconstructing and documenting the fire's virtual source, point of origin, area, and direction of travel. However, if the pattern is clear enough, simple geometric extension of the V sides suffices to establish the virtual origin.

The virtual origin of a fire is located below the floor level when the area of the fuel source is large compared with the energy released by the fuel, as illustrated in previous examples. Likewise, a fuel releasing a high energy over a small area will produce a virtual origin above the floor level (Karlsson and Quintiere 2000). An example of a high-energy release over a small area is a small gasoline pool fire.

5.5.3 TRACING THE FIRE

The fire investigator's task would be quite easy if he or she were present for the duration of the incident. Unfortunately, fire scenes are often cold and in disarray after the extinguishment and subsequent overhaul to assure that the fire will not **rekindle**. The investigator's role then becomes one of reconstructing the sequence of the fire backward to its area and point of origin. A firm understanding of fire behavior becomes imperative during this examination and documentation of the fire scene.

rekindle ■ A return to flaming combustion after apparent but incomplete extinguishment (NFPA 2017, pt. 3.3.155).

The ability to trace the fire's behavior and growth is important to the investigation. Like an experienced tracker, the investigator relies on pattern damage as trail markers of the fire's path. Based on experience, the following rules or characteristics of fire behavior are offered to help the investigator understand and interpret this pattern damage (DeHaan and Icove 2012, chap. 7).

radiation ■ Heat transfer by way of electromagnetic energy (NFPA 2017, pt. 3.3.153).

- *Fire's Tendency to Burn Upward:* A fire plume's hot gases, including flames, are much lighter than the surrounding air and therefore will rise. In the absence of strong winds or physical barriers, such as noncombustible ceilings, that divert flames, fire will tend to burn upward. **Radiation** from the plume will cause some downward and outward travel.

- *Ignition of Combustible Materials:* Combustible materials in the path of the plume's flames will be ignited, thereby increasing the extent and intensity of the fire by increasing the heat release rate. The more intense the fire grows, the faster it will rise and spread.

- *Potential for Flashover:* A flame plume that is large enough to reach the ceiling of a compartment is likely to trigger full involvement of a room and increase the chances for flashover to occur. If there is not more fuel above or beside the initial plume's flame to be ignited by convected or radiated heat, or if the initial fire is too small to create the necessary heat flux on those fuels, the fire will be self-limiting and often will burn itself out.

- *Location and Distribution of Fuel Load:* In evaluating a fire's progress through a room, the investigator must establish what fuels were present and where they were located. This fuel load includes not only the structure itself but its furnishings; contents; and wall, floor, and ceiling coverings; as well as combustible roofing materials, which feed a fire and offer it paths and directions of travel.

- *Lateral Flame Spread:* Variations on the upward spread of the fire plume will occur when air currents deflect the flame, when horizontal surfaces block the vertical travel, or when radiation from established flames ignites nearby surfaces. If fuel is present in these new areas, it will ignite and spread the flames laterally.

- *Vertical Flame Spread:* Natural (buoyancy-driven) upward, vertical spread is enhanced when the fire plume finds chimney-like configurations. Stairways, elevators, utility shafts, air ducts, and interiors of walls all offer openings for carrying flames generated elsewhere. Fires may burn more intensely because of the enhanced draft.

- *Downward Flame Spread:* Flames may spread downward whenever there is suitable fuel in the area. Combustible wall coverings, particularly paneling, encourage the travel of fire downward as well as outward. Fire plumes may ignite portions of ceilings, roof coverings, draperies, and lighting fixtures, which can fall onto ignitable fuels below and start new fires that quickly join the main fire overhead, a process called fall-down or drop-down. Radiant heat and momentum flow of hot gases can also cause downward spread under appropriate conditions. An energetic fire can produce radiant heat sufficient to ignite adjacent floor surfaces. The momentum flow of ceiling jets from such fires can extend downward on nearby walls.

- *Impact of Radiation:* Fire plumes that are large enough to intersect with ceilings will usually form ceiling jets that extend radially along the ceiling surface. Radiation from overhead ceiling jets or hot gas layers can ignite floor coverings, furniture, and walls even at some distance, creating new points of fire origin. The investigator is cautioned to take into account what fuel packages were present in the room from the standpoint of their potential ignitability and heat release rate contributions.

- *Impact of Suppression Efforts:* Suppression efforts can also greatly influence fire spread, so the investigator must remember to confer with the fire suppression personnel present about direct consequences of their actions in extinguishing the fire. Positive-pressure ventilation (PPV) or an active attack on one face of a fire may force it back into other areas that may or may not already have been involved and push the fire down and even under obstructions such as doors and cabinets. The investigator should interview the firefighters and obtain details on how water was applied, because this important information is rarely entered into a fire department's narrative of the fire.

- *Behavior of Heat and Smoke Plumes:* Because of their buoyancy, heat and smoke plumes tend to flow through a room or structure much like a liquid—upward in relatively straight paths and outward around barriers.
- *Impact of Fire Vectors:* The total fire damage to an object observed after a fire is the result of both the intensity of the heat applied to that object and the duration of that exposure. Both factors may vary considerably during the fire.
- *Impact of Plume's Radiant Heat Flux:* The highest-temperature area of a plume will produce the highest radiant heat flux and will, therefore, affect a surface faster and more deeply than will cooler areas. This pattern can show the investigator where a flame plume contacted a surface or in which direction it was moving (because it will lose heat to the surface and cool as it moves across).
- *Impact of the Plume's Placement:* The contribution that fire plume placement makes to the growth process in a room depends not only on its size (heat release rate) and direction of travel but also on its location in the room—in the center, against a wall, in a rear corner, away from ventilation sources, or close to a ventilation opening.

Fire investigation and reconstruction of a fire's growth pattern back to its origin are based on the fact that fire plumes form patterns of damage that are, to a large extent, predictable. With an understanding of fire plume behavior, combustion properties, and general fire behavior, the investigator can prepare to examine a fire scene for these particular indicators. As with the application of the scientific method, each indicator is an independent test for direction of travel, intensity, duration of heat application, or point of origin. There is no one indicator that proves the origin or cause of a fire. All indicators must be evaluated together, and yet they may not all agree. Finally, the application of fire vectoring can also enrich and buttress the opinion rendered as to the original location of the fire plume.

5.6 Fire Burn Pattern Tests

Fire testing can produce all types of fire pattern damage phenomena (Table 5-1) including demarcations, surface effects, penetrations, and loss of materials. Fire testing is one method for expanding the range of knowledge about recognizing and interpreting fire patterns.

With the assistance of NIST, the Federal Emergency Management Agency's US Fire Administration (FEMA/USFA), and the US Tennessee Valley Authority (TVA), police in Florence, Alabama conducted validation testing to explore fire pattern generation. The tests used two forms of structures, a vacant single-family dwelling and a multiple-use assembly building (FEMA 1997; Icove 1995). While the US TVA Police study concentrated on extending the results of fire pattern burn testing on larger-scale structures, NIST and FEMA worked down the street on the single-family dwelling scenarios. Additional full-scale fire tests were reported by Carman (2008, 2009, and 2010), supplemented by post-fire computer modeling.

The primary goals of the project test included demonstrating the production of fire burn patterns, exploring fire scene evidence and documentation techniques, and validating basic fire modeling—all concepts that form the basics of forensic fire scene reconstruction.

5.6.1 FIRE TESTING GOALS

The objectives for conducting the test burns on a multiple-use facility included the simulation of arson fires using plastic containers of ignitable liquids, because arsonists often use these containers when setting fires to structures (Icove et al. 1992). Often, when a burned,

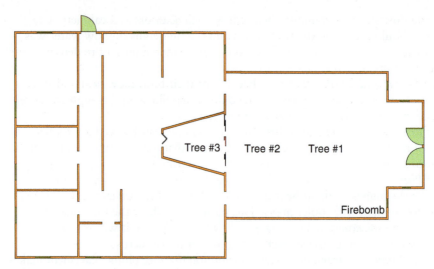

FIGURE 5-29 Floor plan of structure used to simulate the use of a typical firebomb placed in the corner of the room as indicated. *Courtesy of David J. Icove, University of Tennessee.*

self-extinguished firebomb is found, investigators ask the questions: How long did the device burn? What damage can be expected? and Where is the best place to collect evidence of the device once it is damaged?

To simulate the arson, a typical firebomb consisting of a 3.8-L (1-gal) plastic container filled with unleaded gasoline was placed in the corner of the multiple-use facility's main assembly room, as shown in the floor plan in Figure 5-29. The main room was carpeted with institutional-grade synthetic carpeting.

The firebomb was remotely ignited with an electric match. Thermocouple data for the test showed that the resulting fire lasted approximately 300 seconds and then self-extinguished, leaving a 0.46-m (1.5-ft)-diameter circular burned area. Three thermocouple trees recorded the room-temperature profiles, as shown in Figure 5-30.

FIGURE 5-30 Three thermocouple trees recorded the room temperature profiles after the firebomb was remotely ignited with an electric match.

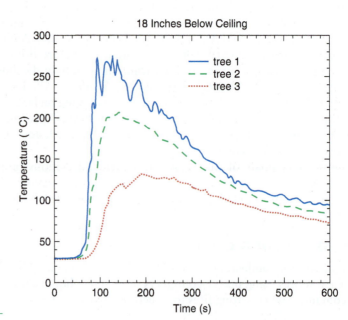

The pre- and post-fire damage patterns are depicted schematically and photographically in Figures 5-31a and b. The exact location of the firebomb and its subsequent burning pool diameter are indicated. The plastic jug melted quickly, so the majority of the fire occurred when its contents were released to burn as a pool fire on the floor. Figure 5-31b illustrates the fire patterns from demarcations, surface effects, penetrations, and loss of material. The schematic uses the relative damages revealed on the exposed surfaces to form isochar lines corresponding to nearly equal char depths. These isochar lines are useful in assisting in the placement and interpretation of fire vectors. The lines also document the ignitable liquid burn patterns found on carpeted and other floor surfaces.

Estimated Heat Release Rate

The peak estimated heat release rate, $\dot{Q}$, for the gasoline pool fire can be calculated using the standard heat release equation:

Heat release rate	$\dot{Q}$	$= \dot{m}'' \Delta h_c A$
Area of the buring pool	A	$= (3.1415/4)(0.457^2) = 0.164 \text{ m}^2$
Mass flux for gasoline	$\dot{m}''$	$= 0.036 \text{ kg/(m}^2 \cdot \text{s)}$
Heat of combustion for gasoline	Δh_c	$= 43.7 \text{ mJ/kg}$
Heat release rate	$\dot{Q}$	$= (0.036)(43700)(0.164) = 258 \text{ kW}$

The real-world estimate for the heat release rate would be between 200 and 300 kW.

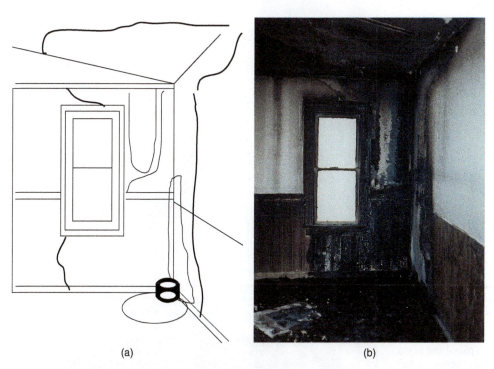

(a)   (b)

FIGURE 5-31 The post-fire pattern damage from the firebomb test depicted both (a) schematically and (b) photographically. (a) Dark lines indicate major demarcations of burned/unburned areas. Light lines indicate isochar demarcations. (b) The wall finish above the wainscoting was painted drywall and played no significant role in vertical flame spread. Colored lines can be used to delineate areas of surface deposit, penetration, and consumption. *Courtesy of David J. Icove, University of Tennessee.*

5.6.2 VIRTUAL ORIGIN

The investigator can use a fire vector analysis of this firebomb test case to better understand and interpret the combined movement and intensity of plumes that created the fire pattern damage shown in Figure 5-32. The vectors originated from an area above where the firebomb was located on the floor, which corresponded to the theoretical virtual origin of the fire plume.

The calculation for the location of the virtual origin confirms this observation. As previously calculated in Example 5-3, the heat release rate for a 0.46-m (1.5-ft)-diameter gasoline fire is approximately 258 kW. The calculation for virtual origin, as taken from the Heskestad equation, is as follows:

Virtual origin	$Z_0 = 0.083 \, \dot{Q}^{2/5} - 1.02 \, D$
Equivalent diameter	$D = 0.457 \text{ m}$
Total heat release rate	$\dot{Q} = 258 \text{ kW}$
Virtual origin	$Z_0 = (0.083)(258)^{2/5} - (1.02)(0.457)$
	$= 0.766 - 0.466 = 0.3 \text{ m (1 ft)}$

For this case example, Z_0 is determined to be 0.3 m (1 ft), which is above the floor level, as documented in the vector diagram in Figure 5-32. As stated previously, research has shown that a fuel releasing a high energy over a small area, as in this example, may produce a virtual origin above the floor level (Karlsson and Quintiere 2000).

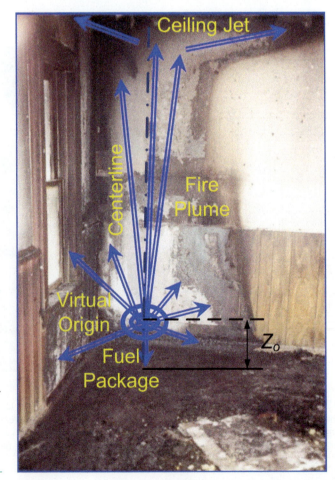

FIGURE 5-32 Fire vector analysis of the firebomb test case assists in understanding and interpreting the fire plume and points to an area above the floor that corresponds to the plume's theoretical virtual origin. *Courtesy of David J. Icove, University of Tennessee.*

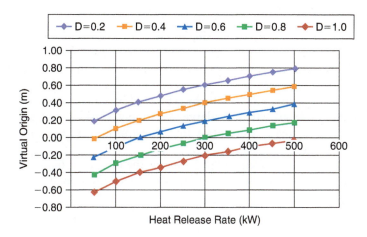

FIGURE 5-33 Plot of the relationship of the virtual origin with changes to the heat release rate and effective diameter of the burning fuel. *Courtesy of Icove and DeHaan (2006).*

A more detailed analysis of the relationship of the virtual origin with changes to the heat release rate and effective diameter of the burning fuel is plotted in Figure 5-33. This plot explores the prediction of the Heskestad equation when comparing fire plumes whose virtual origin may be above or below the burning fuel surface.

For example, a combustible fire with a high heat release rate and small-diameter fuel package will typically have a positive value for the virtual origin, indicating it is located along the centerline above the burning surface of the fuel package. This relationship can be further explored in the graph plotting the relationship of the virtual origin with changes in the heat release rate and effective diameter of the burning fuel.

5.6.3 FLAME HEIGHT

The *NFPA 921*, 2004 edition, flame height calculation (NFPA 2004) takes into account the placement of the fire within the compartment, particularly in corners. By observation of the damage caused by the fire plume as well as its positive virtual origin above the floor, we can assume that the flame height at least touched the ceiling, which, based upon measurements taken at the scene, is 3.18 m (10.43 ft) high.

Total heat release rate	$\dot{Q} = 258\ \text{kW}$
Flame height	$H_f = 0.174(k\dot{Q})^{2/5}$
In a corner ($k = 4$)	$H_f = (0.174)(4 \times 258)^{2/5}$
	$= 2.79\ \text{m}\ (9.15\ \text{ft})$
Including the virtual origin	$H_{\text{total}} = Z_0 + H_f$
	$= 0.299 + 2.79 = 3.09\ \text{m}\ (10.14\ \text{ft})$
	(about 3 m, or 10 ft)

This value corresponds to a greater-than-ceiling height, thus creating the conditions for a ceiling jet across the ceiling. Therefore, the fire plume was high enough to reach the ceiling and radially disperse ceiling jets extending out from the centerline, a behavior that was observed during the test.

5.6.4 FIRE DURATION

It is useful in fire scene reconstruction to determine the initial growth period. In validating estimates of fire duration, it is always helpful to have historical testing, actual loss history data, and realistic fire models.

When comparing the development of real-life fires with models, the investigator relies on observations, documentation, analysis of historical fire test data, and similar cases that relate to the fire under study. A wealth of information is available from handbooks available in the fire protection engineering field (SFPE 2008, sec. 3-1).

Fire duration was one of the key questions addressed in the firebomb test case. After the firebomb ignited, the plastic jug melted, releasing its contents of gasoline into a circular pool of burning liquid. The question then arose: How long could the pool of gasoline be expected to burn? The question of whether the surface under the spill was nonporous concrete or a carpeted material is addressed in a later section.

The burning duration of pool fires can usually be estimated based on the steady-state mass burning rate, assuming rapid growth and a large fuel supply. Gasoline has a density of 740 kg/m^3 (0.74 kg/L). The steady-state mass loss rate (mass flux) of gasoline is 0.036 $kg/(m^2 \cdot s)$ (SFPE 2008, fig. 5-1.2[a]).

The following calculation is the working hypothesis for the estimated burning duration of the gasoline, assuming that it would self-extinguish after all the available fuel was consumed.

Mass of gasoline	$m = (1 \text{ gal})(3.785 \text{ L/gal})(740 \text{ g/L}) = 2.7 \text{ kg}$
Mass buring rate for gasoline	$\dot{m}'' = 0.036 \text{ kg}/(m^2 \cdot s)$
Burning area	$A = \pi r^2 = (3.1416)(0.23 \text{ m})^2 = 0.166 \text{ m}^2$
Burning area	$\dot{m} = A\dot{m}'' = (0.166 \text{ m}^2)[0.036 \text{ kg}/(m^2 \cdot s)]$
	$= 0.00598 \text{ kg/s}$
Approximate buring duration	$= \dot{m}/m = 2.7 \text{ kg}/0.00598 \text{ kg/s} = 451 \text{ s}$

The real-world estimate for the average burning duration should be 7 to 8 minutes. Comparison of this result with the time–temperature curve (5-30), confirms that this time frame is consistent with the actual test results.

5.6.5 REGRESSION RATES

A flammable liquid pool will burn from the top down at a fairly predictable rate, called its *regression rate*, depending on its chemical composition and physical properties if all other factors (e.g., pool diameter and depth) are constant. A thin layer of liquid will burn away very quickly, often so quickly that only the most transient thermal effects will be observed. The depth of a pool is determined by the quantity of liquid, its physical properties (viscosity), and the nature of the surface.

On a level, smooth nonporous surface, if not otherwise limited, a low-viscosity liquid like gasoline will form a pool approximately 1 mm or less deep. On a porous surface the liquid will tend to penetrate as far as it can and then spread horizontally by gravity flow and capillary action. The amount of liquid and the depth of the porous material, the porosity of the substrate, and the rate at which the liquid is poured will determine the size of the pool. On carpeted floors, as a rough guideline, the thickness of carpet can be used as a maximum pool depth, because saturated carpet represents a pool whose depth equals the thickness of the carpet and of any porous pad beneath (DeHaan 1995).

The surface area of the liquid pool is an important variable. A large quantity of gasoline dripping slowly from a leaking gas tank may produce a visible pool on soil or sand not much larger than the diameter of the individual drops but many feet deep. The same quantity dumped quickly onto the same ground may produce a much shallower pool of great diameter. A similar volume of liquid can generate a shallow layer (film) in an arc over a large area. The viscosity and surface tension of the liquid and the speed with which the material is ejected will determine the nature (thickness) of this film. Testing may be needed to establish the bounding conditions of maximum and minimum areas.

Once the liquid is ignited, the rate of burning per unit area (mass flux) is controlled by the amount of heat that can reach the surface of the pool and the size of the perimeter through which air can be entrained. The mass flux depends on the fuel and the size of the pool. For gasoline pools of 0.05 to 0.2 m in diameter the minimum regression rate is 1 to 2 mm/min. (Blinov, in Drysdale 2011). For very small pools, the rate is much higher owing to the laminar flame structure. The heat effects or scorching beneath the burning pool of gasoline are superficial because there is insufficient time and heat flux to produce them. Because the fire size is driven by the evaporation rate per area (mass flux), the larger the pool in surface area, the larger the fire (the greater the heat release rate, $\dot{Q}$). Gasoline pools over 1 m in diameter have a maximum regression rate of 3 to 4 mm/min owing to the limitations of turbulent mixing in the plume (Blinov, in Drysdale 2011).

The flame produces a variety of effects on nearby surfaces depending on the geometry and nature of heat application. Because the fuel-covered substrate is being cooled by evaporation of the liquid fuel in contact with it, its temperature cannot be more than a few degrees hotter than the boiling point of the liquid and so will not do much more than scorch the surface directly under the pool. Low-melting-point materials like synthetics can melt as well as scorch. The areas of carpet or floor immediately outside the pool will be exposed to the radiant heat of the plume during the fire. Without the protection of the evaporating liquid, materials will melt and scorch, particularly if small or thin (carpet fibers). Materials in direct contact with the flame front will be scorched and ignited or at least charred.

Thermal effects of materials near the flame front often produce what is called a *halo* or *ring effect* around the outside of the pool, as shown in tests by Putorti, McElroy, and Madrzykowski (2001). If the substrate is ignitable, a ring of damage may extend some distance from the pool. Eventually, the center of the protected area may be burned as the protective layer of liquid fuel evaporates. In traditional carpets (wool or nylon) this area will be noticeable, and sufficient residues of the liquid fuel may survive in the center of the burned area to be recovered and identified. If the fire burns itself out or is quickly extinguished by a sprinkler system or oxygen depletion, the pool area can be roughly estimated from the dimensions of the burned margins. If the fire is sustained by the carpet, or if the fire (externally) reaches flashover, the area of burned carpet can grow well beyond the area of the original liquid pool. This is particularly true for the new generation of synthetic fiber carpets with polypropylene backing and polypropylene face yarn pile (DeHaan and Icove 2012).

Wool or nylon carpets with jute backing will tend to self-extinguish, but polypropylene will not. Combustion tests have shown that flames on these types of carpets can propagate at a rate of approximately 0.5 to 1 m²/hr (5 to 11 ft²/hr), generating very small flames at the margins of the burning area. Such carpets will pass the methenamine tablet test (*ASTM D2859-16)* (ASTM 2016), because its igniting flame is about 50 W and of brief duration (similar to that of a dropped match); but if there is any significant additional heat flux from a larger ignition source (wad of paper) or a continuously burning object like a piece of furniture, these can propagate a fire over a large area if given enough time (DeHaan and Icove 2012).

5.6.6 NIJ-FUNDED RESEARCH

The National Institute of Justice (NIJ) funded research (Mealy, Benfer, and Gottuk 2011) on the fire dynamics and forensic analysis of liquid fuel fires that explored fluid depths, substrates, burning rates, and impact on ignition delay times. The researchers documented the statistical bounds of spill sizes and depths caused by flammable and combustible fuels including gasoline, kerosene, and denatured alcohol. They also examined spill depths affected by the type of substrates, including vinyl, carpet, plywood, concrete (smooth, brushed, and coated), and oriented strand board.

For spill depth, the researchers conducted a statistical analysis of fluid depths of common liquid types except lube oil on smooth substrates, reporting an average depth of 0.72 mm (0.028 in.) with a standard deviation of 0.34 mm (0.013 in.). Spill depths ranged from 0.22 mm (0.0087 in.) up to 2.4 mm (0.094 in.) depending on the specific liquid/substrate scenario.

Research confirmed two factors governing the spread of a fuel's spill depth—the surface tension of the liquid and the surface characteristics of the substrate on which it is spilled. Because the surface tensions of most fuels are relatively similar, the dominant variable is the substrate's surface topography, which can have an impact on the spill's overall spread and equilibrium spill depth.

The researchers confirmed that the mass burning rates of a fuel are different when the fuel is spilled onto surfaces of differing thermal properties. For each fire, the highest burning rates occurred on the vinyl flooring, and the lowest on concrete. No correlation could be found between burning rates and any specific thermal property of the substrates (i.e., thermal conductivity, **thermal inertia**, thermal effusivity, and thermal diffusivity).

thermal inertia ▪ The properties of a material that characterize its rate of surface temperature rise when exposed to heat; related to the product of the material's thermal conductivity (k), its density (ρ), and its heat capacity (c) (NFPA 2017, pt. 3.3.186).

Finally, these researchers found that the ignition delay time—the time between the initial spill and its ignition—affects the peak mass burning rate. In general, the 300-second ignition delay tests resulted in larger areas with reduced peak mass burning rates per unit area. However, the differences in the average increase in spill area from the 30-second to the 300-second ignition delay times ranged from 8 to 76 percent, with an average value of 36 percent. The percent decrease in the average peak heat release rates ranged from 25 to 74 percent, with an average of 52 percent, for the 30-second and 300-second ignition delay times, respectively. The effects resulting from delayed ignition could not be fully explained from the data, but substrate cooling and evaporative fuel losses were shown to account for some changes in peak mass burning rate.

5.6.7 ADJUSTMENTS TO FIRE DURATION

A comparison of the calculated burning duration of 451 seconds in the previously described firebomb test (Icove 1995) with the actual burning duration shown in Figure 5-30 showed that the actual duration was less than the estimated duration. This working hypothesis had to be modified to account for the carpet present rather than the concrete floor assumed in the initial calculation.

Experiments on carpet saturated with pentane, a component of gasoline, showed that its rate of evaporation (nonburning) is 1.5 times higher than that for a freestanding pool at the same temperature (DeHaan 1995). The steady-state mass loss rate by evaporation of gasoline saturated into carpet is approximately 1.5 times the freestanding value of 0.036, or 0.054 kg/(m^2 · s), assuming in this case that the thermal degradation of the carpet does not affect the mass transfer. Because the combustion processes will progress in the same manner as evaporation on this carpet, the recalculated burning duration for a carpeted surface gave a corrected estimate of 316 seconds and a heat release rate of 387 kW.

Knowledge of the burning characteristics of common flammable and combustible liquids on various surfaces, including those of pool fires such as the one in this test case, is crucial in fire testing and analysis. Synthetic carpets may melt and reduce the mass flux. Also, heat release rate contributions from the molten plastic container pool and carpet were not included. These would be expected to add to the heat release rate and possibly to reduce the duration of the fire.

NIST research on flammable and combustible liquid spill and burn patterns reported that the peak spill fire heat release rates for thin layers of burning liquids on nonporous surfaces were only 12.5 percent to 25 percent of those from equivalent deep-pool fires. The peak heat release rates for fires on carpeted surfaces were found to be approximately equal to those for equivalent pool fires (Putorti, McElroy, and Madrzykowski 2001). Because the nature of the carpet substrates was not reported in these tests, the carpet's contribution cannot be assessed.

In small liquid pool fires, researchers have reported that after the ignition of the fuel, the mass burning rate will increase until a steady rate is reached (Hayasaka 1997). Research and validation experiments on burning rates of liquid fuels on carpet by Ma et al. (2004) indicate that the phenomenon is possibly more complex, particularly regarding the role the carpet plays in supplying fuel to the fire. Ma noted that several factors affect carpet fires: the capillary, or wick, effect of its fibers; evaporation, combustion, and heat transfer; and mass transfer–limited combustion. He surmised that the carpet has two conflicting roles on the mass burning rate: (1) as an insulating material that blocks heat transfer losses to the depth of the pool and increases the mass burning rate along with resulting higher temperatures and (2) as a porous medium that decreases the mass burning rate owing to an insufficient capillary effect. A thin fuel layer on a hard surface such as concrete or wood, whose conductivity is greater than that of the liquid fuel, will result in greater conductive heat transfer losses. Ma pointed out that the reports of observations that liquid fires burn more severely on carpets than on smooth uncarpeted floors or ground can be explained. Carpet enhances the mass burning rate at the earlier stages of burning because it insulates the fabric pile, making the burning liquid fuel appear to behave as a steady deep-pool fire.

5.6.8 FLAME HEIGHT ADJUSTMENT FOR FIRE LOCATION

The flame height is a function of the fire location within the room. As shown, the flame height depends on the fire's placement either in the center ($k = 1$), against the wall ($k = 2$), or in the corner ($k = 4$) of the compartment.

In the initial approach, the corner of the test in Figure 5-31 was assumed to have full impact on the flame height, and a total flame height of 3.1 m (10.1 ft) was predicted. With the new heat release rate of 387 kW and the corner configuration, the new flame height estimate would be recalculated to be 3.28 m plus the virtual origin of 0.43 m, or 3.71 m (12.2 ft). The damage to the corner of the ceiling above the fire demonstrated that a sufficient flame plume was entrained in the corner to cause such penetration. The additional fire from the combustible wall covering (wainscoting) added an unknown factor to the plume generation.

5.6.9 POOL FIRES AND DAMAGE TO SUBSTRATES

When a flammable liquid burns, it does so by evaporating vapors from the liquid, creating a layer of vapor denser than air. Brownian motion at elevated temperatures causes this layer to have a finite thickness and to diffuse into overlying air to form a steep concentration gradient with distance from the liquid surface (DeHaan 1995). Wherever this gradient is within the flammable range of the vapors, a flame can be supported. A **diffusion flame** is one supported by fuel vapors diffusing from the fuel surface into the surrounding air/oxygen.

diffusion flame ■ A flame in which fuel and air mix or diffuse together at the region of combustion (NFPA 2017, pt. 3.3.48).

The distance between the fuel surface and the flame front varies with the temperature and vapor pressure of the fuel. Radiant heat from the layer of flame travels in all directions. Some of the heat radiated downward is absorbed by the fuel, keeping the temperature high enough that there is a continual supply of vapors to support a flame. Some heat is transferred through the fuel into the substrate beneath and is absorbed, increasing the temperature of the substrate. Owing to contact between the substrate and the liquid fuel, heat is transferred to the fuel and then distributed through the fuel, if it is a deep enough layer, by convective circulation.

The temperature of the surface under the pool will not be more than a few degrees above the boiling point of the liquid overlying it. If the fuel's boiling-point temperature is low enough (<200°C, 390°F), the liquid can burn off without any visible effect if the surface is smooth with no pores, joints, or seams, and has a relatively high decomposition temperature. The higher the boiling point of the liquid, the greater the chances of thermal damage to the floor, such as pyrolysis (scorching), melting, or both. In a burning pool of fuel, the radiant heat at the edges absorbed by the substrate may produce localized scorching or other heat effects. If a fuel contains a mixture of compounds with different boiling points, the low-boiling liquid will tend to burn off first, leaving the higher-boiling compounds to continue to heat.

A mixture like gasoline covers the range of boiling points 40°C to 150°C (100°F to 300°F). As the mixture burns, the boiling point of the residue increases, and therefore the limiting temperature factor increases. At 250°C (450°F), wood surfaces will be only scorched, but some synthetic floor coverings can be significantly damaged. Synthetic carpet fibers can also melt and reduce the mass transfer rate of the liquid fuel as the fire progresses. Field fire tests demonstrating the absence of significant thermal effects on wood with gasoline pools have been published (DeHaan 2007).

As reflected in this case example, the final hypothesis noted for this test is the consumption of the gasoline in the time–temperature curve, leveling out approximately 400 seconds after ignition, which is consistent with the estimate. This result demonstrates the effects of the use of flammable liquids in arson and other fire-related crimes—a very rapid increase in localized temperature followed by a rapid consumption to self-extinguishment.

Expert conclusions or opinions on the strength of these hypotheses rest partially on the use of accepted and historically proven fire testing techniques that validate this methodology and can easily be replicated. Additionally, this methodology and similar studies have been peer reviewed and published (DeHaan 1995; Ma et al. 2004; Icove and DeHaan 2006). There are established error rates for applying this methodology specifically to known variables such as room size and fire development times. See Mealy, Benfer, and Gottuk (2011) and Wolfe, Mealy, and Gottuk (2009) for research into the application of fire dynamics to the forensic analysis of liquid-fuel and limited-ventilation compartment fires. Standardized methods are also maintained by independent and unbiased organizations for applying and interpreting these relationships.

Summary

Fire scenes must be accurately examined for the origin and cause. In order to complete that task, fire investigators need to have a basic understanding of the underlying principles of fire dynamics that directly relate to the damage caused by the fire, particularly the damage formed by fire patterns. Fire scene examinations are best approached from a three-dimensional viewpoint, since two-dimensional interpretations of damage may lead the investigator to a wrong hypothesis as to the fire's origin and cause.

The combined disciplines of physics, thermodynamics, chemistry, heat transfer, and fluid mechanics assist the investigator in making accurate determinations of a fire's origin, intensity, growth, direction of travel, duration, and extinguishment. Fire investigators can benefit from published research involving the application of the expertise that exists in the area of fire dynamics; however, many fire investigators do not have access to all these resources.

Following an investigative protocol is an expectation of courts as a result of the *Daubert*, *Kumho Tire*, and *Benfield* decisions. Reconstructing the pre-fire scene as completely as possible using a step-by-step plan is critical to evaluating fire patterns accurately. This includes not only physically relocating fuel packages in their original locations but also identifying wall, floor and ceiling coverings, determining window and door openings, and conducting a fire engineering analysis for a reconstruction of fire spread.

Review Questions

1. What is overhaul and why is it critical that it be kept to a minimum?
2. What basic fire behaviors are revealed by post-fire indicators?
3. Name three ways suppression efforts can affect fire spread and post-fire indicators.
4. What is the most common search pattern for structure fires and what are four of its advantages?
5. Why is the documentation and reconstruction of fuel load so important?
6. What is a heat horizon and how does it help establish direction of development of a structure fire?
7. Name three ways ventilation openings can affect fire patters in a room fire.
8. How does window glass provide useful information to a fire investigator?
9. Why is a contents inventory important in a fire investigation?

References

Alpert, R. 1972. "Calculation of Response Time of Ceiling-mounted Fire Detectors." *Fire Technology* 8 (3): 181–95, doi: 10.1007/bf02590543.

Alpert, R. J., and E. J. Ward. 1984. "Evaluation of Unsprinklered Fire Hazards." *Fire Safety Journal* 2, No. 2 (1984): 127–43.

ASTM 2014. *ASTM C1396/C1396M-14a: Standard Specification for Gypsum Board*. West Conshohocken, PA: ASTM International.

———. 2016. *ASTM D2859-16. 2016. Standard Test Method for Ignition Characteristics of Finished Textile Floor Covering Materials*. West Conshohocken, PA: ASTM International.

Audouin, L., G. Kolb, J. L. Torero, and J. M. Most. 1995. "Average Centreline Temperatures of a Buoyant Pool Fire Obtained by Image Processing of Video Recordings." *Fire Safety Journal* 24 (2): 167–87, doi: 10.1016/0379-7112(95)00021-k.

Babrauskas, V. 1980. "Flame Lengths under Ceilings." *Fire and Materials* 4 (3): 119–26, doi: 10.1002/fam.810040304.

———. 2004. *Glass Breakage in Fires*. Issaquah, WA: Fire Science and Technology Inc.

———. 2005. "Charring Rate of Wood as a Tool for Fire Investigations." *Fire Safety Journal* 40 (6): 528–54, doi: 10.1016/j.firesaf.2005.05.006.

Babrauskas, V. and J. Krasny. 1985. *Fire Behavior of Upholstered Furniture.* NBS Monograph 173. Gaithersburg, MD: US Department of Commerce, National Bureau of Standards.

Bessey, G. E. 1950. "Investigations on Building Fires. Part II: The Visible Changes in Concrete or Mortar Exposed to High Temperatures." *Technical Paper No. 4.* Garston, England: Department of Scientific and Industrial Research, Building Research Station.

Beyler, C. L. 1986. "Fire Plumes and Ceiling Jets." *Fire Safety Journal* 11 (1–2): 53–75, doi: 10.1016/0379-7112(86)90052-4.

———. 2008. "Fire Hazard Calculations for Large, Open Hydrocarbon Fires." In *SFPE Handbook of Fire Protection Engineering,* 4th ed., ed. P. J. DiNenno. Quincy, MA: National Fire Protection Association.

Bostrom, L. 2005. "Methodology for Measurement of Spalling of Concrete." Paper presented at Fire and Materials 2005, 9th International Conference, January 31–February 1, San Francisco, CA.

Buchanan, A. H. 2001. *Structural Design for Fire Safety.* Chichester, England: Wiley.

Butler, C. P. 1971. "Notes on Charring Rates in Wood." *Fire Research Notes 896.* London: Joint Fire Research Organization. Borehamwood, England: Fire Research Station.

Canfield, D. 1984. "Causes of Spalling of Concrete at Elevated Temperatures." *Fire and Arson Investigator* 34 (4): 22–23.

Carman, S. W. 2008. "Improving the Understanding of Post-flashover Fire Behavior." Paper presented at the International Symposium on Fire Investigation Science and Technology, May 19–21, Cincinnati, OH.

———. 2009. "Progressive Burn Pattern Developments in Post-flashover Fires." Paper presented at Fire and Materials 2009, 11th International Conference, January 26–28, San Francisco, CA.

———. 2010. "Clean Burn Fire Patterns: A New Perspective for Interpretation." Paper presented at Interflam, July 5–7, Nottingham, UK.

Chakrabarti, B., T. Yates, and A. Lewry. 1996. "Effects of Fire Damage on Natural Stonework in Buildings." *Construction and Building Materials* 10 (7): 539–44.

Chu Nguong, N. 2004. "Calcination of Gypsum Plasterboard under Fire Exposure." Master's thesis, University of Canterbury, Christchurch, New Zealand (*Fire Engineering Research Report 04/6*).

Cox, G., and R. Chitty. 1982. "Some Stochastic Properties of Fire Plumes." *Fire and Materials* 6 (3–4): 127–34, doi: 10.1002/fam.810060306.

DeHaan, J. D. 1987. "Are Localized Burns Proof of Flammable Liquid Accelerants?" *Fire and Arson Investigator* 38 (1): 45–49.

———. 1995. "The Reconstruction of Fires Involving Highly Flammable Hydrocarbon Liquids." PhD diss., University of Strathclyde, Glasgow, Scotland, UK.

———. 2007. *Kirk's Fire Investigation.* 6th ed. Upper Saddle River, NJ: Pearson-Prentice Hall.

———. 2012. "Sustained Combustion of Bodies: Some Observations." *Journal of Forensic Science*, May 4, doi: 10.1111/j.1556-4029.2012.02190.x.

DeHaan, J. D., S. J. Campbell, and S. Nurbakhsh. 1999. "Combustion of Animal Fat and Its Implications for the Consumption of Human Bodies in Fires." *Science & Justice* 39 (1): 27–38, doi: 10.1016/s1355-0306(99)72011-3.

DeHaan, J. D., and D. J. Icove 2012. *Kirk's Fire Investigation.* 7th ed. Upper Saddle River, NJ: Pearson-Prentice Hall.

DeHaan, J. D., and E. J. Pope. 2007. "Combustion Properties of Human and Large Animal Remains." Paper presented at 11th International Fire Science and Engineering Conference, Interflam 2007, September 3–5, London, UK.

Drysdale, D. 2011. *An Introduction to Fire Dynamics,* 3rd ed. Chichester, West Sussex, UK: Wiley.

Fang, J. B., and J. N. Breese. 1980. *Fire Development in Residential Basement Rooms.* Gaithersburg, MD: National Bureau of Standards.

FEMA. 1997. "USFA Fire Burn Pattern Tests." *Report FA 178.* Emmitsburg, MD: Federal Emergency Management Agency, US Fire Administration.

Harris, R. J. 1983. *The Investigation and Control of Gas Explosions in Buildings and Heating Plants.* London: British Gas Corp.

Harris, R. J., M. R. Marshall, and D. J. Moppett. 1977. "The Response of Glass Windows to Explosion Pressures." Published as IChemE Symposium Series No. 49, April 5–7.

Harrison, R. 2004. "Smoke Control in Atrium Buildings: A Study of the Thermal Spill Plume." In *Fire Engineering Research Report 04/1*, ed. M. Spearpoint. Christchurch, New Zealand: University of Canterbury.

Harrison, R., and M. Spearpoint. 2007. "The Balcony Spill Plume: Entrainment of Air into a Flow from a Compartment Opening to a Higher Projecting Balcony." *Fire Technology* 43 (4): 301–17, doi: 10.1007/s10694-007-0019-3.

Hasemi, Y., and M. Nishihata. 1989. "Fuel Shape Effects on the Deterministic Properties of Turbulent Diffusion Flames." Paper presented at Fire Safety Science, Second International Symposium, Washington, DC.

Hayasaka, H. 1997. "Unsteady Burning Rates of Small Pool Fires." In *Proceedings of 5th Symposium on Fire Safety Science,* ed. Y. Hasemi. Tsukuba, Japan.

Hertz, K. D., and L. S. Sorensen. 2005. "Test Method for Spalling of Fire-Exposed Concrete." *Fire Safety Journal* 40: 466–76.

Heskestad, G. H. 1982. *Engineering Relations for Fire Plumes.* SFPE Technology Report 82-8. Boston: Society of Fire Protection Engineers.

———. 1983. "Virtual Origins of Fire Plumes." *Fire Safety Journal* 5 (2): 109–14, doi: 10.1016/0379-7112(83)90003-6.

———. 2008. "Fire Plumes, Flame Height, and Air Entrainment." Chapter 2-1 in *SFPE Handbook of Fire Protection Engineering,* ed. P. J. DiNenno. Quincy, MA: National Fire Protection Association, Society of Fire Protection Engineers.

Hietaniemi, J. 2005. "Probabilistic Simulation of Glass Fracture and Fallout in Fire." *VTT Working Papers 41,* ESPOO 2005. Finland: VTT Building and Transport.

Holleyhead, R. 1999. "Ignition of Solid Materials and Furniture by Lighted Cigarettes. A Review." *Science & Justice* 39 (2): 75–102.

Hopkins, R. L., G. E. Gorbett, and P. M. Kennedy. 2007. "Fire Pattern Persistence and Predictability on Interior Finish and Construction Materials During Pre- and Post-Flashover Compartment Fires." Paper presented at Fire and Materials 2007, 10th International Conference, January 29–31, San Francisco, CA.

Icove, D. J. 1995. "Fire Scene Reconstruction." Paper presented at the First International Symposium on the Forensic Aspects of Arson Investigations, July 31, Fairfax, VA.

Icove, D. J., and J. D. DeHaan. 2006. "Hourglass Burn Patterns: A Scientific Explanation for Their Formation." Paper presented at the International Symposium on Fire Investigation Science and Technology, June 26–28, Cincinnati, OH.

Icove, D. J., J. E. Douglas, G. Gary, T. G. Huff, and P. A. Smerick. 1992. "Arson." In *Crime Classification Manual,* ed. J. E. Douglas, A. W. Burgess, A. G. Burgess, and R. K. Ressler. New York: Macmillan.

Iqbal, N., and M. H. Salley. 2004. *Fire Dynamics Tools (Fdts): Quantitative Fire Hazard Analysis Methods for the U.S. Nuclear Regulatory Commission Fire Protection Inspection Program.* Washington, DC: Nuclear Regulatory Commission.

Jansson, R. 2006. Thermal Stresses Cause Spalling. *Brand Posten SP, Swedish National Testing and Research Institute* 33: 24–25.

Jia, F., E. R. Galea, and M. K. Patel. 1999. "Numerical Simulation of the Mass Loss Process in Pyrolyzing Char Materials." *Fire and Materials* 23: 71–78.

Karlsson, B., and J. G. Quintiere. 2000. *Enclosure Fire Dynamics.* Boca Raton, FL: CRC Press.

Kennedy, J., and P. Kennedy. 1985. *Fires and Explosions: Determining the Cause and Origin.* Chicago, IL: Investigations Institute.

Kennedy, P. M. 2004. "Fire Pattern Analysis in Origin Determination." Paper presented at the International Symposium on Fire Investigation Science and Technology, Cincinnati, OH.

Khoury, G. A. 2000. "Effect of Fire on Concrete and Concrete Structures." *Progress in Structural Engineering Materials* 2: 429–42.

König, J., and L. Walleij. 2000. "Timber Frame Assemblies Exposed to Standard and Parametric Fires. Part 2: A Design Model for Standard Fire Exposure." *Report No. 100010001.* Stockholm, Sweden: Swedish Institute for Wood Technology Research.

Lau, P. W., C. R. White, and I. Van Zeeland. 1999. "Modelling the Charring Behavior of Structural Lumber." *Fire and Materials* 23: 209–16.

Lawson, J. R. 1977. *An Evaluation of Fire Properties of Generic Gypsum Board Products.* Gaithersburg, MD: National Bureau of Standards.

Lentini, J. J. 1992. "Behavior of Glass at Elevated Temperatures." *Journal of Forensic Sciences* 37 (5): 1358–62.

Ma, T. S., M. Olenick, M. S. Klassen, R. J. Roby, and L. J. Torero. 2004. "Burning Rate of Liquid Fuel on Carpet (Porous Media)." *Fire Technology* 40 (3): 227–46.

Mann, D. C., and N. D. Putaansuu. 2006. "Alternative Sampling Methods to Collect Ignitable Liquid Resides from Non-Porous Areas Such As Concrete." *Fire and Arson Investigator* 57 (1): 43–46.

McCaffrey, B. J. 1979. *Purely Buoyant Diffusion Flames: Some Experimental Results (Final Report).* Washington, DC: National Bureau of Standards.

McGraw, J. R., and F. W. Mowrer. 1999. "Flammability of Painted Gypsum Wallboard Subjected to Fire Heat Fluxes." Paper presented at Interflam 1999, June 29–July 1, Edinburgh, Scotland, UK.

Mealy, C. L., M. E. Benfer, and D. T. Gottuk. 2011. *Fire Dynamics and Forensic Analysis of Liquid Fuel Fires.* Baltimore, MD: Hughes Associates, Inc.

Merck Co. 1989. *Merck Index.* 11th ed. 1989. Rahway, NJ: Merck Co.

Milke, J. A., and F. W. Mowrer. 2001. "Application of Fire Behavior and Compartment Fire Models Seminar." Paper presented at the Tennessee Valley Society of Fire Protection Engineers (TVSFPE), September 27–28, Oak Ridge, TN.

Mitler, H. E., and J. A. Rockett. 1987. *Users' Guide to FIRST, a Comprehensive Single-Room Fire Model.* Gaithersburg, MD: National Bureau of Standards.

Moodie, K., and S. F. Jagger. 1992. "The King's Cross Fire: Results and Analysis from the Scale Model Tests." *Fire Safety Journal* 18 (1): 83–103, doi: 10.1016/0379-7112(92)90049-i.

Morgan, H. P., and N. R. Marshall. 1975. "Smoke Hazards in Covered Multi-Level Shopping Malls: An Experimentally Based Theory for Smoke Production." *BRE Current Paper* 48/75: 23. Garston, England, UK: Building Research Establishment.

Mowrer, F. W. 1998. *Window Breakage Induced by Exterior Fires.* Washington, DC: US Department of Commerce.

———. 2001. "Calcination of Gypsum Wallboard in Fire." Paper presented at the NFPA World Fire Safety Congress, May 13–17, Anaheim, CA.

Newman, J. S. 1993. "Integrated Approach to Flammability Evaluation of Polyurethane Wall/Ceiling Materials." *Journal of Cellular Plastics* 29 (5), doi: 10.1177/0021955X9302900535.

NFPA. 1949. *The Firemen's Responsibility in Arson Detection.* Quincy, MA: National Fire Protection Association.

———. 2004. *NFPA 921: Guide for Fire and Explosion Investigations.* Quincy, MA: National Fire Protection Association.

———. 2008. *NFPA Fire Protection Handbook*. 20th ed. Quincy, MA: National Fire Protection Association.

———. 2014. *NFPA 1033: Standard for Professional Qualifications for Fire Investigator*. Quincy, MA: National Fire Protection Association.

———. 2015. *NFPA 92: Standard for Smoke Control Systems*. Quincy, MA: National Fire Protection Association.

———. 2016. *NFPA 53: Recommended Practice on Materials, Equipment, and Systems Used on Oxygen-Enriched Atmospheres*. Quincy, MA: National Fire Protection Association.

———. 2017. *NFPA 921: Guide for Fire and Explosion Investigations*. Quincy, MA: National Fire Protection Association.

NIST. 1991. *Users' Guide to BREAK1, the Berkeley Algorithm for Breaking Window Glass in a Compartment Fire*. Gaithersburg, MD: National Institute of Standards and Technology.

NPL. 2000. *Guides to Good Practices in Corrosion Control*. National Physical Laboratory, Queens Road, Teddington, Middlesex TW11 0LW.

Ogle, R. A., and J. L. Schumacher. 1998. "Fire Patterns on Upholstered Furniture: Smoldering Versus Flaming Combustion." *Fire Technology* 34 (3): 247–65.

Orloff, L., A. T. Modak, and R. L. Alpert. 1977. "Burning of Large-Scale Vertical Surfaces." *Symposium (International) on Combustion* 16 (1): 1345–54, doi: 10.1016/s0082-0784(77)80420-7.

Parker, T. W., and R. W. Nurse. 1950. "Investigations on Building Fires. Part I: The Estimation of the Maximum Temperature Attained in Building Fires from Examination of the Debris." *National Building Studies*, Technical Paper no. 4: 1–5. Building Research Station, Garston, England: Department of Scientific and Industrial Research.

Perry, R. H., and D. W. Green, eds. 1984. *Perry's Chemical Engineers' Handbook*. 6th ed. New York: McGraw-Hill.

Putorti Jr., A. D., J. A. McElroy, and D. Madrzykowski. 2001. *Flammable and Combustible Liquid Spill/Burn Patterns*. Rockville, MD: National Institute of Standards and Technology.

Quintiere, J. G. 1998. *Principles of Fire Behavior*. Albany, N.Y.: Delmar.

———. 2006. *Fundamentals of Fire Phenomena*. West Sussex, England, UK: Wiley.

Quintiere, J. G., and B. S. Grove. 1998. *Correlations for Fire Plumes*. (NIST-GCR-98-744). Gaithersburg, MD: National Institute of Standards and Technology.

Richardson, J. K., L. R. Richardson, J. R. Mehaffey, and C. A. Richardson. 2000. What Users Want Fire Model Developers to Address. *Fire Protection Engineering* Spring: 22–25.

Sanderson, J. L. 1995. "Tests Results Add Further Doubt to the Reliability of Concrete Spalling as an Indicator." *Fire Findings* 3 (4): 1–3.

———. 2002. "Depth of Char: Consider Elevation Measurements for Greater Precision." *Fire Findings* 10, no. 2 (Spring): 6.

Schroeder, R. A., and R. B. Williamson. 2001. "Application of Materials Science to Fire Investigation." Paper presented at Fire and Materials 2001, 7th International Conference, January 22–24, San Francisco, CA.

———. 2003. "Post-fire Analysis of Construction Materials: Gypsum Wallboard." Paper presented at Fire and Materials 2001, 8th International Conference, January 28–29, San Francisco, CA.

SFPE. 2008. *SFPE Handbook of Fire Protection Engineering*. 4th ed. Quincy, MA: National Fire Protection Association, Society of Fire Protection Engineers.

Shields, T. J., G. W. H. Silcock, and M. F. Flood. 2001. "Performance of a Single Glazing Assembly Exposed to Enclosure Corner Fires of Increasing Severity." *Fire and Materials* 22: 123–52.

Short, N. R., S. E. Guise, and J. A. Purkiss. 1996. "Assessment of Fire-Damaged Concrete Using Color Analysis." *InterFlam '96 Proceedings*. London: Interscience.

Silcock, G. W. H., and T. J. Shields. 2001. "Relating Char Depth to Fire Severity Conditions." *Fire and Materials* 25: 9–11.

Smith, D.W. 1997. "The Firefighter's Role in Preserving the Fire Scene." *Fire Engineering* 150 (1): 103–109.

Smith, F. P. 1991. "Concrete Spalling: Controlled Fire Test and Review." *Journal of Forensic Science* 31 (1): 67–75.

Spearpoint, M. J., and J. G. Quintiere. 2001. "Predicting the Piloted Ignition of Wood in the Cone Calorimeter Using an Integral Model: Effect of Species, Grain Orientation and Heat Flux." *Fire Safety Journal* 36 (4): 391–415, doi: 10.1016/s0379-7112(00)00055-2.

Steckler, K. D., J. G. Quintiere, and W. J. Rinkinen. 1982. "Flow Induced by Fire in a Compartment." *Symposium (International) on Combustion* 19 (1): 913–20, doi: 10.1016/s0082-0784(82)80267-1.

Stratton, B. J. 2005. "Determining Flame Height and Flame Pulsation Frequency and Estimating Heat Release Rate from 3D Flame Reconstruction." Master's thesis, University of Canterbury, Christchurch, New Zealand (*Fire Engineering Research Report 05/2*).

Takeda, H., and J. R. Mehaffey. 1998. "WALL2D: A Model for Predicting Heat Transfer Through Wood-Stud Walls Exposed to Fire." *Fire and Materials* 22: 133–40.

Tanaka, T. J., S. P. Nowlen, and D. J. Anderson. 1996. *Circuit Bridging of Components by Smoke. S. N. Laboratory*. Albuquerque, New Mexico: US Nuclear Regulatory Commission.

Tewarson, A. 2008. "Generation of Heat and Gaseous, Liquid, and Solid Products in Fires." Chapter 3-4 in *SFPE Handbook of Fire Protection Engineering*, ed. P. J. DiNenno. Quincy, MA: National Fire Protection Association, Society of Fire Protection Engineers.

Thomas, G. 2002. "Thermal Properties of Gypsum Plasterboard at High Temperatures." *Fire and Materials* 26 (1): 37–45, doi: 10.1002/fam.786.

Tobin, W. A., and K. L. Monson. 1989. "Collapsed Spring Observations in Arson Investigations: A Critical Metallurgical Evaluation." *Fire Technology* 25 (4): 317–35.

Wallace, M., and J. D. DeHaan. 2000. "Overhauling for Successful Fire Investigation." *Fire Engineering* (December): 73–75.

Wolfe, A. J., C. L. Mealy, and D. Gottuk. 2009. *Fire Dynamics and Forensic Analysis of Limited Ventilation Compartment Fires*. National Institute of Justice: 194.

Wu, Y., and D. D. Drysdale. 1996. *Study of Upward Flame Spread on Inclined Surfaces*. Edinburgh, UK: Health & Safety Executive.

You, H-Z. 1984. "An Investigation of Fire Plume Impingement on a Horizontal Ceiling. 1: Plume Region." *Fire and Materials* 8 (1): 28–39.

Zukoski, E. E. 1978. "Development of a Stratified Ceiling Layer in the Early Stages of a Closed-Room Fire." *Fire and Materials* 2 (2): 54–62, doi: 10.1002/fam.810020203.

Zukoski, E. E., B. M. Cetegen, and T. Kubota. 1985. "Visible Structure of Buoyant Diffusion Flames." *Symposium (International) on Combustion* 20 (1): 361–66, doi: 10.1016/s0082-0784(85)80522-1.

Legal References

Daubert v. Merrell Dow Pharmaceuticals Inc., 509 U.S. 579 (1993); 113 S. Ct. 2756, 215 L. Ed. 2d 469.

Daubert v. Merrell Dow Pharmaceuticals Inc. (Daubert II), 43 F.3d 1311, 1317 (9th Cir. 1995).

Kumho Tire Co. v. Carmichael, 526 U.S. 137 (1999).

Michigan Millers Mutual Insurance Corporation v. Benfield, 902 F. Supp 1509 (M.D. Fla. 1995).

6

Fire Scene Documentation

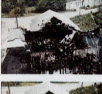
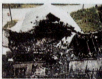
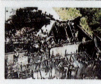
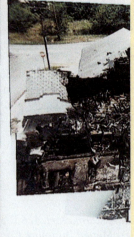
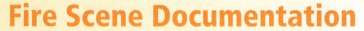

Courtesy of David J. Icove,
University of Tennessee.

ambient, *p. 397*	**char,** *p. 378*	**soot,** *p. 376*
annealing, *p. 402*	**fire patterns,** *p. 365*	**spoliation,** *p. 405*
arc-fault mapping, *p. 378*	**fuel load,** *p. 379*	**thermal inertia,** *p. 390*
arcing through char, *p. 378*	**heat release rate (HRR),** *p. 390*	**ventilation,** *p. 365*
calcination, *p. 398*	**isochar,** *p. 428*	
chain of evidence **(chain of custody),** *p. 433*	**overhaul,** *p. 375*	
	plume, *p. 391*	

OBJECTIVES

After reading this chapter, you should be able to:

- Define and outline proper fire scene documentation.
- Illustrate the fire scene and its reconstruction.
- Employ proper tools to record the scene.
- Recognize and minimize the possibility of spoliation when processing a fire scene.

Fire scenes often contain complex information that must be thoroughly documented. A single photograph and scene diagram are not sufficient to capture vital information on fire dynamics, building construction, fire indicators, evidence collection, and avenues of escape for the building's occupants.

Comprehensive documentation with an emphasis on a systematic set of guidelines includes forensic photography, measurements, sketches, drawings, and analysis. The purposes of forensic fire scene documentation are to record visual observations, to authenticate physical evidence found at the scene, and to ensure the integrity of the scene delayering process.

6.1 National Protocols

The systematic documentation of a fire scene from its initial stages plays an essential role in the effort to record and preserve the events and evidence for all parties involved, particularly for forensic and other experts who are retained later use for criminal, civil, or administrative matters. Systematic documentation ensures that an independent, qualified investigator examining the evidence can arrive at the same opinions as the documenting investigator. Additionally, a failure to systematically document a scene can have severe consequences in litigation when *Daubert* (1993 and 1995) or similar types of challenges are raised.

POST-INCIDENT INVESTIGATION STANDARD: 4.6.1 *NFPA 1033*, 2014 EDITION

TASK:

Gather reports and records, given no special tools, equipment, or materials, so that all gathered documents are applicable to the investigation, complete and authentic; the chain of custody is maintained, and the material is admissible in a legal proceeding.

PERFORMANCE OUTCOME:

The investigator will gather reports/records, given no special tools or equipment, so that all gathered documents are appropriate to the investigation, complete and authentic, and the chain of custody is maintained.

CONDITIONS:

Given several different sources of reports and records, the investigator will complete the listed task.

TASK STEPS:

1. Review provided materials
2. Request and document request for needed materials
3. Select documentation acceptable to the courts
4. Document steps to maintain chain of custody of requested documents

Source: Derived and updated from Washington State Patrol, Form No. 3000-420-081 (Sept. 2014) Fire Protection Bureau, Standards and Accreditation, Olympia, Washington http://www.wsp.wa.gov/fire/docs/cert /fire_invest.pdf

POST-INCIDENT INVESTIGATION STANDARD:
4.6.2 *NFPA 1033*, 2014 EDITION

TASK:

Evaluate the investigative file, given all available file information, so that areas for further investigation are identified, the relationship between gathered documents and information is interpreted, and corroborative evidence and information discrepancies are discovered.

PERFORMANCE OUTCOME:

The investigator will evaluate the investigative file.

CONDITIONS:

Given all available fire information.

TASK STEPS:

1. Evaluate the investigative file and identify areas for further investigation
2. Correctly interpret the relationship between the gathered documents and available information
3. Determine appropriate corroborative evidence
4. Appropriately document any discrepancies found in the investigative file

Source: Derived and updated from Washington State Patrol, Form No. 3000-420-081 (Sept. 2014) Fire Protection Bureau, Standards and Accreditation, Olympia, Washington http://www.wsp.wa.gov/fire/docs/cert/fire_invest.pdf

PRESENTATION STANDARD:
4.7.1 *NFPA 1033*, 2014 EDITION

TASK:

Prepare a written investigation report, given investigative findings, documentation, and a specific audience, so that the report accurately reflects the investigative findings, is concise, expresses the investigator's opinion, contains facts and data that the investigator relies on in rendering an opinion, contains the reasoning of the investigator by which each opinion was reached and meets the needs or requirements for the intended audience(s).

PERFORMANCE OUTCOME:

The investigators will hand-write an initial investigation report, including an opinion as to the cause of the fire.

CONDITIONS:

Given investigation findings, documentation, an identified audience, forms, note pad, and authorization from the prosecutor to include the investigator's opinion in the report.

TASK STEPS:

1. Review provided investigation information and incident reports
2. Ask the assistant investigator follow-up questions, if necessary
3. Write initial investigation report using provided materials
4. Include opinion of fire cause, properly marked as opinion
5. Review the report for grammar and accuracy
6. Submit the report to the intended audience

Source: Derived and updated from Washington State Patrol, Form No. 3000-420-081 (Sept. 2014) Fire Protection Bureau, Standards and Accreditation, Olympia, Washington http://www.wsp.wa.gov/fire/docs/cert/fire_invest.pdf

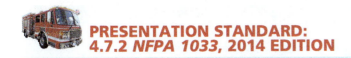

Several national protocols cite the need for systematic documentation of fire scenes, including two protocols by the US Department of Justice and the National Fire Protection Association (NFPA). A one-page synopsis of these protocols, guides, and standards appears in Table 6-1 (Icove and Haynes 2007; Icove and Dalton 2008).

US Department of Justice

The National Institute of Justice (NIJ), which serves as the applied research and technology agency of the US Department of Justice, developed a peer-reviewed national protocol for fire investigation. The NIJ's (2000) *Fire and Arson Scene Evidence: A Guide for Public Safety Personnel* was the product of their Technical Working Group on Fire/Arson Investigation, which consisted of 31 national experts from law enforcement, prosecution, defense, and fire investigation communities. Two of the authors of this text (DeHaan and Icove) participated in the preparation and editing of the NIJ guide.

The intent of the NIJ guide is to educate as many public sector personnel as possible, mainly fire, police, and emergency medical, to the process of identifying, documenting, collecting, and preserving critical physical evidence at fire scenes. This document has become the most widely distributed public guide on fire scene processing since the 1980 historic publication by the National Bureau of Standards (NBS; forerunner of the National Institute of Standards and Technology), *Fire Investigation Handbook* (NBS 1980).

National Fire Protection Association

The NFPA's *Guide for Fire Incident Field Notes*, *NFPA 906*, first published in 1988, and republished in 1998, is a standardized protocol for recording field notes of fire scenes (NFPA 1998). The NIJ's 2000 guide cites *NFPA 906* and includes the data collection forms in its appendix. These forms have been merged into *NFPA 921* (NFPA 2017).

TABLE 6-1 Summary of Guidelines, Protocols, and Standards in a Comprehensive Fire Investigation

Instructions: Check the appropriate block to indicate the presence or absence of the following information.

YES	NO	
☐	☐	Scene secured (*NFPA 1033, 4.2.1*)
☐	☐	Scene safety assessment conducted (*OSHA, 29 CFR Section 1910*)
☐	☐	Exterior survey conducted (*NFPA 1033, 4.2.2; NFPA 906-2*)
☐	☐	Interior survey conducted (*NFPA 1033, 4.2.3; NFPA 906-2*)
☐	☐	Burn patterns interpreted (*NFPA 1033, 4.2.4; NFPA 906-2*)
☐	☐	Burn patterns correlated (*NFPA 1033, 4.2.5; NFPA 906-2*)
☐	☐	Fire debris examined and removed (*NFPA 1033, 4.2.6; ASTM E1188; ASTM E1459*)
☐	☐	Area(s) of origin reconstructed (*NFPA 1033, 4.2.7*)
☐	☐	Building performance inspected (*NFPA 1033, 4.2.8*)
☐	☐	Effects of explosions discriminated from other damage (*NFPA 1033, 4.2.9*)
☐	☐	Scene diagrammed (*NFPA 1033, 4.3.1; NFPA 906-9*)
☐	☐	Scene photographed (*NFPA 1033, 4.3.2; NFPA 906-8; ASTM E 1188*)
☐	☐	Investigative notes taken and preserved (*NFPA 1033, 4.3.3; NFPA 906*)
☐	☐	Eyewitness evidence identified, preserved, collected, packaged (*NIJ Eyewitness Evidence Guide*)
☐	☐	Evidence (physical, electronic, digital) identified, preserved, collected, packaged (*NFPA 1033, 4.4.1, 4.4.2; NFPA 906-7; ASTM E 620; ASTM E 860; ASTM E1188; ASTM E1459; NIJ Electronic Crime Scene Investigation Guide; FBI Guidelines for Imaging Technologies*)
☐	☐	Evidence properly selected for analysis (*NFPA 1033, 4.4.3; NFPA 906-7; ASTM E620; ASTM E1492*)
☐	☐	Chain of custody documented (*NFPA 1033, 4.4.4; NFPA 906-7*)
☐	☐	Evidence properly disposed (*NFPA 1033, 4.4.5*)
☐	☐	Interview plan developed (*NFPA 1033, 4.5.1*)
☐	☐	Interviews/interrogations properly conducted (*NFPA 1033, 4.5.2; NFPA 906-6*)
☐	☐	Investigative information properly inventoried (*NFPA 906-0*)
☐	☐	Investigative information properly analyzed/correlated (*NFPA 1033, 4.5.3; ASTM E620*)
☐	☐	Investigative information properly obtained/documented (*NFPA 1033, 4.6.1; NFPA 906-1, 906-10, 906-11*)
☐	☐	Investigative information in file is interpreted/corroborated (*NFPA 1033, 4.6.2*)
☐	☐	Investigative information on victims/casualties documented (*NFPA 906-5, NIJ Death Investigation Guide*)
☐	☐	Investigative information need for fire modeling documented (*NFPA 921, ASTM E 1355, ASTM E 1472, ASTM E 1591, ASTM E 1895*)
☐	☐	Investigative information need for determining occurrence of room flashover documented (*NFPA 555*)
☐	☐	Expert resources matched to needs, causation (*NFPA 1033, 4.6.3*)
☐	☐	Motive/opportunity evidence established (*NFPA 1033, 4.6.4*)
☐	☐	Person(s)/product(s) identified for responsibility (*NFPA 1033, 4.6.5*)
☐	☐	Concise written report prepared (*NFPA 1033, 4.7.1; ASTM E 620; ASTM E678; ASTM E1020; ASTM E1188; ASTM E1492; ASTM E1459; ASTM E1546*)
☐	☐	Investigative findings verbally presented (*NFPA 1033, 4.7.2*)
☐	☐	Testimony clearly presented at legal proceedings (*NFPA 1033, 4.7.3*)
☐	☐	Public informational presentations are accurate (*NFPA 1033, 4.7.4*)

Source: (Icove and Haynes 2007; Icove and Dalton 2008)

TABLE 6-2	Forms Used in Assuring the Collection of Uniform and Complete Field Data for Constructing Written Reports

FORM	NAME	DESCRIPTION
921-1	Fire Incident Field Notes	Collects general identification and contact information
921-2	Structure Fires	Used for documenting structure fires
921-3	Motor Vehicle Fires	Used for documenting vehicle fire inspections
921-4	Wildland Fires	Used for documenting grass, brush, or wildland fires
921-5	Casualties	Records information on persons injured or killed in the fire
921-6	Evidence	Documents and records recovered, seized, and released evidence
921-7	Photographs	Logs the descriptions of all photographs taken by the investigators
921-8	Electrical Panel	Records information as to the position and identification of circuit breakers in an electrical distribution panel
FFSR/Kirk's	Fire Modeling	Data for compartment fire modeling

Sources: Derived from NFPA 1998; NFPA 2011; and *Kirk's Fire Investigation,* 7th ed. (DeHaan and Icove 2012).

These data collection forms constitute an organized investigative protocol to be used by fire company officers, incident commanders, fire marshals, and private investigators. These forms serve as an official procedure for collecting and recording preliminary information needed to prepare a formal incident or comprehensive investigative report and for constructing a compartment fire model.

The reports cover structure, vehicle, and wildland fires; information on casualties, witnesses, evidence, photographs, and sketches; and documentary data on insurance and public records. A cover case management form is used to track the progress of the investigation. Maintenance of the updated and expanded *NFPA 906* forms is now the responsibility of NFPA's Technical Committee on Fire Investigations, which also oversees *NFPA 921*.

See Table 6-2 for a synopsis of documentation techniques.

6.2 Systematic Documentation

Fire investigators should adopt a *systematic procedure*, or *protocol*, for documenting, through sketches, photographs, and witness statements, the examination of a fire scene as well as for recording the chain of custody of all evidence removed.

A systematic four-phase process (Icove and Gohar 1980) was first introduced with the publication of the NBS (1980) *Fire Investigation Handbook*. This process recommends a careful documentation of the fire scene in the following four phases.

- *Phase 1:* Exterior
- *Phase 2:* Interior
- *Phase 3:* Investigative
- *Phase 4:* Panoramic or specialized photography

Table 6-3 shows the recommended updated guidance and purpose for this systematic documentation philosophy. This approach covers fire investigations without any preconception as to whether the fire was accidental, natural, or incendiary in cause.

TABLE 6-3		Systematic Documentation Techniques in Fire Investigation	
STEP	**TECHNIQUE**	**GUIDANCE**	**PURPOSE**
1	Exterior	■ Photograph perimeter and exterior of property. ■ Sketch exterior. ■ Use GPS to obtain location.	■ Establishes venue and location of fire scene in relation to surrounding visual landmarks ■ Documents exposure damage to adjacent properties ■ Reveals structural conditions, failures, violations, or deficiencies ■ Establishes extent of fire damage to exterior of scene ■ Establishes egress and condition of doors and windows ■ Documents and preserves possible physical evidence remote from the fire
2	Interior	■ Record and sketch extent of fire damage potential ignition sources, and data needed for fire reconstruction and modeling.	■ Traces fire travel and development from exterior to suspected point(s) of fire origin ■ Documents heat transfer damage, heat and smoke stratification levels, and breaches of structural elements ■ Documents condition of power utility and distribution, furnace, water heater, and heat-producing appliances ■ Documents position and damage to windows, doors, stairwells, and crawl space access points ■ Documents fire protection equipment locations and operation (sprinklers, heat and smoke detectors, extinguishers) ■ Documents readings on clocks and utility equipment ■ Documents alarm and arc fault information
3	Investigative	■ Document clearing of debris and evidence prior to removal, fire burn and charring patterns, packaged evidence.	■ Assists in recording fire pattern and plume damage, isochar lines ■ Establishes condition of physical evidence, utilities, distribution, and protection equipment (breakers, relief valves) ■ Documents integrity of the chain of custody of evidence
4	Panoramic specialized	■ Produce multidimensional sketches. ■ Capture evidence using forensic light sources or special recovery techniques.	■ Provides clearer peripheral views of exterior and interiors ■ Establishes photograph viewpoints of witnesses ■ Documents and preserves critical evidence

Source: Updated from Icove and Gohar 1980.

Agencies that use the *NFPA 921* field or similar-styled notes often copy the blank forms directly from the standard and bind them into packets that are placed into case jackets. Several additional copies of the witness statement form are often included for multiple interviews. Many agencies use a cover sheet for their investigative notes, which is used as a working document for both investigator and supervisor. The form typically includes check boxes indicating whether a form is contained in the case file, the date when it was completed, and remarks as to its status. The disposition of evidence, court-imposed deadlines, and other significant pieces of information may be noted in the activity section of the report.

Another high-level case document is Form 921-1, "Fire Incident Field Notes" (Figure 6-1). This form records how an agency was notified of the incident, the conditions on arrival, the owner/occupant of the property, other agencies involved, and an estimated total financial loss. Also documented are the time of arrival, the basis for an investigator's legal authority to enter the scene, and the time the scene was released.

Form 921-2, "Structure Fire Field Notes" (Figure 6-2), offers the investigator a tool for documenting the type of property, geographic area, address, construction techniques, security, alarm protection, and utilities. Documenting the security at the time of the fire is an important consideration in arson cases, where the issue of exclusive opportunity is raised, along with the condition of doors, windows, and protection systems. Also important is documentation of the condition of doors, windows, and evidence found as part of the external documentation, noting **fire patterns** emanating from the doors or windows (or the lack of them) that may later provide critical information relative to fire development, **ventilation**, and timeline. The location and distances of window glass displaced from the structure or vehicle are documented during the exterior examination.

The "Vehicle Inspection Field Notes" (Form 921-3; Figure 6-3), "Wildfire Notes" (Form 921-4; Figure 6-4), "Casualty Field Notes" (Form 921-5; Figure 6-5), "Evidence Form" (Form 921-6; Figure 6-6), "Photograph Log" (Form 921-7; Figure 6-7), and "Electrical Panel Documentation" (Form 921-8; Figure 6-8) are used to further document the various aspects of the fire investigation.

The weather conditions and history (NFPA 2017, pt. 28.3.1) prior to the fire incident sometimes become important, especially when there are high winds, temperature fluctuations, or lightning. The National Weather Service, Office of Climate, Water, and Weather Services, has a forensic services program to support investigations. Certified climatological records including radar images, satellite photos, and surface analysis can be obtained from the National Weather Service headquarters in Silver Spring, Maryland. Alternative free and low-cost weather notification and historical systems available in the United States provide radar and severe-weather notifications. One popular website is Weather Underground (wunderground.com), which provides historical weather data for many US locations.

The location of *lightning strikes* is important information when addressing the possibility that lightning caused a particular fire (NFPA 2017, pt. 9.12.8). The US National Lightning Detection Network locates strikes across the United States. For a fee, the private firm Vaisala (vaisala.com) will provide a report on all lightning strikes in a particular area for a given time frame and supply data and custom software.

fire patterns ■ The visible or measurable physical changes, or identifiable shapes, formed by a fire effect or group of fire effects (*NFPA 921*, 2017 ed., pt. 3.3.70).

ventilation ■ Circulation of air in any space by natural wind or convection or by fans blowing air into or exhausting air out of a building; a firefighting operation of removing smoke and heat from the structure by opening windows and doors or making holes in the roof (*NFPA 921*, 2017 ed., pt. 3.3.199).

FIRE INCIDENT FIELD NOTES

Agency: _____   File No: _____

TYPE OF OCCUPANCY

Location/Address	
Property Description	Structure	Residential	Commercial	Vehicle	Wildland	Other
Other Relevant Info	

WEATHER CONDITIONS

| Indicate Relevant Weather Information | Visibility | Rel. humidity | GPS | Elevation | Lightning |
| Temperature | Wind direction | Wind speed | Precipitation |

OWNER

Name		DOB
d/b/a (if applicable)	
Address	
Telephone	Home	Business	Cellular

OCCUPANT

Name		DOB
d/b/a (if applicable)	
Permanent Address	
Temporary Address	
Telephone	Home	Business	Cellular

DISCOVERED BY

Incident Discovered by	Name		DOB
Address	
Telephone	Home	Business	Cellular

© 2010 National Fire Protection Association   NFPA 921 (p. 1 of 2)

FIRE INCIDENT FIELD NOTES (Continued)

File No: _____

REPORTED BY

Incident Reported by	Name		DOB
Address	
Telephone	Home	Business	Cellular

INVESTIGATION INITIATION

Request Date and Time	Date of request	Time of request
Investigation Requested by	Agency name	Contact person/Telephone no.
Request Received by	Agency name	Contact person/Telephone no.

SCENE INFORMATION

Arrival Information	Date	Time	Comments
Scene Secured	Yes	No	Securing agency	Manner of security
Authority to Enter	Contemporaneous to exigency	Consent	Warrant
		Written	Verbal	Admin.	Crim.	Other
Departure Information	Date	Time	Comments

OTHER AGENCIES INVOLVED

	Dept. or Agency Name	Incident No.	Contact Person/Phone
Primary Fire Department			
Secondary Fire Department(s)			
Law Enforcement			
Private Investigators			

ADDITIONAL REMARKS

© 2010 National Fire Protection Association   NFPA 921 (p. 2 of 2)

FIGURE 6-1 The *NFPA 921-1* "Fire Incident Field Notes" form offers the investigator a tool to record information on the type of occupancy, weather conditions, owner and occupant, person discovering the fire, how the investigation was initiated, and scene information. *Reproduced with permission from NFPA 921-2017, Guide for Fire and Explosion Investigations, Copyright © 2016, National Fire Protection Association. This reprinted material is not the complete and official position of the NFPA on the referenced subject, which is represented only by the standard in its entirety which may be obtained through the NFPA web site www.nfpa.org.*

STRUCTURE FIRE

Agency: _____ Case number: _____

TYPE OF OCCUPANCY

Residential	Single family	Multifamily	Commercial	Governmental
Church	School	Other:		

Estimated age: _____ Height (stories): _____ Length: _____ Width: _____

PROPERTY STATUS

Occupied at time of fire? ☐ Yes ☐ No   Unoccupied at time of fire? ☐ Yes ☐ No   Vacant at time of fire? ☐ Yes ☐ No

Name of person last in structure prior to fire: _____   Time and date in structure: _____   Exited via which door/egress: _____

Remarks: _____

BUILDING CONSTRUCTION

Foundation Type	Basement	Crawl space	Slab	Other:
Material	Masonry	Concrete	Stone	Other:
Exterior Covering	Wood	Brick/Stone	Vinyl	Asphalt	Metal	Concrete	Other:
Roof	Asphalt	Wood	Tile	Metal			Other:
Type of Construction	Wood frame	Balloon	Heavy timber	Ordinary	Fire resistive	Non-combustible	Other:

ALARM/PROTECTION/SECURITY

Sprinklers ☐ Yes ☐ No   Standpipes ☐ Yes ☐ No   Security camera(s) ☐ Yes ☐ No

Smoke detectors ☐ Yes ☐ No   Hardwired ☐ Yes ☐ No   Battery ☐ Yes ☐ No

Were batteries in place? ☐ Yes ☐ No   Location(s): _____

Hidden keys ☐ Yes ☐ No   where: _____   Security bars: Windows? ☐ Yes ☐ No   Doors? ☐ Yes ☐ No

Remarks: _____

© 2010 National Fire Protection Association   NFPA 921 (p. 1 of 2)

STRUCTURE FIRE (Continued)

CONDITION OF DOORS/WINDOWS

Doors	Locked	Unlocked but closed	Open
	Forced entry? ☐ Yes ☐ No	Who forced if known?	
Windows	Secure	Unlocked but closed	Open	Broken
	Broken by first responders? ☐ Yes ☐ No	Remarks:	

FIRE DEPARTMENT OBSERVATIONS

Name of first on scene: _____   Department: _____

General observations: _____

Obstacles to extinguishment: _____   First-In Report attached? ☐ Yes ☐ No

UTILITIES

Electric	☐ On	☐ Off	☐ None	☐ Overhead	☐ Underground
	Company:	Contact:		Telephone:	
Gas/Fuel	☐ On	☐ Off	☐ None	☐ Natural	☐ LP	☐ Oil
	Company:	Contact:		Telephone:	
Water	Company:	Contact:		Telephone:	
Telephone	Company:	Contact:		Telephone:	
Other	Company:	Contact:		Telephone:	

COMMENTS:

_____

© 2010 National Fire Protection Association   NFPA 921 (p. 2 of 2)

FIGURE 6-2 The *NFPA 921-2* "Structure Fire Field Notes" form collects occupancy, property status, building construction, alarm protection and security, condition of doors and windows, fire department observations, and utilities information. *Reproduced with permission from NFPA 921-2017, Guide for Fire and Explosion Investigations, Copyright © 2016, National Fire Protection Association. This reprinted material is not the complete and official position of the NFPA on the referenced subject, which is represented only by the standard in its entirety which may be obtained through the NFPA web site www.nfpa.org.*

VEHICLE INSPECTION FIELD NOTES

Job # _____ File # _____

Insured _____ Date of Occurrence _____

Address (City, State) _____ Date of Assignment _____

Loss Location _____ Date of Receipt _____

_____ Insp Location _____

Stolen? ☐ Yes ☐ No   Recovered by _____ Time of Inspection _____

Police Report _____ Fire Report _____

# of Keys _____ Alarm System? ☐ Yes ☐ No   Alarm Type _____

Hidden Keys? ☐ Yes ☐ No   Location _____

VEHICLE

Make _____ Model _____ Year _____

VIN _____ Odometer _____

EXTERIOR

Tires	Tire Type	Wheel Type	Tire Tread Depth	Lugs	Missing
LF					
LR					
RR					
RF					
SP					

Doors	Glass Y/N	Window UP/DOWN	Locked Y/N	Open/Closed	Prior Damage
LF					
LR					
RR					
RF					

Body Panels	Construction	Condition	Prior Damage
F Bumper			
Grill			
LF Fender			
LR Quarter			
R Bumper			
RR Quarter			
RF Fender			
Hood			
Roof			
Trunk			

UNDER HOOD	Intact	Missing	Parts Missing	Condition
Engine				
Battery				
Belts & Hoses				
Wiring				
Accessories				

FLUIDS	Level	Condition	Sample Taken
Oil			
Transmission			
Radiator			
Pwr Steer			
Brake			
Clutch			

ATS 851B, 8/97   NFPA 921 (p. 1 of 2)

VEHICLE INSPECTION FIELD NOTES (Continued)

Job # _____

INTERIOR	Intact	Missing	Parts Missing	Condition
Dash Pod				
Glove Box				
Strg Column				
Ignition				
Front Seat				
Rear Seat				
Rear Deck				

Make/Model _____

	Sample Taken
Stereo	
Speakers	
Accessories	

FLOOR	
LF	
LR	
RR	
RL	

PERSONAL EFFECTS IN THE INTERIOR

TRUNK OR CARGO AREA

AFTERMARKET ITEMS NOT PREVIOUSLY DESCRIBED

ATS 851B, 8/97   NFPA 921 (p. 2 of 2)

FIGURE 6-3 The *NFPA 921-3* "Vehicle Inspection Field Notes" form collects vehicle description, owner/operator, exterior/interior, security, and area of fire origin information. *Reprinted with permission from NFPA 921: Guide for Fire and Explosion Investigations, 2011 Edition. Copyright © 2011, National Fire Protection Association, Quincy, MA 02269. This reprinted material is not the complete and official position of the National Fire Protection Association on the referenced subject, which is represented only by the standard in its entirety.*

WILDFIRE NOTES

Agency: _____   File number: _____

PROPERTY DESCRIPTION

_____
_____
_____

Fire damage:	Other properties involved:
❏ Less than acre _____ No. acres	
Security:	Comments:
❏ Open ❏ Fenced ❏ Locked gate	

FIRE SPREAD FACTORS

| Type fire: | Factors: | Comments: |
| ❏ Ground ❏ Crown | ❏ Wind ❏ Terrain | |

AREA OF ORIGIN

_____
_____
_____

PEOPLE IN AREA

| At time of fire: | Comments: |
| ❏ Yes ❏ No   ❏ Undetermined | |

IGNITION SEQUENCE

Heat of ignition: _____

Material ignited: _____

Ignition factor: _____

If equipment involved: Make: _____   Model: _____   Serial no.: _____

Comments: _____
_____
_____
_____

© 2010 National Fire Protection Association   NFPA 921

FIGURE 6-4 The *NFPA 921-4* "Wildfire Notes" form collects property, fire spread factors, area of origin, people in the area, and ignition sequence information. *Reproduced with permission from NFPA 921-2017, Guide for Fire and Explosion Investigations, Copyright © 2016, National Fire Protection Association. This reprinted material is not the complete and official position of the NFPA on the referenced subject, which is represented only by the standard in its entirety which may be obtained through the NFPA web site www.nfpa.org.*

CASUALTY FIELD NOTES

DESCRIPTION

Agency: _____ Incident date: _____ Case number: _____

Name: _____ DOB: _____ Sex/Race: _____

Address: _____ Phone: _____

Other identifiers: _____

Description of clothing and jewelry: _____

Occupation: _____ Place of employment: _____

Marital status: _____

Victim's doctor: _____ Victim's dentist: _____

Smoker: ☐ Yes ☐ No ☐ Unknown

CASUALTY TREATMENT

Treated at scene: ☐ Yes ☐ No   By: _____

Transported to: _____ Remarks: _____

SEVERITY OF INJURY

☐ Minor ☐ Moderate ☐ Severe ☐ Fatal

Describe injury: _____

NEXT OF KIN

Name: _____ Address: _____ Phone: _____

Relationship: _____ Notified on ___ / ___ / ___ By: _____

FATALITY INFORMATION

Where was victim initially found: _____

Who located victim: _____

Body position when initially found: _____

Victim's appearance: _____

Body removed by: _____ To: _____

Photographed in place: ☐ Yes ☐ No   Significant blood present under/near victim: ☐ Yes ☐ No

MEDICAL EXAMINER/CORONER

Agency: _____ Location: _____

Date of examination: ___ / ___ / ___

Autopsy requested: ☐ Yes ☐ No   Autopsy completed: ☐ Yes ☐ No   Copy attached: ☐ Yes ☐ No

Full body x-rays: ☐ Yes ☐ No   Other x-rays: _____

Identification made from: ☐ Physical appearance ☐ Dental records ☐ Fingerprints ☐ Prior injury comparison

☐ Other: _____

Condition of trachea: _____

Evidence of pre-fire injury: ☐ Yes ☐ No   Type/location: _____

Blood samples taken: ☐ Yes ☐ No   Other specimens collected: _____

CO level: _____ Blood alcohol: _____ Other: _____

Cause of death: _____

COMPLETE BODY DIAGRAM ON REVERSE

© 2010 National Fire Protection Association   NFPA 921 (p. 1 of 2)

CASUALTY FIELD NOTES (Continued)

REMARKS

_____
_____
_____
_____

BODY DIAGRAM

Indicate parts of body injured: ☐ None ☐ Blisters (red marker) ☐ Burns (black marker)

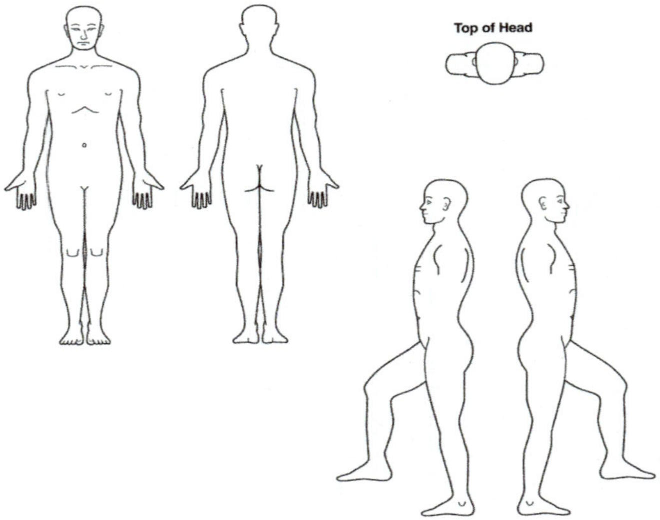

Top of Head

Fire Investigation Data Sheet/Attachment: _____
Body Diagram   Initials: _____

© 2010 National Fire Protection Association   NFPA 921 (p. 2 of 2)

FIGURE 6-5 The *NFPA 921-5* "Casualty Field Notes" form collects the name and description of the injured or deceased person, treatment, next of kin, medical examiner/coroner, and body diagram information. *Reproduced with permission from NFPA 921-2017, Guide for Fire and Explosion Investigations, Copyright © 2016, National Fire Protection Association. This reprinted material is not the complete and official position of the NFPA on the referenced subject, which is represented only by the standard in its entirety which may be obtained through the NFPA web site www.nfpa.org.*

EVIDENCE FORM

Date of incident: ___ / ___ / ___ Storage location: _____ Case #: _____

Item No.	Description	Location		
			Destroyed	Released
			Destroyed	Released
			Destroyed	Released
			Destroyed	Released
			Destroyed	Released
			Destroyed	Released
			Destroyed	Released
			Destroyed	Released
			Destroyed	Released
			Destroyed	Released

How was evidence received? Date received: ___ / ___ / ___ Date stored: ___ / ___ / ___

☐ Removed from scene by investigator.

☐ Received by investigator from: _____ Name, Company, or Dept.

Received via: ☐ UPS ☐ FedEx ☐ Airborne ☐ U.S. Mail ☐ In person ☐ Freight ____ Name of Company

☐ Other: _____ Describe

Received by _____ Case Investigator

LOCATION EVIDENCE REMOVED

Owner _____ State ___ Zip ___ Phone ___

Company _____ Address 2 ___

Address 1 _____ City ___

City _____ State ___ Zip ___ Phone ___

© 2010 National Fire Protection Association NFPA 921 (p. 1 of 2)

EVIDENCE FORM (Continued)

INTERNAL EXAMINATION

Investigator	Date Pulled	Date Examined	Date Returned

EXAMINATION BY OTHERS

Name _____ Date of Examination ___

Company _____

Address _____

City ___ State ___ Zip ___ Phone ___

Authorized by _____

Investigator's Authorization _____ Date ___

EVIDENCE DESTRUCTION

Authorized by _____ Date ___

Investigator's Authorization _____ Date ___

Destroyed by _____ Date ___

Name _____ Date of Examination ___

Company _____

Address _____

City ___ State ___ Zip ___ Phone ___

Authorized by _____

Investigator's Authorization _____ Date ___

EVIDENCE RELEASE

Signature of Person Receiving Evidence _____

Person Receiving Evidence (Please Print) _____ Date ___

Company Name _____

Address _____

City ___ State ___ Zip Code ___

Authorized by _____ Date ___

Investigator's Authorization _____ Date ___

Released via _____

Name _____ Date of Examination ___

Company _____

Address _____

City ___ State ___ Zip ___ Phone ___

Authorized by _____

Investigator's Authorization _____ Date ___

REMARKS

_____

© 2010 National Fire Protection Association NFPA 921 (p. 2 of 2)

FIGURE 6-6 The *NFPA 921-6 "Evidence Form"* collects the information on the disposition of items collected, released, and destroyed from a fire scene. *Reproduced with permission from NFPA 921-2017, Guide for Fire and Explosion Investigations, Copyright © 2016, National Fire Protection Association. This reprinted material is not the complete and official position of the NFPA on the referenced subject, which is represented only by the standard in its entirety which may be obtained through the NFPA web site www.nfpa.org.*

PHOTOGRAPH LOG

Roll #: _____   Exposures: _____

Case #: _____   Date: _____

Camera make/type: _____   Film type: _____ Film speed: _____ ASA: _____

Number	Description	Location
1)		
2)		
3)		
4)		
5)		
6)		
7)		
8)		
9)		
10)		
11)		
12)		
13)		
14)		
15)		
16)		
17)		
18)		
19)		
20)		
21)		
22)		
23)		
24)		
25)		
26)		
27)		
28)		
29)		
30)		
31)		
32)		
33)		
34)		
35)		
36)		

Photos taken by: _____   Initials: _____

NFPA 921

FIGURE 6-7 The *NFPA 921-7* "Photograph Log" collects the information on the description and location of which each photograph is taken and by whom at a fire scene. The form should be modified to include digital photo data such as medium identification and image number. *Reprinted with permission from NFPA 921-2017: Guide for Fire and Explosion Investigations, Copyright © 2016, National Fire Protection Association, Quincy, MA 02269. This reprinted material is not the complete and official position of the National Fire Protection Association on the referenced subject, which is represented only by the standard in its entirety.*

ELECTRICAL PANEL DOCUMENTATION

Fire location: Date: Case #:

Panel location: Main size: Fuses: ☐
                                                                         Circuit breakers: ☐

LEFT BANK

#	Rating Amps	Labeled Circuit	Status
1	—		—
3	—		—
5	—		—
7	—		—
9	—		—
11	—		—
13	—		—
15	—		—
17	—		—
19	—		—
21	—		—
23	—		—
25	—		—
27	—		—
29	—		—

Notes:

RIGHT BANK

#	Rating Amps	Labeled Circuit	Status
2	—		—
4	—		—
6	—		—
8	—		—
10	—		—
12	—		—
14	—		—
16	—		—
18	—		—
20	—		—
22	—		—
24	—		—
26	—		—
28	—		—
30	—		—

Notes:

Documented by:

© 2010 National Fire Protection Association   NFPA 921

FIGURE 6-8 The *NFPA 921-8 "Electrical Panel Documentation"* form collects the information on the location of the electrical panel and the condition of circuit breakers along with their amperage rating and status. *Reprinted with permission from NFPA 921-2017: Guide for Fire and Explosion Investigations, Copyright © 2016, National Fire Protection Association, Quincy, MA 02269. This reprinted material is not the complete and official position of the National Fire Protection Association on the referenced subject, which is represented only by the standard in its entirety.*

6.2.1 EXTERIOR

The first step in the documentation process after securing the fire ground (NFPA 2014, pt. 4.2.1) is inspecting and recording details of the exterior of the structure, vehicle, forest, wildland, or boat (NFPA 2014, pt. 4.2.2).

While circling the exterior of the structure or vehicle, the investigator can make a cursory field search for additional evidence, noting that fire patterns emanating from the doors or windows may provide critical information relative to the fire's development, ventilation, and timeline. The exterior inspections should also reveal the extent of fire damage, collapse, structural conditions, failures, code violations, deficiencies, or potential safety concerns. This step establishes the location of the fire scene in relation to surrounding visual landmarks and documents exposure damage to adjacent properties from the fire. In large investigations, an overhead crane, aerial ladder truck, or aircraft can be used to obtain panoramic photographs of the scene.

If there has been an explosion, the investigator must measure and document, by both diagramming and photographing, the points to which fragments of glass or structure were thrown. These concepts are discussed in later sections.

When considering sources of ignition, the condition of the utilities at the time of the fire may indicate whether the owner/occupant(s) was (were) living in the structure. If

TASK:

Conduct an exterior survey, given standard equipment and tools, so that evidence is preserved, fire damage is interpreted, hazards are identified to avoid injuries, accessibility to the property is determined, and all potential means of ingress/egress are discovered.

PERFORMANCE OUTCOME:

Remaining alert for safety hazards, the investigator will conduct a 360-degree exterior survey of the scene. The investigator will identify entry/exit points, items of potential evidence, and post-fire indicators. The investigator will also indicate on a photo log where exterior photos are taken, if any, using the following task steps.

CONDITIONS:

Given a fire scene, a note pad, and a photo log.

TASK STEPS:

1. Locate fire scene
2. Proceed 360 degrees around the scene
3. Enter on the photo log where photos would be taken
4. Ribbon potential evidence items
5. Ribbon or mark entry/exit points
6. Document observations

Source: Derived and updated from Washington State Patrol, Form No. 3000-420-081 (Sept. 2014) Fire Protection Bureau, Standards and Accreditation, Olympia, Washington http://www.wsp.wa.gov/fire/docs/cert/fire_invest.pdf

instructions to disconnect the utilities were given prior to the fire, it is important to identify and document who gave those instructions and why they were given. Determining when gas and electric services were cut off (and by whom) during fire suppression is also important. If electrical power interruptions or surges are suspected, neighbors who share the same power service should be canvassed.

6.2.2 INTERIOR

The second phase of the documentation process involves documenting interior damage by showing the extent and progress of the fire through the room(s), area(s), and suspected point(s) of fire origin (NFPA 2014, pt. 4.2.3). Pictures and sketches made prior to excavating the fire debris serve to document the conditions of the scene found on the investigator's arrival. As long as there is legal authority for entry, all undamaged areas of the building should be examined and documented for comparison and hypothesis formulation.

Documentation of Damage

While conducting the interior examination, the investigator documents damage or lack of damage to all rooms, including heat and smoke stratification levels, smoke deposits, heat transfer effects, and breaches of structural elements (walls, floors, ceilings, and doors). The investigator may find it useful to map out and delineate the areas of damage corresponding to the pattern types described in Table 6-2, with color-coded chalk or tape on the surfaces themselves, followed by photography. Areas of surface deposit demarcations sometimes referred to as smoke horizons, thermal effects, penetrations, and loss of material can also be outlined using colored markers on sketches or photographs. One

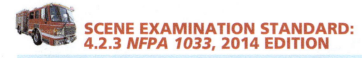

TASK:

Conduct an interior survey, given standard equipment and tools, so that areas of potential evidentiary value requiring further examination are identified and preserved, the evidentiary value of contents is determined, and hazards are identified to avoid injuries.

PERFORMANCE OUTCOME:

Remaining alert for safety hazards, the investigator will conduct a 360-degree interior survey of the scene. The investigator will identify entry/exit points, items of potential evidence, and post-fire indicators. The investigator will also indicate on a photo log where interior photos are taken, if any, using the following task steps.

CONDITIONS:

Given a fire scene, a note pad, and a photo log.

TASK STEPS:

1. Locate fire scene
2. Proceed 360 degrees around the scene; observe and document effects of fire
3. Enter on the photo log where photos would be taken
4. Ribbon potential evidence items
5. Ribbon or mark entry/exit points
6. Document observations, including presence or absence of normal building contents

Source: Derived and updated from Washington State Patrol, Form No. 3000-420-081 (Sept. 2014) Fire Protection Bureau, Standards and Accreditation, Olympia, Washington http://www.wsp.wa.gov/fire/docs/cert/fire_invest.pdf

system might be to use yellow lines to outline areas of surface deposits, green lines for thermal effects, blue lines for penetrations, and red lines to outline areas where the material has been consumed completely.

This phase includes examination and documentation of the condition of power utility and distribution, furnace, water heater, and heat-producing appliances, as well as the contents and conditions of the rooms. The investigator should document the location of the HVAC system and the condition of the unit, ductwork, and filters. The thickness of window glass, the sizes of windows, and whether they are single or double-glazed must also be noted and documented. The sill height and soffit depth of each door and window in the rooms involved must be noted, as well as their opening dimensions and whether they were open during the fire or broken sometime later.

Structural Features

The design and construction of the ceiling may play a key role in spread of smoke or fire, or detection. A smooth, sloping ceiling may direct smoke away from a detector, whereas one with exposed beams or one with deep decorative bays may channel smoke or fire in a preferred direction or prevent it from spreading at all (see Figure 6-9). Because ceilings often suffer major damage during a fire or during **overhaul**, it is important to document similar undamaged rooms in the building when practical. Otherwise, occupants or maintenance staff should be interviewed about such features. Such features may also be documented using prefire photos, videos, or building plans.

The type, location, and operation of HVAC components are also important. In one case, an accidental fire originating in a chair took the life of the sole occupant of a room designated as the smoking room for the facility. The midmorning fire was well advanced

overhaul ■ A firefighting term involving the process of final extinguishment after the main body of the fire has been knocked down. All traces of fire must be extinguished at this time (*NFPA 921*, 2017 ed., pt. 3.3.135).

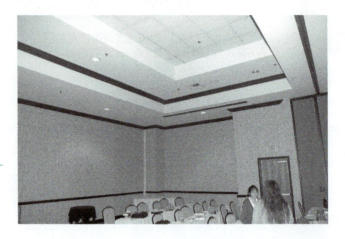

FIGURE 6-9 Complex ceiling structures, such as those in this hotel conference room, will affect fire and smoke spread. This photo captures the structural features as well as ventilator, sprinkler, and alarm sensor locations. *Courtesy of John Houde.*

before it was detected by a staff member on the floor above who saw smoke rising past the window of her room and went to investigate. The question ultimately was, "Why did the fire get so large and yet the smoke detector in the hall on the ceiling just outside the open door to the room failed to function?" No smoke was seen in the hallway as staff rushed to the room, and the detector was hardwired to an alarm system. It was discovered that an exhaust fan in the room's window was left on and its cubic feet per minute (CFM) rating was sufficient to draw enough smoke-laden air from the limited fire in the room away from the door, preventing its detection outside.

Even passive elements of HVAC systems can play a role. The void space above many suspended ceilings acts as an open air-return plenum, allowing smoke and hot gases to spread quickly. See Figure 6-10 for an example. The filters and condensers on HVAC systems should be checked for **soot** or pyrolysis products.

soot ■ Black particles of carbon produced in a flame (*NFPA 921*, 2017 ed., pt. 3.3.173).

Fire Protection Systems

It is also important to document for later evaluation the fire protection equipment (e.g., fire alarms, smoke detectors, automatic suppression systems, fire doors, thermally operated safety devices, and the presence or lack of compartmentation) that would have helped contain the fire as well as alert the occupants (NFPA 2014, pt. 4.2.8). Documentation includes function and location. The time readings on electric and mechanical clocks may document the approximate times that they were damaged and halted by heat or by interruption of power.

The investigator will perform a post-fire inspection of a scene and indicate on a floor plan the location and condition detection and alarm system, HVAC, utilities, and suppression system (NFPA 2014, pt. 4.2.8).

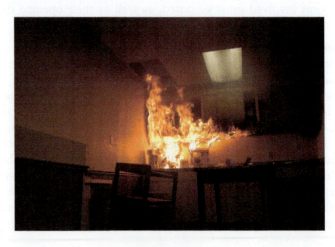

FIGURE 6-10 An air-return plenum vent opening in this kitchen allowed very rapid extension into the ceiling space and faster-than-expected collapse of the suspended ceiling. *Courtesy of Jamie Novak, Novak Investigations and St. Paul Fire Dept.*

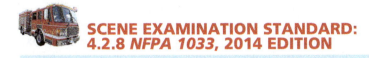

SCENE EXAMINATION STANDARD:
4.2.8 *NFPA 1033*, 2014 EDITION

TASK:

Inspect the performance of building systems, including detection, suppression, HVAC, utilities, and building compartmentation, given standard and special equipment and tools, so that a determination can be made as to the need for expert resources, an operating systems impact on fire growth and spread is considered in identifying origin areas, defeated and/or failed systems are identified, and the system's potential as a fire cause is recognized.

PERFORMANCE OUTCOME:

The investigator will perform a post-fire inspection of a scene and indicate on a floor plan the location and condition of each of the following: detection system, HVAC, utilities, and suppression system. The investigator will identify which expert resources, if any, would be needed to confirm that any of the systems were found defective or defeated.

CONDITIONS:

Given a fire scene, adequate portable lighting, tools, note pad, and a general suppression briefing.

TASK STEPS:

1. Locate the fire scene; identify and inspect exterior utilities
2. Locate and inspect detection systems
3. Locate and inspect HVAC systems
4. Locate and inspect suppression systems
5. Report which, if any, expert resources would be needed
6. Report which, if any, and how systems inspected were defective and/or defeated
7. Evaluate and report the impact of suppression effort on building system

Source: Derived and updated from Washington State Patrol, Form No. 3000-420-081 (Sept. 2014) Fire Protection Bureau, Standards and Accreditation, Olympia, Washington http://www.wsp.wa.gov/fire/docs/cert /fire_invest.pdf

Documentation needs to include the position, type, and operability of smoke, heat, and carbon monoxide (CO) detectors and sprinkler systems. This is important, because NFPA studies show that almost all US households have at least one smoke alarm, yet during the period 2000–2004, no smoke alarms were present or none operated in almost half (46 percent) of the reported home fires (Ahrens 2007). Also during this time period, 43 percent of all home fire deaths resulted from fires in homes with no smoke alarms, and 22 percent of such deaths occurred in homes in which smoke alarms were present but simply did not operate.

Investigations of fatal fires often found that batteries had been removed for use in toys or remote controls or to prevent false alarms from being triggered by cooking or even bathroom steam. Hardwired detectors can be disconnected from unmonitored systems or covered with tape or plastic film to prevent alarms. The condition, fusing temperature, and orifice size of any open sprinkler heads should also be documented and the head(s) preserved as evidence, including exemplars of unfused sprinkler head.

The data systems in modern fire alarm systems can be electronically examined to capture the time, sequence, and zone of alarms or sprinkler activations. The zones and manner of activation should be established for alarm sensors. Someone knowledgeable about the alarm system should be consulted for assistance. Even systems that are not remotely monitored have a battery-powered memory of recent activations that can be downloaded.

Arc-Fault Mapping

Arc-fault mapping (NFPA 2017, pt. 9.11.7) provides a way of locating a possible area of origin of a fire by tracing the wiring from its power source (such as the breaker or fuse box) and mapping the locations of all failures of the wire (because wires can be caused to fail by fire effects even when non-energized). The failures are then characterized as arcing (energized) or melting (non-energized) by their gross appearance. The locations of the arcing phenomena farthest downstream along a circuit from the power source are indicators of the point at which the fire first attacked the wiring, as illustrated in Figure 6-11. These failures, then, may be very useful in indicating a possible area of origin. Dr. Robert J. Svare (1988) pioneered this approach, which has been tested in numerous live-burn structure tests.

When a flame or heat attacks an insulated electrical cable, the insulation begins to pyrolyze and degrade. When rubber, cloth, or some plastic insulation **chars**, the carbonaceous residue becomes conductive, and current can pass if the conductor is energized and a return path established (sometimes called **arcing through char**). With PVC, a temperature of 120°C (248°F) is sufficient to initiate an arc-tracking process and allow a current to begin to flow (Babrauskas 2006). The resistance decreases as the insulation degrades further. In either case, current begins to flow between the hot, or energized, wire and the neutral or ground (or to a grounded conduit, appliance, or junction box). This increased current creates heat that further chars the insulation, providing even better current flow.

Because of the resistance provided by the charred insulation, this condition is not the same as a direct short or fault, which has nearly zero resistance. This can produce a variety of arc-damaged areas along the conductor—ranging from small craters to beads of molten metal. Because the conductors are not bonded together, they are free to move, so these current flows are usually very short in duration, in many cases too short to cause overcurrent protective devices (OCPDs) to function. This means that arcing can occur at many places along a single energized wire and multiple times until the OCPD trips or the wire is severed by melting (sometimes called *fusing*). Once the wire is separated, no current can flow beyond that point.

NFPA 921 (2017, pt. 9.11, 7.5.1) cautions that testing of fires in single compartments show arcs that are frequently in the area of the fire's origin. However there is ongoing research on correlating arc frequency and the fire's origin. The technique requires diligent and careful tracing of wiring and circuits, because the source of the energy has to be established and the nature of the failure accurately evaluated. *NFPA 921* suggests the documentation of the electrical distribution panel using a form similar to that previously shown in Figure 6-8 (NFPA 2017, pt. 9.6).

In buildings protected by zone alarm systems, arc-fault indicators can be used together with data from the alarm system (alarm, sensor, or sprinkler activation) to estimate areas of possible origin. This approach may not be of use in extensively collapsed or fire-damaged buildings where the relationship and tracing of wires cannot be established accurately.

arc-fault mapping ■ The systematic evaluation of the electrical circuit configuration, spatial relationship of the circuit components, and identification of electrical arc sites to assist in the identification of the area of origin and analysis of the fire's spread (*NFPA 921*, 2017 ed., pt. 3.3.9).

char ■ Carbonaceous material that has been burned or pyrolyzed and has a blackened appearance (*NFPA 921*, 2017 ed., pt. 3.3.29).

arcing through char ■ Arcing associated with a matrix of charred material (e.g., charred conductor insulation) that acts as a semiconductive medium (*NFPA 921*, 2017 ed., pt. 3.3.11).

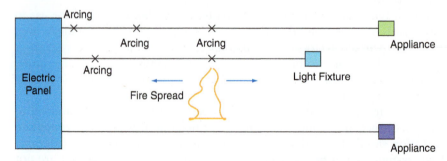

FIGURE 6-11 Mapping the locations of arcing failures farthest downstream along a circuit from the power source, which are indicators of the point at which the fire first attacked the wiring.

6.2.3 INVESTIGATIVE

Systematic investigation concentrates on the debris clearing operations, **fuel loads**, char and burn patterns, potential ignition sources, and position of evidence prior to its removal from the fire scene as well as expert services (NFPA 2014, pts. 4.2.6 and 4.2.7, 4.6.3). Evidence of any crimes associated with the fire such as burglary, theft, and homicide should also be documented.

fuel load ■ The total quantity of combustible contents of a building, space, or fire area, including interior finish and trim, expressed in heat units or the equivalent weight in wood (*NFPA 921*, 2017 ed., pt. 3.3.93).

SCENE EXAMINATION STANDARD: 4.2.6 *NFPA 1033*, 2014 EDITION

TASK:

Examine and remove fire debris, given standard equipment and tools, so that all debris is checked for fire cause evidence, the ignition source(s) is identified, and evidence is preserved without investigator-inflicted damage or contamination.

PERFORMANCE OUTCOME:

The investigator will, in protective clothing, dig out an origin area that will contain an ignition source and item(s) of evidence.

CONDITIONS:

Given a fire scene, tools, and evidence collection containers that investigator will demonstrate and be able to complete the tasks as listed below.

TASK STEPS:

1. Locate fire scene
2. Locate area of origin
3. Locate, identify, and protect items of evidence
4. Remove fire debris and locate ignition source
5. Evidence collected and preserved without investigator-inflicted damage or contamination

Source: Derived and updated from Washington State Patrol, Form No. 3000-420-081 (Sept. 2014) Fire Protection Bureau, Standards and Accreditation, Olympia, Washington http://www.wsp.wa.gov/fire/docs/cert /fire_invest.pdf

SCENE EXAMINATION STANDARD: 4.2.7 *NFPA 1033*, 2014 EDITION

TASK:

Reconstruct the area of origin, given standard and, if needed, special equipment and tools, as well as sufficient personnel, so that all protected areas and fire patterns are identified and correlated to contents or structural remains, items potentially critical to cause determination and photo documentation are returned to their pre-fire location, and the point(s) of origin is discovered.

PERFORMANCE OUTCOME:

The investigator will identify protected areas, locate and replace items moved during fire suppression activities to their pre-fire location, and indicate on a photo log what photos should be taken to document reconstruction.

CONDITIONS:

Given a fire scene, tools, burned items, a fire suppression briefing, an assistant, photo logs, and wearing protective clothing.

(Continued)

POST-INCIDENT INVESTIGATION STANDARD: 4.6.3 *NFPA 1033*, 2014 EDITION

TASK:

Coordinate expert resources, given the investigative file, reports, and documents, so that the expert's competencies are matched to the specific investigation needs, financial expenditures are justified, and utilization clearly furthers the investigation toward the goals of determining cause or affixing responsibility.

PERFORMANCE OUTCOME:

The investigator will coordinate expert resources by evaluating investigative files, reports, and documents, expert witness backgrounds and competencies, and fee schedules in order to match expert competencies with specific investigation needs

CONDITIONS:

Given investigative files, expert witness backgrounds and local/regional resources, competencies, and fee schedules, the investigator will complete the listed task.

TASK STEPS:

1. Review provided materials
2. Document need for specific experts
3. Justify costs for each expert witness selected
4. Document how the selected expert witnesses will assist in the determination of causation or affixing responsibility

Source: Derived and updated from Washington State Patrol, Form No. 3000-420-081 (Sept. 2014) Fire Protection Bureau, Standards and Accreditation, Olympia, Washington http://www.wsp.wa.gov/fire/docs/cert /fire_invest.pdf

Until photographically recorded and supported by fire scene notes, nothing should be moved, including bodies of victims. Investigative photographs ensure the integrity of the probe and custody of evidence.

Requirements for Taking and Retaining Notes

The investigator is required to construct, take, and retain investigative notes regarding the incident (NFPA 2014, pt. 4.3.3).

Casualties

Information on casualties (NFPA 2014, pt. 4.4.1) is recorded on the "Casualty Field Notes" form (Figure 6-5). This report includes a description of the victim, type of injury,

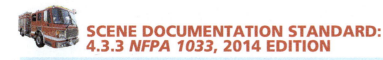

SCENE DOCUMENTATION STANDARD:
4.3.3 *NFPA 1033*, 2014 EDITION

TASK:

Construct investigative notes—given a fire scene, available document (e.g., pre-fire plans and inspection reports), and interview information, so that the notes are accurate, provide further documentation of the scene, and represent complete documentation of the scene findings.

PERFORMANCE OUTCOME:

The investigator will review investigation documents, determine, if any, conflicting information, and identify other information that may be needed to document scene findings.

CONDITIONS:

Given an investigation file including interviews, photos, suppression report, and any available pre-fire information.

TASK STEPS:

1. Document investigative notes
2. Review file documents for completeness, relevant data, and accuracy of findings
3. Identify conflicting information
4. Determine and/or recommend needed follow-up information to corroborate or dispute investigative findings

Source: Derived and updated from Washington State Patrol, Form No. 3000-420-081 (Sept. 2014) Fire Protection Bureau, Standards and Accreditation, Olympia, Washington http://www.wsp.wa.gov/fire/docs/cert/fire_invest.pdf

circumstances, treatment received, disposition of the body and its examination, next of kin, and other appropriate remarks. This information should be collected on all injured parties, not just on fatalities.

This form currently does not include general information about the victim obtained at autopsies such as burn injuries, tests for blood alcohol, hydrogen cyanide, carboxyhemoglobin levels, and other conditions often documented in fire death investigations. Note that the Health Insurance Portability and Accountability Act (HIPAA) regulations (*45 CFR 160* and *164*, subparts A and E) restrict access to some information.

Witnesses

Information from witnesses (NFPA 2014, pts. 4.5.1, 4.5.2 and 4.5.3) is documented in field notes taken by the investigator, including identification, home and work addresses, contact information, and expected testimony.

INTERVIEW/INTERROGATION STANDARD:
4.5.1 *NFPA 1033*, 2014 EDITION

TASK:

Develop an interview plan, given no special tools or equipment, so that the plan reflects a strategy to further determine the fire cause and affix responsibility and includes a relevant questioning strategy for each individual to be interviewed that promotes the efficient use of the investigator's time.

PERFORMANCE OUTCOME:

The investigator will develop two interview plans that assist in fire cause and suspect determination.

(Continued)

INTERVIEW/INTERROGATION STANDARD: 4.5.2 *NFPA 1033*, 2014 EDITION

NFPA 921 identifies witness information as one of the primary sources of information to be considered by investigators in determining a fire's origin and cause (NFPA 2017, pts. 18 and 19). It is imperative to interview as many witnesses to a fire as possible, including fire and police personnel, as soon as possible while the information is fresh and untainted. *NFPA 921* cautions that the rate of fire growth as solely determined by witness

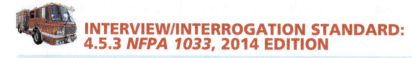

INTERVIEW/INTERROGATION STANDARD: 4.5.3 *NFPA 1033*, 2014 EDITION

TASK:

Evaluate interview information, given interview transcripts or notes and incident data, so that all interview data is individually analyzed and correlated with all other interviews, corroborative and conflicting information is documented, and new leads are developed.

PERFORMANCE OUTCOME:

The investigator will evaluate, analyze, and correlate interview information to determine if the information is corroborative or conflictive in nature and develop new investigative leads.

CONDITIONS:

Given incident information, interview transcripts, and note paper, the investigator will be able to complete the listed task.

TASK STEPS:

1. Review provided information
2. Correlate information into corroborative or conflicting groups
3. Document new investigative leads
4. List follow-up names and contact numbers

Source: Derived and updated from Washington State Patrol, Form No. 3000-420-081 (Sept. 2014) Fire Protection Bureau, Standards and Accreditation, Olympia, Washington http://www.wsp.wa.gov/fire/docs/cert /fire_invest.pdf

---

statements may be subjective. It notes that often the time of discovery is considerably later than the time of actual ignition, and witnesses report the fire growth observed from time of discovery not ignition (NFPA 2017, pt. 5.10.1.4).

In cases involving on-scene witnesses, thorough interviews may reveal additional information relating to the initial stages of the fire and the environmental conditions at the time (rain, wind, extreme cold, etc.). In most cases, survivors can provide information on pre-fire conditions; fire and smoke development; fuel package location and orientation; activities of victims and suspects before, during, and after discovery of the fire; actions resulting in their survival; and critical fire events such as flashover, structural failure, window breakage, alarm sounding, first observation of smoke, first observation of flame, fire department arrival, and contact with others in the building (NFPA 2017, pt. 11.8.5).

Furthermore, it is important to document details of the position of the witnesses in relation to the fire scene when recording their visual observations, especially when using witness-viewpoint photographs (NFPA 2017, pt. 16.2.8.10). This process can be enhanced by walking witnesses through the scene when safe or back to the location from which they witnessed the fire. This can help establish or confirm lines of sight and prompt more complete statements.

EXAMPLE 6-1 ■ Systematic Analysis of Witness Statements

On January 16, 2007, a fire at the Castle West Apartments, a 129-unit wood-framed three-level apartment building in Colorado Springs, Colorado, resulted in two deaths, thirteen injured occupants, six injured firefighters, and an estimated $6 million loss. The building did not have automatic sprinklers or a monitored/addressable fire alarm system and had emergency lighting only in hallways and stairs, and only battery-operated smoke detectors in hallways and in some units.

The multiagency investigation team interviewed witnesses from 96 occupied units of the 129 units, 24 of which were vacant. These interviews resulted in coverage of more than 90 percent of the total occupied units.

To minimize confirmation bias, a study by ATF's Fire Research Laboratory (Geiman and Lord 2011) mapped the mosaics of the individual observations of the witness interviews onto the floor plans of the three levels. The result was an open-ended protocol of essential questions to ask witnesses that increased their independent reliability and corrected for many of the factors that would lead to confirmation bias introduced either consciously or subconsciously by the interviewer.

The results of the analysis demonstrated the survivability of victims. Figure 6-12 shows that almost all the occupants on Level A (first floor) successfully exited their apartment building. The analysis of the individual observations of smoke and fire by occupants exiting the building helped independently isolate the area of fire origin to the north wing of the building on Levels B and C, as seen in Figure 6-13 from the study.

The study concluded that this approach provides a systematic analytical tool for fire investigators to use in testing fire origin hypotheses. This methodology reduces the potential for confirmation bias by both the investigators and witnesses when a consistent protocol of open-ended questions is applied in mass interviews. Encoding the interviews into a text retrieval system allows for later content analysis of the witness information. Finally, the simple graphical presentation of the investigation overlaid on the building plan assists in interpreting the results of the analysis and provides positive demonstrative evidence for inclusion in reports and potential legal proceedings.

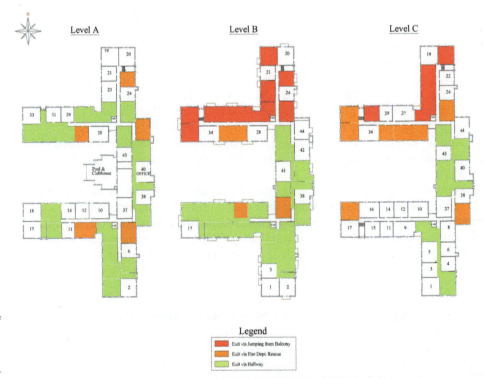

FIGURE 6-12 Three-level plan of the apartment complex showing the egress modes of the occupants via jumping from the balcony, rescue by the fire department, and simple unaided egress. *Courtesy of the Fire Research Laboratory, US Department of Justice, Bureau of Alcohol, Tobacco, Firearms and Explosives.*

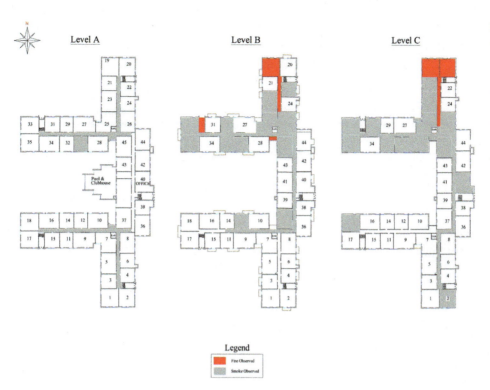

FIGURE 6-13 Three-level plan of the apartment complex showing the observations by escaping occupants of smoke and flame. *Courtesy of the Fire Research Laboratory, US Department of Justice, Bureau of Alcohol, Tobacco, Firearms and Explosives.*

Evidence Collection and Preservation

The chain of custody is intended to trace the item of evidence from its discovery, collection, preservation, and finally to court, and eventual disposal (NFPA 2014, pt. 4.3.1, 4.4.2, 4.4.3, 4.4.4, and 4.4.5; NFPA 2017, pt. 17).

EVIDENCE COLLECTION/PRESERVATION STANDARD: 4.4.1; 4.4.2 *NFPA 1033*, 2014 EDITION

TASKS:

Utilize proper procedures for managing victims and fatalities, given protocol and appropriate personnel. Locate, collect, label, package, and store evidence, given standard tools or special tools and equipment and evidence collection materials, so that it is properly identified, preserved, collected, packaged, and stored for use in testing, legal, or other proceedings and examinations, ensuring cross-contamination and investigator-inflicted damage to evidentiary items is avoided and the chain of custody is established.

PERFORMANCE OUTCOME:

The investigator will collect and package two different types of identified evidence, maintaining chain of custody and avoiding contamination. The investigator will ensure evidence related to victims is discovered and preserved following proper protocol.

CONDITIONS:

Given several types of evidence, needed evidence collection supplies and appropriate forms.

TASK STEPS:

1. Identify two different types of evidence
2. Select and collect one of each of the two types of evidence

(Continued)

3. Package selected/collected items
4. Document the process in field notes
5. Identify what type of evidence testing would be requested (if any)
6. Evidence related to victims is discovered and preserved following proper protocol
7. Document and report fire-related fatalities with appropriate forms

Source: Derived and updated from Washington State Patrol, Form No. 3000-420-081 (Sept. 2014) Fire Protection Bureau, Standards and Accreditation, Olympia, Washington http://www.wsp.wa.gov/fire/docs/cert /fire_invest.pdf

EVIDENCE COLLECTION/PRESERVATION STANDARD: 4.4.3 *NFPA 1033*, 2014 EDITION

TASK:

Select evidence for analysis, given all information from the investigation, so that items for analysis support specific investigative needs.

PERFORMANCE OUTCOME:

The investigator will review an investigation report, select one item of evidence, and fill out a standard crime lab analysis request form indicating specific test(s) requested.

CONDITIONS:

Given an investigation report, several different types of evidence, and a standard crime lab analysis request form.

TASK STEPS:

1. Review the investigation report
2. Select one appropriate item of evidence
3. Fill out the crime lab analysis request form completely

Source: Derived and updated from Washington State Patrol, Form No. 3000-420-081 (Sept. 2014) Fire Protection Bureau, Standards and Accreditation, Olympia, Washington http://www.wsp.wa.gov/fire/docs/cert /fire_invest.pdf

EVIDENCE COLLECTION/PRESERVATION STANDARD: 4.4.4 *NFPA 1033*, 2014 EDITION

TASK:

Maintain a chain of custody, given standard investigative tools; marking tools, and evidence tags or logs, so that written documentation exists for each piece of evidence and evidence is secured.

PERFORMANCE OUTCOME:

The investigator will mark, package, and log six items of evidence.

CONDITIONS:

Given equipment, forms, tags, and six items of evidence.

EVIDENCE COLLECTION/PRESERVATION STANDARD: 4.4.5 *NFPA 1033*, 2014 EDITION

TASK:

Dispose of evidence, given jurisdictional or agency regulations and file information, so that the disposal is timely, safely conducted, and in compliance with jurisdictional or agency requirements.

PERFORMANCE OUTCOME:

The investigator will dispose of evidence in a timely and safe manner and document the disposal of evidence.

CONDITIONS:

Given incident information, model evidence policy, evidence, and evidence disposal forms, the investigator will complete the listed task.

TASK STEPS:

1. Review provided information
2. Identify evidence subject to disposal
3. Dispose of evidence according to the model evidence policy
4. Document the disposal using the provided forms

Source: Derived and updated from Washington State Patrol, Form No. 3000-420-081 (Sept. 2014) Fire Protection Bureau, Standards and Accreditation, Olympia, Washington http://www.wsp.wa.gov/fire/docs/cert/fire_invest.pdf

Its purpose is to authenticate the evidence as it is found as well as to prevent its loss or destruction. The documentation includes photographing the evidence at its discovery and preparing a written list itemizing the transfer of the evidence once it leaves the scene, as on the Evidence form (Figure 6-6). Such documentation will demonstrate compliance with guidelines such as *ASTM E1188: Standard Practice for Collection and Preservation of Information and Physical Items by a Technical Investigator* (ASTM 2011b).

Photography

Photographs (NFPA 2014, pt. 4.3.2; NFPA 2017, pt. 16.2) should include not only overall views but also close-ups of critical evidence and intermediate establishing shots when necessary.

Photos should record the scene as found, during debris clearance, after clearance, and with furnishings replaced in their pre-fire positions. An accurate photo log (NFPA 2017, pt. 16.3(4)) is nearly as important as the photos themselves to ensure that the investigator can correctly reconstruct the scene days, weeks, or months later when called on.

SCENE DOCUMENTATION STANDARD:
4.3.2 *NFPA 1033*, 2014 EDITION

TASK:

Photographically document the scene, given standard tools and equipment, so that the scene is accurately depicted and the photographs support scene findings.

PERFORMANCE OUTCOME:

The investigator will photograph an interior scene and provide a photo log and photo rough sketch of the photos taken. (Use 35mm camera or a high-resolution digital camera. The use of video camera systems to supplement visual documentation can be utilized and is encouraged.)

CONDITIONS:

Given a fire scene, a 35mm camera and flash, film, note pad, and measuring devices. (Note: outside photos already taken.)

TASK STEPS:

1. Locate and size up the scene
2. Photograph from the outside of the room to the inside
3. Photograph items of evidence without size references
4. Photograph items of evidence with size reference
5. Document photos taken on a photo rough sketch and photo log

Source: Derived and updated from Washington State Patrol, Form No. 3000-420-081 (Sept. 2014) Fire Protection Bureau, Standards and Accreditation, Olympia, Washington http://www.wsp.wa.gov/fire/docs/cert /fire_invest.pdf

The Photograph Log form (Figure 6-7) is used to record the description, frame, roll, or image storage card, and digital image number of each photograph taken at the fire scene. Investigators should follow a similar systematic documentation scheme for fire scene photographic images taken with video recorders. The form is designed to be filled out as the photographs are taken. The frame and roll (or photo) image numbers are used later on the fire scene sketch to indicate the location and direction from which they were taken. Each roll of film, digital image, and videotape that is preserved by duplicate archived media should be documented on a separate form. The Remarks field is used to document the disposition of the film, archived media, and videotapes. Close-up photos of evidence should be accompanied by overall, orientation, or panoramic shots. Photography is discussed in more detail in a later section of this chapter.

Sketching

Fire scene sketches, diagrams, and drawings (NFPA 2014, pt. 4.3.1; NFPA 2017, pt. 16.4), whether or not to scale, are important supplements to photographs. They graphically portray the fire scene and items of evidence, pertinent contents, significant fire patterns, and area(s) or point(s) of origin (NFPA 2014, pt. 4.3.1) as recorded by the investigator.

A typical sketch is a simple two-dimensional drawing of the fire scene that includes all major dimensions of rooms, compartments, buildings, vehicles, and curtilage, where applicable. Square-grid paper is available in many sizes at business and school supply stores. These sketches may range from rough exterior building outlines or room contents to detailed floor plans. Sketches of the distribution of window glass fragments are critical to later reconstruction of explosion events (NFPA 2017, pt. 6.2.13.1.6). They must include distances and angular direction data.

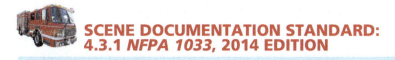

SCENE DOCUMENTATION STANDARD: 4.3.1 *NFPA 1033*, 2014 EDITION

TASK:

Diagram the scene, given standard tools and equipment, so that the scene is accurately represented and evidence, pertinent contents, significant patterns, and area(s) or point(s) of origin are identified.

PERFORMANCE OUTCOME:

The investigator will diagram (rough sketch) the fire scene. The diagram shall include at least one item of evidence, one item of pertinent contents, one significant burn pattern, and one area or point of origin.

CONDITIONS:

Given a safe and secure fire scene, a note pad, measuring devices, and an assistant, if requested.

TASK STEPS:

1. Locate and size up the fire scene
2. Diagram the fire scene to include each of the following:
   a. Relative locations, dimensions, rooms, stairs, doors, and windows
   b. At least one item of evidence with location dimensions indicated
   c. At least one item of pertinent contents with location and dimensions indicated
   d. At least one burn pattern with location identified
   e. At least one area or point of origin with size indicated
   f. The investigator's name, date, and scene number or location

Source: Derived and updated from Washington State Patrol, Form No. 3000-420-081 (Sept. 2014) Fire Protection Bureau, Standards and Accreditation, Olympia, Washington http://www.wsp.wa.gov/fire/docs/cert /fire_invest.pdf

Documentary Records

Insurance information and documentary records (NFPA 2014, pt. 4.6.1) are required to be collected to ensure that a thorough investigation is conducted, particularly when there are multiple policyholders, as in the case of commercial buildings. Care should be taken to evaluate, catalog accurately, and secure these incident, property, business, and personal documentary records (NFPA 2014, pt. 4.6.2).

Compartment Fire Modeling Data

The documentation needed for compartment fire modeling exceeds the data normally collected by investigators. These additional details are listed on the Room Fire Data form. Information on the compartment needed for the model includes room dimensions, construction, surface materials, interior finish, openings in doors and windows, HVAC, event timeline, and fuel packages (NFPA 2017, pt. 16.4.5.6.1). This information is critical to hypothesis formation and testing in all fire reconstructions, even if computer modeling is not planned. It is especially important that height information, not just the floor plan, be accurately and fully recorded. For example, any places where the ceiling height changes must be clearly identified because slope, deep beams, and architectural features can affect hot gas flow and layer development.

Physical Evidence

Physical evidence (NFPA 2014, pt. 4.4.2; NFPA 2017, pt. 17) is sometimes called the silent witness because it can provide reliable answers to questions that other investigative techniques cannot address, fill in details, and corroborate other information. The investigative phase of systematic investigation combines all the essential elements of forensic evidence collected from the fire scene.

Generally accepted forensic guidelines are designed to prevent contamination, loss, or destruction of the evidence and to provide a reliable chain of custody for that evidence. For instance, when there is an object with dried blood on it, the object itself should be collected whenever possible and allowed to air-dry before packaging. Bloody objects should be placed into individual sealed paper bags, boxes, or envelopes after drying and kept dry and refrigerated if possible. Ordinary plastic bags should not be used, since they will not allow the sample to ventilate. Investigators should be aware of the safety issues involving blood-borne pathogens (NFPA 2017, pt. A.13.4.2.1).

All firearms should be placed into individual manila envelopes, and rifles should be tagged. Firearms should be hand-carried to the laboratory. Special handling instructions include the collecting technique, unloading and noting the cylinder position in revolvers, and recording the serial number, make, and model of the weapon. Fire debris or containers containing volatile liquids must be sealed in appropriate packaging to prevent loss or contamination and kept cool to minimize evaporation.

Handheld Laser Measurement Techniques

Investigators often find themselves documenting the measurements of several rooms within a structure. This is a cumbersome, time-consuming task that can be inaccurate. Measuring tapes are most efficient when used by two persons. Handheld devices are beneficial when a single person is responsible for measuring distances.

With the introduction of low-cost accurate handheld laser devices, an investigator can now measure not only the distance but also the area and volume of a room. Published specifications for devices sold for less than $100 report an accuracy of ±6.35 mm (1/4 in.) at 30.48 m (100 ft). The typical range of these devices is 0.6 to 30 m (2 to 100 ft), they can be switched to read in English or metric units, and they operate on low-cost 9 V batteries (Stanley 2012).

Ignition Matrix™

Today, more than ever before, fire investigators face the challenge of identifying all potential ignition sources in the area of origin and then eliminating them, down to one (based on reasonable data or methods). The scientific method of fire investigation requires that an investigator reach a defensible conclusion by demonstrating not only how this source could have started the fire but also how all other reasonably possible sources have been excluded. If two or more ignition sources are deemed possible at the end of the investigation, the cause has to be declared to be undetermined. Demonstrating these conclusions can be difficult, especially in a concise yet comprehensive manner.

The ignition matrix™ approach forces the investigator to consider a comprehensive range of alternative hypotheses and consider each one on the basis of factors such as **heat release rate (HRR)**, heat flux, separation distances, **thermal inertia**, and routes of fire spread. A completed matrix offers a concise demonstration that all potential ignition sources have been considered and all but one, presumably, eliminated. A matrix is also more easily verified than the traditional item-by-item list, improving the investigator's own review process. This comprehensive approach is not the casual process of elimination that *NFPA* (NFPA 2017, pt. 19.6.5). It is an exhaustive approach reflecting the true intent of the scientific method.

The process begins with a detailed evaluation and sketch of the suspected area of origin. All identified first fuels and possible ignition sources are documented. The *Bilancia Ignition Matrix™* entails exhaustive pairwise comparisons designed to systematically evaluate numerous ignition sources and also to document how each was or was not competent to ignite a particular first fuel. The suggested ignition matrix™ is merely a grid on paper. In that layout, each square represents a pairwise assessment of the interaction between an energy source and a first fuel.

heat release rate (HRR) ■ (HRR) The rate at which heat energy is generated by burning (*NFPA 921*, 2017 ed., pt. 3.3.105).

thermal inertia ■ The properties of a material that characterize its rate of surface temperature rise when exposed to heat; related to the product of the material's thermal conductivity (k), its density (ρ), and its heat capacity (c).

Each combination is then evaluated on four primary values:

1. Is this ignition source competent to ignite this fuel?
2. Is this ignition source close enough to this fuel to be capable of igniting it?
3. Is there evidence of ignition?
4. Is there a pathway for a fire ignited in this first fuel to ignite the main fuel?

Comments or notes can be included and applied to each evaluation. These notes might include one or more of the following:

- This source was not energized (appliance or power cord) or not in use (candle).
- "Too far away" or "Depends on duration being adequate," or "Unknown—must test exemplar."
- Physical or visual evidence of burning; ignition was witnessed or recorded in video.
- **Plume** developed from first fuel sufficient, or flashover produced ignition.

plume ∎ The column of hot gases, flames, and smoke rising above a fire; also called *convection column*, *thermal updraft*, or *thermal column* (*NFPA 921*, 2017 ed., pt. 3.3.141).

Finally, the matrix can be color-coded to indicate which combinations are capable, which are excluded, and which need further data. This color legend might be Red—Competent and close, Blue—Not competent, and Yellow— Competent but ruled out.

Forming Opinions

The investigator is responsible for an opinion concerning origin, cause, or responsibility for the fire (NFPA 2014, pt. 4.6.4 and 4.6.5)

POST-INCIDENT INVESTIGATION STANDARD: 4.6.5 *NFPA 1033*, 2014 EDITION

TASK:

Formulate an opinion concerning origin, cause, or responsibility for the fire, given all investigative findings, so that the opinion regarding origin, cause, or responsibility for a fire is supported by the data, facts, records, reports, documents, and evidence.

PERFORMANCE OUTCOME:

The investigator will formulate an opinion of the person and/or product responsibility for the fire.

CONDITIONS:

Given a complete fire investigation file, including records, documents, and evidence, the investigator will complete the listed task.

TASK STEPS:

1. Review provided materials
2. Formulate and document an opinion as to the person and/or product responsibility

Source: Derived and updated from Washington State Patrol, Form No. 3000-420-081 (Sept. 2014) Fire Protection Bureau, Standards and Accreditation, Olympia, Washington http://www.wsp.wa.gov/fire/docs/cert/fire_invest.pdf

6.2.4 PANORAMIC PHOTOGRAPHY

Photographic Stitching

A majority of the photographs taken at fire scenes focus on fire patterns and other evidence. But a simple photo may not capture information around the perimeter of a room. In structure fires, an aerial view, perspective view, panoramic view of the building, or a combination of all three can reveal the overall impact of the fire on the structure, including

TASK:

Establish evidence as to motive and/or opportunity, given an incendiary fire, so that the evidence is supported by documentation and meets the evidentiary requirements of the jurisdiction.

PERFORMANCE OUTCOME:

The investigator will establish motive and/or opportunity of an incendiary fire through the use of prudent and complete investigation files, determining if the evidence meets legal requirements.

CONDITIONS:

Given a complete incendiary fire investigation file and evidence log, the investigator will determine motive and/or opportunity and determine the legal value of provided evidence.

TASK STEPS:

1. Review provided materials
2. Determine and document the motive and/or opportunity of the incendiary fire
3. List supporting documents that establish motive
4. Document evidence used to determine motive
5. Document legal value of evidence provided

Source: Derived and updated from Washington State Patrol, Form No. 3000-420-081 (Sept. 2014) Fire Protection Bureau, Standards and Accreditation, Olympia, Washington http://www.wsp.wa.gov/fire/docs/cert/fire_invest.pdf

how the building itself was breached by both the fire and efforts to extinguish the blaze. An example of a *panoramic photograph* of a fire scene created by stitching several photographs together is shown in Figure 6-14.

The creation of panoramic images to improve scene review and illustration for court is not new. Panoramic (scanning slit) cameras have been around for more than 100 years, but they were rarely used, because the specialized equipment was heavy, yet delicate. Panoramic cameras, popular in the late 1800s, were sometimes used to capture the ravaging effects of fires. Many present-day cameras simply crop the top and bottom portions of the image, creating a false appearance of a panoramic photograph.

Super-wide-angle and 360° rotating cameras are now available, but they are costly (Curtin 2011). Human vision typically captures a 170° view of a room, but a typical 50 mm camera lens captures only about one-fifth of that field of view. An investigator attempting to capture fire patterns around a room needs some type of panoramic technology.

At its simplest, constructing a panoramic photograph can consist of using a steady tripod, taking a series of overlapping photographs, and then physically overlaying prints to form a mosaic view of the fire scene. Overlaying several photographic shots in the form of a mosaic can compensate for the lack of a true panoramic photograph. For best results a lens with 35 to 55 mm focal length is used, because wide-angle (<35 mm) and telephoto lenses introduce unwanted distortions. Once an investigator has become familiar with the results and limitations of the camera, he or she should work on developing an expertise with panoramic photography (see Figure 6-15).

Simple paste-ups of overlapping images are acceptable, but there are always perspective-shift distortions between views that can disorient the viewer. The advent of panoramic view stitching in computer photo editing programs has made it possible to create seamless, perspective-corrected panoramic images from a series of simple still photos without specialized cameras such as digital scanning cameras, which are discussed in detail later in this chapter.

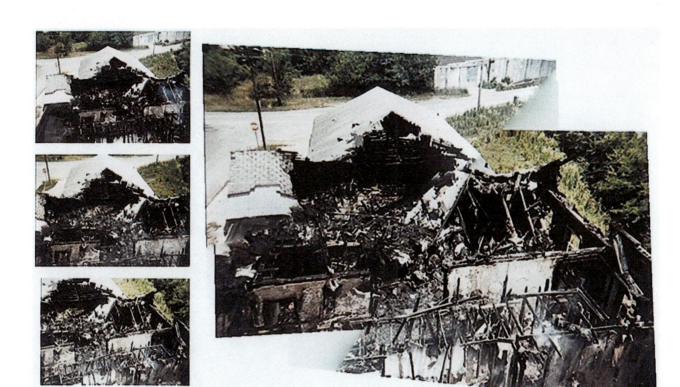

FIGURE 6-14 Construction of a panoramic view using individual photographs and stitching software. *Courtesy of David J. Icove, University of Tennessee.*

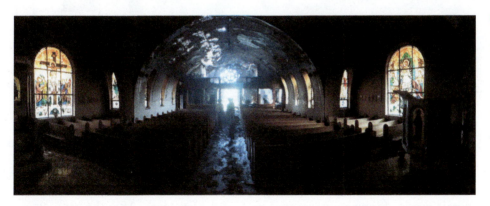

FIGURE 6-15 Separate sequential photos stitched together using an Apple IPad panoramic capture software of a church fire. *Courtesy of Det. Aaron Allen, Knox County Sheriff's Office, Tennessee, Fire Investigation Unit.*

EXAMPLE 6-2 ■ The School Fire

Large multi-room school fires with massive structural destruction are difficult to reconstruct. A fire scene reconstruction was conducted of a large school fire that occurred some years ago in the Southeast. A majority of the contents and walls had been removed and placed outside the structure prior to examination of the scene.

The fire scene was reconstructed using a combination of eyewitness statements, raw news videos, scene analysis, and knowledge of plume geometry. Investigation revealed that a fire started on the school office floor adjacent to filing cabinets where student records were stored.

A methodical examination of the debris, the dynamic time sequence of the fire's movement, and the damage caused by the fire confirmed the office to be the room of fire origin. A careful fire scene analysis of pattern damage revealed a roughly elliptical

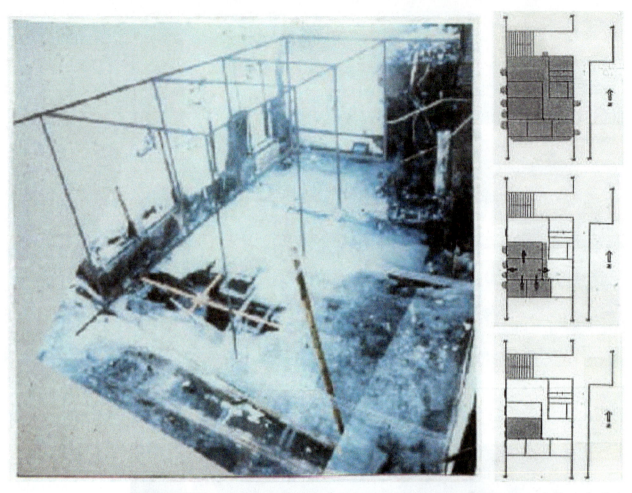

FIGURE 6-16 The panoramic photo overlay from Example 6-2 with graphic chart tape on a plastic overlay that shows missing walls and area of fire origin. Floor plans on right show (bottom to top) the successive fire spread as seen through exterior windows. *Courtesy of David J. Icove, University of Tennessee.*

penetration at the floor of the office where the fire originated. The apparent point of fire origin was at the center of this elliptical pattern.

Yellow chalk was used to sketch on the floor the location of the desk, cabinets, and walls. These chalk lines were photographed from the second floor and displayed as a mosaic overlay forming a panoramic view of the fire scene. After the panoramic photos were pieced together, the walls were marked using graphic chart tape on a plastic overlay. Plastic overlays are important for courtroom presentation, because they can be removed if objections are raised to their use. A photograph of this exhibit with the overlay present is shown to the left of the schematic floor plans in Figure 6-16. Ghost walls can today be inserted using the graphics packages described previously. Such displays can also be helpful in confirming witness observations.

One of the most persuasive visual exhibits offering a perspective view is a scale model for courtroom presentations. The overall dimensions of the building being re-created must be carefully defined and accurately captured. Architectural firms often have technicians on staff who can prepare these models. A removable roof on the model should be included to provide access to the building's interior layout.

Specialized photographic techniques can involve the use of forensic (alternate) light sources and suitable filters, ultraviolet or infrared films or imaging systems, and close-up (macro) photography or other techniques to preserve physical evidence such as fingerprints. Some of these are discussed in later sections of this chapter.

Total Station Survey Mapping

A new generation of computer-driven surveying technology is now being used for mapping of large interior and exterior scenes. A single reference location is selected and located using a *global positioning system* (GPS) integrated with a *geographic information system* (GIS). The laser sighting unit is then trained on individual features—corners of rooms, curb lines, or evidence locations. The computer notes each feature's direction, angle of elevation, and distance. The program then draws a plan of the scene with extremely accurate dimensions [error of ±1 cm (±0.39 in.) at 150 m (492 ft) is typical] even without reflector posts. Systems by Leica, Sokkia, and Topcon that have been used by traffic accident investigation teams in many police jurisdictions for years are now being used by some major arson investigation agencies.

Laser Scanning Systems

Laser scanners combine the accuracy of total station measurements with the completeness of panoramic digital photography. Three-dimensional (3D) laser scanners use LIDAR (LIght Detection And Ranging) technology to quickly capture millions of measurements at a scene (NFPA 2017, pt. 16.4.5.6). Most scanners are integrated with a high-resolution digital camera or are coupled with an external digital camera to capture colors and textures of surfaces. This information is then mapped onto the laser measurements to produce a fully navigable 3D virtual reality (VR) (called a *point cloud*) of data of any interior or exterior scene. A scene can be scanned from multiple locations and the images registered or stitched together to produce a comprehensive and visually stunning 3D data collection. Any measurement in three dimensions can later be extracted from the data using the software provided with the system.

Laser scanners have become more widely used and lower in cost. Several manufacturers now offer PC-driven scanners that are placed in a room or at an outdoor scene and scan a laser beam vertically and rotate horizontally (using mirrors), taking distance and angular deflection measurements at the rate of several to many thousand per second. Distance may be measured by time of flight (TOF), in which the delay time between a pulsed output and its returned reflection determines distance, or phase shift, in which the beam is continuous and the interference between outgoing and returned light waves determines distance. Phase-shift scanners emit a continuous laser beam, and the phase difference between outgoing and returning sine waves determines the distance to an object. Both kinds of systems employ a mirror to direct the beam vertically around a scene while motors drive the scanner to rotate horizontally. Data are typically collected at a rate of tens of thousands of measurements per second.

Several manufacturers now offer high-speed laser scanners that are widely used and are lower in cost. The technology firm 3rd Tech Inc. has developed a laser-scanning device that uses a time-of-flight 5 MW laser range finder that, when mounted on a photographer's or surveyor's tripod, will scan an entire room, taking 25,000 measurements per second (3rd Tech 2012).

Leica Geosystems (Leica 2012) offers the ScanStation laser scanner, which uses a pulsed green class 3R laser to capture high-accuracy measurements both indoors and outside, regardless of lighting conditions. Their Cyclone software outputs data that are compatible with most third-party computer-aided drafting (CAD) products and can also quickly produce a fully immersive and measurable 3D environment called Leica TruView that is sharable with free viewing software. Faro (2017) is a 3D imaging system using laser and imaging technologies. The firm markets portable CMMs (coordinate measuring machines) along with 3D imaging equipment used in forensic fire, crime, and accident scenes.

The data from these scans can be analyzed and displayed in many ways. After the registration process is completed in a computer lab, the 3D VR image can be rotated and viewed from any angle or any scanner setup position. Outlines, wireframes, and diagrams can be created. Hotspot links to close-up photos, lab reports, notes, or chain-of-custody information can be added. Additional distance and angle measurements can be taken and recorded at any time. The Department of Justice (DOJ); crime labs; and police, security, and fire agencies use scanner technology. A number of manufacturers offer laser scanners with different capabilities and limitations (Leica 2012; 3rd Tech 2012; Riegl 2012, and Faro 2017).

Selection considerations for laser scanners include:

Accuracy (resolution):   Each time the laser measures a distance, it records a point (scan spot). After all measurements have been merged, the scanner forms a "point cloud," which allows further viewing and analysis. Point spacing (equivalent to the dpi rating of digital images) can be adjusted by the scanner technician to provide the necessary detail for a given project's needs in relation to distance from the target area. Leica Geosystems has announced the introduction of a new tool that validates the accuracy of forensic 3D laser scans generated by the Leica Geosystems ScanStation C10. The new validation tool is designed specifically to help crime laboratories and crime scene units achieve ISO/IEC 17020 and 17025 accreditations. The twin-target pole, placed at the scene in various locations to allow precise calibration and measurements, has a design distance of 1.700 m between the two targets.

In order to achieve National Institute of Standards and Technology (NIST) trace-ability, Leica Geosystems has contracted with the Large-Scale Coordinate Metrology Group at NIST to perform individual calibrations on specific Leica Geosystems twin-target poles by carefully measuring multiple times between the target centers on each end of the pole (artifact) using a wavelength-compensated helium–neon linear interferometer. NIST then applies serial numbers to each target system and generates a Report of Calibration that is provided to Leica Geosystems customers. "It's the 3D laser scanning equivalent of introducing a scale into a crime scene photograph to provide a control," said Tony Grissim, Leica Geosystems Public Safety and Forensic Account Manager. "The provable accuracy of 3D laser scanner measurements to a known standard is key to forensic credibility in the courtroom, and our new NIST traceable twin-target pole has the added benefit of supporting the ISO/IEC requirements for quality systems and quality control" (Leica 2011).

Court acceptability: Of critical importance to the users of scan data in forensic cases is the technique's successful admissibility in court. As with other forensic tools, the user must be able to explain the device's scientific foundation and validate the accuracy of the measurement. In addition to NIST and ISO, *ASTM E2544-11a: Standard Terminology for Three-Dimensional (3D) Imaging Systems* (ASTM 2011c) offer users assistance with validation should a *Daubert* challenge be executed. Courts repeatedly rule in favor of accepting laser-scanned data and animations that have been developed using scanners as the basis for data collection, analysis, and visualization.

Distance range: Some scanners have a minimum range of 2 m (6.6 ft), so their usefulness for small spaces needs to be considered. Others have a maximum range of 16 m (52 ft), so they have limited use in large indoor scenes or exterior scenes. Distance upper limits are dependent on the reflectivity of the target [e.g., 300 m (980 ft) at 90 percent reflectivity versus 134 m (440 ft) at 18 percent reflectivity], so the conditions of the scene and nature of the target are crucial. Ranges are offered up to 280 m (900 ft), but the resolution and accuracy will naturally decline.

Wavelength: Some wavelengths perform better with dark (charred) surfaces, which is a concern to fire investigators. Some wavelengths encounter interference with **ambient** light and suffer from a condition called "day blindness" and thus require the scanned area to be darkened. Others (e.g., Leica) will work in daylight or full darkness.

Accuracy (distance):   Accuracy of distance measurements depends on the type (TOF or phase shift) and range. Accuracy is typically on the order of 4 to 7 mm (0.16 to 0.28 in.) at 50 m (160 ft).

Field of view: Some scanners will scan from vertical (90° up to almost 90° down); others can scan only from 45° up to 45° down and require a rescan to capture information from directly overhead.

Scan rate: Most systems will complete a 360° high-resolution scan of a room in 12 to 30 minutes, taking 4000 to 50,000 measurements per second for TOF, and 500,000 points per second for phase-based systems.

Safety: All systems use a Class I laser, so eye safety is a concern. Some systems are designed (by scan rate) so that duration of exposure to an unprotected eye will not exceed the federal safety limits. Others require eye protection for users or others in the room.

Ease of "registration" or stitching: Most scenes require scanning from at least two positions. Systems (software) vary in the ease with which integration of these data sets can be done. Some systems produce a data format that can be entered directly in AutoCAD and similar drafting programs.

ambient ■ Someone's or something's surroundings, especially as they pertain to the local environment; for example, ambient air and ambient temperature (*NFPA 921*, 2017 ed., pt. 3.3.5).

Such scanners are somewhat expensive, but they permit rapid, extremely accurate measurement of all critical features in a fire scene, such as room dimensions, ventilation openings, and structural features (beams, sloping ceilings, and ductwork). For users who do not have their own scanning system, both public and private sources offer technicians for single-use deployments. The captured images can be revisited at any time to conduct additional measurements. Data from some software systems can be imported into CAD systems for rendering to fixed images or creating a physical model. Readers are encouraged to contact vendors or manufacturer websites (listed at Resource Central) for detailed information. Depending on the wavelength of their lasers, laser scanners can capture variations in surface condition (reflectivity) that may not be apparent in standard color photographs. Compare the false-color laser scan of a burned test cubicle with a color photo of the same scene in the following test study.

EXAMPLE 6-3 ■ Wildland Fire Scene Reconstruction

Problem. Reconstruct a wildland fire scene two years post-extinguishment. Several factors contributed and need to be considered including a wind event, a damaged tree, and a subsequent wire strike. The suspected tree was cut into sections and stored as evidence.

Solution. The steep site was accessed, and the terrain at the scene was laser scanned (Figure 6-17a). An expert arborist assisted with reconstruction of the eight tree sections, via the 3D computer terrain model (Figure 6-17b). The scene and the reconstructed tree were scanned separately with a Leica Geosystems scanner, which produced several million measurements.

Conclusion. A visually and spatially accurate 3D model depicting the tree in position prior to wind damage, wire strike, and fire was produced (Figure 6-17c). Case study courtesy of Precision Simulations Inc. and Kirk McKinzie CFI.

One benefit of scanning a scene is that it can complement the use of the NIST Fire Dynamics Simulator (FDS) fire model. Should a particular scene be scanned and a subsequent 3D model

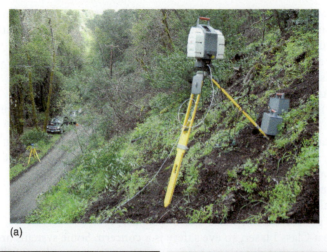

(a)

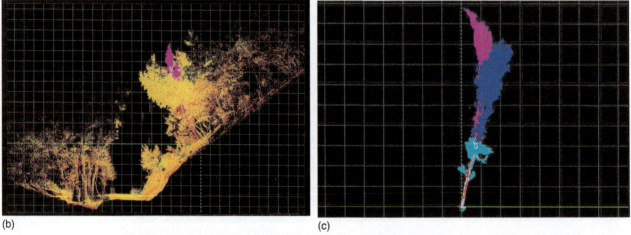

(b)   (c)

FIGURE 6-17 (a) The scanner and steep terrain near the area of fire origin, two years postfire. (b) The main trunk, limbs, and branch structure reassembled in the elevation model. (c) Once the tree was accurately reassembled, it was rotated and properly positioned in elevation, plan, and orientation in the 3D forensic computer model/scene. *Data collection, registration, and images courtesy of Craig Fries, Precision Simulations Inc.*

constructed, a rapid and exceptionally accurate set of input data can expedite development of models for fire propagation, carbon monoxide, oxygen, heat release, and temperature studies.

An area for future study is of the fire patterns associated with **calcination**. One theory that deserves consideration and study is the possibility that reflectance data from scans of gypsum surfaces that have been exposed to heat energy may provide quantifiable heat flux data. The correlation between laser reflectance at a variety of reflectance levels must be established. Paint, paper, smoke, bare gypsum, and variations in penetrating calcination each have their own reflectance qualities, and there may be a correlative heat flux factor/index relation.

Conclusion. Speed, accuracy, and portability make 3D terrestrial and airborne scanners a natural choice for important scene documentation. With *NFPA 921* and *NFPA 1033* requiring the most complete documentation with the most advanced technology, it is inevitable that 3D laser scanners will be increasingly used at fire scenes.

calcination ■ A fire effect realized in gypsum products, including wallboard, as a result of exposure to heat that drives off free and chemically bound water (*NFPA 921*, 2014 ed., pt. 3.3.23).

6.3 Application of Criminalistics at Fire Scenes

Criminalistics is the application of scientific techniques in collecting and analyzing physical evidence in criminal cases. Criminalistics examines physical evidence; human behavior; physical dynamics of force, impact, and transfer; and the reconstruction of scenes in both physical and dynamic aspects to link them to a common origin, identify them, or use them in the reconstruction of events. This becomes especially important when the scene is complex or serious (involving deaths or injuries), and every avenue of information seeking must be explored. Evidence may include physical items such as debris or incendiary devices, witness interviews, casualty injuries or postmortems, and fire scene photographs and sketches.

There is a set of generally accepted forensic guidelines for collecting and preserving physical evidence recovered from fires during a fire scene investigation (DeHaan and Icove 2012).

As a simple example, an investigator arrives at a crime scene to find a broken window, an unlatched door, and blood smears—all visible evidence and easily documented. The reconstruction of this evidence would determine whether the door was originally locked and its window broken by mechanical force (determined by glass fracture patterns to have come from the outside), and the intruder cut himself/herself on the glass and, while fumbling for the lock and latch, left blood smears behind on the door.

Laboratory analysis of the blood or any fingerprints left on the door, glass, or latch could identify the intruder. Glass found on the clothing could be compared with window glass from the door to confirm a two-way transfer (suspect blood to scene, scene glass to suspect), and the distribution of cuts or abrasions (and glass/paint fragments) would confirm the method of entry.

6.3.1 GRIDDING

Methodical techniques for assisting in forensic evidence collection and documentation have been widely used by archaeologists when processing field sites. Fire investigators can adopt similar searching and photographic techniques (Bailey 2012). There are several accepted methods for *gridding* and documenting scenes (DeHaan and Icove 2012, chap. 7). Measurements of the location of recovered physical evidence must be reliable and accurate to allow the reconstruction of distances and relationships. Several convenient methods for recording measurements are shown in Figure 6-18.

Coordinate systems aligned perpendicular to major structural walls can aid in the placement of grid lines, especially when the zero point is a corner, usually on the bottom or top left-hand side. *Triangulation* measures distances to an item of interest within a room from two fixed points. *Angular displacement* uses one fixed point and a compass direction and is most appropriate for large outdoor scenes (Wilkinson 2001). A handheld GPS device can be used to establish the location of the fixed reference point as well as compass directions, or for mapping large scenes.

A *grid system* is well suited for large-scale scenes such as explosions, where shrapnel and other evidence are hurled away from a central location. A grid system can also be used in small scenes, for example, quadrants within a vehicle. A baseline and distance system can also be used for large outdoor scenes, particularly explosions, where there are no natural rectilinear baselines.

Although most scenes can be layered and examined room-by-room, some scenes require more carefully controlled examination. This is particularly true at fire death scenes, where the location of small items is very important, particularly in the vicinity of the body. Using techniques developed in archaeology, the investigator divides the scene into grid squares using the walls as reference base lines. Rope, string, or even chalk can be used to mark out grids. Squares within the grid typically are marked using letters along

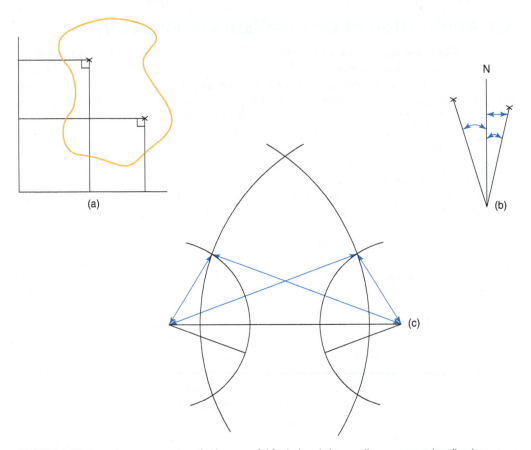

FIGURE 6-18 Several measurement methods are useful for indoor (where walls can serve as baselines) or outdoor scenes. (a) Right-angle transect: baselines at right angles (established with GPS and compass outdoors). (b) Azimuth/baseline: single baseline (in north–south or east–west orientation). Locations are noted by angle and distance from a reference point. (c) Intersecting arcs from two fixed reference points.

one axis and numerals along the other. Using alphanumeric coordinate identifiers simplifies and reduces the possibility of inadvertently switching the coordinates. These grids may be 0.5 to 0.8 m (2 to 3 ft) square in critical areas and as large as 3 × 3 m (10 × 10 ft) in surrounding areas with lighter debris concentrations.

Debris is removed from each grid square, layer-by-layer, for manual/visual inspection and sieving. Material (including evidence) recovered from each grid is kept in a bag, can, or envelope identified by corresponding number/letter. This ensures that at a later stage the evidence can be placed back to within 0.30 m (1 ft) of its original location. Although time consuming, labor intensive, and costly, this method is the best way of finding and documenting evidence that permits physical reconstruction after the scene has been completely searched.

Iso-damage curves have been used by archaeologists in documenting the impact of fires on historic monuments and have application to the documentation of the thermal impact of modern-day fires. For example, one study evaluated damage sustained by the Parthenon from a fire set by Celts in CE 267 (Tassios 2002). Based on observed burn pattern damage, the study determined that there had been more intense thermal damage within the interior section of the structure than on the exterior. The investigation by Tassios used nondestructive pulse velocity measurements to correlate three quantitative criteria corresponding to the thermal damage.

6.3.2 DOCUMENTATION OF WALLS AND CEILINGS

Although most investigators are diligent about identifying floor coverings and assessing their potential contributions to fire spread, the same diligence is not always utilized in documenting wall and ceiling materials and coverings. The nature and thickness of walls, ceilings, and their coverings are important for accurate reconstruction of the event.

In some cases, noncombustible walls of concrete, masonry, or stucco will not contribute to the fire spread, but their low thermal conductivity and large thermal mass may affect some stages of the fire's development. Plaster, whether with metal or wood lath, will dehydrate and fail, allowing fire to penetrate into ceilings or wall cavities. Modern gypsum board will resist fire spread for some time if properly installed (typically 15 to 20 min of direct fire exposure) before it collapses. X- or fire-rated gypsum wallboard is 16 mm (⅝ in.) or thicker and contains fiberglass fibers to strengthen the gypsum. As a result, it will withstand 30 minutes or longer of direct fire contact (White and Dietenberger 2010).

Walls and ceilings can be made of solid wood, plywood paneling, fiberboard (high density like Masonite or low density like Celotex), particleboard, OSB (oriented-strand board), or even metal. Each affects fire spread differently. Noncombustible walls can be covered with combustible materials. Thin plywood paneling or low-density cellulose can speed up fire spread. Karlsson and Quintiere (2000) estimated that lining a room or covering a ceiling with low-density fiberboard would cut the development-to-flashover time in half compared with that for the same room with noncombustible walls or ceilings. If adequately ventilated, these materials will almost guarantee a flashover fire and can be destroyed so completely as to make their detection difficult.

Fire resistance ratings (1 hr, 2 hr, etc.) are based on laboratory test exposure to a furnace fire whose growth is programmed on a standard time–temperature curve to make the test reproducible, as described in *ASTM E119* (ASTM 2016; see Figure 6-19). These tests do not necessarily replicate real-world compartment fires and are not intended to predict failure times in such fires. Such fire testing results can often be used as confidence levels for expected performance.

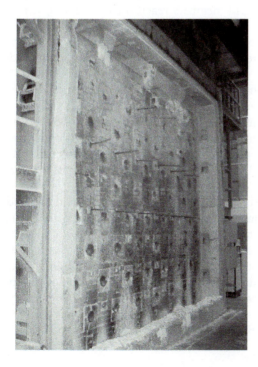

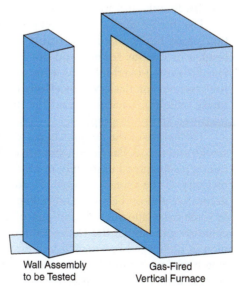

Wall Assembly to be Tested

Gas-Fired Vertical Furnace

FIGURE 6-19 The *ASTM E119* test for wall or floor assemblies uses a large vertical or horizontal gas-fired furnace. The test assembly is built against the open face of the furnace, which is operated according to a set time–temperature curve. *Courtesy of NIST.*

The investigator must be familiar with these materials and how they are installed. Irregular squiggles or zigzag lines of charred adhesive on cement or plasterboard walls indicate that the paneling was glued at one time. Remnants of the paneling will usually survive at the toe plate or behind baseboards, plumbing, or electrical fixtures. The small nails used to secure paneling or cellulose tiles are very different from those used to secure gypsum board.

Wood or metal furring strips may be used to install tiles on walls or ceilings. Their presence should be taken as a cue to search out and identify the sometimes fragmentary remains of combustible walls or ceilings. Wall or ceiling tiles are sometimes installed only with dabs of cement on the backside, so patterns of large dark dots on remaining surfaces should be carefully examined. Samples of unburned wall covering should be measured, identified, and retained for later confirmation.

In a case of one of the authors' experience, post-fire scene photos showed only bare studs, with gypsum board on only one (exterior) face of a common wall. Careful searching revealed that the wall facing the room of origin was covered only in thin plywood veneer paneling that had burned nearly completely and contributed to an extremely intense and fast-growing fire (*Commonwealth of Pennsylvania v. Paul S. Camiolo* 1999).

Although not common in modern structures, the presence of combustible ceilings should not be dismissed. Low-density cellulose ceiling tiles were widely used for many years prior to about 1960. They can be 0.3 m × 0.3 m (12 in. × 12 in.) tiles or 0.61 m × 1.22 m (2 ft × 4 ft) panels. Decorative-edged tongue-and-groove pine or fir boards (sometimes called *beadboard*) were widely used in the late nineteenth to early twentieth centuries for walls and ceilings. Polystyrene ceiling tiles have been widely installed during remodeling of older structures. Such linings will add dramatically to the fuel load and increase the rate of fire development in the room (cutting time to flashover by as much as half, per Karlsson and Quintiere 2000).

The nature and thickness of ceiling materials must be noted. Retaining samples for later testing is strongly recommended. Suspended ceilings are very common in commercial structures, as they can lower ceilings and conceal electrical, plumbing, and HVAC services. These ceilings, although usually noncombustible, allow fire gases to penetrate the large plenum area they offer and spread throughout the concealed space. They typically fail as the steel wires or lightweight steel grid members reach their **annealing** temperatures and lose their tensile strength. This can occur in as little as 10 minutes once the flames reach the ceiling. For additional examples and discussion, see the NIST experiments as a result of their study into the fire at the Cook County Administration Building (Madrzykowski and Walton 2004).

The interior dimensions of all rooms involved in the fire (by flame or smoke penetration) must be recorded (preferably to the nearest ±50 mm (±2 in.). This includes the heights of various rooms (and not assuming all rooms in a structure to be the same). Height is often overlooked as a measurement, but is critical when evaluating the size of fire required for flashover or effects of a given initial fire size, estimating smoke-filling rates, visibility, tenability, and the like. Unusual features such as skylights should be measured and photographed.

The nature of the design, shape, and slant of the ceiling itself will affect the spread of smoke and fire. A flat (level), smooth ceiling will allow the smoke and hot gases from the ceiling jet to spread uniformly in all directions; a pitched (slanted) ceiling will direct the majority of the spread upward. Headers above doors, exposed structural beams—even decorative add-on beams—and ceiling-mounted ductwork will limit spread dramatically, in some cases allowing the buildup of a sufficient hot gas layer on the side of the room containing the initial fire to the point of transition to flashover. Open ceiling joists (common in unfinished basements) will direct most of the accumulating hot gases along their length while dramatically reducing (if not preventing) transverse spread into adjacent joist spaces. Such features must be measured and documented.

annealing ■ Loss of temper in metal caused by heating.

Efforts should be made to find pre-fire photos or videos that show the character of the ceiling and walls, as the action of fire and subsequent extinguishment and overhaul activity may have obliterated signs of wall and ceiling coverings. Failing that, interviews should be conducted with owners, occupants, guests, customers, visitors, maintenance personnel, and the like, asking them to describe ceiling and wall finish (as well as type and placement of furniture). Examination and documentation of undamaged areas of the building may reveal the original structural features.

6.3.3 LAYERING

At scenes where there has been significant destruction and collapse of furniture, walls, or ceilings, investigators would be well-advised to process at least the most critical portions in *layers* (NFPA 2017, pts. 18.3.2, 25.5.5, 25.5.7.1). Most evidence of the critical early stages of a fire will be buried beneath the debris from the collapsed ceiling and roof.

In the collection and interpretation of empirical data during this analytical process, NFPA 921 recommends many careful and professional recovery techniques during scene investigations. In addition to NFPA 921, several expert treatises in the fire investigation field recommend "grid-based" searches, particularly for the recovery of victims and evidence (NFPA 2017, pt. 25.5.7).

For example, *Kirk's Fire Investigation* recommends the use of the quadrant method in vehicle fire investigations where sections of a vehicle under examination are successively divided and subdivided. These grid-based searches have expanded as a systematic methodology using matrices for origin determination in compartment fires.

However, the science of grid- and matrix-based examinations of fire scenes is based upon scientifically grounded approaches commonly used in the field of archaeology (Lally 2006; Icove, Welborn, Vonarx, Adams, Lally, and Huff 2006), the study of ancient human activity through the recovery and analysis of artifacts, charred debris (Pichler et al. 2013), human remains (Olson 2009), and architecture left behind (Ide 1997; Harrison 2013; Braadbaart et al. 2012). Physical evidence created during fire events has been known to survive the ravages of time, whether it is hours, days, years, or centuries before being uncovered, as shown in Figure 6-20.

Undamaged areas of the building may be surveyed to establish what types of materials to expect. The roof structure can be photographed and its direction of collapse noted, and then it can be removed. Roof or ceiling insulation can then be removed noting whether it is loose (blown-in) fiberglass, mineral wool, or cellulose; batting; or rolled insulation. Samples should be taken for later identification if ignition or spread through the insulation is considered possible.

The ceiling material can then be identified: gypsum wallboard, lath and plaster (wire or wood lath makes a difference in manner and time of collapse), ceiling tile, plywood, or wood plank. An investigator should never assume that all insulation, ceiling, or lining materials are consistent throughout even a small residence, because repairs, renovations, or additions will usually be made with materials available at the time.

Light fixtures, furnishings, and victims will be found under the ceiling material. Most of the critical evidence will be found between the ceiling and the floor covering, but even here, the sequence of positioning may be of importance. Window glass will tend to break and collapse when the temperatures or heat flux become high enough during the fire's development. This usually occurs after the smoke products have condensed on the glass, and the fracture pattern would be expected to be thermal rather than mechanical (unless the glass is toughened safety glass). Glass falling inward may fall on furnishings or floors that are already fire damaged. If a window is broken before the fire reaches it, the fracture pattern will be mechanical in appearance, and the glass, bearing few or no soot deposits, may fall and protect unburned materials beneath. Radiant heat in a subsequent post-flashover may melt and char even protected material beneath the glass. Breakage of glass in locations where fire exposure does not seem to have been sufficiently intense must be examined for other causes.

The location of first collapse of ceiling or wall covering may be estimated by careful examination of the debris at this stage, and should be photographed before further excavation. As the furnishings are documented and removed, the nature of floors and floor coverings can be determined. The distribution of carpet, tile, bare wood, composite floor coverings, and vinyl or asbestos (tile or sheet) should be noted. Comparison samples of carpet, floor covering, and underlayment should be taken in areas of suspected origin.

Testing has shown that carpet fiber content cannot accurately be estimated from observation alone. Using a match or lighter flame will reveal only whether the face yarn is synthetic or natural fiber with the application of *NFPA 705* (NFPA 2009) and other tests. Fire tests have further demonstrated that a carpet may not support flame spread alone but if installed over a particular type of pad, may burn readily. It is always best to recover and preserve a small [at least 0.15 m × 0.15 m (6 in. × 6 in.)] sample of unburned carpet and pad for later identification. Samples can be recovered in most scenes from under large furniture or appliances or in protected corners of the room. These samples can help forensic testing by being used as a comparison to establish what volatiles they contain or may yield on burning.

Regarding the process of layering, archaeologists use a systematic approach of coordinate systems that account for not only the location but also the depths where objects are found. Their excavations are carried out layer by layer, so the depth of each object is known. This approach can be helpful when layering debris at fire scenes that has fallen onto an area of fire origin. Such cases include multistory buildings, where collapsed floors bury important evidence. In some cases fallen debris often preserves evidence on lower floors.

As previously noted, it is important to place these layers spatially in the documentation process. If forensic evidence collection and documentation are viewed as a scientific endeavor, the use of archaeological techniques will only enhance this effort. In both fire scene investigations and archaeological excavations, it is important to document the physical structures, three-dimensional layers of stratified debris, and the location of critical evidence that is preserved, altered, or destroyed by the excavation process. These surfaces are known as *units of stratification*.

The standard of care in the archaeological community for scene excavations is the use of the *Harris Matrix*, named after British archaeologist Dr. Edward Cecil Harris, who invented it in 1973 (Harris 2014). This matrix documentation technique shows the chronological relationships (temporal sequences) in a stratified sequence of layers excavated at a site in logically presented and abstracted form (Icove et al. 2014). For a download of the English and translated versions of the textbook *Principles of Archaeological Stratigraphy* by Dr. Harris, see: http://www.harrismatrix.com/harrisbook.html

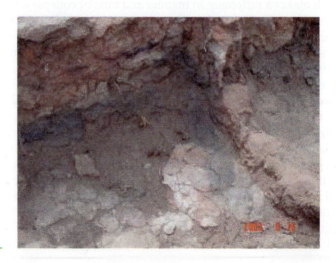

FIGURE 6-20 An example of typical fire debris found on interior wall in archeological excavations at Mesa Portales (LA145165). *Courtesy of Joe Lally*

Standards promoted by *NFPA 921* and ASTM International's *ASTM E860* (ASTM 2013b) point out the importance of identifying the location of evidence, safely collecting it without altering it, and preserving evidence that is of forensic value. This process maintains the integrity of the process through comprehensive documentation and disposition of evidence found during the delayering processes in fire investigations.

The loss of critical evidence is defined by *NFPA 921* (NFPA 2017, pt. 3.3.167) as **spoliation**, which is the "Loss, destruction, or material alteration of an object or document that is evidence or potential evidence in a legal proceeding by one who has the responsibility for its preservation." Clearly, the use of the Harris Matrix in documenting evidence can do much to ensure that spoliation is minimized, preserving the integrity of the investigation.

A properly documented delayering process at fire scenes is essential in understanding the progress of a fire, especially during death investigations where the position of the body and other relevant evidence is often buried under layers of fire debris. The authors recommend the adoption of the Harris Matrix approach by forensic fire investigators, because it is already a worldwide standardized archaeological approach employed in documenting the delayering and temporal succession of evidence found at both present-day and ancient fire scenes, and on archaeological sites in general. Its use in documenting evidence can do much to ensure that spoliation is minimized, preserving the integrity of the investigation.

The Harris Matrix has gained wide acceptance in the archaeological community. For example, in Belgium the Harris Matrix has been added to a set of universal requirements to be fulfilled during the processing of every archaeological site excavation and will soon be required by law (Harris 2014).

Figure 6-21 is a hypothetical application of the Harris Matrix in a fire scene examination. In the formal process, layers and surfaces define the major elements of the schematic drawing and resulting matrix. In terms of fire scenes, the layers are dimensionally thick, while the surfaces represent thinner physical items such as flooring materials.

In this hypothetical case, careful excavation reveals that evidence is discovered over and under the deceased victim trapped in fire debris within Layer 8 of the interior of a building. The victim is within the interior wall (Layers 2 and 3) under debris (Layer 4), including the roof (Layer 5). The earthen floor (Layer 9) is beneath the victim. The exterior debris consists of exterior (Layer 1), construction materials (Layers 6 and 7), and the earthen layer (Layer 9). The stone wall (Layer 2) and backfill (Layer 3) both rest on the footer (Layer 10) beneath the wall.

The Harris Matrix can also address surfaces discovered during excavation. In this case, a surface number for the interface between Layers 2, 3, and 10 defines the relationship

spoliation ■ Loss, destruction, or material alteration of an object or document that is evidence or potential evidence in a legal proceeding by one who has the responsibility for its preservation (*NFPA 921*, 2017 ed., pt. 3.3.178).

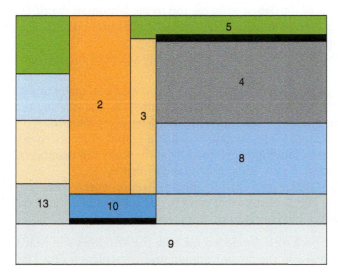

FIGURE 6-21 A hypothetical application of the Harris Matrix in a fire scene examination.

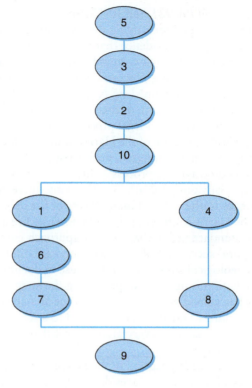

FIGURE 6-22 A schematic representation of the hypothetical fire scene from Figure 6-21.

to Layers 1 and 4. A surface appears under Layer 10 and over Layers 1 and 4. For the sake of preventing confusion, Figure 6-22 illustrates the layers, but they are not reflected in the Matrix diagram.

This is only a simplified generic case and does not relate to an actual incident. The integrity of an investigation may be called into question without this form of documentation. However, there are several advantages for using the Harris Matrix approach in the forensic processing of fire scenes. The following advantages underscore the importance of adherence to methodologies borrowed from the allied field of archaeology:

- Preserves the Chronology of the Excavation – The methodology records the order in which these events occurred and the reverse order in which they should have been excavated.
- Three-Dimensional Documentation – Previous fire scene excavation techniques used simple gridded zones of the debris from the top to the bottom of the surface. This layered approach preserves the three-dimensional representation of evidence with regard to stratigraphic relationships.
- Time-Proven Methodology – The method is already accepted and proven to be reliable within the scientific community.
- Maintains the Integrity of the Process – The method assists in maintaining the integrity of the forensic fire scene investigation by documenting the layering process. Photographic documentation of the process can also deter any concerns.
- Produces a Visual Record – The method provides a graphical record to document and compare. The use of multiple investigators at the scene can maintain the same context of structural materials, soils, debris, and evidence.
- Universal Training – Wherever a fire investigator lives or works, there are competent archaeology schools and programs that can provide systematic training on the use and implementation of the Harris Matrix approach.

There are computer packages, developed for both the Windows and Mac OSX operating systems that can assist in the documentation and construction of a Harris Matrix

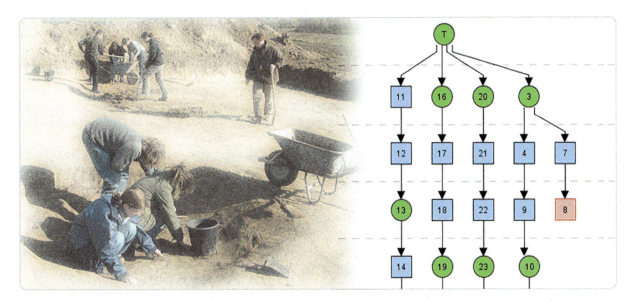

FIGURE 6-23 Harris Matrix Composer (HMC, Version 2.0b), the program builds and administers a representation of an archaeological stratification in the form of a Harris Matrix. *Source: Vienna Institute for Archaeological Science, University of Vienna*

(Figure 6-23). Called the Harris Matrix Composer (HMC, Version 2.0b), the program builds and administers a representation of an archaeological stratification in the form of a Harris Matrix (Harris 2016).

Researchers are continuously exploring the complex relationships for Harris Matrices. The science of graph theories continues to explore the application of this approach.

6.3.4 SIEVING

In the ashes, all evidence seems to be the same shades of white, gray, or black, and it is not readily distinguishable from fire debris. A manual and visual search may overlook evidence critical to a complete reconstruction. Wet sieving of the debris affords a better chance of detecting small items such as glass fragments, projectiles, keys, or jewelry that may go unnoticed in dry ash. Bone fragments that are highly calcined by fire exposure can disintegrate if exposed to water, so areas around hands and feet of burned bodies should be manually searched and dry sieved.

Sieving (NFPA 2017, pt. 25.5.7.2) is most effective when done with at least three sieve frames stacked together using 25-, 12.7-, and 6.35-mm (1-, 0.5-, and 0.25-in.) mesh. Some examiners will use a fourth sieve with window screen if searching for tiny tooth or bone fragments. Debris is placed in the correct grid and agitated, or a garden hose or hose reel line is used to wash debris through the sieves. The debris should never be pushed through by hand, because that can shatter bones and teeth.

Wet sieving for general evidence is preferred, because the water washes off the gray ash and makes small objects visible by color or reflectance. If the objects recovered can be visually identified, they can be placed directly into evidence bags. Items that cannot be readily identified should be kept in a separate container, labeled as to grid of recovery, until they can be properly analyzed.

6.3.5 PRESERVATION

Fire exposure causes materials to become fragile and brittle, so preservation (NFPA 2014, pts. 4.2.1, 4.2.2, 4.2.3, and 4.4.1; NFPA 2017, pt. 17.3; ASTM 2011b) is key to their survival. This is especially true of copper wiring and electrical insulation and components.

Recovery starts with thorough photographic documentation before an attempt is made to move the object.

Wiring can be preserved on 1 × 4 lumber 4 to 8 ft long, affixed with cable ties or wraps with the ends numbered and distances from a reference point labeled on the wood. Fragile wiring or components can be protected with cling wrap. Smaller lengths of wiring or wiring from an appliance can be tie-wrapped to a piece of corrugated cardboard. Colored or numbered tape can be used around ends of wires to denote the circuit to which they were connected.

When a scene is gridded off for searching, numbered tarps (plastic) can be used for materials recovered from each grid. If the scene is not gridded off, a separate tarp can be used for each room or each sector of a scene. Large plastic tarps can be marked off with waterproof tape to produce a full-scale reproduction of the room. This technique has been used to reconstruct positions of furniture and other evidence, and even for court display (Rich 2007).

6.3.6 IMPRESSION EVIDENCE

Impression evidence is a general term for the transfer of pattern or contour information from one surface to another. Fingerprints and shoe prints are commonly found forms of impression evidence (NFPA 2017, pts. 17.5.3 and 27.7.4).

Photography is the primary means of documenting most impressions, but care must be taken not to distort the image in the photograph. Whenever possible, the object bearing the impression should be recovered and submitted to the lab. The object is always preferable to a photo or cast, but if the object is not removable, photos with scales, or casting or lifting by adhesive or electrostatic lifter, will be necessary.

Items bearing tool marks should also be collected and individually wrapped in paper packages to protect their surfaces. Similar collection guidelines apply to the suspected tools. Wrap each tool separately to prevent shifting or damage during submission to the laboratory. Place each tool in a separate envelope or box with a folded sheet of paper over the end of the tool to minimize damage and loss of trace evidence adhering to the surfaces and to prevent rusting.

Transfer may take the form of a harder material making an impression on a softer material on contact. For example, a shoe may make an impression in soft clay outside a window. Transfer can also occur when a transfer medium preserves the two-dimensional shape of contoured surfaces that come into contact with it. A dusty shoe can leave an identifiable print on a clean surface, and a clean shoe can remove dust from a dirty surface and leave the same information.

Designed by the American Board of Forensic Odontology (ABFO), the ABFO L-shaped No. 2 scale, measuring 10 cm × 10 cm, has become the standard scale for recording through photography fingerprints, wounds, blood spatters, and similar small evidence. The three circles are useful in compensating for distortion resulting from photographs taken from oblique camera angles.

A larger scale, shown in Figure 6-24, is ideal for shoe prints, because it helps prevent distortion (LeMay 2002). Originally made to FBI specifications, the "Bureau Scale," as it is referred to, contains a 15 cm × 30 cm L-shaped scale. Alternating black and white bands provide a visual reference, and circled crosshairs assist in checking and correcting perspective distortion in photographs.

Fingerprints

A finger touching a clean surface like glass or metal can leave a reproduction of its friction ridge contours on the surface by the transfer of the nearly invisible oils, fats, and sweat secretions normally found on the skin. Such patterns are often called *latent* because they are not readily visible to the unaided eye and require some sort of physical, chemical, or optical treatment to make them visible and recordable (and comparable to "inked" record prints).

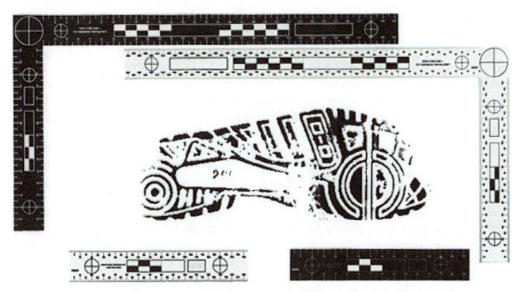

FIGURE 6-24 An example of a forensic photographic scale alongside impression evidence for a shoe by the transfer of pattern or contour information from one surface to another. © *Safariland, Courtesy of Forensics Source™ by Permission.*

The skin can also be contaminated with blood, food, grease, or paint that leaves behind a visible or *patent* impression. Even though the skin is pliable and deforms on contact with most other materials, it can deform soft materials such as cheese, chocolate, solvent- or heat-softened plastic or paint, and window putty and leave a three-dimensional or molded "plastic" impression of its ridge detail. The same considerations apply to other deformable materials like rubber shoe soles, gloves, tires, or cloth; each may deform softer materials or leave a pattern on harder ones through transfer of some intermediate medium or even residues of itself.

Impressions of friction ridge features from fingers, palms, and feet can and do survive fires. The multitude of chemical, physical, and optical techniques available today to enhance fingerprints (both latent and patent) has made it possible to recover prints from difficult, textured, or contaminated surfaces. Heat alone can cause the constituents in skin oils to darken or even react with the surface beneath, producing a patent impression from a latent one (DeHaan and Icove 2012; Lennard 2007; Deans 2006.

If fire exposure has not been so severe as to melt or severely char the base material, there is a good chance of fingerprint transfer. Handling must be very careful and kept to an absolute minimum. The material must be transported very carefully to the lab (preferably by hand) using containers or devices that minimize contact with potential print-bearing surfaces.

Water contamination from condensation, hose stream, or environmental exposure once meant that prints on paper or cardboard would be impossible to develop (because the amino acids detected by ninhydrin processing are water soluble). The advent of physical developer (which reacts with the fatty constituents that are not water soluble) made it possible to process wet paper or cardboard. Small-particle reagent (SPR) allows processing on nonporous surfaces like metal, glass, and fiberglass even while still wet. Forensic light sources (multiple wavelength, high intensity) and a variety of chemicals and powders make it possible to recover prints from textured or contaminated surfaces. Fingerprint experts such as Jack Deans have documented that modern optical, chemical, and physical methods are capable of developing latents on all manner of surfaces after fire exposure (Deans 2006; Bleay, Bradshaw, and Moore 2006; DeHaan and Icove 2012, chap. 14).

Soot can often be washed off smooth metal or glass surfaces with running water, leaving behind prints developed by the soot carbon to be photographed or lifted. A recent Malaysian study assessed the effectiveness of soot removal techniques on glass fire debris without affecting the fingerprints found on the evidence (Ahmad et al. 2011).

Fingerprints in blood can be enhanced with amido black or leucocrystal violet (LCV) sprays, which react chemically with blood to form a dark blue–purple-colored product. The solvent for the LCV has been seen to help rinse overlying soot away from the surface. In one case where two fires had been set in a house, the LCV solution washed soot away, revealing blood spatters on walls where a resident had been bludgeoned to death some two years previously (the fires having been subsequently set to simulate drug gang activity).

Charred or burned paper documents are important to a fire scene examination, particularly when business records and important documents are involved. Fragile fire-damaged documents should be placed on soft cotton sheets in rigid containers and hand-carried to the laboratory for examination. Papers should not be treated with any lacquer or coating if they are to be processed for identification or comparison.

Although the foot traffic of emergency personnel, tires of vehicles, water, or structural changes often compromise shoe prints, shoe prints can survive fires if left on surfaces that have not been destroyed by fire or heat. Shoe prints left behind on doors that are forcibly kicked in may actually be enhanced by the action of the fire. In the example case shown in Figure 6-25, the dusty shoe print was lightened by heat exposure, and the wood around it scorched, increasing its contrast and readability.

Shoe prints, like fingerprints, link a person or persons with a scene. Shoe prints can offer information about where someone entered or left a room or building, where he/she went, and in what sequence. Paper or cardboard can bear latent shoe impressions (detected and preserved using a physical developer chemical treatment even after water exposure) or patent impressions in soil, dust, or blood.

6.3.7 TRACE EVIDENCE FOUND ON CLOTHING AND SHOES

Trace evidence (NFPA 2017, pts. 17.5.3 and 25.5.7.3) such as soil, glass, paint chips, metal fragments, chemicals, and hairs and fibers may cling to the shoes or clothing of a suspect. Liquids may also soak into the clothing or remain on the bottom of the individual's shoes. Glass, plasterboard, sawdust, and metal shavings have all been found embedded in shoes to offer a link with a scene (as long as comparison samples are recovered). Footwear and clothing can also absorb residues of flammable liquid or chemical accelerants used in arson attacks.

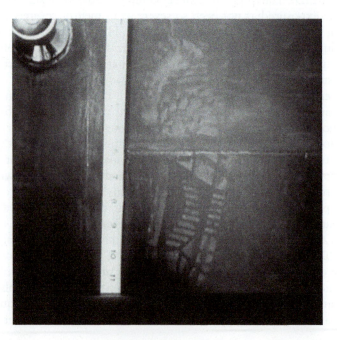

FIGURE 6-25 Shoe prints left behind on doors that are forcibly kicked in may be enhanced by the action of the fire. In this case the dusty shoe print was lightened by heat exposure, and the wood around it scorched, increasing its contrast and readability. *Photo by Joe Konefal, Shingle Springs, California.*

A New Zealand study illustrated the necessity of quickly analyzing clothing and shoes of suspected arsonists for the presence of ignitable liquids. The study found that detectable amounts of petrol were transferred to the clothing and shoes of a person during the action of pouring it around the room. This study also addressed the pouring heights and floor surfaces. Results of the study showed that petrol was always transferred to the shoes and often transferred to both the upper and the lower clothing, but a sample must be seized and properly packaged quickly (Coulson and Morgan-Smith 2000; Coulson et al. 2008). Tests using a carbon strip extraction method found that 10 mL (0.34 oz or 2 tsp) of gasoline on clothing worn continuously, evaporated much more quickly than on the same clothing left on the lab bench at 20°C to 25°C (68°F to 77°F) and was barely detectable after only four hours of wear (Coulson et al. 2008). Clothing must be recovered and packaged soon after exposure.

Solvents used in glues holding footwear together (particularly athletic shoes) can interfere with identification of ignitable liquid residues, as they can produce false positives (some manufacturers have been known to use gasoline as a substitute glue solvent). Preservation of shoes separately from other evidence and from each other in vapor-tight containers is essential to prevent cross-contamination (Lentini, Dolan, and Cherry 2000). Owing to the unpredictable presence of gasoline and other ignitable liquids in footwear, many forensic laboratories are reluctant to analyze them.

An Australian transfer study examined the possibility of a natural occurrence of petrol residues tracked inside a vehicle on the shoes of drivers or passengers. The results showed that small quantities of petrol (500 μL) could be detected after 24 hours, but evaporation prevented it from being discovered after one week on the shoes. The researchers concluded that it would be significant if fresh or slightly evaporated petrol is found on the car carpet (Cavanagh-Steer et al. 2005).

A separate study by the same Australian researchers found that car carpets, since they may be manufactured from petroleum feed stocks, might decompose when heated and produce volatile organic compounds that produce background interference when testing for the presence of petrol. The researchers found, however, that these components produced chromatographic patterns that were distinguished from those produced by petrol. Both studies underscore the necessity to obtain reference samples to eliminate or account for background interference (Cavanagh, Pasquier, and Lennard 2002).

In field experiments, Armstrong et al. (2004) poured a specified amount of gasoline at designated locations. The subject then stepped into the pour location and walked the length of the testing area. Gasoline on contaminated footwear was found no farther than two steps away from the site of the pour on carpet.

The general forensic guidelines for handling items of clothing stipulate that they should be marked directly on the waistband, pocket, and collar with the investigator's initials and date found. If being preserved for blood or trace evidence, these items must be packed separately into clean paper bags, with each item wrapped separately in clean paper. If they are damp (water or blood), they must be allowed to air-dry before being packaged. Clothing should only be handled by someone wearing clear nitrite or latex gloves to prevent DNA transfer cross contamination.

If flammable liquid residues are suspected to be present, the clothing must be sealed separately in vapor-tight cans or sealed nylon or AMPAC FireDebris™ bags. AMPAC Fire Debris polymer for fire debris packaging, useful in a wide variety of applications for evidence collection, was reintroduced into the US market in July 2010 and is being evaluated. Preliminary tests showed that heat-sealed AMPAC FireDebris™ bags will preserve even light hydrocarbons and will not introduce foreign trace volatiles (AAFS 2011). When properly heat-sealed, these airtight and puncture-resistant polyester pouches are ideal for packaging and storing chemicals, controlled substances, and related paraphernalia while preventing cross contamination and protecting individuals from exposure to dangerous substances. (See www.ampaconline.com.)

When dealing with glass, the investigator should collect as many fragments as possible and place them in paper bags, boxes, or envelopes for later physical reconstruction or reassembly. The fragments should be packaged so that their movement within the containers is kept to a minimum. Paint chips, particularly those at least 1.5 cm^2 (0.5 in.^{2}) large should be placed in pillboxes, paper envelopes, cellophane, or plastic bags and carefully sealed. Smaller glass or paint chips should be placed in a folded paper bindle and then sealed in a paper envelope. All trace evidence must be kept separate from any control or comparison samples to avoid cross contamination.

Trace evidence includes hairs and fibers. Loose hair combings and clumps of fibers cut from various areas should be packaged separately in pillboxes, paper envelopes, cellophane, or plastic bags. The outside of the container should be sealed and labeled. Hairs from pets in structures may also be transferred to persons, so comparison samples may be suggested. Comparison samples from victims or suspects may reveal a direct or indirect relationship.

6.3.8 DEBRIS CONTAINING SUSPECTED VOLATILES

Items containing suspected ignitable liquids should be sealed in clean metal cans, glass jars, or specialized polymeric (AMPAC FireDebris or nylon) bags that have been developed for fire debris preservation. Common polyethylene plastic or paper bags should not be used because they are porous and allow evaporation or cross contamination and may contain volatile chemicals that may contaminate the evidence, resulting in false-positive or false-negative results when subjected to laboratory analysis. The container should be filled no more than three-fourths full, using clean tools to prevent contamination. Clean disposable plastic, isoprene, or latex gloves should be worn when collecting the debris and then discarded after each sample is taken.

Investigators should seek to collect and preserve comparison samples of uncontaminated flammable and combustible liquids from the scene. Samples of suspected liquids measuring up to 1 pt should be sealed in Teflon-sealed glass vials, glass bottles, or jars with Bakelite or metal tops (preferably with Teflon seals), or metal cans. Comparison samples should be carefully labeled as to their source if they are not submitted in their original containers. They must be stored and shipped separately from scene samples to avoid any chance of contamination.

Per *ASTM E1459* (ASTM 2013d), the collecting officer should label each container with a brief description of the contents and the location from which the sample was collected. Collectors are cautioned not to use rubber stoppers or jars with rubber seals because gasoline, paint thinners, and other volatile liquids compromise the sample by dissolving the seals. Any odor present or reading obtained on a hydrocarbon detector should be noted prior to sealing the container. Plastic bottles are inappropriate containers for debris, liquid, or comparison samples. Techniques available for collecting liquids from concrete floors include using absorbents such as flour, sweeping compounds, and calcium carbonate or "kitty litter" (Tontarski 1985; Mann and Putaansuu 2006; Nowlan et al. 2007). Investigators should remember to submit a sample of the type of absorbent material used along with their scene samples for laboratory analysis (Stauffer, Dolan, and Newman 2008, 170).

Samples containing garden soil should be frozen as soon as possible to minimize possible degradation of hydrocarbons by microbial action and kept frozen until submission to the laboratory. All other samples should be kept as cool as possible and submitted to a testing laboratory as soon as possible. Further details are included in *Kirk's Fire Investigation,* 7th ed. (DeHaan and Icove 2012).

6.3.9 UV DETECTION OF PETROLEUM ACCELERANTS

Since the 1950s, *ultraviolet (UV) fluorescence* has been touted as a way of discovering deposits of some hydrocarbon liquids at fire scenes. Unfortunately, simple fluorescence observation (observing the visible light emitted when some materials are exposed to UV) is not reliable for that purpose. Many materials naturally fluoresce, and pyrolysis produces a large number of complex aromatic hydrocarbons as breakdown products that fluoresce and obscure and interfere with any fluorescence from "foreign" accelerants. Some flammable liquids produce no fluorescence at all.

A reported innovation promises some success in using UV light, but it involves two electronic manipulations. If the UV source is pulsed rapidly and the electronic detector is gated so it observes only the target after a preset delay, the decay time of most pyrolysis products can be discriminated from those of petroleum products. Another method is to use an image-intensified charge-coupled device (CCD) detector to look at emissions (fluorescence) at wavelengths and intensities not visible to the unaided eye. A time-resolved fluorescence system pulsed laser offers a promising future for the UV detection of stains of ignitable liquid (Saitoh and Takeuchi 2006).

6.3.10 DIGITAL MICROSCOPES

Many investigators carry an eye loupe or linen tester magnifier to scenes to enable them to examine small objects, but capturing those images requires an interface to capture the image data (which may be critical if the object is likely to change with time owing to evaporation, handling, or storage). A handheld digital microscope (MiScope) is available that combines built-in LED lighting, precision optics, and a digital movie camera (Zarbeco 2012). The microscope offers 40X to 140X magnification (field of view 6 × 8 mm to 1.5 × 2 mm), and the image is fed directly to a laptop computer via a USB port for examination, capture, and labeling as still, movie, or time-lapse images. It is available for less than $300. A high-resolution version (MiScope MP offering 12X to 140X magnification with 2.3-μm resolution) is available for under $700 (see Figure 6-26).

6.3.11 PORTABLE X-RAY SYSTEMS

Laboratory x-ray systems such as Faxitron (2012) have been used by crime labs and engineering labs for many years to evaluate evidence of all types after recovery. These are similar to medical x-ray systems using variable voltages and exposure times to suit a wide variety of target materials.

Portable x-ray systems have been used for some years by bomb disposal squads to evaluate suspected devices in situ, but the recent developments in spoliation issues have made on-scene x-ray examination more effective for the fire investigator. One such system is a battery-powered x-ray system weighing less than 2.5 kg (5 lb). The XR150 system by Golden Engineering (Golden 2012) uses electrically generated pulses of X-rays of very short duration (50 ns) but very high power (150 kV) (see Figures 6-27 and 6-28). The images are accumulated based on the type and thickness of the material (1 to 2 pulses for

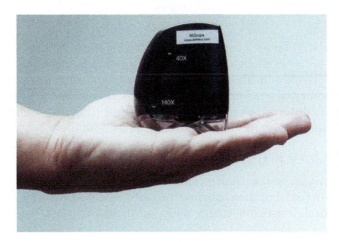

FIGURE 6-26 A handheld digital microscope (magnification 40X–140X) has built-in LED lighting. Its images are displayed on a laptop computer and captured as movie or still images. *Courtesy of Zarbeco LLC.*

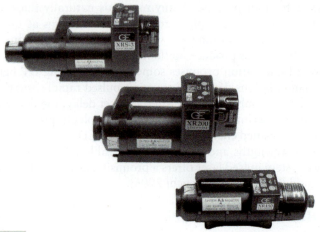

FIGURE 6-27 A portable x-ray unit can take images of electrical equipment and appliances at a scene using a 150 kV x-ray source. *Courtesy of Golden Engineering Inc.*

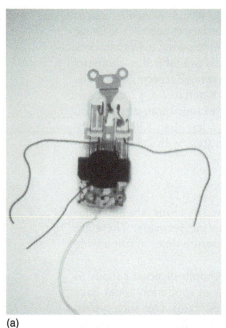

(a)

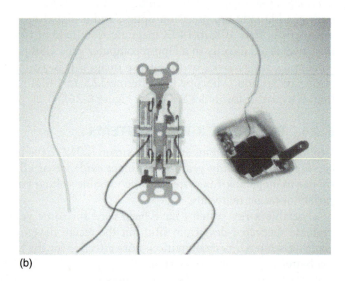

(b)

FIGURE 6-28 (a) Its image can be captured on film, fluoroscope screen, or digital devices. *Courtesy of Golden Engineering Inc.* (b) A typical x-ray of a household receptacle is shown on the left, plug-in power supply on right. *Courtesy of Golden Engineering Inc.*

paper envelopes, 100 for steel up to 1 cm (0.4 in.) thick. Images can be produced on a "green screen" fluoroscope, a "live" digital image system, or on a conventional 20 cm × 25 cm (8 in. × 10 in.) Polaroid film sheet. These devices allow a trained and qualified investigator to assess the internal condition of electrical devices, appliances, or mechanical systems before they are disturbed or removed from the scene (thus minimizing risk of damage or loss). Such systems are currently available for under $5000.

6.3.12 PORTABLE X-RAY FLUORESCENCE

Another valuable technique, x-ray fluorescence elemental analysis (NFPA 2017, pt. 17.10.2.5), long used in the laboratory, can now be performed on a portable handheld unit the size of a power drill. It uses low-energy x-ray (10 to 40 kV) beams focused on a nearby surface to identify all but the lightest elements in one scan of a few seconds. It can be used to help detect and identify chemical incendiaries, low explosives, bromine-based flame retardants, chemical treatments, coatings, and fragments of solids of all types (Innovxsys 2012).

ThermoFisher Scientific (2012) also produces a handheld x-ray fluorescence instrument for elemental analysis. The object or surface to be tested is brought into contact with the window of its Niton XL device. A 2 W x-ray tube is triggered, and a spectrum of the elements present is displayed on the built-in screen or (via USB connection or integrated Bluetooth communications) transferred directly to a PC or other storage device. The standard system permits identification of elements from chlorine to uranium. A helium purge of the detector extends its sensitivity down to magnesium, making it very useful for characterizing possible residues of incendiary or inorganic explosive materials. The Niton system also permits the choice of full-area analysis or a 3-mm "small-spot" analysis. An optional internal digital camera permits documentation of the sample being analyzed.

6.3.13 INFRARED VIDEO THERMAL IMAGING

Pioneered by Inframetrics, which was acquired by FLIR Systems (FLIR 2012), false-color infrared video recording has been used in industrial and military applications for more than a decade to remotely and quickly survey high-tension line insulators for heating from leakage currents, transformers for overheating, and chemical delivery pipes and storage tanks for leaks, and to measure operating temperatures of surfaces of aircraft or vehicles.

As applied to fire research, infrared video thermal imaging allows remote and accurate measurement of the surface temperatures of fuel surfaces or masses of hot gases or of the external surfaces of walls, windows, or other structural elements as they are exposed to fires.

A very early version was used by Helmut Brosz in 1991 in monitoring fire development in compartments. Although DeHaan (1995, 1999) used Inframetrics equipment to measure the surface temperatures of carpet during the evaporation of volatile fuels, very few papers on the topic have been published in the fire research literature. Infrared video imaging can distinguish areas of a surface whose temperatures differ by only 0.25°C (0.5°F) in static images. Its applicability to capturing transient events such as the chaotic movement of the high-temperature flames in post-flashover fires has been demonstrated (DeHaan 2001).

The high cost of the necessary equipment has been reduced significantly in recent years with the dramatically increased power of low-cost computer components. Hopefully, more researchers will use this type of technology to study surface temperatures that currently are impractical to measure accurately using traditional hard-wire thermocouple devices. Several versions are made today by FLIR Systems (FLIR 2012).

6.3.14 MRI AND CT IMAGING

Progress in magnetic resonance imaging (MRI) and computerized tomography (CT, or multiple-position x-ray imaging) has been rapid. MRI and multiple-slice CT have established the presence or absence of fractured bones and reconstruction of impact injuries as well as documented the presence of surgical implants in the examination of a very badly charred body (Thali et al. 2003).

These techniques have also been suggested for use in examination of melted or charred artifacts from fire scenes where nondestructive testing for pockets of liquid or similar non-radiopaque inclusions would be desirable. Although expensive, these techniques may provide answers where X-rays cannot.

6.3.15 DNA RECOVERY

Recent work by the Forensic Science Centre at the University of Strathclyde has shown that owing to the STR (short tandem repeat) methods now available for deoxyribonucleic acid (DNA) analysis, identifiable DNA from saliva can be found on the necks of gasoline-filled Molotov cocktails (petrol bombs). Using both sterilized bottles with 50 µL (2 drops) of saliva deposited on the exterior and a random selection of bottles that had been drunk from, researchers recovered identifiable DNA even after gasoline had been poured in and a wick inserted. When the devices were thrown to explode and burn, identifiable (4 to 7 loci) DNA was found on about 50 percent of the bottle necks, and full DNA profiles were identifiable on another 25 percent of the burned bottles (Mann, Nic Daéid, and Linacre 2003).

Sometimes a suspect has set a fire to cover up or destroy possible evidence of a homicide, and bloodstain patterns spattered on surfaces are removed for later DNA analysis. Research by ATF Fire Research Laboratory shows that DNA can be recovered from these fire scenes, even in some cases when the blood spatter or stains have been subjected to elevated temperatures (Tontarski et al. 2009).

The ATF Laboratory found that in simulated multi-room fires, bloodstain patterns remained visible and intact inside the structure and on furnishings unless the surface that held the blood was totally burned away. For the most part, the recovered DNA seemed to be unaffected by the heat until the temperature was 800°C (1500°F) or greater. At this temperature, no DNA profiles were obtained.

ATF cautions that in cases when presumptive chemical tests for the presence of blood were conducted prior to DNA testing, there could be a failure to obtain useful typing results. They recommend that recovery of DNA is most successful where the blood is removed by methods using either swabbing or cutting/scraping.

6.4 Photography

Fire investigators should both photograph and sketch carefully even the seemingly least significant fire scene detail. *NPFA 921* notes that photography, whether still or video, is the most efficient reminder of what a fire investigator saw while examining the fire scene. Photography is used to substantiate witness statements, document reports, provide documentary exhibits for courtroom presentations, and ensure the integrity of the debris delayering process (NFPA 2014, pt. 4.3.2). Critical evidence, including complex fire patterns, may also be more visible later than when originally examined (NFPA 2017, pt. 16.2.1).

Other standards of care also mention how photography should be used in documenting fire scenes. *ASTM E1020,* pt. 5.1.2 (ASTM 2013c), states that investigators must take photographs "that accurately and fairly identify and depict the scene, the items, or systems involved in the incident, and the post-incident conditions." *ASTM E1020* also provides additional guidance in that "photographs should be taken from many directions and should include overall site views, overall item and system views, intermediate views, and close-up views."

Photography, especially digital, is a very inexpensive investigative step in documenting fire scenes. Some benchmark estimates vary as to the actual average direct costs of performing a preliminary scene investigation, yet photography may be the least costly (Icove, Wherry, and Schroeder 1998). In present-day digital cameras (to be discussed later in detail), a 10-gigabyte (GB) photographic image can be stored as a 4.5 megabyte (MB) JPEG image. Therefore, a 1 GB digital storage card will hold about 200 images. With digital storage cards for cameras retailing at about $1.00/GB, the cost per image would be $0.005 (half a cent).

Fire investigators are required by *NFPA 1033* (NFPA 2014, pt. 4.3.2) to be knowledgeable in photographic documentation of fire scenes. Fire investigators are usually not required to qualify as expert photographers, but they must be able to understand and utilize their equipment to the maximum benefit (Berrin 1977). Thus, the following items should be included as minimum equipment for forensic fire scene photography.

6.4.1 DOCUMENTATION AND STORAGE

The "Photograph Log" form (Figure 6-7) is used to record the description, frame, and unique storage media number (for example, the serial number of digital memory card, CD-ROM, or DVD) of each photograph or video taken at the fire scene. The form is designed to be filled out as the photographs are taken. The frame and storage media numbers are later used on the fire scene sketch or separate photographic log to indicate the location and direction from which they were taken. The documentation should include a brief caption that permits an independent reviewer correctly to identify the object of interest and the position from which the photos were taken. Each storage media number should be documented on a separate form. The "Remarks" field is used to document the disposition of the medium used to store the images or videos.

The fire scene sketch or diagram should contain the image or video number within a circle on the sketch showing the position and viewpoint from which the image was captured. Figure 16.4.2(d) in *NFPA 921* illustrates this technique, which is invaluable for later assessing witness and fire investigator observations (NFPA 2017, pt. 16.4.2).

At the time of the investigation, a descriptive photographic index should be completed using the log shown in Figure 6-7 or a similar photo log. The photographic index or log, complete with narrative, should be included in the investigation report.

6.4.2 FILM CAMERAS AND FORMATS

The most versatile cameras traditionally available to fire investigators were 35 mm single-lens reflex with focal-plane or between-the-lens shutter systems (Berrin 1977). Single-lens reflex cameras are expensive but allow for close-ups and specialized scene photography and introduce little distortion. Viewfinder cameras are low cost but introduce parallax errors and cannot perform many useful photographic functions.

With the introduction of electronically operated shutter systems, both 35 mm film and digital-format cameras have become the recommended standard for fire investigation photography (NFPA 2017, pt. 16.2.3; Peige and Williams 1977). Competitive pricing has placed the cost of many acceptable units below $100.

Many versatile film cameras have been updated by outfitting them with digital camera backs, which allows them to take high-resolution digital photographs. Two suppliers of such digital camera backs are Phase One (2012) and Mamiya Leaf (2012).

Economic considerations play a key role in deciding on a film format over less expensive digital images. However, if the choice is to use film, especially as a backup camera, the standard 35 mm color film is the nearly universal choice for fire scene photography over black-and-white film. Black-and-white photography of fire scenes has been all but abandoned owing to its inability to record important colored fire and burn patterns (Kodak 1968).

Print film requires development and costly printing of photographs. Some investigators may choose to use color slide films having an American National Standards institute (ASA) rating between 100 and 500 to maintain resolution. In some processing laboratories, at development time the customer can choose prints, negatives, slides, or scanned images delivered on CD-ROM.

6.4.3 DIGITAL CAMERAS

Newer and higher-resolution digital cameras are introduced each year. Resolution of image quality is often measured in millions of pixels (megapixels). The current minimum acceptable resolution is upward of 10 megapixels, which is still less than the resolution available using standard film photography. The higher the number of pixels is, the better the quality of the image. Many cameras will capture 6 megapixels per image on a flash card or similar downloadable medium.

Computer technology has made dramatic improvements in the capabilities of even relatively low-cost digital cameras. Today's cameras offer image capture quality of 15 MB or higher, with more than 5 GB flash storage memory readily available. Digital cameras are now available with SLR lens-and-shutter assemblies, so traditional photographic equipment can still be used.

One of the most useful innovations is the incorporation of a microphone and sound recording chip into the camera. With each photo taken, the photographer can dictate a description of the photo up to 20 seconds in length. The chip can then be downloaded and the narration converted to a printed photo log. This eliminates the need to set the camera down and make a log entry with each photo (or to try to later re-create a photo log from memory after viewing the photos).

These features are available on the Nikon D100, Sony 727 and 828, and some Olympus digital cameras. For those who prefer to use a film camera, small voice-activated digital voice recorders are available at low cost from retailers such as Radio Shack. These can record up to 1 hour on a single chip in a device the size of a half-pack of cigarettes without the use of fragile tape cassettes.

The improper use of digital cameras in investigative photography may undermine the viability of a case, owing mainly to evidentiary considerations. Investigators are advised to adhere to a standard protocol for preserving digital images. Some agencies preserve images on their original media (CD or flash cards), whereas others save original images on disk drive memory and make copies for any medium or any digital image processing.

As with all photographs, the courtroom tests for authentication must be met: each image used must be a "true and accurate representation" and "relevant to the testimony" to the fire investigation, particularly under *Federal Rules of Evidence 403* (Lipson 2000). Systematic handling and processing of digital images is the only method for assuring their long-term acceptability (NFPA 2017, pt. 16.2.3.4).

Computer operator error and unforeseen crashes can cause digital images to be lost forever, so precautions are necessary. It is often impractical and costly to store high-resolution images permanently on some media or flash cards; they must be copied onto another medium. Two copies of the original electronic/magnetic medium should be made and placed in the case file in the same manner as an audio or video recording. A third copy is used as a working copy. Images should not be compressed, as this causes loss of detail and clarity. Copies should also be placed on external hard drives and stored off site. Operating systems, programs, and file formats change and render some files unreadable. Some investigators use two cameras at critical scenes (print and digital) and take duplicate photos to ensure that some images are always available, even years after the fire.

Digital cameras and their electronic images are useful in the production of preliminary photographs of fire scenes or final investigative reports, as the images can easily be processed to lighten, darken, or enhance features and easily transferred to printed documents. They are also helpful in producing panoramic views of fire scenes, as discussed previously. However, file compression and other manipulations may reduce the quality of the images and introduce suspicions of manipulation of the photo's content.

Digital images can be coded or watermarked while being recorded to demonstrate they are "as taken," an unmodified original. The ease and low per-image cost of digital photography tempts some investigators to take far more photos at scenes than are really necessary or justified. Investigators should consider what information they are attempting to capture with any particular photograph before taking any image.

6.4.4 DIGITAL IMAGE PROCESSING

In addition to easy-to-use computer image software for creating panoramic photos from a series of still photos, digital scanning cameras are also now available. With these technologies, investigators have realized the advantage of panoramic views, especially for briefing clients and making courtroom presentations.

Several packages, both for purchase as well as at no cost (freeware), are available for constructing stitched views of both interiors and exteriors of structures. The packages can also be used to photograph large outdoor areas, particularly wildland fires. During this process, a series of photos with overlapping edges are taken from a single viewpoint using a normal focal length lens (35 to 55 mm), and the software easily stitches the images together. Distortion is minimized if the photos are taken using a leveled rotating-head tripod, with 15 to 20 photos for a full rotation.

Adobe Photoshop is a commercial program with a function called Photomerge that quickly and easily stitches several overlapping photographic images into one (Adobe 2011).

The Roxio Panorama Assistant program is part of Roxio's Creator software that will match features in a series of photos (scanned or digital) to produce a single panoramic scan (Roxio 2012). Photos must be cropped so that all images are exactly the same size, and they are manually overlapped before being merged digitally. The system produces only end-to-end panoramas.

A more advanced system is the Graphical User Interface for Panorama Tools (PTGui), a panoramic stitching software developed for both the Windows and Mac OSX operating systems. PTGui (2012), based on the successful Panorama Tools (PT) program developed by Bernhard Vogl, allows the creation of spherical, cylindrical, or flat interactive panoramas from any number of source images. Figure 6-15 illustrates an example of a PTGui 150° panorama of a large industrial fire scene. This software supports JPEG, TIFF, PNG, and BMP source images. The computer mouse can be used to move the images to change yaw, roll, and pitch with corrected perspective in real time.

In a typical application, 16 photos taken of a large, complex fire scene using a hand-held manual 35 mm camera are scanned and stored as separate files then opened in PTGui with the 360° single-row panorama editor selected. The latest version of PTGui is 10.0.15, and a full trial version can be downloaded.

Select Hewlett Packard (HP) digital cameras can also capture panorama-ready images and produce them immediately (Deng and Zhang 2012). HP digital cameras offer both in-camera panorama preview and in-camera panorama stitching. With the in-camera panorama preview, up to five photos can later be combined into one seamless image once they are downloaded to a computer for photo stitching. With in-camera panorama stitching, up to five single shots are stitched together within the camera to create one seamless image without having to be downloaded to a computer.

Another digital scanning approach to panoramic or three-dimensional photography was the iPIX (2012) camera system. Its 180° fish-eye lens and tripod mount are compatible with many film or digital 35 mm cameras. Mounted on a tripod, the camera takes a photo, and then rotates to take a second picture in the opposite direction. Fish-eye lenses produce severe distortion when images are viewed directly, but the images are imported into the iPIX software, which corrects the distortion and seamlessly stitches the two images together. The result is a fully immersive, navigable computer image. The iPIX software then permits interactive examination or illustration of fire patterns or explosion damage around the entire periphery of a room. This process requires that the special equipment be available at the scene. It has been used successfully by a number of US police agencies.

Panoscan of Van Nuys, California, offers a scanning digital camera that can complete a 360° scan of a room in 8 seconds with high resolution and great dynamic range. Its images are readily viewable as a flat panorama or as a virtual reality movie on QuickTime VR, Flash Panoramas, Immervision JAVA, and other imaging software. Developed for both the Windows and Mac OSX operating systems, Panoscan also offers a photogrammetric capacity using two scans at different heights with specialized software (PanoMatrix), allowing accurate measurements of any scene, indoors or out. The system is fully portable.

QuickTime VR (also known as QuickTime Virtual Reality or QTVR) is an image format for use with the Apple media player QuickTime Player. QTVR is used to both create and view panoramic photos. There are software installable plug-ins for use with both the stand-alone QuickTime Player and a Web browser (QuickTime 2012). Data are saved in DXF format for use in AutoCAD, Maya, and other CAD programs. Measurements (with an accuracy of fractions of an inch over a 25-ft radius) can be made or added to the file at any time. Some advanced digital image systems allow the user to interactively browse the scene and can even link to views in adjacent rooms. Full 360° immersive images allow viewing of floors, ceilings, and walls in any direction. Images can then be linked together or linked to traditional photographs and renderings as well as to audio or other file types.

Panoramic photographs can be used to establish *viewpoint photographs*. This type of photography can be used to document what a witness might have seen or not seen from a particular location. The peripheral vision or field of view of the normal human eye is not readily duplicated by a normal camera lens, so panoramic imaging is sometimes the only way to replicate the view a witness may have had.

Crime Scene Virtual Tour (CSVT 2012) Version 3.0 uses the Java Virtual Machine (Sun Java) software to produce a fully integrated virtual scanned image with links to floor plans, close-up still photos, and investigative notes. With CSVT, users can immerse themselves in the scene, get accurate measurements of important objects from any angle, measure the distance of any two points, and generate documentation.

The GigaPan System (2012) is a derivative of NASA technology that can capture thousands of digital images and weave them into a single uniform high-resolution picture. The process allows users to share and explore gigapixel panoramas. A gigapixel image is a digital image composed of one billion pixels (1,000 megapixels), which is more than 150 times the graphic information captured by a 6 megapixel digital camera. The technology sold by GigaPan is the product of collaboration between Carnegie Mellon University and NASA Ames Intelligent Robotics Group, with support from Google. GigaPan sells automatic stepping panning heads for ordinary cameras that make it easy to capture gigapixel panoramas that can later be combined with GigaPan Stitch software.

6.4.5 HIGH DYNAMIC RANGE PHOTOGRAPHY

High dynamic range imaging (HDR) photography is a technique that increases the range between the lightest and darkest areas of an image captured by a digital camera, allowing details to be revealed in areas that are too dark or shaded. It has been suggested that fire scene photography could benefit from the use of HDR (Kimball 2012; Howard 2010).

HDR involves taking three or more images of the same scene at different shutter speeds or apertures and combining them into a single image using a processing algorithm. The final image shows details in both the shadows and highlights. The image processing algorithms are available in many programs, including Adobe Photoshop. The algorithms that produce HDR images use the static metadata stored in each digital image, also known as the *exchangeable image file format* (EXIF) information, that reveal information such as the camera's make and model, orientation, shutter speed, aperture, focal length, metering mode, and ISO settings.

HDR technologies are also used in other visualization programs, such as the Spheron-VR's SceneCenter forensic visual content management software (Spheron 2012). Scene-Center documentation allows virtual access to documentation from a crime scene through its presentation in court. It also allows for 3D photogrammetric measurement.

6.4.6 DIGITAL IMAGING GUIDELINES

The first draft of "Definitions and Guidelines for the Use of Imaging Technologies in the Criminal Justice System" was published in October 1999 in *Forensic Science Communications* (FBI 1999). The guidelines were prepared by the Scientific Working Group on Imaging Technology (SWGIT 2002; FBI 2004) and cover the "documentation of policies and procedures of personnel engaged in the capture, storage, processing, analysis, transmission, or output of imagery in the criminal justice system to ensure that their use of images and imaging technologies are governed by documented policies and procedures."

Table 6-4 lists the current approved guidelines issued by the SWGIT, now known as the "Guidelines for the Use of Imaging Technologies in the Criminal Justice System." These guidelines cover imaging technologies, recommended policies, best practices, and techniques for photographing specific impression evidence. These resource documents are available on the websites for the FBI (fbi.gov) and the International Association for Identification (theiai.org).

Agencies or individuals using either simple or complex photography should develop a standard operating procedure and departmental policy. The SWGIT procedures recommend preserving original images by storing and maintaining them in an unaltered state and in their original uncompressed file formats. Duplicates or copies should be used for working images. Original images should be preserved in one of the following durable formats: silver-based (non-instant) film, write-once compact recordable disks (CDRs), or digital versatile recordable disks (DVD-Rs).

If image processing techniques are used on the original image, they should be documented with standard operating procedures. These procedures should be visually verifiable and include cropping, dodging, burning, color balancing, and contrast adjustment. Advanced techniques include increasing the visibility of the image through multi-image averaging, integration, or Fourier analysis. Other techniques include cropping, overlaying, and creating panoramic views from individual series of photographs. An image processing log is recommended so that the process can be replicated later, if required.

A chain of custody should be maintained for the media on which original images are recorded. This chain of custody should document the identity of the personnel who had custody and control of the digital image file from the point of capture to archiving.

When compressing images into formats such as JPEGs, investigators should maintain as high a resolution as possible to avoid degrading the image. Image capture devices should render an accurate representation of the images. Different applications will dictate different standards of accuracy.

Training is important when using imaging technologies. Formal uniform training programs should be established, documented, and maintained. Proficiency testing will ensure that camera equipment, software, and media keep pace with hardware or software updates.

TABLE 6-4	Recommended Guidelines and Best Practices in Forensic Photography by the Scientific Working Group on Imaging Technology

SECTION	DESCRIPTION
Section 1	Use of Imaging Technologies in the Criminal Justice System
Section 2	Considerations for Managers
Section 3	Guidelines for Field Applications of Imaging Technologies in the Criminal Justice System
Section 4	Recommendations and Guidelines for Using Closed-Circuit Television Security Systems in Commercial Institutions
Section 5	Recommendations and Guidelines for the Use of Digital Image Processing in the Criminal Justice System
Section 6	Guidelines and Recommendations for Training in Imaging Technologies in the Criminal Justice System
Section 7	Recommendations and Guidelines for the Use of Forensic Video Processing in the Criminal Justice System
Section 8	General Guidelines for Capturing Latent Impressions Using a Digital Camera
Section 9	General Guidelines for Photographing Tire Impressions
Section 10	General Guidelines for Photographing Footwear Impressions
Section 11	Best Practices for Documenting Image Enhancement
Section 12	Best Practices for Practitioners of Forensic Image Analysis

Source: Forensic Science Communications (FBI 2004).

6.4.7 LIGHTING

No matter what camera is used, lighting plays an important role in fire scene photography (NFPA 2017, pt. 16.2.3.7). Intensely burned areas tend to absorb light from natural or artificial sources. Powerful electronic flashes are useful for lighting char details in dark scenes. Some built-in flashes on film and digital cameras do not have enough power to adequately illuminate large fire scenes, so provisions should be made for external flash connections.

Sometimes, burn patterns can best be photographed using an oblique flash to light the area of interest. Therefore, a camera should be selected that allows for an externally connected flash unit for oblique or remote illumination of the scene (NFPA 2017, pt. 16.2.3.7.2).

A major problem for interior fire scenes or exterior scenes at night is the provision of suitable lighting. Quartz-halogen work lights are widely used, but they have limited coverage and produce glare and blind spots. One new innovation uses a halogen–metal halide lamp inside a translucent balloon mounted on an extendable mast. An Airstar (2012) balloon creates uniform white glare-free light over a large area. These balloons range in size from 200 W to 4000 W and with masts from 1.8 to 9 m (6 to 36 ft) in height and can cover areas from 200 m² (2100 ft²) to 10,000 m² (108,000 ft²).

6.4.8 ACCESSORIES

Many attachments are available for cameras; however, for the sake of simplicity, it is recommended that non-expert investigators limit their use. The maximum effectiveness of the single lens provided with the camera (typically, 50- to 55-mm focal length) is for normal room and exterior view photos. Close-up (18 to 35 mm) and telephoto (100 to 400 mm) are for specialized applications, but they can introduce optical distortions. Furthermore, the use of filters and interchangeable lens configurations might disqualify photographs or slides used in courtroom presentations when investigators cannot authoritatively qualify their uses, advantages, deficiencies, or effects (Icove and Gohar 1980). A clear filter to protect the lens is the only recommended filter for fire scene photography (NFPA 2017, pt. 16.2.3.6). Some photographers prefer using polarizing or UV filters (which do not affect the color of the image) in place of clear filters.

The single most recommended accessory for photographing fire scenes is a sturdy tripod. This simple device enables the photographing of scenes with clear detail when low-lighting conditions demand longer shutter exposures. Also, a tripod allows the optimization of depth of field according to available lighting conditions. For example, an aperture setting of f/16 will usually produce a depth of field ranging from 0.91 m (3 ft) to 3.05 m (10 ft) when the camera is focused on a point 1.8 m (6 ft) from the lens. As previously discussed, panoramic scenes are most easily recorded when using a tripod. Longer exposure times may be needed to accommodate smaller aperture settings, and any exposure longer than 1/30 second is subject to tremors if the camera is handheld.

6.4.9 MEASURING AND IMAGE CALIBRATION DEVICES

Measuring and image calibration devices are used to provide additional information in both processing and interpretation. These devices should be used uniformly from case to case. Even though fire and explosion investigation guidelines recommend the use of an 18 percent grayscale calibration card), there are many advantages to using a color calibration card. With the move toward the universal use of color photography for fire scenes, the investigator should consider the use of a combined color and grayscale calibration card.

A *color and grayscale calibration card* bearing the agency name, case number, date, and time should be photographed on the first frame and last frame of each roll of film, digital camera memory card, or video camera recording. With this technique, variations in color accuracy can be detected in both film and digital images, and professional film processing laboratories will calibrate their equipment using these cards to ensure that the best color calibrations and gray scales are met. Also, color printers, like Xerox (2012), can be calibrated and corrected to ensure the proper colors are used in the graphics display and commercial printing process. Figure 6-29 shows an example of a commercially available card with the essential calibration and documentation information.

Forensics Source (2012) produces a 15-cm (6-in.) scale that is printed on 18 percent gray low-reflection plastic so that even close-up digital images can include grayscale calibration. The International Association of Arson Investigators (IAAI) also produces a similar plastic 6-in. ruler as a promotion for their CFITrainer program.

Calibration cards also have measuring devices (rulers) on their edges to document distances and sizes of objects photographed. Other measurement devices include longer folding rulers and yellow numbered tent cards to identify the location of individual points of interest or forensic evidence. Bright-colored pointers can be used to indicate important features or document direction of fire travel.

6.4.10 AERIAL PHOTOGRAPHY

In rural areas, the US Soil Conservation Service has *aerial photos* (also known as *orthophotoquads*) of a majority of the farmlands within its area of responsibility. These photos are at various resolutions (NFPA 2017, pt. 27.7.4). Aerial photographs do not always need to be taken from aircraft. Perspective photographs, as seen in Example 6-1, can be taken from higher floors of adjacent buildings. Photos taken from the elevated platform of a fire truck can be useful, providing a closer look at the overall pattern of damage, as seen in Figure 6-30(b).

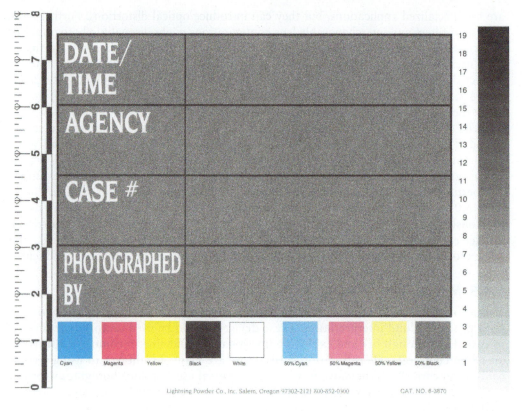

FIGURE 6-29 Commercially available grayscale and color calibration chart suitable for use in forensic fire scene documentation. *© Safariland, Courtesy of Forensics Source™ by Permission.*

Satellite and commercial aerial photos are widely available at a modest cost. Many cities and counties use aerial survey to search for non-permitted construction. Care must be taken in using commercial databases (e.g., Google Earth, Bing), as street addresses are not always up to date in data files. Users must also confirm that the image was recent enough that it accurately reflects the prefire conditions.

A developing, low-cost form of aerial photography uses field-deployable remote-controlled drones and helicopters to survey fire scenes at low altitudes. Figures 6-30(a)–(c) show examples of aerial photographic imagery produced by the helicopters courtesy of the Mesa County Sheriff's Office (MCSO) Unmanned Flight Program.

One commercial product is the Draganflyer X8 UAV helicopter (Draganfly 2012), which is battery operated and can be equipped with one of four optional cameras: high-resolution still (with remote zoom, shutter control, and tilt), high-definition video, low-light black-and-white video, or infrared camera.

The helicopter's size—only 25.4 cm (10 in.) high and 99 cm (39 in.) wide including rotors—enables it to move in very close quarters. Because it is battery-powered, the helicopter has a flight time of around 20 minutes. Batteries are easily changed, so that repeat flights are possible. There is an optional capability for live video feed, allowing the operator and/or others on the ground to monitor the imagery simultaneously.

The firm Infinite Jib (2012) is a distributor for the Droidworkx Airframe multirotor helicopter, which can deliver low-altitude imagery suitable for fire scene photography. The current ready-to-fly units consist of the EYE-Droid 4, 6, and 8 models and cost up to $13,000 each.

6.4.11 PHOTOGRAMMETRY

Photogrammetry, the science of extracting measurement data from photographs, was unaffordable for the typical fire investigator but has become more accessible in recent

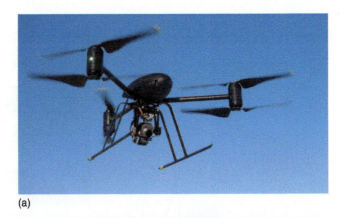

(a)

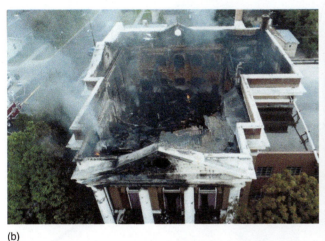

(b)

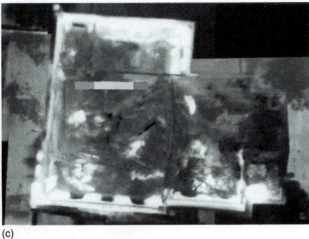

(c)

FIGURE 6-30 (a) Helicopter with mounted camera, (b) aerial image, and (c) FLIR image. *Courtesy of MCSO Unmanned Flight Program.*

years through affordable, user-friendly computer software (NFPA 2017, pt. 16.4.5.6). In photogrammetry, two or more photographs are taken and used to extract absolute coordinates and distance measurements from key features in those images (see Figure 6-31). Close-range photogrammetry programs compensate for the shortening of object lines due to perspective that is present in nearly all photographs, thus allowing users to obtain accurate measurements and create realistic models (Eos 2012).

For example, the walking distance from a deceased victim in a bed to the doorway threshold may be crucial in an investigation. Photogrammetry can capture measurement data in large or complex scenes where tape measure and notepad are inadequate or too time consuming. It also allows investigators to measure evidence that may have been moved or cleaned up or no longer exists at the scene. Photogrammetry has been in use in North America, Europe, and Australia for many years for accident scenes and major crimes, and has been proposed for use in advanced fire investigations. In one case in the United States, the technique was first used forensically to reconstruct a model of a kitchen area to enhance a V burn pattern on three dimensions (King and Ebert 2002).

Some photogrammetry programs allow users to map two-dimensional images over three-dimensional surfaces that have been created, to provide photorealistic models with perspective-corrected phototextures. There is a wide range of software programs for calculating these measurements and constructing three-dimensional models from two-dimensional photographs. Figure 6-32 shows an example of the use of photogrammetry

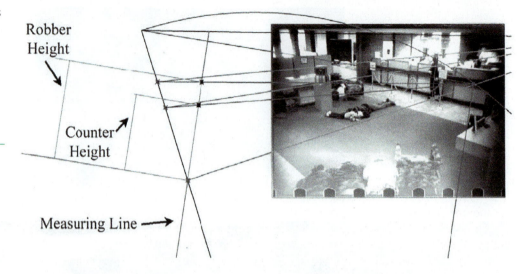

FIGURE 6-31 Illlustrates an example of a photogrammetric analysis conducted to determine the height of a subject depicted in a bank robbery surveillance photograph. *Source: Federal Bureau of Investigation, Washington, DC.*

Robber Height

Counter Height

Measuring Line

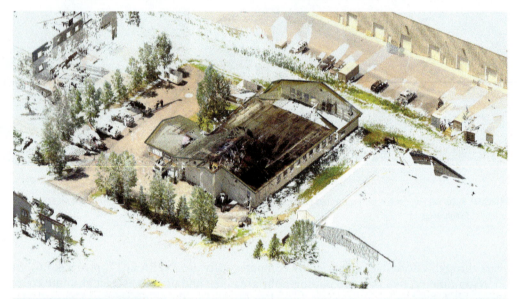

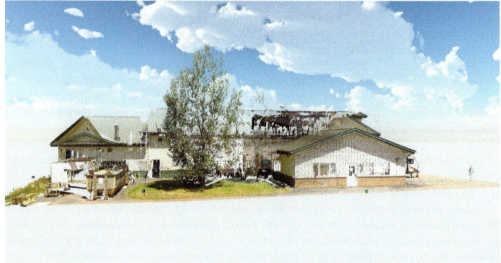

FIGURE 6-32 An example of the use of photogrammetry to combine several two-dimensional images to construct a three-dimensional view. *Compliments of Robert Toth, IAAI-CFI® - IRIS Fire Investigations Inc.*

to construct a three-dimensional view of the exterior of a building using two-dimensional photographs.

6.4.12 DIGITAL SCANNING CAMERAS

One new innovation combining the capabilities of both panoramic photography and photogrammetry is the digital scanning camera, such as the previously mentioned Panoscan (Panoscan 2012) or Spheron VR model. Photogrammetry capability is available on the Panoscan and the other systems. After the area is captured in a single scan, the camera is elevated on a vertically extendable mast that allows the camera to capture an image from the same position in the room but from a view line some 0.5 m higher, and the area is scanned again. The two images are then combined digitally (the Panoscan system uses proprietary software called PanoMetric) to produce a stereoptic virtual reality in which any measurement can then be taken with millimeter precision.

The core of the system is a specialized digital camera that works much like the moving-slit film cameras of a century ago but uses a high-resolution image converter and a specialized lens-and-shutter system to capture in each vertical "slice" an image of about 170° vertically.

The camera automatically rotates, so that the final image is a spherical high-resolution image. (The maximum vertical resolution is 5200 pixels and the total image capture can be up to 50 megapixels.) The dynamic range of image capture is up to 26 f-stops, so information from very dark areas to those in full sunlight is captured in a single pass. This is an extension of the high dynamic range technology described earlier.

6.5 Sketching

Fire scene sketches and diagrams, whether to scale or not, are important supplements to photographs and can assist the investigator in documenting evidence of fire growth, scene conditions, and other details of the fire scene (NFPA 2017, pt. 16.4; NFPA 2014, pt. 4.3.1).

A sketch graphically portrays the fire scene and items of evidence as recorded by the investigator. Investigators use this valuable documentation technique when drawing simple two-dimensional sketches of fire scenes. These sketches may range from rough exterior building outlines to detailed floor plans. Sketches allow the investigator to illustrate relationships between objects that cannot be captured via photography, such as those in separate rooms, under or behind large furniture, or visible only from overhead or via cross section.

6.5.1 GENERAL GUIDELINES

Good scene sketches do not require highly artistic skill. Even informal hand-drawn representations can capture locations and relationships between items that cannot be shown in photographs. Forensic fire scene sketches serve many purposes and should include the following information and elements of the fire scene (NFPA 2014, pt. 4.3.1; NFPA 2017, pts. 16.4.4 (A) through (D); and (NFPA 2012).

- The investigator's full name, rank, agency, case number, and the date/time when the sketch was prepared along with the full names of other individuals involved in constructing the sketch
- The location and geographic orientation of the fire scene (north arrow). Latitude and longitude using GPS data may be very helpful for rural scenes to determine jurisdiction boundaries (state, county, township, etc.) or to relocate the scene accurately
- The outline and scaled dimensions of the building, room, vehicle, or area(s) of interest, including the compass orientation. Note that if the scale is approximated, this should be indicated by the phrase "Not to Scale" on the sketch or drawing.

- A legend identifying and describing all symbols and their meanings, the scale, and other significant information used on the sketch or diagram (see *NFPA 170, 2012 ed.: Standard for Fire Safety and Emergency Symbols*)

Sketches are very useful for recording the following:

- The locations of pertinent evidence or critical features such as fire patterns and plume damage
- The locations and dimensions of all major fuel packages and competent sources of ignition involved in the fire
- Locations and travel distances of possible points of entry and exit of victims and suspects through simple measurement, laser-assisted measurements, and GPS coordinate data
- Conditions, security (locked or unlocked), and dimensions of windows, doors, floors, ceilings, and wall surfaces including sill and soffit heights for later use in fire scene reconstruction and analysis
- The detailed locations of the arc fault sites in arc survey diagrams (NFPA 2017, pt. 18.4.5.2).
- In some instances, multiple sketches using the same overall dimensions are necessary. Several separate types of evidence can be preserved in this manner including **isochars**, plume damage, and sample (evidence) collection sites. A sketch can often reveal characteristics not readily obvious in a photograph.
- The areas of surface demarcations, thermal effects, penetrations, and loss of material can also be outlined using colored markers on sketches or photographs. For example, one system uses yellow lines to outline areas of surface deposits, green lines for thermal effects, blue lines for penetrations, and red lines for areas where the material has been consumed completely. Background patterns (lines, cross-hatching) can be used in computer diagrams.
- A sketch is usually initially drawn by hand and sometimes followed up with a computer-assisted drawing. An effective hand-sketching tool is a grooved grid pad on which the pencil lead follows a slight indentation on a plastic surface (Accu-Line 2012) (see Figure 6-33).

A reliable fire scene sketching program, Visio, by Microsoft Corporation, is sufficient to produce accurate representations of structures (Visio 2012). The Microsoft website provides an add-on crime scene package for Visio at no charge. Experienced investigators have developed templates for use in fire scene analysis. Figure 6-34 shows an example of a typical fire scene diagram produced using Visio.

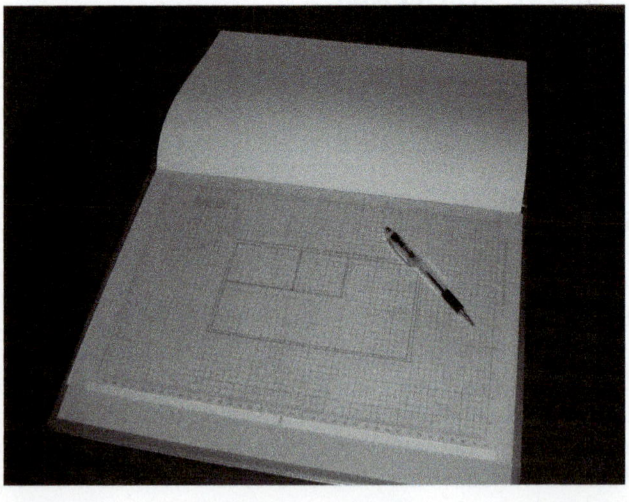

isochar ■ A line on a diagram connecting points of equal char depth (*NFPA 921*, 2017 ed., pt. 3.3.121).

FIGURE 6-33 New tools such as this Accu-line drawing aid make manual sketching easier. *Courtesy of David J. Icove, University of Tennessee.*

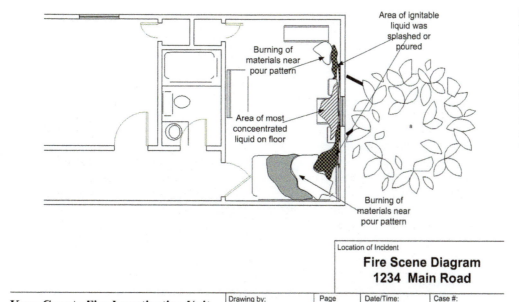

FIGURE 6-34 A typical fire scene diagram using a sketching program sufficient to produce accurate representations of burn patterns, location of evidence, and other details. *Courtesy of Det. Michael Dalton (ret.), Knox County Sheriff's Office.*

Area of ignitable liquid was splashed or poured

Burning of materials near pour pattern

Area of most conceentrated liquid on floor

Burning of materials near pour pattern

| Location of Incident |
| **Fire Scene Diagram** |
| **1234 Main Road** |

| **Knox County Fire Investigation Unit** | Drawing by: Mike Dalton | Page 3 of 5 | Date/Time: 8-26-02 1735 hrs | Case #: 012345 |

6.5.2 GPS MAPPING

Magellan (2012) has improved on an innovative approach to mapping large scenes using handheld GPS units. Using a GPS device (the Mobile Mapper CE) the size of a cell phone with GPS Differential software extension, the examiner walks to various points at the scene and keys in a code (ArcPad) denoting a particular set of features. The data are then downloaded and processed by specialized software (Mobile Mapper Office) to produce a plot of the scene accurate to ±0.5 m (depending on the number of satellites in "view" and the stabilization time at each location).

Such a device allow the mapping of large and complex scenes where view lines for Total Station surveying would be obscured by terrain or features (trees, equipment, etc.). The handheld device contains all the usual features of GIS/GPS location systems.

6.5.3 TWO- AND THREE-DIMENSIONAL SKETCHES

With the advent of CAD tools, two- and three-dimensional sketches can now be used for courtroom exhibits. Figure 6-35 shows an example of this technique. Plastic overlays can also be placed over the large sketches, which can be annotated in court using either prepared overlays or impromptu markings on the overlays. Using a convenient coordinate system allows the accurate placement of critical evidence such as the orientation of torsos of victims, fire plumes, and evidence locations.

Trimble Navigation Limited's SketchUp (Trimble 2016), available in both a free and a for-purchase version, allows the user to construct two- and three-dimensional buildings using simple commands. SketchUp works with the Windows and Mac OSX operating systems.

A special application of sketching is to copy an overhead or plan view of the scene onto several clear (transparency) sheets. Each sheet can be used to record a different indicator such as fire travel vectors, char depths, calcination, and furniture patterns. The overlays then can be compared with one another or with the original floor plan to illustrate convergence on a possible area of origin. Putting sketches on separate sheets avoids the problem of having too much detail in a single diagram.

Inclement weather can affect the survivability of field notes. HTRI Forensics of Newberg, Oregon (HTRI 2012), distributes two products using special writing paper

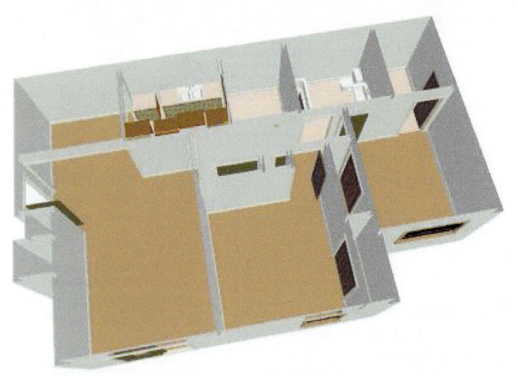

FIGURE 6-35 Construction of a three-dimensional view using an architectural rendering program. *Courtesy of David J. Icove, University of Tennessee.*

called "Rite in the Rain." The Field Investigation Field Notes contains blank pages necessary for a full investigation report, including the *Bilancia Ignition Matrix*™ (Bilancia 2012), as shown in Figure 6-36. A smaller Fire Incident Report pocket notebook is designed for use by first responders responsible for collecting initial data on fire investigations.

6.6 Establishment of Time

Several natural processes can be used to establish one of the most difficult factors in scene investigation—the passage of time. These processes include evaporation, warming, cooling, drying, and melting.

6.6.1 EVAPORATION

One of the most critical factors in fire reconstruction is determining the use or presence of accelerants. Estimating the evaporation of accelerants may provide important insight as to the passage of time and the dynamics of the resulting fire. The evaporation rate of a liquid depends on its vapor pressure (which is temperature dependent), the temperature and nature of the surface on which it is deposited, its surface area, and the circulation of air around it.

Vapor pressure is a fundamental physical property of all liquids and solids. It is the pressure that would be generated by the material if it were placed in a vacuum and allowed to come to equilibrium. Vapor pressure is a measure of how volatile the material is (i.e., how easily it vaporizes). Because vapor pressure is temperature-dependent, the higher the temperature is, the higher the vapor pressure. It is the temperature of the liquid (or of the surface on which it is spread) that is critical, not necessarily the ambient temperature of the room. A pan of acetone on a hot stove will evaporate very quickly even in a cold room.

Heat sources / Fuels	Clock radio	Cell phone charger	Cigarette	Candle	Compact fluorescent lamp	Plug-in room refresher
Lace night table cover	1. yes (a) 2. yes close 3. no (d) 4. yes path	1. yes (a, c) 2. not close 3. 4. yes	1. 2. yes close 3. no evid. 4.	**1. yes comp** **2. yes** **3. yes** **4. yes**	1. yes (a, c) 2. yes 3. no (d) 4. yes gravity	1. yes (a) 2. not close 3. no (d) 4.
Sheets or bed covers	1. no (c) 2. not close 3. no (d) 4. yes gravity	1. yes (a, c) 2. yes close 3. no (d) 4. yes	1. 2. not close 3. no evid. 4.	1. yes comp 2. not close 3. 4.	1. yes (a, c) 2. no 3. no (d) 4. no	1. yes (a) 2. yes close 3. 4.
Curtains	1. no (c) 2. not close 3. no (d) 4. yes path	1. yes (a, c) 2. yes close 3. no (d) 4. yes	1. 2. not close 3. no evid. 4.	1. yes comp 2. not close 3. 4.	1. yes (a, c) 2. no 3. no (d) 4. yes shade	1. yes (a) 2. yes close 3. no (d) 4.
Plastic decorative flowers	1. no (c) 2. not close 3. no (d) 4.	1. yes (a, c) 2. not close 3. no (d) 4. no	1. not comp. 2. 3. no evid. 4.	**1. yes comp** **2. yes close** **3. yes** **4. yes**	1. no (a, c) 2. no 3. no (d) 4. yes shade	1. no (a, c) 2. not close 3. no (d) 4. no
Lamp shade	1. yes comp 2. not close 3. no (d) 4. yes path	1. yes (a, c) 2. not close 3. no (d) 4. no	1. 2. not close 3. no evid. 4.	1. yes comp 2. not close 3. indirect 4. yes path	1. no (a, c) 2. yes close 3. no (d) 4. yes	1. no (c) 2. not close 3. no (d) 4. no

1. Competent ignition source Y/N?
2. Proximity, ignition close to fuel Y/N?
3. Evidence of ignition Y/N?
4. Initial fuel path to fuel load Y/N?

Color legend
Red = Competent and close
Blue = Not competent
Yellow = Competent but ruled out
White = Uninvestigated

Codes
P = plume or flashover
W = witnessed
F = open flame
N = not energized

Notes
a. *if the device failed*
b. *if fuel was cellulosic with a breeze*
c. *only with open flame*
d. *device was intact*

FIGURE 6-36 Ignition Matrix™ —identified fuels along vertical axis; ignition sources along horizontal. *Courtesy of Lou Bilancia, Synnovation Engineering Inc. Copyright 2008–17. All rights reserved. Used with permission.*

Vapor pressure is also highly dependent on molecular weight. The lower the molecular weight of a substance, the higher its vapor pressure, and the faster it will evaporate. The physical form of the material is also critical. A very thin film of volatile liquid on a surface will evaporate more quickly than a deep pool. Volatile liquids on porous surfaces like cloth or carpet will evaporate more quickly than they will from a free-standing pool of the same size. The larger the size of the pool and the more air movement there is around the pool, the faster the total evaporation (DeHaan 1999).

A complex mixture like gasoline contains more than 200 compounds, some of which, like pentane, are very volatile and evaporate very quickly. Others, like trimethylbenzene, evaporate very slowly and will persist for a long time. When such a liquid is poured out, the lightest, most volatile compounds will represent the entire bulk of the initial vapors generated. Thus, it is the presence of toluene, pentane, and other volatile components that controls the ignitability of the vapors being generated. Components like octane or heavier hydrocarbons slowly evaporate at room temperatures. The vapors created by evaporation are easily distinguished from the residues of the liquid based on their gas chromatographic profiles.

This process means that partially evaporated gasoline will have a very different gas chromatographic profile than fresh gasoline. Simple evaporation and burning of gasoline result in the same disproportionate loss of the lighter, more volatile components. The process is accelerated by the added heat flux from the flames. This property can be used to estimate the relative time of exposure. Gasoline that is present in fire debris as a contaminant from gas-powered firefighting equipment or intentionally added after the fire will have far more volatiles than would be expected from residues after normal evaporation or combustion. Partial evaporation of gasoline will reduce the effective vapor pressure of the remaining liquid by the loss of the most volatile components. This can change the flash point of the remaining liquid and ignitability of the product (Stevick et al. 2011).

Changing the physical form of a liquid by placing it on an absorbent wick or aerosolizing it (changing it to a mist by releasing it under pressure) will increase its vapor pressure and make even its heavier components evaporate more quickly or make them more readily ignitable. If evaporation is a concern, from the standpoint of either creating a risk by evaporation of a liquid fuel or reconstructing time factors (time since release), several factors must be documented. These factors include accurate identification of the material itself; the temperature of ambient air, surfaces, or the liquid itself at the time of release; and the nature of surfaces on which it was spread (liquids evaporate much more quickly from thin materials like clothing with free air movement than from thick porous materials like shoes).

The predominant air conditions are also critical: high temperatures, direct sun, wind, mechanical movement by fans, HVAC systems, and movement of equipment, vehicles, or people all increase the evaporation rate. Evaporation of flammable liquids from evidence that could be significant in establishing the cause of the fire or linking a person with the scene needs to be arrested by sealing the evidence in an appropriate vapor-tight container and keeping it as cool as possible to reduce further losses. On the container, the investigator should note the time at which it was sealed.

6.6.2 DRYING

Drying is usually closely related to evaporation (as in the drying of water from clothing), but when blood or other complex liquids are involved, other processes may occur. Blood, for instance, changes chemistry, color, and viscosity as it dries, becoming darker and stickier (if it is drying as a pool on a nonporous surface). Documentation of the drying state of blood involves more than simple photography, as the texture needs to be assessed, usually using a sterile cotton swab (which would be used in its eventual collection in any event). The time at which this observation is made must also be recorded. The same considerations apply to paint, adhesives, plastic resins, or other materials that change mechanically as they dry. Also, the ambient temperature must be noted if drying is a critical concern.

6.6.3 COOLING

Cooling and *melting* are time indicators that play roles in crime scene investigation (such as still partly frozen ice cream on the counter) but occasionally are useful in fire reconstruction. The cooling (or lack thereof) of materials directly exposed to fire can be assessed by direct contact, thermal imaging, or temperature probe. Inexpensive digital thermometers that are good from −45°C to 200°C (−50°F to 400°F) are available from kitchen and housewares stores. Once again, ambient conditions of wind, rain, sun, standing or running water, and the like, need to be recorded at the same time.

Cooling of a body is a routine estimate in death investigations but is often ignored in fires. That is unfortunate, because the death and the fire need not have occurred at the same time. An adult human body, once cooled to room temperature, must be exposed to heat (even from a fire) for a significant period of time before its internal core temperature rises. The thermal inertia of human tissue is similar to that of pine wood or polyethylene plastic. The internal temperature (rectal or liver) of a body at a fire scene should be recorded not for estimation of the time of death interval as much as for exclusion of situations in which the victim was dead for many hours prior to the fire. Recent work by DeHaan reports on experiments with the sustained combustion of human bodies (DeHaan 2012; Schmidt and Symes 2008, chap. 1).

6.7 Spoliation

The fire scene is often the most important piece of evidence in forensic analysis and reconstruction, particularly when the fire clearly will result in criminal and/or civil litigation. The major concern of fire investigators is the preservation of evidence to prevent its destruction or alteration before it is submitted for competent examination and analysis. *NFPA 921* (NFPA 2017, pt. 12.3.4.2) restates the *ASTM E860* (ASTM 2013b, pt. 3.3) standard that spoliation is the "loss, destruction, or material alteration of an object or document that is evidence or potential evidence in a legal proceeding by one who has the responsibility for its preservation." Both *NFPA 921* (NFPA 2017, pt. 12.3.5.1) and ASTM E860 (ASTM 2013b), caution that spoliation may occur during initial and subsequent fire scene processing, particularly when the movement or the alteration of the debris at the fire scene may significantly impair the opportunity of other interested parties to obtain the same evidentiary value from the evidence as did any prior investigator.

The inherent problem with spoliation is that intentional or negligent destruction or alteration of evidence not only may be the subject of pending litigation but also could be considered in future litigation. Failure to prevent spoliation can result in disallowance of testimony, sanctions, or other civil or criminal remedies (Burnette 2012). Published standards (*ASTM E860*) establish practices for examining and testing items of evidence that may or may not be involved in product liability litigation. This evidence may include equipment, items, or components that will not be returned to service. In laboratory examinations where the evidence will be altered or destroyed, all persons involved in the present or potential cases should be given the opportunity to express their opinions, to provide input on any proposed examination protocol, and to be present at the testing.

ASTM E860 refers to other ASTM practices, including those concerning the reporting of opinions *ASTM E620* (ASTM 2011a), evaluation of technical data *ASTM E678* (ASTM 2013a), reporting of incidents *ASTM E1020* (ASTM 2013c), and collection/preservation of evidence *ASTM E1188* (ASTM 2011b). For example, *ASTM E1188*, sec. 4.1, states that the investigator should "obtain statements as early as feasible from all individuals associated with the event and recovery activity" (ASTM 2011b). *ASTM E1188* also guides the investigator in maintaining a **chain of evidence (chain of custody)** by identifying and uniquely labeling evidence as to the location, time and date, and name of collector.

chain of evidence (chain of custody) ■ The chronological documentation, or paper trail, showing the seizure, custody, control, transfer, analysis, and disposition of physical or electronic evidence.

When the evidence is subject to in-place or later laboratory examination by a coordinated and informed group of affected parties, these processes must be documented and photographed. These tests or examinations may consist of disassembly or destructive testing (*ASTM E1188*, sec. 4.3). Disposal of evidence should also be coordinated with ample notification of all parties and clients.

Both *NFPA 921* and *ASTM E860* provide guidance to fire investigators on their responsibilities in minimizing spoliation of evidence (NFPA 2017, pt. 12.3.5.1; ASTM 2013b, pt. 5.2 et seq.):

- Immediately inform their client that there was a need to secure and preserve crucial evidence;
- Recommend that their client notify all other interested parties which may have a standing or exposure to the potential civil litigation; and
- Cease all destructive disassembly and testing until all other interested parties are given the opportunity to participate in and record the results of the examination and potential destructive testing.

Guidelines for avoiding sanctions for spoliation of evidence include conducting an immediate investigation, giving timely notification to potential defendants, and arranging for long-term preservation of the evidence collected (Sweeney and Perdew 2005). The realization that the fire scene cannot be preserved throughout litigation is an incentive to allow interested parties to take steps to identify and preserve other relevant evidence. *NFPA 921* defines an *interested party* as "any person, entity, or organization, including their representatives, with statutory obligations or whose legal rights or interests may be affected by the investigation of a specific incident" (NFPA 2017, pt. 3.3.167).

Table 6-5 summarizes relevant fundamental case citations and opinions. Fire investigators should keep up to date on legal issues surrounding the problem of spoliation and how to guard against violating its principles and practices. When questions arise, a legal advisor or prosecutor should be consulted for clarification or advice. Thorough documentation with photography and detailed notes is the best protection against problems arising from accidental damage during storage and transport.

TABLE 6-5	Summary of Case Citations and Opinions on Spoliation of Evidence

PRINCIPLE	CASE CITATION	DISCUSSION
Definition	*County of Solano v. Delancy,* 264 Cal. Rptr. 721, 724 (Cal. Ct. App. 1989)	Failure to preserve property for another's use in a pending or future litigation
	Miller v. Montgomery County, 494 A.2d 761 (Md. Ct. Spec. App. 1985)	Destruction, mutilation, or alteration of evidence by a party to an action
Dismissal	*Allstate Insurance Co. v. Sunbeam Corp.,* 865 F. Supp. 1267 (N.D. Ill. 1994)	Dismissal of action as result of spoliation by deliberate or malicious conduct
	Transamerica Insurance Group v. Maytag Inc., 650 N.E. 3d 169 (Ohio App. 1994)	Dismissal of action for failure to preserve all evidence prior to suit
Duty to preserve evidence	*California v. Trombetta,* 479, 488–89 (1984)	Duty to preserve exculpatory evidence that will play a role in suspect's defense
Exclusion of expert testimony	*Bright v. Ford Motor Co.,* 578 N.E. 2d 547 (Ohio App. 1990)	Exclusion of expert testimony for failure to protect evidence prejudicial to innocent party
	Cincinnati Insurance Co. v. General Motors Corp., 1994 Ohio App. LEXIS 4960 (Ottawa County Oct. 28, 1994)	In product liability actions, expert testimony may be precluded as a sanction for spoliation of evidence
	Travelers Insurance Co. v. Dayton Power and Light Co., 663 N.E. 2d 1383 (Ohio Misc, 1996)	Negligent or inadvertent destruction of evidence sufficient for sanctions excluding deposition testimony of expert witness
	Travelers Insurance Co. v. Knight Electric Co., 1992 Ohio App. LEXIS 6664 (Stark County Dec. 21, 1992)	Opinion evidence of plaintiff's expert struck because physical evidence no longer available
Evidentiary inferences	*State of Ohio v. Strub,* 355 N.E. 2d 819 (Ohio App. 1975)	Attempts to suppress evidence indicating consciousness of guilt
	U.S. v. Mendez-Ortiz, 810 F.2d 76 (6th Cir. 1986)	Inference that evidence unfavorable to spoliator's cause was intentionally spoliated or destroyed
Independent torts	*Continental Insurance Co. v. Herman,* 576 So. 2d 313 (Fla. 3rd DCA 1991)	Independent actions for intentional or negligent spoliation of evidence
	Smith v. Howard Johnson Co. Inc., 615 N.E. 2d 1037 (Ohio 1993)	Existence of cause of action in tort for interference with or destruction of evidence
Criminal statutes	Ohio Statute, Section 2921.32	"Obstructing justice" by destroying or concealing physical evidence of the crime or act

Source: Derived from information given by Burnette (2012).

Summary

Fire scenes often contain complex information that must be thoroughly documented, because a single photograph and scene diagram are not sufficient to capture vital information on fire dynamics, building construction, evidence collection, and avenues of escape for the building's occupants.

Fire scenes are documented through a comprehensive protocol of forensic photography, sketches, drawings, and evidence collection. Various computer-assisted photographic and sketching technologies can help ensure accurate and representational diagramming. Comprehensive documentation aids the primary investigation and any subsequent investigations or inquiries, and minimizes charges of spoliation. Documentation offers support for any opinions offered and makes effective peer or technical review possible. Finally, documentation demonstrates that the investigator has followed required professional guidelines.

Review Questions

1. Discuss the methods used to document a fire scene.
2. Discuss who is interviewed at fire scenes and why.
3. Discuss observation of various burn items and observed damage, burn patterns, and times.

Suggested Classroom Exercises

1. Fire investigators apply the basic principles of combustion of common fuels and the dynamics of fire and flame. Obtain a copy of a fire investigation report and photographs, and cite as many of the rules of fire behavior documented in the report as possible.

2. In the fire investigation report obtained in the previous exercise, isolate as many fire behavior indicators as possible. Determine if the burning fuel created plume-induced charring, and point out several of these indicators.

References

AAFS. 2011. *Fire Debris Workshop*. Chicago, IL: American Academy of Forensic Science.

Accu-Line. 2012. *Accu-Line Industries, USA*. Retrieved January 31, 2012, from https://www.acculine.com.

Adobe. 2011. *Adobe Photoshop*. Retrieved January 31, 2012, from www.adobe.com/PhotoshopFamily.

Ahmad, U. K., Y. S. Mei, M. S. Bahari, N. S. Huat, and V. K. Paramasivam. 2011. "The Effectiveness of Soot Removal Techniques for the Recovery of Fingerprints on Glass Fire Debris in Petrol Bomb Cases." *Malaysian Journal of Analytical Sciences* 15 (2): 191–201.

Ahrens, M. 2007. *U.S. Experience with Smoke Alarms and Other Fire Detection/Alarm Equipment*. Quincy, MA: National Fire Protection Association.

Airstar. 2012. *Airstar Space Lighting USA*. Retrieved January 31, 2012, from http://airstarlight.us.

Armstrong, A., V. Babrauskas, D. L. Holmes, C. Martin, R. Powell, S. Riggs, and L. D. Young. 2004. "The Evaluation of the Extent of Transporting or 'Tracking' an Identifiable Ignitable Liquid (Gasoline) Throughout Fire Scenes During the Investigative Process." *Journal of Forensic Sciences* 49 (4): 741–48.

ASTM. 2011a. *E620-11: Standard Practice for Reporting Opinions of Scientific or Technical Experts*. West Conshohocken, PA: ASTM International.

———. 2011b. *E1188-11: Standard Practice for Collection and Preservation of Information and Physical Items by a Technical Investigator*. West Conshohocken, PA: ASTM International.

———. 2011c. *E2544-11a: Standard Terminology for Three-Dimensional (3D) Imaging Systems*. West Conshohocken, PA: ASTM International.

———. 2013a. *E678-07: Standard Practice for Evaluation of Scientific or Technical Data*. West Conshohocken, PA: ASTM International.

———. 2013b. *E860-07(2013)e1: Standard Practice for Examining and Preparing Items That Are or May Become Involved in Criminal or Civil Litigation*. West Conshohocken, PA: ASTM International.

———. 2013c. *E1020-13e1: Standard Practice for Reporting Incidents That May Involve Criminal or Civil Litigation*. West Conshohocken, PA: ASTM International.

———. 2013d. *E1459-13: Standard Guide for Physical Evidence Labeling and Related Documentation*. West Conshohocken, PA: ASTM International.

———. 2016. *E119-16a: Standard Test Methods for Fire Tests of Building Construction and Materials*. West Conshohocken, PA: ASTM International.

Babrauskas, V. 2006. "Mechanisms and Modes for Ignition of Low-Voltage, PVC-Insulated Electrotechnical Products." *Fire and Materials* 30: 151–74.

Bailey, C. 2012. *One Stop Shop in Structural Fire Engineering*. Retrieved January 31, 2012, from http://www.mace.manchester.ac.uk/project/research/structures/strucfire.

Berrin, E. R. 1977. "Investigative Photography." *Technology Report 77-1*. Bethesda, MD: Society of Fire Protection Engineers.

Bilancia. 2012. *Bilancia Ignition Matrix™*. Retrieved January 31, 2012, from http://www.ignitionmatrix.com.

Bleay, S. M., G. Bradshaw, and J. E. Moore. 2006. *Fingerprint Development and Imaging Newsletter: Special Edition*. Publication No. 26/06. Home Office Scientific Development Branch, UK, April.

Braadbaart, F., I. Poole, H. D. J. Huisman, and van B. Os. (2012). "Fuel, Fire and Heat: An Experimental Approach to Highlight the Potential of Studying Ash and Char Remains from Archaeological Contexts." *Journal of Archaeological Science*, 39(4), 836–47. doi: http://dx.doi.org/10.1016/j.jas.2011.10.009.

Burnette, G. E. 2012. *Spoliation of Evidence*. Tallahassee, FL: Guy E. Burnette, Jr, P.A.

Cavanagh, K., E. Du Pasquier, and C. Lennard. 2002. "Background Interference from Car Carpets: The Evidential Value of Petrol Residues in Cases of Suspected Vehicle Arson." *Forensic Science International* 125 (1): 22–36, doi: 10.1016/s0379-0738(01)00610-7.

Cavanagh-Steer, K., E. Du Pasquier, C. Roux, and C. Lennard. 2005. "The Transfer and Persistence of Petrol on Car Carpets." *Forensic Science International* 147 (1): 71–79, doi: 10.1016/j.forsciint.2004.04.081.

Coulson, S., R. Morgan-Smith, S. Mitchell, and T. McBriar. 2008. "An Investigation into the Presence of Petrol on the Clothing and Shoes of Members of the Public." *Forensic Science International* 175 (1): 44–54, doi: 10.1016/j.forsciint.2007.05.005.

Coulson, S. A., and R. K. Morgan-Smith. 2000. "The Transfer of Petrol on to Clothing and Shoes While Pouring Petrol Around a Room." *Forensic Science International* 112 (2–3): 135–41, doi: 10.1016/s0379-0738(00)00179-1.

CSVT. 2012. *Crime Scene Virtual Tour*. Retrieved January 31, 2012, from http://crime-scenevr.com/index.html/.

Curtin, D. P. 2011. *Curtin's On-Line Library of Digital Photography*. Retrieved January 30, 2012, from http://www.shortcourses.com/.

Deans, J. 2006. "Recovery of Fingerprints from Fire Scenes and Associated Evidence." *Science and Justice* 46 (3): 153–68.

DeHaan, J. D. 1995. "The Reconstruction of Fires Involving Highly Flammable Hydrocarbon Liquids." PhD diss., University of Strathclyde, Glasgow, Scotland, UK.

———. 1999. "The Influence of Temperature, Pool Size, and Substrate on the Evaporation Rates of Flammable Liquids." *Proceedings of InterFlam 99, June 29–July 1, Edinburgh, UK*. Greenwich, UK: Interscience.

———. 2001. "Full-Scale Compartment Fire Tests." *CAC News* (Second Quarter): 14–21.

———. 2012. "Sustained Combustion of Bodies: Some Observations." *Journal of Forensic Science*, May 4, doi: 10.1111/j.1556-4029.2012.02190.x.

DeHaan, J. D., and D. J. Icove. 2012. *Kirk's Fire Investigation*. 7th ed. Upper Saddle River, NJ: Pearson-Prentice Hall.

Deng, Y., and T. Zhang. 2012. *Generating Panorama Photos*. Palo Alto, CA: Hewlett-Packard Labs.

Draganfly. 2012. *DraganFlyerX8: Fire Investigation*. Retrieved January 31, 2012, from http://www.draganfly.com/uav-helicopter/draganflyer-x8/applications/government.php.

Eos. 2012. *Eos Systems: Imaging and Measurement Technology*. Retrieved January 31, 2012, from http://www.eossystems.com.

Faro. 2017. Retrieved May 6, 2017, from www.faro.com.

Faxitron. 2012. *Faxitron Bioptics: Forensic Analysis*. Retrieved January 31, 2012, from http://faxitron.com/scientific-industrial/forensics.html.

FBI. 1999. "Definitions and Guidelines for the Use of Imaging Technologies in the Criminal Justice System." *Forensic Science Communications* 1 (3).

———. 2004. "Scientific Working Group on Imaging Technology (SWGIT) References/Resources." *Forensic Science Communications* (March).

———. 2005. "Best Practices for Forensic Image Analysis." Forensic Science Communications. Vol 7, No. 4. Federal Bureau of Investigation, Washington, DC.

———. 2005. "Best Practices for Forensic Image Analysis." Forensic Science Communications. Vol 7, No. 4. Federal Bureau of Investigation, Washington, DC.

FLIR. 2012. *FLIR: The World Leader in Thermal Imaging*. Retrieved January 31, 2012, from http://www.flir.com/US/.

Forensics Source. 2012. *Crime Scene Documentation: Photo ID Cards*. Retrieved January 31, 2012, from http://www.forensicssource.com/ProductList.aspx?CategoryName=Crime-Scene-Documentation-Photo-ID-Cards.

Geiman, J. A., and J. M. Lord. 2011. "Systematic Analysis of Witness Statements for Fire Investigation." *Fire Technology*, 1–13, doi: 10.1007/s10694-010-0208-3.

GigaPan. 2012. *GigaPan Systems*. Retrieved January 31, 2012, from http://gigapan.org.

Golden. 2012. *Golden Engineering, Inc.: Manufacturer of Lightweight Portable X-Ray Machines*. Retrieved January 31, 2012, from http://www.goldenengineering.com.

Harris, E. C., ed. 2014. *Practices in Archaeological Stratigraphy*. Amsterdam: Elsevier.

Harris, E. C. 2016. *Harris Matrix.Com: Home of Archaeology's Premier Stratigraphy System*. Retrieved August 31, 2016, from http://www.harrismatrix.com.

Harrison, K. 2013. "The Application of Forensic Fire Investigation Techniques in the Archaeological Record." *Journal of Archaeological Science* 40 (2): 955–59. doi: http://dx.doi.org/10.1016/j.jas.2012.08.030.

Hewitt, Terry-Dawn. 1997. "A Primer on the Law of Spoliation of Evidence in Canada." *Fire & Arson Investigator* 48, no. 1 (September): 17–21.

Howard, J. 2010. *Practical HDRI: High Dynamic Range Imaging for Photographers*. 2nd ed. Santa Barbara, CA: Rocky Nook.

HTRI. 2012. *HTRI Forensics: The Cross-Technology Integration Specialists*. Retrieved January 31, 2012, from www.htriforensics.com.

Icove, D. J., and M. W. Dalton. 2008. "A Comprehensive Prosecution Report Format for Arson Cases." International Symposium on Fire Investigation Science and Technology, ISFI 2008, Cincinnati, OH, May 19–21, 2008.

Icove, D. J., and M. M. Gohar. 1980. "Fire Investigation Photography." In *Fire Investigation Handbook*, ed. F. L. Brannigan, R. G. Bright, and N. H. Jason. NBS Handbook 123. Washington, DC: National Bureau of Standards, US Department of Commerce.

Icove, D. J., and G. A. Haynes. 2007. "Guidelines for Conducting Peer Reviews of Complex Fire Investigations." Fire and Materials Conference, San Francisco, California, January 29–31, 2007. (Updated References, October 2, 2011)

Icove, D. J., J. R. Lally, L. K. Miller, and E. C. Harris. 2014. "The Use of the 'Harris Matrix' in Fire Scene Documentation." Paper presented at the International Symposium on Fire Investigation Science and Technology, College Park, MD, September 22–24, 2014.

Icove, D. J., H. E. Welborn, A. J. Vonarx, E. C. Adams, J. R. Lally, and T. G. Huff. 2006. "Scientific Investigation and Modeling of Prehistoric Structural Fires at Chevelon Pueblo." Paper presented at the International Symposium on Fire Investigation Science and Technology.

Icove, D. J., V. B. Wherry, and J. D. Schroeder. 1998. *Combating Arson-for-Profit: Advanced Techniques for Investigators*. 2nd ed. Columbus, OH: Battelle Press.

Ide, R. H. 1997. "Investigative Excavation at Fire Scenes." *Science & Justice* 37 (3): 210–2.

Infinite Jib. 2012. *Droidworkx Airframe Multi-rotor Helicopter*. Retrieved January 31, 2012, from http://www.infinitejib.com.

Innovxsys. 2012. *Olympus Inspection and Measurement Systems*. Retrieved January 31, 2012, from http://www.olympus-ims.com/en/innovx-xrf-xrd.

iPIX. 2012. *Minds-Eye-View, Inc.* Retrieved January 31, 2012, from http://www.ipix.com.

Karlsson, B., and J. G. Quintiere. 2000. *Enclosure Fire Dynamics*. Boca Raton, FL: CRC Press.

Kimball, C. 2012. *Fire Photographer Magazine*. Retrieved January 31, 2012, from http://firephotomagazine.com.

King, C. G., and J. I. Ebert. 2002. "Integrating Archaeology and Photogrammetry with Fire Investigation." *Fire Engineering* (February): 79.

Kodak. 1968. *Basic Police Photography*. Publication no. M77. Rochester, NY: Eastman Kodak Co.

Lally, J. R. 2006. "Prehistoric Arson Cases." *Fire and Arson Investigator*, pp. 22–24.

Leica. 2011. *Leica Geosystems Introduces NIST Traceable Targets for 3D Laser Scanning of Crime Scenes to Support ISO Accreditation*. Retrieved January 31, 2012, from www.leicageosystems.us/forensic.

———. 2012. *Leica Geosystems*. Retrieved January 31, 2012, from http://www.leicageosystems.us.

LeMay, J. 2002. "Using Scales in Photography." *Law Enforcement Technology* 29 (10): 142.

Lennard, C. 2007. "Fingerprint Detection: Current Capabilities." *Australian Journal of Forensic Sciences* 39 (2): 55–71, doi: 10.1080/00450610701650021.

Lentini, J. J., J. A. Dolan, and C. Cherry. 2000. "The Petroleum-Laced Background." *Journal of Forensic Science* 45 (5): 968–89.

Lipson, A. S. 2000. *Is It Admissible?* Costa Mesa, CA: James.

Madrzykowski, D., and W. D. Walton. 2004. "Cook County Administration Building Fire, October 17, 2003." *NIST SP 1021*. Gaithersburg, MD: National Institute of Standards and Technology.

Magellan. 2012. *Magellan Mobile Mapper CE*. Retrieved January 31, 2012, from http://www.magellangps.com.

Mamiya Leaf. 2012. *Mamiya Leaf Imaging, Ltd.* Retrieved January 31, 2012, from http://www.mamiyaleaf.com.

Mann, D. C., and N. D. Putaansuu. 2006. "Alternative Sampling Methods to Collect Ignitable Liquid Resides from Non-Porous Areas Such As Concrete." *Fire and Arson Investigator,* 57 (1): 43–46.

Mann, J., N. Nic Daéid, and A. Linacre. 2003. "An Investigation into the Persistence of DNA on Petrol Bombs." *Proceedings of the European Academy of Forensic Sciences*, Istanbul.

NBS. 1980. *Fire Investigation Handbook*. NBS Handbook 123, edited by F. L. Brannigan, R. G. Bright, and N. H. Jason. Washington, DC: National Bureau of Standards, US Department of Commerce.

NFPA. 1998. *NFPA 906: Guide for Fire Incident Field Notes*. Quincy, MA: National Fire Protection Association.

———. 2009. *NFPA 705: Recommended Practice for a Field Flame Test for Textiles and Films*. Quincy, MA: National Fire Protection Association.

———. 2012. *NFPA 170: Standard for Fire Safety and Emergency Symbols*. Quincy, MA: National Fire Protection Association.

———. 2014. *NFPA 1033: Standard for Professional Qualifications for Fire Investigator*. Quincy, MA: National Fire Protection Association.

———. 2017. *NFPA 921: Guide for Fire and Explosion Investigations*. Quincy, MA: National Fire Protection Association.

NIJ. 2000. "Fire and Arson Scene Evidence: A Guide for Public Safety Personnel." (O. o. J. Programs, Trans.) *Technical Working Group on Fire/Arson Scene Investigation (TWGFASI)* (pp. 48). Washington, DC: National Institute of Justice.

Nowlan, M., A. W. Stuart, G. J. Basara, and P. M. L. Sandercock. 2007. "Use of a Solid Absorbent and an Accelerant Detection Canine for the Detection of Ignitable Liquids Burned in a Structure Fire." *Journal of Forensic Sciences* 52 (3): 643–48, doi: 10.1111/j.1556-4029.2007.00408.x.

Olson, G. 2009. *Recovery of Human Remains in a Fatal Fire Setting Using Archaeological Methods*. Ottawa, Canada: Canadian Police Research Centre.

Panoscan. 2012. *Panoscan: A Breakthrough in Panoramic Capture*. Retrieved January 31, 2012, from http://www.panoscan.com.

Peige, J. D., and C. E. Williams. 1977. *Photography for the Fire Service*. Oklahoma City, OK: Oklahoma State University.

Phase One. 2012. *Phase One IQ Photography*. Retrieved January 31, 2012, from http://www.phaseone.com.

Pichler, T., K. Nicolussi, G. Goldenberg, K. Hanke, K. Kovács, and A. Thurner. 2013. "Charcoal from a Prehistoric Copper Mine in the Austrian Alps: Dendrochronological and Dendrological Data, Demand for Wood and Forest Utilization." *Journal of Archaeological Science* 40(2): 992–1002. doi: http://dx.doi.org/10.1016/j.jas.2012.09.008.

PTGui. 2012. *PTGui: Create High Quality Panoramic Images*. Retrieved January 31, 2012, from http://www.ptgui.com.

QuickTime. 2012. *QuickTime 7*. Retrieved January 31, 2012, from http://www.apple.com/quicktime.

Rich, L. 2007. *Rooms to Go*. Personal communication.

Riegl. 2012. *Riegl Laser Measurement Systems*. Retrieved January 31, 2012, from http://www.riegl.com.

Roxio. 2012. *Roxio Creator 2011 Digital Media Suite*. Retrieved January 31, 2012, from http://www.roxio.com.

Saitoh, N., and S. Takeuchi. 2006. "Fluorescence Imaging of Petroleum Accelerants by Time-Resolved Spectroscopy with a Pulsed Nd-YAG Laser." *Forensic Science International* 163 (1–2): 38–50, doi: 10.1016/j.forsciint.2005.10.025.

Schmidt, C. W., and S. A. Symes, eds. 2008. *The Analysis of Burned Human Remains*. London: Academic Press.

Spheron. 2012. *Spheron VR Virtual Technologies*. Retrieved January 31, 2012, from http://www.spheron.com.

Stanley. 2012. *Stanley FatMax Electronic Distance Measuring Tool*. Retrieved January 31, 2012, from http://www.stanleytools.com.

Stauffer, E., J. A. Dolan, and R. Newman. 2008. *Fire Debris Analysis*. Boston, MA: Academic Press.

Stevick, G., J. Zicherman, D. Rondinone, and A. Sagle. 2011. "Failure Analysis and Prevention of Fires and Explosions with Plastic Gasoline Containers." *Journal of Failure Analysis and Prevention* 11(5): 455–65, doi: 10.1007/s11668-011-9462-z.

Svare, R. J. 1988. "Determining Fire Point-of-Origin and Progression by Examination of Damage in the Single Phase, Alternating Current Electrical System." Paper presented at the International Arson Investigation Delegation to the People's Republic of China and Hong Kong.

Sweeney, G. O., and P. R. Perdew. 2005. "Spoliation of Evidence: Responding to Fire Scene Destruction." *Illinois Bar Journal* 93 (July): 358–67.

SWGIT. 2002. *Guidelines for the Use of Imaging Technologies in the Criminal Justice System. Version 2.3 2002.06.06*. Hollywood, FL: International Association for Identification, Scientific Working Group on Imaging Technologies.

Tassios, T. P. 2002. "Monumental Fires." *Fire Technology* 38 (3): 11–17.

Thali, M. J., K. Yen, W. Schweitzer, P. Vock, C. Ozdoba, and R. Dirnhofer. 2003. "Into the Decomposed Body: Forensic Digital Autopsy Using Multislice-Computed Tomography." *Forensic Science International* 134 (2–3): 109–14, doi: 10.1016/s0379-0738(03)00137-3.

ThermoFisher. 2012. *ThermoFisher Scientific*. Retrieved January 31, 2012, from http://www.thermofisher.com.

3rd Tech. 2012. *3rdTech, Inc.: Advanced Imaging and 3D Products for Law Enforcement and Security Applications*. Retrieved January 30, 2012, from http://www.3rdtech.com.

Tontarski, K. L., K. A. Hoskins, T. G. Watkins, L. Brun-Conti, and A. L. Michaud. 2009. "Chemical Enhancement Techniques of Bloodstain Patterns and DNA Recovery After Fire Exposure." *Journal of Forensic Sciences* 54 (1): 37–48, doi: 10.1111/j.1556-4029.2008.00904.x.

Tontarski, R. E. 1985. "Using Absorbents to Collect Hydrocarbon Accelerants from Concrete." *Journal of Forensic Sciences* 30 (4): 1230–32.

Trimble. 2016. *Google SketchUp: 3D Modeling for Everyone*. Retrieved September 1, 2016, from http://www.sketchup.com.

Visio. 2012. *Microsoft Visio 2000 Crime Scenes Add-In Available for Download*. Retrieved January 31, 2012, from http://support.microsoft.com/kb/274454.

White, R. H., and M. A. Dietenberger. 2010. "Fire Safety of Wood Construction." Chap. 18 in *Wood Handbook*. Madison, WI: US Department of Agriculture, Forest Products Laboratory. Retrieved from http://www.fpl.fs.fed.us/documnts/fplgtr/fplgtr190.

Wilkinson, P. 2001. "Archaeological Survey Site Grids." *Practical Archaeology* 5 (Winter): 21–27.

Xerox. 2012. *PhaserMatch 4.0: Xerox Professional Color Matching*. Retrieved January 31, 2012, from http://www.office.xerox.com/latest/PMSDS-07.PDF.

Zarbeco. 2012. *Zarbeco: Portable and Powerful Digital Imaging Solutions*. Retrieved January 31, 2012, from http://www.zarbeco.com.

Legal References

Commonwealth of Pennsylvania v. Paul S. Camiolo, Montgomery County, No. 1233 of 1999.

Daubert v. Merrell Dow Pharmaceuticals Inc. 509 U.S. 579 (1993); 113 S. Ct. 2756, 215 L. Ed. 2d 469.

Daubert v. Merrell Dow Pharmaceuticals Inc. (Daubert II), 43 F.3d 1311, 1317 (9th Cir. 1995).

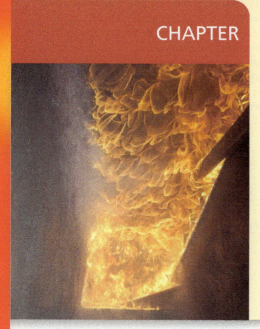

Courtesy of Jamie Novak, Novak Investigations and St. Paul Fire Dept.

KEY TERMS

alligatoring, *p. 480*

annealing, *p. 486*

area of origin, *p. 443*

area of transition, *p. 507*

backing, *p. 501*

calcination, *p. 485*

chain of evidence (chain of custody), *p. 459*

char depth, *p. 478*

clean burn, *p. 480*

crazing, *p. 490*

crowning, *p. 501*

drop-down, *p. 444*

fire patterns, *p. 463*

flanking, *p. 501*

ghost marks, *p. 484*

heat horizon, *p. 471*

hot-plate ignition (hot surface ignition), *p. 523*

hot set, *p. 518*

ignitable liquid, *p. 456*

indicators, *p. 463*

ladder fuels, *p. 500*

rekindle, *p. 514*

salvage, *p. 497*

smoke horizon, *p. 471*

spot fires, *p. 511*

trailer, *p. 494*

OBJECTIVES

After reading this chapter, you should be able to:

- Describe the investigative methodology for determining the origins and causes of structural, wildland, and vehicle fires.
- Understand and explain the systematic documentation of the fire scene through photography, sketching, evidence collection and preservation, and use of timelines.
- Understand the general principles of fire behavior including fire spread and burn patterns.
- Identify the major challenges associated with investigating fires in structures, wildlands, and vehicles.

The goals of fire scene investigations of structures, wildlands, and vehicles are the same: to determine the cause and origin of the fire. Key components of the investigation include the following:

- Examination of the fire scene
- Collection and preservation of physical evidence
- Documentation via photographs, diagrams, maps, evidence collection
- Reconstruction of the fire scene
- Evaluation and analysis of available data, test possible hypotheses
- Determination of origin and cause

Following *Daubert, Kumho Tire, Benfield,* and other decisions regarding admissibility of expert witnesses and their opinions, the expectation of courts is an investigation using the scientific method. The investigation focuses on answering the following questions:

- Where did the fire start?
- What was the cause of the fire (i.e., how was the fire started)?
- What was the initial fuel and means of ignition? What was ignited? What ignited it? How did first fuel and ignition source come together?
- Was the fire accidental or intentional?
- If the fire was intentionally set, what was the motive?
- If the fire was accidental, what factors contributed to its ignition or spread?
- If life was lost, what contributed to the death? Was it the rapidity of the fire spread or the toxic gases and smoke? Why or how did others survive?
- How did fire protection equipment or systems function to minimize losses or fail to protect the property?

PART 1: General Principles

7.1 General Principles of Fire Investigation

The origin and cause of a fire is usually not known until well into the investigation; therefore, every fire scene must be approached as a potential crime scene for purposes of documentation and evidence collection. Arson is a most difficult crime to prove because it is often not apparent until the investigation is nearly complete. The investigator must not prejudge the cause of any fire and must consider the cause of every fire to be undetermined until completion of the collection of evidence, examination, and documentation. Failure to consider a presumption of innocence may lead to wrongful prosecution.

With an understanding of the basic principles of combustion of common fuels and the dynamics of heat transfer, fire, and flame, the investigator can apply those principles to more complex situations involving combinations of fuels and their structural arrangement.

7.1.1 GENERAL CONSIDERATIONS

Even accidental fires may have far-reaching consequences from a liability standpoint, and the physical evidence may be just as crucial to investigators from regulatory agencies or the insurance industry. [See *ASTM E860* (ASTM 2013a), *E1188* (ASTM 2011), and *E1459* (ASTM 2013b)] for guidance on preserving evidence.) There are also concerns of spoliation of evidence in civil cases where evidence critical to establishing what caused a fire and what did not has been destroyed or removed by the public-sector investigator.

This caution extends *both* to the security of the scene and to the initial dealings with occupants and all witnesses in that individual accounts of what happened should be carefully cross-checked and verified. The scene *must* remain in the custody of the fire or police department from the time of the fire to ensure the integrity of the scene and its evidence.

It is the responsibility of the fire department to ensure continuity of possession. If that custody has not been maintained, a search warrant must be obtained or the owner's permission secured before any evidence can be rightfully recovered.

It is vital that the investigator be willing to do a complete investigation before he or she begins. It must be appreciated that this may entail many hours of difficult and unpleasant effort, sometimes under less-than-ideal conditions. Custody and control of the scene must be retained until the investigation is complete. Supreme Court decisions have made it clear that security of the scene must be strictly maintained both before and during the investigation. The investigator must be willing to examine *every* fire systematically and thoroughly, paying close attention to small details. The scene must be sketched and photographed to preserve its appearance for later court inspection. These sketches and photos must be accompanied by careful notes and an adequate report to permit an accurate reconstruction at any later time. Because so many fires are arson caused, the fire investigator must be careful to examine every fire scene for things that look out of place—objects that do not belong in the area in which they are found or are in positions that do not appear to be normal or logical. Because of the tremendous damage that many structure fires cause, it is attention to small details and such vague properties as "out of place" that can make the difference between a successfully identified fire origin and the frustrating opinion "undetermined cause."

7.1.2 INTERVIEWS WITH WITNESSES

While the investigation relies on application of the scientific method, the gathering of information from witnesses requires the art of communication. Just like fires, no two witnesses are exactly the same. They may be traumatized or excited, helpful or obstructive. The investigator must be skillful in adopting a demeanor and approach that will encourage the free flow of information and enable an accurate picture to be drawn. It is as important to identify and properly react to the genuine concerns of fire victims as it is to recognize suspicious behavior.

The investigator should attempt to discreetly canvass the neighborhood for witnesses to the fire or people with knowledge as to the structure, its owners, occupants, or its past history. He or she should determine who was in the building last and when and, most important, what the furnishings and contents of the building were and how they were distributed. The combustible contents of a structure have the largest single effect on burn patterns, and the pre-fire fuel load must be identified.

Civilian witnesses to the earliest stages of a fire or explosion can offer information to the investigator that may be impossible to establish in any other way, especially in cases where there is extensive destruction before the fire can be reported or where fire service response is delayed. Their observations could include the following: what was on fire when the fire was noticed, where in the building they first saw fire and/or smoke, how they first become aware of the fire (explosion, smell, sound of breaking glass, smoke or fire alarm, etc.), what unusual smells, sounds, vehicles, or people they noticed just before the fire. When these interviews are conducted, it may help to walk with the witnesses to where they said they were to see if lines of vision are unobstructed. Sometimes the process of re-creating witness position and path triggers additional memories. These interviews will go a long way to helping the investigator establish the starting conditions, that is, what the scene looked like at the start of the fire, a step essential to accurately interpreting the indicators.

7.1.3 INTERVIEWS WITH PUBLIC SAFETY OFFICIALS

Because the suppression activities can affect fire patterns inside, the investigator should determine where the structure was entered and what attacks were made on the fire. Were windows and doors open, closed, or locked upon arrival? Were entry paths blocked? Were doors or windows blocked open (to improve draft)? If so, how was entry made? Did anyone try the lock before forcing the door? It must be remembered that an arsonist usually has to gain entry to a building in the same way as a burglar or other criminal. Signs of forced entry, such as damaged locks or doorjambs or broken windows, are sometimes overlooked by fire investigators who are focused on the fire and its aftermath. Where were attempts made to ventilate the structure to aid in suppression? Were tactics like positive-pressure ventilation used? Because such operations can dramatically affect the course, intensity, and time factors of a fire, the investigator must be made aware of their use and of the response of the fire.

The observations of the first-in firefighters are often crucial to the reconstruction of a fire. What was on fire and what was not? Was the fire localized on one side of the room, just at floor level, just at ceiling level, or was everything on fire (i.e., post-flashover)? Was the smoke so thick one could not tell? More departments are using thermal imaging cameras, and that information may be useful in establishing where the hottest part of the fire was. With the use of protective clothing and self-contained breathing apparatus (SCBA), observations of temperature and odor will usually be very limited, so visual observations will be most important. If the time of entry can be established from the radio log or arrival times of other units, a timeline may be reliably established to at least trace the development of the fire from that point. Fire crews should also be asked about their use or refueling of any gasoline-powered tools or equipment, precautions taken, and locations of use or refueling.

The fire crews can also offer important information as to the weather conditions (wind, temperature, humidity) and the nature of the utilities. Were the gas, electricity, phone, and cable TV in service? Who disconnected them? Did any of the occupants or witnesses speak to the firefighters? What did they say regarding the fire, the building, its contents, or the activities of people around the building recently? The sum total of information gathered by the firefighters combined with their own observations often offers the key to the entire investigation. The skill is to gather the details, compare them with other witnesses' accounts, and make accurate assessments and records in order that conclusions can be properly presented. Many fire departments today request a "debriefing" report from every firefighter who attended, describing what was seen and done.

7.1.4 FIRE PATTERNS

The effects of smoke, hot gases, heat, and flames on materials form the fire patterns that investigators use to trace the course of the fire and, by reversing that process, establish the **area of origin** of the fire. Fire patterns reflect the intensity and duration of thermal exposure. These effects can be generally categorized as follows:

- Surface deposits (with no irreversible effects on substrate)
- Surface thermal effects—scorching or melting, discoloration
- Charring—surface
- Penetration—charring below surface
- Consumption—charring completely through a material or its actual destruction

If no thermal effect is observed on a surface, the investigator can conclude it was not exposed to enough heat to induce any chemical change. In general, the observed changes reflect the intensity of the applied heat flux—the higher the heat flux, the higher the surface temperature (dependent, of course, on the thermal inertia of the surface). In general, the deeper the penetration of the changes, the longer the *duration* of the exposure. The higher the heat flux (or the higher the temperature of the exposed surface), the faster heat is conducted into the material. The total observed damage is the result of both intensity and duration, so both must be taken into account.

7.1.5 TRACING THE COURSE OF THE FIRE

Fire scenes are nearly always cold and badly burned. Thus, the investigator must reconstruct the sequence of the fire backward from what is visible afterward to its point of origin. With few exceptions, fires, however large, start with a small flame, such as a

area of origin ■ A structure, part of a structure, or general geographic location within a fire scene, in which the *"point of origin"* of a fire or explosion is reasonably believed to be located (*NFPA 921*, 2017 ed., pt. 3.3.12; see *also* pt. *3.3.142, Point of Origin*).

match, candle, or lighter, or a spark of some type. The investigator must determine the point and source of ignition in order to determine the cause of the fire. The primary exceptions are fires where the first fuel ignited is a flammable gas or vapor.

The following are key principles of fire behavior:

- Hot gases (including flames) are much lighter than the surrounding air and therefore rise. In the absence of strong winds or physical barriers like ceilings that force hot gases to travel elsewhere, smoke and hot gases will always move upward.
- Due to heat transfer processes in the buoyant flame plume, fire will move upward more rapidly than horizontally or downward with some downward progression as a result of radiant heat and fall-down.
- Combustible materials in the path of the flames will be ignited, thereby increasing the extent and intensity of the fire. The more intense (higher heat release rate) the fire, the faster it will rise and spread.
- If there is not more fuel above or beside the initial flame to be ignited by convected or radiated heat, or if the initial fire is too small to create the necessary heat flux on those fuels, the fire will be self-limiting and often will burn itself out. A flame plume that is large enough to reach the ceiling of a compartment is likely to trigger full involvement of a room, for it is charging the upper gas layer in the room with gases that have not cooled by mixing or radiative losses as much as gases in a shorter plume. As a result, the hot gas layer maintains a higher temperature and is more likely to reach its critical temperature (~600°C or 1,150°F in a typical room), which then induces flashover or full-room involvement.
- The fuel load of the room or structure has a significant impact on the development of a fire. The fuel load includes not only the structure itself but also the furnishings and contents, and the wall, floor, and ceiling coverings that feed a fire and offer it paths and directions with optimum fuel conditions. In evaluating a fire's progress through a room or structure, the investigator must establish what fuels were present and where they were located. The chemical nature of the fuels and their physical forms will affect their ignitability and their expected heat release rate. In the reconstruction of a fire, the fuel load is not just the total number of joules or Btu's of heat that can be generated but the rate at which that heat is released.
- Variations on the upward spread of fire or smoke will occur when air currents deflect the flame, when horizontal surfaces block the vertical travel, or when radiation from established flames ignites nearby surfaces. If fuel is present in these new areas, it will ignite and spread the flames laterally.
- Upward, vertical spread is enhanced when the fire finds chimneylike configurations. Stairways, elevators, utility shafts, air ducts, and interiors of walls and hollow support columns offer openings for carrying flames generated elsewhere, and fires may burn more intensely because of the enhanced draft.
- Downward spread will occur whenever there is suitable fuel in the area. Fire will burn downward across a solid fuel but at a rate that is a tiny fraction of its upward spread rate. Combustible wall coverings, particularly paneling, encourage the travel of fire downward as well as outward. Burning portions of ceiling and roof coverings, draperies, and lighting fixtures can fall onto ignitable fuels below and start new fires called fall-down or **drop-down** fires that quickly join the main fire overhead. Radiation from rollover fires or very hot gas layers can ignite floor coverings, furniture, and walls even at some distance, creating new areas of fire. The resulting fire patterns can be complex to interpret, and, once again, the investigator must remember to take into account what fuel packages were present from the standpoint of their potential heat release rate contributions.
- Suppression efforts can enhance fire spread. Positive-pressure ventilation (PPV) or an active hose stream attack on one face of a fire may force it back into other areas

drop-down ■ The spread of fire by the dropping or falling of burning materials. Synonymous with "fall-down" (*NFPA 921*, 2017 ed., pt. 3.3.49).

that may or may not have already been involved, and push fire down, even under obstructions such as doors or cabinets. The investigator must remember those unusual conditions and check with the firefighters present.

- Fire tends to flow through a room or structure much like a liquid—upward in relatively straight paths and outward and around barriers.
- Ventilation from open doors, windows, or vents, or forced by heating, ventilating, and air conditioning (HVAC) systems or PPV fans can affect fire growth and movement as much as fuel arrangement. All ventilation must be documented.
- The hot gas layer in a room can reach its critical intensity (producing a heat flux of >20 kW/m^2) if the fire is large enough to overcome the leaks of hot gases due to openings or due to radiant and conductive losses. As seen in the 1985 Bradford (UK) football stadium fire, even a compartment that is open on three sides can develop flashover conditions when the fire gets big enough.
- Fire intensity in a post-flashover room is often greatest around ventilation sources. Thus, damage occurs more quickly around door sills, windows, or other openings where fresh air can be drawn into the room and can even reach walls opposite the opening.
- The total fire damage to an object is the result of both the intensity of heat applied to that object and the duration of the exposure (with the realization that intensity of heat varies considerably during a fire and that all the exposure may not have occurred at the same time).

7.1.6 IMPLICATIONS FOR THE FIRE INVESTIGATOR

Fire investigation and the reconstruction of a fire's growth pattern back to its origin are based on the fact that fires form patterns of damage that are, to a large extent, predictable. With an understanding of combustion properties, heat transfer, and general fire behavior, the investigator can reliably examine a fire scene for specific indicators. Using each indicator as an independent test for direction of travel, intensity or duration of heat application, or point of origin, the investigator can approximate the fire's development.

Every fire forms a pattern determined by the configuration of the room or structure, the availability of fuel, and ventilation effects. Because of the upward-reaching tendency of flames, a conical form of fire damage is most common, with the apex at the bottom being a source of fire, possibly a point of origin, and the fire rising and spreading out from there. This pattern will be altered by the presence of obstructions or the availability (or lack) of fuel in an area. Thus, interior fires often appear to have very complex patterns as the result of complex structural arrangement rather than any unusual property of the fire.

The task of the investigator is to identify the origin (the point or space where the fire began), examine that space for possible ignition sources, and identify the fuel first ignited at the origin, even by elimination, to establish a causal link between the ignition source and the final destructive fire. If the investigator cannot identify the fuel first ignited, the ignition source competent to ignite that fuel, and the circumstances that brought that fuel and that ignition source together, the cause cannot be conclusively established. This determination is not limited to the identification of physical residues of both fuel and ignition source, but may depend on the hypothesis testing of observed fire behavior and damage.

7.1.7 ANALYSIS AND HYPOTHESIS TESTING

The investigator must be aware of any tendency to prejudge the origin and cause of any fire. The fire scene investigation is carried out to identify the origin of the fire (where it started), and its cause (what burned at the area of origin and what caused the fuel to ignite). Careful evaluation of the indicators should result in an accurate determination of at least an area, if not a point, of origin and a hypothesis of the direction, intensity, and duration of the fire. Without at least a definable general area or origin, no reliable evaluation of ignition sources can be carried out.

In the vicinity of the origin, the presence of the first fuel ignited and a possible ignition source should have been detected. The investigator must be able to define and defend the chain of events from the event that brought the first fuel and ignition source together to the spread of the fire, based on knowledge of the location and size of major fuel packages and relevant fire dynamics. The amount of damage visible must correspond to the heat release rate that would be expected from those packages.

The scientific method demands that all reasonably possible alternative hypotheses be evaluated; tested against test data, scene evidence, or witness information; and eliminated to demonstrate the reliability of the final conclusion. It is also necessary to be sure all data critical to such testing are collected and documented.

Even in the absence of an incendiary device, the crime of arson can be proven in the absence of *all* logically possible accidental and natural causes at the point of origin. This methodology is sometimes called a *negative corpus*, since a complete positive corpus for the crime of arson includes proof of burning, proof of incendiary cause, and proof of absence of natural and accidental causes. The term negative corpus has no recognized definition but *implies* that the corpus of the crime (or event) has not been proven. This is *not* to say it is permissible to conclude a fire is an arson simply because too much damage was done or because no accidental source could be identified. While some investigators treat negative corpus as a catchall, it is a very difficult case to *prove* and should be relied upon only in the most special circumstances. Negative corpus cases are accepted in some jurisdictions and not in others, so the investigator should confer with local prosecutors before pursuing such cases.

The thorough investigator also considers all possible alternative explanations for the fire and evaluates the evidence, whether physical or testimonial, in deciding whether those alternatives are excluded. Application of the *Bilancia Ignition Matrix*™ will result in consideration of likely first fires and ignition sources. Such consideration and elimination of alternative scenarios is a primary element of the scientific method of fire investigation.

Careful engineering analysis including fire modeling may be useful in testing and eliminating hypotheses. If alternative explanations cannot be excluded, additional information either from the scene or from research or testing can clarify the energies, times, or conditions for each hypothesis. Based on additional data, it may be possible to exclude other hypotheses and make it easier to defend the final conclusion. Termed *affirmative exclusion* instead of *negative corpus*, this reasoning can be applied in cases where the first fuel ignited and source of ignition cannot be positively demonstrated if the scientific reasoning and assessment can be shown to be sound.

It is not possible to identify the cause of every fire. Depending on the extent of damage to the structure, there may not be enough information to reliably conclude the actual cause. If all possible explanations cannot be excluded, then the professional investigator must recognize his or her limitations, as well as the limitations of the evidence, and realize that it is time to admit that the cause is undetermined.

7.2 General Considerations

7.2.1 PROTECTED AREAS

Protected areas (i.e., areas that have not been damaged by the flames) are sometimes as significant as areas that are badly charred. Areas shielded by an appliance, piece of furniture, or waste basket may assist the fire investigator in (1) establishing the locations of objects and (2) identifying the general type of the object. For example, a bucket that

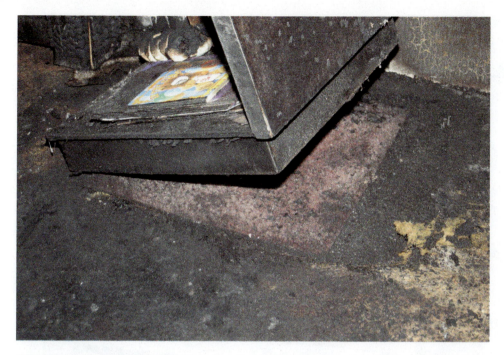

FIGURE 7-1 Protected areas of the carpet show the locations of furniture during the fire. *Courtesy of Jamie Novak, Novak Investigations and St. Paul Fire Dept.*

originally contained liquid accelerant (or a metal wastebasket where a discarded cigarette ignited the contents) might be placed on the floor in the fire area, and its location would be proved. Delineation is generally so accurate that the size and shape of the bottom of the object is readily determined and compared with any suspect item that is located.

The greatest damage will be at points where active flame or radiant heat existed for an appreciable time. Because flames burn upward, floor areas do not receive as much active flame as other fuels. Flames will char by radiant heat in most instances, but it is often noted that areas of the floor are totally undamaged though surrounded by damaged areas (Sanderson 2001). These areas tend to have a definite form (e.g., circular or rectangular) and invariably show clearly the location of an object sitting on the floor at the time of the fire (see Figure 7-1). The object may be combustible and show the effect as well as though it were noncombustible. Cardboard cartons often serve to protect the floor under them, because the bottom of the carton does not burn well due to poor ventilation, even when the remainder of the carton is totally destroyed.

In fires that approached flashover, protected areas on the floor can reveal the locations of furniture or victims that were moved, or even combustibles, like paper or cardboard, that were consumed during the later stages of the fire, as in Figures 7-2 and 7-3. These objects are frequently removed during the firefighting or in clearing the area afterward and will only occasionally be found still sitting in the original position. When undamaged areas are found, it is up to the investigator to determine what object protected the floor and where it is now. Objects are most often removed during suppression or overhaul, but sometimes, the perpetrator removes the remains of a container or delay device after the fire. Thus, it is important for the scene to be secured from all persons until the investigation is complete.

In a fire where a metal wastebasket or trash can forms a protected area, if there is not much fuel in the can or the fire is prolonged, fire may heat the bottom of the can and scorch the floor beneath. In most cases, the bottom of the container will protect the area

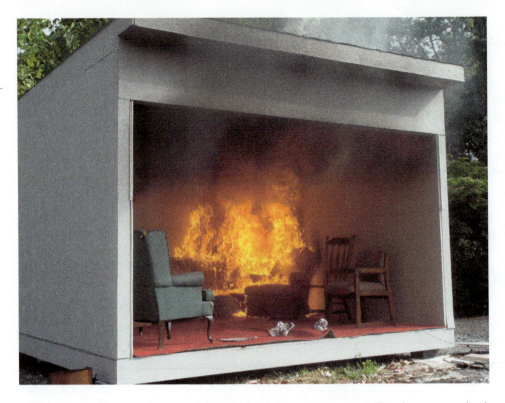

under it as well as retain manufacturer data. Its position may then be accurately determined if the floor is discolored or charred around it. A fire starting inside a plastic wastebasket will tend to cause collapse uniformly around the perimeter. A fire involving a container from outside will usually cause asymmetric melting (greater on the side facing the oncoming fire).

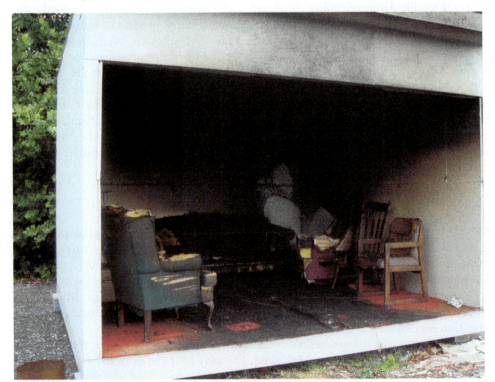

FIGURE 7-3 Test fire from Fig. 7-2 after extinguishment. Note protected areas beneath chairs as well as newspapers on floor in front. *Courtesy of David J. Icove, University of Tennessee.*

By examining the arrangement adjacent to the trash container and the extent of fire in this region, the investigator may be able to assign the source of the fire to this origin or to rule it out. Without the knowledge of the exact location of the container, this is likely to be impossible or very difficult. Often, a fan-shaped char pattern will occur on a wall just over the source of the fire, with its lower boundary at the height of such a trash container. This circumstance is frequently the best evidence of the trash container as the origin of the blaze. When a plastic gasoline container is ignited in a fire, it burns or melts from the top down. If there is liquid fuel left in it, the fuel will be trapped between the folds of the collapsing container. Some liquid may leak out when the mass is overturned, or it may be detected by a visible or audible sloshing.

Scrutiny of protected areas on walls yield clues to fire cause, origin and spread. The location of an item of furniture that is no longer present can often be determined accurately from such an area, as shown in Figures 7-4 and 7-5. The opposite effect is also observed occasionally in instances where the furniture burned and collapsed; instead of protecting the wall behind it, it enhanced the burn. Such protection effects will not necessarily serve to locate the position of a specific piece of furniture, because the marginal dimensions are lost, but they can, at times, contribute significant knowledge of the fire origin, when considered along with the general fire pattern. Localized floor penetrations are often caused by combustible furniture burning for prolonged periods.

A combination of the two effects is also sometimes seen. When a piece of furniture is afire, it may both protect the wall behind it and, by intensifying the local fire, increase the amount of wall damage on the sides and above the item. This is especially important when the fire started in the furniture in question. Ventilation effects can also produce low burns, even in the absence of localized fuel packages.

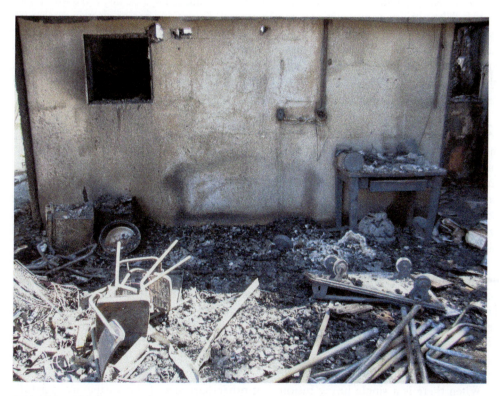

FIGURE 7-4 This fire occurred on a covered patio (assuring plenty of ventilation) and burned post-flashover. The outline of the completely destroyed sofa (and likely origin) is still visible on the stucco wall. *Courtesy of Derrick Fire Investigations.*

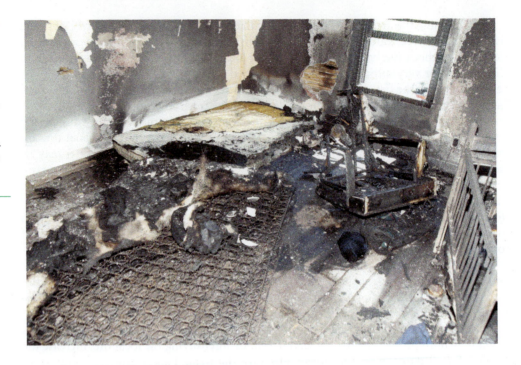

FIGURE 7-5 Protected area on left wall shows there was a mattress in place at the time of the fire. Damaged area on right wall and damaged area of mattress in foreground shows the mattress was overturned during firefighting. *Courtesy of Jamie Novak, Novak Investigations and St. Paul Fire Dept.*

7.2.2 UTILITIES

The condition of the utilities servicing the building should always be inspected and documented. When utility companies respond to a scene to remove gas or electric meters (to ensure the safety of scene investigators), they should be asked to evaluate the service for signs of tampering, bypassing, damage, or malfunction. The investigator should determine when power, gas, telephone, cable TV, and the like were cut off and by whom. Sometimes a planned fire will be betrayed by the owner's cutting off costly services several days before the structure was destroyed.

7.2.3 ELECTRICAL IGNITION SOURCES

Checking out an electrical system in a burned structure is often the most frustrating portion of the entire examination. Wires, conduits, and remains of fixtures are often scattered throughout the rubble. This can include the utilities, appliances, and electrical wiring, both fixed and power cords. Wires will generally lack insulation, as this will have been burned off in the fire. Because wiring is most commonly of copper that, when heated, is readily oxidized to copper oxide, the blackened and brittle condition of the wires will make them difficult to handle when attempting to trace them.

The most significant item to look for in such an instance is not just a mass of damaged wire but rather fused copper in localized areas. Such fused masses are most likely to occur near switches, outlets, and similar connections, and at the fuse box. At any of these places it is common to find wires with rounded, fused ends, which demonstrates that there was arcing, almost certainly by short-circuiting. When there are numerous such fused ends it is unlikely that a fire origin has been found, but rather that the breakers failed to shut off current when wires farther away from the breaker or fuse box shorted together as the insulation failed in the fire.

When there is a single heavy fusion, but other portions of the wiring are generally intact, this single point becomes highly suspect as a *possible* source of ignition. Normally, in such an instance, the fuse is blown or the breaker is open, indicating that this short circuit occurred and triggered the safety mechanism. Protective devices respond to a direct short and usually interrupt power before a fire can be started. High-resistance connections, on the other hand, can create enough heat for long periods of time without drawing enough current to trip protective devices. These long-term heat sources are much more likely to ignite ordinary fuels than momentary short-circuit arcs. Examination of the fuse box or circuit breaker panel to determine which circuits have been tripped may be helpful in eliminating areas and the circuits that serve them.

Wire within a metal conduit will rarely short except when the conduit is heated sufficiently by an external fire to char the wire's insulation. If a short circuit is formed within a conduit from any cause, it must be a high-energy one to penetrate to the exterior and start a fire, although such events are not unknown [involving unprotected circuits, high-current applications (>40 A), failed overcurrent protection devices, or three-phase wiring]. Starting a fire requires that the conduit itself be heated. In a very rare instance, it might be heated above the ignition temperature of some material in contact with it, which could become ignited. The high heat conductivity of the metal conduit is actually a very good protection against starting of fires from wires enclosed in the conduit.

Zinc die casts used in conduit connectors have relatively low melting points and will melt in a fire surrounding the conduit. The heat of the fire may also remove the insulation, so that molten zinc will contact copper. When this occurs, the zinc and copper will form brass. Either the molten zinc or the brass formed may complete a short circuit between wires not previously in contact. This effect is not a cause of the fire but the result of an external fire. The presence of brass within a conduit or spilled from a broken conduit is good evidence of an external fire that led to its formation.

7.2.4 ARC MAPPING

The plotting of electric arcing in electrical wiring found at a fire scene is valuable in testing hypotheses about possible areas of origin. A map of arc faults can be overlaid on diagrams of other indicators. If the electric circuit involved can be traced back to its power source, the location of the arc fault (which caused the overcurrent device to trip or the conductors to part) farthest from the power source is likely to be the area closest to the origin. This assumes that the wiring was equally exposed to the fire. Wiring concealed in walls will be affected much later than exposed power cords. Arc-fault mapping is not used to establish whether an electrical fault caused the fire but as an indicator of area of origin. For guidance on arc mapping, refer to the latest edition of NFPA 921, pt. 9.11.7 (NFPA 2017).

7.2.5 APPLIANCE CONDITION

The appearance of an appliance that started a fire is different from that of one that was in a fire, but the differences can be difficult to spot. The external fire will damage any appliance by burning the enamel, discoloring and corroding the steel, and otherwise distorting or warping it. If the fire is external to the appliance, whatever damage it suffers will show uniformity, or at least agreement, with the fire patterns on walls, furniture, or other appliances in the vicinity. The appliance is much less likely to be damaged internally if the cabinet or housing is noncombustible. If the appliance started the fire, it will be damaged more internally than externally and will usually have some local damage or effect that is quite distinct from the general damage pattern. Because fires are easily blamed on a faulty oven or a maladjusted furnace, incendiary fires are sometimes ignited in the vicinity of such appliances to throw the investigator off the track.

In most such instances, the arsonist will pour a flammable liquid around and under the appliance and then ignite it. In such instances, it is normal for the liquid to penetrate below the appliance and to give a burn far below that which is possible for the appliance itself. Gas appliances and fireplaces will usually lead to fire above the base level of the normal combustion, not to a region under the floor. Burns below this level of support may be traceable to a failure or defect of the gas supply or firebox or to improper installation.

In some instances, there may be penetration of the floor under a fireplace or stove/heater due to the dropping of hot materials onto the combustible floor through gaps in the firebox. Burning to the floor level is not normal for a fire escaping from an appliance unless there is very obvious and severe damage to the unit itself.

The investigator will need to determine if there were defects in the appliance. Misuse of any heat-producing appliance can cause a fire, and any fire in the vicinity should be considered suspect and investigated with extraordinary care. A portable x-ray system, such as those used by bomb squads, can be used to examine appliances and connectors at the scene. Such examinations may reveal useful information without destructive dismantling.

One cause of accidental fires that is often related to appliances is the formation of "self-heating charcoal" by prolonged exposure of a wood surface to heat. The investigator should consider this as a possibility whenever wood is exposed to even moderate temperatures [over 105°C (220°F), or so)] in conditions where ventilation is excluded or very limited. The lower the temperature, the longer it takes for a sufficient mass of such charring to form, and the less likely its formation will occur at all. Wood exposed to temperatures below 300°C (600°F) for a long time is characteristically dull- or flat-finished, with a sunken appearance. Char that has penetrated completely through the wood structures involved and is much deeper than the known circumstances of the fire should be further examined. This phenomenon has been thought to turn even large wooden structural members completely to charcoal over a period of months or years before finally igniting them. Post-suppression and prolonged smoldering can also produce deep destruction.

7.2.6 TRASH

Trash accumulations found at a fire scene can contribute information to the fire investigation as they can be an ignition source, especially when doused with a liquid accelerant. However, they also can be set on fire by accident. Both possibilities must be considered before deciding that a trash pile was used by an arsonist. If liquid flammables were poured on the trash, some of the liquid may be recovered and identified, in which case, strong evidence of arson is available. When a trash pile appears to be an origin or possible origin of the fire, it is important to search both for ignitable liquids, as well as ignition sources and for clues that the ignition could have been accidental.

7.2.7 DETECTION SYSTEMS MAPPING

In a large compartment or a building protected by fire alarm or sprinkler systems, the investigator should document detectors or sprinkler heads triggered during the fire on a map of the building. This map can reveal the most energetic (if not the first) stages of the fire. When the times of their responses are included, a sequence of the fire's spread may be reconstructed. Many alarm systems have a data chip that can be read after the fire that reveals the time of functioning of connected systems and the sequence of various alarm functions. When contacted, alarm companies can provide information about alarm settings, functions, and history.

The sprinkler system and its connections should be examined and documented. Fire investigators should be familiar with system components and signs of tampering or inoperability.

7.2.8 INTERIOR FIRES FROM EXTERIOR SOURCES

Fires within structures do not always originate inside the building. Structural fires can start from:

- a fire in an adjacent building spread by radiant heat or burning debris,
- grass or brush fires exterior to the building,

- trash fires that are out of control, or
- arson by trash or accelerant ignition against the side of the structure, under porches, or around doors.

When the fire is initially outside the building, it may involve exterior surfaces and never penetrate to the interior. Such a fire pattern is obvious and the cause simple to determine. However, special circumstances may exist. For example, an open door or window, combined with wind and burning fragments from a nearby fire, may start a fire on the interior with no burning of the exterior structure. This fire would have an interior origin that would be traced in the conventional manner. Radiation from a large nearby fire can ignite the interior of a building through windows and doors before the exterior is ignited. In this case, the determination of cause depends on demonstrating the existence of a nearby fire, the wind, the opening, and the absence of any other reasonable interior cause. While these types of fires are not common, they can be quite challenging to the investigator, because they prompt reports of multiple fire origins from witnesses and firefighters.

7.2.9 ROOF AND ATTIC FIRES

Airborne burning materials, like tree branches, falling on combustible roofs are a common type of transmission of fire from an exterior source. These types of fires threaten residential areas surrounded by brush or timber and have caused heavy destruction in fires in San Diego, San Bernardino, Orange, and Los Angeles counties in California. One such fire spread caused the destructive Oakland Hills fire that destroyed 2,500 homes and 500 apartment units in a single day in 1991. The investigator must consider variations in the mode of transmission of fire from point to point depending on the ambient conditions as well as environmental conditions.

In residences, it is not uncommon for a roof to burn away or for a combined attic-roof fire to occur. For this reason, attic and roof fires are often confused and can lead to misinterpretation. A roof-started fire is totally different in behavior from an attic-started fire. In both instances, the absence of fire on a lower level will define the fire as being one or the other, but often it is difficult to determine which.

An attic fire is started under the roof and will usually involve all the roof that is accessible to the spread of flames beneath it. Thus, it is likely that the entire roof is either burned away or that destruction is very widespread. Widespread burning in the attic is indicative of this type of fire.

A roof fire, in contrast, must have been ignited from the exterior, otherwise it would have developed as an attic fire. Sparks from chimneys, or similar causes, may ignite leaf debris, shingles, or shakes on a roof, resulting in an exterior fire. This fire will follow the usual inverted-cone pattern on an inclined roof and will ultimately penetrate the roof into the attic below. At this point the main distinction between an attic-started and a roof-started fire becomes apparent. The first hole that burns through the roof ventilates the fire, drawing air upward through the hole, which generally confines the fire to the exterior and to parts of the roof immediately adjacent to the hole. Here, air is being drawn from the attic to the fire, which in some instances suffices to prevent a secondary spread as an attic fire. The major burn is usually on the outside of the roof, not under it, although in some steep roofs fire can spread internally up along the inside pitch of the roof. If enough of the roof is involved, of course, structural collapse can spread the fire down into the living space, eventually causing a total burnout.

In an attic fire, there is almost always a great deal of burning under all parts of the roof before the roof is breached. Because upward ventilation is limited, spread of the fire is inevitable. Fire spread on the underside of a combustible roof assembly (plywood or wood lattice) can be very rapid and difficult to extinguish. After a hole is chopped in the roof to ventilate the fire under it, that fire can then be controlled much more easily because

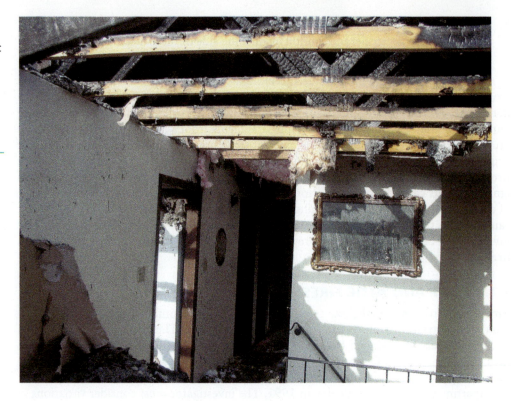

FIGURE 7-6 Ceiling joists exhibit typical top-down burning in this attic fire where there is a relative absence of damage to worn contents below. *Courtesy of Greg Lampkin, Knox County Sheriff's Office, Tennessee, Fire Investigation Unit.*

the flames are funneled toward the hole that ventilates them. Figure 7-6 illustrates the burned-from-the-top-down appearance of ceiling joists after a typical attic fire.

Although the destruction may not be significantly different in the roof and attic fires, the investigations differ, because the roof fire is caused by external ignition, while the attic fire is ignited within the structure.

7.2.10 TIMELINES

Every fire has a life cycle—from the time a heat source first comes into contact with the first fuel to its extinguishment. The timeline for this cycle is defined by the following time factors: (1) ignition time, (2) incipient fire duration, (3) response time, and (4) extinguishment time. The nature of the ignition source and the nature of the first fuel control the ignition time and incipient fire. The fire growth is controlled by the fuel, its arrangement, and the ventilation conditions. These factors can be estimated from test data from existing research or specialized tests or case history as part of the hypothesis testing.

As seen on the modeling data form in the chapter on documentation, establishing a timeline includes hard times linked directly or indirectly to an accurate and reliable clock or timing device and soft times linked to someone last in the vicinity, alarm set or activation times, time of detection by witnesses, time of 9-1-1 call, arrival time, and sometimes time of control or extinguishment. Soft times are estimates of clock time or duration by witnesses or engineering analysis of known fire behaviors. Timelines can be used to test and exclude some scenarios such as smoky self-heating processes or instantaneous ignition by discarded cigarette and suggest other scenarios. The successful use of a timeline depends on the investigator's knowledge of time factors in all manner of fires. Timelines can be reconstructed from fire or police dispatch recordings, 9-1-1 calls, or from videos of events from security and surveillance cameras, cell phones, or police, fire, or public transport windshield.

7.3 Collection and Preservation of Evidence

A complete fire scene evidence kit should be carried and available at all fire scenes. Briefly, an evidence kit has a number of containers for various kinds of physical evidence and the tools that may be required to recover them. Evidence recognition, recovery, and preservation all follow rules of plain common sense. Preservation of evidence means just that—*preserve* it until it reaches the laboratory or the court. Preservation, via proper collection and packaging, means the evidence is not allowed to change by evaporating, breaking, spoiling, or being contaminated. Think about the limitations of the evidence being picked up and package it accordingly.

If it is a volatile liquid you suspect, you do not want it to evaporate, so package it in an airtight can or jar and keep it cool and sealed. If it is an organic—blood, tissue, soil, or hair—you do not want to let it decompose by mildewing or developing mold. If you allow such material to air dry at room temperature, package it in clean paper containers, and keep it dry and cool, it will stay intact. With fragile objects, avoid further breakage by packing them in suitable containers and hand-carrying them to the lab. Minute trace evidence, which is easily lost or contaminated, is best preserved by placing it in a clean container of suitable size and sealing it. Comparison samples of any floor coverings involved in the fire's origin should be taken (preferably from areas not damaged by fire) not only to aid laboratory analysis for volatiles but also to help reconstruct the potential contributions the carpet and pad could make to the fuel load in the room and the spread of fire.

Table 7-1 lists some common evidence types and collection and preservation methods. Guidelines for evidence collection are the subject of *ASTM E1188* and *E1459*.

TABLE 7-1	Physical Evidence Collection and Preservation		
EVIDENCE TYPE	**SAMPLE AMOUNT DESIRED**	**PACKAGING**	**SPECIAL HANDLING**
Checks, letters, and other documents	All	▪ Place in manila envelope; do not fold; wrap securely.	▪ Do not handle with bare hands.
Fire debris with suspected accelerants	All	▪ Seal in clean empty metal paint can, Kapak (by Ampac) or nylon bag, or glass jar; fill container no more than 3/4 full.	▪ Label as to origin and collecting investigator; keep cool.
Flammable liquids	All (up to 500 ml; 1 pt)	▪ Seal in glass bottle, jar with Bakelite or metal top with Teflon liner, or metal can.	▪ Do not use rubber stoppers or jars with rubber seals; do not use plastic bottles.
Charred or burned paper or cardboard	All	▪ Pack loosely on soft cotton; hand-carry to laboratory.	▪ Pack in rigid container; mark FRAGILE; do not treat with lacquer or other coating.
Clothing	All	▪ Mark directly on clothing in waistband, pocket, or coat collar with initials and date; pack in clean paper bags; wrap each item separately in paper; do not use plastic bags; on outside of container indicate nature of item, date obtained, and investigator's name.	▪ If clothing is wet with water or blood, hang to air dry before packaging to prevent putrefaction; fold neatly with clean paper between folds, and refrigerate if possible. If there are residues of ignitable liquids, seal in metal can or Kapak bag. Freeze if possible.

| TABLE 7-1 | Physical Evidence Collection and Preservation (*Continued*) |

EVIDENCE TYPE	SAMPLE AMOUNT DESIRED	PACKAGING	SPECIAL HANDLING
Hairs and fibers	Any loose hairs or fibers. Comparisons: clumps of 10 to 20 closely cut pubic or head hairs from various areas	■ Pill box, paper envelope or bindle, cellophane or plastic bag; seal carefully.	■ On outside of container: label as to type of material, where found, date, investigator's name.
Paint chips	At least 100 mm² (1/2 in.²) of flake; entire object if small	■ Pill box, paper bindle, or envelope; seal carefully.	■ Obtain control sample from outside transfer area.
Soil	At least 25 g (1 oz)	■ Plastic bag or jar. If suspected of containing volatiles, seal in glass jar or metal can and freeze.	■ Collect several samples from area.
Tools	All	■ Wrap each tool separately to prevent shifting and loss of trace evidence.	■ Secure envelope or folded sheet of paper carefully over end of tool to prevent damage and loss of adhering paints, etc.
Tool marks	Send in tool if found; submit all items having tool mark scratches.	■ After marks have been protected, wrap with wrapping paper and place in envelope or box.	■ Cover marks with soft paper, tape in place; keep from rusting.
Dry blood stains	As much as possible; submit object if possible	■ Use paper bags, boxes, bindles, or envelopes; seal to prevent loss of scrapings; keep dry; do not use plastic bags; refrigerate if possible.	■ On outside of container: type of specimen, date secured, investigator's name, and where found.
Glass fragments	As much as possible	■ Box, paper bags, bindle, or envelope; pack and seal to avoid movement in container.	■ On outside of container: type of specimen, date, investigator's name, and number. Keep evidence separated from control sample.
Firearms	All	■ Place revolvers and automatics in cardboard box or manila envelope; tag rifles; hand-carry to laboratory.	■ Unload: note cylinder position; if automatic, do not handle side of magazine—possible fingerprints in this location; note serial number and make of weapon.
Latent fingerprints	All	■ Secure in rigid container so surfaces do not rub on packaging. Clean paper envelope OK for porous objects. Keep dry and cool.	■ Allow to air-dry if damp. Keep immersed in water if recovered from water.

ignitable liquid ■ Any liquid or the liquid phase of any material that is capable of fueling a fire, including a flammable liquid, combustible liquid, or any other material that can be liquefied and burned (*NFPA 921,* 2017 ed., pt. 3.3.111).

7.3.1 DEBRIS SUSPECTED OF CONTAINING VOLATILES

The most commonly submitted form of arson evidence is solid debris suspected of containing the residue of **ignitable liquids.** The major concern here is to prevent the evaporation of volatile liquids. Collection of all physical evidence must be carried out with full realization of the chances of contamination. Due to the sensitivity of laboratory methods, invisible traces of volatiles transferred by the tools, gloves, or even the boots of the investigator can compromise the value of such trace evidence.

The investigator must:

- Carefully clean trowels, scoops, brooms, and brushes in clean running water using detergent and water between scenes and between collection sites at the same scene.
- Clean and wipe tools with a clean paper towel between samples.
- Wear clean disposable plastic or latex gloves and then change them before collecting debris.
- Always use a container similar in size to the amount of debris and collect *more* than you think the laboratory will need.

No matter how strongly it smells of accelerant, more debris is always preferred. Debris can best be preserved in clean metal friction-lid paint cans, which are reasonably airtight and unbreakable. The cans come in a variety of sizes, they are easily opened and resealed, and the top can easily be punched for insertion of a sampling syringe. They can be lined or unlined, but unlined cans tend to rust very quickly, so lined cans (used for water-based paints) are preferable. Today's linings contain no significant volatile residues.

The second choice for containing debris suspected of containing volatiles is the familiar Mason jar, which is airtight and transparent, permitting ready visual examination of the contents, and has a metal top for easy sampling. The third choice is a glass jar or bottle with a metal or Bakelite cap or a Teflon liner. Plastic caps, rubber seals, or stoppers should never be used when a liquid sample of suspected material is submitted. Gasoline, paint thinner, and other common volatile hydrocarbons will attack and dissolve such closures. Do not fill any container more than three-quarters full of debris to leave a headspace for sampling.

Two types of polymeric bags have been found suitable for packaging most volatile evidence. Bags made of nylon film (sold by Grand River) or special polyester film (Kapak™ sold by Ampac) have been found to retain even the lightest hydrocarbons for moderate lengths of time. They will allow the loss of methyl and ethyl alcohols, however, and debris suspected of containing these unusual accelerants should be sealed in metal cans or glass jars. For most debris, however, such bags provide a convenient, low-cost, and unbreakable alternative container (DeHaan and Skalsky 1981). The polyester bags are heat-sealable and provide even greater integrity to the evidence container than a tape seal (Mann 2000). Any polymeric bag can be penetrated by sharp debris, so care must be used (Demers-Kohl et al. 1994). Because of a minute chance of contamination during manufacturing of some cans and bags, a sample container from each batch should be tested for the presence of trace hydrocarbons before they are issued for use (Kinard and Midkiff 1991).

A common household plastic container should be used as a last resort. Polypropylene jars are permissible, but never polystyrene, which is readily soluble in gasoline. Polyethylene plastic bags, caps for coffee cans, and wrapping films are permeable to some hydrocarbons and allow them to escape (or cross-contamination to occur) before analysis can be attempted and should not be used for arson debris. Paper and polyethylene bags also allow cross-contamination, as external volatiles can permeate them and be absorbed by evidence within. For large, awkward items, large plastic bags may be the only packaging alternative. In such cases, the evidence should be double-bagged and taken to the laboratory as soon as possible, and be kept as cool as possible in the interim.

Refrigeration and even freezing is recommended for all arson fire debris except for glass jars containing wet debris that can expand and shatter the container if frozen. Freezing is especially important when soil is collected for ignitable liquid residues, as the bacteria in garden soil can decompose petroleum products if stored at room temperatures (Mann and Gresham 1990).

7.3.2 OTHER SOLID EVIDENCE

Chemicals from clandestine drug laboratories and most chemical incendiary mixtures are corrosive and care must be taken to ensure they are *not* packaged in metal cans, which can be destroyed by the chemical action. When such corrosives are suspected, the debris may be packaged in glass jars (then kept upright to avoid contact between the lid and debris) or in nylon or polyester bags, which are then sealed in cans.

Nonporous materials such as glass do not retain volatile petroleum distillates, but wrappers, labels, and associated debris may offer absorbent surfaces to retain enough for characterization in the lab. If bottle fragments are found from a suspected Molotov cocktail, locate the neck and base of the bottle sides and label, and package all of it to prevent further breakage. The neck often retains portions of the cloth wick, the base bears manufacturer's data to identify the bottle, and the sides and label may bear usable latent fingerprints. The neck may also bear saliva with identifiable DNA.

Newly developed techniques using lasers, chemicals, and physical developers are now making it possible to recover identifiable latent prints from objects that have been exposed to gasoline, water, or even fire. Unless an object has been heavily damaged by direct exposure to fire, there is a chance that latents and DNA can be recovered (Tontarski et al. 2009; Nic Daéid 2014). The crime laboratory should be contacted for advice before dismissing the possibility of prints, because prints have been identified on glass bottles, plastic jugs, and metal cans even after fire exposure (Deans 2006; Nic Daéid 2003; Nic Daéid 2014; Tontarski et al. 2009).

7.3.3 LIQUIDS

Uncontaminated flammable liquids from the scene are the best kind of evidence for laboratory analysis. If the liquid is still in its original container, as long as that container can be properly sealed, it may be left in the original container. Otherwise, transfer liquids by eyedropper (pipette) or syringe to a clean sealable container. Do *not* use a bottle with a rubber stopper or a jar with a rubber sealing ring for any liquid hydrocarbon. It will dissolve the rubber and leak out. A small quantity of liquid in debris may be recovered directly with an eyedropper or by absorbing it into a pad of clean absorbent cloth, gauze, or cotton wool, and then sealing it in a suitable airtight container.

When flammable liquids are suspected in concrete, samples can be collected from cracks or expansion joints, but often, a better method is to wet-broom the suspected area and then spread a quantity of absorbent material. The best absorbent is clay-type kitty litter, although diatomaceous earth or even flour can be used. This layer is allowed to stand for 20 to 30 minutes and then recovered into a clean metal can using a clean putty knife and brush for laboratory analysis (Tontarski 1985; Mann and Putaansuu 2006). A control sample of the unused absorbent must be sealed in a separate can. The cleanliness of the absorbent (and any collection tools used) is critical to the value of this evidence. The use of hazardous material recovery pads is not recommended due to the possible contamination of such pads by exposure to volatile materials in the environment. Chemically aggressive absorbents such as activated charcoal are not recommended due to their susceptibility for external contamination.

7.3.4 TESTING OF HANDS

Liquid hydrocarbon fuels can be absorbed into the skin after even brief exposure, but the warmth of living tissue causes rapid desorption of such volatiles. Over the years, a number of methods have been suggested for testing of hands of suspects in arson investigations. Canines have often alerted to hands contaminated with gasoline even after some time has elapsed, but the trace amounts present make recovery for laboratory analysis very difficult. Methods such as swabbing with a dry or solvent-wetted cotton gauze are useless for recovering such traces. The best system is to place a clean disposable PVC or latex glove on each of the suspect's hands or to secure a polyester or nylon fire debris bag around the hand with a rubber band at the wrist, enclosing an activated carbon recovery device (such as a carbon strip or solid-phase microextraction (SPME) device) in the bag for 15 to 20 minutes. The warmth of the skin will cause the absorbed volatiles to evaporate into the glove or bag (assisted by exposure to a heating lamp), where they are sampled by the activated carbon. After the subject removes his or her hand, the glove or bag is sealed with the sampling device inside and forwarded to the lab for analysis. Tests indicate that for this testing to yield positive results, it must be done within an hour or two of contact with gasoline (Almirall et al. 2000; Darrer et al. 2000).

Swabbing of the hands of suspects in explosives cases using dry cotton-tipped swabs [such as those in gunshot residue (GSR) kits] or ones wetted with distilled water or methyl or isopropyl alcohol (but *not* with the acid supplied with the GSR kit) can capture traces of either organic or inorganic explosives. Fingernail scrapings using clean, flat wooden toothpicks are collected and sealed in clean glass or plastic vials. This technique is particularly valuable for soft organic explosives such as dynamite or C-4.

7.3.5 TESTING OF CLOTHING

Rapid pouring of an ignitable liquid onto a hard surface often causes spattering onto nearby shoes and pants cuffs. Arsonists may also step into the liquid after it is poured. The gas chromatographic profile of such transfers will be different from that from vapor contact alone. Because such volatiles are lost within a few hours (1 to 6) if the garment is worn, residues on clothing can help identify the perpetrator. Clothing of a suspect should be seized as soon as possible and packaged *separately* in appropriate sealed containers until tested by the lab.

A New Zealand study illustrated the desirability of analyzing clothing and shoes of suspected arsonists for the presence of ignitable liquids. The study found that detectable amounts of gasoline were transferred to the clothing and shoes of a person during the action of pouring it around the room, with various pouring heights and floor surfaces. Results of the study showed that gasoline was always transferred to the shoes and often transferred to both the upper and lower clothing but that the seizure and proper packaging must take place quickly (Coulson and Morgan-Smith 2000). In tests using a carbon strip extraction method, it was found that 10 ml (0.34 oz. or 2 tsp) of gasoline on clothing worn continuously evaporated much more quickly than on the same clothing left on the lab bench at 20°C to 25°C (68°F to 77°F) and was barely detectable after only 4 hours of wear (Morgan-Smith 2000). Clothing must be recovered and packaged soon after exposure.

A second New Zealand study further examined a potential defense argument that the gasoline residues located on a suspect's clothing came from a legitimate source. The study showed that it is extremely unlikely to have detectable levels of gasoline on clothing and shoes following the activity of filling a vehicle with fuel, without the spillage of any noticeable amount of fuel onto the clothing and shoes. The study found it possible for gasoline to be detected on the shoes of people after using a gasoline-powered mower to cut their lawns. The study further underscored that the time delays between commission of the crime and seizure of the suspect's clothing need to be taken into account when considering the possibility of evaporation of any volatile residues from the suspect's clothing (Coulson et al. 2008).

7.3.6 CHAIN OF EVIDENCE

No matter what kind of material is recovered or how carefully it is preserved, it is valueless as evidence if it has not been maintained and documented completely. The **chain of evidence (chain of custody)** is a record of the existence and the whereabouts of the item from the time it is discovered at the scene to the moment it is yielded to the court. This documentation of an item is in the form of a written record, usually on the sealed evidence package, that lists every person who has had custody or possession of the item. The list must include the dates and times of transfer and the signature of anyone involved in that transfer (see *ASTM E1459*). The documentation starts with the photography of the item

chain of evidence (chain of custody) ■ Written documentation of possession of items of physical evidence from their recovery to their submission in court.

in place at the scene and records *all* people who handle the evidence or its sealed container. The number of people handling evidence should be kept to a minimum to minimize chances for damage and to reduce the number of people who must be ready to testify in court as to the existence of the evidence, for each person is then a link in this crucial chain.

An evidence log is an accurate, complete list of all items of evidence recovered from a scene or location. Many agencies prefer to use a preprinted form, as suggested in the chapter on documentation. The form provides a checklist for recording what was recovered, from where, and by whom, and also that the item was documented by photograph and diagram before recovery. If more than one person is recovering evidence at a scene, it is preferable that the evidence log for a scene be maintained by one person to avoid duplicate or conflicting numbering. It is the responsibility of the person recovering the item to ensure that each item is properly packaged and labeled or tagged, and that the photos and diagram entries have been made. An evidence log is a useful supplement to the custody list on the item itself.

If the chain of custody is broken, it cannot be restored, the evidence is valueless to the court, and the case may well be lost. A complete, well-documented chain allows the court to admit evidence that can be verified, allowing the investigator to say, "Yes, this is the device I recovered from the scene. I know that because here is where I marked it, here is the container in which I sealed it." The importance of the chain of evidence to a successful fire investigation cannot be overemphasized.

PART 2: Structural Fires

7.4 Examination of a Fire Scene

Every fire scene investigation follows a certain protocol or logical sequence that will vary slightly depending on the circumstances of the individual fire and its investigation. If a fire investigator is fortunate enough to arrive at the scene while the fire is still underway, first contact should be made with the fire officials present. The ranking fire official can provide information as to the time of alarm, time of arrival, and time required for control, as well as the names of owners, occupants, and witnesses. Copies of all relevant departmental reports should be requested. The firefighters will be able to provide valuable information as to the extent of involvement of the structure, behavior of the fire, unusual odors, and whether any explosions took place.

7.4.1 SEARCH PATTERNS AND PRACTICES

As described earlier in this chapter, before beginning the actual search for evidence, the investigator should examine the exterior of the structure from all sides. This walk-around survey will give a fair idea of the limits of the fire damage, the areas of heaviest damage, and the possibilities of an external source of ignition (such as a trash fire) or reveal obvious forcible entry. View lines can be established at this stage. What was visible to passers-by or neighbors? Which neighbors have a view of the scene? After the survey is completed, it is useful for the investigator to step back from the immediate scene for a moment and determine what areas *surrounding* the structure must be searched as well—for example, along likely paths of entry or exit and the areas under windows or around doors. If a tall adjoining building is not available, it is often helpful to use an aerial snorkel or ladder unit to get immediately above the fire scene to facilitate observing, charting, and photographing the damage. Figure 7-7 illustrates the value of an overhead photo from an aerial ladder—showing the location of the most damage.

Once an accurate idea of the scene limits is in mind, a perimeter is established, preferably by means of a physical barrier such as rope, banner, or barricades. All personnel not

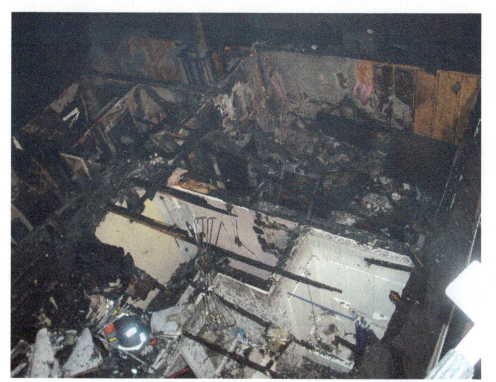

FIGURE 7-7 Photo from aerial ladder shows extent of damage. *Courtesy of Greg Lampkin, Knox County Sheriff's Office, Tennessee, Fire Investigation Unit.*

essential to the search are then kept outside that perimeter for the duration of the scene examination. This perimeter method provides both scene security and a good starting place for the search that follows, because it sets the outer limits of the search pattern. Documentation also begins before the search, normally at the outer perimeter, in the form of photos, notes, and sketches. Some investigators find it useful to prepare a rough floor plan at this stage to help plan the investigation and begin to put the scene features into context.

Most structure fires lend themselves to a spiral search pattern, beginning at the outer perimeter and working toward the center of the fire. The search pattern will, of course, depend on the size and shape of the area to be searched and the time and number of people available to do the search. The exterior areas of the scene must be carefully examined for shoe and tire impressions that do not appear to be those of fire or police personnel or their vehicles, discarded tools (e.g., from a forced entry), fuel containers, beer or soft drink containers, matchbooks, or shards of glass from windows. If an explosion preceded or accompanied the fire, the exterior search will focus on any fragments of the structure or explosive device. Because the trajectory these fragments followed must be reconstructed to establish the seat of the explosion, it is vital that the location and distribution of any such fragments be carefully charted on the crime scene sketch. Special attention should be paid to the distribution and distance of dispersal of all window glass. This process minimizes the chances of destroying evidence that was damaged by the fire or explosion before its relationship to the scene has been assessed. As the investigator works through the scene, the process is one of tracing the flow of the fire back to its origin and cause, which is often (but not always, for reasons to be discussed) in the area most damaged. Indicators of direction of movement will be discussed in an upcoming section. Large scenes may require division into sectors that are then searched in sequence, as dictated by access or exigencies (limitations). An example is shown in Figure 7-8.

As a general rule, anything that looks out of place should be checked. Does the item belong to the scene? Is it clean and fresh, as if recently dropped there, or stained and weathered, as if exposed for many weeks? Is the grass underneath it still green? Anything

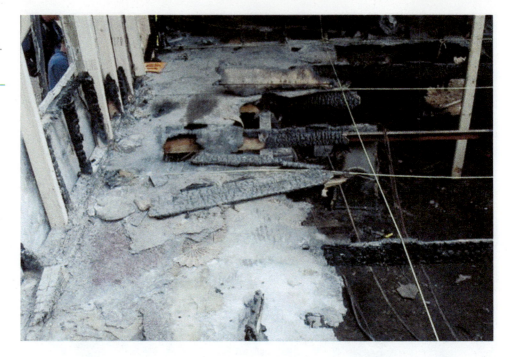

FIGURE 7-8 String grid divides this large scene into sectors for searching. *Courtesy of Kyle Binkowski, Fire Cause Analysis.*

that looks odd or out of place should be charted on the scene sketch, photographed in place, and then collected. It is always easier to disregard collected items if proven later to be unrelated to the fire than to try to recover important items once they have been left behind. *All* collected objects should be considered potential sources of latent fingerprints and therefore must not be handled directly by more than one person, and must be packaged to minimize damage and contamination by others' handling them. Vinyl or latex gloves prevent contact with chemical or biological hazards and minimize (but not always prevent) deposition of fingerprints or DNA.

Proceeding toward the building itself, the investigator looks for signs of attempted forced entry, such as tool marks, fresh damage to door or window frames, broken locks, or broken windows. Are there signs of prior efforts at extinguishing the fire—a garden hose or an empty fire extinguisher? If so, an attempt should be made to find the people responsible, because they may have valuable eyewitness information to offer about the early stages of the fire. Documentation should include photos supported by notes or diagrams showing the presence or *absence* of signs of forced entry at all possible access areas, as well as signs of activity—tire impressions, shoeprints, extinguishers, and the like. All external areas of the structure must be photographed before disturbing them.

No matter what the nature of the structure or the extent of the fire damage, nearly every thorough fire investigation starts in the least damaged areas and progresses toward the most heavily damaged areas, in other words, starts with the areas of *least* confusion and disruption and proceeds to those *most* disrupted by fire or explosion. This process helps establish the starting conditions in the fire damaged areas by showing the investigator what wall and ceiling finishes were like, as well as furnishings. As the investigator works through the scene, the process is one of tracing the flow of the fire back to its origin and cause. It can be thought of as a search for what material was first ignited and the source of heat that ignited it.

Logic and knowledge of basic fire dynamics are the most important tools. Materials exposed to a violent fire can do some unusual things and exhibit unexpected properties, but the fundamental precepts of matter, energy, and heat transfer cannot be violated. There must be fuel, oxidizer, and energy in appropriate forms and amounts before there will be fire. The combination of fuel and energy that the investigation indicates as the source of the fire must meet the scientific and fire engineering requirements of energy release, fuel, and oxygen supply. As fuel packages and potential ignition sources are discovered they should be plotted on a detailed scene diagram. For the reasons we have discussed, the area most heavily damaged is not always the area of origin, because the intensity and duration factors will be influenced by fuel load, manner of ignition, ventilation, and fire suppression activities. The investigator must take all these into account when evaluating the damage pattern in the search for the origin.

7.4.2 FIRE BEHAVIOR INDICATORS

Indicators are the visible, and usually measurable, changes to the surfaces and materials of a fire scene produced by smoke, heat, or flames. Because they are produced by predictable physical processes, they can be used to re-create the path of the fire's development, the location of fuel packages, the nature of ventilation, and sometimes the height, intensity, and duration of the flames. There are many indicators that the investigator can use in reconstructing the path of the fire. None of them are precise. None of them are foolproof. None should be relied on to the exclusion of all others. Depending on the nature of the structure and the extent of the fire, it may not be possible to apply some indicators. The most accurate origin determinations are accomplished by applying a number of different indicators independently and then combining the results as a series of "overlays." The investigator examines the structure methodically, checking and recording one fire indicator at a time. Each search will reveal some useful information about the direction of fire travel (sometimes called "arrows") and the relative intensity in each area. After several such surveys, stacking the indicators up against each other will reveal points of similarity and agreement. Further searches can then be concentrated in the general area of suspected origin indicated by the combination of indicators.

indicators ■ Observable (and usually measurable) changes in appearance caused by heat, flame, or smoke.

Some indicators of fire travel result from the deposit of soot and other combustion products on exposed surfaces without any chemical changes. Most other indicators are produced by heat-induced changes to surfaces. The intensity and duration of the heat applied will dictate the nature and depth of those changes. Because indicators of damage (or relative lack of damage) form patterns, and are created by a combination of smoke, heat, and flames, they are sometimes called **fire patterns**. The diagnostic signs most often used to indicate fire intensity and direction of travel are outlined in the following sections.

fire patterns ■ The visible or measurable physical changes, or identifiable shapes, formed by a fire effect or group of fire effects (*NFPA 921*, 2017 ed., pt. 3.3.74).

Burn Patterns

Burn patterns are created when applied heat fluxes are above the critical thresholds to scorch, melt, char or ignite a surface. Where the fire's destruction did and did not take place constitutes the burn pattern. Burn patterns are the cornerstone of all fire investigation because of their universal applicability. Data from a fire scene include the evaluation of any and all heat transfer patterns. In seriously damaged structures, the question "Where was the destruction most complete?" may accomplish the same end. We know that fire *generally* travels upward and outward, leaving, in the absence of barriers or unusual fuel conditions, a V-shaped or conical pattern in the structure it leaves behind. In the absence of active suppression, fire will usually have time to burn longer at its point of origin than at places subsequently involved by spreading flames. As a result, destruction will be more extensive in that area, all other things being equal. These include fuel loads and ventilation, however, which are rarely equal throughout an entire scene. Figures 7-9A–D illustrate patterns in a bedroom fire originating from a wastebasket fire.

One of the factors that is not always equal is fire suppression. Fires are attacked at what appear to be their most critical areas—where other buildings are threatened, where victims are trapped, where dangerous contents are to be protected, and so forth. Occasionally, suppression will be focused on the very area of a structure in which the fire was started, and even though the rest of the building is destroyed, the area of origin may be the most intact. That is why interviews of the suppression crews are so important to revealing where the fire was attacked and with what tactic.

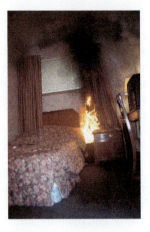

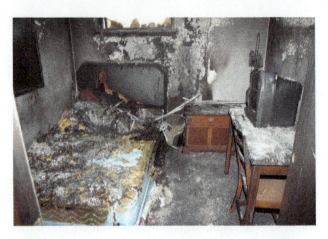

FIGURE 7-9A Small waste-basket fire quickly spreads to drapery and bedding. *Courtesy of Jamie Novak, Novak Investigations and St. Paul Fire Dept.*

FIGURE 7-9B "V" patterns on wall and headboard point back toward wastebasket. Note thermal patterns at margins of pattern (charring to scorching to no damage). *Courtesy of Jamie Novak, Novak Investigations and St. Paul Fire Dept.*

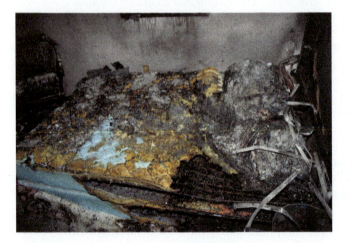

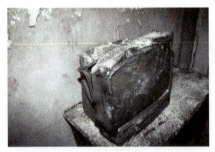

FIGURE 7-9C Damage pattern on bed (including partially collapsed springs) becomes more intense toward origin (lower right corner). *Courtesy of Jamie Novak, Novak Investigations and St. Paul Fire Dept.*

FIGURE 7-9D TV set shows more collapse and glass fracturing on side facing growing fire as fire grows and spreads around corner from bed. *Courtesy of Jamie Novak, Novak Investigations and St. Paul Fire Dept.*

Burn patterns that can be used to indicate the direction of fire spread can be observed on structural elements, wall surfaces, or even furnishings remaining in the building. In order to prevent destruction of burn patterns that can be used as evidence, overhaul of the structure needs to be minimum. Application of heat to a material causes changes first only to its surface and if sustained, changes to its bulk. By applying the principles of heat transfer and the structure of flame plumes, the investigator can understand how patterns were formed.

The temperatures in a flame and smoke plume decrease with height in the plume or distance from the centerline, as shown in Figure 7-10. Because the radiant heat flux intensity is controlled by the temperature of the source, we can see why the pattern of damage from a moderate-sized fire to an adjacent noncombustible vertical surface is often in the form of an inverted "V" (as depicted in Figure 7-11). As room air is entrained into the rising flame and smoke plume it will be spread out as it rises, but it will also be diluted

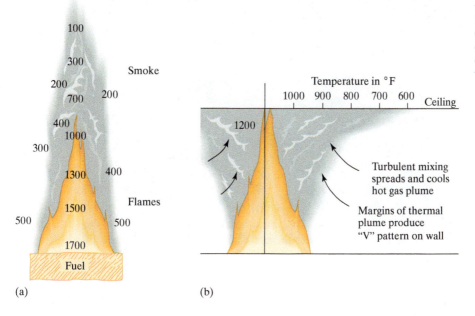

(a)

(b)

FIGURE 7-10 Temperature distribution of gases in a buoyant plume (a) unrestricted (b) under ceiling (temperatures in degrees Fahrenheit).

In diagram (a):

Smoke

100

300

200

700   200

400

1000

300

1300   400

Flames

1500

500   500

1700

Fuel

In diagram (b):

Temperature in °F

1000 900 800 700 600

Ceiling

1200

Turbulent mixing spreads and cools hot gas plume

Margins of thermal plume produce "V" pattern on wall

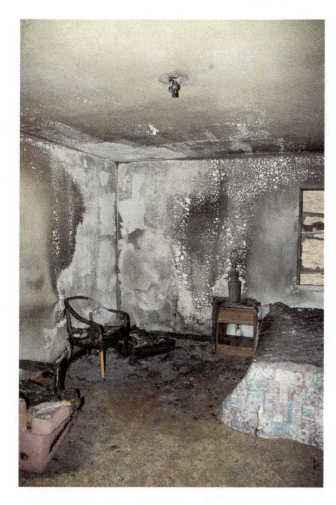

FIGURE 7-11 Energetic fire on chair in corner produced an hourglass pattern on a noncombustible and on the ceiling as a result of the corner configuration. Note gradations of thermal damage. *Courtesy of Jamie Novak, Novak Investigations and St. Paul Fire Dept.*

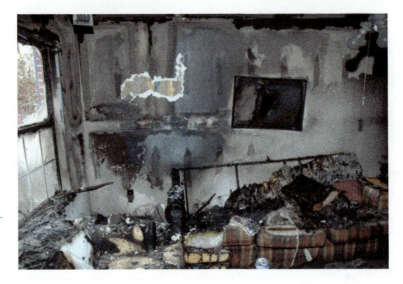

FIGURE 7-12 Fire that started at the end of the sofa produced a "V" pattern of damage on the wall behind the sofa and on the sofa. Note clean burn on drywall, thermal transfer pattern on side wall, and enhancement of ceiling damage as a result of corner effect. *Courtesy of Greg Lampkin, Knox County Sheriff's Office, Tennessee, Fire Investigation Unit.*

and cooled. If the adjacent surface is very susceptible to thermal changes or if combustion products are deposited as the gases cool, there may be a pattern resembling an hourglass or a "V" in outline (Icove and DeHaan 2006). The overall pattern most often resembles a "V" or "U" with its apex pointing toward the heat source.

Wherever the total heat flux onto the wall is below the critical intensity needed to affect the surface, there will be a *line of demarcation* for that heat pattern. Areas outside that demarcation will not be visibly affected. This process is driven by the buoyant flow of the hot gases, so the "V" (or inverted "V") is produced on vertical surfaces, not on horizontal ones. Because the gases cool as they move away from the centerline of the plume, damage patterns to horizontal surfaces above the fire will tend to be circular, with a "bull's-eye" of the most damage directly above the fire.

Figure 7-12 illustrates a typical "V" pattern on a wall as a result of a localized fire. Notice how the pattern spreads out naturally, with the apex of the "V" right at the origin of the fire. Although it is sometimes the case that the more vertical the sides of the "V," the faster the initial fire (and therefore the more suspicious), one can appreciate that the nature of any wall covering or vertical target surface, size of the fuel package, height of the ceiling, and conditions of ventilation determine the shape of the pattern. The angle and width of the "V" are not dependent on the rapidity of ignition of the initial fuel but on the fire properties of the target surfaces.

The "V" pattern associated with most fires is a result of several factors, one being that the natural plume shape of a large fire is a cone. The interaction of the plume with a wall or a ceiling is the major factor in producing a pattern. The shape of this cone depends on the size of the fire with respect to a ceiling that tends to flatten and spread it horizontally. A vertical wall intersecting this cone may then display a vertical cross section of the cone. If a fire is located some distance away from the wall, the cone does not intersect the fire cone at its base, so a shallow "U" or "V" pattern may appear, as in Figure 7-13. The ceiling directly above a large fuel package may exhibit a circular bull's-eye pattern of damage (unless bounded by nearby walls), with the center reflecting the effects of the highest temperature gases, and succeeding rings of less damage. Because hot gases moving across a surface lose some of their heat by convective transfer, they cool, producing less damage as they move away. If the fire is located against a wall, the circular pattern is interrupted by the wall to form a semicircle (as in Figure 7-13).

A small fire of low energy and limited duration will typically display a triangular, inverted-"V" or "A" pattern of damage to a nearby adjoining wall. This is especially true if the wall or its covering is not readily ignitable. If the wall covering is very combustible,

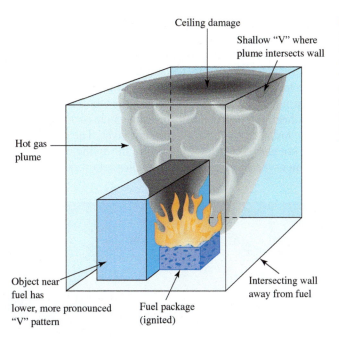

Ceiling damage

Shallow "V" where plume intersects wall

Hot gas plume

Object near fuel has lower, more pronounced "V" pattern

Fuel package (ignited)

Intersecting wall away from fuel

FIGURE 7-13 A fuel package burning in a room may produce a circular burn on the ceiling if the plume is large and energetic enough. Vertical surfaces intersecting the plume may have areas of plume-induced charring.

the flame travel can be almost vertical. If the wall covering has been destroyed, the "V" pattern is often recorded on the wall studs still remaining, as in Figure 7-14. Because the sides of an object exposed to an encroaching flame will be more heavily burned than the protected sides, and the buoyancy of the hot gases causes them to rise as they flow horizontally, the object will often have a beveled appearance that is more pronounced on the side and edges facing the oncoming fire, as illustrated in Figure 7-15. If a fire is traveling very rapidly, the hot gases will flow over recessed areas on the downwind side, leaving relatively undamaged areas on the side away from the fire.

Furniture will also exhibit burn patterns of use in determining point of origin and direction of spread, because an object, whether upholstered or not, will generally be burned more extensively on the surfaces exposed to an oncoming fire. In large combustible objects, significant portions of a "V" pattern may be visible, as in Figure 7-16. If the original location of the furniture can be established by observation or by witnesses, the patterns can be incorporated into the overall pattern observed in the room.

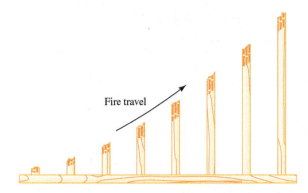

Fire travel

FIGURE 7-14 Even if the wall covering is destroyed, the "V" pattern is often reflected in the remaining structural members.

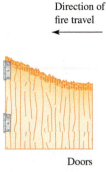

Direction of fire travel

Doors

FIGURE 7-15 Beveling of exposed combustible surfaces indicates that fire moved from right to left.

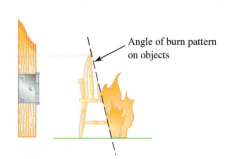

Angle of burn pattern on objects

FIGURE 7-16 The "V" pattern can be reflected in large items of furniture.

The photos of a nonaccelerated test fire in Figures 7-17A–B demonstrate a number of these features, including the "V" pattern on the corner walls, as well as on both sofas. The paint and paper have been burned off the walls and the ceiling in the corner around the origin. Radiant heat damage to the left side of the TV stand and the armchair shows more intense heat coming from the left. The fire was approaching flashover when it was extinguished, so the carpet in the corner where the fire began and the wood floor beneath it were very badly burned by radiant heat. The carpet and furnishings closer to the photographer were just being affected by the radiant heat from the hot gas layer. The header formed by a structural beam restrained the hot gas layer from flowing into the dining room. The protected area on the right (far) wall shows where the back of the smaller sofa was in contact with it.

FIGURE 7-17A Overall photo of scene shows floor-to-ceiling plume damage in the corner, floor-level damage between the sofas, and higher damage farther away. *Courtesy of Kellie Sullivan, Marin County Fire Department, Woodacre, CA.*

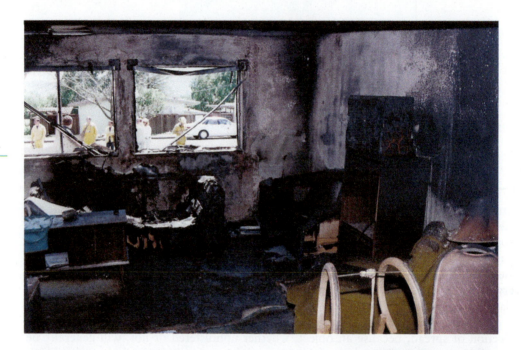

FIGURE 7-17B After removal of the sofas, the protected area on the wall shows the location of the sofa back. Radiant heat damage to the left front corner of the chair was produced by the sofa fire. The "V" pattern from the sofa includes the left side of the TV and stand. Note the damage to the floor caused by radiant heat ignition of all-synthetic carpet and pad. No ignitable liquids were used. *Courtesy of Kellie Sullivan, Marin County Fire Department, Woodacre, CA.*

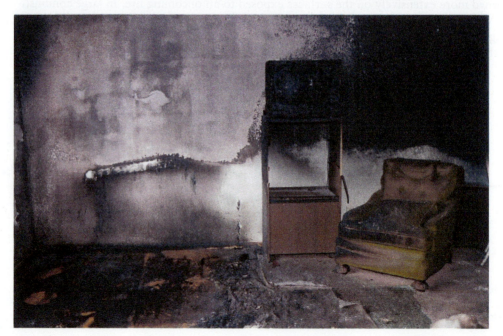

Beveling of exposed edges occurs when heat is applied and the temperatures of edges and corners rise faster than those of adjacent flat surfaces (because of their more limited thermal capacity, they cannot lose heat as quickly to the interior). That is why the edges are easier to ignite than a flat surface and, once ignited, burn more quickly. This predictable behavior allows the investigator to use such beveling to re-create the direction of travel of the fire gases. Directional travel can produce cross-sectional beveling of exposed wood elements that can indicate the direction of the flow of hot gases around them. Such beveling, then, can be used to plot pointers or arrows of fire spread direction on a plan of the building.

This beveling effect can be very useful in establishing the direction of burn-through of floors. Because of the complexity of most structure fires, it is not enough to record the fact that the floor has been burned through in a particular area. It must be determined whether the floor has been burned from underneath or from the top. It is obvious that joists will protect the flooring immediately above them when the fire burns from underneath, but all the flooring surrounding the hole will be destroyed first if the fire is burning downward.

After these indicators of direction of fire spread (sometimes called *vector* or *arrow patterns*) have been observed throughout the structure, they can be combined with observations of relative char depth and the heights of heat and smoke horizons in various rooms to map out the fire's approximate course of travel (NFPA 2014). The combination of direction and intensity indicators is sometimes referred to as *vector analysis*. These vectors can be mapped out on a floor plan to help establish a likely area of origin. This information must be considered in light of what is known about the suppression efforts that occurred at the scene.

It is well known that venting a burning building or actively attacking it on one side can force fire to reverse its course and attack new areas or reburn previously affected areas. It has been observed that if a fire starts in one room and spreads to another with a larger fuel load, the subsequent extension of the second fire can obliterate the direction indicators on adjoining walls, making it look as if the fire started in the second room. Ventilation through windows, whether wind-driven or from PPV fans during suppression, is a critical factor in evaluating burn patterns and fire behavior (Kerber and Madrzykowski 2009).

Heat Level (Heat Horizon)

As hot gases are released into a room their buoyancy causes them to rise to the ceiling, and then their accumulating mass and momentum causes them to start to flow outward. When hot gases flow across a surface, the flame front is always at a marked acute angle to the surface because of the physical properties of the density-driven flow. In the same manner as when a dam bursts, and the gravity-driven flow of the "wall" of water causes it to flow with its face at an angle to the ground (as illustrated in Figure 7-18), the same occurs with hot gases. If the flame front comes into contact with vertical surfaces, it produces a characteristic "front" that will tell the investigator the direction of flame spread at that point at some time during the fire.

As the hot gases continue to accumulate they fill the room from the top down, producing a hot gas layer. In large rooms or with very large (high HRR) fires, there may be times when the gas accumulates (in a corner, for instance) in a deeper layer immediately above the fire than it does in the rest of the room; eventually the layer will fill the room

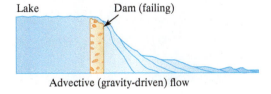

Lake   Dam (failing)

Advective (gravity-driven) flow

FIGURE 7-18 Advective (gravity-driven) flow of water released from a collapsing dam assumes an acute angle from the ground.

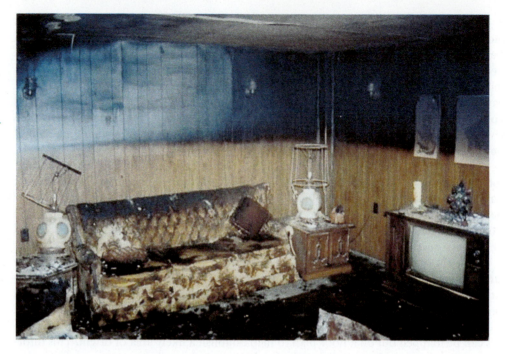

FIGURE 7-19 A uniform hot gas layer ignited paneling near its entry to the room and scorched the paneling across the room. *Courtesy of Det. Michael Dalton (ret.), Knox County Sheriff's Office.*

to a uniform height throughout (except near ventilation openings, where it rises) (see Figure 7-19). The larger the fire or the smaller the room, the faster this hot gas layer deepens until it can begin spilling out windows or under headers into adjacent rooms. As the hot gas layer spills out into adjacent rooms it begins to fill those rooms from the ceiling downward. This produces "shallower" layers in other rooms, with the "deepest" layer in the room of origin. This process produces a characteristic stair-step pattern of smoke or heat damage that will help trace the flow of the fire, as shown in Figure 7-20.

The height of significant levels of heat (i.e., the depth of the hot gas layer described earlier) in a room is revealed by the charring, burning, blistering, or discoloration of paint

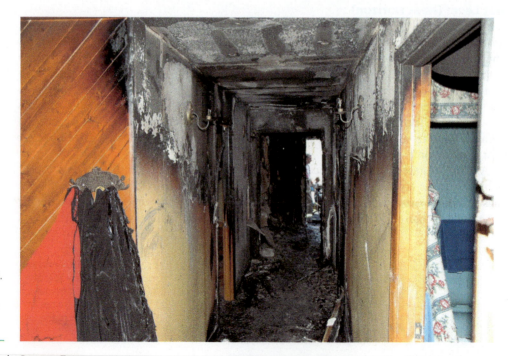

FIGURE 7-20 Fire moving down this hall from the far end produced a stair-step or rising heat horizon pattern. Note damage to paneling in the next room on the left. *Courtesy of Greg Lampkin, Knox County Sheriff's Office, Tennessee, Fire Investigation Unit.*

or wall coverings. The **heat horizon** will generally be level, that is, of uniform height from the floor when the atmosphere in the room is fairly static. Changes in level indicate points of ventilation, such as open windows or doors or breaks in the walls or floor. Typical questions for the fire investigator include the following:

- Do such points of ventilation agree with the known history of the fire, or do they indicate that an attempt was made to encourage fire spread by opening walls, ceilings, or floors prior to the fire?
- Are there signs of such intentional venting?
- If windows or doors were open, were they known to be open before the fire?
- Were the windows or doors damaged before the fire or during it?

The heat level will often drop markedly in the vicinity of the point of origin or when there is combustible material ignited lower down or along the base of the wall. Low burns can also be produced by combustion of floor coverings during full involvement of the room. As the hot gas layer deepens, the heat level will sink from near the ceiling as the fire grows. At flashover with involvement of floor coverings, the heat level will be at or near floor level (bases of walls). Ignition of a premixed quantity of natural gas, LP gas, or flammable liquid vapors in a room tends to produce a *scorching* of wall surfaces that is uniform from floor to ceiling, while post-flashover burning usually produces deeper burning with its longer duration. In rooms not involved in fire, the heat level may be revealed by the distribution of melted objects—candles, plastic fixtures, even appliances—in the room.

The temperature of the heat source determines the intensity of heat flux it produces. Therefore, the temperature profiles will produce commensurate effects. As hot gases move across a solid surface some of their heat is lost by convective transfer, so they cool as they move away from the primary contact point. This produces a gradation of effects, as shown in Figure 7-21, which allows testing of hypotheses about contact and movement.

Smoke Level (Smoke Horizon)

Even when there is no heat effect on a surface, surface deposits can reveal the **smoke horizon**, the height at which smoke has stained the walls and windows of a room, which reflects the nature and extent of the fire and the amount of ventilation. Smoke staining can occur even in rooms that have not been damaged by the flames themselves. Such staining is produced by the condensation of liquid products of incomplete combustion (pyrolysis products) and the deposition of soot. As with heat levels, smoke levels will change at points of ventilation and therefore may be useful in estimating which doors and windows were open during the fire.

The smoke level may also be useful in assessing the cause of fire deaths. For instance, it may be possible to estimate if a person of a certain height would have been able to see an exit if standing in the room during the fire or whether he or she would have been overcome by the cloud of hot toxic gases accompanying the smoke. Occasionally, victims who did not stand up during a smoky fire escaped, while people who did were quickly overcome. The heat and smoke levels throughout a building are most conveniently charted on a separate scene sketch for later comparison with other data.

Buoyant flow of hot smoke can produce a backsplash or mushrooming effect if the hot gases have sufficient momentum when they encounter a wall. Just as water waves pile up against a breakwater, hot smoke can pile up against a wall, producing a drop-down of the smoke horizon (sometimes called *momentum flow*). Flow through a door often leaves a void or clear area on the "downstream" side of the header, as illustrated in Figure 7-22.

Low Burns and Penetration

The lowest point of burning in a structure or room must be examined carefully, for it may offer evidence of the cause of the fire, as well as its origin. Fires ignited in a room's normal

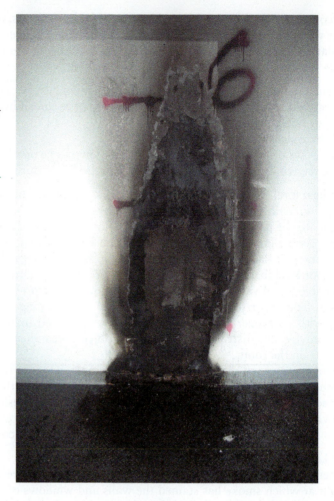

FIGURE 7-21 Gradations of thermal damage on this wall show the intensity of the plume as it cooled from the centerline out and vertically. Smoke deposits (nonthermal) surround the upper portions of the pattern. *Courtesy of Jamie Novak, Novak Investigations and St. Paul Fire Dept.*

fuel load most rapidly burn vertically upward from their point of ignition, leaving the floors and lower reaches of the walls much less damaged than the ceiling and upper walls. Any localized area with a floor burned or a wall burned right down to the floor require investigation. The burn does not mean that the fire is incendiary in origin but that high temperatures or high heat fluxes were encountered at floor level. Combustible floor

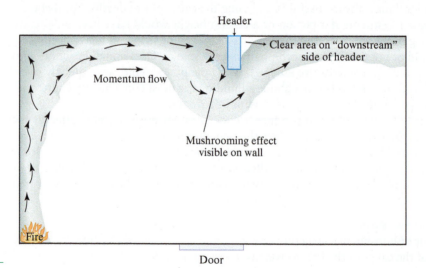

Header

Clear area on "downstream" side of header

Momentum flow

Mushrooming effect visible on wall

Fire

Door

FIGURE 7-22 Momentum flow and doorway flow, leaving clear area "downstream." Deeper layer exists in room of origin.

coverings, post-flashover burning, fall-down, or collapse may have caused it to burn. Each possible hypothesis has to be tested and eliminated.

During the free-burning phase of a room fire after flashover, the radiant heat is extremely intense (120 to 150 kW/m^2), and the combustion in the room becomes unstable and extremely turbulent. The intense radiant heat causes ignition of floor coverings and the floors themselves, producing a generalized although not always uniform burning. Synthetic carpet and pad materials melt and ignite readily upon exposure to these post-flashover radiant heat fluxes.

In a post-flashover fire, when the size of the fire is controlled by ventilation, the most intense burning will be in the vicinity of ventilation openings (see Figures 7-23A and B). The very high flame temperatures of burning carpet, pad, and floor materials can be sustained as long as there is fuel—much longer than the typical flammable liquid fire—and can

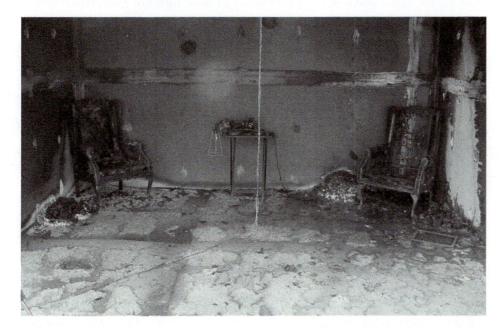

FIGURE 7-23A Extensive melting of synthetic carpet caused by radiant heat (pre-flashover). Notice the pattern is very irregular. "Clean burn" on right wall is due to ventilation (fresh air drawn into fire at floor level). *Courtesy of SA/CFI Michael A. Marquardt, ATF, Department of the Treasury, Grand Rapids, MI.*

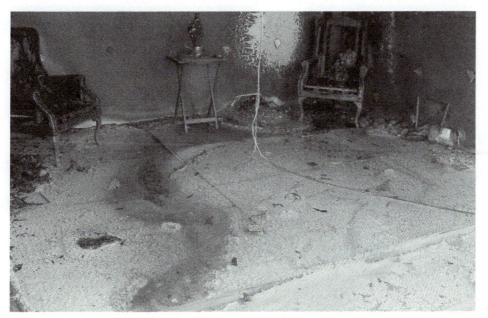

FIGURE 7-23B The same carpet in a room fire ignited with gasoline shows similar irregular melting. Charred and scorched area shows location of gasoline pour. "Clean burn" beside the chair is a ventilation effect as the energetic gasoline fire beside the chair entrains fresh air from the front of the room. *Courtesy of SA/CFI Michael A. Marquardt, ATF, Department of the Treasury, Grand Rapids, MI.*

induce fire damage down to floor level. Even before flashover occurs, the room is exposed to high heat fluxes across a wide area, producing a generalized although not always uniform scorching and melting. Localized low burns surrounded by large areas of undamaged floor are unusual and deserve close attention. The pre-fire conditions of the floor are important because even combustible trash or clothing will protect the floor covering from radiant heat, leaving the exposed areas to be damaged by the full brunt of the post-flashover fire.

Figure 7-23 shows two identically furnished rooms, one accelerated with gasoline, the other ignited by open flame, that were extinguished just as flashover occurred [with ceiling and floor temperatures of 815°C (1500°F)]. Note that the synthetic carpets melted in both rooms in an irregular fashion, probably due to their non-uniform contact with the floor (from curling). The pour pattern of the gasoline is still visible but would be obscured once the carpet and floor were fully ignited by post-flashover radiant heat. Figures 7-24A–D illustrate the flames and post-fire patterns of a gasoline trailer in a carpeted room.

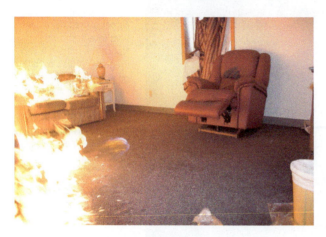

FIGURE 7-24A Ignition of gasoline trailer from door to sofa. Note flash (blue) flame extending through vapor layer from pool. *Courtesy of Jamie Novak, Novak Investigations and St. Paul Fire Dept.*

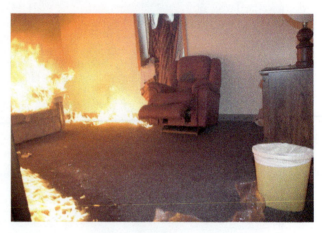

FIGURE 7-24B Seconds later, flames have traveled along trailer against the base of the wall to recliner. *Courtesy of Jamie Novak, Novak Investigations and St. Paul Fire Dept.*

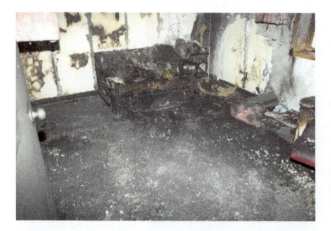

FIGURE 7-24C Fire extinguished just before flashover. Post-fire (after removal of some of the suspended ceiling). Trailer pattern on carpet barely visible on the left. Uniform damage across the sofa and to floor level to walls to left and right is not consistent with limited damage to other furnishings. *Courtesy of Jamie Novak, Novak Investigations and St. Paul Fire Dept.*

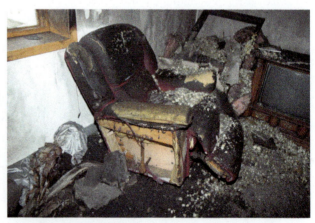

FIGURE 7-24D Damage to left side of recliner down to floor level should prompt further exam. Drapery collapse may have caused this, but residues of the gasoline trailer in the carpet would betray an arson cause. *Courtesy of Jamie Novak, Novak Investigations and St. Paul Fire Dept.*

One possible cause of low burns is the ignition of a pool or trailer of ignitable liquid on the floor. When localized burn damage extends down a wall to the floor surface, it may indicate that an ignitable liquid was used, because other sources of intense local combustion, such as trash, usually do not burn right to floor level. The flames from a pile of flammable trash burn upward in the typical convective cone from the fuel surface and contact the wall higher than floor level. Sustained combustion of a pile of cellulosic clothing, bedding, or furniture that has collapsed onto a wood floor, however, has been seen to cause penetrations through floors. Ignitable liquids alone will not burn long enough to achieve generalized penetrations of wood floors. However, a liquid can soak into the crack that separates the wall from the floor and take the fire to the very bottom of the wall. A puddle or trail of flammable liquid is the most commonly detected arson device.

The use of these liquids often produces effects that are most characteristic if the room has not gone to flashover. Because corners are usually dead air spaces that are destroyed last in accidental fires, it is unusual fire behavior if the corners of a room are burned out *before* other exposed areas of the room are damaged. Post-flashover fires, however, can generate so much radiant heat and be so turbulent that destruction can extend into the corners and even down stairs, as shown in Figures 7-25A–C. Older structures may have uneven floors, and any liquid poured on them in quantity seeks out the lowest surface. Such pools of poured liquid provide a longer-duration fire with potential to create more localized damage.

The behavior of ignitable liquids in a fire follows certain physical rules, which investigators must appreciate if they are to detect such accelerated fires. These physical rules include the following:

- Liquids (and their vapors) flow downhill, seeking out the lowest available surface. They can flow under doors and even under the toeplate of wood-frame partition walls.
- Liquids will seep into seams or cracks in a floor and, from there, provide a reservoir of liquid to sustain more prolonged burning and localized charring.
- Very volatile liquids (camp fuel, acetone, alcohols, lacquer thinners, and even gasoline) will flash quickly off a nonporous surface. [In burn tests of 1- to 4-L (1- to 4-qt) quantities, which produced a freestanding pool less than 0.5 mm deep, a regression rate of 0.5 to 1 mm/min (0.02 to 0.04 in./min) and a total burn time of about 1 min was expected and observed] (DeHaan 1995).
- Because of the low-boiling-point liquids involved, such fires produce minimal surface scorching compared with the relatively deep charring induced by burning an overturned cardboard box filled with crumpled newspaper.
- Only the reservoirs along cracks and seams provide fuel for deep charring. Scorching and some sooting of the floor surfaces surrounding the pool are likely, particularly on the downwind side of a pool burning in a draft.

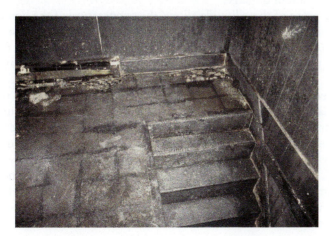

FIGURE 7-25A Post-flashover fire deeply charred all exposed surfaces down to floor level. *Courtesy of Jamie Novak, Novak Investigations and St. Paul Fire Dept.*

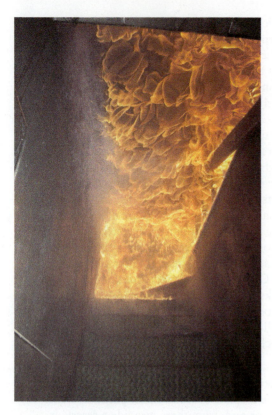

FIGURE 7-25B View looking up the stairwell shows ignition of the top step. *Courtesy of Jamie Novak, Novak Investigations and St. Paul Fire Dept.*

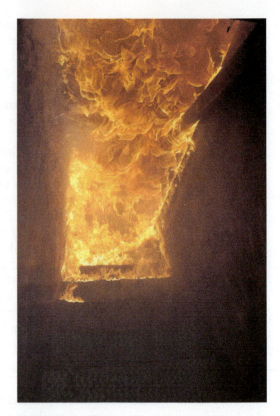

FIGURE 7-25C View looking up the stairwell shows ignition of lower steps. *Courtesy of Jamie Novak, Novak Investigations and St. Paul Fire Dept.*

- The floor under the pool may be discolored by the solvent action of the liquid or damaged by the brief exposure to flames as the last of the liquid boils off. Flooring with very low thermal damage thresholds such as modern vinyl sheet flooring may be scorched or distorted by a burning gasoline pool.
- Less-volatile fuels with a higher boiling-point range such as paint thinner or kerosene will exhibit different effects. Recall that it is the vapors of liquid fuels that burn rather than the liquids themselves. The more radiant flames from these fuels produce a more pronounced charring on the floor surface *surrounding* the liquid pool, often producing a halo or ring of damage.
- The higher boiling point of these liquids allows the temperature of the liquid pool to rise enough that the floor surface beneath the pool may be scorched. These liquids can form deeper pools on nonporous surfaces and burn more slowly than the volatile fuels and have more time to spread into floors and penetrate crevices and porous edges.
- The resulting pattern can be a deep ring of char damage around the edges of a lightly charred area that defines, to some extent, the liquid pool (as in Figure 7-26). However, a similar pattern can be created by the burning of thermoplastic materials (including upholstery) that melted and burned as a semimolten pool. Residues of unburned polymer should be found adhered to the floor in such cases.
- When first ignited, any liquid fuel burning on a carpet will produce a pronounced ring or halo of damage on the adjacent carpet pile, leaving the carpet pile in the center of the pour undamaged (the pile acts as a wick) until the liquid is nearly consumed (DeHaan 1995).

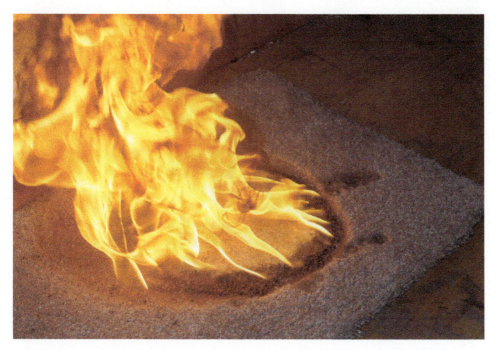

FIGURE 7-26 Halo pattern around a pour of gasoline on a carpet in an arson fire. Note the unburned carpet in the center of the pool. *Courtesy of Jamie Novak, Novak Investigations and St. Paul Fire Dept.*

- When that last liquid is burned, the center of the pool will scorch, char, and ignite. On some carpets, this sequence will leave a charred area surrounded by a more deeply charred halo.
- On carpet, the size of the damaged area is not always a reliable indicator of how much fuel was involved or even how large the liquid pool was prior to ignition because carpets vary greatly in the amount of penetration (into the pad) and the response of the carpet to radiant heat from the flames (Putorti, McElroy, and Madrzykowski 2001).
- Data and observations from tests of similar carpet and pad can support conclusions about pool size versus quantity and fire behavior.
- New all-synthetic carpets can self-sustain combustion and produce extensive burn patterns that bear no similarity to the original pool of liquid fuel that ignited them (DeHaan 1999).

Oxygen masks and cannulas fed by clear plastic tubing are becoming common in residences today. If the oxygen-saturated tubing is ignited, a blowtorch effect rapidly burns the tubing away, leaving behind a narrow trailer of burn damage (see Figure 7-27).

Floor Burns and Penetrations

The investigator must be aware of the effects of radiant heat from burning fuel packages, or from masses of hot gases in a post-flashover room or moving through ventilation openings such as doors and windows (DeHaan 1987; Gudmann and Dillon 1988; Albers 2002). The mixing of fuel-rich hot gases with fresh oxygen-rich air as they leave such openings produces very-high-temperature flames and enhanced radiant heat output, causing enhanced thermal damage. Floors can be charred and even ignited at heat fluxes of 20 kW/m^2 or greater even if no fuel is on fire in the immediate vicinity.

Due to the effects of radiant heat from burning surfaces and combustion of fall-down fuels, it is not sound practice merely to clear a room of its burned contents and rely on the burn patterns on the floor as indicators of fire location. Post-flashover burning is intense but non-uniform and unstable and can produce floor burns that bear no relationship to fuel locations. Synthetic carpets and pads melt in such exposures, leaving irregular pools of melting and burning residue and equally irregular areas of exposed floor (Powell 1992;

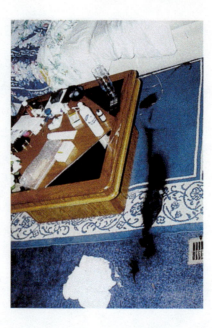

FIGURE 7-27 Linear burn pattern on carpet from burning oxygen cannula tubing. *Courtesy of Det. Michael Dalton (ret.), Knox County Sheriff's Office.*

Lentini 1992b; DeHaan 1992). The ignition of floors and floor coverings can melt aluminum threshold strips that tests have shown will not be melted by ignitable liquid fires alone. The sustained flames of the burning floor coverings add to the radiant heat input from the room fire and can overwhelm the high thermal conductivity of the aluminum.

Often, the investigator is tempted to identify any burning through a wooden floor as having been caused by the ignition of a flammable liquid. As discussed previously, fire burns downward into a solid fuel very slowly. While penetrations can be caused by a liquid's seeping into the seams and joints of a leaky floor and then being ignited along the seams or underneath, this is usually not the cause. Penetration is more likely to occur due to the radiant heat from a prolonged post-flashover room fire; from the sustained burning of a substantial fuel package like a sofa, bed, or overstuffed chair; or from prolonged burning of other fuels that fall onto the floor from above while still burning energetically. Sustained smoldering combustion of such fuels as draperies or upholstered furniture has been observed to cause isolated, localized penetration down through a wood floor.

Other fuels burning from underneath must also be considered. Unusual floor construction, fuel materials stored on the next floor down, or unusual air draft conditions can all contribute to floor penetration. Floor penetrations are more common in post-flashover room fires in the vicinity of ventilation openings. The beveling effect of the burn pattern helps in establishing whether the fire came from above or below as it penetrated the floor.

Isolated burns can be produced by burning fall-down fuels (as in Figure 7-28), that is, the investigator must be careful about ascribing an ignitable liquid cause. Once again, a sketch of the fire scene is made with the extent and distribution of any low burns or floor penetrations recorded on it. This is retained for later comparison with the other indicators. Observations must also be made of any possible fall-down sources—cabinets, draperies, light fixtures, wall paneling, and ceiling materials.

7.4.3 CHAR DEPTH

char depth ■ The measurement of pyrolytic or combustion damage to a wood surface compared with its original surface height.

The depth to which the pyrolysis action of fire has converted an organic material (usually wood) to its volatile fractions and charcoal is called the **char depth**. Heat applied to wood surfaces causes progressive destruction of the cellulose and other organic constituents of the wood. This charring will progress through a layer of wood at a somewhat predictable

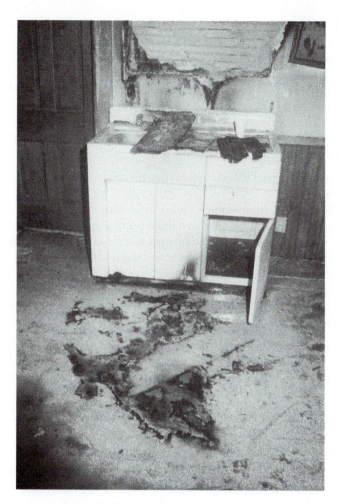

FIGURE 7-28 Isolated burns on kitchen floor resulting from fall-down of cabinet (and its contents) above the sink. Note "low burn" on front of cabinet from fall-down fire. *Courtesy of Jamie Novak, Novak Investigations and St. Paul Fire Dept.*

rate. The char rate of structural wood [which is often cited as being on the order of 2.5 cm (1 in.) in 45 minutes] is, first of all, *not* a linear phenomenon. That is, wood chars very quickly for the first few fractions of an inch and then at a much slower rate, presumably due to an insulation effect of the newly formed char and to reduced air/fuel interaction. It is only an average rate that can be projected, so any attempt to interpolate short times of fire exposure precisely based on fractions of an inch of char depth is seriously misleading.

Most significantly, it is not the time of burning, but the *intensity* of the heating (which varies locally and with time to a great degree) that most affects the char rate. The higher the intensity of the applied heat, the faster the charring, and the deeper the resulting char in a given amount of time (Drysdale 1999; Babrauskas 2004). Anything that affects the intensity, such as ventilation or localized fuel, will affect the char depth. Different species of wood will also char at somewhat different rates. The density of the wood is a major factor in char depth, as it is with regard to the rate of spread of a fire. The same wood will char at different rates on faces cut across its grain than on faces cut with it (and create different char patterns) due to the differences in heat conductivity and transport of fluids within the wood.

The adherence of the char is also an extremely important variable with certain species such as redwood. Variations of exposure created when char flakes off in some areas and adheres in others further complicate the relationship between char depth and fire exposure. Edges and corners cannot lose heat to the interior of a fuel mass as well as flat surfaces and will char more quickly. This difference in heat loss can produce cross-sectional beveling on exposed wood members that can indicate the direction of flow of hot fire gases around them. Even the dimensions may have an influence because of their variable effects on heat capacity and conductivity. To complicate the practical picture further, misinterpretation may follow because water may have been applied in one area in fighting the fire, inhibiting charring there, while water may not have been applied in another area close by, although the general fire intensity was similar.

Although char depth cannot be used to establish precise times of fire exposure, it can be used, if applied systematically, to assess the *relative* fire exposure throughout a structure. When testing for depth of char, remember the following:

- Measure depth from the original wood surface, not the existing char layer (which may often be impossible).
- Use whatever small-diameter, blunt-tipped tool is most convenient to test for the depth at which intact wood remains. (A sharp knife point should be avoided, because it tends to easily penetrate into undamaged wood; some investigators prefer a tire tread-depth gauge or plastic caliper, because it has a blunt wire indicator.)
- Use the same tool throughout the scene.
- Take char depth readings on similar wood surfaces at the same level(s) throughout—for instance, waist height, head height, and knee height—logging all observations on an appropriate sketch of the scene.

Some investigators prefer to plot an *isochar* diagram of the scene by connecting points of similar char depth. The resulting contours (resembling the isotherms of a weather map) outline the areas of deepest charring. These areas can then be correlated to fuel packages and ventilation sources. Remember, with *all* else being equal, char depth is most likely to be at its maximum at or near the fire's point of origin (where it burned longer) *or* near another localized source of fuel or ventilation (where it could burn more intensely). Distribution of char depth *must* be correlated to the fuel load and ventilation to be of any value.

Variations in char depth may be of use in positioning fuel packages and establishing ventilation conditions. Due to the rapid combustion of wood in high heat flux exposures and the production of such exposures around ventilation points such as doors or windows in post-flashover fires, floor penetrations in or near door openings in such fires have no value in indicating placement of accelerants. In a post-flashover room fire, the interior of the room may be burning in an oxygen-deficient condition except around ventilation sources. There may be deeper charring or **clean burn** patterns around such vent openings or in the flow path of incoming fresh air. Analyses of post-flashover rooms by Carman (2009) revealed that ventilation effects not only enhance combustion around ventilation points but also can produce clean-burn patterns of fire damage across the room from the ventilation source. This may give the appearance of a "V" pattern where there was no localized fuel package

Appearance of Char Surface

The appearance of the char surface may be indicative of the fire conditions. Many investigators rely on a rule that says that large, shiny blisters of char (**alligatoring**) indicate a fast-moving, rapidly burning fire, while small, dull checkering indicates a slow-burning fire—without realizing that many of the factors mentioned previously affect surface appearance as well as char depth. While a deeply seated, flat, or "baked"-appearing char is most often produced by prolonged heating, it can also be produced by a short-duration fire under some fire conditions (very intense fire with limited ventilation).

One observation is that charring of wood surfaces in oxygen-deficient conditions (such as the underside of a wood floor deck) may be more likely to produce flattened, dull, sharp-edged char. This char formation is caused by heat-driven shrinkage. Insufficient oxygen reduces the combustion rate of the exposed margins. One study by Ettling

clean burn ■ A distinct and visible fire effect generally apparent on noncombustible surfaces after combustible layers (such as soot, paint, and paper) have been burned away. The effect may also appear where soot has failed to be deposited because of high surface temperatures (*NFPA 921*, 2017 ed., pt. 3.3.31).

alligatoring ■ Rectangular patterns of char formed on burned wood.

showed a relationship between temperature of exposure and size of char blisters (on one species of wood)—the higher the temperature, the smaller the blisters. However, oven exposure at a constant temperature for various times caused differences (Ettling 1990). In a real fire where both times and temperatures are unknown, one cannot reliably assess the effects of both. Exposure to low [below 300°C (600°F)] oven temperatures did produce a characteristic sunken appearance of the wood surface with infrequent cracks or fissures that wandered over the surface in Ettling's study.

One indicator that may be more useful is the appearance of the charred wood in cross section. The thermal changes in wood occur at characteristic temperatures of short duration. An intense heat exposure produces a sharp, steep gradient between a high-temperature layer and unaffected material below in a poor conductor like wood. Spearpoint and Quintiere (2001) confirmed such gradients in wood. The transmittal of heat through the wood has less time to occur in a sudden, fast-developing fire, and the resulting pyrolysis zone is very narrow. As a result, there is often a sharp line of demarcation between the charred and unburned layers of the wood. When a charred beam is cut lengthwise, the gradation between the charred layer and underlying undamaged wood is more gradual with a prolonged, slowly developing fire. No matter how reliable an indicator such gradients may be regarding the speed of development of a fire, a fast-developing fire may or may not be accelerated depending on what fuels are found in the room and how it was ignited. An accidental fire involving direct-flame ignition of a polyurethane mattress can produce flashover in a room just as quickly as intentionally ignited gasoline.

Surface Effects

Radiant heat fluxes on the order of 10 kW/m^2 [or prolonged contact with hot gases over 150°C (300°F)] will cause surface thermal effects such as scorching of wood or thermosetting polymers or melting of thermoplastic coatings. Higher heat fluxes or high temperatures will induce charring even without ignition. Such indicators need to be documented as to type, location, and depth. Comparison samples of undamaged materials are needed to allow identification and establishment of critical heat fluxes or temperatures.

Displacement of Walls and Floors

Extensive overhaul and dismantling of the structure may make it impossible to determine whether walls, floors, or ceilings were moved by the effects of an explosion prior to or during the fire. The amount of material moved and the degree of fragmentation of the resulting pieces are the critical observations. Walls may be dislodged at their tops, at their bottoms, or both, depending on the directional effects of the developing blast or its reflections, or simply because one edge of the wall was fastened into the rest of the structure more rigidly than another.

The majority of the examination for displacement is easiest to carry out during the examination of the exterior, but damage is sometimes readily detected upon checking the interior. Window glass is the most readily broken structural material and may be thrown large distances by an explosion. Diffuse vapor/air explosions may not break window panes but may knock them free of their frames and toss them intact some distance away. All materials moved by an explosion should be carefully charted and compared against their original positions so that the direction of force can be assessed. If the structure collapsed or was razed, careful examination of the floors or foundations where the sole plates of the walls were attached sometimes may yield indications of sudden disruption. The investigator must measure and document the displacement of all structural elements.

7.4.4 SPALLING

Spalling, the chipping or crumbling of a concrete, plaster, or masonry surface, can be caused by the effects of heating, by mechanical pressure, or by a combination of both. Concrete is an aggregate of sand and gravel held together by a crystalline matrix (cement) containing a considerable quantity of water of hydration. When exposed to heat, some of this water is released from both the crystalline matrix and the aggregate (gravel), and the material loses its integrity and crumbles. While concrete is very strong in compression, it is relatively weak in tension. As a result, heating may cause some types of sand or gravel aggregate to expand more than others, which puts the cement matrix into tension, resulting in failure. This material property is a variable that many experiments in inducing spalling have overlooked (Sanderson 1995; Smith 1993; Midkiff 1990).

Moisture trapped in the porous structure of concrete or masonry is also evaporated into steam by heating. Forces generated by the expanding steam then can disrupt the cement, causing it to crumble. The inclusion of polypropylene fibers in concrete can provide pressure relief as the fibers melt during fire exposure, reducing spalling. This steam expansion is especially true of recently poured (green) concrete and masonry.

Heat expansion of steel reinforcing components within a concrete floor, beam, or column can also cause failure of the covering concrete. Steel reinforcing rods have a higher rate of thermal expansion than concrete, so steel components, if not buried deeply enough, can heat, expand, and distort to displace overlying concrete, compromising the mechanical strength of the beam, column, or floor. Other forms of mechanical stress can cause spalling of concrete or masonry, especially high mechanical pressures or the shock of rapid cooling of a superheated concrete surface by a stream of cold water. Although these other causes can contribute to spalling, by far the most common cause of spalling of structural concrete in structure fires is localized heating as a result of some ordinary fuel load in the immediate area.

The formation of the crumbling surface is quite variable and depends on the nature of the aggregate used, the age of the concrete, the amount of mechanical restraint as in prestressed panels or reinforced slabs, and the rapidity of the rise in temperature, as well as the temperature itself (Canfield 1984). Because spalling can be triggered by thermal expansion, it is important to consider the physics of heat transfer from a fire on a concrete surface into that concrete. As shown in Figure 7-29, the radiant heat from the flames first raises the temperature of the fuel, causing faster evaporation. Some heat will pass through the liquid and raise the temperature of the surface beneath the pool. Excess heat from the surface is quickly transferred to the liquid, keeping the maximum temperature of the surface at or just above the boiling point of the liquid. As we have seen, the boiling point of gasoline (a mixture) is from 40°C to 150°C (100°F to 300°F); therefore, the temperature of the concrete beneath a burning pool of gasoline can never be much higher than 150°C (300°F), which is not high enough to trigger the thermal expansion *usually* needed for spalling. The duration of a flammable liquid fire on concrete is also very short (typically 1 to 2 minutes). That is not enough time for a significant amount of heat to penetrate concrete with its limited thermal conductivity.

As a fire indicator, spalling can indicate the presence of a significant fuel load of ordinary combustibles, as well as sources of intense localized heating such as a chemical

FIGURE 7-29 Radiant heat from ignitable liquid fire on a concrete surface causes evaporation of liquid fuel and warms the surface beneath. The temperature of the surface outside the pool will rise as radiant heat is absorbed by the concrete. The temperature of the surface beneath the pool is limited by the boiling point of the liquid in contact with it.

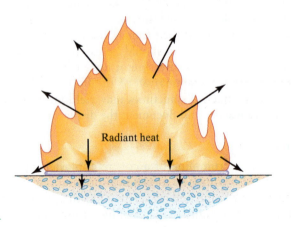

Radiant heat

incendiary (Béland 1993). A flammable liquid burns only at its top surface and along its edges while protecting the area immediately beneath the pool from high temperatures. As a result, spalling is often more pronounced along the outside edges of the burning pool. Free-standing pools rarely burn long enough to induce much radiant heat into the surface, with minimal expansion effects. After the main pool of liquid is consumed, flames may continue at cracks, holes, seams, and expansion joints where pockets of fuel have collected. As a result, spalling tends to be more pronounced in the vicinity of such irregularities.

If a heavier petroleum distillate fuel such as kerosene is burning, its higher boiling-point range will permit higher temperatures beneath the pool, and more persistent, more radiant flames will result. Such flames *may* have more pronounced effects on the concrete, but such fuels are also unlikely to be used as accelerants. Edges of spall patterns may be stained or discolored from the tarry residues of such combustion, but such discoloration is not proof of the involvement of flammable liquids, because such staining has been observed in tests where only normal combustibles were burned. Sometimes, localized spalling was much more likely if the floor was covered with carpet or tile. In such instances, the localized burning induced by a gasoline spill was more likely to involve prolonged burning of the combustible floor covering. This combustion would involve no protective pool of liquid and was more likely to induce spalling than a pour of liquid alone. Note that the depth of spalling has no relationship to the quantity or type of liquid fuel involved.

Spalling is more likely to be produced over large, unprotected areas of concrete floors by radiant heat developed by normal fire progression, especially where there is extensive collapse or fall-down. See Figures 7-30 A and B and 7-31 A–C for the results of an experiment contrasting the effects of a gasoline fire and a wood bonfire on the same type of concrete (note the staining around spalled areas on the wood-fire concrete). The symmetry and location of spalled areas must be carefully considered. Even localized spalling, when accompanied by staining, may not be the result of a flammable liquid.

An ultraviolet light (or various wavelengths of visible light) from a forensic light source played on a concrete surface may aid in detecting ignitable liquid residues as a result of their fluorescence. An early reference addressed this technique (Thaman 1978). While this suggestion has not been investigated in depth, the presence of fluorescent compounds in asphalts, greases, and other petroleum products indicates that they would be present in the pyrolysis products of many complex synthetics. Such compounds would be expected to fluoresce in the same manner as the petroleum distillates and thereby interfere with their detection by producing false positives. Preliminary field tests have revealed few useful patterns on real-world surfaces that would indicate the presence of ignitable

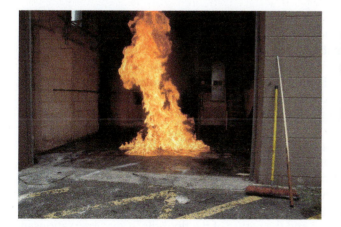

FIGURE 7-30A Spalling test on interior concrete floor. Pool fire of white gas. *Courtesy of Jamie Novak, Novak Investigations and St. Paul Fire Dept.*

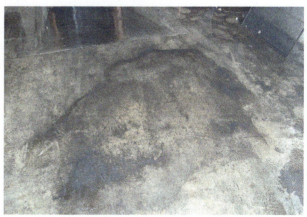

FIGURE 7-30B After self-extinguishment, some staining around margins, but no spalling. *Courtesy of Jamie Novak, Novak Investigations and St. Paul Fire Dept.*

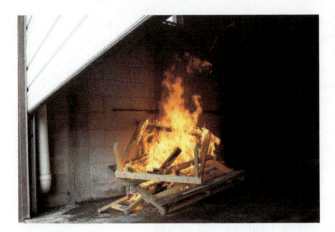

FIGURE 7-31A Spalling test on interior concrete floor. Large wood-fueled bonfire. No ignitable liquids. *Courtesy of Jamie Novak, Novak Investigations and St. Paul Fire Dept.*

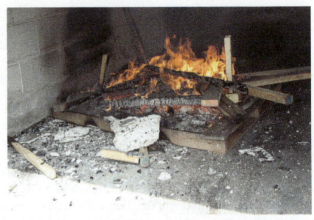

FIGURE 7-31B Prolonged burning promoted explosive spalling during fire. *Courtesy of Jamie Novak, Novak Investigations and St. Paul Fire Dept.*

FIGURE 7-31C Post-fire appearance. Note extensive spalling (especially nearest ventilation source—door to left). Note "pool-shaped" discoloration on concrete. *Courtesy of Jamie Novak, Novak Investigations and St. Paul Fire Dept.*

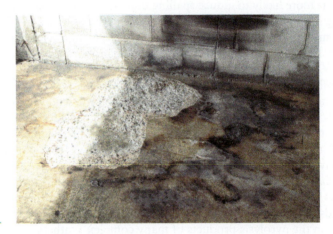

liquids. A new generation of pulsed-laser fluorescence detectors holds promise for distinguishing pyrolysis products from ignitable liquid residues, but they await validation (Saitoh and Takeuchi 2006).

Ghost Marks

Localized spalling of concrete surfaces often takes place in conjunction with **ghost marks**, another diagnostic sign of flammable liquid fires on floors covered with vinyl or asphalt tiles. When asphalt tile squares are affixed to concrete surfaces, they are glued down with a more-or-less continuous layer of tarry adhesive. When a petroleum-based flammable liquid is poured on such a floor and set afire, the heat and solvent action tends to curl the tiles up at the edges. Liquid on the surface then seeps between the tiles and, in some cases, partially dissolves the adhesive. As the fire progresses toward full room involvement, the combination of flammable liquid and adhesive provides fuel for the flames, which tend to be more intense at the seams than in surrounding areas. As a result, more of the adhesive is destroyed, and the underlying concrete floor may be locally discolored and is more likely to be spalled. The adhesive in these areas will be burned off the surface leaving *subsurface* staining in the concrete along a grid pattern corresponding to the seams between the tiles. Depending on the fire conditions and the nature of the floor tile, some observations in experimental room fires are that tiles will shrink even in the absence of flammable liquids, exposing the floor at the joints to higher heat fluxes and producing similar *general* effects. In these cases, the residues of the adhesive tend to remain on the surface of the concrete.

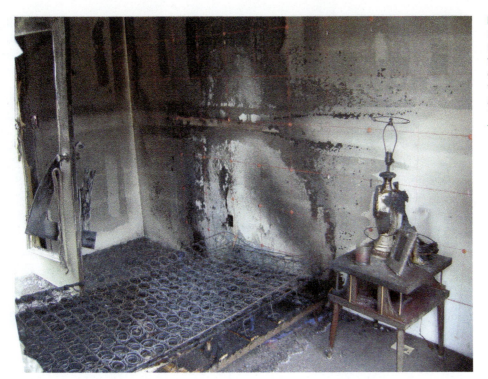

FIGURE 7-32 A technique using chalk string marked walls at intervals to measure depth of calcination of gypsum wallboard. *Courtesy of David J. Icove, University of Tennessee.*

Very faint subsurface staining has been observed on concrete that had a tile floor over it but no fire damage (as in Figure 7-32). This staining was thought to be a result of the solvent action of the floor-wax–stripping solvent used for many years in the room as it soaked between the tiles. Once again, the observation of such a feature across a wide, general expanse of floor rather than in small, isolated, or discrete areas should indicate by hypothesis testing that it was the result of some general feature of the room and not the result of a release of massive quantities of a flammable liquid.

Ghost marks, then, should not be considered to be proof of the use of a flammable liquid, but taken in proper context may be an indicator of such an accelerant. Samples of flooring and adjacent framing should always be taken for lab analysis.

Calcination of Gypsum Board

As we have seen previously, gypsum wallboard consists of a layer of calcium sulfate (plaster) between layers of heavy paper. The calcium sulfate is normally in the dihydrate form (two molecules of water per molecule). When exposed to heat, this water of crystallization is lost through **calcination** in two major steps at predictable temperatures [52°C to 80°C (125°F to 175°F) and 130°C to 190°C (266°F to 375°F)]. In wallboard, each dehydration is detectable as a loss of mechanical strength (penetration resistance) when a probe is pushed into the surface. In addition, as the paper and paint burn off the exposed surface, the combustion products appear to condense in the outermost portion of the gypsum. As heating continues, this layer migrates through the matrix, resulting in a visible color change from gray to white, as seen in Figure 7-33. As the gypsum is heated and dehydrated it shrinks, cracks, and loses its mechanical strength until it is completely dehydrated to a fragile powdery substance.

Mann and Putaansuu recently reported on a series of tests using a cone calorimeter to reproducibly heat samples of gypsum wallboard, after which the amount of dehydration was measured using FTIR, and penetration depth with a modified tire tread-depth gauge (Mann and Putannsuu 2006). These tests indicated that probe penetration with 0.87 kg/mm^2 (6 lb)

calcination ■ A fire effect realized in gypsum products, including wallboard, as a result of exposure to heat that drives off free and chemically bound water (*NFPA 921*, 2017 ed., pt. 3.3.24).

FIGURE 7-33 Calcination of gypsum drywall advancing from fire exposure (fire on right side). *Courtesy of Jamie Novak, Novak Investigations and St. Paul Fire Dept.*

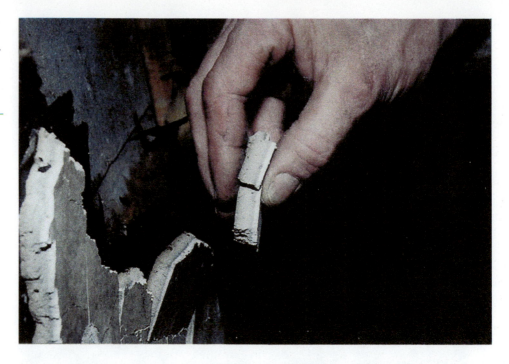

of force followed the depth of the interface between the fully hydrated layer and the hemihydrate form, as the anhydrous and hemihydrated forms offered less resistance than did the fully hydrated form. Color changes, however, did not. It was suggested that the deposition and migration of colored combustion products have numerous variables.

Mann and Putaansuu (2006) reported that similar testing of fiberglass-reinforced (X-rated) gypsum board revealed similar linear results between penetration depth, exposure time, and depth of dehydration. The presence of the fibers or vermiculite reduces the shrinkage of the gypsum and the formation of cracks that weaken the material. If applied systematically with some care to ensure reproducible force applications [0.87 to 1.03 kg/mm^2 (6 to 10 lb)], this technique does yield reliable data on the duration of typical fire exposures for these products. Mann and Putaansuu reported that the visible "smoke layer" position correlates well to the depth of the anhydrous/hemihydrate interface due to changes in porosity caused by dehydration (but not the actual depth of the hydrated layer).

There may be two or three discrete changes in color (white to gray to white), possibly as a result of the two steps of the dehydration or the chemistry of the condensed pyrolysis products. The colors of interest are transitions between gray and white. Other colors such as pink, blue, or green have no causal link to the fire, because they have been linked to impurities in the gypsum. Data on this color phenomenon are still fairly limited (Posey and Posey 1983). Because gypsum is usually a uniform manufactured product with a predictable and uniform thermal conductivity, the depth of thermal effects should be directly related to the duration of exposure, with the caveat that extreme radiant heat fluxes will cause faster buildup of surface effects. Air pockets or voids in gypsum may also give rise to erroneous estimates. A thorough survey of a room can allow the mapping of areas with the highest "penetrations" corresponding to the locations of the most severe heating (from fuel packages, plumes, or ventilation effects). Kennedy, Kennedy, and Hopkins (2003) have examined the processes of heat effects on drywall and have also demonstrated the reliability of calcination observations.

Annealed Furniture Springs

annealing ■ Loss of temper in metal caused by heating.

As a steel wire spring is heated it will reach a temperature, well below its melting point, at which it loses its springiness, or its *temper*. This temperature is called its **annealing** temperature. At temperatures of about 600°C to 650°C (1100°F to 1200°F) the spring will collapse if there is any weight on it and may even collapse of its own weight. This temperature-related indicator may be of assistance to the investigator in establishing whether a fire developed within an upholstered sofa or bed or enveloped it from without. A smoldering fire developing slowly within the upholstery of a sofa or bed often produces a localized area of intense heat. The springs in this localized area will often be more collapsed or extended if they are in suspension than those springs around the margins. When furniture is enveloped by an external fire, heating may be less intense, and the general degree of spring collapse is often less marked than from a long-burning internal fire. In a prolonged post-flashover fire, however, collapse will often be total no matter what the origin of the fire.

One useful indicator of spring collapse is directional, in that the collapse of springs may be more pronounced in the corner or side facing an oncoming fire, if the resulting destruction is not complete and ventilation is fairly uniform. Temperatures adequate to cause collapse of springs by loss of temper can be produced by both flammable liquids and by ordinary combustibles, so their collapse cannot be reliably used to demonstrate an incendiary origin (Tobin and Monson 1989). Springs often taper away, appearing to have been melted by fire exposure. This tapering is due to repeated exposure to turbulent flames and not to intense heat from an incendiary mixture. Such appearances are more often noted in structures gutted by fire (Lentini, Smith, and Henderson 1992). Objects lying on the springs or debris falling onto them during the fire will cause more collapse, and any interpretation of indicators from spring collapse must keep such limitations in mind. Like other fire-direction indicators, spring collapse should be noted and photographed as part of the general scene search.

7.4.5 GLASS

Found in virtually all structures, glass has properties that make it a valuable indicator to the investigator. First, although it looks and generally acts like a solid, it is in fact a super cooled liquid. As a result, when exposed to stress, glass is elastic and will actually bend to a substantial degree before breaking. When a large object strikes a normal (i.e., non-reinforced, non-tempered) glass window, the pane bows out until its elastic limit is reached, whereupon it shatters. This reaction results in two sets of fracture lines, radial and concentric, as shown in Figure 7-34.

The edges of mechanically broken glass will almost always bear a series of curved, *conchoidal* fracture lines produced by the release of internal stress within the glass when it breaks. These conchoidal fracture lines are roughly perpendicular to one side of the

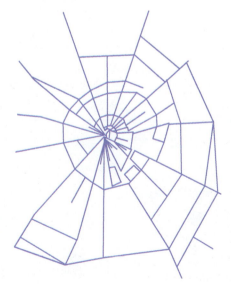

FIGURE 7-34 Typical mechanical impact fracture allowing the development of radial and concentric fracture pattern.

FIGURE 7-35 Conchoidal fracture lines on the edges of glass fragments can reveal the direction of the impact. *Courtesy of Jamie Novak, Novak Investigations and St. Paul Fire Dept.*

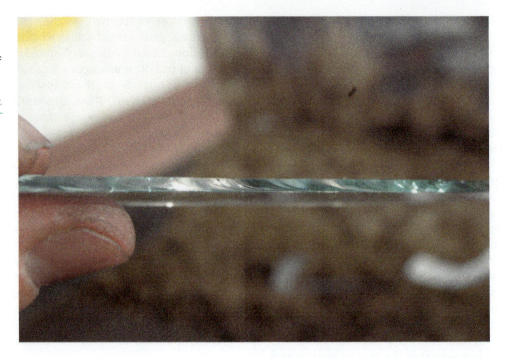

glass and curve around to be roughly parallel to the other, as shown in Figure 7-35. These lines can reveal the side of the pane from which the breaking force came. It is vital to know whether one is dealing with a radial fracture or a concentric fracture. For this reason, it is best that as much of the broken window as is practical be recovered and submitted to the laboratory for reconstruction.

Glass can also break as a result of stress produced by non-uniform heating. The resulting fractures tend to curve randomly about the pane as opposed to mechanically caused fractures, which are almost always straight lines, and the fracture edges bear little or no conchoidal lines, usually being almost mirror smooth, as in Figure 7-36. Glass expands

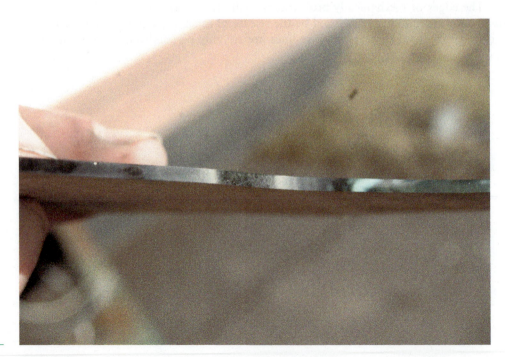

FIGURE 7-36 Edges of thermally fractured glass reveal virtually no conchoidal fracture lines. *Courtesy of Jamie Novak, Novak Investigations and St. Paul Fire Dept.*

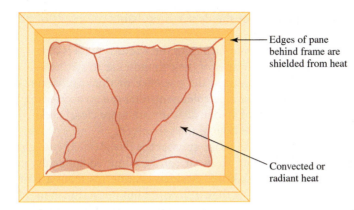

FIGURE 7-37 Radiant or convected heat on the central portion of the glass pane causes thermal expansion of heated portion. The portion behind the molding or frame is in shadow and "sees" no heat and does not expand. When tensile stress becomes sufficient, the glass breaks, typically in fractures roughly parallel to the frame.

Edges of pane behind frame are shielded from heat

Convected or radiant heat

when heated, so convected or radiant heat raises the temperature of the exposed portion of the glass pane, and it expands. The portion of the pane behind or in the frame or molding is protected or shadowed and sees no heat, and because of its poor thermal conductivity, maintains its starting temperature and size. Tensile stress builds up until the tensile strength of the glass is exceeded, and the pane cracks, usually roughly parallel to the framed edges as shown in Figure 7-37.

This process can be predicted by mathematical modeling in terms of temperature differences (Skelly 1990). Studies of this process have shown that it is dependent on the strength and type of glass; ordinary window glass breaks when there is a temperature difference of about 70°C (126°F) (Pagni and Joshi 1991). This breakage can occur in any glass object that is subjected to uneven heating and may reflect the direction from which heat approached. Thick glass can shatter due to a sufficient temperature difference between the side facing the fire and the one facing away from it. Double-glazed windows fail in sequence; the pane facing the fire fails first, then shields the other pane until it falls out of the frame. If the glass simply cracks and does not fall away, the outer pane may survive even through flashover (Nic Daéid 2003).

Not only can one determine whether the glass was broken by mechanical or thermal stress, but from the presence or absence of soot, char, or ash deposits on the broken edges, one can tell if the breakage occurred before or after the fire (Figure 7-38). The location of the glass in the fire debris is important in interpreting its evidential information. Glass with relatively little soot found on the carpet of a room, for instance, with all fire debris on top of it would be a strong indication that the window was broken before or very early

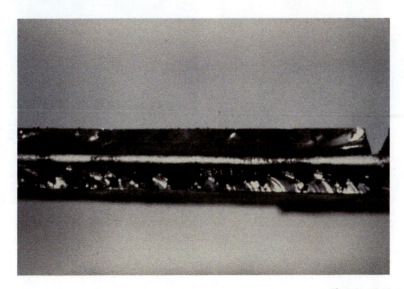

FIGURE 7-38 Broken edges of glass fragments reveal deposits of soot and ash consistent with having been broken before the onset of the fire. *Courtesy of the State of California, Department of Justice, Bureau of Forensic Services.*

on in the fire. Glass found lying on top of the debris is probably the result of breakage during suppression or overhaul.

The appearance of deposits on the inside surface of the window glass is of less evidential value than was previously thought. Because of the common use of synthetic materials in upholstery and in wall and floor coverings, the presence of thick, oily soot can no longer be used as an indicator of the use of a petroleum distillate as an accelerant. Unfortunately, the color, density, and tenacity of smoke deposits are more closely related to the degree of ventilation of the fire than to the type of fuels involved.

Glass breakage often occurs just as the room approaches flashover. If enough cracks develop that the glass can actually fall out, fresh air can be admitted suddenly, possibly triggering a backdraft coincident with flashover. Sudden heating (as from a flammable liquid accelerant) may induce more cracking than a slow fire but not so much more that it will be detectable by post-fire examination of the fragments. If such heating occurs very quickly, the glass pane usually simply shatters (Lentini 1992a). Crazed glass, in which the pattern of partial-thickness fractures or cracks (Figures 7-39A and B), resembling a complex road map in the glass, was once thought to be indicative of a very rapid buildup of heat sometime during the fire.

crazing ■ Stress cracks in glass as the result of rapid cooling.

Laboratory tests have shown that **crazing**, like cratering (pitting of the surface in small circular defects), is caused by a spray of water hitting a window already heated by fire exposure, usually during suppression (Lentini 1992a). Narrow slivers or long shards of glass indicate that some type of explosion took place. The presence of heavy soot or varnish on splinters of glass indicates that the explosion took place late in the fire, most probably as a result of a smoke or backdraft explosion. Glass can also be broken and projected some distance from the window if struck by a straight-stream hose. Absence of soot, or a very faint coating, indicates an explosion early in the fire, possibly caused by an explosive device or fuel/vapor deflagration.

The appearance of the glass can reveal a great deal about the nature of the fire or explosion; it can tell even more if its location in the debris is carefully noted and photographed before it is disturbed. Broken glass scattered by an explosion should be charted (with dimensions) and photographed during the exterior examination, and this documentation can be supplemented with observations of the glass remaining in and around the window frame. Tempered glass, found in vehicles and many structure doors, is made by

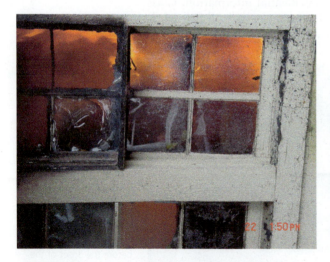

FIGURE 7-39A A glass window fractured and softened by heat exposure during an ordinary combustible fire (post-flashover). Crazing was caused by suppression water spray. *Courtesy of Jamie Novak, Novak Investigations and St. Paul Fire Dept.*

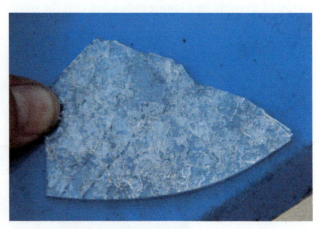

FIGURE 7-39B Close-up of crazed glass. *Courtesy of Jamie Novak, Novak Investigations and St. Paul Fire Dept.*

treating the glass with chemicals or heat during manufacture, which results in glass sheet that is much more resistant to mechanical breakage. When it does break, it shatters into thousands of small cubic blocks. In general, it is not possible to reconstruct such a window or to determine whether it was broken by mechanical or thermal shock. One exception is in vehicles or metal-framed glass doors where there is often a rigid frame that holds the peripheral fragments in their original configuration even after the collapse of the majority of the glass. The fracture pattern remaining can sometimes allow discrimination between mechanical and thermal fractures.

Melting glass, whether it is part of a window, furnishings, or electrical lamps, can be useful in indicating the direction of fire travel. Heat causes glass to expand on the surface being heated, which often causes a window to bend or "belly-in" toward the source of heat. When it finally melts at a temperature of approximately 750°C (1400°F), glass will soften on the side facing the heat first, and so it will sag or flow in that direction as it loses structural strength. Windows in aluminum frames may react to heat-induced distortion of the frame rather than the glass. Observed tests show that although normal single-glazed windows more often fall inward toward the heat, they *can* fall outward as well.

An electric light bulb is first evacuated and then filled with an inert gas, often nitrogen (except for very low-wattage lamps, which is evacuated). When a light bulb is heated, the expanding gas inside creates overpressure, which balloons out the first area of the bulb to soften in the advancing flame. This blowout points back in the direction from which the fire came, because the side facing the oncoming flame will usually be the first to soften as seen in Figure 7-40. Other glass objects in the structure—containers, mirrors, and the like—will indicate not only what temperatures were developed but also from which direction the flames came—but only if they remain undisturbed until they are photographed and examined. Glass bottles, for instance, may be much more intricately fractured on the side facing the heat source even if they appear to be intact. They can shatter, however, if any attempt is made to move them.

Melting Points of Materials

Plastics are often the materials first affected in a fire. Many plastics begin to soften and melt at low temperatures of 100°C to 200°C (212°F to 400°F), and others decompose at

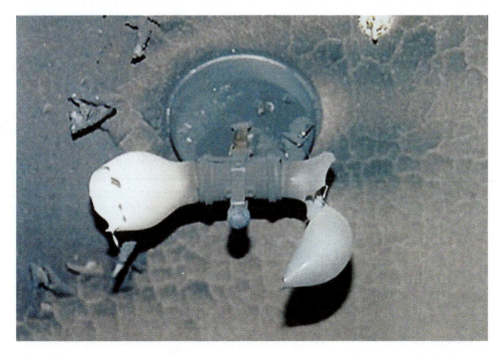

FIGURE 7-40 The blowout on this light bulb faces the oncoming flames and indicates the left to right direction of fire travel. *Courtesy of Det. Michael Dalton (ret.), Knox County Sheriff's Office.*

similar temperatures. The melting behavior of glass mentioned in the previous section is diagnostic of the conditions created within a structure. The melting point of glass varies depending on its composition. Ordinary soda-lime glass used in most windows has a melting point of about 700°C to 800°C (1300°F to 1400°F), a temperature that is reached in many wood-fueled structure fires.

Metals are often useful as additional indicators of the intensity of a fire. When a fire scene is examined, previously molten aluminum residues are often found. Because this metal melts at a comparatively low temperature, 660°C (1220°F), this is not unexpected or indicative of a particularly unusual fire when found. Its high thermal conductivity means that localized flames are unlikely to melt thick metal components. This is especially true of flammable liquid fires, whose typical durations are so short that even low-melting-point metals are likely to be affected.

Zinc/aluminum die-cast fittings, sometimes called pot metal, have a very low melting point [380°C (718°F)] and are very common in fire scenes (Gilchrist 1937). A more useful indicator is melting brass or copper. Depending on its composition, brass melts over a range of 875°C to 980°C (1625°F to 1780°F). Its presence in a burned structure is not unusual, but it may assist in establishing which parts of a room reached higher temperatures than other parts. Copper, commonly present as water piping and electrical wiring, will occasionally melt in the hottest structure fires, its melting point being 1080°C (1981°F). In their extensive study of buildings totally burned during an urban firestorm, Lentini, Smith, and Henderson discovered melted brass and copper fittings in many of the ruins. These included copper water pipe (although water service to the area was interrupted during the fire, water should still have been present in these lines). This demonstrated that such melted materials in individual fire-gutted scenes (so-called black holes) cannot be linked to the use of an accelerant (Lentini, Smith, and Henderson 1992).

The flame temperatures produced by flammable liquids burning as a pool in air are not necessarily higher than those produced by ordinary combustible fuels, so the presence of melted metals should not be taken as proof of the presence of liquid accelerants. Molten aluminum can interact with copper and dissolve in it to form a bimetallic alloy. This alloy can have any percentage of copper and aluminum, but at a ratio of 67 percent aluminum and 33 percent copper, it forms a eutectic metal alloy with a melting point of only 548°C (1013°F), below that of either original metal. Molten aluminum can therefore attack and dissolve away heated copper conductors in electrical systems and appliances (Béland, Ray, and Tremblay 1987).

Zinc falling onto heated steel can cause penetrations by a similar alloying process. Cast iron, which melts in the range of 1200°C to 1450°C (2200°F to 2700°F), is sometimes found melted in the ashes and rubble of heavily burned heavy-timber structures. Because well-ventilated wood and charcoal fires can produce temperatures on the order of 1300°C (2400°F), such melting may occur by strictly thermal processes (Henderson 1986). It has also been suggested that carbon monoxide combustion and actual reductive smelting of the cast iron may play a part. It has recently been suggested that black iron can alloy with calcium salts to form a eutectic with a relatively low melting point.

Whenever any residues of a molten metal are found at a fire scene, they can help establish the minimum temperature occurring at that spot in the structure. While such melted metals cannot and should not be used as proof that the fire was incendiary, the fire investigator should note their presence, extent, and distribution. This information can help to establish differences between temperatures produced by normally fueled and ventilated accidental fires and those produced by enhanced draft conditions or unusual fuel loads from chemical accelerants in incendiary fires.

Copper and, to a lesser extent, copper alloys are very susceptible to oxidation when heated in air. This reaction results in the formation of black copper oxide on the surface of the metal. If the heating and exposure to air are continued long enough, the entire object, for instance, wire, may be changed to oxide. The degree of oxidation of exposed copper wiring can serve as an indicator of the conditions existing at the point of exposure. Copper wire carried in conduit is not so subject to oxidation because of the limited access to air and the general reducing (rather than oxidizing) atmosphere resulting from the decomposition of insulation materials. The surface of copper wire and other conductors may turn green as the hydrogen chloride gas (HCl) released by the pyrolysis of the PVC insulation turns the metal to copper chloride.

Clean Burn

When a noncombustible surface is exposed to soot and pyrolysis products, they condense on it. If that surface is heated sufficiently, those materials can be burned off, leaving a clean burn. The surface temperatures needed to accomplish this are flame temperatures [>500°C (1000°F)]. Therefore, a clean burn indicates direct flame contact of some duration. The flames may be from a fuel package playing on the surface or from incursion of fresh air into an underventilated post-flashover room.

7.4.6 MYTHS AND MISCONCEPTIONS ABOUT INDICATORS

A number of indicators traditionally linked to incendiary fires have been shown to be unreliable.

Evidence (Documentary or Witnesses) of an Abnormally Fast Rate of Fire Spread or Collapse

Fact: Fires are rarely seen from the moment of their ignition, and so the actual rate of fire development is rarely known. The furnishings in use today will also support more energetic, much faster growing fires than most people appreciate. The pre-fire fuel loads and their placement are critical to evaluating fire spread. Lightweight construction techniques often used today in commercial and residential structures can lead to much more rapid penetration and collapse of floors, ceilings, and roofs than occur with traditional techniques (Earls 2009).

Evidence of Abnormally High Temperatures (Melted Metals, etc.)

Fact: Flame temperatures of flammable liquid fires are about the same as temperatures of wood-fueled fires. Higher temperatures [in excess of 1000°C (2000°F)] can be produced by the combustion of many synthetic materials, and post-flashover fires can create temperatures of that magnitude from floor to ceiling in modern furnished rooms in the absence of any flammable liquids.

Spalling of Concrete

Fact: Radiant heat from sustained fires in ordinary fuels and structural collapse are much more likely to transfer enough heat into concrete to cause it to spall than is the heat from short-lived fires of pools of flammable liquids. Temperatures and heat fluxes under pools of flammable liquids are too low to induce sufficient heating to cause most concrete to spall. Flammable liquids on floor coverings can induce sufficiently energetic burning of those coverings to induce spalling.

Crazing of Glass

Fact: Thermal stress can cause glass to fracture, but rapid buildup of such thermal stress (thermal shock) causes rapid failure, often producing shattering of the glass, rather than the intricate partial-thickness patterns associated with crazing. Such patterns are produced when glass heated by fire exposure is suddenly cooled (usually by hose stream during suppression).

Irregular Damage to Floors and Floor Coverings

Fact: Heat fluxes on floors in post-flashover room fires are not only very high, they are not constant, driven by extremely turbulent mixing between the combustion gases and air coming into the room through doors and windows. As a result, the post-fire damage is often more intense around these ventilation openings. The reaction of synthetic carpets and pads to such radiant heat causes irregular melting and combustion. Fall-down or collapse of overhead structural materials can cause irregular, intense floor-level damage even in the absence of flashover conditions.

Black, Heavy, Oily Soot on Windows/Black Dense Smoke

Fact: Black, dense smoke is a result of the type of fuel burning in a room and the efficiency of the combustion. Modern synthetic materials are almost always petroleum-based and, when burned in a typical fire, release large quantities of black soot and dark pyrolysis products.

Annealing of Steel Springs and Steel Structural Materials

Fact: Steel loses its temper and tensile strength at temperatures above 500°C (1000°F). Such temperatures can be produced by smoldering or flaming combustion of ordinary upholstery materials. Ignitable liquid accelerants are not required.

Floor-to-Ceiling Heat Damage

Fact: As the temperature of the hot gas layer in a room exceeds 600°C (1150°F), the radiant heat flux exceeds that needed to char and ignite all exposed fuel surfaces. Due to the large surface area of the hot gas layer, shadowed or protected areas beneath furniture may not be adequate to prevent ignition of carpets under furniture.

Deep Char

Fact: The rate at which wood chars is dependent on many factors (type of wood, nature of finish, etc.) but especially on the intensity of the radiant heat (heat flux) falling on it. Direct flame exposure can cause wood to char at twice the rate at which it chars at ignition, and wood in a post-flashover fire can char at 10 times the rate at which it chars at ignition.

Progression to Flashover

Fact: Today's furniture with its synthetic fabrics and padding is capable of producing very high heat release rates. (A single modern recliner fully involved produces as much heat per second as a half-gallon of gasoline poured on the floor and ignited.) Although modern furnishings are more resistant to smoldering heat sources, they are more susceptible to open-flame ignition and, once alight, can cause the spread of a fire in a 3-m × 4-m (10-ft × 14-ft) room to flashover in 5 to 8 minutes in the absence of any ignitable liquids.

Alligatoring (Shiny or White)

Fact: The surface appearance of charred wood is dependent on the nature of the wood and ventilation conditions during its combustion. The presence of white ash on charred surfaces is the result of prolonged burning in a well-ventilated fire, resulting in complete combustion of carbonaceous residues, leaving behind the light-colored oxides of inorganic compounds.

7.4.7 ARSON EVIDENCE

There are many other observations that will be made in the course of the scene examination that may reveal the fire's origin and cause. Incendiary fire cause may be revealed by obvious indicators such as separate multiple points of origin, the presence of **trailers** of flammable liquid or paper or rags connecting areas of intense burning, or the remains of timing or ignition devices.

trailer ■ Solid or liquid fuel used to intentionally spread or accelerate the spread of a fire from one area to another (*NFPA 921*, 2017 ed., pt. 3.3.193).

Trailers

What appear to be trailers may be artifacts of normal fuel combustion, as illustrated in Figure 7-41. Arsonists often use multiple "sets" or ignition sources to ensure maximum destruction. Very often, unless the devices are carefully synchronized, the first devices ignite a fire that interferes with the operation of later ones. They may be found incompletely burned and readily identified. What appear to be multiple points of origin must be carefully evaluated so as to eliminate their cause by fall-down of draperies or lighting

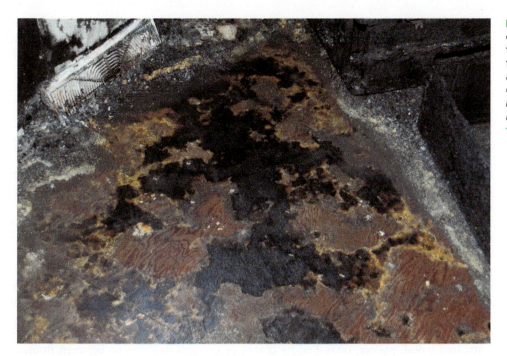

FIGURE 7-41 Irregular char pattern on a wood floor caused by post-flashover fire, set by ignitable liquid on furniture. *Courtesy of Jamie Novak, Novak Investigations and St. Paul Fire Dept.*

fixtures, by lightning or power surges (causing multiple failures of appliances), or even by radiant heat or hot fire gases traveling across a room or between rooms.

Containers

Containers are commonly found at fire scenes. While most of them will be normal contents of the house, such as paint cans and household supplies, they may have contained flammables that could be associated with arson and, if not, may still provide useful information. If the can contained a liquid, from a small amount up to a full can, and it was tightly sealed and heated, exposure to heat would cause it to bulge and split around one or more seams. If the liquid was flammable, it would have boiled out of the can and contributed substantially to the total fuel. If such a can is not bulged or burst, it is an indication that it was either totally empty or that the cap was loose. Under some circumstances, lightly soldered cans may selectively heat from radiant fire above them, so that the solder softens and allows escape of the contents without showing a bulge. When arson is suspected, it is essential that all such containers be collected and submitted for laboratory examination, with care being taken to preserve possible latent fingerprints.

Contents Inventory

All portions of the structure should be carefully inventoried and documented by the investigator, whether or not the contents were damaged by the fire. This process serves two purposes. First, it is for the protection of the investigators, who may be called on to prove the appearance and contents of the scene at the time of their possession. This is especially important when the contents are of high monetary value. Second, it ascertains the contents of the structure at the time of the fire. A post-fire inventory should be carefully checked against an inventory prepared by the owner or tenant. Removal of a building's contents before a fire is a strong indication that the fire was planned. The investigator must be sensitive to the absence of major appliances, tools, equipment, stock, guns, clothing, jewelry, memorabilia, antiques, sports equipment, and pets. In cases of insurance fraud, junk or cheap goods may be substituted for valuable goods or stock (which has been stored elsewhere or sold).

We have illustrated in a number of instances how the fuel load in a structure affects the fire pattern. A thorough inventory of the burned structure provides the investigator with a clear and complete picture of the fuel load in the building at the time of the fire. Objects that could contribute significantly to the fuel load of each room—sofas, upholstered chairs, drapes, carpets, and the like—should be marked on a sketch of the scene. If the contents are removed during overhaul, the investigator may seek the assistance of the owner or tenant in identifying what furniture was present and where it was located before the fire.

Ignitable Liquids

Although it is possible to set large, very destructive structure fires without the use of ignitable liquids, by far the most commonly *detected* arson means is the pouring or spilling of an ignitable liquid (usually a petroleum product) onto the floor and contents of a room followed by direct ignition with a match. Ignitable liquids are used as accelerants because they are cheap, easily available, and volatile and therefore easily ignited. Because of the frequent use of ignitable liquids, the investigator who is able to locate identifiable residues of such liquids will be more effective in detecting incendiary fires.

Whenever an ignitable liquid is exposed to the high temperatures of a fire, it is going to vaporize quickly even if it does not burn. When the post-fire debris is being examined, only liquid that has been protected from the flames and high temperatures will remain. This protection can be afforded by absorbent materials such as carpet, upholstery, untreated wood, plaster, or soil or by cracks or crevices in floors or between floors and baseboards. Water used to extinguish most fires tends to protect residues from evaporation for some time. Whenever localized burn patterns are discovered on walls, floors, or floor coverings, nearby debris should be checked for the odors of common flammable liquids. The appearance of burn patterns is often enhanced by cleaning the floor with a broom and then flushing with water. The pattern can then be photographed and sketched as needed. Seams, crevices, and other protected areas can then be checked for distinctive smells by nose or portable hydrocarbon detector (Figure 7-42).

Many investigators rely on olfactory detection of volatile fuels, and some have a very sensitive and accurate sense of smell. There are several drawbacks, however. First, the

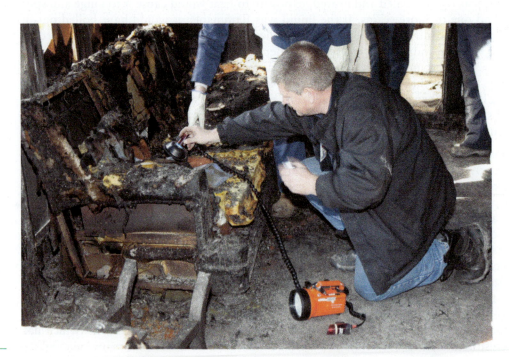

FIGURE 7-42 Electric hydrocarbon detector uses a solid-state sensor that vapors enter by passive diffusion. Operator must move the sensor slowly. *Courtesy of Jamie Novak, Novak Investigations and St. Paul Fire Dept.*

human nose is very subjective in its perception of odors and can be "fooled" into false reactions. The human nose fatigues quickly, and inhalation of some vapors can render the nose incapable of detecting other odors. The fire scene also contains toxic gases and vapors that should not be inhaled in high concentrations.

If a floor is porous or leaky, some of the accelerant may have seeped through and penetrated the soil underneath. Water and debris falling onto the soil then trap the volatiles for later detection. Specially trained canines have proved their value in locating areas of debris where ignitable liquid residues can be identified by laboratory analysis. While not substitutes for a complete, professional investigation, trained canines can help expedite the scene examination for likely areas to sample.

The flame temperatures produced by accelerants such as gasoline burning in air are not significantly higher than those produced by ordinary combustibles (and in some cases are lower). Ignitable liquid accelerants are noteworthy because of their potential for rapid combustion, localized damage, and unusual distribution. Liquid accelerants can burn at low levels in a room and in protected areas, leaving burn patterns that are often distinguishable from those produced by ordinary fuels (barring overwhelming subsequent fire damage such as post-flashover burning or collapse).

Some ignitable liquids do not have a characteristic odor, and some do not cause an electronic detector or a canine to react. It is also possible for a sustained fire to consume all liquid fuels used as accelerants. Other materials, such as crumpled newspaper, waxed paper, and plastic packing materials can very easily accelerate a fire and leave little residue detectable by chemical or even visual examination. When indications are that an ignitable liquid has been used, it is important to recover samples of the flooring and nearby associated debris for laboratory testing no matter what odors are present. Water-soluble flammable liquids such as methanol, acetone, or ethanol are diluted and may be washed away by the application of hose streams during suppression or debris removal. Empty containers of such solvents should warn of their possible use as accelerants.

The presence of unusual, pour, or pool patterns of floor damage are not necessarily proof that ignitable liquid accelerants were used. Laboratory tests are needed to confirm hypotheses. This is especially true if there has been structural collapse or post-flashover burning.

Minimizing time and exposure minimizes the chances of contamination of the scene (accidental or intentional) from spurious sources of ignitable liquids (such as from equipment used for **salvage**) and provides the best chance of detection. When the debris dries out, sun and high temperatures will evaporate even protected residues in a matter of days. Some residues have been detected in soil under houses a few weeks after a fire. Finding of liquids under the house suggests that large quantities were used. While cold, wet weather may aid in the retention of ignitable liquid residues, it may adversely affect burn patterns and other evidence exposed to the elements.

salvage ■ Procedures to reduce incidental losses from smoke, water, and weather following fires, generally by removal or covering of contents.

If the burn pattern is on a carpet or rug, it is often useful to brush it vigorously with a clean, stiff broom—after carefully visually examining it for the presence of trace evidence (adhering glass fragments or plastic, paper, or fabric from an incendiary device)—to remove loose debris and enhance the burn pattern for examination. The carpet and any pad can then be sampled for lab testing. The resulting burn pattern may be enhanced by sweeping away loose debris and then flushing with clean water. Residues may be found between the tiles remaining, under baseboards, or soaked into the wood sub-floor. In a multiple-layer floor covering, residues of ignitable liquids with evidentiary significance are not going to be found in the lowest layers if they are not found in the ones above.

No matter from where laboratory samples are to be taken, two things must be kept in mind: First, volatile liquids are driven off by high temperatures; therefore, they are *not* likely to be found in the areas of deepest char. Rather, they are more likely to be found in places where the liquids would be protected from the heat. Second, many building and upholstery products involved in fires today are synthetic materials that share the same petroleum-based origin as most accelerants.

Taking comparison samples is important to ensure that the lab will be able to distinguish minute traces of accelerants from the semi-volatile decomposition products of synthetics. A quantity of undamaged material should be collected from a nearby area that does not appear to have been contaminated with accelerant. Even in badly damaged structures, comparison samples of floor coverings may be found under appliances, bookcases, or large furniture. Because these scene samples cannot be guaranteed to be free from accelerants, they cannot be considered to be *control blanks* and should be considered and labeled as *comparison samples*. True control blanks would have to come from a non-contaminated source such as a retail store, manufacturer, or identical unburned vehicle.

Detectors—Electronic and Canine

Sniffers or, more properly, portable hydrocarbon detectors, are used in many investigations. Although many varieties of detectors are available, they should not be used to the exclusion of other tests examining appearance or odor. Like the human olfactory system, detectors can be overwhelmed or fatigued by continued exposure to high levels of volatile fuels. They may not be sensitive at all to some common accelerants (odorless charcoal lighter seems to be the most elusive) and thus yield false negatives when there really is an ignitable liquid present. Most of them are sensitive to an oxidizable gas or vapor, including the carbon monoxide (CO), ammonia (NH_3), methane (CH_4), and methyl alcohol (CH_3OH) vapors produced by the destructive distillation of wood and give false positives. Many modern sniffers rely on an electronic detection element that is not as sensitive to pyrolysis products or water vapor as were older designs. One successful approach is to use two matched detectors, one of which is located in a burned reference area while the other is used to examine a burned target area. The difference between the two signals is then more likely to be significant and less likely to indicate simple volatile pyrolysis products.

Accelerant-detection canines, typically trained to detect one drop of partially evaporated gasoline or paint thinner, have a detection limit on the order of 0.1 part per million (ppm) [0.1 microliter (μL) in a 1-L can] in samples with a clean background. The presence of burned debris (particularly carpet and pad) can reduce this sensitivity significantly, but at scenes dogs have been able to discriminate traces of ignitable liquid from fire debris more successfully than the human nose, and they carry out a search of a scene much more quickly than a person. As with drug-detection dogs, their positive alerts can be used as probable cause to search a person or take a sample from a fire scene, but their positive indications should *not* be accepted as proof of the presence of accelerants.

Dogs cannot discriminate between gasoline used as an accelerant and volatile traces of carpet adhesives or insecticide sprays. Only a proper laboratory analysis can specifically identify the material, and only then can it be put into context with the scene findings, for an accelerant must be identified by its intended use, not by its mere detection (Gialamas 1994). Because of the variety of petroleum products that can be detected at trace levels in normal household items, the investigator must be careful not to put too much value on detection at very low concentrations unless proper comparison samples are collected (Lentini, Cherry, and Dolan 2000; DeHaan 2003).

Areas of wood surrounding a char pattern should be chiseled or pried up and tested with a sniffer or the nose. Areas yielding any sort of response can then be cut out and sealed in appropriate containers for laboratory testing. When all the areas have been checked and sampled, the containers can be left in place, labeled with numbered cards, and the entire area then photographed to record graphically the disposition of the samples recovered.

PART 3: Wildland Fires

7.5 Wildland Fires

Fires in open land covered with grass, brush, or timber are often termed *wildland fires*. Although they are often terrifying in their destructive power and intimidating in their coverage, they begin, like almost every other fire, with suitable fuel and a small, localized source of ignition. In some respects, the investigation of a wildland fire is simpler than that of a structure fire, because the fuels involved are generally limited to naturally occurring vegetation. They are ignited by some finite source of heat—natural, such as lightning; accidental, such as a discarded match; or incendiary, with an intentional ignition device. Some evidence of the source of ignition will remain unless, as in a fire started with a lighter, the source has been removed from the scene.

The causes of wildland fires are more varied than for structure fires. The California Department of Forestry and Fire Protection (CDF), which annually responds to an average of over 5,500 wildland fires in its direct protection area, reported 11 major categories for identified causes, as shown in Table 7-2.

Unlike with structure fires, however, there are complications in retracing the progression of the fire by variable environmental conditions—fuels, wind, weather, and terrain. The large scale of many wildland fires results in major firefighting efforts that can disturb or destroy delicate evidence. Because of the fire, an area of interest may remain inaccessible to the investigator for days, during which time the evidence is exposed to the elements, further diminishing its value. All fire investigations require thorough and systematic examination of the suspected area of origin and logical and analytical assessment of the evidence found, and wildland fires are no exception. The investigator who understands fuels, fire behavior, and the effects of environmental conditions is in a better position to interpret the subtle and sometimes delicate signs of fire patterns in wildland fires, and therefore is better able to identify the origin and cause, no matter what type of fire is involved.

TABLE 7-2	Wildland Fire Causes in California, 2006–2008			
CAUSE	**2006**	**2007**	**2008**	**PERCENT (3-yr)**
Arson	319	227	220	6.4
Campfire	113	41	23	1.5
Debris burning	455	490	431	11.5
Equipment use	1,237	489	401	17.7
Lightning	237	126	332	5.8
Miscellaneous	627	1,061	1,115	23.3
Playing with fire	40	12	8	0.5
Power line	130	27	20	1.5
Railroad	19	0	4	0.2
Smoking	87	84	62	1.9
Undetermined	986	969	908	23.8
Vehicle	555	84	69	5.9
Total	4,805	3,610	3,593	100.0

Source: 2006–2008 Historical Wildfire Activity Statistics (Redbooks) (Sacramento, CA: California Department of Forestry and Fire Protection, 2008a and 2008b).

7.5.1 FIRE SPREAD

The spread of a wildland fire (and thereby the means of retracing its development back to a point of origin) involves consideration of many more factors than the typical structure fire. These factors include the following:

- Topography such as slope (and the local winds slopes can engender) and aspect (fuels on south-facing slopes in the Northern Hemisphere are exposed to more sun than those on the north-facing slopes and are therefore drier and able to support larger, faster-moving fires),
- Terrain (natural noncombustible barriers of rock or bare soil versus chimneys (defiles) that can draw fires faster upward,
- Weather conditions including wind direction, speed, and variability, as well as temperatures and relative humidity. Because these conditions affect both ignition and spread, they must be documented for times before and during the fires as thoroughly as possible, and
- Fuels can be extremely varied and must be documented (both in the fire area and in adjoining areas). While the names of fuels can vary, the general categories are displayed in Table 7-3.

Each category of fuel supports a different type of fire. The duff and surface litter most often burn as a slow smoldering fire, only contributing when strong winds can kick up burning embers to produce airborne fire brands. Grasses, shrubs, and slash can all support fast-moving flaming fires that can ignite the **ladder fuels** (Rothermel 1992).

The crown, being a porous array of fine fuel elements surrounded by air, can support extremely fast burning, intense, flaming fires. The canopy can be nonhomogenous, as well. Ladder fuels are the bridge that can connect fires started in ground litter to the canopy or connect a crown fire to the next susceptible fuel array. The oncoming fire first evaporates (by radiant or convective transfer) the water in the exposed foliage, then evaporates the volatiles present, and then pyrolyzes the hemicellulose, cellulose, and lignin components into combustible gases (Johnson 1992).

ladder fuels ■ Intermediate-height fuels between the ground litter and the crowns of trees overhead.

TABLE 7-3	Fuel Categories in Wildland Fires
CATEGORY	**EXAMPLE**
Duff	Decomposed organic layer (humus) on the soil
Ground or surface litter	Dropped leaves Dropped branches Needles and twigs
Ladder fuels	Intermediate-height grasses Shrubs [less than 2 m (6 ft) in height] Seedlings Small trees Lower branches Loose bark
Crown	Canopy of foliage leaves, needles, and fine twigs (more than 2 m above ground)
Slash	Branches and foliage left as heavy ground cover after logging operations[a]

[a]From R. C. Rothermel, *How to Predict the Spread and Intensity* of Forest and Range Fires, Gen. Tech. Rep. INT-143 (Ogden, UT: US Dept. of Agriculture, National Wildfire Coordinating Group, June 1983), 10–12.

The seasonal stage of the foliage (green or live, mature, cured or dead) has a significant effect on the fuel moisture and thereby on the fuel's ignitability and rate of spread of the fire. The volumes and arrangements of fuels (continuous, intermittent, or isolated) also are important variables that the investigator must consider. Rothermel (1992) has offered guidance regarding the interpretive complexities of these factors and has developed nomograms for predicting the effects of numerous such variables on fire behavior. Anderson (1982) published a photographic guide to identify the fuel model of various fuel arrays.

The wildland fire investigator must be prepared to take all these factors into account when evaluating the spread of a large fire with the intent of backtracking it to its origin and then evaluating various ignition mechanisms there. The proper investigation therefore entails the determination and documentation of as many of these factors as possible.

7.5.2 FUELS

By definition, wildland fires consume grass, brush, and timber but will also involve structures and even vehicles and equipment as subsidiary fuels. Although the basic fuels are all cellulosic in nature, they can vary considerably in their fire behavior because of their volume, density, arrangement, and moisture content. Short dry grasses, for instance, tend to flash over once, contributing little to the fire (except to carry it into denser fuels), while short green grasses may not burn at all during their first exposure to the fire but will dry out, ready to provide fuel for a reburn of the same area. Long dry grasses may be burned off at their tops if the fire is passing quickly across dense growth. The remaining grass stems then provide fuel for a second or following burn. If a slow-moving fire moves into tall grass, it is more likely to burn the stems away near the ground, allowing the tops to fall. This behavior is most often seen in areas where the fire is **backing** into the wind or down a hill or **flanking** (moving laterally at roughly right angles to its major direction of progression).

Brush and heavy timber may also burn in the same ways. Fire may flash across and upward through the leaves and finer twigs (called **crowning**), leaving heavier portions to ignite later as fire conditions change. This condition is especially notable downwind and uphill from a fast-moving fire, in the area sometimes called the *head* for obvious reasons. Radiant and convective heat from an intense nearby fire can raise the temperature of an entire bush or tree or its volatile resins to its ignition temperature, whereupon it explodes in flames.

Fire Spread

The nature of the fuels will have considerable effect on the spread of the fire and its intensity. The higher resin content of firs and pines causes them to burn faster and more fiercely than many hardwoods. Few trees are resistant to the intense flames of a fully developed forest fire. Some, like the firs, will die when the *cambium*, the living layer of cells just beneath the bark, is breached even though damage to the rest of the tree may be slight. The critical temperature for cambium death is about 60°C (140°F), so as a general rule, the thicker the bark, the greater the tree's resistance to fire death (Johnson 1992). A few trees, like the giant redwoods of the Pacific Coast, resist even serious fires with a thick, almost noncombustible bark. Some species actually *require* a fire to open their cones to allow the sowing of new seedlings.

Finely divided cellulosic fuels, such as grasses with a high surface-to-mass ratio, will ignite easily when dry and allow the spread of fire by fast flashing across the tops or by slow, creeping, smoldering spread along the ground. In semiarid regions, the brush, sometimes termed *chaparral*, protects its living cells from death via evaporation by developing a high oil or grease content in the wood. The high oil or grease content shields the cells

backing ■ Slow extension of a fire downslope or into wind in the opposite direction of its main spread.

flanking ■ Lateral spread of fire in a direction at right angles to the main direction of fire growth.

crowning ■ Rapid extension of fire through the porous array of leaves, needles, and fine fuels above 2 m.

from the hot, dry environment allowing the cells to maintain a normal moisture level. The oils or greases in the brush, however, provide an exceptionally high-quality fuel for a fire. A fire in cellulosic fuel develops extremely high temperatures that cause the oils of nearby plants to volatilize at a rapid rate, generating clouds of flammable vapors. The passage of a fire through such brush is awesome in its ferocity.

Moisture Content

The general response of wildland fuels to changes in relative humidity is categorized in terms of the time required to equilibrate. Small-diameter fuels (grasses, foliage, twigs) are considered to be "<1-hour" fuels. Larger diameter branches are "1–10 hour" fuels. Timber is rated 10–100 hours.

The moisture content of fuels is of more interest to the wildland fire investigator than to the structure fire specialist, because it can vary considerably with the environment. Fuels having excessive surface moisture will be more resistant to ignition on the first pass of a fire. The heat generated can evaporate the moisture, thereby preparing the fuel for more ready ignition if the fire alters its course and reburns the same area. The same holds true to a lesser extent for internal moisture content. This is water trapped within the plant (fuel moisture) that reaches equilibrium with the humidity of the surrounding air through the life processes of the plant's living cells. Dramatic changes in the temperature and humidity in the surrounding air can affect this cellular water, only at a much slower rate than the surface moisture.

The passage of fire or even hot gases can reduce the moisture content of leaves, brush, and needles to materially increase their combustibility in a short time. The relationship is more complex with living cellulosic materials, because wind and sun exposure can accelerate moisture losses. Fuels that are difficult to ignite with "weak" sources such as cigarettes in still air at moderate temperatures and humidity become much more susceptible with increases in atmospheric temperature and wind speed or decreases in humidity (National Wildfire Coordinating Group 2005). Weather and exposure conditions in the area of origin just prior to the start of the fire are therefore very important data to have.

Measuring the Intensity of Wildland Fire

The intensity of a wildland fire is often measured in kilowatts per meter of a fire line. Intensity can range from 40 kW/m for a smoldering fire in duff to 100 to 800 kW/m for backing fires in surface or ladder fuels, 200 to 15,000 kW/m for advancing head fires, and up to 30,000 kW/m for a single-front crown fire in timber (Johnson 1992). Crown fires have been measured to produce peak incident heat fluxes of 40 to 150 kW/m^2 at distances of 10 m (33 ft) from experimental fires in stands of 10-m tall jack pine–black spruce trees (Stocks et al. 2004). The durations of these peak exposures were typically 30 to 90 seconds.

7.5.3 FIRE BEHAVIOR

Virtually all wildland and grass fires begin as a small source of flame or smoldering fire—match, cigarette, electrical arcs, hot fragments or embers, lightning—that kindles easily ignitable fuels in the area. As the small fire exposes sources of fuel, its growth and direction of travel will depend on availability of fuel, direction and strength of wind, and the slope of the surrounding terrain. A small fire burning through uniformly distributed fuel on level ground will grow slowly in every direction in which fuel is available if there is no external wind, as illustrated in Figure 7-43. Hot gases generated by the fire rise at the center of the fire and draw in air from all directions along the ground. The fire must then back into surrounding fuel against its own induced draft, and its growth rate is limited as a result.

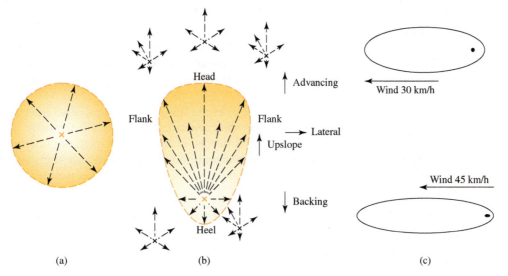

FIGURE 7-43 (a) Typical fire spread in uniform ground cover with no wind on level ground. (b) Fire spread in uniform fuel on moderate slope with no prevailing wind. Although some spot fires may occur downslope from the origin, they will predominantly be upslope. (c) The higher the wind velocity, the more elongated the fire area becomes and the closer the origin to the upwind heel.

(a) (b) (c)

If this same small fire and fuel are arranged on a slope, convective entrainment draws more air from the bottom of the incline, and the spread of the fire is then enhanced by both this draft and the exposure of more fuel to hot gases and flames on the uphill side of the fire. The fire progresses more rapidly up the slope and travels predominantly in this direction, following the available fuel. This progression gives the fire direction, and the head of this advancing flame front grows in energy as it moves into more and more fuel. The draft caused by the fire grows in strength as the fire grows, thus perpetuating the development in a chain reaction. Fire winds are those induced by the buoyancy or convective entrainment of the fire plume. In a large wildland fire, this draft or entrainment effect is great, and a very strong wind is created by the fire itself. In a fully developed fire, this can become a firestorm of superheated gases and flames igniting all fuels in its path. As a result of these dynamics, the fire not only spreads uphill in a fan-shaped pattern, it can also progress downhill (by radiant heating or direct flame contact). If sufficient suitable fuel is available, the fire will back slowly down the slope, even against a fire-caused draft. Burning embers, falling timber, and loose, burning debris can also fall downhill, starting secondary fires, sometimes at a significant distance from the actual fire.

Effect of Wind

Natural winds driven by high- and low-pressure atmospheric areas are called *meteorological winds*. Any prevailing atmospheric wind will affect the progress of the fire, particularly during its erratic, early development stages. It will force the flames and hot gases in one direction or spread an uphill fire sideways across the slope, modifying its fan-shaped pattern of general development. The higher the wind speed, the narrower the elliptical burn pattern becomes, with the origin becoming closer to the downwind end (as shown in Figure 7-43) (Johnson 1992). Very strong winds can force a fire downhill or cause a fire to reburn previously flashed-over areas where unburned fuel remains.

An external wind will have the greatest effect on the downwind edges and tops of the forest, as it is quickly dissipated by the porous canopy. Warm, dry winds flowing across a mountain ridge can produce very strong downslope winds on the leeward side (especially in valleys and passes). These are sometimes called *foehn winds* (referred to locally as Chinook or Santa Ana winds) and have been responsible for many major firestorms (Rothermel 1992). Diurnal winds are caused by daytime solar heating and nighttime cooling. They flow upslope during sunny days and downslope after sunset.

Effect of Tall Fuels

The growth of fires in tall fuels [>2 m (7 ft)] becomes more complex than growth in structures fires because the fire grows through a porous array of small fuel elements—leaves, needles, twigs—rather than across a simple surface. As the buoyant (upward) flow and wind-driven flow carries flames through the foliage the fire can quickly grow to enormous intensity, a process called crowning.

These slow-moving (essentially backing) fires are low in energy and often leave a lot of unburned or slightly burned material on the ground and on vertically arranged fuels above the average flame heights. These lightly burned materials are sometimes referred to as *color*. This phenomenon is commonly seen in an origin area, with the fire starting with low intensity at ground level and then transitioning into higher fuels as it moves away from its origin.

- Ambient meteorological wind will modify the pattern by adding an additional spreading component, so that the fan-shaped pattern on the hillside will deflect to one direction or the other, and a predominant direction of travel will be created on level ground.
- In the circumstance of a strong downhill wind, the fire will burn downhill only to the degree that the ambient wind can overcome the fire's own tendency to burn uphill.
- In a fire having an extended perimeter, the direction of burning may vary locally in almost any direction, depending on the interdependence of the fuel, topography of the terrain, the air currents created by the fire itself, and the ambient wind.
- High winds tend to produce long, narrow burn patterns.

Fully developed crown fires in timber can reach heat release rates of 30 MW/m of fire line (Johnson 1992). This intensity causes remote ignition by radiant heating and generation of wind-driven flaming brands.

7.5.4 DETERMINATION OF ORIGIN

Once these factors are identified, the investigation can then focus on what actions and series of events brought the ignition source and first fuel together to cause the fire and the identity of the responsible party. The investigator must document the terrain, weather conditions, and fuel distribution. The determination of area of origin is generally carried out by examining the fire scene for indicators of direction of fire travel. Once a pattern of these directional indicators can be established, it can be used to point back toward the area of origin. Such interpretive signs should be used strictly as indicators—none are foolproof, none are fail-safe. With the complexity of exterior fire behavior, modified as it is by weather, fuel distribution, terrain, and suppression activities, it is the *predominant pattern* of indicators that must be sought out, not a single isolated one here or there.

Investigation Methodology

The most widely accepted protocol for wildland fire investigation today is described in the NWCG manual *Wildfire Origin and Cause Determination Handbook* (National Wildfire Coordinating Group 2005). It is the foundation for the FI 210 course, "Wildfire Origin and Cause Determination," offered nationally by a wide variety of state and federal agencies in the United States, Canada, Australia, and other countries.

Prior to the start of the scene examination, the investigator must be prepared with knowledge of the local area including topographical maps, people with reliable local knowledge, and even fire histories of previous events in the area. Prior to scene arrival, the investigator can record observations (weather conditions, fire and smoke conditions, equipment, vehicles, and people in the area) and assess available manpower and expertise. On arrival, the investigator must assure that the suspected area of origin is protected (from vehicles, foot traffic, retardant or water drops, water runoff). Interviews with witnesses are a critical first step to minimize wasted search time.

First Evaluation

Almost every wildland fire will have been observed in the early stages of its development by someone—camper, sightseer, hiker, ranger, pilot, or firefighter. Although these people may not be easy to find, it will be much easier than spending days trekking over the later-burned areas spotting indicators of fire direction. All subsequent investigation is then limited to the general locality that witnesses indicate was first burned regardless of how far it spread later.

The investigation should follow a logical scheme that allows thorough and accurate determination while preserving the evidence remaining (not to mention the investigator's time). Several of the first firefighters present should be questioned as to wind direction and weather conditions, as well as to the extent, location, and behavior of the fire. First-in fire companies are often aware of where the fire appears to have begun. They are often trained to protect such areas (which may have already burned out) with flags or barrier tape (National Wildlife Coordinating Group 2005). Interviews with local residents or law enforcement witnesses may help establish an area of origin or identify unusual vehicular or pedestrian traffic or equipment use in the area.

Other Sources of Information

Infrared photography or video imaging from aircraft has been used to map wildland fires and detect hot spots within a fire area. If these are taken over a time interval, the progression of the fire can be retraced via these images. Images from earth-resources satellites can show smoke movement as well as thermal images. These images, when combined with topographic and weather maps of the fire area, may permit retracing the fire's development back toward its origin and eliminating certain mechanisms of fire spread.

Establishing multiple origins that are separate in place but coincidental in time and that could not be the result of natural fire progression by airborne embers would go a long way to demonstrating an incendiary origin for those fires. In the Oakland Hills fire of 1991, infrared imaging from a C130 aircraft and mapping via global positioning satellite (GPS) and transponders allowed the rapid assessment of the fire's extension (through fog, smoke, and darkness) and its damage (Public Works Journal 1992). American Defense Support Program (DSP) satellites today offer a 10-second "revisit" rate of a target area, allowing for minute-by-minute detection and monitoring of wildland fire events (Pack et al. 2000). The use of remote-controlled surveillance drones is also reportedly being evaluated by DSP researchers.

The Scene Search

The scene search involves a perimeter search and then a more focused search of areas closer to the apparent area of origin.

Perimeter Search

First, the general area of the first-observed fire is surveyed to determine the outer perimeter of the search area. The general area is mapped out on a rough sketch; a topographic map showing hills, valleys, and similar features of the area may be very helpful at this time. This general origin area can be identified through witness statements, fire behavior observations, or gross indicators of direction. The outer portions of the secured area (away from the apparent origin) are searched by whatever systematic pattern best suits the terrain.

These early sweeps are for general indicators, observing the larger, more obvious signs (sometimes called *macro-scale* indicators, to be described later), if possible, working from one side or flank of the burn pattern to the other. Indicators can then be mapped onto a drawing of the scene as they are found. It is recommended that the perimeter of this general area of origin be searched twice, from opposite directions.

The shape of the burn pattern often helps investigators focus on a likely area of origin. Depending on the nature of the terrain and the extent of the fire, a fan-shaped or V-shaped pattern may be visible from a short distance away. The apex of this pattern can then be

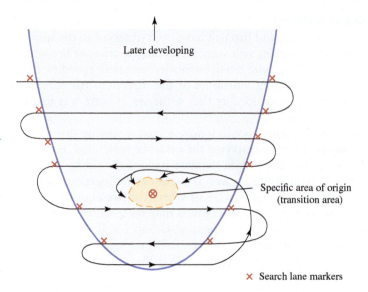

FIGURE 7-44 Typical "V" pattern of burn on hillside with suggested search pattern. This pattern starts from outside the margins of the burn pattern and works progressively toward the earliest portions of the fire.

Later developing

Specific area of origin (transition area)

× Search lane markers

selected as the focal point for the search pattern (see Figure 7-44). A barricade of rope, twine, or plastic banner is arranged to control access and limit further damage to the physical evidence from personnel, vehicles, or the heavy equipment so common to wildland fires.

The perimeter search should focus on the macro indicators and examination of adjacent *unburned* areas to establish pre-fire fuel type and distribution. Unless the scene is very large, this search can be done on foot, slowly, methodically, observing and recording. Photographs should be taken of all significant indicators (macro and micro). It may be helpful to keep track of the searching process by using visible markers or flags (color-coded to reflect advancing fire progression, lateral progression, flanking, backing, and items of evidence). A standardized color flag system has been developed to note fire movement and evidence location, as seen in Table 7-4.

These markers can help keep track of the fire spread and provide a visual reference of the overall fire scene (National Wildfire Coordinating Group 2005). Keeping a written fire-spread map that corresponds to this flagging system is also a good idea. Remember that the direction determinations you make are based on the indicators you have found, not on the flags added.

Focused Search

The search can then progress to areas of interest closer to the apparent area of origin. As the investigator's search approaches the specific area of origin, there is often a change in the burn pattern indicators being examined, from the larger-scale indicators to the indicators (called *micro-scale* indicators) characteristic of the origin area. The focus is not on a single spot but on a small area of several square feet or yards. Wherever fires of

TABLE 7-4	Standardized Color Flag System
FLAG COLOR	**INDICATOR**
Red	Advancing fire spread
Yellow	Lateral (flanking) fire spread
Blue	Backing fire spread
Green, white, other	Physical evidence

multiple origin merged, the areas of erratic fire travel around each will remain. These areas contain the small indicators and remaining physical evidence.

It is always best to minimize all traffic in these areas until an inch-by-inch examination can be carried out. Burn indicators on larger brush and trees will usually not be usable unless the fire took on a direction and some intensity. In the area surrounding the point of origin, the smaller indicators in this specific origin area may show considerable variation as the fire sought fuel and responded to the conditions of wind and topography. For this reason, once the area of origin has been located, it is usually necessary for the examination to be carried out on hands and knees looking at individual pebbles, leaves, and twigs for the resulting signs, and, ultimately, for the cause of the original ignition.

As the **area of transition** (to directional spread) is detected, the investigator should proceed slowly *around* the area, but doing so from outside the burn itself or the suspected area of origin. The most common method is to grid or lane this area off, using twine on stakes. Because the transition from random to directional (driven by wind, fuel, or terrain) may be very subtle, it is easier to overrun the origin if it is approached from the backing or heel area; approaching from the advancing area is recommended. Each lane or grid can then be searched visually, with magnification like a handheld or headband magnifier or 2X–3X magnifying glasses and a magnet. The detail search is often carried out using a straightedge (ruler) to help focus the visual examination.

The debris is then swept with a handheld magnet in a plastic bag to collect iron-containing debris. A sensitive metal detector may be swept over the suspected area to locate metal vehicle or tool components, or ignition devices. A small kitchen baster, photographer's bulb, or blowing by mouth can be used to direct small puffs of air to move surface debris and light ash. Heavier covering debris can be moved using a soft paint brush, tweezers, or long forceps. If the ash layer is deep, it will need to be removed by gently blowing it away after the first search, possibly revealing additional indicators beneath.

Suppression and control efforts can vastly complicate the reconstruction of a wildland fire. Bulldozers can build firebreaks to divert normal progress. Tanker air drops can cool off areas, allowing nearby areas to burn. Secondary backfires or burnouts may be set deliberately to deprive the main fire of fuel and can dramatically affect the appearance of burn indicators. Wind and rain may quickly compromise many useful indicators, so the investigation should be carried as soon as it can safely begin.

area of transition ■
Mixture of fire directional indicators in a wildlands fire.

Burn Indicators

Because the effects of the nature of fuels and fire conditions in a wildland fire are fairly predictable, there are a number of fairly reliable indicators that can be used to determine the direction of fire spread past a given point.

Charring of a tree trunk, plant stem, or fence post is deeper on the side facing the oncoming fire. Char depth can be checked with a knife blade, pencil point, ice pick, or screwdriver. It is strictly a comparative indicator, so absolute depth is of little consequence (Figure 7-45).

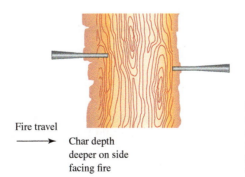

Fire travel →

Char depth deeper on side facing fire

FIGURE 7-45 Char depth will usually be deeper on the side (with uniform fuel) facing the fire.

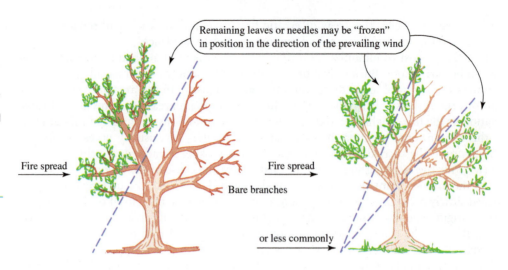

FIGURE 7-46 Partial combustion of trees and bushes can reveal the fire spread. Fire will progress upward as it moves forward through the foliage, leaving an angled interface between burned and unburned portions. Remaining leaves or needles may be frozen in position in the direction of the prevailing wind.

Remaining leaves or needles may be "frozen" in position in the direction of the prevailing wind

Fire spread

Fire spread

Bare branches

or less commonly

Destruction of a bush or tree may be more extensive on the side facing the fire (Figure 7-46). Fire will progress upward as it moves forward through the foliage, leaving an interface between burned and unburned portions as the buoyancy of hot gases causes the flame front to rise as it moves forward.

The beveling effect of a fast-moving fire may influence the appearance of branches or twigs remaining upright. Twigs and branches facing the fire may have flat or rounded ends, while those facing away from it (downwind) will be tapered or pointed, as shown in Figure 7-47.

A fast-moving fire creates a draft around large objects, which creates an angled pattern around tree trunks, posts, and plant stems as shown in Figure 7-48. On foliage crowns, this angle of fire pattern may also be evident when the tree or burn is viewed from the side. It may reflect the fire behavior of the flames coming in low and exiting high.

Fast-moving (either fire- or wind-driven) fires moving past large-diameter vertical tree trunks or power poles create a low-pressure area on the downwind side. This low-pressure area draws the passing flames from local fuels into a vertical vortex, creating a

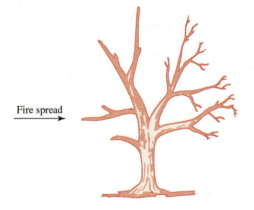

Fire spread

FIGURE 7-47 Beveling effects of oncoming fire blunt the ends of branches facing the fire and taper those away from it.

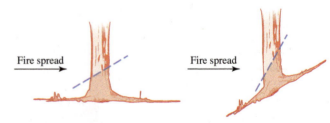

Fire spread

Fire spread

FIGURE 7-48 In a fast-moving fire, the fire pattern on a tree will start lower on the trunk side facing the oncoming fire, even on a slope. The charred area *may* wrap completely around and extend up the back side. (See Figure 7-49.)

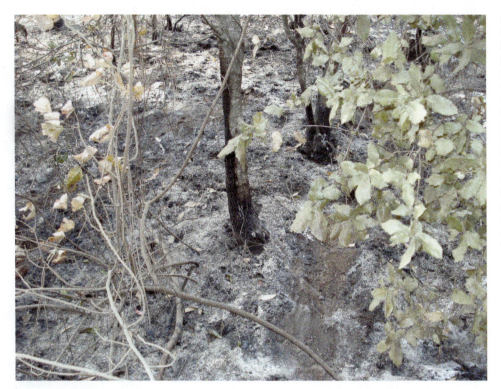

FIGURE 7-49 This fire (moving from right to left) induced a low-pressure zone on the leeward side of the center tree trunk, which caused the formation of a laminar flame entraining the flames in the ground cover at its base. This flame lasted longer than the passing flame front and produced much higher burn damage on the downwind side. *Used with permission of Donna Deaton, Deaton Investigation, LLC.*

laminar flame. The laminar flame lasts longer than the passing flame front and can induce significant fire damage to the downwind side, extending several times the height of the flame front (Gutsel and Johnson 1996). A very slow-moving fire, especially one that is backing against the wind or down a slope, will create a burn pattern *approximately* parallel to the ground (as depicted in Figure 7-50A).

Burn patterns can be influenced by local fuel load such as needles, leaves, and debris around the base of the tree, leaving a pattern higher on the side facing the oncoming fire or the upslope side (which catches such debris). This may also be the result of momentum flow of the fire against the vertical surface. Wind-driven (either from fire plume convection or atmospheric wind) fires often produce a rising char pattern on the leeward side of the trunk or pole, as in Figure 7-50B.

If the vertical stem is burned away, the remaining stump will be beveled or cupped on the side facing the fire, as shown in Figure 7-51. This will be true even for stems of weeds. When the back of the hand is brushed lightly against such stubble, the beveled tops allow the skin to pass smoothly across in the same direction as the fire but resist with sharp points a hand passing in the opposite direction.

Rocks, signs, and other noncombustibles will show greater heat discoloration (staining) on the side facing the fire, as pictured in Figures 7-52A and B. Lichen, moss, and close-growing grass may survive on the side away from the fire. Extensive exposure may burn all soot off (leaving a light-colored or white surface) on the side facing the oncoming fire.

Large rocks, walls, and large objects provide a barrier to the flow of the flames. The area downwind of the obstacle may escape damage completely or be burned later as the fire changes direction (Figure 7-53). Intense flame contact may cause spalling of stone or concrete on the upwind or facing side.

Tall weeds and grasses, when burned by a slow-moving fire (particularly as it spreads laterally along the flanks or backs downslope or against the wind), will be undercut by the

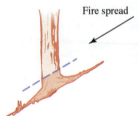

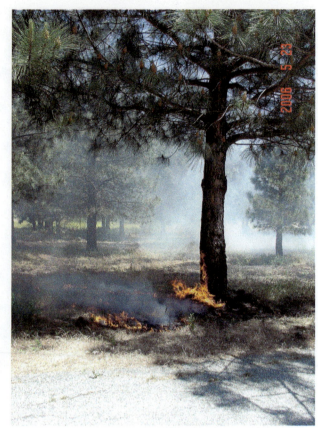

FIGURE 7-50A In a slow-moving or "backing" fire, the burn pattern will be *roughly* parallel to the ground. Wind-driven patterns often exhibit a rising char pattern on the leeward side. Accumulations of ground litter may produce char patterns on the upslope side of tree trunks and utility poles.

FIGURE 7-50B Observed low-intensity test fire moving from right to left in light ground fuel with a light (5 mph) wind. Char pattern is higher on the leeward (downwind) side of the trunks. *Courtesy of Marion Matthews, US Forest Service.*

fire moving along the ground. The stems, if vertical, will then fall toward the fire with the heads of grass stems pointing back toward the fire origin, as in Figure 7-54. This effect is highly dependent on the wind conditions prior to and during the fire. Tall grass that is already matted down pointing away from the fire will fall in that direction, so there may be conflicting directions from such indicators.

The height of remaining stems and grasses is roughly proportional to the speed of the fire. The effect is dependent on the moisture content of the plants and will not be visible in areas that have reburned.

In the immediate vicinity of the origin, the fire will not have developed any particular direction, and so the indicators will be variable or contradictory. Fuels in the form of

FIGURE 7-51 Beveling or cupping on vertical stems or stumps will point back in the direction of the fire's origin.

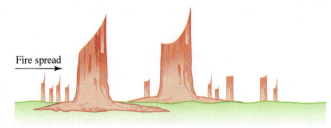

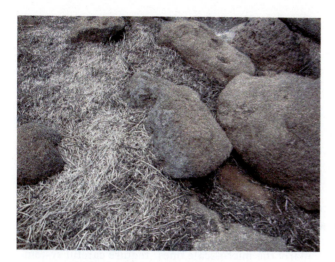

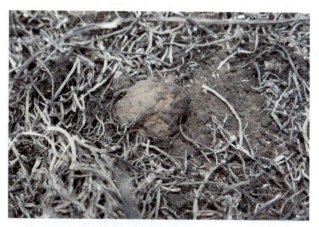

FIGURE 7-52A Deposits left on upper left sides of large rocks as a result of observed fire spread (through coarse grass) from top to bottom. *Courtesy of Marion Matthews US Forest Service.*

FIGURE 7-52B Micro-scale indicator deposits on small stone amid burned grass confirm that the fire was moving from right to left. *Used with permission of Donna Deaton, Deaton Investigations, LLC.*

grasses or weeds may still be upright or only partially burned. Large fuel may be burned only at its base with fire extending into upper branches only as the fire moves away from its origin.

Extension of a fire beyond a barrier, for example, a road or river, will cause the appearance of a brand new origin. This is particularly true when the new fire is started by airborne embers or burning debris (brands) from an established fire. (Such new fires are sometimes called **spot fires**; see Figure 7-55.)

By their quantity and distribution, ashes can indicate the direction of wind and the amount and nature of fuels present. If the fire is very recent, the white ash formed by the fire's impact on the facing side (with more complete combustion) can be compared with

spot fires ■ Fires started by airborne embers some distance away from the main body of the fire.

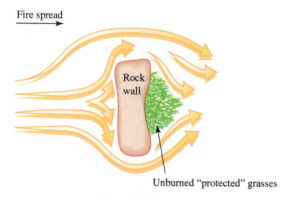

FIGURE 7-53 The flow of a fast-moving fire around a large obstacle often leaves protected vegetation on the downwind or "lee" side of the obstacle.

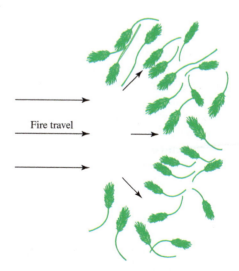

FIGURE 7-54 Tall stems of grass or weeds point predominantly back toward the source of the fire in the absence of a strong prevailing wind.

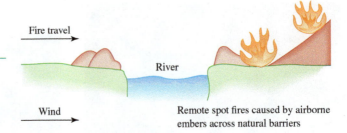

FIGURE 7-55 Remote spot fires caused by airborne embers across natural barriers.

Fire travel

River

Wind

Remote spot fires caused by airborne embers across natural barriers

the darker area of less intense fire on the leeward side. Viewing the overall fire scene from the origin may reveal the white ash deposits on exposed surfaces. Wind or rain will remove such deposits.

Most of these indicators (particularly the micro-scale ones) require careful systematic *comparison* of one side of an object with the other, not an assessment of absolute condition. Ventilation and venturi effects in high-wind conditions or around/under objects not in full contact with the ground may produce contradictory indicators. Because wind conditions change as the fire grows or responds to slope and terrain, the investigator must consider the totality of indicators observed before concluding direction of fire spread. Reliance on a single indicator is not good practice, as it may be misleading.

Once the area has been thoroughly examined, with direction indicators carefully flagged and noted on the sketches, it is often beneficial for the investigator to stop for a few moments and reevaluate what has been found. Questions such as the following can be helpful:

- What patterns do the indicators reflect?
- What features of the terrain, weather, or the fuel load could affect the development of those patterns?
- Do there appear to be multiple origins that grew into one large fire?
- What area of origin appears to be consistent with those patterns?
- What firefighting tactics were used in the area that could have produced patterns of their own—backfires, or retardant or water drops?

There may be disparities in the indicators that were not apparent during the actual search that need to be resolved. For example, until the fire develops direction as a result of wind, fuel, or terrain, it will often extend erratically in several directions, producing a pattern of contradictory direction indicators. This specific origin area could be the point of origin. Once the point of origin has been located and the first fuel identified (and possibly an ignition source detected), the origin needs to be thoroughly documented with photographs. A sampling of the specific indicators by class needs to be photographed, documented in the photo log, and their location measured from a previously selected main reference point. This information can then be used to draw a to-scale scene diagram that corresponds with the photographic record and re-creates the origin determination process.

Documentation

The recommended minimum documentation for wildland fire investigation should include a comprehensive narrative report, photographs of burn pattern indicators used, maps, diagrams, witness statements, weather information, and forensic lab analysis reports (if applicable).

Photographs provide a clear understanding of what was seen, done, and used, and preserve critical data for review later by the investigator. A photo log describing the

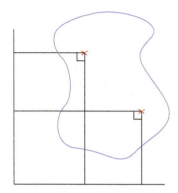

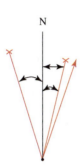

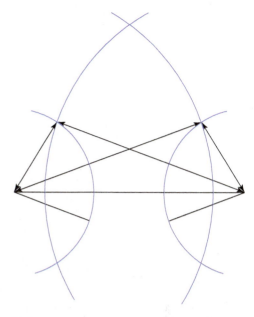

FIGURE 7-56A Right-angle transect: baselines at right angles with endpoints set by GPS and compass. Baselines are marked by string, paint, or metal tape.

FIGURE 7-56B Azimuth/baseline: single baseline (in N–S or E–W orientation) (set via compass and/or GPS). Locations noted by angle and distance from baseline or reference point.

FIGURE 7-56C Intersecting arcs from two fixed reference points.

FIGURE 7-56 Methods for baseline reference at wildland fire scenes.

subject of each photo and direction in which the photo was taken may be in the form of a scene diagram with symbols (numbered to show frame [image] number, or negative/roll number) with an arrow to show direction, or a numbered list.

Diagrams show the location of indicators used, witnesses, and evidence collected. They must include date, location, compass, initials of preparer, and documentation of dimensions and topographic features (White 2004). Measurements can be in one of three formats, as shown in Figure 7-56. GPS coordinates can be used to establish locations of evidence and possible areas of origin. These coordinates can be used to create reports and diagrams and to confirm jurisdiction.

There are several computer-aided drawing systems designed for use in wildland fire investigations. These include standardized symbols and plotting methods.

7.5.5 SOURCES OF IGNITION FOR WILDLAND FIRES

The next step in the investigation of the wildland fire is to determine the cause when possible. In some instances, this may be impossible because the evidence has been destroyed. It is always necessary to make a reasonable search for the physical remains of the ignition source and to establish a defensible cause. Ascribing such cause to unknown factors should be only a last resort. The causes of outdoor fires are well known in general. The National Wildfire Coordinating Group (NWCG) maintains records of wildland fires in the United States. Human-caused fires account for approximately 80 percent of all wildfires annually (National Wildfire Coordinating Group 2005). The California Department of Forestry reports that in over 12,000 wildland fires over a three-year period, in the average year, the leading identified causes (in descending order of occurrence) were equipment use (tractors, chain saws, weed cutters, etc.), debris burning, arson, vehicles (trucks and cars), lightning, smoking, campfire, power line, playing with fire, and railroad (California Department of Forestry and Fire Protection 2008a). The following are examples of some of the possible causes:

- Unextinguished fires (including discarded unextinguished coals) left by campers, hunters, and others.
- Carelessness with smoking materials, including burning tobacco and matches.
- Trash burning and, in some areas, controlled grass and brush burning (including airborne firebrands).
- Sparks (hot exhaust particles) from vehicles, especially locomotives or other motor-driven equipment.
- Lightning, a major cause of timber fires.
- Power transmission lines and equipment, including birds and mammals that may come into contact with the power, short-circuit it, and catch fire, falling into nearby fuel.
- Arsonists, who may use a variety of devices but generally use a lighter or match.
- Firearms, which under certain circumstances may blow sparks of burning powder into dry vegetation, and steel-core and tracer bullets.
- Spontaneous combustion, limited to very specific types of circumstances.
- Overheated machinery, which may be in contact with combustibles.
- Sparks from any source, such as impacts of metal with rock.
- Discharges of static electricity.
- **Rekindling** of smoldering embers from previous controlled fires, whether they were barbecues, campfires, or previously burned timber slash or debris piles, or small (possibly unreported) brush fires. These are sometimes referred to as *holdovers*. These have been reported to have time frames of up to and exceeding 12 months (Steensland 2008).
- *Sleepers,* which are old trees or stumps containing much rotted wood internally in which a smoldering fire has been previously induced. Because of their unique burning characteristics, fire may persist in them for long periods, documented in some instances to be as much as nine months.
- Miscellaneous objects sometimes found in trash, including clear glass (cylindrical or lens-shaped in cross section) or concave reflective surfaces that can focus the sun's rays. These are rarely responsible for wildland fires but should be considered.

rekindle ■ A return to flaming combustion after apparent but incomplete extinguishment (*NFPA 921*, 2017 ed., pt. 3.3.155).

The search for cause includes examining the ground cover for ignition sources, looking for things that do not belong, and noting circumstances like proximity of roads, trails, railroads, or signs of recent equipment use (freshly cut weeds, recent gouges in road or stone surfaces). A follow-up search from a different direction or a second examination can reveal additional information.

The nature of the fuel at the origin and the relevant characteristics of the proposed ignition source must be evaluated together. Because most wildland fires involve cellulosic fuels, either open flames or hot (glowing) sources must be considered as competent.

Power Lines

Power lines often generate fires. Power lines may initiate a fire in the following ways:

- Transformer short circuits and malfunctions—perhaps one of the more common and dangerous situations, causing overheated oil or molten metal droplets to fall into ignitable fuel,
- Leakage over dirty insulators and supports when moist, giving rise to "pole top" fires,
- Fallen wires that arc with the ground or objects on it,
- Arcing between conductors that accidentally come into contact (typically in high winds),
- Grounding of in-place conductors by external objects such as fallen trees, branches, or birds,

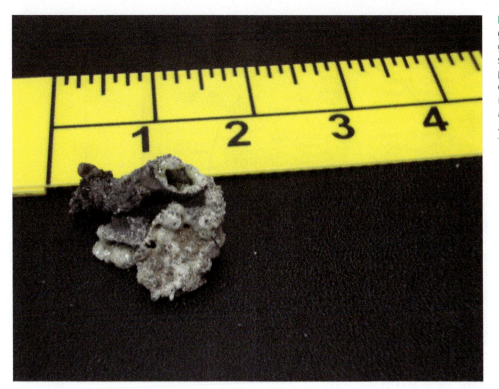

FIGURE 7-57 Small fulgurites of soil fused into a glassy mass by a ground strike of a high-voltage power line. Larger ones can be produced by lightning strikes. *Courtesy of Marion Matthews, US Forest Service.*

- Unprotected fuses dropping hot metal,
- Tree limbs coming into contact with conductors, and
- Animals coming into contact with equipment and shorting it out.

Despite the hazard of power lines as a source of ignition, careful analytical investigation can determine that the fires were started by other means, such as failure of associated power pole equipment like transformers, fuses, breakers, and switches. High-voltage conductors that come into contact with soil can produce glassy fulgurites, which are produced by the high-temperature fusion of minerals in the soil (see Figure 7-57). They will be found just below the surface of the soil by detail search and sifting.

Lightning, Another Common Cause of Timber and Grass Fires

Lightning strikes can shatter or explode trees or limbs, peel bark from trees, split rock, or fuse soil or sand into glassy fulgurites at the point of contact as seen in Figure 7-57. Evidence of lightning strikes may be available from witnesses.

The tremendous heat generated by the passage of lightning through wood can ignite even massive timbers under some circumstances. Reports of lightning in an area can be compared against lightning data accumulated by the National Oceanographic and Atmospheric Administration (NOAA), which operates a National Lightning Detection Network reporting system. There is also a private firm, Vaisala Inc., that employs more than 100 sensing stations in the lower 48 United States and a global positioning system. This network can locate lightning strikes (to the earth) to an accuracy of 500 m (1,500 ft).

A report recording the time, intensity, polarity, and location of all strikes for a particular location for a requested time period is available online for a fee. See Figure 7-58 for an example. This service is reportedly 90 percent accurate (multiple reports can sometimes reveal a strike not reported in a single report). Lightning can also strike wire or metal fences, buried pipes or cables, and underground storage tanks, causing direct ignition or ignition remote from the actual strike. See Figure 7-59 for an example of a lightning strike on a tree.

FIGURE 7-58 StrikeNet map of lightning strikes in area, color-coded to differentiate those between 0200-0300 and 0300-0400. *Courtesy of Vaisala, Inc., Tucson, AZ.*

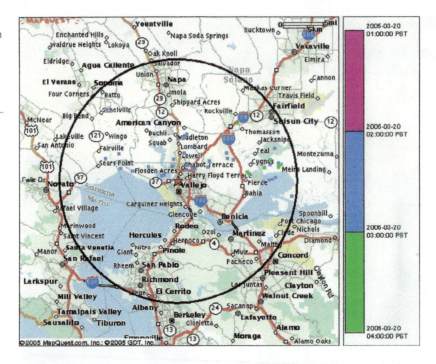

Burning or Hot Fragments

Fragments from a disintegrating catalytic converter are small and may escape detection, but they may have a characteristic ceramic honeycomb appearance in which the cells may be square, rectangular, or hexagonal in shape. Small spherical pellets are also often used. The rare metals used in them, such as platinum or iridium, can be readily identified in the

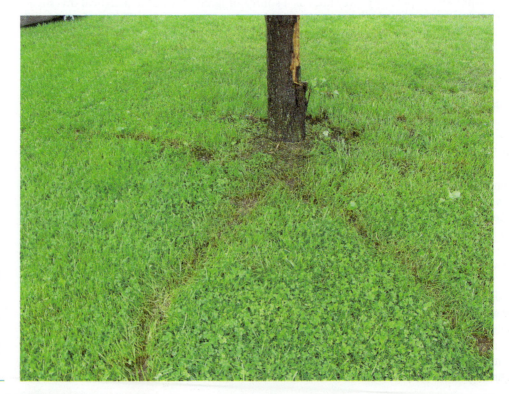

FIGURE 7-59 Lightning striking this tree stripped its bark and charred surface grass along its roots. *Courtesy of Greg Lampkin, Knox County Sheriff's Office, Tennessee, Fire Investigation Unit.*

laboratory. Fragments or sparks of burning carbon from the eductor tubes of diesel locomotive engines are nondescript in appearance but tend to be dense and may burrow through layers of dry leaves or grass before igniting them. Some exhaust fragments (especially those from gasoline engines) contain iron residues that can permit their recovery using a strong permanent magnet (Bernardo 1979). Fragments of automobile or railroad equipment and welding slag will also be recovered with a magnet.

Campfires

Campfires can ignite wildland fires through direct flame contact, aerial sparks (embers), improper disposal or covering of ashes and coals, or even direct ignition of hidden pockets of combustible duff or buried roots. Ignition is usually close to the campfire site, and proof of mechanism and improper care or extinguishment will be an important element of the case. Shoe prints or food containers may reveal recent use. Hot wood or charcoal coals can retain their heat for extended periods of time (1 to 2 days) and may be buried or discarded away from the main campsite.

Cigarettes

Cigarettes discarded while still smoldering represent a competent ignition source for grasses under some conditions. The relative humidity has to be low (<22 percent) and ambient temperature over 26°C (80°F) to produce the low fuel moisture necessary (Countryman 1983). The lower the humidity, the lower the fuel moisture and the more likely that ignition will occur. The fuel has to be loose enough to permit rapid burrowing of the burning cigarette and good contact between the exposed coal and suitable fuel. Surrounding fuel has to be sufficiently dense to sustain the fire spread. Ignition is more likely if the cigarette lands coal-end down or facing into the wind.

Incendiary Fires

Incendiarism cannot be overlooked as a significant cause of wildland fires, especially in rural and urban-wildland interface areas. During a thorough search through a fire scene, obvious signs of recent activity should be noted. Cans, bottles, tire and shoe impressions, weapons, and mechanical delay devices may all survive even the most awesome of conflagrations. An eye should be kept open for these during all phases of a scene search. Ignition devices are probably more common in wildland arsons, where one may need many more minutes to flee the area than in urban structure arsons.

Unless the fire has been set with a pocket lighter, the remains of the ignition device often are recoverable from the point of origin. Cigarettes have rarely been seen to ignite grasses or brush when the relative humidity of the surrounding air was above 22 percent. Relative humidity lower than 22 percent can produce fuel moistures below 14 to 15 percent, at which the low heat release rate of a smoldering cigarette can ignite fine fuels such as grasses and needles (duff) (Babrauskas 2003). Weather data for several days prior to the fire are critical for proper testing of hypotheses involving any wildland ignition source.

Multiple points of origin are indicators of incendiarism, although there are accidental circumstances that could account for such fires. An overheated catalytic converter spitting glowing remnants of its matrix, or a stuck brake shoe or failed bearing on a railroad car spewing bits of hot metal over some distances, are examples. Glowing particles of carbon from diesel locomotive engines can be thrown some distance from their moving source to ignite multiple fires along the right-of-way. Witnesses may see small fires along the right-of-way following the passage of railroad equipment.

Because readily ignitable fuels are present in such quantities in wildland, the use of a flammable liquid such as gasoline or kerosene as an accelerant is uncommon. Unusual odors or the appearance of trailers between points of origin should always be carefully examined.

Devices may be used to ignite remote spot fires, to delay detection and suppression, or to delay ignition of the set itself. The most effective remote ignition sets consist of a bundle of matches wired or taped to a cigarette. A rock or steel washer may be added for additional weight if the device is to be thrown any distance. Once ignited, the device can be thrown from a passing car deep into a brush-covered ravine or similar inaccessible location. Many devices can be set in a short period of time. Some will not land on suitable fuel, but those that do can ignite serious fires with little evidence with which to link a suspect to the crime.

Searches of nearby roadsides in the vicinity of a fire have revealed similar serial devices that were unsuccessful and therefore undamaged by ensuing fire. Such devices may bear fingerprints and trace evidence that can be associated with a suspect. Shoe prints and tire prints from such locations have successfully linked a suspect to a general fire area. Wrapping a rock with paper, tissues, or cloth and throwing the ignited bundle into brush can also kindle fires with little traceable evidence remaining.

Incendiary devices are used by fire services for starting backfires. These can range from commercially made pyrotechnic devices with a cardboard cylinder and a fuse to table-tennis balls filled with gasoline/diesel mixture. They have occasionally been stolen or misappropriated from fire agencies. Kerosene-fueled drip torches are often used to start intentional backfires but have also been misused.

Elaborate time-delay devices are very rare in wildland fire arsons. Concave shaving mirrors have been used to start remote fires, sometimes with more than a year's passing before the focused rays by chance fell onto suitable fuel. Other time delays may have been used and have escaped detection and analysis, just as in the case of structural arson sets. Arsonists will generally stay with a device for an entire season if it proves successful, thus creating a signature for linking incidents together and eliminating copycat scenes.

As mentioned previously, the most common time-delay device is a bundle of matches or a matchbook affixed to a burning cigarette. When such a device is found, it is vital that it not be disturbed until it has been fully documented via appropriate sketches and photographs. The appearance and length of ash can indicate if a cigarette was being smoked and discarded, whether it was burned in place by an encroaching fire, or if it was ignited and left deliberately (with malice). The brand of cigarette and the conditions of burning have a great effect on burning time.

Tests by the California Department of Forestry demonstrated burn rates of 4 to 8 mm/min (0.16 to 0.33 in./min) for various cigarettes burning horizontally in still air. These rates were faster when the cigarette was burning vertically upward and when burning in the direction of an external wind. Total burn times were on the order of 10 to 15 minutes (Eichmann 1980). The brand of cigarette can often be determined if the butt end (with or without a filter) remains unburned. Bourhill's manual for such identifications remains a valuable resource (Bourhill 1995). The introduction of reduced ignition propensity cigarettes is likely to reduce the number of fires ignited accidentally or deliberately with cigarettes but not to eliminate them from consideration.

hot set ■ Direct ignition of available fuels with an open flame (match or lighter).

Devices that do not provide time-delay ignition are sometimes called **hot sets**. The direct application of flame from a match or lighter to available fuels is almost certainly responsible for a large percentage of wildland arsons. When the source of flame is removed by the arsonist, establishing the cause of the fire will depend on thorough elimination of all other possible causes and extremely careful searching and documentation including documentation of sources that were considered and eliminated (Ford 2002). Hot sets that may leave identifiable remains include dropped matches and cigarettes, rescue flares, flaming arrows, or lighted road flares or fusees. The remains of matches and cigarettes tend to stay on top of other ash and debris but are easily destroyed by weather or persons searching the scene.

Road flares leave a cakey, white, or pastel-colored residue of characteristic appearance (and chemical composition) and usually a wooden end plug and plastic striker cap. The plug and cap often survive even a major fire if they are protected, and the length of the original flare can be estimated from the size of the plug and the amount of residue left behind. Figure 7-60 shows the characteristically bright-white and pastel residue of a common emergency road flare used to start a grass fire. The components of the flare can vary with manufacturer and age.

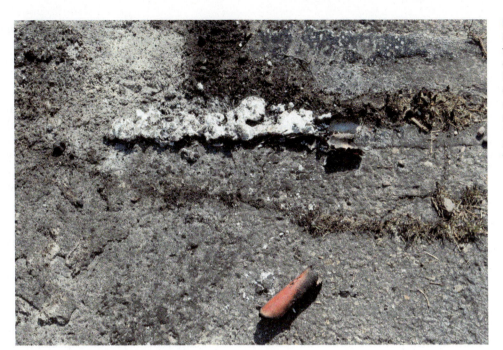

FIGURE 7-60 Top: Intact debris from a road flare (fusee). The hollow cardboard end cap is at lower right; the plastic cap is melted and burned. *Courtesy of Greg Lampkin, Knox County Sheriff's Office, Tennessee, Fire Investigation Unit.*

Modeling

Computer models have been developed for predicting growth and intensity of wildland fires given known fuel, weather, and topography information. The most commonly used programs—Behave, Behave Plus, and FARSITE—can generate predictions of large-scale time lines and behavior patterns (Andrews and Bevins 1999). Like computer fire models for room fires, they have been used for hypothesis testing, but they should not be counted on to provide "proof" of how and where a particular fire was ignited. They await validation for forensic application.

Given the complexity of wildland fire dynamics, it is not surprising that accurate modeling has been a difficult challenge. Some programs for two-dimensional, wind-driven spread on grasslands have been validated by fire tests (Mell et al. 2006). The advent of ever-more powerful computers has aided the development of limited models of crown fires (Meroney 2004). NIST is also evaluating the Fire Dynamics Simulator (FDS) for use in predicting fire spread in wildland-urban interface fires where trees and shrubs present the initial fire-spread mechanism, and structures are ignited by radiant heat from those sources (Evans et al. 2004). Sullivan has compiled a comprehensive account of wildland fire modeling in the years 1990–2007, and the reader is referred there for more detailed information (Sullivan 2009).

7.5.6 COLLECTION AND PRESERVATION OF PHYSICAL EVIDENCE

The documentation of the appearance of the wildland fire scene and its related evidence by sketching and photography is as important as it is in structure fires. Considering the fragile nature of important evidence and the vagaries of the environment, it is all the more surprising that some agencies do not routinely document their fire evidence in this way. Some situations peculiar to wildland fire evidence should be reemphasized, however.

Cigarettes, Matchbooks, and Other Fragile Evidence

When recovering cigarettes or matchbooks, remember that spraying them with lacquer or some other preservative will generally make it impossible for the laboratory to test for latent fingerprints, to obtain saliva-borne DNA typing results, or to conduct brand identification or physical comparison tests. It is best to photograph the object in place and then package it between layers of loosely fluffed cotton wool in a rigid box for hand transmittal to the laboratory.

One recommended technique for collecting fragile evidence, such as cigarettes or matchbooks, which permits recovery of parts of evidence buried in the ash beneath, is to dig into the ash and underlying soil using a sharp-edged, flat-bladed garden trowel and loosen the soil under the object in a rectangular area. After this is done, a clean rectangle of sheet metal is worked carefully through the soil without disturbing the surface debris. The sheet metal is worked all the way under the soil platform and then used to lift the soil, ash, and object together. The entire mass is then transferred to a properly sized and padded evidence box. If the soil is very hard, water can be introduced to the trenches around the target and allowed to stand to soften the soil. On rocky surfaces, it may be possible to lift only the ash layer with the sheet metal.

Shoe and Tire Impressions

Shoe and tire impressions should be photographed using low-angle oblique lighting and a ruler or scale near (not *in*) the impression. (Placing a scale in or across an impression can obscure critical details.) If at all possible, the impression should then be cast using plaster, dental stone, paraffin, or other suitable casting agent.

Charred Matches

Matches that are completely charred are probably not useful as evidence (except to demonstrate their presence), but if any unburned cardboard remains, an attempt can be made to match it to a matchbook.

Debris Suspected of Containing Volatiles

Debris suspected of containing volatiles should be sealed in appropriately sized cans, jars, or polyester or nylon bags. Polyethylene plastic or paper bags must not be used.

Containers

All containers much be securely sealed to prevent loss or contamination, and the chain of evidence must be recorded on it in ink. The date, time, and location of recovery and the name of the person recovering the evidence must be on the package as well.

Weather Data

A critical item of evidence that is not found at the scene itself and is sometimes overlooked is weather-related data. This should be obtained as soon as possible, either from first-on-scene fire suppression personnel, websites such as Weather Underground (www.wunderground.com) or NOAA, nearby Remote Automated Weather Stations (RAWS) (http://raws.fam.nwcg.gov/), or collected firsthand using either a handheld digital weather recorder or a belt weather kit (shown in Figure 7-61).

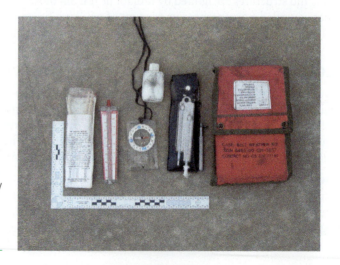

FIGURE 7-61 "Belt" weather kit: Pitot-type wind gauge (anemometer), compass, water bottle, psychrometer (wet/dry bulb humidity gauge), and case. *Courtesy of US Forest Service (photo by author).*

The RAWS system uses remote sensor stations that automatically send weather data via satellite every hour to the National Weather Service's Weather Information Management System. There are approximately 2,200 RAWS sites across the United States.

Weather data should be taken from outside the burn but as close to the suspected origin as possible and as close to the estimated/known ignition time as possible. Handheld devices can be used to record temperature, relative (air) humidity, and wind speed. Weather data can provide a critical source of information with which to assess fire behavior, rate of spread, and fire intensity through the use of nomogram fire calculations or computer models. Such analysis can support burn pattern interpretation and scientifically corroborate or exclude possible ignition sources.

PART 4: Vehicle Fires

7.6 Vehicle Fires

All types of motor vehicles contain substantial quantities of ignitable liquids for fuels; electrical and mechanical systems to provide ignition sources; and combustible plastic and metal components and cargo, which provide fuel loads. Vehicle fires can be accidental or incendiary in origin. And, arsonists will often try to simulate such accidental fires to escape detection.

The NFPA has estimated that US fire departments respond to an average of over 287,000 fires in highway vehicles per year, which cause some $1.3 billion in direct property damage each year, an estimated 1,525 injuries, and 480 deaths to civilians (Ahrens 2010). Vehicle fire investigators must be familiar with fuels, ignition sources, and dynamics as encountered in vehicles if they are to carry out correct investigations. We shall describe the fuels, fuel systems, and ignition sources and then discuss the investigation.

7.6.1 FUNCTIONAL ELEMENTS

Fuel Tanks

The fuel tanks of most autos or light trucks contain flammable and potentially explosive gasoline and gasoline vapors (diesel, biodiesel, LPG, or CNG are, of course, also encountered). Firefighting experience and laboratory tests reveal that, contrary to expectations, fuel tanks very rarely explode during a vehicle fire. It is nearly impossible to ignite the gasoline inside a tank because its vapors are much heavier than air and tend to fill the tank completely to the top. Except at extremely low ambient temperatures, the vapor pressure of gasoline is such that it tends to form a mixture with residual air in the tank that is well above the explosive limit and cannot be ignited. It follows that fire will not ordinarily invade an open gasoline tank but will be limited to the outside of any openings where there is sufficient air for combustion. Gasoline vapors outside an open fuel filler neck can usually be ignited with an open flame, to create a steady, torch-like flame longer than a foot (30 cm) or so in length. Propagation into the tank to cause an explosion is almost impossible unless the tank has so little fuel in it that an equilibrium vapor pressure is not reached. A closed vapor recovery system, when exposed to a fire, can release vapor under pressure, creating a torch-like effect, sometimes in locations remote from the tank itself.

When exposed to a general fire, the soldered seams and fittings of a metal tank may melt and separate, releasing fuel (sometimes under considerable pressure) to fuel the fire.

Pressure built up by vaporizing fuel can split the tank or blow the filler cap off of either metal or polymeric tanks. Accidents can, and frequently do, lead to rupture of the fuel tank by mechanical force, producing a very hazardous spill. Because most large trucks use diesel engines, their fuel presents less of a hazard when spilled at ordinary temperatures, but in a general fire, diesel fuel can vaporize to form explosive vapor mixtures. In addition, some vehicles are being fitted with LPG (liquefied petroleum gas) or CNG (compressed natural gas) fuel systems, and a number of fires have been caused by even small leaks or poor filling practices that resulted in explosive vapor mixtures in or around the vehicle.

To minimize fabrication costs and vehicle weight, manufacturers are using polymeric tanks in more and more vehicles today. They are strong and puncture-resistant, but unlike metal tanks, they are subject to cracking and can melt or burn through in an enveloping fire, releasing their contents quickly, giving the appearance of an accelerated fire. Under rare conditions, polymeric tanks can fail explosively as a result of a boiling-liquid, expanding-vapor explosion (BLEVE).

Fuel Tank Connections

Because regular fuel tanks are mechanically strong and usually well protected, the tanks themselves are rarely involved in accidental fires (except in severe crashes). The filler spouts of many tanks have flexible rubber connections that can crack or loosen and allow fuel to spill into trunks and passenger compartments.

CNG vehicles may have a glass-fiber-wrapped polymeric tank that can fail explosively in a general vehicle fire. Topping off the tank often leads to overfilling, creating hazardous spills beneath the vehicle. In older vehicles, fuel filler leaks could introduce fuel into the trunk or even the passenger or engine compartment. Overfilling may cause excess fuel to be siphoned into the vapor recovery canister in the engine compartment. This canister, often filled with charcoal, is designed to trap fuel vapors, which are then drawn into the engine to be burned. Liquid fuel in this canister can pose a fire hazard.

The flexible connectors (hoses) on metal fuel lines are subject to splitting or cracking with age or loosening due to abuse or improper service repairs, causing a fuel spill hazard. Many manufacturers have adopted the use of nylon fuel lines and polymeric connectors. Physical damage, exposure to severe heat conditions, or improper service procedures can result in these cracking, splitting, or leaking, which can result in a fire hazard. It was observed that a polymeric fuel line, ignited by accidental contact with an exhaust header, burned the length of the car to the fuel tank, with the fuel in the line supporting the fire.

Fuel Pumps, Fuel Lines, and Carburetors

The fuel pumps on many older cars are mechanical ones, mounted on the side of the engine, that function only when the engine is turning over. Most imported cars and newer domestic cars are fitted with high-capacity electric pumps that are pumping whenever the ignition is on. Because most electric pumps push better than they pull, they are most often mounted at or near the tank (and many are enclosed in the tank itself). Without a proper interlock to oil pressure or engine-speed sensors or with failure of the interlock safety, such pumps can pump a great deal of fuel out through a loose or ruptured fuel line even though the engine may not be running. Some new vehicles have two pumps to produce high pressure—one in the tank and a second one closer to the engine. If a fuel line is compromised by external fire or mechanical impact (collision), gasoline may siphon out of the tank by gravity even if the fuel pump is inoperative. Although the amount of gasoline in the carburetor itself or in the fuel injection lines (rails) may be small, the fuel lines of some cars are positioned over electrical components or the exhaust manifold, and loose connections pose a hazard for a large fire. If a fire is limited to the fuel in the carburetor or fuel rail, the fire will generally be limited to moderate damage of the air cleaner, hood, and engine wiring and rarely be transmitted to other parts of the vehicle.

Fuel Injection Systems

Most fuel injection systems are electronically controlled and are found on nearly all newer gasoline-fueled vehicles. These systems provide additional fire risks because their fuel delivery lines carry gasoline at pressures from 25 to 100 psi (150 to 700 kPa). Even a pinhole leak in a line or minor crack in a fitting allows gasoline to be atomized and sprayed around the engine compartment at high pressures, quickly producing an explosive vapor mixture requiring only a suitable electrical arc to ignite. The fuel rail is the metal tubing that distributes the fuel to individual injectors on each cylinder or, in older vehicles, directly to the throttle body. It usually has a high-pressure (delivery) side and a low-pressure (return) line. Such systems can leak at the gaskets or seals at the injectors or the connectors.

Vehicle Fuels

Today, more vehicles use gaseous fuels rather than liquid ones. Propane (sometimes called LPG) is stored in a vehicle as a liquid in a pressurized metal tank at pressures of approximately 75 psi. The fuel is delivered to the motor as a liquid, which evaporates quickly to a clean-burning gaseous fuel. Natural gas may be encountered (especially in large commercial or passenger vehicles) as compressed gas (CNG) with tank pressures of 2,400 to 3,600 psi (16,500 to 24,800 kPa). These tanks may be of steel or glass-fiber composites.

Gasoline is the most common fuel used in automobiles. The fuel with the lowest flash point is often thought to be the first fuel ignited. However, gasoline's properties render it somewhat less likely to ignite upon contact with a hot surface, referred to as **hot-plate ignition**, than are other heavier combustible liquids such as hydraulic fluids and lubricating oils. Tests performed by auto manufacturers and fire investigators have shown that gasoline seldom ignites at hot-plate temperatures near the listed *autoignition temperature (AIT)* and, in the under-hood environment, requires surface temperatures between 590°C and 730°C (1100°F to 1350°F) to reliably ignite. These temperatures may be attained at the exhaust manifolds, but only after extreme and sustained engine load or severe mechanical malfunction (timing and mixture), or on the surfaces of turbochargers or catalytic converters.

Textures of hot surfaces including crevices and cracks may reduce the required temperature. The rough undersides of hot cast exhaust manifolds may offer better chances of ignition. Leaks of burning combustion gases around loose spark plugs or faulty manifold gaskets offer a chance of flame ignition.

hot-plate ignition (hot surface ignition) ■ Temperature of a metal test plate at which liquid fuel ignites on contact.

Other Combustible Liquids

The residence or contact time between a fuel and a hot surface is critical, as are the nature of the surface and the quantity of fuel. Hot-surface ignition of transmission oil [460°C to 600°C (860°F to 1112°F)] or steering or brake fluid [540°C to 570°C (1000°F to 1060°F)] is much more likely than open hot-surface ignition of gasoline. Of course, in a severe collision, all these fluids may be released.

Antifreeze is not often thought to be combustible, but pure ethylene glycol has a flash point of 111°C (232°F) and an AIT of 398°C (748°F), and the values for propylene glycol are even lower (NFPA 2001). If antifreeze, often, a 50/50 mix of ethylene glycol and water, is allowed to pool on top of an engine, the water can boil away until the pure glycol can form a vapor ignitable by heated surfaces [530°C to 570°C (986°F to 1058°F)] or by arcing within the distributor, alternator, faulty spark plug leads, fan motor, or other electrical equipment (Higgins 1993). The surface temperatures of exhaust manifolds, turbochargers and catalytic converters may be in excess of the 398°C (748°F) required to ignite ethylene glycol, and the high boiling point of the glycols slows their evaporation to give more time for energy transfer and mixing. Ignition of a 50/50 ethylene glycol–water mixture sprayed directly onto a hot exhaust manifold has been reported, although documented cases of such ignition are very rare.

Brake fluid, which is usually a heavy glycol mix, and automatic transmission fluid (ATF) and power steering fluid, which are light lubricating oil–grade petroleum distillates, also represent potential fuels ignitable by hot surfaces (Cope 2009). Such fluids may be present in reservoirs, including polymeric ones that can leak, fracture, or melt, or in pressurized lines. If these lines suffer even a small puncture or leak, the fluid is sprayed out in an easily ignitable aerosol. These fluids have low ignition temperatures and can be ignited if sprayed onto hot exhaust components or disc brake rotors, or if they come into contact with electrical arc sources.

Gasoline, by contrast, is not readily ignited by contact with the exterior of a hot exhaust manifold, due in part to its volatility, but other more viscous, less volatile fuels with similar AITs, such as diesel fuel or motor oil, are ignited. The normal maximum temperature for an exhaust manifold of 550°C (1020°F) is not adequate for hot-surface ignition of gasoline (petrol), while temperatures above 395°C (743°F) can ignite DOT 3 brake fluid or automatic transmission fluid dripped onto its exterior (March 1993).

Many fluids in vehicles are at elevated pressures. The release of any ignitable fluid under pressure produces an aerosol mist that is much more readily ignitable than the bulk liquid. Operating fluids are usually at elevated temperatures as well, making them easier to ignite upon release.

Transmission or torque converter failure can produce internal heat sufficient to vaporize transmission fluid. This vaporization may produce internal pressures that result in fluid being expelled from vents, seals, or dipstick tubes. When the fluid or its aerosol contacts heated exhaust components, it can ignite. Post-fire indicators of this event include low transmission fluid level combined with a darkened oil color, particulate contamination, or a strong burned odor. Heat transfer patterns from transmission fluid fires tend to be at the bottom of the compartment near the transmission tunnel or at the base of the radiator where the fluid can leak from cooler connections. Confirmation of the failure may require removal and disassembly of both the transmission and the torque converter (Suefert 1995).

Engine Fuel-System Fires

Engine fuel-system fires tend to show heat effects in the upper part of the engine compartment, and particularly on the hood, where a series of rings or halos of pyrolyzed paint and metal oxidized to different degrees may indicate a localized fire from such a fuel source. Such fires also tend to produce white oxidation (high-temperature) patterns on the firewall, inner fenders, or strut towers. Whenever the fuel system is pressurized, leaks elsewhere in the delivery lines may allow fuel to spill beneath the vehicle to be ignited there. Leaks may occur from loosened connections and failures of the lines due to corrosion, aging, splitting, vibration, or mechanical damage such as crushing or contact against moving parts, as illustrated in Figure 7-62 (Suefert 1995).

Many connectors today are made of plastic. Some modern vehicles have fuel lines entirely made of plastic that can burn away completely, so they may not be detectable post-fire. In-line fuel filters made of metal, plastic, or glass and metal can fracture or separate to produce fuel leaks. O-ring seals in fuel injection systems degrade from heat, pressure, or fuel additives (or improper installation) and release fuel under pressure. Fires on the top of the engine are most likely to be fuel fires, while fires near the firewall (bulkhead) or wheel wells are more likely to be brake fluid or automatic transmission fluid fires. Lines can be cut and even ignited by contact with moving parts such as pulleys, belts, or drive shafts. Because of the complex routing of their hoses, power steering and coolant systems cannot be generalized as to origin location.

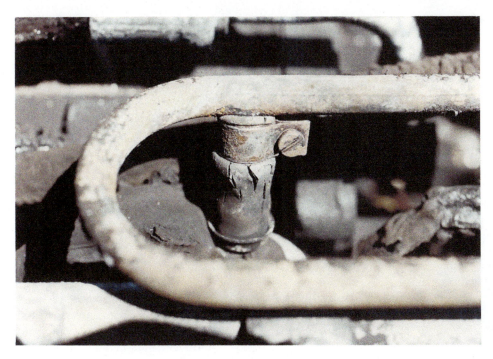

FIGURE 7-62 A rubber fuel line, connecting a fuel injector to the fuel rail, cracked from age and sprayed gasoline on the top of an engine. *Courtesy of Bloom Fire Investigation, Grants Pass, OR.*

Once ignited, the hoses, vacuum lines, and plastic-insulated wires of modern vehicles provide a great deal of fuel to support a fire. Very few of the polymeric materials in engine compartments are fire-resistant. Many vacuum system and vapor recovery hoses use plastic connectors that can fracture, melt, or simply add to the fuel load. The modern vehicle has many fresh-air, heating, and air-conditioning ducts of synthetic materials that originate in the engine compartment and penetrate the firewall, as shown in Figure 7-63. These are, in turn, connected to polymeric fan enclosures. While they are not ignited by glowing ignition sources, all these can support flaming ignition once ignited and allow flames to readily penetrate into the passenger compartment.

Fires in these enclosures and ducts may be ignited by failure of fan motors or by fires in the engine compartment (Suefert 1995). Fire entering the interior through the large openings created by failure of polymeric enclosures will impinge on plastic dashboard components and spread readily into the interior. If the fire progresses to the point where window glass is exposed to fire, side window glass, being tempered, is especially vulnerable to thermal-shock failure. If the window glass breaks, there can be sufficient ventilation to allow the fire to *eventually* involve all combustible interior components. Fire thus transmitted into the passenger compartment may be revealed by fire damage coming from the defroster vents between the windshield and top of the dashboard. Engine compartment, tire, or brake fluid fires can ignite the polymeric fender liners used on many cars. These fires can extend under front fenders and attack side windows, door seals, and the lower front corners of windshields (Marley and DeHaan 1994).

Electrical Systems

The general principles of electrical fire causation are just as applicable in vehicle circuits as in structural ones. Although the operating voltage of most autos and light trucks today is only 12 V, and the currents (in most fused circuits) are limited to a few amps, electrical

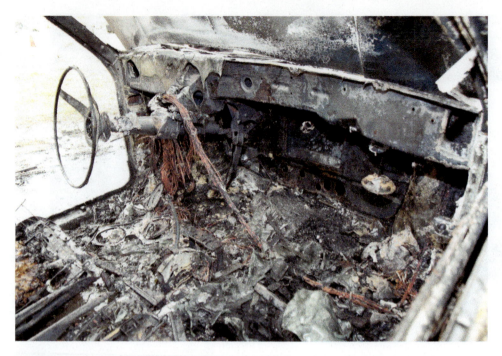

FIGURE 7-63 Penetrations of the "firewall" in modern vehicle. *Courtesy of Jamie Novak, Novak Investigations and St. Paul Fire Dept.*

causes of vehicle fires cannot be dismissed out of hand. Most power on vehicles is direct current, so arcing, once established, will not self-extinguish, as often seen in alternating current events. Trucks and commercial vehicles commonly have 24-V systems for starting and charging systems.

Most vehicles today have a single energized conductor connected to the positive battery terminal, with the return path provided by the metal vehicle frame and components. This is called a negative-ground system, because the negative post of the battery is connected to the vehicle's frame. American cars made before 1955 often used a 6-V positive-ground system. This frame-ground system means that an energized conductor coming into contact with any metal component can cause current flow.

The high-capacity cables fitted to the battery connections can carry sufficient amperage to start fires of the cable insulation, starter, and related electrical fittings. In short circuits of these or high-current circuits of the horn, cooling fans, cigarette lighter, or lighting equipment, the temperatures developed will cause smoking or even flaming combustion of the insulation and any connectors or terminals. These circuits are usually energized even when the key is in its off position, but all but the starter are often protected by a fusible link—a special wire connector. There is no overcurrent protection on the starter circuit. If this circuit shorts to start a fire near combustible components (fender underliners, splash shields, ducts, hoses, etc.), a large fire can develop quickly. Attempts to deliberately cause such electrical fires in the protected wiring in a series of modern vehicles, however, invariably caused the overcurrent devices in the vehicles to interrupt the power before ignition could occur (Marley and Dehaan 1994). Relays control many of the higher-current accessories like blower motors in newer cars, so there is less chance for a high-current fault to occur to initiate a fire.

Ignition switches which have unfused "hot" wires and ground connections in close proximity have been linked to fires started when carbon tracking allowed current to flow continuously between contacts in the switch and eventually to degrade and ignite the plastic housing (Bloom and Bloom 1997). Some vehicle fires have been linked to corrosion of fittings associated with speed control of activation switches on master brake cylinders (Morrill 2006). When large, energized, unfused conductors can come into contact with grounded metal components, a massive current flow can result, with the accompanying increased likelihood of ignition.

One form of grounded metal component that is easily overlooked is the steel braid wrapping in high-pressure hydraulic and brake lines. Chafing of these lines against metal edges (such as starter cable terminals) can abrade the protective rubber coating and allow contact as shown in Figures 7-64A and 7-64B. The hot electric arc produced quickly chars the rubber liner, allowing a leak of the ignitable fluid and the potential for a very destructive fire fueled first by the fluid, then by the rubber lines. As with any other kind of fire investigation, the first fuel ignited has to be identified, and the chain of reactions has to be demonstrated. Just having a source of heat, no matter how intense, will not result in a fire unless an adequate supply of a suitable fuel is present and the mechanism for enough heat transfer from that source to that fuel can be shown.

The newest generation of theft protection devices includes keyless entry and starting (with an encoded transponder), remote locking and unlocking, and specially coded ignition keys. Their contribution to fires and investigations is unknown at this time.

Although the current standard for automotive electrical systems is 12 VDC, negative ground, recently developed technology suggests that more efficient higher-voltage systems will be implemented on most automobiles in the near future. These systems will likely employ a 42 V alternator/starter motor combination that will be installed in the flywheel area. Many trucks and other diesel-powered vehicles use 24 V systems. Electric- and hybrid electric-gas-powered vehicles are already in service. The high wattage capabilities of such electrical systems (including batteries that can keep mechanical systems operational) can create fire hazards after crashes. The power for electric propulsion motors is 600 VDC with high-current batteries. This power is supplied in two conductors (with brightly colored insulation—blue, orange, or green) separate from the vehicle's lighting and control systems (NFPA 2014).

Many modified vehicles use high-current accessories (such as audio systems or hydraulic pumps) in an unsafe fashion, and wiring may be exposed to all manner of crushing and chafing hazards that can compromise the insulation. The same care should be exercised in examining such vehicles as one would employ in examining an older house for dangerous modifications. It is obvious that modern vehicles are often fitted with power accessories such as power seats, power windows, seat heaters, telephones, and even

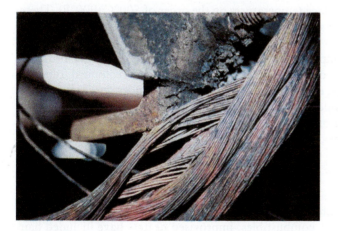

FIGURE 7-64A The vibrations of a farm tractor caused chafing to the battery cables, resulting in a dead short. *Courtesy of Tim Yandell, Public Agency Training Council.*

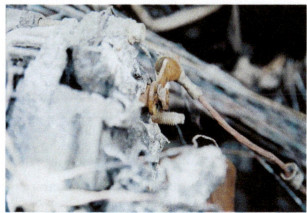

FIGURE 7-64B The main alternator connector on this vehicle failed, causing a significant engine fire. *Courtesy of Tim Yandell, Public Agency Training Council.*

portable computers and video systems. All these add to the complexity of the fire scene even if they do not usually add to the fire hazards when properly installed.

One additional source of electrical fire hazard is the battery. In normal use, it presents no fire hazard, but when it is receiving a charging current, considerable volumes of explosive hydrogen gas are generated. An explosion will result from an arc (even between the cells of the battery) or other source of ignition, and a fire may follow if the charging continues. Explosions unaccompanied by fire are the rule, and even these are rare. Symptoms of malfunction will usually be apparent to the operator. Extra batteries may be concealed in the vehicle to power hydraulic lift systems or high-power sound systems in modified vehicles. Some vehicles have their operational batteries in trunks or beneath cargo floors. Some accessories require the use of inverters to convert the 12 VDC of the vehicle to 120 VAC. Such inverters can fail, causing fires.

Miscellaneous Causes

The NFPA estimates that some 50 percent of highway vehicle fires are caused by mechanical failures or malfunctions and 24 percent are caused by electrical failures or malfunctions. Other identified causes include misuse (11 percent), intentional ignition (8 percent), and collision or overturn (3 percent) (NFPA 2010b).

Turbochargers

Many vehicles (both gasoline- and diesel-fueled cars and trucks) are fitted with turbochargers that redirect the exhaust gases to a housing to spin an impeller. This impeller then helps push air into the intake system. Such turbocharger housings operate at very high external temperatures and also, because of their very high rotational speeds, are subject to bearing failures that can produce hot-fragment ignition as the bearing, housing, and rotor fail. Bearing failure can also result in the ignition of the lubricating oil supplied to the center bearing under pressure.

Catalytic Converters

Catalytic converters have been fitted to domestic (US) cars since 1975 and to light trucks since 1984. These units convert hydrocarbons, carbon monoxide (CO), and nitrogen oxides (NOx) to less-toxic compounds by chemical conversion using a metallic catalyst like platinum or palladium in a porous ceramic foam or in loose beads. Under normal operating conditions, these converters operate at internal temperatures between 600°C to 650°C (1100°F to 1200°F) with external surface temperatures of approximately 300°C (575°F). If the converter is misused or the vehicle is not maintained properly, the converter can develop internal temperatures that can exceed the melting point of the ceramic matrix, 1250°C (2300°F), and surface temperatures on the order of 500°C (900°F). These radiative sources can ignite combustible materials under the vehicle or in contact with the floorpan above them.

Some vehicles have been completely burned when carelessly parked in dry brush or leaves with the hot converter in contact with the combustible litter. Prolonged idling of some converter-equipped vehicles, especially where air circulation under the car is limited, can produce sufficiently high temperatures that floor coverings and upholstery within the vehicle can be ignited by radiant or conducted heat. The newer-generation catalytic converters use smaller, often multiple, reactors whose surface temperatures are much lower than those of the 1980s. They also tend to be shielded better and much less likely to ignite fires inside or below the vehicle by contact with ignitable fuels.

Block and Other Heaters

In cold climates built-in block heaters or accessory block heaters (OEM and aftermarket) have been known to fail and ignite combustibles. Improvised heaters have included hair dryers, electric blankets, and trouble (service) lamps. Considering the damp conditions that may be present, each of these presents new ignition risks that should be considered (see Figures 7-65A and B).

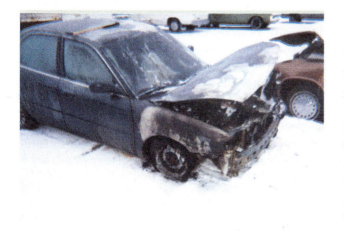

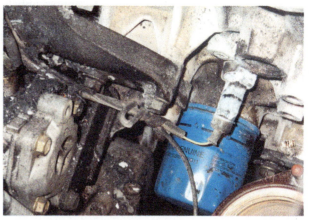

FIGURE 7-65A Fire in engine compartment could have had several possible causes. This one was a challenge because the vehicle was parked and off at the time of the fire. *Courtesy of Peter Brosz, Brosz & Associates Forensic Services, Inc.; Professor Helmut Brosz, Institute of Forensic Electro-Pathology.*

FIGURE 7-65B Engine block heater (above oil filter) failed and caused the fire. *Courtesy of Peter Brosz, Brosz & Associates Forensic Services, Inc.; Professor Helmut Brosz, Institute of Forensic Electro-Pathology.*

Rags

Other types of common carelessness cannot be ignored as fire causes. Rags have been left in the engine compartment or on top of exhaust pipes and mufflers during servicing, only to ignite when the exhaust system reached its operating temperature [as much as 550°C (1000°F)]. The burning rag then spreads the fire to other combustible materials. It matters little whether the rag is oily or not because it is the rag that will be ignited by contact with the hot surface. Improperly installed hydraulic lines can come into contact with moving engine parts to cause penetration and loss of ignitable fluid, as shown in Figure 7-66. Overflows from leaking overfilled or overheated transmission, power steering, or brake systems can flow or spray onto hot surfaces, causing ignitions.

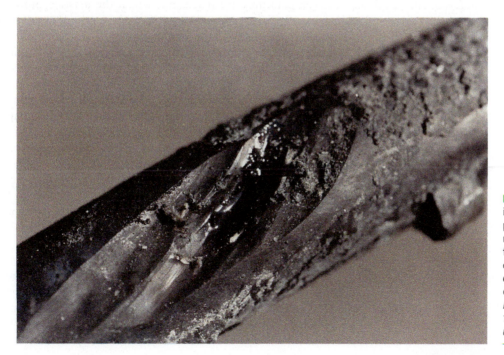

FIGURE 7-66 An improperly installed power steering line rubbed against an engine fan belt and sprayed its contents, causing an engine compartment fire. *Courtesy of Greg Lampkin, Knox County Sheriff's Office, Tennessee, Fire Investigation Unit.*

Tires

Drivers can be almost unbelievably insensitive to the condition of their tires, especially those on trailers. A deflated tire, when run against the road surface mile after mile, develops great frictional heat. This heat can build up sufficiently to ignite the tire, the hydraulic system of the brakes, and even the vehicle or its cargo, sometimes with disastrous results. Such a situation is most serious. The movement of the vehicle usually aids in dissipating the heat being developed, but when the driver finally stops to inspect the problem, the heat can ignite the tires to flaming combustion. Although tires under these conditions require a great deal of heat to ignite, once ignited they are extremely difficult to extinguish. Once burning, the oily char of rubber repels water, and the insulative properties of the rubber prevent cooling by conduction. Even a driver prepared with a portable fire extinguisher may be unable to prevent a disastrous fire. Single large tires on industrial (earth-moving) equipment have been measured to produce maximum fires of 3 MW (at 90 minutes after ignition by a diesel fuel fire) (Ingason and Hammarstrom 1992).

7.6.2 CONSIDERATIONS FOR FIRE INVESTIGATION

Many accidental vehicle fires occur in the first few minutes after being shut off. When the circulation of air, oil, and coolant is stopped, the external temperatures of many engine components (exhaust manifolds and systems, turbocharger housings, and the like) rise. Furthermore, with the cessation of movement and fan circulation, concentrations of ignitable vapors, which had been dispersed or diluted to safe concentrations, can accumulate to above their lower explosive limit. The combination of higher temperatures and higher concentrations of vapors, including pyrolysis products from smoldering plastics, can result in ignition. These situations may be preceded by unusual odors, noises, mists, or electrical fluctuations, which can paralyze an engine management computer and cause stalling, so the driver should be asked specifically about any peculiarities that may have indicated such problems. These fires normally begin with a smoldering ignition that then goes on to flaming combustion to engulf the car, so the time frame for development is some minutes.

Electrical shorts developing in the maze of wiring and myriad components have a rich source of fuel available once temperatures are reached at which the plastics and resins begin to pyrolyze and ignite. These initial stages take many seconds or minutes to develop. Depending on the initial fuel and ventilation conditions, an accidental fire may not be visible for many minutes to someone outside the vehicle. A fire accelerated with a flammable liquid would be expected to be visible as open flames almost immediately after ignition, especially if a door, window, hatchback, or sunroof was open. However, a fire ignited only by a direct flame in a closed car may not be visible from a distance for some minutes.

The investigator should exercise great care in deciding what amount of damage is consistent with an accelerated fire versus that from an accidental fire. Normally, the time factor of fire development is usually a significant diagnostic sign of accidental origin. If a reliable witness observed the progress of the fire and can establish that the vehicle was totally involved in flames within 5 minutes or so of its arrival or last occupancy, it is a very strong indication that the fire was set with the use of an accelerant. Accidental fires usually require considerably longer to start, develop into flaming combustion, and spread than do accelerated fires. In the absence of a reliable eyewitness or videotape, it is very dangerous to estimate speed of development.

If the vehicle was being driven (or had just been parked) when it caught fire, the driver and any passengers should be interviewed to gain information about possible mechanical problems. Questions should include the following: How long was the car driven just prior to the fire? When was it last fueled? When and where was it last serviced? Were there any problems with starting, steering, or shifting? Were there any unusual smells? Did the car overheat recently? Were there any noises just prior to the fire?

Were there any electrical events—lights coming on, instrument readings surging, accessories or controls not working properly, and so forth? The owner should also be interviewed about modifications, special equipment, or recent repairs.

7.6.3 COMBUSTIBLE MATERIALS

The upholstery of seats, carpeting, headliners, and side panels represent a significant fuel load in every car or light truck. Modern cars make extensive use of vinyl plastics, polyurethane foam rubber, nylon carpeting, and polyester and cotton seat fabrics. All these products are combustible to a greater or lesser extent and thus provide fuel for fires started by direct accidental ignition with any open flame, as well as for fires started in other portions of the vehicle. It is estimated that some 20 percent (by weight) of a modern auto consists of combustible fabrics, plastics, polymers, and rubber. This constitutes on the order of 228 to 273 kg (500 to 600 lb) of fuel load, which is responsible for the fire damage to the vehicle, no matter how it is first ignited (Allen et al. 1984).

Although no recent published data are available, it is clear that today's vehicles use considerably more combustible plastic and synthetic components than these data reflect. Most of the interior, including seat backs, instrument panels, dashboards, and side panels, are readily combustible. Unlike in earlier cars, polymeric materials are used throughout—including exterior body panels, structural components, and even suspension and drivetrain—not just in the upholstery. Before an investigator concludes that a component has been stripped off a car before it was burned, he or she must make sure that it has not simply burned up with the rest of the fuel.

7.6.4 MOTOR VEHICLE SAFETY STANDARD 302

It is a common misconception that the plastic upholstery materials in automobiles have to be flame retardant or pass ignition tests. In fact, the only applicable fire performance test is US Motor Vehicle Safety Standard No. 302 (MVSS-302), which applies to all nonmetal parts of vehicle interiors (Krasny, Parker and Babrauskas 2000). It is an open-flame, horizontal-spread test that is very easy to pass, as it was designed in response to vehicle fires in which the headliners ignited and dripped flaming residues onto occupants. It has been in effect since 1972 without change and has been found to have had no measurable effect on the incidence or severity of fire injuries to passengers. The MVSS-302 test does not accurately reflect the fire performance of fabrics in real fires in vehicles, and replacement tests are being evaluated (Spearpoint et al. 2005). There are no tests for flammability of seat padding, which is almost universally polyurethane foam. Tests have demonstrated that even a modest open flame applied to the underside of a vehicle seat cushion will result in rapid involvement of the seat and potentially full involvement of the interior of the vehicle. It has been suggested that materials used in higher-value cars today include more fire-resistant compounds, but this has not been confirmed by testing (Barnett 2007).

7.6.5 MISCELLANEOUS IGNITION MECHANISMS

Accidental fires today rarely start from cigarettes lying in the crevices of seats, due to the almost universal use of thermoplastic fabrics and urethane foam padding. (Of course, accumulations of cellulosic trash—facial tissues, newspapers, food wrappers—pose the same risks of smoldering ignition as they do in homes.) Although such trash fires are usually limited to smoldering, they can occasionally produce (if cellulosic fuels are present and if properly ventilated) flaming combustion that spreads quickly through the rest of the car. Pillows, blankets, and other nonstandard accessories provide the same risks to vehicles as they do to dwellings, because they may be subject to both flaming and smoldering ignition sources (DeHaan 1993). Foam rubber in later-model cars is more fire resistant to smoldering (versus open-flame) ignition than the latex foam and cotton padding used in earlier cars. Because of the variation in fire susceptibility, if there is reason to believe that a fire was started accidentally, it may be necessary to obtain a duplicate car from a wrecking yard and test various means of ignition directly.

Virtually all synthetic materials used in modern car interiors are susceptible to flame ignition (e.g., a match flame). Most are thermoplastics, which means they melt as they burn, and the burning droplets of material then fall onto other ignitable surfaces and spread the fire very quickly. The flame temperatures and heat fluxes of such plastic fires exceed those of a gasoline fire and can mimic many of the same effects. Studies by Hirschler, Hoffmann, and Kroll showed that nearly all plastic vehicle components in passenger compartments had short ignition times and high heat release rates when tested using cone calorimetry (Hirschler, Hoffmann, and Kroll 2002).

7.6.6 VEHICLE ARSON

The NFPA estimated that incendiary fires accounted for 9 percent of all reported highway vehicle fires (NFPA). Fires accounted for 4 percent of the 33,602,500 total calls. Of these, 2,560, or 78 percent of all fire deaths, occurred in the home, a decrease of 6.7 percent. Another 445 civilians died in highway vehicle fires, which represents 13.6 percent of all deaths. Many civilian injuries are not reported to the fire service, and the actual numbers may be higher (NFPA 2015).

Many US jurisdictions do not investigate vehicle fires, so this percentage should be considered very conservative. Until recently, vehicular arson was quite rare, because a predominant motive, insurance fraud, was of minimal economic benefit to the arsonist. Unlike real property that can be traded back and forth to inflate its insured value prior to the fire, most motor vehicles are insured on the basis of their actual cash value—that is, their replacement cost less a substantial amount for depreciation. If a vehicle is burned, the payoff on the policy is usually based on Kelley Blue Book figures for that make and model, with credits added for accessories and reductions made for high mileage. Because these values are often quite low compared with the actual resale value of the car or its components, it does not often pay the arsonist to burn his or her own vehicle. Motives are discussed in more detail in a later section of this chapter.

7.6.7 CONSIDERATIONS FOR FIRE INVESTIGATION

Setting fire to a modern vehicle does not require the use of an ignitable liquid accelerant. Any direct flame source of moderate size (a burning crumpled sheet of newspaper) under the seat or under the instrument panel can result in a fast-spreading, destructive fire inside a modern vehicle if there is ventilation. Whether an accelerant is used or not, ventilation is critical. Newer vehicles are sufficiently airtight that if the windows and doors are all closed, a fire in the passenger compartment will usually self-extinguish unless a window (or sunroof) fails from thermal shock early in the fire.

7.6.8 PROTOCOL FOR VEHICLE EXAMINATION

As in structure fires, the protocol for vehicle examination follows the same logical steps—documentation and examination of exterior, interior, and specialized evidence features. The procedure is outlined in Figure 7-67 as a general checklist protocol.

Safety

As in structure fires, safety is an important consideration in vehicle examinations. Before beginning the examination, the investigator must be sure that all batteries are disconnected, air bags (steering wheel, passenger dash, side curtain, side impact, and seat backs) are disabled or discharged (see Figure 7-68) pressurized fuel containers (LP or CNG) are sealed, and hydraulic cylinders (shock absorbers, bumpers, tailgate assists) are cooled. There are also risks from leaking fuel, broken glass, torn metal, and toxic gases from continuing smoldering. More components are made of carbon fiber, and burned carbon fiber

Motor Vehicle Fires

AGENCY	FILE NUMBER

VEHICLE DESCRIPTION

Year	Make	Model	License # ST Expiration
Color(s)		VIN#	

OWNER/OCCUPANT

Owner's Name	Owner Address	Owner Phone#
Operator Name/License#	Operator Address	Operator Phone#

EXTERIOR

Prior Damage		Fire Damage	
Tread Depth	Wheel Type	Lug Nuts Present and Number	
Condition of Glass			
Tires/Wheels (Missing, Match, Condition)			
Parts Missing			

FUEL SYSTEM

Prior Damage		Fire Damage	
Type Fuel	Condition of Tank	Filler Cap Condition	Fuel Line Condition

ENGINE COMPARTMENT

Prior Damage		Fire Damage	
Fluid Levels OIL	TRANSMISSION	RADIATOR	OTHER
Parts Missing			

INTERIOR

Prior Damage		Fire Damage	
AirBags Present	Sound systems and accessory		
Ignition system			Keys in Ignition Yes or No
Personal Content Missing			
Accessories Missing			
Odometer Reading	Service Sticker Information		

VEHICLE SECURITY

Alarm	Doors and Trunk Locked	Window Position

ORIGIN/IGNITION SEQUENCE

Area
Heat Source
Material Ignitied
Ignition Factor

Odometer Reading	Service Sticker Information

Field Fire Investigation Report Forms v6-10

FIGURE 7-67 Vehicle fire inspection data sheet. *Courtesy of Det. Mike Dalton (ret.), Knox County Sheriff's Office.*

(Continued)

Motor Vehicle Fires

AGENCY	FILE NUMBER

Items found in Vehicle

Personal Effects	
Trunk/Cargo Area Contents	
Aftermarket Items	
Airbags In Place/Missing	
Personal Effects	

NOTES

DIAGRAM

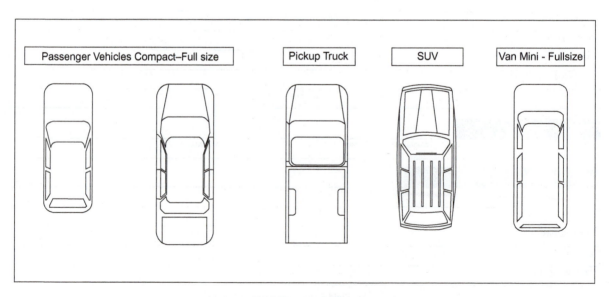

Passenger Vehicles Compact–Full size   Pickup Truck   SUV   Van Mini - Fullsize

Field Fire Investigation Report Forms v6-10

FIGURE 7-67 (*Continued*)

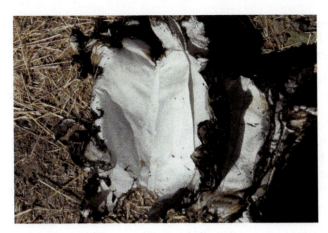

FIGURE 7-68 Partially burned air bag indicates that it functioned during the fire. *Courtesy of Jamie Novak, Novak Investigations and St. Paul Fire Dept.*

has been linked to inhalation injuries (Bell 1980). If the vehicle is lifted to allow examination of its underside, it must be securely based on proper jackstands (or service rack) before anyone gets underneath. Although it may be necessary to use a forklift to position a vehicle for examination, it is violation of OSHA standards to have any person under a vehicle being supported by a forklift.

Stay Safe

Safety is as important a consideration in vehicle examinations as it is in structure fires!

Photography and Sketches

The vehicle should be thoroughly photographed inside and out before any disturbance. Photos should capture front, rear and both sides, plus quarter views. If possible, it is preferable to examine the vehicle at the fire scene. There, the distribution of glass can be measured and documented. Air bag explosions are very unlikely to throw glass fragments more than a few feet even to the rear of the car, but the directionality of fragment distribution from such devices should be considered. Glass fragments found more than 2 m (6 ft) away are most likely to have been thrown there by a gas or vapor explosion within the vehicle. Smoke explosions are very rare in vehicle fires, so such glass will be soot-free, indicating an explosion prior to onset of fire, so the condition of the glass should be documented. Components that have fallen off from fire damage or fire suppression (or rescue) can be documented in situ.

The rectangular outline of most vehicles, with two or three separate areas of concern, lends itself to dividing the vehicle into quadrants, as shown in Figure 7-69: four in the engine compartment, four to six in the passenger compartment, and one in the trunk (and one for the underside!). Depending on the vehicle, separate quadrants can be considered for the console and dash/instrument panel. A photo showing number tags or a plan-view diagram showing the quadrant designations will make examination and note-taking easier.

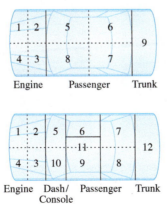

FIGURE 7-69 Quadrant system for examining and documenting vehicles: four in engine compartment, four to six in passenger compartment, one or two in trunk, one for the underside. Quadrants can be added for console and instrument panel.

Be sure to provide full documentation of the appearance of the vehicle by means of both photographs and sketches at all stages of all the scene examination. If the vehicle has not been gutted, document which portions are more heavily damaged.

Importance of Scene Preservation

It is always preferable to examine a burned car or truck before it is moved or disturbed in any way. Valuable evidence is often destroyed when the vehicle is towed to another location for examination (see before and after Figures 7-70A and 7-70B). Because most vehicle arsons take place, conveniently enough, in lonely, deserted areas protected from witnesses by trees or heavy brush, leaving the vehicle in situ is rarely a problem of public safety or even inconvenience.

Figure 7-70C shows a good example of the value of scene preservation. Had the utility trailer (foreground) been moved, the origin and cause of the much more serious and costly fire in the motorhome would have been very difficult to establish. Access to the vehicle should be tightly restricted until the exterior examination is completed. Shoe prints of the perpetrator(s) (and sometimes those of the owner!) may be found around the car if there is soft soil. Another vehicle may have been present to retrieve the arsonists or to tow or push the vehicle to be burned to its final resting place. Tire impressions may be invaluable in reconstructing the crime or identifying the second vehicle and should be preserved by photography and casting, if possible.

Exterior Examination

Portions of the vehicle that may fall off during any fire—gas cap, door handles, side mirrors, grillwork, headlamps, and the like—should be present in the debris near or under

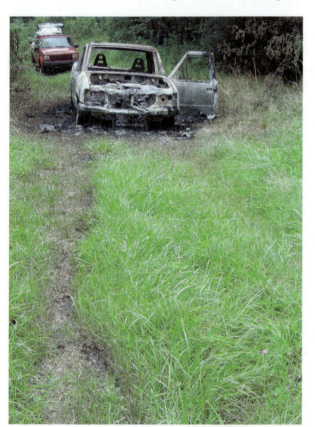

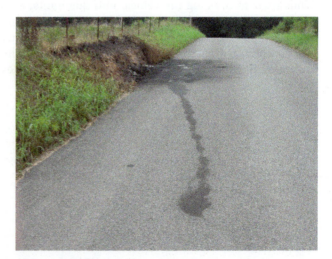

FIGURES 7-70A AND B Even if the vehicle has been moved, the scene of the fire should be examined and documented. Evidence of arson may also be found there. *Courtesy of Greg Lampkin, Knox County Sheriff's Office, Tennessee, Fire Investigation Unit.*

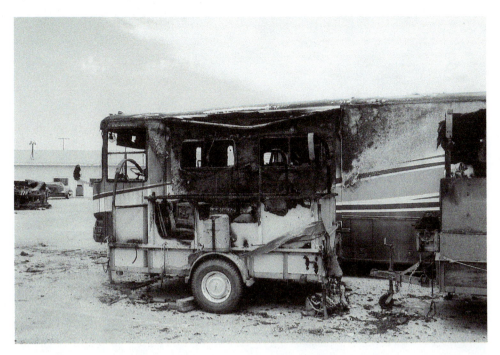

FIGURE 7-70C Destructive fire in a motorhome caused by radiant heating from fire in the utility trailer parked alongside. Notice contiguous "V" pattern on both vehicles. *Courtesy Chris J. Bloom, CJB Fire Consultant, White City, OR.*

the car if the vehicle was not stripped prior to the fire. It is important to remember that in the interest of saving weight, substantial portions of the exterior trim and major body panels of current vehicles are being made from synthetic materials, which can burn almost completely away.

Cans or jars used to carry an accelerant or the remains of initiating devices such as safety flares may be found under the car or nearby. All such evidence must be photographed in place before it is recovered. Latent fingerprints can survive on the smoother surfaces of jars and cans, and this evidence should not be handled excessively before an examination is conducted. Plastic side mirrors and door handles may melt off early and should be considered for latent print examination.

Evidence of Stripping

From the outside of the vehicle it should be possible to determine whether it was stripped prior to being burned. Most vehicle arsonists cannot resist removing the more salable items from a car or truck before burning it, thinking all signs of their removal will be destroyed anyway. Many vehicles are burned to destroy the physical evidence relating to the original crime of theft and stripping. Are all mechanical components present and properly installed? Are the wheels and tires correct for the car? Are all the lug nuts present and tight? Most people will not bother to replace all the lug nuts when putting junk tires and wheels on a car. Even when the tires are badly burned, the portion of the tread in contact with the road will not be burned, as shown in Figure 7-71. The tread pattern and depth can be established from these unburned "pads." Do they match the tires that the owner says were on the car?

Considerations for Fire Investigation

Although it can happen if there are multiple duct penetrations of the firewall or sufficient combustible materials in contact with the firewall, an accidental fire in the engine compartment of a front-engine car is less likely to travel into the passenger compartment than an intentional fire (Bell 1980). Recent changes in automobile design have resulted in less separation between the luggage and passenger compartments. As a result, fire established in one area is more likely to spread to the other than in earlier cars, no matter what the cause of the fire.

Determine whether the windows were rolled up or down (being aware that position of electric windows may be impossible to establish). (Is the greatest amount of broken

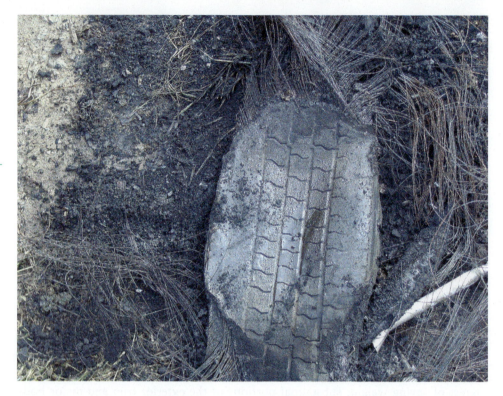

window glass down inside the door or inside or outside the car?) Examine the nature of char patterns on the outside of the body. If an accelerant was poured over a vehicle, splash and drip patterns like those in structures may be detected on exterior painted surfaces as discoloration, scorching, checkering, or blistering of the paint, as shown in Figure 7-72. Weather stripping and rubber seals are usually ignited.

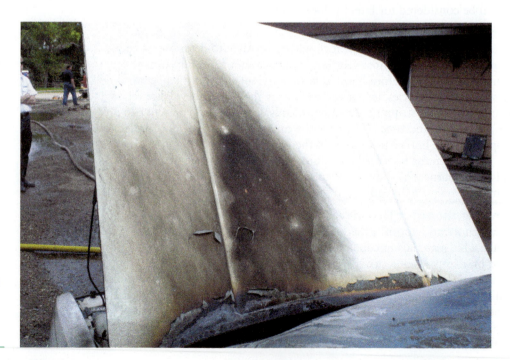

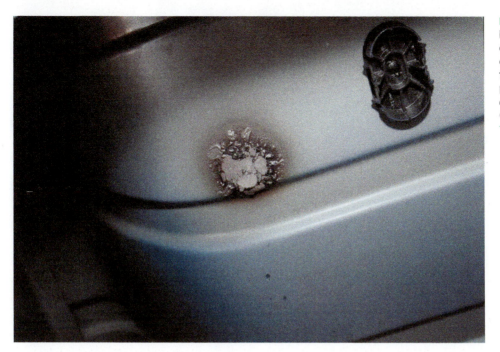

FIGURE 7-73 Gasoline burning in a footwell often produces localized charring or blistering on the underside of the body pan. *Courtesy of Tim Yandell, Public Agency Training Council.*

Examination of the vehicle's underside is important. The paint or undercoating on the underside of a footwell floor pan is likely to be blistered or charred if a fire was ignited on the floor with a flammable liquid in that area, as shown in Figure 7-73 (Riggs 2009).

Fire tests have revealed that plastic and pot-metal fuel door latches can fail at relatively low temperatures, allowing spring-loaded fuel doors to pop open. Filler caps are often made of plastic today; these can melt and fall into the filler neck or burn off completely. Internal pressure can push a heat-softened cap off the filler tube. The investigator must be careful to examine the filler tube and tank before concluding that the cap was removed deliberately.

Char discoloration and oxidization patterns on the painted metal surfaces of the body and fracture patterns to the windshield glass may help reveal the direction of fire spread. If a fire starts in the engine compartment, heat conducted through body panels causes damage to paint layers that decreases in a radial pattern as the heat moves away from its original source. Fire progressing from an engine compartment into the passenger compartment will usually cause the windshield to fail at its lower edge first, with the most intense fracturing and delamination occurring there, as illustrated in Figure 7-74. Fire starting in the passenger compartment will tend to form a hot gas layer near the roof that attacks the windshield from the top and causes patterns of damage that radiate out into adjoining body panels, as shown in Figures 7-75A and B.

During a car fire, electrical connections can be made by the charring of switches, relays, and insulation. With a battery in place, headlights, wipers, horn, gas door releases, and even the starter have been seen to operate. If the vehicle is left in gear, the starter may move the vehicle some distance while burning, unless the handbrake is engaged (Marley and DeHaan 1994). Fires ignited in pressurized fluids can produce localized areas of damage from fire plume impact. Fuel leaks from hoses or fuel rails may cause hot spots on engines, firewalls, or frame components. Transmission fluid fires will often be concentrated around the dipstick/filler tube or the housing below. (There may be oily residues adhering to nearby metal surfaces from such fires.) Many petroleum products fluoresce under ultraviolet (UV) or short-wavelength visible light, so examination with a forensic light source *may* be useful in spotting localized deposits.

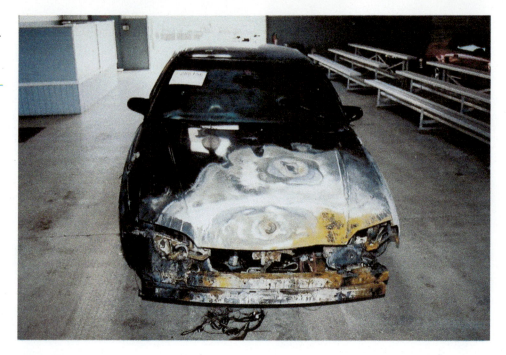

FIGURE 7-74 Engine compartment fire pattern. *Courtesy of Jamie Novak, Novak Investigations and St. Paul Fire Dept.*

Because of the large quantity of combustible fuels present in the modern car, the duration and intensity of an extensive fire cannot be related back to the presence or absence of a flammable liquid accelerant. The accelerant serves mainly to ensure ignition of the substantial natural fuel load (Nicol and Overley 1963). Figure 7-76 illustrates the extensive combustion of combustible automotive components—aluminum deck lids, plastic trim, composite panels, and light-steel-alloy hoods—in nonaccelerated fires in modern vehicles. Pouring gasoline on the outside of a closed modern car produces surprisingly little damage.

Paint will scorch or blister, plastic trim will melt or char, and weather stripping may be ignited. Tests of modern vehicles conducted in 1992, however, showed that even a modest flaming ignition source beneath a seat would result in full involvement of the interior within 2 minutes of ignition, whether the windows were open or not (Marley and DeHaan 1994).

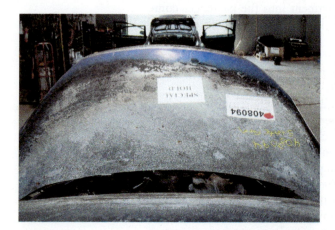

FIGURE 7-75A Concentric passenger compartment fire pattern on hood. *Courtesy of Jamie Novak, Novak Investigations and St. Paul Fire Dept.*

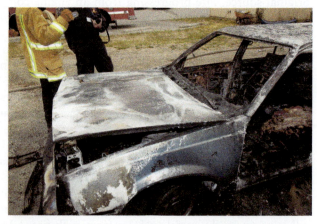

FIGURE 7-75B Concentric passenger compartment fire pattern on hood. *Courtesy of Tim Yandell, Public Agency Training Council.*

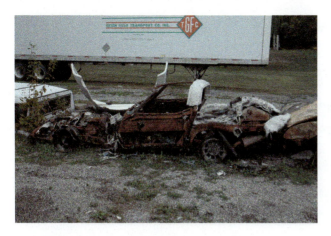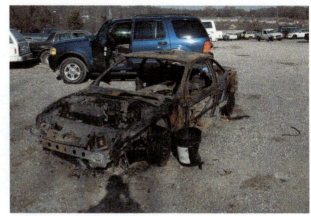

FIGURE 7-76 Extensive destruction of light-alloy and plastic components in a nonaccelerated vehicle fire.
Courtesy of Greg Lampkin, Knox County Sheriff's Office, Tennessee, Fire Investigation Unit.

The interior of a vehicle can be thought of as a compartment that will undergo the same development as the room fire. If provided adequate ventilation, fires inside vehicles with their rich fuel load can progress to intense, full post-flashover fires with the same high temperatures (over 1000°C) as a well-furnished room (DeHaan and Fisher 2003). Because a vehicle is dimensionally smaller, it will undergo the process even more quickly than a typical room. The maximum heat release rate for a fully involved modern automobile ranges from 1.5 MW to 8 MW, with newer cars exhibiting larger heat release rates (Mangs 2004a and 2004b). Partial enclosures such as canopies, roofs, or parking garages produce larger fires that can readily spread to adjacent vehicles in as little as 8 minutes.

Direct exposure to fire can cause not only tires to burst but also shock absorbers, gas-filled suspension and hatchback struts, driveshafts, and bumper (collision) impact absorbers to explode, sometimes with dangerous force. Fire-weakened assemblies have also been known to explode as they cool after a fire. Such explosions can inflict damage that could be misinterpreted by an investigator, as well as pose a safety risk to fire suppression personnel and investigators.

Vehicle Identification Number

Before proceeding to the interior examination, the vehicle identification number (VIN) plate should be located and the identity and ownership of the vehicle determined. It is not beyond the realm of imagination that one vehicle was substituted for another to defraud an insurance carrier. The National Insurance Crime Bureau (NICB, www.nicb.org) and the Alliance of Automobile Manufacturers (AAM, www.autoalliance.org) produce guides to the location and interpretation of vehicle identification data plates. The NICB or the Canadian Automobile Theft Bureau (CATB) can also assist qualified members with locating "confidential" identification numbers hidden on every modern vehicle if the VIN plate has been destroyed.

Interior Examination of the Vehicle

As previously noted, the vehicle can best be examined in quadrants—four in the engine compartment and at least four in the passenger compartment. Each quadrant can then be evaluated and documented for fire damage, fuel sources, and ignition sources using the ignition matrix concept (Morrill 2006). Fire damage can include total or partial destruction as well as direction and intensity indicators. Because stolen vehicles are often at least partially stripped before they are burned, the most marketable components and accessories should be accounted for in the passenger compartment, including the stereo, CB, CD/DVD player, seats, navigation system, radar detector, air bags, and the like. They may be melted

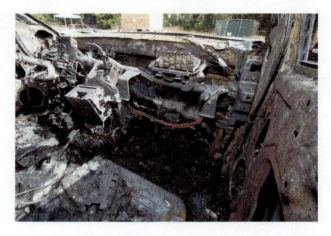

and badly damaged, but some remains should be on the floor beneath the mounting brackets. The seats are very valuable and a frequent target of strip-and-burn auto thieves. The air bag(s) will be triggered by the heat of the fire, but some remains of the deployed bag or its base plate should remain, as shown in Figure 7-77. Because air bags are very expensive, they are often stolen for resale. Air bags functioning during a fire may give bystanders the impression that an explosive device was present. The gas generated in an air bag is non-flammable nitrogen. The remains of a deployed air bag may be found outside the car.

If the owner is claiming a loss of valuable personal property with the vehicle—tools, clothing, fishing tackle, and so on—the metal pieces of such items should survive even the most complete conflagration. The jack and the spare tire (or at least its metal bead wires, belting, and valve) should still be identifiable. The ignition lock should be located even if it has melted and fallen from its mounting hole. Sometimes a key will still be found in the ignition switch (as in Figure 7-78). Signs of tampering with, forcible damage to, or removal of the ignition switch and steering lock should be eliminated.

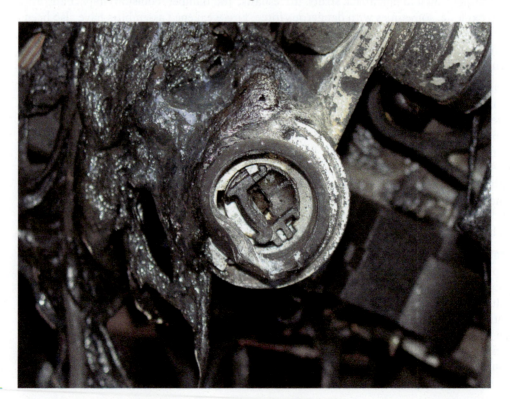

Upholstery

If the seat upholstery has not burned completely, it will behave in much the same way as household furniture, and its examination for relative consumption and direction of burning may be carried out in the same way. Most vehicles use a pad of foam rubber over a network of metal springs. This pad is covered in turn by a vinyl, leather, or polyester fabric covering. The foam rubber can vary considerably in its flammability characteristics, and if none remains unburned, it may be necessary to secure a control sample from a duplicate vehicle for laboratory testing. It tends to burn completely away in a well-ventilated fire in 10 to 30 minutes, no matter how the fire was started.

Accelerants and Other Liquids

If a liquid accelerant was used in excess, unburned liquid may be found soaked into the upholstery, carpets, and carpet padding or even pooled in low spots of the body pan (Service and Lewis 2001). If the doors and windows are fully closed, the fire may self-extinguish, leaving raw unburned accelerant, as pictured in Figure 7-79.

One study reported that the thick soot on the interior of window glass contained identifiable residues of the ignitable liquids used to burn two vehicles in test burns, but the duration and maximum temperatures reached were not cited (Sutherland and Byers 1998). It is often the case that fire went undetected and the vehicle burned to completion, with *all* combustibles within the vehicle completely consumed, including accelerants. In such cases, flammable liquid that leaked through and soaked into the soil under the vehicle may yet be detectable.

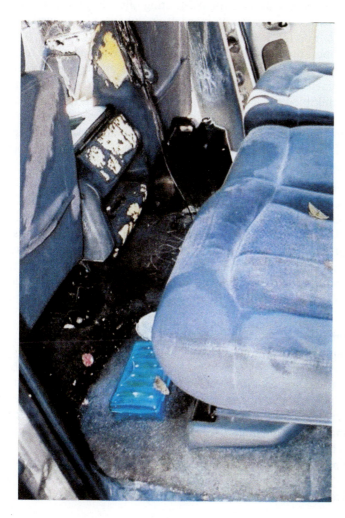

FIGURE 7-79 Windows and doors were closed after gasoline was ignited in front seat. Fire self-extinguished, leaving raw gasoline on the rear seat. *Courtesy of Tim Yandell, Public Agency Training Council.*

When the vehicle is moved, the debris and soil under it should be examined carefully, using a hydrocarbon detector if possible. Samples should be collected and sealed in airtight metal cans or glass jars if there are any indications of flammable liquids. A leaking fuel tank can simulate such conditions, and a control sample of the fuel should be taken in most instances. Electric fuel pumps *may* continue to pump as long as the ignition is on and will empty the entire tank under the car if the electrical system remains intact and there has been no severe mechanical impact that would have triggered the interrupter fitted to some cars. In many vehicles there is an interlock, so the loss of oil pressure or electrical signal from a stopped engine will shut the fuel pump off as well.

Interior Debris

Portions of timing and ignition devices may be discovered in the interior debris. Safety flares make excellent ignition devices (and they are innocuously present in most vehicles) but a careful search can reveal their wooden end plugs and white or gray lumpy residues. Paper matches survive even substantial fires if they are resting on a noncombustible surface, and are worth looking for. Crumpled paper makes a good, fast initial fire.

Fire from a small plastic bag of potato chips provides more than enough heat to ignite the upholstery in a modern car and yet burns away to an amorphous, unrecognizable carbonaceous ash. The oils in the chips produce a prolonged, intense fire because they are distributed on a thin, porous, combustible wick. The residue is easily overlooked and, even if discovered, may be dismissed as accidental. The vegetable oils present, however, may be identifiable in the carpet if it is analyzed by gas chromatography/mass spectrometry (GC/MS) by the same method as used for self-heating oils. Fires under seats can also be accidental—from hot work done recently, rags left on exhaust pipes, overheated converters, or service lights left on inside the vehicle.

Sometimes, an attempt is made to simulate an accidental fire by loosening fuel lines or drain plugs or disconnecting them completely. All such plugs and connectors should be accounted for and examined for the presence of loosening or fresh tool marks indicating recent tampering. One multiple-vehicle arson involved the removal of fuel tank caps from a line of diesel tractor-trailer trucks. The fuel tanks were connected by means of fuel-soaked rag trailers, and the series of tanks was ignited by floating a plastic cup with a small firecracker and blackpowder in each. The resulting fires destroyed a number of the vehicles, despite the failure of most of the rag trailers.

Mechanical Condition

If it is possible, the mechanical condition of the vehicle prior to the fire should be established. Mechanical problems may provide a motive for "selling" the vehicle to the insurance company, as well as a possible cause of an accidental fire. Observations should include whether the battery is in place and connected and whether the engine's electrical connections are still intact. Even if the wires melt or burn away, the metal connectors generally remain. Are all the engine components and accessories present? Do the water, oil, and transmission fluid levels indicate the vehicle was operational at the time of the fire?

Mechanical Examination

Disassembly of the engine or gearbox may reveal the operational status, which can then be compared against the owner's statements. Engine oil and transmission fluid should be drained. Simple observations for condition and contaminants can be carried out by eye, but such fluids can also be laboratory tested to reveal mechanical malfunctions prior to the fire. If the owner claims the vehicle to be complete and operational, a check of the engine compartment may reveal missing, disconnected, or out-of-place components that would render the vehicle inoperative (Suefert 1993). Accidental fires involving the automatic transmission or power steering unit during operation usually produce severe damage inside the unit, as fluid is expelled. External fires do not cause the same kind of internal damage. Analysis of the oil or fluid may reveal the mechanical state of the unit.

Theft and Other Non-fire Damage

Non-fire-related body damage should be documented and compared against the owner's description of the condition of the vehicle. Previous damage may be detectable from part numbers or inventory. Body damage that is costly to repair the condition but makes the car unsalable and may be reason for destroying the car by fire. As in the investigation of structural fires, it is important that the investigator look for anything that seems unusual and out of place. No matter how clever the vehicle arsonist is, it is very difficult to arrange a destructive fire that can pass for an accident without modifying the vehicle or adding something to it to help it burn.

If the vehicle was found burned and the owner claims the vehicle had been stolen, there are additional avenues of inquiry. The scene where the vehicle was found (even if the vehicle has already been removed) should be examined as a potential crime scene for shoe and tire impressions, tools, accelerant containers, and means of ignition (matchbooks, lighters, flare striker caps). The area should be canvassed for possible witnesses who can help establish time factors or information about people or vehicles in the area at the time of the fire. The person who found the vehicle (or reported the fire) should be interviewed as to how they came to be in that location. The owner should be interviewed about the circumstances of the loss (Who last drove the vehicle and when? Was the vehicle locked? Was the alarm set? What were the vehicle contents? At what time and location was the vehicle last seen? At what time was the theft discovered? At what time was it reported?). The status of keys for the vehicle and access by others should be established. Modern theft or GPS/navigational systems may provide data about the movements of the vehicle prior to the fire. Some vehicles are also equipped with event data (black box) recorders that capture vehicle operational data before a crash! These recorders require specialized equipment and expertise for access. A ASTM monograph describes the examination of vehicle data (black box) recorders from accident vehicles (ASTM 2009).

Interviews

Wendt has published a comprehensive outline for interviewing the victim of a vehicle theft and fire (Wendt 1998). Interviewees may include the vehicle's owner, driver, occupants, and mechanic. Responding police and fire personnel are also important sources of information.

NHTSA Information

The National Highway Traffic Safety Administration (NHTSA) should be consulted for recalls or problems associated with the type of vehicle involved. One must be very careful not to assume that a recall *proves* the fire in question was caused by the failure reported! Such recalls must be included as a testable hypothesis in complete investigation (www.nhtsa.gov).

Vehicle Fire Tests

Considerable experience has been gained from laboratory tests involving the burning of complete automobiles under various conditions. These tests reveal that, for the most part, the amount of structural damage done to the exterior of the vehicle does not bear a direct relationship to whether the fire is of incendiary or accidental origin. Some tests have revealed that temperatures near the roof of a burning car reach as high as 1000°C (1860°F) at some stage of a fire no matter what the means of ignition (Hrynchuk 1998). This is more than sufficient to warp sheet metal and melt glass and aluminum trim. As a result, body and roof panels buckle and warp, window glass melts and icicles, and seat springs lose their temper at temperatures developed in slow-burning accidental fires as well as in fast, accelerant-fueled fires. Similarly, the color, density, and appearance of soot and pyrolysis products on remaining windows depend largely on the upholstery materials present and the degree of ventilation present during the fire. Although the amount of structural damage will, of course, be generally related to the intensity and duration of the fire, those features are not necessarily determined by whether or not the fire was incendiary. One series of tests indicated that, in fact, more complete damage can result from a slow-developing accidental fire that has more time to bring more of the entire mass of the vehicle up to high temperatures than from a fast-moving gasoline fire (Nicol and Overley 1963).

7.7 Motorhomes and Other Recreational Vehicles

A recreational vehicle is defined as a motor vehicle containing living quarters for recreation, camping, travel, or seasonal use. Recreational vehicles come in different styles, shapes, sizes, and with different accessories. They range from a simple tent trailer to a bus-chassis motorhome. The basic designs are the camping trailer, truck camper, travel trailer, fifth wheel, park trailer, and the motorhome.

7.7.1 CHARACTERISTICS OF MOTORHOMES

Most motorhomes are constructed and assembled from four distinct and important components, often made by different manufacturers: the unit's engine; the transmission; the chassis; and the remaining portions of the unit, including the assembly and installation of appliances and furnishings. It is not uncommon for there to be several fire investigators examining the remaining debris, each one representing the individual interests of each manufacturer involved.

Motorhomes are categorized into three distinct classes: Class A, Class B, and Class C. Class A motorhomes are the largest units and are designed and built from the ground up. Class B motorhomes are van conversions that have been altered to accept appliances and furnishings for the living space. Class C motorhomes are units that incorporate a van cab portion, with an attached body, usually with an over-the-cab sleeping area.

7.7.2 FIRE RISK

Motorhomes are subject to a combination of the risks of accidental fires of vehicular origin with those peculiar to the heating, cooking, and living conditions found in dwellings. Because the interiors of these vehicles are used for day-to-day living, the hazards of cooking and smoking materials are as present as they are in a stationary dwelling. Many such vehicles have moderate-capacity electrical systems of 12 V, so electrical fires, while not completely impossible, are quite rare. Some vehicles have large-capacity, complex electrical systems of 24 V, which provide higher risks. In addition, many of them are fitted with a parallel 120 VAC system to operate lights, heaters, radios, and the like when they are connected to an outside source of AC power or to a portable generator mounted within the vehicle. Many of the same appliances found in the home will be found in the motorhome. High-current devices such as televisions, toasters, and microwave ovens are common, as well as their attendant risks of misuse.

7.7.3 PROPANE TANKS

Most such vehicles also include a propane (or LPG) tank to provide fuel for the heater, stove, refrigerator, and even generator with the attendant hazards of explosions from spills and leaks. If factory equipped, the recreational vehicle will be fitted with either DOT or ASME tanks, steel and/or copper piping, rubber hose connections with brass fittings, valves, and the appliances they serve, including a refrigerator, furnace, stove, and even a generator. The size of the propane tanks can vary from 5-gallon tanks on trailers to upward of 80-gallon tanks on the more expensive motorhomes and bus conversions. There is no guarantee that propane systems will be properly installed in amateur conversions. One explosion, costing 12 lives, involved a modified motorhome. The cause was traced to an improperly installed LP tank that leaked its contents into the vehicle until it was ignited by an electric arc or open flame as the vehicle proceeded down the highway (McGill 1995).

All propane tanks are equipped with some type of a pressure-relief valve, which is designed to vent the contents of the tank at a certain pressure. When the propane tank heats up due to flame impingement, the pressure inside it increases. When the pressure inside becomes greater than the pressure-relief valve setting, the valve opens and rapidly expels the contents away from the motorhome and tank. This expulsion will continue until either (1) the pressure inside the tank is less than the pressure-relief valve setting, at which time the valve will close again, or (2) the valve expels all the contents of the tank during the fire.

Many motorhomes and travel trailers today are fitted with propane detectors. The location of these must be carefully assessed, for thermal currents in the vehicle may move the fuel/air vapor away from the detector. Recall that the density of an ignitable propane/air mixture is very close to that of air, so it will not settle like pure propane.

Manufacturers use plastics, synthetic fabrics, foam rubber, and particleboard to save both cost and weight. The structural elements are most often a skeleton of aluminum tubing to which is riveted an exterior aluminum or fiberglass skin. Plywood or synthetic paneling is fitted to the inside, and thermal and sound insulation is made of fiberglass or polystyrene or polyurethane foam sandwiched between those layers. Once the main fabric of such a vehicle is ignited, there is little to prevent it from being completely destroyed. While the vehicle is burning, formaldehyde and various cyanogens are released from the interior finishes, sometimes with fatal results to any occupants. Although most reputable manufacturers strive to make their vehicles as safe as possible, there is no code applicable to custom conversion facilities. The fire investigator must be alert to the possibility of finding patently hazardous practices and products in such vehicles.

7.7.4 CONSIDERATIONS FOR FIRE INVESTIGATION

Almost every fire involving a recreational vehicle will develop very quickly due to the lightweight construction utilizing foams, resins, plastics, and other highly combustible materials. The federal standards for allowable flame spread rate are on a scale from 25 to 200, with 200 being the maximum allowed. Due to the lightweight construction methods and materials employed, a flame spread rating of 200 is allowed for recreational vehicle construction. Because of the materials involved, when a small fire occurs, it develops rapidly and quickly involves the gasoline or diesel fuel tanks and the propane system. It is not uncommon for a small fire to completely consume a recreational vehicle down to the frame within 12 minutes (Bloom and Bloom 1997 and 2007).

When investigating fires in such vehicles, the investigator should expect substantial destruction of their structural elements, with consequent loss of evidence that would normally permit a reconstruction of the fire sequence. Within the limitations of the construction materials involved, diagnostic signs of fires caused by electrical failures, smoking materials, heating systems, and arson remain largely as they are described elsewhere in this book. The investigator must be aware of the extensive fire damage resulting from the construction of such vehicles, as shown in Figures 7-80 and 7-81.

Photographs should be taken at every step prior to, during, and after the investigation (including the general scene). This is to allow documentation and reconstruction of the scene as found. Valuable information that was not readily apparent during the initial examination could easily become visible after the photographs are developed.

When examining the remains of a motorhome, it is also important to examine the scene where the fire occurred, because critical evidence may have dropped off and away from the vehicle during the fire and its suppression. It is most important when inspecting the unit, unless it is absolutely necessary to move them, to leave the remains undisturbed.

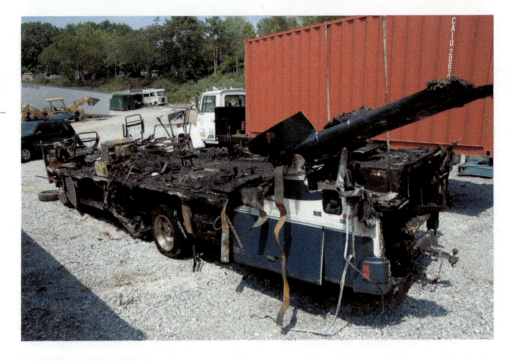

FIGURE 7-80 Remains of a Class A motorhome ready for examination. *Courtesy of Greg Lampkin, Knox County Sheriff's Office, Tennessee, Fire Investigation Unit.*

If items or debris need to be moved to allow for an examination, only professionally accepted practices for the documentation and removal of the debris should be employed. When the unit needs to be moved from the scene location to a storage facility, the unit should be moved via a flat-bed towing truck and tarp-wrapped, if at all possible, to minimize potential loss or damage to components (Bloom and Bloom 1997). Because of the enormous variety of styles of fittings and interior finishes, it is often helpful to locate and inspect an exemplar unit of the same type, floor plan, and age. Photos or videos taken by owners or passers-by may capture vital data, as illustrated in Figure 7-82.

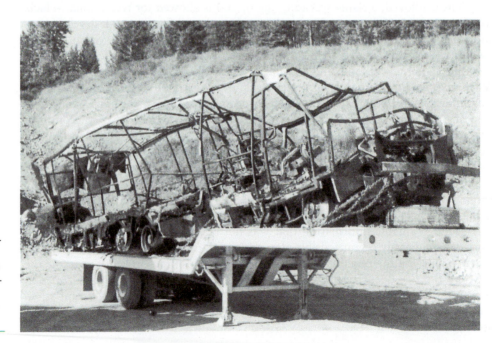

FIGURE 7-81 The remains of a large motorhome being properly transported on a flat-bed carrier. Total destruction resulted from an accidental origin. *Courtesy of Joe and Chris J. Bloom, Bloom Fire Investigation, Grants Pass, OR.*

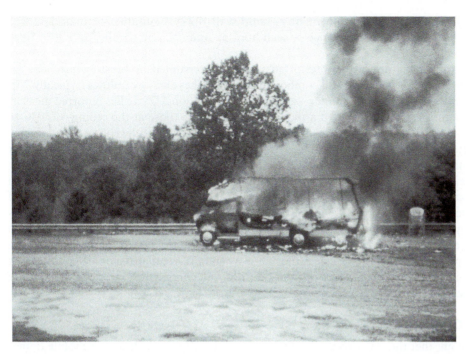

FIGURE 7-82 A passerby recorded this accidental fire in a Class C motorhome, which destroyed the vehicle. Such recordings preserve indicators such as direction of fire travel, time involved, suppression attempts, and wind direction. *Courtesy of Joe and Chris J. Bloom, Bloom Fire Investigation, Grants Pass, OR.*

PART 5: Manufactured Housing

7.8 Manufactured Housing

7.8.1 CONSTRUCTION AND MATERIALS

In many respects, the structure and materials of mobile or manufactured homes (sometimes called *modular* homes), the causes of fires within them, and the problems of investigating such fires are similar to those just discussed in regard to recreational vehicle fires. Structurally, manufactured homes are most often built on a heavy steel frame supported on three axles. A wooden floor structure of plywood or particleboard provides a base for the erection of a wooden or metal framework upon which the exterior aluminum or wooden sheathing is installed. The interior walls are often framed (as are exterior walls) with 2-in. × 3-in. wood studs and then covered with plywood, wood paneling, or more recently, gypsum board specially designed to resist the flexing and vibration induced by moving. Insulation is often fiberglass batting in the roof and exterior walls.

The interior finish in many such mobile homes is similar to the paneling of motorhomes and thus poses a high risk of rapid fire development. The occurrence of fully involved (post-flashover) fires seems to be much more common in mobile homes, and the time to flashover is much reduced over that seen in most standard buildings. The small-dimension wood members burn quickly and allow more rapid structural collapse than in a structure of standard construction. With the advent of *NFPA 501B: Manufactured Housing* (imposed by the US Department of Housing and Urban Development on manufactured homes starting in 1976), the speed and severity of development of fires has been notably reduced (Earls 2001).

The date of manufacture of the structure being investigated is therefore critical to estimating what the materials and construction would be (as well as smoke detectors and the like). The recent development of gypsum wall finishes suitable for manufactured housing has made fire performance of such housing more closely parallel to that of fixed structures.

The tubular nature of the interior structure uninterrupted by firestops provides for rapid fire spread throughout, and combustible wall finishes and low ceilings (typically 7 ft) provide for extremely rapid buildup and flashover conditions. Davie has reported measuring temperatures at floor level of a mobile home equal to those at the ceiling—750°C to 1000°C (1400°F to 1800°F). This is due to the size and shape of the rooms, the combustible nature of wall and flooring materials used, and the reflective properties of the outer walls and roof (Davie 1988).

The development of fires in such structures to post-flashover follows the same pattern as in fixed structures but happens more quickly. The location, thickness, and spacing of the structural members and the installation of electrical and heating equipment are considerably more variable in mobile homes than in conventional structures. (Walls are often framed and erected after carpet is laid across the entire floor area, for instance.) The motion produced when the vehicle is moved or when fans, ventilators, or air-conditioning units are operated can chafe wire insulation or loosen connections far more than would be expected in fixed structures.

7.8.2 CONSIDERATIONS FOR FIRE INVESTIGATION

It is thought that the small rooms and narrow hallways typically found in mobile homes contribute to the rapid development of flashover and unusual burn patterns, such as those observed in Figure 7-83, where the most intense fire was to the floor and wall to the right of the bed and not at the origin. The minimal insulation and conductive roof covering (typically aluminum or steel sheathing) may allow fire damage to the roof to record the development of fire in the rooms beneath.

An investigator should be wary of placing too much importance on the presence of complex burn patterns on the floors of a heavily damaged mobile home. The combustible floor materials and wall coverings and high fuel loads combine to produce intense post-flashover fires that in some cases can penetrate the floors under furniture as well as in

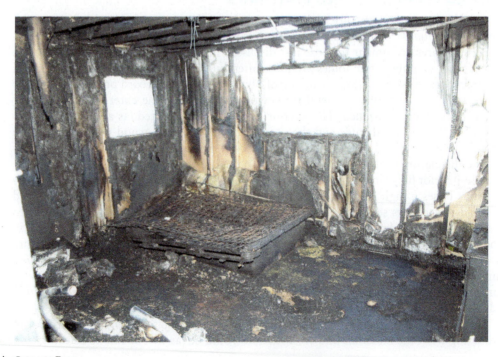

FIGURE 7-83 Fire in the bedroom of this mobile home started near the floor to the left of the bed. The dynamics of air entrained from the entry door during post-flashover burning caused a false "V" of severe burn to the right of the bed. *Courtesy of Jamie Novak, Novak Investigations and St. Paul Fire Dept.*

exposed floor areas. (Pre-fire degradation of floors from water incursion will accelerate floor combustion and failure.) Rapid failure of single-glazed windows adds ventilation sources. Post-flashover burning (especially when synthetic carpet and pad are involved) will produce irregular burn patterns on floors. Although the fire in a mobile home behaves in a manner consistent with basic scientific and engineering principles, the investigator must be careful not to use the same criteria for evaluating indicators of time and estimating fuel effects as used in evaluating fires in buildings of standard construction.

When investigating fires in mobile homes, the investigator should expect substantial destruction of their structural elements, with consequent loss of evidence that would normally permit a reconstruction of the fire sequence. Within the limitations of the construction materials involved, diagnostic signs of fires caused by electrical failures, smoking materials, heating systems, and arson remain largely as they are described elsewhere in this book.

7.9 Heavy Equipment

Motorized equipment such as tractors, loaders, earthmovers, forklifts, harvesters, and the like can pose special fire risks. If not cleaned properly, agricultural equipment can accumulate thick layers of cellulosic dusts that can ignite from hot surfaces (as shown in Figure 7-84). Excess dusts and fibers can accumulate in moving parts to cause frictional heating in belts, bearings, and gearsets. Improperly maintained hydraulic and oil systems cause special problems, as they operate at very high pressures when in use.

The extremely fine aerosol mists that are created at such leaks are readily ignited by hot surfaces or electric arcs. Vibration causes loosening of fittings and fracturing of rigid pipes—all leading to loss of fluids under pressure. Fires started from hydraulic or other fluid leaks can spread very quickly to engulf the equipment. Fires started in solid dusts grow more slowly but can be ignited for some time after the equipment is shut off and left unattended. Either ignition can lead to a major fire involving expensive equipment. The

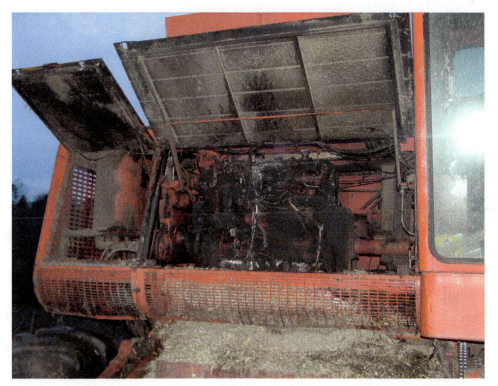

FIGURE 7-84 Fire in harvester caused by accumulation of combustible dust. *Courtesy of Greg Lampkin, Knox County Sheriff's Office, Tennessee, Fire Investigation Unit.*

size of combustible components is a factor in determining the size of the resulting fire. Heat release rates as high as 3 MW have been observed in tests of single earthmover tires [ignited by a pool of diesel fuel beneath the tire (Hammarstrom 2008)]. Large tanks of diesel fuel or hydraulic oil (or propane cylinders to aid in cold-weather starting) can also contribute to the fire's intensity and duration. The investigator must be very familiar with the specialized equipment used in such vehicles before attempting to determine the origin and cause of major fires.

PART 6: Boats and Ships

7.10 Boats and Ships

Pleasure boats are more like automobiles in their relative fire hazards and susceptibility than dwellings or larger ships. The boat and the automobile most often have a gasoline-powered motor, gasoline tank, and electrically driven accessories. There is one major difference that makes the boat fire more destructive and much more difficult to investigate than the auto fire, namely, all the flammables are enclosed in a more-or-less tub-shaped container—the hull. Certain terms peculiar to vessels are helpful to the fire investigator in conducting interviews and are shown in Table 7-5.

Leaking gasoline or its vapors will settle into the bottom of the hull, where they remain unless circulated by drafts from the engine fan or bilge pump. Comparable leakage in an automobile is generally to an open or well-ventilated exterior. This is the basic

TABLE 7-5	Terms for Ship Construction which are Helpful to the Fire Investigator
Hull:	Main body of a vessel—may be steel, aluminum, wood fiberglass, concrete
Deck:	Horizontal element separating levels
Bulkhead:	Vertical partition separating compartments
Bridge:	Location from which the vessel is steered and controlled
Cockpit:	In small boats, the opening in the deck from which the vessel is steered
Ladder:	Vertical access between decks
Passageway:	Horizontal access between compartments (hallway)
Porthole:	Transparent windows from a compartment through hull
Galley:	Kitchen area
Boat:	Smaller water vehicle (sometimes defined as capable of being carried by a ship)
Ship:	Larger, oceangoing vessel

Source: F. Herrera, "Investigation of Boat Fires," *California Fire/Arson Investigator* (January 2005): 10–11.

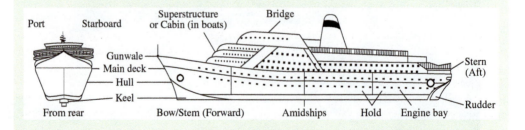

reason for the greater danger and likelihood of explosion of fuel vapors in a boat. In addition, many boats are made of wood or fiberglass, while the automobile does not usually consist of such a combustible container.

A gasoline fire in a wooden or fiberglass container is a far more formidable occurrence than the same fire in a steel conveyance. Wooden decks and cabins are likely to be burned completely, and the hull is likely to be burned down to the waterline. Fire patterns are therefore obscured or destroyed, and points of origin are often not identifiable. Smaller rooms and the presence of all-wood interiors will produce more intense, faster growing fires than normally found in the larger, gypsum-wallboard finished compartments of buildings. With larger wooden vessels that have considerable secondary interior structure, patterns will be found that are in every way comparable to those in any other similar wood-framed structure.

In addition to sources of gasoline vapors, boats may have heaters or stoves that are fueled by kerosene, alcohol, or liquid propane (LP) gas. Each of these poses risks of accidental fires and must be considered when investigating these fires; LP gas can settle into the hull like gasoline vapors, and kerosene or alcohol stoves can spill or leak, producing pools of ignitable fuel. The electrical systems may include separate systems for 120 VAC and 12 or 28 VDC power.

On newer vessels, these electrical systems must meet the requirements of the US Federal Boat Safety Act of 1971, but earlier ones need meet no requirements, and modifications may or may not have been done correctly. This same act requires flame arrestors, appropriate fuel lines, and other safety equipment. Minimizing the risk of fire and loss of life on such crafts is the focus of *NFPA 302: Fire Protection Standard for Pleasure and Commercial Craft* (NFPA 2010a). Like standards for structures, such guides can only describe recommended (or required) practices, not capture the content and fire risks as seen in real-world occupancies.

The investigation of boat fires involves the evaluation not only of the presence of such features but also their operability and effectiveness (e.g., flame arrestors may be present but are compromised by a hole punched through them by a careless mechanic). One survey of small-vessel fires reported that 55 percent were caused by wiring and appliances (both AC and DC), 24 percent were caused by overheating of engines or transmissions, 8 percent by fuel leaks, and 1 percent by stoves (Herrera 2005). Some vessels combine entirely combustible (exposed wood) structure and linings with large windows and numerous household ignition sources and corroded and contaminated electrical fittings, leading to a high risk of very intense, destructive fires.

7.10.1 SHIPS

Although large steel-framed ships would not be expected to burn, it is fortunate that most fire investigators are not called on to examine such fire scenes frequently, because such ships and their flammable contents can burn with incredible ferocity and massive destruction. This destructiveness is based largely on three factors: fuel load, spread of fire by conduction, and inhibited access to firefighters, which are all peculiar to large steel ships.

Although the steel structure itself is not readily ignitable, a considerable fuel load is present in the ship's interior finishes, furnishings, cargo, and fuel. The interior finishes and furnishings represent the same degree of combustibility hazard as comparable furnishings in a dwelling. A large cargo of freight, however, imposes its own flammability characteristics on the ship. In bulk shipping of products like wood chips, grain, coal, and natural fibers, smoldering fires are common and are very difficult to extinguish.

Water tends to wet only the top layers and not penetrate, and extinguishing gases are expensive. In most cases, the holds with the smoldering cargo are sealed and left, hoping the fire will self-extinguish. Unfortunately, due to the low oxygen limits for smoldering combustion, considerable combustion can occur, creating heat and combustible gases that are trapped in the hold. When fresh air is admitted, a backdraft or smoke explosion can

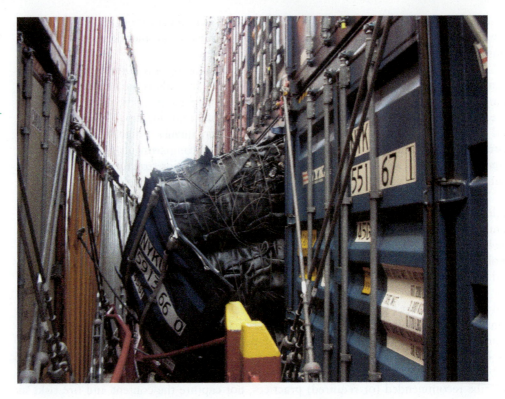

FIGURE 7-85 Explosion in a container mid-voyage caused by leakage from used gasoline tanks being shipped for recycling. *Courtesy of Kyle Binkowski, Fire Cause Analysis.*

result with disastrous effect. Self-heating of bulk cargoes is also a problem, particularly in hot climates. Steam, nitrogen, or carbon dioxide gas injection is sometimes used to suppress cargo compartment fires. Cargo itself (see A. D. Sapp et al., "Arson Aboard Naval Ships: Characteristics of Offenses and Offenders," NCAVC, 1995) can contain flammable or explosive vapors, as illustrated in Figure 7-85

Explosive dust suspensions are encountered during loading and unloading of flour, sulfur, and similar finely powdered products. Such products as ammonium nitrate, used for chemical and fertilizer production, are well recognized for their hazardous properties, and special precautions are required (Hadden, Jervis, and Rein 2009).

7.10.2 TANKERS

Tankers, often loaded with very large quantities of fuel, generally of petroleum origin, might be expected to be subject to enormously increased hazards. The main cargo of a tanker while contained is no more dangerous than is the gasoline tank on an automobile and for the same reason. Bulk cargo may be contained in freestanding containers or in open holds. Many tanks are provided with inert gas (such as nitrogen) systems to exclude air from the ullage spaces. However, the danger of a fuel spill above board, where the vapors can mix with air, creates a hazard similar to that produced by a fuel spill in the exterior in any other environment. Ignitable liquid cargoes require that special precautions be taken. Far more serious hazards are associated with a rupture in the hull of a tanker that releases great quantities of fuel or with tanks that have been unloaded, where air can mix with the fuel vapors, forming an explosive mixture.

7.10.3 SHIP CONSTRUCTION AND FIREFIGHTING TECHNIQUES

Once a fire has started, by whatever cause, extinguishment is very difficult and hazardous. The modern welded-steel ship can be thought of as a huge box girder with the steel plates of the sides, bottom, and main deck forming the four sides. This box is strengthened by steel girders forming the keel or "backbone" and the frames or "ribs." It is separated into many smaller compartments by the lower decks and transverse bulkheads (Swanson 1941). These elements are part of the strengthening substructure and are also all steel (or aluminum in some ships). Unlike a fire in a frame or masonry structure, fire in one compartment of a ship is not thermally insulated from neighboring compartments. The steel plates conduct heat quickly and efficiently to other adjacent or overhead compartments. Combustibles in these compartments quickly reach their ignition points and contribute to the fire spread. Damage may be more extensive in compartments above or alongside the point of origin than in the actual compartment where the fire started. Tunnels and vertical chases for electrical and hydraulic systems provide chimneys for the spread of fire by convection or even direct flame impingement.

Standard firefighting practice in dwellings often calls for getting above the fire to ventilate it and thereby to cool it. In a steel-compartmented ship, access above the fire is often restricted, and entry may not be achieved by anything less than an oxyacetylene torch. In such conditions, the spread of fire upward through a ship may not be preventable, and efforts will be directed at removing cargo and reducing loss of life.

Fires aboard very large modern cruise ships combine firefighting difficulties with huge life safety concerns in which over 5,000 passengers may be at risk (Nicholson 2007). Fires on such ships have been started by discarded smoking materials, welding repairs, laundry fires, and arson. *NFPA 301* and the International Maritime Organization (IMO) *Convention for Safety of Life at Sea* (SOLAS) (1992) are the predominant codes for such ships (NFPA 2008).

Idle vessels are often moored side by side or berthed alongside disused piers, where fire can spread from pier to ship or from ship to ship by radiant heat, flaming debris, or direct flame contact. The investigator must be aware of the mobility of such vessels (before and after the fire) and that the fire may not have been an isolated occurrence. The original location of the vessel must be determined as part of the investigation. Because of the unusual nature of the fire conditions aboard such vessels, the investigator is directed to seek the assistance of specialists in this area (Stuart 1979).

7.10.4 MOTIVES FOR VEHICLE AND MARINE ARSON

As in any other kind of fire investigation, the intimation of a possible motive for arson may provide a significant turning point for any vehicle fire investigation. Although proof of motivation is not necessary for the conviction of an arsonist, it can pull all the pieces of an investigation together.

Insurance fraud, either involving the owner directly or the financial institution that is carrying the loan, is certainly a consideration. The fuel crisis of the 1970s and 2006–2009 prompted many owners of large, gasoline-thirsty vehicles to dispose of them. Government-imposed requirements for mandatory emission-control modifications may also force owners to abandon vehicles.

Depressions in the general economy in the 1980s (and currently) forced people to acknowledge that they had paid too much for a vehicle or that the monthly payments were too high to maintain. With a substantial increase in the number of leased cars; changes in the tax deduction bases for cars, trucks, and other vehicles; and changes in the marketability of expensive or fuel-inefficient cars of recent vintage, vehicular arson is more common today than ever before. Faced with a substantial payoff due on a leased car or truck or when stuck with a relatively new vehicle whose resale value has plummeted, an individual or a company may see "selling" it to the insurance or leasing company as a convenient way out.

Large diesel tractors routinely cost over $150,000 today, and a major engine rebuild can cost over $20,000. If a company or private trucker is operating on a thin margin, the loss of the vehicle to a convenient fire may be the solution to financial problems. Vehicles are also subject to arson motivated by a number of other reasons—spite or hatred, intimidation, vandalism, concealment of a crime, or even pyromania. Vehicles stolen for joyriding, for parts, or for the commission of other crimes are often burned to destroy fingerprints or other associative evidence.

Inquiries as to the purchase price of the vehicle, standing loan balance, and monthly payments should be accompanied by a determination of the fiscal well-being of the owner. Are there indications of reduced income, unemployment, business losses, or gambling debts? If a vehicle is mechanically unreliable or inoperative, it is more likely to be a candidate for arson. The same holds true if the vehicle is no longer used or has outlived its usefulness. Domestic problems are sometimes behind the destruction of an automobile, recreational vehicle, or pleasure boat. A vehicle that has sentimental value to one partner may be destroyed by the other as a gesture of spite or anger. Any indications of marital difficulties should prompt a closer examination of the circumstances of the fire. As with other fires, the investigator must always be careful to keep motive and proof of cause separate and distinct determinations.

With fires in large commercial ships, any of the same reasons that prompt the burning of land-based properties can hold true. Business-related motivations can include intimidation, elimination of competition, labor unrest, or the concealment of other crimes, particularly theft, pilferage of cargo, and smuggling of goods or drugs. The financial motivations are even stronger when entire fleets are idled by international trade or monetary reversals. The thorough investigator must consider all possibilities when the values of vehicles and their cargoes reach into the thousands or millions of dollars, thus providing rich rewards to those clever enough to escape detection. Fires have been set aboard military vessels to delay deployments (Sapp et al. 1995).

At the same time, the investigator must remember that a motive alone does not change a fire of undetermined cause into an arson. The origin and cause of a fire is established from careful data collection and proper analysis of the evidence at the scene. There are many ignition sources in the average vehicle or vessel, rich fuel loads, and many ways for accidental fires to ignite. The investigator has to be just as diligent in establishing the first fuel ignited (suitable in both type and quantity), a competent heat source, and the mechanism for contact in these fires as in a structure fire before concluding the cause of the fire. If not suppressed shortly after ignition, these fires can result in such complete destruction of the vehicle or vessel and evidence of the fire that an origin and cause cannot be reliably established.

See Chapter 11 on "Arson Crime Scene Analysis" for a detailed discussion on motives for arson.

Summary

In fire scene investigations of structures, wildlands, and vehicles, the investigator methodically searches the fire scene for evidence and data to determine the cause and origin of the fire.

The key components of the investigation include the following:

- Examination of the fire scene
- Collection and preservation of physical evidence
- Documentation via photographs, diagrams, maps, evidence collection
- Reconstruction of the fire scene.
- Evaluation and analysis of available data, testing of possible hypotheses
- Determination of origin and cause

Although the process fire investigation is similar for structures, wildlands and motor vehicles, the investigator does have different elements to consider.

- In structure fires, the investigator must consider the many types of building material that may have enhanced the development of the fire, the type and location of ventilation sources, as well as those of fuel packages.
- In wildland fires, fire spread is dependent on topography, ground cover, and weather conditions. Fire scene search, burn patterns, and documentation techniques differ from those of structure and motor vehicle fires.
- In motor vehicle fires, combustible interiors, ignitable liquid heat sources, moving parts, and complex electrical and hydraulic systems and accessories present a challenge for the fire investigator. Although a fire along a roadside suggests that a careless smoker may have caused it, without finding the residue of the match or cigarette, there is the possibility that sparks from a vehicle exhaust, deliberate hot set, or other source could have played a part.

To quote Sir Arthur Conan Doyle, "I have devised seven separate explanations, each of which would cover the facts as far as we know them. But which of these is correct can only be determined by the fresh information which we shall no doubt find waiting for us." (The Adventure of the Copper Beeches)

The fire scene investigation is like an onion with many layers to unpeel. One piece of evidence may yield another piece of evidence. Initial conclusions often need to be tweaked with a new finding. Final conclusions must be based on fire scene examination, documentation, and reconstruction that are implemented using the scientific method and supported by laboratory testing.

Review Questions

Structural Fires

1. What is overhaul and why is it critical that it be kept to a minimum?
2. What basic fire behaviors are revealed by post-fire indicators?
3. Name three ways suppression efforts can affect fire spread and post-fire indicators.
4. Name five types of information that can be gathered from firefighters.
5. What is the most common search pattern for structure fires and what are four of its advantages?
6. Why is the documentation and reconstruction of fuel load so important?
7. What does the angle of a burn pattern on a wall or furniture reveal about the fire's development?
8. What is a heat horizon and how does it help establish direction of development of a structure fire?
9. Name three ways ventilation openings can affect fire patterns in a room fire.
10. What types of fuels produce the deepest burn patterns on floors?
11. How does the radiant heat flux on a wood surface affect the char rate of the wood?
12. How does window glass provide useful information to a fire investigator?
13. Why is a contents inventory important in a fire investigation?
14. Name four ways a fire scene should be documented.

15. What is the chain of custody and why is it important?

Wildland Fires

1. What are four of the major factors that affect the spread of a wildland fire?
2. Why are weather conditions both before and during a wildland fire very important to the investigator?
3. Name three macro-scale indicators and three micro-scale indicators.
4. What is the most common accidental cause and most common natural cause for wildland fires?
5. What is the area of transition and how is it useful to an investigator?
6. Why is a magnet useful in examining suspected areas of origin?
7. What kinds of physical evidence can be found in wildland fires?
8. What is the critical fuel moisture content for cigarette ignition of grasses and other fine fuels?
9. What is a *hot set* in a wildland fire?
10. Name four ways power lines can ignite wildland fires.

Motor Vehicle Fires

1. What are the most readily ignitable liquids found in a modern auto?
2. How do the boiling points of liquid fuels affect their hot-surface ignitability?
3. Which produces the higher internal temperatures in a modern vehicle fire—a flammable liquid arson or direct ignition of the upholstery—and why?
4. Why is it important to examine the scene of a vehicle fire before the vehicle is removed?
5. How can transmission fluid become ignited?
6. Does extensive combustion of body panels and structural and suspension components indicate an accelerated fire in a modern vehicle? Why or why not?
7. Name five of the items most commonly removed before a stolen vehicle is set afire.
8. Why is it nearly impossible to cause an explosion of a gas tank?
9. Why do recreational vehicle fires develop quickly?
10. What makes extinguishment of a ship fire so difficult?

References

Ahrens, M. 2010. *U.S. Vehicle Fire Trends and Patterns.* Quincy, MA: National Fire Protection Association.

Albers, J. 2002. "Pour Pattern or Product of Combustion?" *California Fire/Arson Investigator* July: 5–10.

Allen, K., et al. 1984. "A Study of Vehicle Fires of Known Ignition Source." *Fire and Arson Investigator* 34 (June): 33–43, 35; (September): 32–44.

Almirall, J. R., et al. 2000. "The Detection and Analysis of Ignitable Liquid Residues Extracted from Human Skin Using SPME/GC." *Journal of Forensic Sciences* 45, no. 2 (March): 453–61.

Anderson, H. E. 1982. "Aids to Determining Fuel Models for Estimating Fire Behavior." Boise, ID: National Wildfire Coordinating Group, April.

Andrews, P. L., and C. D. Bevins. 1999. "BEHAVE Fire Modeling System: Redesign and Expansion." *Fire Management Notes* 59: 16–19.

ASTM. 2009. *Black Box Data from Accident Vehicles: Methods of Retrieval, Translation, and Interpretation.* West. Conshohocken, PA: ASTM.

———. 2011. *E1188-11: Collection and Presentation of Information and Physical Items by a Technical Investigator.* West Conshohocken, PA: ASTM.

———. 2013a. *E860-07(2013)e1: Standard Practice for Examining and Testing Items That Are or May Become Involved in Litigation.* West Conshohocken PA: ASTM.

———. 2013b. *E1459-13: Standard Guide for Physical Evidence Labeling and Related Documentation.* West Conshohocken, PA: ASTM.

Babrauskas, V. 2003. *Ignition Handbook.* Issaquah, WA: Fire Science Publishers.

———. 2004. "Charring Rate of Wood as a Tool for Fire Investigators." Pp. 1155–70 in *Proceedings, Interflam 2004.* London: Interscience Communications.

Barnett, G. 2007. *Automotive Fire Analysis.* 2nd ed. Tucson, AZ: Lawyers & Judges Publishing.

Béland, B. 1993. "Spalling of Concrete." *Fire and Arson Investigator* 44 (September): 26.

Béland, B., C. Ray, and M. Tremblay. 1987. "Copper-Aluminum Interaction in Fire Environments." *Fire and Arson Investigator,* 37 (March). Reprinted from *Fire Technology* 19 (February 1983): 22–30.

Bell, V. L. 1980. *The Potential for Damage from the Accidental Release of Conductive Carbon Fibers from Aircraft Composites.* Hampton, VA: National Aeronautics and Space Administration, Langley Research Center.

Bernardo, L. U. 1979. *Fire Start Potential of Railroad Equipment.* San Dimas, CA: USDA Forest Services.

Bloom, J., and C. Bloom. 1997. "Ford Ignition Switch Overheating and Fires." *Fire and Arson Investigator* 47 (March): 10–11.

———. 2007. *Recreational Vehicle Fire Investigation*. 2nd ed. (DVD). Grants Pass, OR: Bloom Fire Investigation.

Bourhill, R. 1995. *Cigarette Butt Identification Aid.* 16th ed. Colorado Springs, CO: Forensic Science Foundation.

California Department of Forestry and Fire Protection. 2008a. *2006–2008 Fires by Cause Statewide*. Sacramento, CA: Author.

———. 2008b. *2006–2008 Historical Wildfire Activity Statistics (Redbooks)*. Sacramento, CA: California Dept. of Forestry and Protection.

Canfield, D. V. 1984. "Causes of Spalling of Concrete at Elevated Temperatures." *Fire and Arson Investigator* 34 (June).

Carman, S. 2009. "Progressive Burn Pattern Development in Post-Flashover Fires." Pp. 789–800 in *Proceedings Fire and Materials*. San Francisco, CA.

Cope, C. 2009. "Vehicle Engine Compartment Fires." Pp. 561–79 in *Proceedings Fire & Materials 2009*. London: Interscience Communications.

Coulson, S.A., et al. 2008. "An Investigation into the Presence of Petrol on the Clothing and Shoes of Members of the Public." *Forensic Science International* 175: 44–54.

Coulson, S. A., and R. K. Morgan-Smith. 2000. "The Transfer of Petrol onto Clothing and Shoes While Pouring Petrol around a Room." *Forensic Science International* 112, no. 2 (August 14): 135–41.

Countryman, C. 1983. "Ignition of Grass Fuels by Cigarette." *Fire Management Notes* 44: 3, 3–7.

Darrer, M., et al. 2000. "Collection and Persistence of Gasoline on Hands." Paper presented at EAFS, Cracow, Poland, September 2000.

Davie, B. 1988. "The Investigation of Mobile Home Fires." *Fire and Arson Investigator* 39 (September): 51.

Deans, J. 2006. "Recovery of Fingerprints from Fire Scenes and Associated Evidence." *Science and Justice* 40, no. 3: 153–68.

DeHaan, J. D. 1987. "Are Localized Burns Proof of Flammable Liquid Accelerants?" *Fire and Arson Investigator* 38, no. 1.

———. 1992. "Fire: Fatal Intensity." *Fire and Arson Investigator* (September): 55–59.

———. 1993. "A Close Call for a Hot Hudson." *Arizona Arson Investigator*.

———. 1995. "The Reconstruction of Fires Involving Highly Flammable Hydrocarbon Liquids." Ph.D. dissertation, Strathclyde University, Glasgow, Scotland.

———. 1999. "The Consumption of Animal Carcasses and Its Implication for the Combustion of Human Bodies in Fire." *Science and Justice* (January).

———. 2003. "Our Changing World: Part 3 Is More Sensitive Necessarily More Better?" *Fire and Arson Investigator* 53, no. 2 (January).

DeHaan, J. D., and F. L. Fisher. 2003. "The Reconstruction of a Fatal Fire in a Parked Motor Vehicle." *Fire and Arson Investigator* January: 42–46.

DeHaan, J. D., and F. A. Skalsky. 1981. "Evaluation of Kapak Plastic Pouches." *Arson Analysis Newsletter* 5, no. 1.

Demers-Kohl, J., et al. 1994. "An Evaluation of Different Evidence Bags Used for Sampling and Storage of Fire Debris." *Canadian Society of Forensic Science Journal* 27, no. 3.

Drysdale, D. D. 1999. *An Introduction to Fire Dynamics*, 2nd ed. Chichester, UK: Wiley.

Earls, A. R. 2009. "It's Not Lightweight Construction. It's What Happens When Lightweight Construction Meets Fire." *NFPA Journal* July–August: 38–45.

———. 2001. "Manufactured Homes Revisited." *NFPA Journal* March–April: 49–51.

Eichmann, D. A. 1980. "Cigarette Burning Rates." *Fire and Arson Investigator* January–March.

Ettling, B. V. 1990. "The Significance of Alligatoring of Wood Char." *Fire and Arson Investigator* 41 (December).

Evans, D. D., et al. 2004. "Physics-Based Modeling of Community Fires." Pp. 1065–76 in *Proceedings, Interflam 2004*. London: Interscience Communications.

Ford, R. T. 2002. "Proving Hot Start Arson in Wildfires." *Fire and Arson Investigator* April: 42–43.

Gialamas, D. M. 1996. "Enhancement of Fire Scene Investigation Using Accelerant Detection Canines." *Science and Justice* 36 (1): 51–54.

Gilchrist, R. J. 1937. "Die Casting." *The Ohio Engineer* April.

Gudmann, J. C., and D. Dillon. 1988. "Multiple Seats of Fire: The Hot Gas Layer." *Fire and Arson Investigator* 38, no. 3: 61–62.

Gutsel, S. L., and E. A. Johnson. 1996. "How Fire Scars Are Formed: Coupling a Disturbance Process to Its Ecological Effect." *Canadian Journal of Forestry Research* 26, no. 2: 166–74.

Hadden, R., F. Jervis, and G. Rein. 2009. "Investigation of the Fertilizer Fire aboard the Ostedijk." *Fire Safety Science* 9: 1091–1101.

Hammarstrom, R. 2008. "Joint Development of Fire Fighting Systems for Construction Machines." Brand Posten, SP, Boras Sweden, #39, pp. 4–6.

Henderson, R. W. 1986. "Thermodynamics of Ferrous Metals." *National Fire and Arson Report* 4.

Herrera, F. 2005. "Investigation of Boat Fires." *California Fire/Arson Investigator* January: 10–11.

Higgins, M. 1993. "Vehicle Fires: A Practical Approach." *Fire and Arson Investigator* Spring.

Hirschler, M. M., D.J. Hoffmann, and E.C. Kroll. 2002. "Rate of Heat Release for Plastic Materials from Car Interiors." *BCC Flame Retardancy Conference Proceedings,* June.

Hrynchuk, R. J. 1998. "CAFI Vehicle Fire Investigation Techniques: A Report on Vehicle Fire Tests." Canadian Association of Fire Investigators Seminar, Toronto, Ontario, September 30, 1998.

Icove, D. J., and J. D. DeHaan. 2006. "Hourglass Patterns." In *Proceedings of IFSI Conference*, Cincinnati, OH, May.

Ingason, H. and R. Hammarstrom, "3MW from a Single Tyre." Brandposten, SP, Boras, Sweden, #39, P. 6.

Johnson, E. A. 1992. *Fire and Vegetation Dynamics*. Cambridge: Cambridge University Press.

Kennedy, P. M., K. C. Kennedy, and R. L. Hopkins. 2003. "Depth of Calcination Measurement in Fire Origin Analysis." In *Proceedings Fire and Materials 2003*. London: Interscience Communications.

Kerber, S. I., and D. Madrzykowski. 2009. "Fire Fighting Tactics under Wind Driven Fire Conditions: 7-Story Building Experiments." *NIST, TN 1629: NIST Technical Note 1629*. April.

Kinard, W. D., and D. R. Midkiff. 1991. "Arson Evidence Container Evaluation II: Kapak Bags, a New Generation." *Journal of Forensic Sciences* November.

Krasny, F., W. J. Parker, and V. Babrauskas. 2000. *Fire Behavior of Upholstered Furniture and Mattresses*. Norwich, NY: William Andrew.

Lentini, J. J. 1992a. "Behavior of Glass at Elevated Temperatures." *Journal of Forensic Sciences* 37 (September).

———. 1992b. "The Lime Street Fire: Another Perspective." *Fire and Arson Investigator* September: 52–54.

Lentini, J. J., C. Cherry, and J. Dolan. 2000. "Petroleum Laced Background." *Journal of Forensic Sciences* 45, no. 5: 965–89.

Lentini, J. J., D. M. Smith, and R. W. Henderson. 1992. "Baseline Characteristics of Residential Structures Which Have Burned to Completion: The Oakland Experience." *Fire Technology* 28 (August).

Mangs, J. 2004a. *On the Fire Dynamics of Vehicles and Electrical Equipment*. VTT Publication, 521. Helsinki, Finland.

———. 2004b. *VTT Building & Transport* April: 33–35.

Mann, D. C. 2000. "In Search of the Perfect Container for Fire Debris Evidence." *Fire and Arson Investigator* April: 21–25.

Mann, D. C., and W. R. Gresham. 1990. "Microbial Degeneration of Gasoline in Soil." *Journal of Forensic Sciences* 35, no. 4.

Mann, D., and N. Putaansuu. 2006. "Alternative Sampling Methods to Collect Ignitable Liquid Residues from Non-porous Areas Such as Concrete." *Fire and Arson Investigator* 57, no. 1 (July): 43–46.

March, G. 1993. *An Investigation and Evaluation of Fire and Explosion Hazards Resulting from Modern Developments in Vehicle Manufacture*. Newcastle, UK: Tyne and Wear Fire Brigade.

Marley, R. K., and J. D. DeHaan. 1994. *CCAI Vehicle Fire Tests: A Photographic Report*. Sacramento, CA: California Criminalistics Institute.

McGill, L. 1995. *Fire/Explosion Investigator*. Gardnerville, NV.

Mell, W., et al. 2006. *A Physics-Based Approach to Modeling Grassland Fires*. Gaithersburg, MD: BFRL, NIST.

Meroney, R. N. 2004. "Fires in Porous Media: Natural and Urban Canopies." Prepared for NATO Advanced Study Institute: Flow and Transport Processes in Complex Obstructed Geometries, Kiev, Ukraine, May 5–15, 2004.

Midkiff, C. R. 1990. "Spalling of Concrete as an Indicator of Arson." *Fire and Arson Investigator* 41 (December): 42.

Morgan-Smith, R. 2000. "Persistence of Petrol on Clothing." Paper presented at ANZFSS Symposium of Forensic Sciences, Gold Coast, Queensland, Australia.

Morrill, J. 2006. "Analysis of a Ford Speed Control Deactivation Switch Fire." *Fire and Arson Investigator* July: 22–27.

National Wildfire Coordinating Group. 2005. *NWCG Course FI-110: Wildfire Observations and Origin Scene Protection for First Responders*. Boise, ID: NWCG.

NFPA. 2001. *Fire Protection Guide to Hazardous Materials*. Quincy, MA: National Fire Protection Association.

———. 2008. *NFPA 301: Code for Safety to Life from Fire on Merchant Vessels*. Quincy, MA: National Fire Protection Association.

———. 2010a. *NFPA 302: Fire Protection Standard for Pleasure and Commercial Craft*. Quincy, MA: National Fire Protection Association.

———. 2010b. *U.S. Vehicle Fire Trends and Patterns*. Quincy, MA: National Fire Protection Association.

———. 2014. *NFPA 921: Guide for Fire and Explosion Investigations*. Quincy, MA: National Fire Protection Association.

———. 2015. *Fire Loss in United States*. Quincy, MA: National Fire Protection Association.

———. 2017. *NFPA 921: Guide for Fire and Explosion Investigations*. Quincy, MA: National Fire Protection Association.

Nic Daéid, N. 2003. "The ENFSI Fire and Explosion Investigation Working Group and the European Live Burn Tests at Cardington." *Science and Justice* 43, no. 1 (January–March).

———. 2014. *Fire Investigation*. London: Taylor and Francis and CRC Press.

Nicholson, J. 2007. "Cruise Ship Fires." *NFPA Journal* January–February: 37–42.

Nicol, J. D., and L. Overley. 1963. "Combustibility of Automobiles: Results of Total Burning." *Journal of Criminal Law, Criminology and Police Science* 54: 366–68.

Pack, D. W., et al. 2000. "Civilian Class of Surveillance Satellites." *Crosslink*, January: 2–8. El Segundo, CA: Aerospace Corp.

Pagni, P. J., and A. A. Joshi. 1991. "Glass Breaking in Fires." Pp. 791–802 in *Proceedings Third International Symposium on Fire Safety Science*. London: Elsevier Applied Science.

Posey, J. E., and E. P. Posey. 1983. "Using Calcination of Gypsum Wallboard to Reveal Burn Patterns." *Fire and Arson Investigator* 33 (March).

Powell, R. J. 1992. "Testimony Tested by Fire." *Fire and Arson Investigator* (September): 42–51.

Public Works Journal. 1992. "GPS Technology Aids Oakland Hills Fire Efforts." *Public Works Journal* (May 1992). Reprinted in *Arizona Arson Investigator* (August 1993).

Putorti, A., J. A. McElroy, and D. Madrzykowski. 2001. *Flammable and Combustible Liquid Spill/Burn Patterns, NIJ Report 604-00.* Washington, DC: NIJ.

Riggs, S. 2009. *Public Agency Training Council.* Indianapolis, IN.

Rothermel, R. C. 1983. *How to Predict the Spread and Intensity of Forest and Range Fires.* Gen. Tech. Rep. INT-143. Ogden, UT: US Dept. of Agriculture, National Wildfire Coordinating Group.

———. 1992. "How to Predict the Spread and Intensity of Forest and Range Fires." In National Wildfire Coordinating Group, *Fire Behavior Nomograms.* Boise, ID: US Dept. of Agriculture.

Saitoh, N., and S. Takeuchi. 2006. "Floor Scene Imaging of Petroleum Accelerants by Time-Resolved Spectroscopy with a Pulsed Nd-YAG Laser." *Forensic Science International* 163: 38–50.

Sanderson, J. L. 1995. "Tests Add Further Doubt to Concrete Spalling Theories." *Fire Findings* 3 (Fall).

———. 2001. "Science Reconstruction." *Fire Findings,* 9, no. 1 (Winter): 12.

Sapp, A. D., et al. 1995. "Arson Aboard Naval Ships Characteristics of Offenses and Offenders." NCAVC.

Service, A. F., and R. J. Lewis. 2001. "The Forensic Examination of a Fire Damaged Vehicle." *Journal of Forensic Sciences* 46 no. 4: 950–53.

Skelly, M. J. 1990. "An Experimental Investigation of Glass Breakage in Compartment Fires." NIST-GCR-90-578. US Department of Commerce.

Smith, F. P. 1993. "Concrete Spalling: Controlled Fire Tests and Review." *Fire and Arson Investigator* 44 (September): 43.

Spearpoint, M. J., et al. 2005. "Ignition Performance of New and Used Motor Vehicle Upholstery Fabrics." *Fire and Materials* 29, no. 5 (September–October): 265–82.

Spearpoint, M. J., and J. G. Quintiere. 2001. "Predicting the Ignition of Wood in the Cone Calorimeter." *Fire Safety Journal* 36, no. 4: 391–415.

Steensland, P. 2008. "Long-Term Thermal Residency in Woody Debris Piles." Paper presented at International Association of Arson Investigators Annual Training Conference, Denver, CO, May.

Stocks, B. J., et al. 2004. "Crown Fire Behaviour in a Northern Jack Pine–Black Spruce Forest." *Canadian J. Forestry Research* 34: 1548–60.

Stuart, D. V. 1979. "Shipboard Fire Investigation." *Fire and Arson Investigator* 29 (January–March): 55–58.

Suefert, F. J. 1993. "Steal and Burn." *Fire and Arson Investigator,* December: 18–23.

———. 1995. "Automobile Engine Fires." *Fire and Arson Investigator* 45, no. 1 (June): 23–26; "Automobile Engine Fires (Part 2)." *Fire and Arson Investigator* 46, no. 1 (September): 23–26.

Sullivan, A. L. 2009. "Wildland Surface Fire Spread Modelling, 1990–2007: Pt. 1, Physical and Quasi-physical Models," 349–68; Pt. 2, "Empirical and Quasi-empirical Models," 369–86; Pt. 3, "Simulation and Mathematical Analogue Models," 387–403. *International Journal of Wildland Fire* 18.

Sutherland, D., and K. Byers. 1998. "Vehicle Test Burns." *Fire and Arson Investigator* 48 (March): 23–25.

Swanson, W. E. 1941. *Modern Shipfitters Handbook.* New York: Cornell Maritime Press.

Thaman, R. N. 1978. "Laboratory Can Help Investigator Pluck Arson Evidence Out of Debris." *Fire Engineering* 131, no. 8 (August): 48–50, 52.

Tobin, W. A., and K. L. Monson. 1989. "Collapsed Springs in Arson Investigations: A Critical Metallurgical Evaluation." *Fire Technology* 25 (November).

Tontarski, K. L., K. A. Hoskins, T. G. Watkins, L. Brun-Conti, and A. L. Michaud 2009. "Chemical Enhancement Techniques of Bloodstain Patterns and DNA Recovery after Fire Exposure." *Journal of Forensic Sciences* 54 (1): 37–48.

Tontarski, R. E. 1985. "Using Absorbents to Collect Hydrocarbon Accelerants from Concrete." *Journal of Forensic Science,* 30 (4): 1230–1232.

Wendt, G. A. 1998. "Investigating the 'Black Hole' Motor Vehicle Fire." *Fire and Arson Investigator* 49 (October): 11–13.

White, G. L. 2004. "Fire Scene Diagramming for Wildland Fire Investigations." *Fire and Arson Investigator* (October): 31–33.

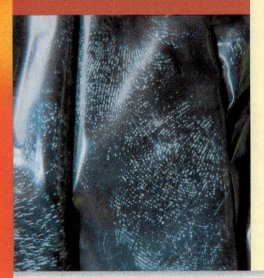

CHAPTER

8

Forensic Laboratory Services

Courtesy of Jack Deans, FFS, MFSSoc, New Scotland Yard (Ret.), Fingerprint Consultant, Gardiner Associates, Ltd.

KEY TERMS

adsorption, *p. 569*

calorimetry, *p. 589*

chromatography, *p. 565*

mass spectrometry, *p. 567*

spoliation, *p. 590*

OBJECTIVES

After reading this chapter, you should be able to:

- Understand the role of laboratory services in fire and explosion investigations.
- Describe the various types of services and tests available from forensic and fire testing laboratories.
- List and identify the common types of evidence found at fire scenes.
- Identify examples of how failure analysis by forensic engineers can be used to help determine fire causation.
- Explain the basic concepts of how volatile accelerants are identified using gas chromatography and mass spectrometry.
- List the various types of techniques used to isolate and identify volatile residues.
- Identify the common types of materials found in chemical incendiaries.
- Search the Internet for the appropriate and up-to-date guidance on standards used by public and private forensic laboratories.
- Recognize the value of fire testing.
- Describe the basic types of fire tests and give examples of each.
- Learn how to interpolate scaled test data to real-world scenarios.
- Appreciate the use of fire test data in the analysis and evaluation of a working hypothesis.

562

8.1 Availability of Laboratory Services

8.1.1 FORENSIC LABORATORIES

Criminalistics laboratories operating under the auspices of the states' departments of justice, public safety, state prosecutor, state police, or law enforcement authority, working in cooperation with city or county laboratories, provide analytic services necessary for comprehensive fire scene investigations. On a national level, the laboratories of the Federal Bureau of Investigation (FBI) and the Bureau of Alcohol, Tobacco, Firearms and Explosives (ATF) provide similar services. In Canada, the Centre of Forensic Sciences in Toronto and Sault St. Marie, the *Laboratoire de sciences judiciaires et de médecine légale* in Montreal, and the Forensic Science and Investigation Service of the Royal Canadian Mounted Police provide fire debris analysis.

With some exceptions, the services from these public laboratories are available at no cost to personnel from public fire or police agencies and to investigators from some semi-private agencies such as transit authorities, public utilities, and railroads. Due to limited laboratory resources, there may be restrictions on which agencies they are permitted to serve. In addition, there may be a case priority scheme in operation that relegates fire-related evidence to low-priority status. Because the priority is often set on the basis of whether there were deaths or injuries or on a court date's having been set, that information should be provided to the lab when the evidence is brought in to ensure fastest possible service time. The investigator should contact the nearest laboratory before its services are needed, so that time is not wasted just in finding a laboratory.

Private investigators, whether retained by public agencies such as public defenders or by private or corporate clients in civil or criminal cases, have a more difficult and costly problem. Although a few public laboratories will service public defenders and even private-sector investigators on a contractual basis, for the most part, private-sector investigators must turn to private laboratories. Many large insurance and engineering firms, in addition to providing laboratory services to their own investigators, offer such services to outside clients on a fee basis. There are also small, private laboratories that can perform appropriate tests on a per-case, per-analysis, or hourly fee basis and provide expert testimony as to their results, with their findings in compliance with standard practices for reporting opinions of scientific or technical experts (ASTM 2011b).

Finally, there are qualified consultants who will evaluate the evidence and provide interpretation and expert testimony while contracting with others for the actual laboratory work. There are many more qualified, private-sector facilities available now than just a few years ago. Many also do work (on a fee basis) for public-sector agencies whose own labs cannot provide timely services.

8.1.2 FIRE TESTING LABORATORIES

Forensic laboratories cannot provide some tests, such as heat release rate testing, flame spread, ignitability, and room (even multiroom) fire tests. Public agencies in the United States may qualify for assistance from the Fire Research Laboratory operated by ATF in Annandale, Maryland. Private laboratories such as Omega Point (Elmendorf, Texas), Southwestern Research Institute (San Antonio, TX), MDE (Seattle, WA), Underwriters Laboratories (Northbrook, IL), Chilworth Pacific Fire Testing, (Kelso, WA), and Western Fire Center (Longview, WA) have provided qualified testing and analysis services.

8.1.3 THE IMPORTANCE OF ACCREDITATION

The most important consideration in choosing a lab is not whether the lab has the necessary equipment but whether the lab has experienced analysts to interpret the data gleaned from testing. The quality of the analysis and interpretation depends on the analysts' understanding of the effects of fire, evaporation, exposure, and even sample collection and storage on physical evidence from fires. Simply having a chart or numerical reading does not do the investigator any good.

The **International Association of Arson Investigators** (IAAI, www.firearson.com) established a Forensic Science Committee to develop guidelines on the analysis and interpretation of fire-related evidence. The ASTM International (formerly known as the American Society for Testing and Materials, www.astm.org) used the IAAI's and others' guidelines as the foundation for test methods, guides, and practices covering many of the techniques used in fire debris analysis, including *ASTM E1618-14 (2014): Standard Test Method for Ignitable Liquid Residues in Extracts from Fire Debris Samples by Gas Chromatography-Mass Spectrometry* (ASTM 2014) and *ASTM E1492-11 (2011): Practice for Receiving, Documenting, Storing, and Retrieving Evidence in a Forensic Science Laboratory* (ASTM 2011c).

The **American Board of Criminalistics** (ABC, www.criminalistics.com) is a collection of professional organizations that represent forensic scientists. Each organization is entitled to one member on the ABC Board of Directors and one member on the ABC Examination Committee. The ABC Board has a certification program for individuals involved in fire debris analysis and other forensic disciplines. Scientists who pass a written exam and who participate in a quality assurance testing program may be designated a Fellow of the ABC (F-ABC) in that specialty.

The **American Society of Crime Laboratory Directors** (ASCLD, www.ascld.org) is a nonprofit professional society of crime laboratory directors and forensic science managers from the United States, Canada, Puerto Rico, Virgin Islands, China, Costa Rica, Finland, Hong Kong, Ireland, Italy, England, Israel, Sweden, Switzerland, New Zealand, Sinapore, Taiwan, Turkey, and Australia. Their professional membership consists of a wide range of individuals whose major responsibilities include the management of a crime laboratory. Their membership consists of biologists, chemists, document examiners, physicists, toxicologists, educators, instructors, and law enforcement officers. ASCLD has established a protocol for accreditation of forensic laboratories that calls for use of standardized methods for analysis and interpretation and record keeping.

The **International Organization for Standardization** (ISO, www.iso.org) develops and publishes international standards. The ISO maintains ISO/IEC 17025, the standard for the Accreditation for Forensic Testing Laboratories, which serves as the general requirements for the competence of testing and calibration laboratories. The ISO/IEC 17025 standard is used by both testing and calibration laboratories and serves as the basis for a laboratory to be deemed technically competent. ISO/IEC 17025 was originally issued in 1999 and updated in 2005 to be in harmony with ISO 9001.

ANSI-ASQ National Accreditation Board (ANAB, www.anab.org) is jointly owned by the American National Standards Institute (ANSI, www.ansi.org) and the American Society for Quality (ASQ, www.asq.org). ANAB serves as the US accreditation body for management systems (for example, ISO 9001) certification bodies, and provides accreditation for ISO/IEC 17025 forensic test agencies and ISO/IEC 17020 forensic inspection agencies. The ANAB accreditation process is based on an assessment of the laboratory, which covers the laboratory's procedures, technical qualifications, and competence for conducting specific testing activities within the scope of the standard. Accreditation cycles cover two to five years, and successful inspections result in the issuance of a certificate of accreditation.

The **American Association for Laboratory Accreditation** (A2LA, www.a2la.org) is a nonprofit, non-governmental, public service, membership society that offers a full range of comprehensive laboratory, laboratory-related accreditation services, and training programs. Their ISO/IEC accreditation programs include ISO/IEC 17025 Testing/Calibration Laboratories, ISO/IEC 17020 Inspection Bodies, ISO/IEC 17043 Proficiency Testing Providers, and ISO/IEC 17065 Product Certification Bodies.

A2LA uses the ISO/IEC 17020 accreditation program for Fire Origin and Cause Investigation. The Forensic Investigations Group, LLC, located in Covington, Louisiana, is A2LA's first commercial, US-based organization to obtain this accreditation.

Active committee membership in one or more professional organizations such as the ASTM International, the IAAI, the National Fire Protection Association (NFPA), or the Society of Fire Protection Engineers (SFPE) lends credibility to a laboratory's report as well as the expert's testimony in support of their work.

8.2 Identification of Volatile Accelerants

The primary lab service provided to fire investigators is the analysis of fire debris for suspected volatile accelerants. In one laboratory study, ignitable liquids both flammable and combustible liquids were found in 49 percent of all arson cases submitted to a major crime laboratory over a 3-year period (DeHaan 1979). Data from a more recent survey verify the same percentages (Babrauskas 2003b). Although fire databases do not include information on the frequency of ignitable liquid use in setting fires, it is the consensus of fire and arson investigators in the United States that more than 50 percent of detected arsons involve the use of accelerants.

The use of ignitable liquids, most commonly petroleum products, has been common throughout the history of twentieth-century incendiarism. Also, ignitable liquids are the first fuel ignited in an estimated 30 percent of all accidental building fires in California (California State Fire Marshal 1995). Many ignitable liquid accelerants are used in excess, and their residues remain for ready detection by instrumental analysis. Accelerants can be used in moderation or on combustible substrates like paper or plastic, and the resulting fire can consume or evaporate all traces of the accelerant.

In a number of structure fire experiments in which a petroleum product such as gasoline had been used to ignite a fire, the debris, even though collected directly after the fire, packaged properly, and analyzed by the best available methods, failed to reveal any accelerant. A negative laboratory finding is not proof that an accelerant was *not* used; it merely fails to establish its presence after the fire. On the other hand, petroleum products are detectable in very low concentrations in a wide variety of consumer products and building materials, so the interpretation of trace levels in debris must take such background volatiles into consideration. Petroleum products change in their physical and chemical properties as they burn or evaporate during and after a fire, so conclusive identification can be a challenge even to experienced laboratory analysts.

8.2.1 GAS CHROMATOGRAPHY

Gas **chromatography** (GC) as an accepted laboratory procedure has been in use for the last 50 years or so. Gas chromatography is used both for the screening of samples to determine which contain adequate volatile ignitable liquids for identification and for the identification itself once the volatile has been isolated. Although gas chromatographs (called GCs) vary considerably in their complexity, their basic principles of operation are quite simple. All types of chromatography are a means of separating mixtures of materials on the basis of slight differences in their physical or chemical properties.

As represented in Figure 8-1, gas chromatography uses a stream of gas (nitrogen or helium) as the carrier to move a mixture of gaseous materials along a long column or tube filled or coated with a separating compound. The components in the mixture interact with the separating compound by alternately dissolving in it and then volatilizing to be swept farther along the column by the carrier. To ensure that all the compounds in the unknown mixture remain in the gaseous state, the whole column is kept in an oven to maintain it at a precisely controlled temperature. The mixture is injected onto the column at one end, and at the other end is a detector, usually a small flame whose electrical properties,

chromatography ■ Chemical procedure that allows the separation of compounds based on differences in their chemical affinities for two materials in different physical states (e.g., gas/liquid, liquid/solid).

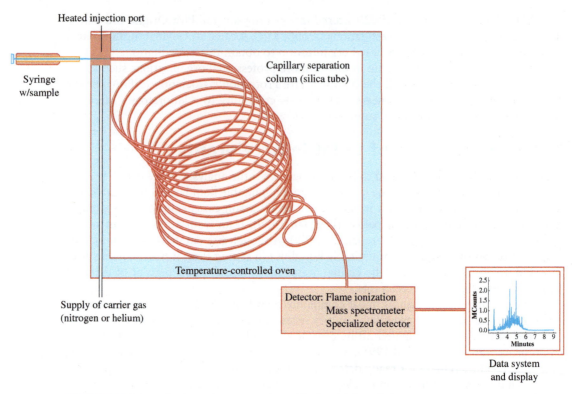

FIGURE 8-1 Schematic of gas chromatograph used for fire debris analysis.

monitored by electronic circuits, change whenever a compound comes off the column in a process called flame ionization detection (FID).

The whole process is analogous to a stream of vehicle traffic routed through a forest. The motorcycles speed right through, zigzagging around the trees, and come out the other side of the forest first to encounter a radar speed trap. The small cars have more trouble finding a path and come out shortly afterward to encounter the same radar. The big cars take a long time to find spaces big enough to allow passage, and they exit after a longer delay, followed by the trucks, which take the longest of all.

In the case of volatile hydrocarbon analysis, the traffic would be the unknown hydrocarbon mixture, and the "forest" would be the GC column. The analyst can adjust the spacing of the "trees" by choosing the correct chemicals for the separating compound and carefully controlling the temperature and carrier flow so that each type of "traffic" comes out in a neat, readily identifiable group. To extend the "forest-traffic" analogy further, the proper choice of GC column and conditions for the hydrocarbons found in fire debris allow the lab to identify the type of "traffic" introduced by analysis of the groups of "vehicles" that result. From simple, insulated box ovens that kept the column at a set temperature, ovens have evolved to models that are programmed to provide steady or increasing temperatures at preset time intervals to maximize the separation of similar compounds. The technology of detectors has progressed from simple thermal detectors to flame detectors that can be made sensitive only to compounds containing specific elements, or to mass spectrometers.

Although the column can be selected to separate a mixture of compounds on the basis of their chemical properties, most separations in volatile accelerant analysis are made on the basis of differences in the boiling points of the various components. Nearly all the components of petroleum distillates of interest are either aliphatic (straight-chain) or aromatic (ring) in structure and thus will have very similar chemical properties within those two groups. A typical separation of a series of aliphatic hydrocarbons is shown in Figure 8-2. In this typical chromatogram, one can see that the heavier a molecule is, the less volatile it is, and the later it will appear on the chromatogram.

Columns for GC analysis of suspected arson residues are usually set up to offer the best separation of components having volatilities between those of pentane (C_5H_{12}) and triacontane ($C_{30}H_{62}$), because that range includes all the commonly encountered petroleum products. Although the mainstay of columns was for many years a packed tubular column, averaging 3 mm (1/8 in.) in diameter and 3 m (10 ft) in length, it has now been supplanted by a new generation of very narrow [0.1 to 0.25 mm (0.004 to 0.01 in.) in diameter] capillary columns of various lengths.

Early capillary columns required very long lengths [50 m (167 ft) or more] to achieve good separations, but these extreme lengths usually required long analysis times. Such columns were used primarily for research or development, in which short analysis times could be sacrificed for sensitivity and selectivity (Jennings 1980).

The newest columns provide extremely high performance on short columns (10 to 25 m, or roughly 33 to 82 ft) using high temperature-programming rates. The result is analysis times that are shorter than those possible with packed columns and faster turnaround times. Capillary columns also use smaller sample sizes than were ever possible with packed columns—an advantage of much merit in forensic work, where the sample size is often critically small. Sensitivity is now in the nanoliter range (10^{-9} liter).

Because gas chromatography is a separation technique, the result of such GC-FID analysis is not a specific identification of each compound but a pattern of peaks that the analyst attempts to match to a reference chromatogram to make the identification. This approach is described in *ASTM E1387-01 (2001): Standard Test Method for Ignitable Liquid Residues in Extracts of Samples of Fire Debris by Gas Chromatograph* (ASTM 2001). Due to the limitations of the GC-FID method, *ASTM E1387* was withdrawn in 2008 and was replaced by the GC-mass spectrometry (GC/MS) method *ASTM E1618-14 (2014)*, described in the next section. GC-FID is still used for special applications such as samples of very low molecular weight.

In addition, progress in computer technology has dramatically improved the data collection and handling in gas chromatography. Runs (and irreplaceable samples) are no longer lost when the recording conditions are not set just right, because the data system collects all the data and then displays whatever portion the analyst specifies. The displayed data can expand or condense portions of the chromatogram to make identification easier. Collected chromatograms are also filed on disks and can be compared against a library of stored chromatograms of known products. Such libraries can be swapped between instruments and even between labs, permitting ready comparison.

8.2.2 GAS CHROMATOGRAPHY/MASS SPECTROMETRY (GC/MS)

Flame ionization detectors (FIDs) are sensitive and stable detectors, but they yield little chemical information about the compounds that pass through to produce a signal. **Mass spectrometry** allows the analyst to break apart each compound into small submolecular pieces and, by counting those pieces, establish the chemical structure of the original molecule. Mass spectrometry is an analytical technique that needs to be fed one compound at a time, while gas chromatography is a separation technique that is good at separating things into groups. Because most of the volatile residues in fire debris involve complex mixtures, coupling the two gives the best tool. While GC/MS has been available for more than 30 years, only recently has it been made small, inexpensive, and user-friendly enough to make it convenient for routine fire debris analysis. It has become the baseline technique for fire debris analysis because it can yield so much more information than GC-FID (Nowicki 1990). In addition to displaying a mass spectrum for each peak, it can be asked to scan for selected ions, those that are characteristic for a particular chemical species of interest, such as the ion having a "weight" of 91, which is characteristic for toluene. This

mass spectrometry ■ Analysis of organic molecules by fragmenting them and separating them by size.

means that the GC/MS can display a chromatogram just for aromatics, for instance, ignoring all the peaks that do not yield that specific ion. This can be accomplished by displaying one ion at a time or by "summing" three or four ions that are characteristic for the species of interest (Gilbert 1998).

The species responsible for the major peaks in the gasoline chromatogram can be identified. The pattern of peaks, their proportions, and the relative concentrations (higher concentrations of aromatics than other species) yields very discriminatory information. This can make it possible to pick out characteristic patterns even amid complex chromatograms with high backgrounds. The counts of separate ions also can be compiled into a single chromatogram called a *total ion chromatogram*, or TIC, which captures the same information as a GC-FID analysis and displays it as a single chromatogram for pattern recognition.

Some particularly difficult samples may require *target compound analysis* (TCA), in which the detection of a set of particular compounds permits identification of a petroleum product among complex background peaks (Sandercock and Pasquier 2003; Rankin and Fletcher 2007). TCA has also been used to compare gasolines with suspected sources. Some particularly difficult samples may require GC/MS/MS, or tandem mass spectrometry. This technique takes the molecular species created by the ionization process of MS and breaks them into even smaller pieces, yielding more specific information. Higher sensitivity is also claimed, but the method has found more application in explosives analysis than in routine fire debris analysis (Sutherland and Penderell 2000; de Vos et al. 2002).

Because of its sensitivity and analytical power (resolution), GC/MS has become the standard forensic technique for fire debris analysis (Stauffer, Dolan, and Newman 2008).

Currently, most forensic GC analyses for suspected accelerants are carried out using a capillary column of moderate length (10 to 25 m; 31 to 76 ft), using dimethyl silicone, phenyl silicone, or an equivalent nonpolar bonded phase, in a programmed temperature range of 50°C to 250°C (122°F to 482°F), and employing a mass spectrometer.

Because the MS detector has to be turned off for the time period when the extraction solvent used is passing through, volatiles such as methanol, ethanol, hexane, acetone, or toluene will not be detected. If such a product is suspected, the lab should be advised so that a GC-FID analysis can be conducted or an appropriate alternative isolation protocol followed such as heated head space or solid-phase microextraction (SPME), which uses no solvent.

8.2.3 SAMPLE HANDLING AND ISOLATION OF VOLATILE RESIDUES

The best containers for debris suspected of containing volatile ignitable liquids are clean, lined metal paint cans, sealable glass jars, or bags of nylon or a suitable copolymer (e.g., nylon/acrylonitrile/methacrylate Kapak made by Ampac). The first step in the examination protocol of such debris is to briefly open the container in the case of bags or jars (this will usually not be necessary) and to inspect the contents.

The nature of the contents may indicate which analytical technique to use or predict interferences likely to be encountered. The contents should be checked to ensure there have been no errors in packaging or labeling that could compromise the value of the evidence. The examination must be brief to minimize losses of volatiles that may be present only at trace levels. Very strong odors of a volatile detected during this examination may indicate that a particular test protocol should be used. The major problem with fire debris analysis is having a small quantity of product mixed with a great deal of solids or liquids that may provide contamination.

Heated Headspace

Because any volatiles present will reach vapor equilibrium in a sealed container, advantage can be taken of the vapors in the air cavity (headspace) of the container. Heating the sample container to 50°C to 60°C (120°F to 140°F) will ensure at least a partial vaporization of heavier hydrocarbons prior to sampling. Some analysts prefer heating the container above 100°C (212°F) to force even higher boiling point materials (such as fuel oil) into the vapor stage. It is the experience of most other analysts, however, that all but the heavy ends of kerosene will be detectable in most samples heated to moderate temperatures (60°C; 140°F) and, more importantly, that excessive temperatures (>80°C; 176°F) encourage the degradation of synthetics (carpet, upholstery, etc.) in the debris. These degradation products add to the complexity of the chromatogram, possibly masking low levels of real accelerants while not contributing significantly to the sensitivity of the method. If a heavy product is suspected, isolation using solvent extraction or dynamic headspace will result in more complete recovery and analysis.

After the sample container has equilibrated at a moderate temperature, it is punctured and a small sample (0.1 to 3 mL) of the headspace vapor is drawn off using a gastight syringe. This vapor is then injected directly into the gas chromatograph. As described in *ASTM E1388-12 (2012): Standard Practice for Sampling of Headspace Vapors from Fire Debris Samples* (ASTM 2012b), positive results of this injection may be adequate to permit characterization of the volatiles present. Positive results also signal the presence of very volatile residues that may be lost by careless handling, or alcohols or ketones that require special handling. Because this technique is not as sensitive as others described, a negative result here merely indicates that no high concentration of volatile exists and that another isolation technique is suggested. The heated headspace technique is fast, convenient, and requires virtually no sample handling, while providing some useful information.

Passive Headspace Diffusion (Charcoal Sampling)

Another technique that capitalizes on the vapor equilibrium in a sealed container while concentrating some of the vapors in a more condensed form is passive **adsorption**. This method includes several similar techniques that rely on the adsorptivity of activated charcoal. Originally developed by forensic scientists in England using a charcoal-coated wire, this technique requires no manipulation of the sample or its original container (Twibell and Home 1977). As originally described, the method called for a coated wire to be inserted into the airspace of the sample container (as shown in Figure 8-2) and allowed to equilibrate for at least 2 hours. The wire was then removed from the container and inserted into the pyrolysis unit of a GC, where it was raised instantly to a very high temperature, driving the adsorbed hydrocarbons off into the column.

adsorption ■ Trapping of gaseous materials on the surface of a solid substrate.

This technique has been adapted in a variety of methods described in *ASTM E1412-12 (2012): Practice for Separation and Concentration of Ignitable Liquid Residues from Fire Debris Samples by Passive Headspace Concentration* (ASTM 2012c). Adaptations include the insertion of a plastic or glass bead coated with activated charcoal, or a sampling tube or bag containing charcoal into the airspace of the container (Juhala 1980; Twibell, Home, and Smalldon 1982). The container is resealed and allowed to equilibrate, usually at room temperature, for 12 to 15 hours or at 60°C to 80°C (140°F to 176°F) for 2 hours. The sampling device is removed, and adsorbed volatiles are extracted from the charcoal with a small quantity of solvent such as pentane, diethyl ether, or carbon disulfide for injection into the GC. Today, a carbon strip is used. These techniques are very sensitive to all types of volatiles, require no heating or manipulation of the samples, and can be repeated again and again because they take up only a small fraction of the volatiles each time. They are suitable for all kinds of debris and are especially valuable for debris that will also be examined for trace evidence or latent fingerprints.

A variant of this technique has become the single most widely used sampling and concentration method for fire debris. In this form, a small strip of activated carbon fiber mat, sometimes called a *C-strip*, is suspended in the container, at room temperature or at moderately elevated temperatures (60°C to 80°C). It is then extracted with carbon disulfide or diethyl ether. The technique has excellent sensitivity [0.1 microliter (µL) under some conditions] and no interferences. It is described in full in *ASTM E1412-12 (2012)*.

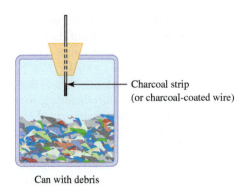

FIGURE 8-2 Passive charcoal strip sampling of fire debris.

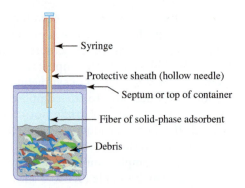

Syringe

Protective sheath (hollow needle)

Septum or top of container

Fiber of solid-phase adsorbent

Debris

FIGURE 8-3 Solid-phase microextraction uses a thin fiber of adsorbent exposed to the headspace of a debris container. The fiber is then placed directly into the injection port of a GC for desorption.

Charcoal strip
(or charcoal-coated wire)

Can with debris

Solid-Phase Microextraction

Solid phase microextraction (SPME), uses a solid-phase adsorbent bonded to a fiber that is inserted into the can of fire debris through a hollow needle, as shown in Figure 8-3. After the fiber has been exposed to the heated contents of the can for 5 to 15 minutes, it is withdrawn and then inserted directly into the injection port of a GC. The heat of the injection port then thermally desorbs the volatiles directly into the GC column. The technique offers extreme simplicity (with no manipulation of the sample or any extract) and low cost, because it involves no solvents and no modifications to existing gas chromatographs (Furton, Almirall, and Bruna 1996). SPME appears to be particularly well suited for isolating petroleum product residues from water and skin tissue (Almirall, Bruna, and Furton 1996; Almirall et al. 2000). The small volume of adsorbent can be overwhelmed by high concentrations of petroleum distillates, causing distortion of the peak pattern in the GC analysis. SPME has the advantage of using no extraction solvent, so all volatiles are readily detectable in a single run. Its limited sample capacity means it is easily overloaded by extended exposure or high concentration, which can lead to distortion of its GC profile (Yoshida, Kaneko, and Suzuki 2008; Lloyd and Edmiston 2003).

Dynamic Headspace (Swept Headspace)

Dynamic headspace, sometimes called the *charcoal trap method*, employs a charcoal or polymeric matrix through which the air from the evidence container is drawn. It was adapted from methods developed for trapping ultralow concentrations of hydrocarbons for environmental monitoring (Chrostowski and Holmes 1979). The sample container is fitted with a modified lid or a septum that allows for the introduction of a heated carrier gas (purified room air or nitrogen). The container is warmed while vapors are drawn off by a low vacuum through a cartridge filter containing activated charcoal or a molecular trapping agent such as Tenax (see Figure 8-4).

After extraction is complete (20 to 45 minutes), the charcoal can be washed with carbon disulfide or a like solvent, and the resulting solution is ready for GC analysis. Tenax or charcoal may be thermally desorbed to avoid the handling of toxic solvents, contamination, or any further dilution. The technique requires the use of traps, commercially prepared or laboratory prepared, and specially built apparatus, described in *ASTM E1413-13 (2013): Standard Practice for Separation and Concentration of Ignitable Liquid Residues from Fire Debris Samples by Dynamic Headspace Concentration* (ASTM 2013b). It is very useful because of its sensitivity (less than 1 μL) and its applicability to all ignitable liquid residues (from gasoline to fuel oil) including alcohols and ketones. The GC analysis of Tenax traps, which are thermally desorbed, has been automated, making

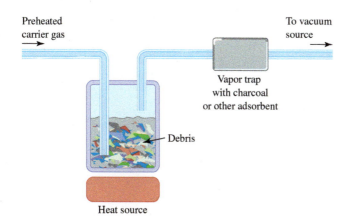

FIGURE 8-4 Swept headspace technique is the most efficient means of collecting volatile hydrocarbons but requires a source of carrier gas, a heat source, and a vapor trap of charcoal or other adsorbent. It is not considered a nondestructive isolation technique.

it more suitable for laboratories with a large caseload. The technique does have the drawback that all the volatiles in a sample can be swept out (and pulled through the trap) if the time and temperature conditions are not monitored closely and are too severe for the sample size. Excessive extraction causes loss of the lighter fractions, and the process can generally be carried out only once on a sample.

Steam Distillation

The oldest separation technique, originating from classical chemistry, requires only modest but specialized distillation equipment. The specimen is removed from its container and boiled with water in a glass flask (as illustrated in Figure 8-5). The steam, carrying the volatiles with it, is condensed and trapped. It is suitable for volatiles that form an *azeotropic* (nonmixing) layer with water; therefore, it cannot be used to recover alcohol or acetone. The technique is suitable for petroleum distillates as heavy as paint thinner; heavier products (e.g., fuel oil) require the use of ethylene glycol, which boils at a higher temperature (Brackett 1955). Light hydrocarbons may be lost in recovery. Detection limits are on the order of 50 μL (for gasoline), so it is not as sensitive as charcoal-trapping methods, but it has the advantage of providing a neat liquid sample with no extraneous solvents (Woycheshin and DeHaan 1978). The method is described in *ASTM E1385-00: Standard Practice for Separation and Concentration of Ignitable Liquid Residues from Fire Debris Samples by Steam Distillation* (ASTM 2009).

Solvent Extraction

Solvent extraction, a direct and simple method for extracting volatiles has been in use for many years. Debris is extracted or washed with a small quantity of *n*-pentane, *n*-hexane, dichloromethane, or carbon disulfide that has been checked to ensure its purity. The liquid extract is filtered and then concentrated by evaporation in a stream of warm air until a small quantity remains for testing, as shown in Figure 8-6.

Solvent extraction is especially suitable for treating small, nonabsorbent specimens like glass, rock, or metal or for washing the interior of containers used to transport ignitable liquid accelerants. It provides good recovery for many petroleum products, especially the heavier ends of kerosene and diesel fuel, but it is not suitable for isolating the lighter petroleum distillates due to evaporative losses. Its overall sensitivity is about the same as for steam distillation with the main drawback being that it will extract residues of partially pyrolyzed carpet or foam rubber, which often interfere with the detection of low levels of hydrocarbons of evidentiary significance (Woychesin and DeHaan 1978). This technique requires only simple glassware and high-purity solvents. It is described in detail in *ASTM E1386-15 (2015): Standard Practice for Separation and Concentration of Ignitable Liquid Residues from Fire Debris Samples by Solvent Extraction* (ASTM 2015c).

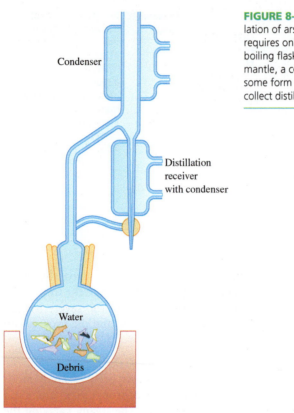

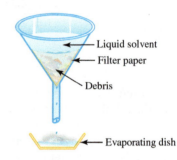

FIGURE 8-5 Steam distillation of arson debris requires only water, a boiling flask, a heating mantle, a condenser, and some form of receiver to collect distillates.

Condenser

Distillation receiver with condenser

Water

Debris

Heating mantle

Liquid solvent

Filter paper

Debris

Evaporating dish

FIGURE 8-6 Solvent extraction is not very sensitive but may be used to extract trace volatiles from non-absorbent materials like metal, glass, or stone.

8.2.4 IDENTIFICATION OF VOLATILE RESIDUES

Once the suspected ignitable liquid residues have been isolated, attention can be turned toward identifying them as precisely as possible. Because recoveries are typically on the order of several microliters, gas chromatography/mass spectrometry will be the technique of first choice because of the quantity of information it yields while consuming 1 μL or less of the sample. The identification of the volatiles (usually a petroleum distillate or product) present is then usually based on a comparison of the pattern of peaks generated in the chromatogram of the unknown against a library of chromatograms of known materials made under the same conditions. A standardized approach to the classification and characterization of volatiles is described in *ASTM E1618-14 (2014): Standard Test Method for Ignitable Liquid Residues in Extracts from Fire Debris Samples by Gas Chromatography-Mass Spectrometry* (ASTM 2014).

Classification of the volatile into one of the basic volatility categories—light, medium, or heavy—is based on the presence of a particular range or sequence of hydrocarbons. The products are further categorized as to their chemical nature—gasoline, true distillates, de-aromatized distillates, isoparaffins, aromatics, naphthenic-paraffinics, *n*-alkanes, oxygenates, and other miscellaneous volatiles—based on the MS data collected. This classification scheme is intended to make description and comparisons easier for the laboratory analyst; but because consumer products may represent different classes of products, and a single product may have more than one consumer designation, the system is not always well understood by investigators. For this reason, it is recommended that when an analyst describes an ignitable liquid residue as a particular classification, examples of some common consumer products should be included, as listed in Table 8-1, which is based on *ASTM E1618-14 (2014)*.

TABLE 8-1	Classification of Ignitable Liquids in Fire Debris		
CLASS	**LIGHT (C$_4$–C$_9$)**	**MEDIUM (C$_8$–C$_{13}$)**	**HEAVY (C$_8$–C$_{20+}$)**
Gasoline (auto)	Fresh gasoline in range C$_4$ to C$_{12}$		
Petroleum distillate	Petroleum ether Some camp fuels	Some charcoal starters Some paint thinners	Kerosene Diesel fuel
De-aromatized distillates	Some camp fuels	Some charcoal starters Some paint thinners	Some charcoal starters Odorless kerosenes
Isoparaffinics	Aviation gas Special solvents	Some copier toners Some paint thinners	Specialty solvents Some copier toners
Aromatic products	Xylene/toluene Some parts cleaners	Some insecticide solvents Parts cleaners Fuel additives	Cleaning solvents
Naphthenics/paraffinics	Solvents	Some charcoal starters Lamp oils	Some lamp oils Some insecticide solvents Industrial solvents
n-Alkane products	Solvents Pentane/hexane	Candle oils Copier toners	Copier toners NCR papers (carbonless forms) Candle oils
Oxygenated solvents	Alcohols/ketones Surfacers Some lacquer thinners Fuel additives	Some lacquer thinners Industrial solvents Turpentines (gum)	
Other: Miscellaneous	Single-component products, blended products		

Adapted from *ASTM Standard E1618-14 (2014): Standard Test Method for Ignitable Liquid Residues in Extracts from Fire Debris Samples by Gas Chromatography-Mass Spectrometry*, copyright ASTM International, 100 Barr Harbor Drive, West Conshohocken, PA 19428. A copy of the complete active standard may be obtained from ASTM, www.astm.org.

A growing number of ignitable liquids are not petroleum distillates and therefore do not lend themselves to a simple distillate classification scheme based on peak pattern alone. For instance, there are aromatic specialty solvents used in insecticides, enamel reducers, and pavement sealers; isoparaffinic mixtures used in consumer products such as "odorless" paint thinners; and naphthenic–paraffinic petroleum products used in lamp oils (and sold as "kerosene" for portable heaters). The GC-FID patterns of these products are not sufficient to permit their identification, and GC/MS is required.

Table 8-1 reflects the use of non-traditional petroleum distillates like naphthenic-paraffinic products in household products. Their peak patterns are not readily differentiated from the patterns generated by some pyrolysis products. Thus, the use of GC/MS is necessary in a larger percentage of cases, because the GC/MS can yield information about what specific chemical species are present. For instance, isoparaffinic hydrocarbon products are used in many consumer products, from copier toners to insect sprays. Because they are not true petroleum distillates, they should not be classified as such, although in some instances they display a boiling point range that fits light or medium distillates. When these products are identified, a list of the consumer products that may contain non-traditional petroleum distillates should be included in the report to give the investigator a clue as to what product may have been used to start the fire or that may have become involved accidentally in the fire. Because the contents of many products are not always described accurately on the labels, comparison samples (preferably in their original containers) of any product in the vicinity of the fire's origin should be collected and submitted for analysis if there is a chance they could have been involved in the fire. Because the analyst is expected to match the GC/MS data from the unknown to that of a known (reference) material, having immediate access to a comparison sample from the scene is very important. This is especially true when the material is an unusual proprietary or specialty solvent.

This classification scheme reflects changing consumer uses and products and a much changed petroleum refining process, as well as improved sensitivity and discrimination of the lab methods used. There is also a desire to provide investigators with the most accurate and meaningful (useful) information. The investigator must strive to understand what these product designations mean and use that information to evaluate various accidental and intentional sources of such residues in fire debris. Special detectors may also be used to gain more information about a volatile. Each requires injection on a separate GC column with a specific detector in place of the FID, but some GCs have the ability to split a single injection onto two separate columns, each with its own detector. Photoionization detection (PID), for example, can be used in parallel with FID because it can be made specific to aromatic, olefinic, or aliphatic hydrocarbons. Another detector, originally intended for the detection of nitrogen- and phosphorus-containing compounds, has been modified to specifically detect the oxygenated volatiles (ketones, alcohols, and ethers) that have become widely used as fuel additives to minimize air pollution (Patterson 1990).When distillation is used to isolate a neat volatile, infrared (IR) spectroscopy can yield considerable information about its chemical structure. About 20 μL of sample is needed for conventional liquid-cell spectrophotometry, but a specialized FTIR microcell has been designed for use as a detector on a GC column when smaller quantities are recovered. While the sensitivity of the method is limited, it can aid in the identification of unusual liquids, complex pyrolysis products, and some natural products (terpenes) (Hipes et al. 1995).

If sufficient quantities of a suspected ignitable liquid are recovered, physical properties like flash point can be measured. Criminal charges against a suspected arsonist may depend on the flammability of the accelerant in his or her possession, and a flash point determination may be required. A precise determination requires a considerable sample and specialized equipment, but a rough estimate can be made by placing several drops of the liquid on a watch glass and placing it in a freezer. On removal from the freezer, the glass will warm up gradually, and a small ignition source passed over the specimen will cause a flash when the flash point is exceeded. If the liquid has a flash point above ambient (usually 25°C; 77°F), the glass can be placed on a hot plate and the sample tested in the same manner. In rare circumstances, steam distillation has been able to recover enough volatile accelerant to permit flash point determination by Setaflash tester, which requires 2 ml of sample [*ASTM D3278-96 (2011); Standard Test Methods for Flash Point of Liquids by Small Scale Closed-Cup Apparatus* (ASTM 2011a)]. Ultraviolet (UV)/visible fluorescence techniques permit extensive characterization of petroleum distillates, and these techniques, along with high-pressure liquid chromatography (HPLC), may be useful in special circumstances because they provide information that supplements gas chromatography, especially for heavy petroleum products (Alexander et al. 1987).

Evaporation and Degradation

Petroleum products behave in a fairly complex but predictable manner when burned or simply exposed to air to evaporate. Due to their higher vapor pressures, the most volatile components evaporate more quickly than those less volatile, and this changes the peak profile of the product when it is subjected to gas chromatography. Gasoline profile changes dramatically as it evaporates, complicating its identification.

When the gasoline is burned, this same process occurs, only much more rapidly. It is not possible to determine whether a petroleum product burned or merely evaporated at room temperature by examination of its chromatogram (Mann 1987). In the case of gasoline, characteristic aromatic compounds are found in residues of gasoline that has evaporated down to less than 3 percent of its original volume. Therefore, evaporated or "weathered" gasoline can still be identified if those key or target compounds are identified in the debris. Unfortunately, this is not true for simple petroleum distillates like mineral spirits (paint thinners). As these substances evaporate, their residues assume more and more of the characteristics of the next heavier class of petroleum distillate. Thus, it is not always possible to conclusively establish the exact nature of the original product.

In addition, petroleum products exposed to moist garden soil can undergo microbiological degradation. This degradation involves the consumption of both aliphatic and aromatic compounds, so the peak profile of gasoline, for instance, can be significantly changed (Mann and Gresham 1990; Kirkbride et al. 1992; Turner and Goodpaster 2009). This degradation is minimized if the samples are kept frozen until analysis.

Evaporation and degradation effects combined with contamination from pyrolysis products in the debris can make the identification of a specific petroleum product from post-fire debris difficult if not impossible. The increased use of non-distillate petroleum products has resulted in GC chromatograms that are not so easily classified or identified.

In most cases, the laboratory can be expected to characterize and distinguish the product or its general family—for example, light (petroleum ether), medium (paint thinners), or heavy (kerosene/diesel) petroleum distillates; lacquer thinners; and so on—from residues left in the debris unless the liquid fuel has been nearly or totally consumed. Any petroleum distillate, when used as an accelerant, can be burned away completely, leaving no readily detectable traces if the fire is hot enough and long enough, and the accelerant is exposed directly to its effects. In most incendiary-caused fires, accelerants are used in excess, and the resulting fires do not burn with sufficient intensity to completely destroy them.

Laboratories are often asked to determine the presence of petroleum distillate accelerants from the soot accumulated on window glass taken from the scene. The appearance of the soot is most directly linked to the state of combustion in the room and the amount of ventilation. Fuel-rich fires produce heavy soot; lean or well-ventilated fires produce little or none. The synthetic fabrics and rubbers that constitute a large percentage of the fuel load in modern structures produce an oily soot very similar chemically to that produced by petroleum distillate accelerants.

It has been suggested that there should be chemical species in the soot produced by gasoline that are characteristic for that fuel and are not produced by any "normal" fuel. It was once thought that the combination of bromine and lead in leaded automotive gasoline would produce soot with a unique elemental profile. Unfortunately, some carpets contain both elements, so there is a potential for background interference (Andrasko et al. 1979). Lead and related additives have been phased out of modern fuels, making them very unlikely to be detected. There are several organic molecules, chiefly polynuclear aromatic hydrocarbons that appear to be produced by burning gasoline but are not produced by burning synthetic materials (Andrasko 1979).

The most extensive work done in this area is that of Pinorini et al, who used GC combined with elemental analysis, x-ray diffraction, and scanning electron microscopy (SEM) to characterize soot from various ignitable liquids and from synthetic fibers and materials (Pinorini et al. 1994). They discovered that under controlled conditions, soot from the liquids could be distinguished from that produced by solid fuels using multiple techniques. Unfortunately, the presence of water from suppression produced nonreproducible condensation of the soot and limited the discrimination value of even the combination of techniques.

Some analysts have reported that freshly made carbon soot will adsorb petroleum distillate fumes from the room air just as activated charcoal adsorbs them in laboratory extractions. If a fire occurs and a too-rich mixture of fuel is present, the soot formed during the early stages may retain enough of the accelerant to permit identification upon extraction of the soot. Occasional analysis of soot on glass from accelerated vehicle fires has been observed, but no systematic study has been reported.

Despite partial evaporation, most common petroleum distillates have a distinctive GC/MS pattern that can be compared with the patterns of known compounds. The experienced analyst will know what the effects of fire and evaporation can be and will take them into account when comparing chromatograms. All petroleum distillates are overlapping cuts or fractions of a continuous spectrum of compounds. Therefore, it is possible for a complex hydrocarbon mixture to be sufficiently affected by fire that its chromatogram cannot readily be identified. It could, for instance, represent a heavily evaporated product such as kerosene, or a relatively undamaged product like a heavier solvent. Today, the introduction of biofuels or synthetic fuels further complicates the interpretation issue. Some of these have unusual gas chromatographic profiles that do not readily fall into the existing classification schemes (Kuk and Spagnola 2008).

Source Identification

As to the identification of a specific source for a product, the range of techniques available now enables the analyst to rule out many potential sources and thereby shorten the list of "possibles." The sophistication of GC/MS and today's data handling systems make it possible to recognize delicate differences in the patterns of GC peaks between products that were thought to be indistinguishable (Armstrong and Wittkower 1978).

Determining the significance of these differences is entirely another matter, requiring extensive field sampling and validation of the reproducibility of patterns detected. As with many mass-produced materials that start from different feedstocks in different manufacturing facilities, changes can be produced by many factors. To complicate matters, when gasoline, for instance, is distributed, it mixes with gasoline from other sources already in storage and transportation facilities, and its composition changes.

Under some circumstances, such as having a liquid gasoline sample that has not undergone significant burning or evaporation, and a small number of potential sources, it is possible to state with some confidence that certain sources can be completely excluded and that another represents a source that is indistinguishable by any of its individual features (Rankin, Wintz, and Everette 2005; Petraco 2008; Barnes et al. 2004). Rather than give the investigator a false lead with a possible identification, the laboratory will usually suggest several alternative identifications in its report. The investigator can evaluate the suggestions and determine which, if any, fit the circumstances best. If the investigator does not clearly understand the identification or characterization, the problem should be discussed with the laboratory before proceeding.

8.2.5 INTERPRETATION OF GC RESULTS

It should be noted that most of the newer isolation techniques, especially when combined with capillary column GC/MS, are more sensitive than the techniques used less than a decade ago. In many cases they are more sensitive than the human nose, often relied upon to screen for the best debris samples at the scene. This means that sample collection may depend not only on the detection of unusual odors but also on the presence of suspicious burn patterns and on aids such as canine detection.

Comparison samples of floor coverings or other fuels involved are much more desirable now than ever before because of the contributions made by the pyrolysis of synthetic materials, binders, and adhesives, which can interfere with the analysis (DeHaan and Bonarius 1988). Recent work has been published by Stauffer exploring the chemical mechanisms of polymer pyrolysis and the contributions each type can make to the GC profile (Stauffer 2003). This work has improved the discrimination of pyrolysis products and petroleum products substantially.

Accuracy of Today's Testing Methods

As the minimum detection level of GC/MS has decreased, analysts have begun to see just what a petroleum-based world we live in. From the volatile products in roofing paper, copy paper, carbonless forms, magazines, and newspaper print, to the solvents in glues and adhesives used in floor coverings and footwear, to residues of dry cleaning solvents, insecticides, and even cleaning agents like the limonene used in "green" grease removers, petroleum products can be detected in a variety of consumer goods today (Lentini, Dolan, and Cherry 2000). Without specific identification of the product and comparison against a reference sample, the mere presence of traces of a volatile petroleum product in fire debris may well be meaningless.

A properly trained dog can detect petroleum products at very low levels with a high degree of accuracy, sometimes at concentrations below even what a qualified lab can properly identify, so there may be samples in which a canine correctly detects traces of gasoline that the lab cannot confirm if it adheres to the accepted standard practices (DeHaan 1994). But a dog is not a replacement for a laboratory. A canine can signal only yes or no and cannot identify the product or discriminate between the residues of carpet glue used to repair a section of carpet from the residues of isoparaffinic solvent used as an accelerant. A laboratory can.

Despite the advice of the IAAI Forensic Science Committee and the NFPA Technical Committee on Fire Investigations (NFPA 2017), a number of courts have admitted evidence of canine alerts as indications of the presence of ignitable liquid accelerants in the absence of laboratory identifications (IAAI Forensic Science and Engineering Committee 1988). Studies have shown that even the best-trained canine teams cannot discriminate all possible pyrolysis products and background contaminants from accelerants and will detect products that do not contain ignitable liquid accelerants (Katz and Midkiff 1998). Without a specific verifiable identification of exactly what is present, the investigator cannot decide the significance of such positive alerts.

It is possible to track gasoline residues into a fire scene. For example, if someone steps in a puddle of gasoline leaking from an electrical generator or spilled from a fuel can outside the scene and then walks through the scene, traces *theoretically* might be found in several adjacent locations. Studies have demonstrated that detectable gasoline residues could be tracked onto clean substrates for a step or two, but not beyond (Armstrong et al. 2004; Kravtsova and Bagby 2007). Transfers by absorption onto clothing of gasoline vapors in a room have also been shown to be remotely possible but very weak (Kuk and Diamond 2005). Exhaust gases from gasoline-powered air fans at fire scenes can contaminate exposed charred material but tests have revealed that although such contamination at trace levels is possible, it is very unlikely to affect waterlogged debris (Lang et al. 2002).

The investigator must ask: Why was this found in these concentrations, and how else might it have gotten there? Fire investigators and forensic analysts need to ask: What is the meaning of this "positive" at the concentration found here? With today's sensitive techniques, the soil gathered from the side of a busy highway will yield identifiable gasoline residues at parts-per-billion levels, just from the traces accumulated from leaks and spills from passing vehicles. Is that finding of any significance? Does that mean that someone poured gasoline along the side of the road and set fire to it to commit arson?

Lentini demonstrated that solvents in floor coatings like stain, varnish, and oil were readily detectable in interior woods for more than 2 years after application (Lentini 2001). Hetzel and Moss detected waterproofing solvent after more than 2 weeks of severe exterior exposure (Hetzel and Moss 2005). A case showed that the gasoline used as a solvent for interior floor varnish some 15 years before the fire was still identifiable when the wood was heated and the volatiles trapped and analyzed by GC/MS. Scientists and investigators of 25 years ago only dreamed about the sensitivity that is available today, but intelligence must be applied to interpret findings accurately. The mere presence of a volatile is no longer sufficient; rather, it is the concentration at which it becomes significant that is critical to its interpretation (DeHaan 2002).

Comparison Samples

With the sensitivity of today's detection methods, including the use of canines and the pervasive use of petroleum products, the investigator must recognize the importance of comparison samples. If debris is collected at a scene for lab analysis, unless there is a broken Molotov cocktail or a can of gasoline lying next to the burned area, comparison samples should be collected. These samples should include the floor covering, any padding or underlay, and the floor beneath, not only near the point of origin but also at another location in the same room, preferably one protected under furniture. If an ignitable liquid is suspected, comparison samples of any solvents, cleaners, or insecticides that may have been stored or used in the vicinity should be collected. This may involve interviewing the owner, tenant, or maintenance staff to ascertain what might have been used in the course of business prior to the fire.

If any material, such as cotton, flour, Fuller's earth, diatomaceous earth, or kitty litter is used to absorb suspected liquid residues, a comparison sample of the absorbent must be submitted in a separate, clean, sealed container. Any item or product used for absorbing suspected ignitable liquids must be tested and shown not to contribute any volatiles that would interfere with GC or GC/MS identification. Ignitable Liquid Absorbent (ILA) was introduced in 2003 but was later found to degrade upon extended storage and contribute volatile breakdown products to the GC analysis (Byron 2004; Mann and Putaansuu 2006; Nowlan et al. 2007).

Activated charcoal or hazmat absorption mats have proven to be such aggressive absorption media that they are easily contaminated by exposure to vehicle exhaust or other atmospheric sources of hydrocarbons. If foams, wetting agents, or other additives are used during suppression, they can affect the chromatographic data obtained from the sample but have not been reported to prevent accurate GC/MS detection and identification (McGee and Lang 2002; Coulson, Morgan-Smith, and Noble 2000; Geraci, Hine, and Shaw 2008). The fire investigator should note the use of any additives in suppression or post-fire hazard control and get a comparison sample.

Detection on Hands

Experts have identified methods for the recovery of volatile products from human skin, particularly from the hands of suspects (Darrer, Jacquernet-Popiloud, and Delemont 2008; Muller, Levy, and Shelef 2011). Volatiles on living skin are rapidly driven off by evaporation or soak into the epidermal and dermal tissues, preventing surface residues. There have been reports of successful detection of ignitable liquid residues by enclosing the hand in a PVC plastic or vinyl glove or polymeric bag with a charcoal strip or SPME collection device and warming the hand gently with a radiant heat lamp (or simply enclosing the hand in a PVC glove and using the glove as the absorbent) (Almirall et al. 2000; Montani, Comment, and Delemont 2010). For this technique to be successful, there has to have been a considerable quantity of fuel on the hand originally, and the collection has to be attempted within 1 to 2 hours of the contact. This short time frame precludes useful testing of suspects taken into custody several hours after contact. Similar testing has been more successful on tissues excised from a body during postmortem and tested in small vials using C-strips. Gasoline and similar volatiles can be detected on shoes and clothing for up to 6 hours if the garments are worn, and longer if they are removed and piled together (Loscalzo, DeForest, and Chao 1980; Kuk and Diamond 2005).

The very nature of fire, fire debris, collection, and analysis means that no one can actually quantify the results of fire debris analysis, but from experience, experiments, and test fires the analyst can establish a feel for the levels detected. The question to be answered then becomes this: Is this material significant at this concentration? The sensitivity and discrimination power of today's fire debris methods is a great tool for the investigator, but it is one that must be used carefully and judiciously if the investigations are to be accurate and just.

8.3 Chemical Incendiaries

Volatile accelerants are not the only arson evidence that is amenable to laboratory testing. A small but significant percentage of all detected arsons use a chemical incendiary as an initiator or primary accelerant (DeHaan 1979). Fortunately, most chemical arson sets leave residues with distinctive chemical properties, although physically the residues may be nondescript and easily overlooked.

Safety flares or fusees are the most commonly used chemical incendiary, presumably because they are effective, predictable, and readily available. Red-burning flares contain strontium nitrate, potassium perchlorate, sulfur, wax, and sawdust (Ellern 1961). Their post-fire residue consists of a lumpy inert mass, white, gray, or greenish-white in color. It is not soluble in water, but exposure to water turns it to a pasty mush.

The residue contains oxides of strontium and various sulfides and sulfates. Although strontium is found in all natural formations of calcium, only flare residues contain strontium salts in nearly pure form. Elemental analysis by emission spectroscopy, atomic absorption, or x-ray analysis will readily reveal these high concentrations of strontium in suspected debris. The igniter-striker button on the cap and the wooden plug in the base of the stick are resistant to burning and may be found in the fire debris, and their manufacturer may be identified by their physical features (Dean 1984).

8.3.1 IMPROVISED MIXTURES

The solid chlorine tablets or powder used for swimming pool purification will react with organic liquids such as the glycols in automotive brake fluid or some hair dressings to produce a very hot flame that lasts for several seconds. This reaction occurs after a time delay that varies with the concentration of the chlorine-based components and the degree of mixing between the solid and liquid phases. The reaction has been studied and a mechanism for the production of ethylene, acetaldehyde, and formaldehyde by the action of the hypochlorite on the ethylene glycol has been suggested and verified (Kirkbride and Kobus 1991). The production of a cloud of readily ignitable vapors would certainly account for the dramatic yellow-orange fireball of flames that occurs in these reactions.

The starting solid compounds are usually not completely consumed and are not immediately water soluble and may be visibly detected after the fire. The presence of hypochlorite salts can be detected by infrared (IR) spectrometry or chemical spot tests to confirm the identity of the oxidizer. Debris containing residues of such chlorine-based products may give off the odor of household bleach when wetted.

Potassium permanganate is used in a variety of chemical incendiary mixtures, including a hypergolic (self-igniting) mixture with glycerin. It is soluble in water and can be washed away. Even a weak water solution of it will have a pronounced red, green, or brown color, depending on the oxidation state of the manganese ion. Such chemical ions are readily identified by chemical test or by IR spectrometry if even a minute chip of the solid chemical is recovered.

Flash powders contain a fine metallic powder, usually aluminum, and an oxidizer such as potassium perchlorate or barium nitrate. Elemental analysis of the powdery residue left after ignition will reveal the aluminum, chlorine, potassium, or barium. The perchlorate or nitrate residues are detectable by micro-chemical test if any trace of the mixture remains unreacted (Meyers 1978). Mixtures of oxidizers (chlorates, nitrates, perchlorates, or sulfates) have been shown to produce extremely hot fires with metallic aluminum or magnesium powders as fuels. With a suitable binder to control combustion rates and prevent aerosolization, these materials will burn progressively and have been used for decades as solid rocket fuels (propellants). In most rocket fuel applications the binder is a rubber, but improvised mixtures have used diesel fuel as a binder. These mixtures have sometimes been referred to as high-temperature accelerants. Tests have demonstrated that such mixtures produce extremely large volumes of hot gases, very high heat fluxes, and extremely high temperatures (of both flame and gases). Even large compartments have been brought to flashover conditions in 2 to 3 minutes by the combustion of about 110 kg (250 lb) of an improvised mix of aluminum and magnesium with potassium nitrate and diesel fuel (Keltner, Hasegawa, and White 1993). Sulfates (of calcium or barium) will also act as oxidizers.

Potassium chlorate is easily identified by chemical or instrumental tests if it can be recovered in its unreacted state. When it reacts in an incendiary mixture, however, its residues are almost entirely chloride salts, which are innocuous and, if recovered from debris, could not be readily identified as having come from a device.

Sugar reacts with sulfuric acid (H_2SO_4) to leave a puffy brown or black ash of elemental carbon. It may have a faint smell of burning marshmallows, but for the most part it is innocuous in appearance and is easily overlooked. The acid present may char wood, paper, or cloth in its concentrated form. It is very soluble in water, but mineral acids like H_2SO_4 do not evaporate, and they remain active and corrosive for some time.

A burning sensation in the skin on contact with debris indicates that the debris should be checked for acids. The pH (acidity) can easily be measured, and chemical tests for sulfate or nitrate ions carried out. Reactive metals such as potassium or sodium can be used as an ignition device because they generate great amounts of heat and gaseous hydrogen on contact with water. The residues will contain potassium hydroxide or sodium hydroxide (lye)—both very strong caustics that can cause skin irritation and burns. The pH of water containing such residues will be very alkaline (basic), and chemical or spectrophotometric tests will reveal the metal present. Residues from these and similar devices are very corrosive to metal. Debris suspected of containing such corrosives should be placed in glass jars with plastic or phenolic lids, or in nylon or polyester/polyolefin bags—not in metal cans, paper bags, or polyethylene bags.

Because white phosphorus ignites on contact with air, it has been used as an incendiary device in the past. Fenian fire is a suspension of crushed white phosphorus in an organic solvent. When the container is smashed, the solvent evaporates, exposing the phosphorus to air with immediate ignition. Elemental analysis of the debris may reveal an elevated concentration of phosphorus, and there are chemical spot tests, although it tends to be a difficult element to detect and confirm. A common source of phosphorus in incendiary mixtures is the household match. Characterization of the components in match heads can be carried out by elemental analysis alone or combined with microscopic analysis using SEM (Andrasko 1978).

A variety of heat- and gas-producing chemical reactions can occur by accidental or intentional combination of household products. Many of these produce only enough heat to evaporate water to create a steam explosion, with no fire or flame. Typical of these are lye (drain cleaner), aluminum foil, and water; dry bleach, sugar and water; or acid and metal. Still other mixtures create flammable gases like acetylene (calcium carbide and water) or hydrogen (mineral acid and zinc) that, if properly ignited, can cause fires as well as explosions. Residues include unreacted starting materials, metallic oxides, chlorides, or sulfates. The heavy soot of acetylene/air combustion may be visible on adjacent target surfaces. Many so-called bottle bombs or acid bombs involve such materials. Capable of producing high temperatures and high-pressure mechanical explosions, they can cause fragmentation injuries, chemical and thermal burns, as well as property damage. Many states and the federal authorities include such chemical mixtures in their explosive device criminal codes today. Fingerprints may survive on the typical 2-L plastic bottles used (Figure 8-7).

8.3.2 LABORATORY METHODS

Recent advances in high-pressure liquid chromatography (HPLC) and the related technique of ion chromatography have made it possible to identify numerous inorganic ions

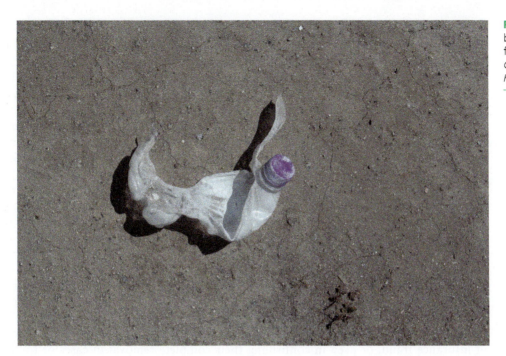

FIGURE 8-7 Bottle bomb remains may bear fingerprints and DNA. *Courtesy of Wayne Moorehead.*

in a water extract of post-fire (or post-blast) debris. As with GC, the characterization of an ion of interest is based on its detection by a suitable detector at a particular retention time as it flows through a separatory column. Single-column analyses are now capable of separating and detecting all the significant anions: Cl^-, ClO_3^-, ClO_4^-, NO_2^-, NO_3^-, SO_4^{2-}, and so on. Others can separate the cations Na^+, K^+, NH_4^+, and even sugars, commonly found in explosive and incendiary materials (Doyle et al. 2000).

Many improvised chemical incendiaries are described in the literature by the US Army's manual *Unconventional Warfare Devices and Techniques* (US Army 1966). Whenever such an incendiary is suspected, samples of nearby materials should be collected for comparison. Sometimes, it is not the presence of a particular element or ion but an elevated concentration with respect to that found in the background that betrays an incendiary. Residues of most chemical incendiaries (sulfates, nitrates, chlorides) are widely dispersed and innocuous in appearance, so selection of negative control areas is not as straightforward as selection of such areas for liquid accelerants. Random selection may be necessary, with chemical analysis revealing areas where no residues are found. Many residues are water soluble, so exposure to rain or suppression water may compromise their detection. Aluminum metal–fueled mixtures have been seen to produce microscopic spheres of aluminum and aluminum oxide, which are visually unlike the residues of unaccelerated combustion (oxidation) of aluminum. SEM may assist identification in such cases.

8.4 Analysis of General Fire Evidence

Considerations related to laboratory analysis of fire evidence include the following:

- Identification of charred or burned materials
- Burned documents
- Failure analysis by forensic engineers
- Evaluation of appliances and wiring
- Miscellaneous laboratory tests
- Spoliation

8.4.1 IDENTIFICATION OF CHARRED OR BURNED MATERIALS

One of the most common questions a fire investigator asks is this: What is (or was) this stuff—and does it belong at the scene? In a fire, many items, both trivial and significant, can be sufficiently damaged that a casual examination will not result in their identification. Plastic, rubber, or metal objects having a relatively low melting point pose typical problems. The identification may be based on the shape of the remaining portion, X-rays, portions of labels or details cast into the object that survive, or a determination of the type of material present.

Even though the plastic or metal can be chemically identified, if only minute amounts remain unburned, this information may not be useful in identifying the material. Some materials, like polyethylene, polystyrene, or zinc diecast, seem to be universal in their applications. Some plastic bottles may be identified by their shape or casting marks, but the knowledge that a puddle of debris is melted polyethylene is of little use in figuring out which of thousands of polyethylene objects it might represent. Glass objects, whether broken by mechanical or thermal shock, can be pieced back together (as shown in Figure 8-8) if there has not been excessive melting of the pieces.

Laboratory identification may consist of visual examination, reassembly, cleaning, or microscopic, chemical, or instrumental tests of considerable complexity, depending on the nature of the material, the quantity recovered, and the extent of damage. By verifying the composition of even partial remains, these services may be crucial in detecting the substitution of less valuable items for heavily insured objects like jewelry, art, or clothes in cases of insurance fraud, or even in confirming their complete removal in cases of fraud or theft. If an ignition or time-delay device is suspected, the laboratory may be able to reconstruct the device. The nature or specific details of the device may then be of use in identifying the perpetrator, linking him or her with the scene, or in interrogating suspects. Figure 8-9 shows an example of a common household object that careful lab examination revealed to have been used as a time-delay device.

8.4.2 BURNED DOCUMENTS

Reconstruction and identification includes fire-damaged documents. Writing paper has an ignition temperature of approximately 250°C (480°F), and single sheets of paper

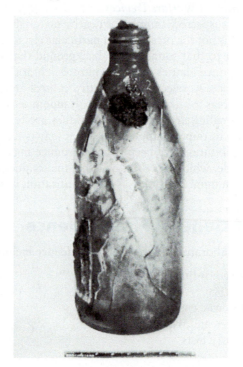

FIGURE 8-8 A suspected incendiary device can be reassembled to help establish the nature of the container and aid in search for fingerprint and trace evidence. *Courtesy of the State of California, Department of Justice, Bureau of Forensic Services.*

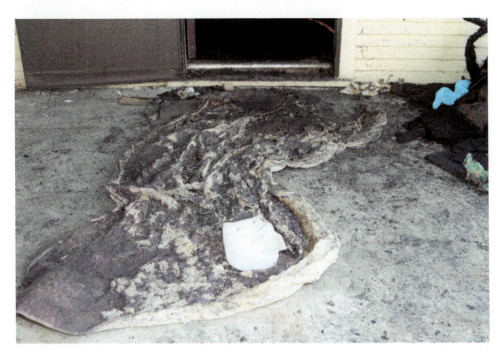

FIGURE 8-9 Plastic milk bottle: Was it a device or innocent "victim"? *Courtesy of Jamie Novak, Novak Investigations and St. Paul Fire Dept.*

exposed to fire in air will readily char and burn almost completely. However, most documents in files, stacks, or books will not burn completely but will char and, if intact, may be identified. Laboratories use UV or IR light, photographic techniques, or treatment with glycerin, mineral oil, or organic solvents to improve the contrast between the paper and the inks. Some clay-coated papers and writing papers with a high percentage of rag content are more resistant to fire and are more easily restored than cheaper wood-pulp papers like newsprint.

Charred papers are fragile. Even fragmentary remains can sometimes be identified, but the more intact the document, the better the chances of identification. Documents should be disturbed as little as possible and carefully eased, using a piece of stiff paper or thin cardboard, onto a cushion of loosely fluffed cotton wool. This cotton should be placed into a rigid box of suitable size and a layer of fluffed cotton wool placed over the documents to keep them in place.

The investigator should not attempt to perform *any* tests in the field. Virtually anything done to a document in the way of coating, spraying, or treating it with solvent will interfere with laboratory tests. Reconstruction of burned documents is best done under controlled laboratory conditions by experienced personnel with proper photographic support in case characters are visible only fleetingly.

8.4.3 FAILURE ANALYSIS BY FORENSIC ENGINEERS

If a mechanical system failed and caused a fire, it may be necessary to determine the causation of the original mechanical fault. A registered mechanical or materials engineer is often able to tell whether a driveshaft or bearing failed as a result of misuse, overloading, poor maintenance, or design error. The failure of hydraulic systems may produce leaks of combustible hydraulic fluid that can contribute to the initiation or spread of a fire, and the experience of a hydraulic engineer may be required.

Because the civil liability of the manufacturer or user of a mechanical system may be in the millions of dollars, it is very important to have an accurate estimation of the condition of that system. Such determinations are beyond the capabilities of most crime laboratory personnel, because they require specialized knowledge of the materials or processes involved in the product's manufacture. A registry of qualified professional engineers is offered in many states to assist investigators.

8.4.4 EVALUATION OF APPLIANCES AND WIRING

Appliance defects and faulty wiring can cause fires. Diagnostic signs require microscopic examinations, metallurgical tests, or continuity and conductance tests that require laboratory examination and interpretation by a specialist. For instance, determination of whether a switch was on or off at the time of the fire requires careful dismantling and examination of the contacts, housing, and switch mechanism.

Due to fire damage, such dissection may easily result in movement of the components and destruction of their precise relationships. X-ray analysis may be used if the contacts and housing are arranged to permit cross-sectional viewing. Twibell and Lomas described a novel resin-casting technique that allows cross-sectioning of the switch unit while ensuring that the components do not move (Twibell and Lomas 1995).

Soft X-rays (of the energies used for medical procedures, 75 to 85 kV) have also been demonstrated to be of value in examining thermal cutoffs (TCOs) used to protect coffeemakers and other similar appliances from overheating, and cartridge-type fuses. Such X-rays can be used to determine their continuity and often to establish the mechanism of their operation or cause of failure. The causes for electrical product failures are sometimes revealed by x-ray examination, as seen in Figure 8-10A–B. In the case of fuses, those that failed due to moderate overcurrents were often differentiable from those that failed in a short circuit (Twibell and Christie 1995). X-rays are also useful in establishing the operability of fire-damaged smoke detectors.

Whether a copper wire was melted by overheating due to excessive current or by the heat of the fire may be determined by the degree of crystallization within the conductor, because the entire cross section of a conductor will be heated by an overcurrent, while the surface of a conductor is likely to be affected to a greater degree than the core if the heat is applied from the exterior.

Some years ago, it was suggested that elemental analysis of the surface of some fire-damaged copper conductors could yield information to determine whether the melting was the cause or result of the fire. Other researchers, however, suggested that the absorption of gases from the ambient atmosphere while the metal was molten do not necessarily reflect the composition of fire gases in the vicinity (Howitt 1998). Others contended that the composition of fire gases, whether they are absorbed or not, do not discriminate between arcing that occurs to cause the fire and arcs that occur as a result of external

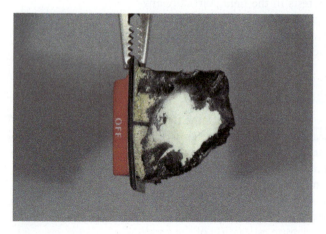

FIGURE 8-10A Fire-damaged switch: on/off or defective? *Courtesy of Helmut Brosz and Peter Brosz, Brosz and Associates.*

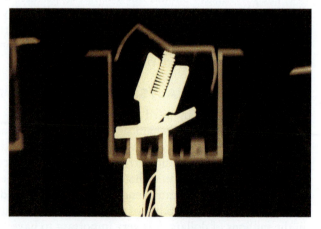

FIGURE 8-10B X-ray of switch reveals internal connections. *Courtesy of Helmut Brosz and Peter Brosz, Brosz and Associates.*

charring (Henderson, Manning, and Barnhill 1998). Because most post-fire indicators are the summation of the fire's effects, testing would have to examine a wide variety of fire exposures. Béland (2004) discussed double-blind tests revealing that diagnosis of fire cause versus fire effect using the Auger emission spectroscopy (AES) elemental profile method was no better than random chance.

There is not a 100 percent reliable means of establishing whether melting of copper conductors was the result of fire exposure or electric overcurrent unless there are very small globules created (Babrauskas 2003a). As a general rule, the finer the droplet size, the higher the energy (and temperature) of the molten copper. Unless there was electric arcing, the conditions needed to produce aerosol-type beads do not exist in normally fueled fires. Even then, proof of electrical activity does not prove the fire was started by an electrical fault, only that the conductor was energized.

Metallurgists can conduct crystallographic tests, but, unfortunately, elemental analysis requires expertise and equipment available only in fairly sophisticated materials- or surface-science laboratories. Elemental analysis by scanning electron microscopy/energy dispersive x-ray spectrometry (SEM/EDS) may be of value in establishing contact between conductors of different metals (e.g., copper wire against a zinc-plated steel receptacle box). This finding may help confirm a particular accidental ignition mechanism (McVicar 1991).

The presence of metallic contaminants on insulators in switches and relays has been linked to arc tracking and electrical equipment fires. SEM/EDS can help identify the nature and origin of such contamination. Recent work by Carey and Howitt on arc faults between copper conductors in fire environments has demonstrated the potential value of microscopic and elemental features (Carey 2009; Howitt and Pugh 2007). Failures such as stress cracking, contamination, microorganism-induced corrosion (MIC), or erosion require analysis by a combination of microscopic, metallurgical, and chemical techniques. These, too, require specialized resources and knowledge not found in public forensic labs.

Although the laboratory specialist can perform tests beyond the capability of the investigator, there are practical limits. It is possible for a fire to be sufficiently hot and prolonged to destroy enough of the diagnostic signs that may have once been present that the required determination cannot be made with any degree of certainty.

Usually, very high localized temperatures produced during the fire may give an indication of the use of an incendiary ignition device or an unusually high fuel load (if post-flashover conditions are considered). These temperatures may be indicated by the melting (or melted state) of various materials in the vicinity. Because small variations in composition may result in considerable differences in melting points, the objects of interest should be identified in the laboratory and their melting points measured directly if at all possible. SEM/EDS has been shown to be of value in establishing the nature of interactions between aluminum and copper in forming eutectic alloys during a fire (Buc, Hoffman, and Finch 2004). SEM can show differences in crystal structure, and when teamed with elemental analysis (SEM/EDS), it can demonstrate mixing of various elements. This finding may be important when melting (of switch or thermostat contacts) or alloying is found. Such melting or alloying may be the result of normal fire exposure or the failure mechanism that caused the fire.

Flash Point

The first ASTM standard for flash point was published in 1918 (Wray 1992) as *ASTM D56-05 (2010): Test Method for Flash Point by Tag Closed Cup Tester* (ASTM 2010). Several years later, two additional test methods were published: *ASTM D92-12b (2012): Test Method for Flash Point by Cleveland Open Cup Tester* (ASTM 2012a), and *ASTM D93-15a (2015): Test Method for Flash Point by Pensky-Martens Closed Cup Tester* (ASTM 2015a). ASTM D93 is one of the most frequently cited in regulations and specifications.

The flash points of materials found at the fire scene, either as part of the scene itself or as part of an incendiary device, should also be determined in a laboratory.

Laboratory-based flash point (FP) determinations are made using one of several types of apparatus:

- Tagliabue (Tag) Closed Cup (FP below 175°F) (80°C)
- Pensky-Martens Closed Cup (FP above 175°F) (80°C)
- Tag Open Cup
- Cleveland Open Cup

The ASTM has established standard methods for the use of these devices (Slye 2008). Many laboratories cannot measure the flash point of a flammable liquid if below ambient (room) temperature. Flash point apparatus most commonly found in analytical labs requires at least 50 mL (2 fl oz), far more than normally recovered as residue from an incendiary device and precludes such analysis. Setaflash Tester, a flash point apparatus approved by ASTM, will accept samples as small as 2 mL (0.08 fl oz) as well as permit subambient measurements.

Melting or Softening Points

Lab methods including thermogravimetric analysis (TGA) or differential scanning calorimetry (DSC) are used to determine the temperatures at which plastics melt or char (see Figure 8-11). For a discussion on DSC see *ASTM D3418-15* (ASTM 2015b). The melting points of even very small samples can be tested using a Mettler Thermometric Hot Stage Microscope.

Mechanical Condition

In reconstructing the scene, visual examination can ascertain whether a door lock mechanism was locked or unlocked at the time of the fire (see Figure 8-12). Lock mechanisms are usually of brass or zinc die cast, both of which have relatively low melting points. As a result, they will often seize at temperatures produced in normal structure fires. When recovered at a scene, they should be photographed in place and then worked to clearly indicate their orientation and photographed in the second position. LP-fueled microtorches

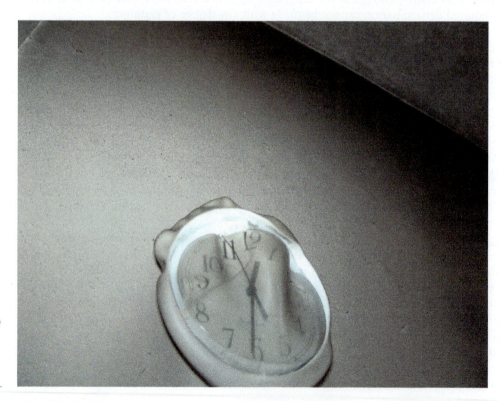

FIGURE 8-11 The softening temperature of the plastic face of this wall clock, if determined by lab analysis, could reveal the temperature of the smoke layer or amount of radiant heat to which it was exposed. *Courtesy of Jamie Novak, Novak Investigations and St. Paul Fire Dept.*

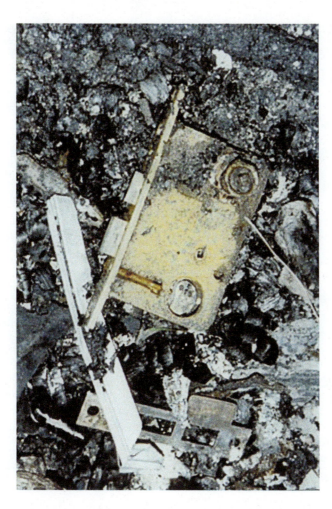

FIGURE 8-12 Door lock assembly. *Courtesy of Det. Michael Dalton (ret.), Knox County Sheriff's Office.*

have been used to melt the internal components of door locks to permit forcible entry while leaving the external housing intact. Internal forensic laboratory examinations of critical door locks should be considered before assuming that the lock was normally inoperative.

If a door was not exposed to too much direct fire, it is possible to figure out if it was open or closed at the time of the fire by examining its hinges. In a closed door, the plates of a typical butt hinge are protected from fire by the door jamb and the edge of the door. The spine of the hinge will be exposed to the fire and will therefore be more heavily damaged than the more protected plates, as shown in Figures 8-13A and B. In contrast, the spine and plates of the hinges of an open door will be exposed to roughly the same amount of heat, and damage will be uniform on both. If the fire was not too extreme, discoloration of the metal and remnants of paint on the hinge may indicate the relative positions of the two plates.

It is possible for the fire damage to be severe enough to erase the diagnostic signs for this determination. Because such fire damage is more likely near the ceiling of a structure, if it is important to know the position of a door, all (usually three) hinges from a door should be recovered and labeled as top, bottom, and middle. Photos of the hinges in place and any protected area on the floor or carpet may also be helpful.

Fire and Smoke Hazards

In accidental fires, the fire test laboratory can assess the contribution of various materials to the fuel load. Carpets, particularly modern ones with polypropylene-blend face yarns, represent a hazard because of their flammability. They have been shown to be ignitable by

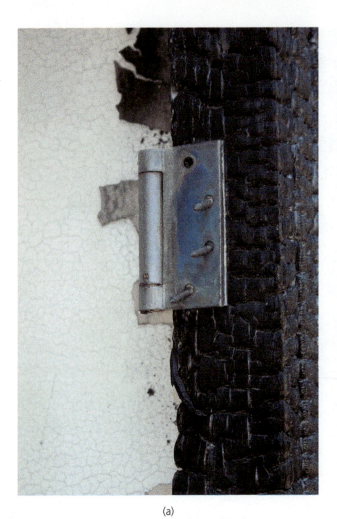 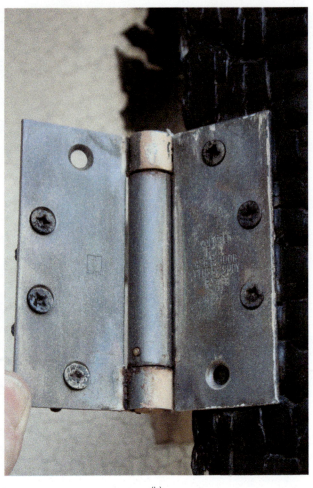

(a)   (b)

FIGURES 8-13A–B As this door hinge is moved, the differential in damage proves it was in the closed position when exposed to the fire. *Courtesy of Greg Lampkin, Knox County Sheriff's Office, Tennessee, Fire Investigation Unit.*

small localized fires and then to spread fire across an entire room over a period of hours. In some states but not all, furnishings must pass flammability tests. Furnishings with either synthetic or cotton coverings and cellulosic, latex, or polyurethane fillings can be a starting point for an accidental fire, depending on the nature of the ignition source. Furniture with synthetic fabrics and padding can spread fire very quickly (i.e., their identification may explain why a fire grew so fast that escape was difficult). If any coverings or fillings remain unburned, it may be possible to identify them, duplicate them, and test the combination for susceptibility to accidental ignition. Such testing, although it can be done informally by most laboratories, requires considerable experience if the results are to be used in civil litigation. Some states have agencies, like California's Department of Consumer Affairs, Bureau of Home Furnishings and Thermal Insulation, that will test such hazards on a contract basis; otherwise, a private consumer or materials laboratory will have to be contacted. By using pyrolysis gas chromatography (pyro GC) or Fourier transform infrared spectrometry (FTIR), forensic labs can identify the fiber constituents of carpets, upholstery, or the rubber (elastomer) in padding. These may be useful in assessing their contributions to ignition or flame spread.

As part of a reconstruction of the cause and manner of death in fatal fires, it may be necessary to determine the origin of toxic gases that caused death, or of heavy smoke that prevented the escape of still-conscious victims from a small fire. Although the production of toxic gases and dense smoke is largely a variable of the temperatures and ventilation during the actual fire, some laboratory tests can evaluate potential hazards. Work of this type has been done to test upholstery materials for closed environments such as airplane interiors, but it is costly and time consuming and may not be available to most fire investigators. The NFPA has developed standard tests for evaluating the fire hazards of interior finishes, and the reader is referred to its publications for specific guidance (DeHaan 1991; Gann and Bryner 2008).

Self-Heating Mechanisms

Self-heating of vegetable oils, fish oils, and many polymers as they dry can lead to ignition. The identification of vegetable oils from fire debris was a major challenge for laboratory analysts due to the thermal destruction that often occurs in the vicinity of the ignition source. In addition, the vegetable oils involved do not have sufficient vapor pressure to be recovered by heating isolation methods.

Stauffer (2005) described sensitive new debris analysis techniques in which the suspected self-heating oils are extracted with a solvent, concentrated, and chemically derivatized. This process causes their fatty acid components to be rendered susceptible to GC/MS characterization by the same methods used for ignitable liquid residues described previously. These techniques are used in many forensic labs (Stauffer 2006; Coulombe 2002; Gambrel and Reardon 2008; Schewenk and Reardon 2009).

In clothes dryer fires, the self-heating of kitchen oils in poorly laundered towels may cause a spontaneous fire. Corn, safflower, and soy oils can self-heat to the point of open flame when the process is initiated by the temperatures of a dry cycle. Analysis of the rinse water of the washing machine that is paired with the dryer is recommended when the dryer contents are suspected of self-heating. While the dryer drum contents may be nothing more than a charred mass, the washing machine rinse water most likely survived the fire intact, preserving traces of the vegetable oil from the original laundered load. Residues in clothes washer pumps and drains reportedly have also been identified (Mann 1999).

Differential scanning **calorimetry**, or critical temperature testing, may reveal self-heating propensities of particular combinations of materials. These tests, however, will require bulk quantities for testing rather than residual amounts.

calorimetry ■ An analytical method used to measure the total heat of combustion of fuels.

8.4.5 FORENSIC EVALUATION OF SMOKE ALARMS

Occupants of a building escaping a fire rely on (1) becoming aware of the fire before it produces untenable conditions, and (2) safely responding to escape. Smoke alarms, when correctly installed and maintained, can provide early notification of the occupants (Kennedy et al. 2004).

Many forensic fire investigations involve determining the role that smoke alarms (ionization, photoelectric, combination, and multi-sensor/multi-criteria) may or may not have played in preventing occupant injuries and casualties. A comprehensive investigation must assess the alarm's history, location in a structure, and a forensic examination of the device after the fire. This examination can assess whether a smoke alarm sounded during a fire, along with its impact on occupant notification and escape.

Worrell discussed techniques for evaluating soot deposits on the components of smoke alarms (Worrell et al. 2001). The mechanical vibration of an operating detector horn causes characteristic patterns of soot deposits called Chladni Figures through a process known as acoustic agglomeration. These patterns can be used in some cases to establish whether the alarm was sounding during the fire. Soot patterns may also reveal if the battery inside was connected or missing (Colwell and Reza 2003).

A competent forensic engineering laboratory may have the proper equipment to determine if the smoke alarm had activated. Other forensic examination criteria may include smoke box sensitivity tests and fire room tests in general accordance with *UL 217 (2015): Single and Multiple Station Smoke Alarms* (Underwriters Laboratories 2015). These UL requirements cover electrically operated single and multiple station smoke alarms intended for open area protection in indoor locations and portable smoke alarms in accordance with *NFPA 72 (2016): National Fire Alarm and Signaling Code* (NFPA 2016); *NFPA 1119 (2015): Standard for Recreational Vehicles* (NFPA 2015b); and *NFPA 302 (2015): Fire Protection Standard for Pleasure and Commercial Motor Craft* (NFPA 2015a).

8.4.6 SPOLIATION

Before any testing is conducted, the investigator needs to consider what effect a test will have on the condition of the evidence. The term **spoliation** refers to any test or examination that will change the condition of the evidence such that other tests cannot be performed. In criminal cases, the concept of nondestructive testing has been well established. See *ASTM E860-07e1 (2013): Standard Practice for Examining and Preparing Items That Are or May Become Involved in Criminal or Civil Litigation* (ASTM 2013a).

An examiner is obligated to retain a sample of evidence if testing is going to be destructive, document the condition of the evidence completely beforehand, or ask that a representative of the opposition be present to observe the test. This principle extends to testing of evidence in civil cases. When testing of evidence is likely to change that evidence such that the opposing party or other interested party cannot test it properly, testing should be delayed until all parties are notified and have an opportunity to nominate a representative to take part in the testing. Failure to notify interested parties may expose the investigator and the examiner to civil penalties, including denial of admissibility of the results of the testing.

8.5 Non–Fire-Related Physical Evidence

The most frequent mistake made by fire investigators is having a single-minded focus on the fire itself and its origin and ignoring other types of physical evidence. It is up to the fire investigator to construct a complete scenario of a fire setter's activities at the scene. These activities are not limited to the setting of the fire itself. Because arson may be used to destroy evidence of other criminal acts, the careful investigator must always be alert to the existence of evidence of normal criminal activity.

Specifically, the fire investigator needs a basic understanding of fingerprints, blood evidence, impression evidence, physical matches, and trace evidence. Note that some of these types of evidence—particularly impression evidence and physical matches—can play a role in reconstructing the fire scene and determining origin and cause for accidental as well as incendiary fires.

8.5.1 FINGERPRINTS

There is no more conclusive proof of identity than a fingerprint, the unique friction ridge patterns on the palmar surfaces of the hands and fingers (or their impressions). Many investigators assume, as do arsonists, that a fire destroys all fingerprints. While it is true that many fingerprints will be lost during a fire, many will survive, even on ignition sources.

Plastic three-dimensional impressions in window putty or *patent* (visible) impressions in paint or blood may remain even after direct exposure to fire. In fact, they may be permanently fixed in place by the heat. Plastic containers used to carry or hold gasoline in an arson fire may be softened sufficiently by the gasoline to allow the plastic to take on the fingerprint impressions of the person holding the container. If a container is not exposed directly to the flames, these plastic impressions may survive. The plastic window attacked with a butane mini-torch shown in Figure 8-14 bore both plastic impressions in the softened plastic and patent impressions in the soot.

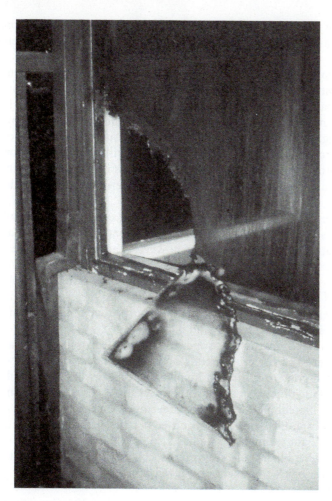

FIGURE 8-14 A plastic window in a school was attacked with a butane mini-torch to permit access. Plastic fingerprint impressions in the softened plastic and patent prints (in soot) were discovered. *Courtesy of Joe Konefal, Shingle Springs, California.*

Latent fingerprints, those requiring some sort of physical or chemical treatment to make them visible, consist basically of five components: water, skin oils, proteins, salts, and contaminants. The water evaporates rapidly or soaks into absorbent surfaces and is usually of little value. Skin oils are the residues normally detected by dusting with a soft brush and fingerprint powder. These oils will remain on hard surfaces for some time or will soak into absorbent materials like paper. They can be evaporated by elevated temperatures, and such dried-out prints may not respond to dusting. The soot produced by a smoky fire such as a gasoline pool may condense on a glass or metal surface to protect the latent prints; however, it may need to be gently brushed or washed in a stream of tap water to reveal the impressions. Exposure to heat may fuse the soot to the ridge details of the print so that the print becomes visible when the excess soot is washed away.

Techniques have been developed for the detection of latent prints that may aid the inspection of fire-related exhibits. Examination using lasers and high-intensity tunable light sources, including UV and IR wavelengths, makes it possible to penetrate contaminants and make prints visible against a variety of backgrounds (Margot and Lennard 1991). Cyanoacrylate ester fuming and a variety of fluorescent dye stains and powders further expand the possibilities of recovery of latent prints (Lee and Gaensslen 1985; Menzel and Duff 1979). These methods permit the development of latent fingerprints on many surfaces thought previously to be incapable of retaining such impressions. These include surfaces such as leather, wood, vinyl plastics, smooth fabrics, and even charred paper and metal.

Proteins degrade to amino acids that are detected by reaction with the chemical ninhydrin. They are easiest to detect when the latent impressions are on clean, light-colored, porous surfaces like paper or cardboard. The proteins can be denatured by high temperatures so that they no longer react, but if the paper has not been charred by the fire, it may be worth testing. However, exposure to water from suppression, from condensation of water vapor from the fire, or from wet weather will dissolve the proteins and amino acids and blur the fingerprints, but the fatty deposits in the latents (skin oils and cosmetics) will not be affected by the water. They can be detected by the physical developer method.

Nonporous surfaces that are or have been wet can be examined using small particle reagent (SPR). The salts are the most fire resistant of all latent fingerprint residues, resisting very high temperatures. Like amino acids, however, they are susceptible to water damage. Salts may react with the inks or coatings on paper or with the metal surfaces of cans. In doing so, they may leave an identifiable patent (visible) print in corrosion. This effect may be enhanced by the heat and moisture of the fire, leaving a visible print requiring no further treatment. Other contaminants that can produce patent prints include cosmetics, food residues, grease, motor oil, and blood.

Fingerprint expert Jack Deans in cooperation with Gardiner Associates (UK) recently conducted a series of fingerprint tests on objects subjected to observed room fires, most of which had gone to full room involvement. Deans has successfully recovered latent prints on plastic bottles by dusting and by cyanoacrylate fuming, on newspaper used as a torch and matchboxes by physical developer, on the paper used as a wick in a Molotov cocktail by ninhydrin, and on other plastic surfaces by vacuum metal deposition and forensic light techniques. He has also developed latent prints on plastic and glass bottles with SPR. He has also reported success in enhancing patent prints in blood and dirt by amido black treatment and forensic light techniques on a variety of surfaces (Deans 2006).

Air temperatures in each of these fire tests were measured at 200°C to 500°C (400°F to 1000°F) at floor level. Suppression of each fire was by normal water hose stream. Any surface that has been protected from direct, prolonged flame contact should be considered as a possible bearer of identifiable prints (Bleay, Bradshaw, and Moore 2006). See Figures 8-15 and 8-16A and B for examples. In addition, Deans reported that the powder from dry chemical fire extinguishers will develop latents on smooth surfaces.

Latent prints have even been recovered from human skin. Recovering such prints requires appropriate skin conditions (smooth, dry, free of hair), and the contact has to have been of adequate duration. Such prints lose detail after a few hours even if the victim is deceased. If a fire victim has not been dead more than a few hours and the skin was not damaged by the fire, a search for such latents should be considered (Graham 1969; Trapecar 2009).

8.5.2 BLOOD

Bloodstains left at a crime scene have much greater evidentiary value now than ever before because of great strides made in analysis of DNA in body fluids, hairs, and tissue. Above 200°C (392°F), the stain degrades and probably cannot be identified even as blood. If the proteins in a blood or semen stain or tissue fragment have not degraded, the evidence can be subjected to DNA typing. DNA analysis has become the primary standard for analysis of blood, saliva, and other body fluids; tissue; and hair. Techniques have been developed for the analysis of increasingly smaller quantities, and databases have been assembled for convicted felons, arrested suspects, and cold cases.

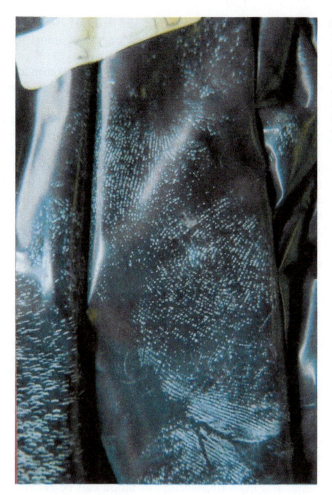

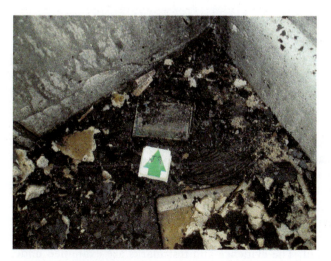

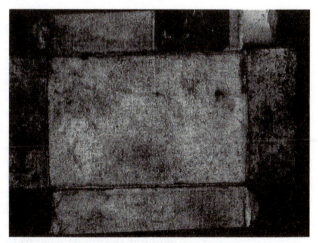

FIGURE 8-15 Enlargement of palm print detail developed on plastic trash bag (post-fire) using cyanoacrylate. *Courtesy of Jack Deans, FFS, MFSSoc, New Scotland Yard (Ret.), Fingerprint Consultant, Gardiner Associates, Ltd.*

FIGURE 8-16A Cardboard matchbox amid burned debris on floor. *Courtesy of Jack Deans, FFS, MFSSoc, New Scotland Yard (Ret.), Fingerprint Consultant, Gardiner Associates, Ltd.*

FIGURE 8-16B Fingerprints developed by physical developer on inner tray of the same box. *Courtesy of Jack Deans, FFS, MFSSoc, New Scotland Yard (Ret.), Fingerprint Consultant, Gardiner Associates, Ltd.*

Mitochondrial DNA allows testing of hairs, bone, and tissue of great antiquity. DNA testing has become a major factor in the solution of crimes, as it can dramatically increase the identifiability of fire victims and fragmentary remains (proven at the Waco and World Trade Center scenes), as well as the link between evidence at a scene or on a victim and a suspect, even when no blood is shed (Di Zinno et al. 1995; Mundorff, Bartelink, and Mar-Casslh 2009).

Advances in extraction and polymerase chain reaction (PCR) and short tandem repeat (STR) DNA analysis methods have led to significant improvement in the DNA analysis of even burned bone (Ye et al. 2004). DNA-typable material is much more resistant to thermal and biological degradation than are the enzymes and protein factors once used. DNA-typable material from saliva was reportedly recovered from the cloth wick from a glass soft-drink bottle subsequently used for a Molotov cocktail (Mann, Nic Daéid, and Linacre 2003).

DNA does not always result in a unique identification, but it does offer a means of associating a stain or tissue fragment with an individual with considerable certainty. If there is any doubt about a suspected stain, it should be collected, kept dry and as cool as possible, and submitted to the laboratory as quickly as possible.

Even in the absence of analysis, bloodstains can be of importance in the reconstruction of murder and assault cases and fire-related activity such as escape attempts. When dried bloodstains are coated with soot and smoke in an ensuing fire, they are easy to overlook and can be very difficult to interpret if detected. A number of chemicals have been used to enhance the visibility of faint or tiny bloodstains at crime scenes. Luminol, for instance, requires complete darkness and continual respraying to make bloodstains visible as glowing images (which are very difficult to photograph).

One chemical more recently introduced, called leuco crystal violet (LCV), reacts with dried blood to form a deep blue-purple stain that is permanent and easily photographed in ordinary room light. The colorless reagent is applied as a wash or a spray (using appropriate safety equipment). The reaction is nearly instantaneous, and the solvent action washes much of the adhering soot away, enhancing the visibility of the stain pattern. Blood spatters, shoeprints, and even fingerprints in blood can be recovered by such enhancement methods. In one case, LCV was used and revealed blood spatters on the walls of a building more than a year after a murder had taken place and after two subsequent fires in the structure.

8.5.3 IMPRESSION EVIDENCE

Often overlooked, impressions made by tools on windows or doors can confirm forced entry (see Figure 8-17), identify points of entry (or attempted entry), and, if tools are recovered, permit identification of the tools responsible. Such tool marks may also be found on desk drawers, filing cabinets, locks, or chains at a scene, confirming that a burglary took place before the fire.

The best kind of tool-mark evidence is the impression itself. After it has been sketched and photographed, the object or suitable portion bearing the impression should be collected. If its size makes recovery impractical, a replica may be cast in silicone rubber (Mikrosil) or dental impression material. Photos of a striated impression are of no use in a laboratory comparison other than to establish the location and orientation of the mark. The submitted tools are tested on a variety of surfaces to duplicate the manner of use and the qualities of the mark-bearing material as closely as possible without risking damage to the tool. The evidence and test marks are examined under 40× to 400× magnification to try to match the striations or contours present. See Figure 8-18 for a typical comparison. Tool impressions can reveal the nature of the tool used to create or modify incendiary devices, and the manner of their use, which can be used to prove intent.

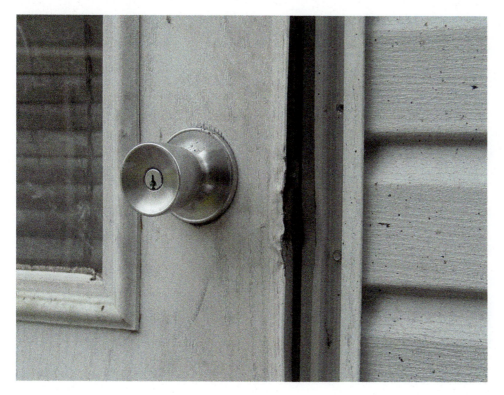

FIGURE 8-17 Doors should also be carefully examined for signs of forcible entry not consistent with the means of entry used by firefighters on the scene, such as this pried and shattered door frame. *Courtesy of Greg Lampkin, Knox County Sheriff's Office, Tennessee, Fire Investigation Unit.*

Impressions of footwear and vehicle tires may be found on the periphery of the fire scene. Shoe prints have also been linked to forcible entry, as shown in Figure 8-19. The visibility of shoe prints left as a transfer of dust or light-colored soil may be enhanced by the scorching or charring of walls or doors. Although prints impressed in soil cannot generally be collected, they are worth photographing in place and possibly casting with

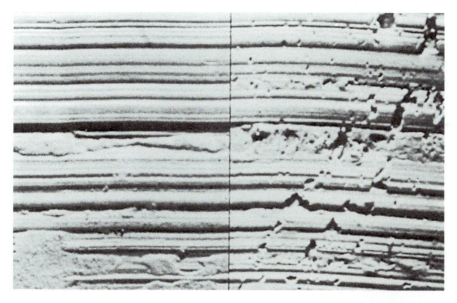

FIGURE 8-18 Tool-mark comparisons provide the potential of linking a suspect and the tools directly with a crime scene. *Courtesy of the State of California, Department of Justice, Bureau of Forensic Services.*

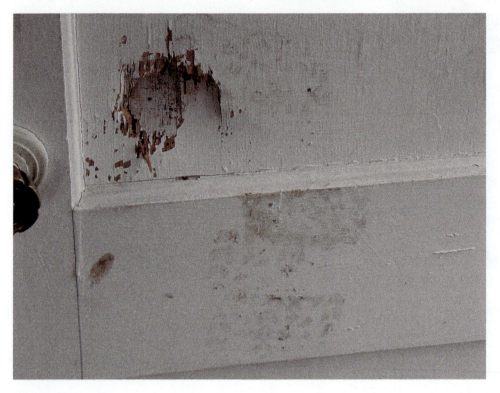

FIGURE 8-19 A shoe print on the door reveals forced entry despite the modest scorching of wood. *Courtesy of Greg Lampkin, Knox County Sheriff's Office, Tennessee, Fire Investigation Unit.*

plaster of Paris. Photographs must be taken using low-angle (oblique) lighting to highlight the three-dimensional details; a scale or ruler must be included in the photo, near and preferably parallel to the impression; and the film plane of the camera must be parallel to the ground to prevent distortion. See Figure 8-20 for a good example. Although particular tires can sometimes be matched to their impressions, it is more common to establish only a correspondence of size and tread pattern. Footwear, due to its characteristic details and slower rate of change, is more amenable to identification and offers a means of placing the subject at the fire scene.

8.5.4 PHYSICAL MATCHES

One of the few conclusive identifications possible with typical evidence is the physical comparison of torn, cut, or broken edges or surfaces with each other to establish a "jigsaw" fit between them. Pieces of glass from shoes or garments have been matched to windows, vehicle lamps, or bottles to connect a victim or suspect with a scene. Wrappings from incendiary or explosive devices have been matched to source materials in the possession of the suspect, as have pieces of tape, wire, wood, and rope. The evidentiary value of such positive identifications is very high, and the investigator must be aware of the possibilities when searching a scene for anything that looks out of place or when searching a suspect's property or vehicle. Close cooperation and communication between the lab and the investigator has produced some excellent evidence.

8.5.5 TRACE EVIDENCE

Trace, or transfer, evidence such as paint, fibers, soil, or glass can be used to link a suspect with a crime scene even in arson cases. Paint can be transferred to clothing or tools when a

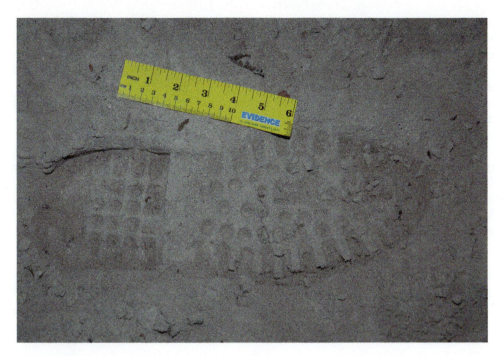

FIGURE 8-20 Good-quality photograph of a shoe impression at a crime scene includes a scale; low-angle, oblique illumination; and carefully focused close-up photography. *Courtesy of Greg Lampkin, Knox County Sheriff's Office, Tennessee, Fire Investigation Unit.*

forcible entry is attempted. Flakes as small as 1 mm (0.04 in.) square are adequate for color or layer sequence comparisons or complete analysis by IR spectroscopy, spectrography, or x-ray analysis. Such properties are generally class characteristics; that is, even a complete correspondence between the chemical properties of known and questioned paints does not imply that the two paints must have come from the same object. Instead, it confirms that they came from the same class of objects painted with the same paint. Multilayered paint chips, however, may be linked to a particular source if they have enough layers to demonstrate a unique origin.

Glass is found in nearly all structures and can reveal a good deal about the events of the crime. It can be broken by either mechanical force or thermally induced stress. Curved fracture ridges on the edges of glass fragments reveal that the breaking force was mechanical. The shape of these conchoidal fracture lines can help establish from which side of the window the force came. The absence of these lines usually means the fracture was caused by thermal stress.

The presence or absence of soot, char, or fire debris on the broken edges can establish whether breakage occurred before or after the fire. When a glass window is broken, minute chips of glass are scattered as much as 3 m (10 ft) away, especially back in the direction of the breaking force. If a subject is standing nearby, minute glass chips may be found in his or her hair, clothes, hat, pockets, or cuffs. Even very small [less than 1 mm (0.04 in.)] fragments can be compared with a suspected origin, such as a bottle or window. This usually results in a class characteristics comparison. Glass is made in large batches that vary little in their physical or chemical properties. But such transfer evidence does not require direct or prolonged contact with the source to make it valuable to the investigator.

Fibers can be transferred from the furnishings of the fire scene to the subject or from the subject's clothes to the scene, particularly at the point of entry. Such two-way transfers can be very useful in linking suspect and scene, even though fibers are usually another type of class characteristic evidence. Fibers are compared by microscopic, chemical, elemental, or spectrophotometric tests. Even the most sophisticated analyses must deal with the fact that synthetic fibers are produced in such large quantities that they are used mainly as corroborative or circumstantial evidence.

In a similar way, soils from shoes or clothing can be compared with soil from a fire scene. This may be especially helpful in a wildland fire where a distinctive or unusual type of natural soil is found in the vicinity of the fire's origin or along an access road. In urban environments, artificial contaminants such as slag, cinders, metal filings, or paint chips may contribute to the uniqueness of a soil. Contact with the soil near a workshop or industrial site may result in the transfer of soils that are unique and very much different from the natural soils nearby. Normally, soil comparisons are of marginal evidential value, but in instances such as those presented here—individual soils, especially artificial ones—do occur and should not be overlooked.

Summary

The forensic scientists or criminalists who examine evidence from fire scenes perform scientific tests, interpret the results, and reconstruct a sequence of events that led to the production of that evidence. The forensic scientist provides an independent evaluation of the evidence that should challenge the interpretation of the evidence as presented by the fire investigator. The role of the laboratory staff is to suggest alternative hypotheses and provide data to support or refute their hypotheses. Forensic scientists must interact with the fire investigators, exchanging information and testing ideas and hypotheses.

The criteria for using fire test information in forensic fire scene reconstructions are whether the test was correctly performed, whether the data were accurately collected and reported, and whether the test was appropriate and applicable to the situation under consideration. Fire tests are designed to collect certain data in a reproducible and valid manner.

The investigator must ask whether the fuels, conditions, and ignition mechanism reproduced the fire in question. Was the test designed to follow a published test protocol such as one from ASTM or NFPA? If so, did it actually follow that protocol? If not, what factors were considered in its design? What variables were considered and how were they controlled? Fuel moisture, fuel mass and quantity, physical state, ambient temperature and humidity, heat flux, and oxygen content all play important roles in ignition, flame spread, and heat release. If it was a custom-designed test, what data could be fairly and accurately collected and analyzed? Was there a planned series of tests to examine the sensitivity and reproducibility of the data? Because of the importance of fire test data in both criminal and civil fire investigations, it is imperative that tests be conducted and data be interpreted without misrepresentation in a balanced, impartial, and reproducible manner.

Review Questions

1. Name four sources of forensic laboratory assistance available to fire investigators.
2. What can elemental analysis offer to a fire investigator?
3. What does the gas chromatograph do?
4. What is the difference between GC/FID and GC/mass spectrometry?
5. Which isolation technique is the most widely used for preparing extracts of fire debris for volatile analysis in forensic labs?
6. Name three of the complications that can arise when a lab attempts an identification of a volatile product in fire debris.
7. Name three different kinds of chemical incendiaries.
8. Under what conditions can latent prints be developed on objects that have been in a fire?
9. What are three ways DNA analysis can assist in an arson investigation?
10. Name three kinds of impression evidence and describe how each can assist in an arson investigation.
11. If the test was intended to replicate an actual event, how closely did the materials, the dimensions, and the ventilation match the original conditions?
12. Find an example of a commercial, academic, or governmental fire testing facility in your state. Visit or call this organization and determine what type of testing it performs.
13. Obtain a collection of at least 10 tests involving the use of a calorimeter from published research.

References

Alexander, J., G. Mashak, N. Kapitan, and J. A. Siegel. 1987. "Fluorescence of Petroleum Products II: Three-Dimensional Fluorescence Plots of Gasolines." *Journal of Forensic Sciences* 32: 72–86.

Almirall, J. R., J. Bruna, and K. G. Furton. 1996. "The Recovery of Accelerants in Aqueous Samples from Fire Debris Using Solid-Phase Microextraction (SPME)." *Science and Justice* 36, no. 4: 283–87.

Almirall, J. R., J. Wang, K. Lothridge, and K. G. Furton. 2000. "The Detection and Analysis of Ignitable Liquid Residues Extracted from Human Skin Using SPME/GC." *Journal of Forensic Sciences* 45, no. 2: 453–61.

Andrasko, J. 1978. "Identification of Burnt Matches by Scanning Electron Microscopy," *Journal of Forensic Sciences* 23, no. 4 (October): 637–42.

———. 1979. "Analysis of Polycyclic Aromatic Hydrocarbons in Soils and Its Application to Forensic Science." Linkoping University, NCJRS: Microfiche Program, Report No. 4, 1979.

Andrasko, J., S. Bendtz, A. C. Maehly, and Linkoping University. 1979. "Practical Experiences with Scanning Electron Microscopy in a Forensic Science Laboratory." Linkoping University, NCJRS—Microfiche Program, Report No. 2.

Armstrong, A., V. Babrauskas, D. L. Holmes, C. Martin, R. Powell, S. Riggs, and L. D. Young. 2004. "The Evaluation of the Extent of Transporting or 'Tracking' an Identifiable Ignitable Liquid (Gasoline) throughout Fire Scenes during the Investigative Process." *Journal of Forensic Sciences* 49, no. 4: 741–46.

Armstrong, A. T., and R. S. Wittkower. 1978. "Identification of Accelerants in Fire Residues by Capillary Column Gas Chromatography." *Journal of Forensic Sciences* 23.

ASTM. 2001. *E1387-01: Standard Test Method for Ignitable Liquid Residues in Extracts of Samples of Fire Debris by Gas Chromatography.* West Conshohocken, PA.

———. 2009. *E1385-00: Standard Practice for Separation and Concentration of Ignitable Liquid Residues from Fire Debris Samples by Steam Distillation.* West Conshohocken, PA: ASTM.

———. 2010. *D56-05: Test Method for Flash Point by Tag Closed Cup Tester.* West Conshohocken, PA: ASTM.

———. 2011a. *D3278-96: Standard Test Methods for Flash Point of Liquids by Small Scale Closed-Cup Apparatus.* West Conshohocken, PA: ASTM.

———. 2011b. *E620-11: Standard Practice for Reporting Opinions of Scientific or Technical Experts.* West Conshohocken, PA: ASTM.

———. 2011c. *E1492-11: Practice for Receiving, Documenting, Storing, and Retrieving Evidence in a Forensic Science Laboratory.* Conshohocken, PA: ASTM.

———. 2012a. *D92-12b: Test Method for Flash Point by Cleveland Open Cup Tester.* West Conshohocken, PA: ASTM.

———. 2012b. *E1388-12: Standard Practice for Sampling of Headspace Vapors from Fire Debris Samples.* West Conshohocken, PA: ASTM.

———. 2012c. *E1412-12: Standard Practice for Separation and Concentration of Ignitable Liquid Residues from Fire Debris Samples by Passive Headspace Concentration with Activated Charcoal.* West Conshohocken, PA: ASTM.

———. 2013a. *E860-07e1: Standard Practice for Examining And Preparing Items That Are Or May Become Involved In Criminal or Civil Litigation.* West Conshohocken, PA: ASTM.

———. 2013b. *E1413-13: Standard Practice for Separation and Concentration of Ignitable Liquid Residues from Fire Debris Samples by Dynamic Headspace Concentration.* West Conshohocken, PA: ASTM.

———. 2014. *E1618-14: Standard Test Method for Ignitable Liquid Residues in Extracts from Samples of Fire Debris by Gas Chromatography–Mass Spectrometry.* West Conshohocken, PA: ASTM.

———. 2015a. *D93-15a: Test Method for Flash Point by Pensky-Martens Closed Cup Tester.* West Conshohocken, PA: ASTM.

———. 2015b. *D3418-15: Standard Test Method for Transition Temperatures and Enthalpies of Fusion and Crystallization of Polymers by Differential Scanning Calorimetry.* West Conshohocken, PA: ASTM.

———. 2015c. *E1386-15: Standard Practice for Separation and Concentration of Ignitable Liquid Residues from Fire Debris Samples by Solvent Extraction.* West Conshohocken, PA: ASTM.

Babrauskas, V. 2003a. "Fires Due to Electric Arcing: Can 'Cause' Beads Be Distinguished from 'Victim' Beads by Physical or Chemical Testing?" In *Proceedings Fire and Materials 2003.* London: Interscience Communications, 2003.

———. 2003b. *Ignition Handbook.* Issaquah, WA: Fire Science Publishers.

Barnes, A. T., J. A. Dolan, R. J. Kuk, and J. A. Siegel. 2004. "Comparison of Gasolines Using Gas Chromatography/Mass Spectrometry on Target Ion Response." *Journal of Forensic Sciences* 49, no. 5: 1018–27.

Béland, B. 2004. "Examination of Arc Beads by Auger Spectroscopy." *Fire and Arson Investigator* 44, no. 4: 20–22.

Bleay, S. M., G. Bradshaw, and J. E. Moore. 2006. "Fingerprinting Development and Imaging Newsletter; Special Edition: Fire Scenes." Publ. 26/06, Home Office Scientific Development Branch, UK, April 2006.

Brackett, J. W. 1955. "Separation of Flammable Material of Petroleum Origin from Evidence Submitted in Cases Involving Fires and Suspected Arson." *Journal of Criminal Law, Criminology and Police Science* 46: 554–58.

Buc, E. C., D. J. Hoffman, and J. Finch. 2004. "Failure Analysis of Brass Connectors Exposed to Fire." Pp. 731–39 in *Proceedings Interflam 2004.* London: Interscience Communications.

Byron, D. E. 2004. "An Introduction to the New Ignitable Liquid Absorbent (ILA)." *Fire and Arson Investigator* January: 31–32

California State Fire Marshal. 1995. *CFIRS Report.* Sacramento, CA, March 1995.

Carey, N. 2009. PhD dissertation, Strathclyde University, Glasgow, November 2009.

Chrostowski, J. E., and R. N. Holmes. 1979. "Collection and Determination of Accelerant Vapors from Arson Debris." *Arson Analysis Newsletter* 3, no. 5: 1–17.

Colwell, J., and A. Reza. 2003. "Use of Soot Patterns to Evaluate Smoke Detector Operability." *Fire and Arson Investigator* July: 42–45.

Coulombe, R. 2002. "Chemical Analysis of Vegetable Oils Following Spontaneous Ignition." *Journal of Forensic Sciences* 47, no. 1: 195–201.

Coulson, S. A., R. K. Morgan-Smith, and D. Noble. 2000. "The Effect of Compressed Air Foam on the Detection of Hydrocarbon Fuels in Fire Debris Samples." *Science and Justice* 40, no. 4: 257–60.

Darrer, M., J. Jacquemet-Popiloud, and O. Delemont. 2008. "Gasoline on Hands: Preliminary Study on Collection and Persistence." *Forensic Science International,* 175 (2008): 171–78.

Dean, W. L. 1984. "Examination of Fire Debris for Flare (Fusee) Residues by Energy Dispersive X-Ray Spectrometry." *Arson Analysis Newsletter* 7.

Deans, J. 2006. "Recovery of Fingerprints from Fire Scenes and Associated Evidence." *Science and Justice* 46, no. 3: 153–68.

DeHaan, J. D. 1979. "Laboratory Aspects of Arson: Accelerants, Devices, and Targets." *Fire and Arson Investigator* 29 (January–March 1979): 39–46.

DeHaan, J. D. 1994. "Canine Accelerant Detection Validation." *CAC News,* Spring 1994.

———. 2002. "Our Changing World: Part 3—Detection Limits: Is More Sensitive Necessarily More Better?" *Fire and Arson Investigator* 52, no. 4.

DeHaan, J. D., and K. Bonarius. 1988. "Pyrolysis Products of Structure Fires." *Journal of the Forensic Science Society* 28, no. 5: 299–309.

DeHaan, N. R. 1991. "Interior Finish." Chap. 4-1 in *Fire Protection Handbook,* 16th ed. Quincy, MA: NFPA.

de Vos, B. J., M. Froneman, E. Rohwer, and D. A. Sutherland. 2002. "Detection of Petrol (Gasoline) in Fire Debris by Gas Chromatography/Mass Spectrometry/Mass Spectrometry (GC/MS/MS)." *Journal of Forensic Sciences* 47, no. 4: 736–42.

Di Zinno, J., D. Fisher, S. Barritt, T. Clayton, P. Gill, M. Holland, D. Lee, C McGuire, J. Raskin, R. Roby, J. Ruderman, and V. Weedn. 1995. "The Waco, Texas, Incident: The Use of DNA to Identify Human Remains." *Fifth International Symposium on Human Identification,* London, England.

Doyle, J. M., M. L. Miller, B. R. McCord, D. A. McCollam, and G. W. Mushrush. 2000. "A Multicomponent Mobile Phase for Ion Chromatography Applied to Separation of Anions from the Residues of Low Explosives." *Analytical Chemistry* 72, no. 10: 2302–7.

Ellern, H. 1961. *Modern Pyrotechnics.* New York: Chemical Publishing.

Furton, K. G., J. R. Almirall, and J. C. Bruna. 1996. "A Novel Method for the Analysis of Gasoline from Fire Debris Using Headspace Solid-Phase Microextraction." *Journal of Forensic Sciences* 41, no. 1: 12–22.

Gambrel, A. K., and M. R. Reardon. 2008. "Extraction, Derivatization and Analysis of Vegetable Oils from Fire Debris." *Journal of Forensic Sciences* 5, no. 6: 1372–80.

Gann, R. G., and N. P. Bryner. 2008. "Combustion Products and Their Effects on Life Safety." Vol. 1, chap. 2 in *Fire Protection Handbook,* 20th ed. Quincy, MA: NFPA.

Geraci, B. S., G. Hine, and W. Shaw. 2008. "CAFS and Its Impact in Fire Scene Investigations." Retrieved from www.firehouse.com.

Gilbert, M. W. 1998. "The Use of Individual Extracted Ion Profiles versus Summed Extracted Ion Profiles in Fire Debris Analysis." *Journal of Forensic Sciences* 43: 871–76.

Graham, D. 1969. "Some Technical Aspects of the Demonstration and Visualization of Fingerprints on Human Skin." *Journal of Forensic Sciences* 14: 1–12.

Henderson, R., C. Manning, and S. Barnhill. 1998. "Questions Concerning the Use of Carbon Content to Identify 'Cause' vs. 'Result' Beads in Fire Investigations." *Fire and Arson Investigator* 48, no. 3: 26–27.

Hetzel, S. S., and R. D. Moss. 2005. "How Long After Waterproofing a Deck Can You Still Isolate an Ignitable Liquid?" *Journal of Forensic Sciences* 50, no. 2: 369–72.

Hipes, S. E., et al. 1995. "Evaluation of the GC-FTIR for the Analysis of Accelerants in the Presence of Background Matrix Materials." *MAFS Newsletter* 20, no. 1: 48–76.

Howitt, D. G. 1998. "The Chemical Composition of Copper Arc Beads: A Red Herring for the Fire Investigator." *Fire and Arson Investigator* 48, no. 3: 34–39.

Howitt, D. G., and S. Pugh. 2007. "Direct Observation of Arcing through Char in Copper Wires." Paper presented at AAFS, Washington DC, February 2007.

IAAI Forensic Science and Engineering Committee. 1988. "Guidelines for Laboratories Performing Chemical and Instrumental Analysis of Fire Debris Samples." *Fire and Arson Investigator* 38, no. 4.

Jennings, W. 1980. *Gas Chromatography with Glass Capillary Columns.* New York: Academic Press, 1980.

Juhala, J. 1980. "A Method of Absorption of Flammable Vapors by Direct Insertion of Activated Charcoal into Debris." *Arson Accelerant Detection Course Manual.* Rockville, MD: US Treasury Department.

Katz, S. R., and C. R. Midkiff. 1998. "Unconfirmed Canine Accelerant Detection: A Reliability Issue in Court." *Journal of Forensic Sciences* 43, no. 2: 329–33.

Keltner, N. R., H. K. Hasegawa, and J. A. White. 1993. "*Investigation of High Temperature Accelerant Fires.*" Pp. 607–20 in *Proceedings, Interflam 1993.* London: Interscience Communications.

Kennedy, K. C., G. E. Gorbett, and P. M. Kennedy. 2004. "Fire Analysis Tool: Revisited Acoustic Soot Agglomeration in Residential Smoke Alarms." Pp. 719–24 in *Proceedings, Interflam 2004.* London: Interscience Communications.

Kirkbride, K. P., and H. J. Kobus. 1991. "The Explosive Reaction between Swimming Pool Chlorine and Brake Fluid." *Journal of Forensic Sciences* 36, no. 3: 902–7.

Kirkbride, K. P., S. M. Yap, S. Andrews, P. E. Pigou, G. Klass, A. C. Dinan, and F. L. Peddie. 1992. "Microbial Degradation of Petroleum Hydrocarbons: Implications for Arson Residue Analysis." *Journal of Forensic Sciences* 37, no. 6: 1585–99.

Kravtsova, Y., and D. Bagby. 2007. "Transfer of Gasoline from Footwear to Flooring Materials: Can This Occur at a Fire Scene?" Paper presented at AAFS, Washington DC, February 2007.

Kuk, R. J., and E. C. Diamond. 2005. "Transference and Adherence of Gasoline Vapors onto Clothing in an Enclosed Room." Paper presented at AAFS, New Orleans, LA, February 2005.

Kuk, R. J., and M. V. Spagnola. 2008. "Alternate Fuels and Their Impact on Fire Debris Analysis." *Journal of Forensic Sciences* 53, no. 5: 1123–29.

Lang, T. L., et al. 2002. *Detection of Exhaust Components from Ventilation Fans*. Toronto: Centre of Forensic Sciences.

Lee, H. C., and R. E. Gaensslen. 1985. "Cyanoacrylate 'Super Glue' Fuming for Latent Fingerprints." *The Identification Officer* Spring.

Lentini, J. J. 2001. "Persistence of Floor Coating Solvents." *Journal of Forensic Sciences* 46, 6: 1470–73.

Lentini, J. J., J. A. Dolan, and C. Cherry. 2000. "The Petroleum-Laced Background." *Journal of Forensic Sciences* 45, no. 5: 968–89.

Lloyd, J. A., and P. L. Edmiston. 2003. "Preferential Extraction of Hydrocarbons from Fire Debris Samples by Solid Phase Microextraction." *Journal of Forensic Sciences* 48, no. 1: 130–36.

Loscalzo, P. J., P. R. DeForest, and J. M. Chao. 1980. "A Study to Determine the Limit of Detectability of Gasoline Vapor from Simulated Arson Residues." *Journal of Forensic Sciences* 25, no. 1: 162–67.

Mann, D. 1999. "Washing Machine Effluent." *Fire Findings* 7, no. 4: 4.

Mann, D. C. 1987. "Comparison of Automotive Gasolines Using Capillary Gas Chromatography (I and II)." *Journal of Forensic Sciences* 32: 616–28.

Mann, D. C., and W. R. Gresham. 1990. "Microbial Degradation of Gasoline in Soil." *Journal of Forensic Sciences* 35, no. 4: 913–23.

Mann, D., and N. Putaansuu. 2006. "Alternative Sampling Methods to Collect Ignitable Liquid Residues from Non-porous Areas Such as Concrete." *Fire and Arson Investigator* 57, no. 1: 43–46.

Mann, J., N. Nic Daéid, and A. Linacre. 2003. "An Investigation into the Persistence of DNA on Petrol Bombs." In *Proceedings European Academy of Forensic Sciences*. Istanbul.

Margot, P., and C. J. Lennard. 1991. *Techniques for Latent Print Development*. Lausanne, Switzerland: University of Lausanne.

McGee, E., and T. L. Lang. 2002. "A Study of the Effects of a Micelle Encapsulator Fire Suppression Agent on Dynamic Headspace Analysis of Fire Debris Samples." *Journal of Forensic Sciences* 47, no. 2: 267–74.

McVicar, M. J. 1991. "The Perforation of a Copper Pipe during a Fire." *The/Le Journal, Canadian Association of Fire Investigators* June: 14–16.

Menzel, E. R., and J. M. Duff. 1979. "Laser Detection of Latent Fingerprints: Treatment with Fluorescers." *Journal of Forensic Sciences* 24: 96–100.

Meyers, R. E. 1978. "A Systematic Approach to the Forensic Examination of Flash Powders." *Journal of Forensic Sciences* 23: 66–73.

Montani, I., S. Comment, and O. Delemont. 2010. "The Sampling of Ignitable Liquids on Suspects' Hands." *Forensic Science International* 194: 15–124.

Muller, D. A. Levy, and R. Shelef. 2011. "Detection of Gasoline on Arson Suspects' Hands." *Forensic Science International*, 206 (1): PP. 150–154.

Mundorff, A. Z., E. J. Bartelink, and E. Mar-Casslh. 2009. "DNA Preservation in Skeletal Elements from the World Trade Center Disaster." *Journal of Forensic Sciences* 54, no. 4: 739–45.

NFPA. 2015a. *NFPA 302: Fire Protection Standard for Pleasure and Commercial Motor Craft*. Quincy, MA: National Fire Protection Association.

———. 2015b. *NFPA 1119: Standard for Recreational Vehicles*. Quincy, MA: National Fire Protection Association.

———. 2016. *NFPA 72: National Fire Alarm and Signaling Code*. Quincy, MA: National Fire Protection Association.

———. 2017. *NFPA 921: Guide for Fire and Explosion Investigations*. Quincy, MA: National Fire Protection Association.

Nowicki, J. 1990. "An Accelerant Classification Scheme Based on Analysis by Gas Chromatography/Mass Spectrometry." *Journal of Forensic Sciences* 35, no. 5.

Nowlan, M., A. W. Stuart, G. J. Basara, and P. M. L. Sandercock. 2007. "Use of a Solid Absorbent and an Accelerant Detection Canine for the Detection of Ignitable Liquids Burned in a Structure Fire." *Journal of Forensic Sciences* 52, no. 3: 643–48.

Patterson, P. L. 1990. "Oxygenate Fingerprints of Gasolines." *DET Report No. 18* October, 8–12.

Petraco, N. D. K. 2008. "Statistical Discrimination of Liquid Gasoline Samples from Casework." Paper presented at AAFS, Washington DC, February 2008.

Pinorini, M. T., C. J. Lennard, P. Margot, I. Dustin, and P. Furrer. 1994. "Soot as an Indicator in Fire Investigations: Physical and Chemical Analysis." *Journal of Forensic Sciences* 39, no. 4: 33–73.

Rankin, J. G., and M. Fletcher. 2007. "Target Compound Analysis for the Individualization of Gasolines." Paper presented at AAFS, Washington DC, February 2007.

Rankin, J. G., J. Wintz, and R. Everette. 2005. "Progress in the Individualization of Gasoline

Residues." Paper presented at AAFS, New Orleans, February 2005.

Sandercock, P., and E. D. Pasquier. 2003. "Chemical Fingerprinting of Unevaporated Gasoline Samples." *Forensic Science International* 134: 1–10.

Schewenk, L. M., and M. R. Reardon. 2009. "Practical Aspects of Analyzing Vegetable Oils in Fire Debris." *Journal of Forensic Sciences* 54, no. 4: 874–80.

Slye, O. M., Jr. 2008. "Flammable and Combustible Liquids." Chap. 5 in *Fire Protection Handbook,* 20th ed. Quincy, MA: NFPA.

Stauffer, E. 2003. "Concept of Pyrolysis for Fire Debris Analysts." *Science and Justice* 43: 29–40.

———. 2005. "A Review of the Analysis of Vegetable Oil Residues from Fire Debris Samples: Spontaneous Ignition, Vegetable Oils, and the Forensic Approach." *Journal of Forensic Sciences* 50, no. 5: 1091–1100.

———. 2006. "A Review of the Analysis of Vegetable Oil Residues from Fire Debris Samples: Analytical Scheme, Interpretation of Results and Future Needs." *Journal of Forensic Sciences* 51, no. 5: 1016–32.

Stauffer, E., J. Dolan, and R. Newman. 2008. *Fire Debris Analysis.* New York: Elsevier/Academic Press.

Sutherland, D. A., and K. C. Penderell. 2000. "GC/MS/MS: An Important Development in Fire Debris Analysis." *Fire and Arson Investigator* October: 21–26.

Trapecar, M. 2009. "Lifting Techniques for Finger Marks on Human Skin: Previous Enhancement by Swedish Black Powder." *Science and Justice* 49, no. 4: 292–95.

Turner, D. A., and J. V. Goodpaster. 2009. "A Comprehensive Study of Degradation of Ignitable Liquids." Paper presented at AAFS, Denver, CO, February 2009.

Twibell, J. D., and C. C. Christie. 1995. "The Forensic Examination of Fuses." *Science and Justice* 35, no. 2: 141–49.

Twibell, J. D., and J. M. Home. 1977. "A Novel Method for the Selective Adsorption of Hydrocarbons from the Headspace of Arson Residues." *Nature* 268.

Twibell, J. D., J. M. Home, and K. W. Smalldon. 1982. "A Comparison of Relative Sensitivities of the Adsorption Wire and Other Methods for the Detection of Accelerant Residues in Fire Debris." *Journal of the Forensic Science Society* 22, no. 2: 155–59.

Twibell, J. D., and S. C. Lomas. 1995. "The Examination of Fire-Damaged Electrical Switches." *Science and Justice* 35, no. 2: 113–16.

Underwriters Laboratories. 2015. *UL 217: Single and Multiple Station Smoke Alarms.* Northbrook, IL: Underwriters Laboratories.

U.S. Army. 1996. "Unconventional Warfare Devices and Techniques." TM 3-201, May 1996.

Worrell, C., R. J. Roby, L. Streit, and J. L. Torero. 2001. "Enhanced Deposition, Acoustic Agglomeration and Chladni Figures in Smoke Detectors." *Fire Technology* 37, no. 4: 343–62.

Woycheshin, S., and J. D. DeHaan. 1978. "An Evaluation of Some Arson Distillation Techniques." *Arson Analysis Newsletter* 2.

Wray, Harry A. 1992. *Manual on Flash Point Standards and Their Use.* West Conshohocken, PA: ASTM.

Ye, J., A. Ji, E. J. Parra, X. Zheng, C. Jiang, X. Zhao, L. Hu, and Z. Tu 2004. "A Simple and Efficient Method for Extracting DNA from Old and Burned Bone." *Journal of Forensic Sciences* 49, no. 4: 754–60.

Yoshida, H., T. Kaneko, and S. Suzuki. 2008. "A Solid-Phase Microextraction Method for the Detection of Ignitable Liquids in Fire Debris." *Journal of Forensic Sciences* 53, no. 3: 668–76.

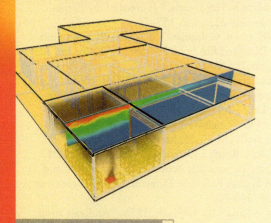

Courtesy of David J. Icove, University of Tennessee

OBJECTIVES

After reading this chapter, you should be able to:

- Identify proper application of fire modeling in fire scene reconstruction.
- Evaluate data necessary for fire model applications.
- Apply fire modeling to case studies.
- Interpret fire modeling results.

Two general types of fire models are used in support of fire investigations, namely, physical models and computational models. The concept of fire modeling as it applies to forensic fire investigation is unique to the last two decades, although models have existed since the 1960s. Previously, fire modeling was centered on explaining the physical phenomena of fires, particularly when applied to verifying existing experimental data. Now, computer modeling is commonplace (DeHaan 2005a, 2005b).

It was the effort of a few fire scientists and engineers working at and associated with the National Institute of Standards and Technology (NIST) in the United States and the Building Research Establishment (BRE), Fire Research Station (FRS) in the United Kingdom, that pushed the acceptability and application of fire modeling out of laboratory conditions and into the world of forensic fire scene reconstruction. The application of these early successes in fire modeling to the field of fire litigation and reconstruction further underscored its usefulness (Bukowski 1991; Babrauskas 1996). Several of the keynote studies that contributed significantly to this effort are described in this text.

The purpose of this chapter is not to make the reader an expert in fire modeling, but to allow him or her to gain a better appreciation for its added value to an investigation. Ample references are provided should more information be needed. This chapter answers the following questions that often arise when fire investigators are confronted with a fire of exceptional scale or impact: (1) What exactly is a fire model? (2) In which aspect of my investigation can fire modeling help? (3) What are the realistic and reliable results of a fire model? (4) Should more than one type of model be used to increase confidence in the results? (5) What is the future of fire modeling?

9.1 History of Fire Modeling

Research by Mitler (1991) at NIST best establishes the historical framework for the application of fire scene modeling. Work in 1927 at the National Bureau of Standards (NBS), the predecessor agency of NIST, was the first attempt to understand and explain in scientific terms the issues surrounding post-flashover compartment fires by relating the room gas temperature to the available mass of fuel being consumed (Inberg 1927).

The first fire model was developed through work in Japan in 1958 to relate the ventilation factor to steady-state fire development (Kawagoe 1958). The second model was constructed in Sweden (Magnusson and Thelandersson 1970), followed by the work of Babrauskas at the University of California, Berkeley (1975).

Historical reasons for developing and applying mathematical fire modeling were also accurately articulated and predicted by NIST (Mitler 1991). A good mathematical fire model of a structure can be helpful by doing the following:

- Avoiding repetitive full-scale testing,
- Helping designers and architects,
- Establishing flammability of materials,
- Increasing the flexibility and reliability of fire codes,
- Identifying needed fire research, and
- Helping in fire investigations and litigation.

The impact of environmental limitations and financial restrictions on fire testing has made fire modeling a valuable supplement to most fire testing programs. Factors such as the placement and combination of fuel items, changes in ventilation, and thickness of materials can be evaluated with fire models, reducing the need for repeated full-scale testing. Fire modeling can also supplement fire testing programs when used as a screening tool for full-scale testing scenarios.

Designers and architects have found modeling useful in assessing the impact of fire on buildings and occupants as they specify new construction methods and materials. New flexible fire performance codes are becoming more generally accepted as modeling introduces alternatives or new designs (such as atrium construction) that traditionally have not been addressed in historical prescriptive codes. Fire modeling can now also address the optimum designs for evacuation of people from buildings during emergencies.

As the science of fire dynamics advances, computational modeling identifies needed new areas of fire research into the phases of growth, flame spread, and flashover. Modeling can aid in gap assessments of certain areas that previously were not fully understood by designers, engineers, researchers, and even fire investigators.

Finally, fire modeling has had significant impact on forensic fire investigations and litigation (DeWitt and Goff 2000; DeHaan and Icove 2012). *NPFA 1033* states that the fire investigator shall have and maintain at a minimum an up-to-date basic knowledge of computer fire modeling beyond the high school level (NFPA 1033, 2014 Ed., pt. 1.3.7). Advancements in these areas are discussed in this chapter.

9.2 Fire Models

fire model ■ A method using mathematical or computer calculations that describes a system or process related to fire development, including fire dynamics, fire spread, occupant exposure, and the effects of fire. The results produced by fire models can be compared with physical and eyewitness evidence to test working hypotheses.

Computer **fire models** have a broad range of applications in the area of fire science and engineering. The fire model works to supplement the information gleaned from forensic evidence, witness interviews, media film footage, and preliminary fire scene examinations. Historically, these fire models, as shown in Table 9-1, have included eight major overlapping categories (Hunt 2000).

TABLE 9-1	Classes of Computer Fire Models and Commonly Cited Examples	
CLASS OF MODEL	**DESCRIPTION**	**EXAMPLE(S)**
Spreadsheet	Calculates mathematical solutions for interpretations of actual case data	FiREDSHEETS, NRC spreadsheets
Zone	Calculates fire environment through two homogeneous zones	FPETool, CFAST, ASET-B, BRANZFIRE, FireMD, BRI2000
Field	Calculates fire environment by solving conservation equations, usually with finite-element mathematics	FDS, JASMINE, FLOW3D, SMARTFIRE, PHOENICS, SOFIE
Post-flashover	Calculates time–temperature history for energy, mass, and species and is useful in evaluating structural integrity in fire exposure	COMPF2, OZone, SFIRE-4
Fire protection performance	Calculates sprinkler and detector response times for specific fire exposures based on the response time index (RTI)	DETACT-QS, DETECT-T2, LAVENT
Thermal and structural response	Calculates structural fire endurance of a building using finite-element calculations	FIRES-T3, HEATING7, TASEF
Smoke movement	Calculates the dispersion of smoke and gaseous species	CONTAM96, Airnet, MFIRE
Egress	Calculates the evacuation times using stochastic modeling using smoke conditions, occupants, and egress variables	Allsafe, buildingEXODUS, EESCAPE, ELVAC, EVACNET, EXIT89, EXITT, EVACS, Simplex, SIMULEX, WAYOUT

Sources: Updated from Bailey 2006; Friedman 1992; and Hunt 2000.

Fire models usually emulate the impact of fires, not the physical fire itself. The two recognized approaches to modeling fires are probabilistic and deterministic. *Probabilistic* models usually center on the application of stochastic mathematics to estimate or predict an outcome (within certain likelihoods), such as human behavior (SFPE 2008, chaps. 3-11 and 3-12). In *deterministic* models, the investigator relies on mathematical relationships that form the underpinnings of the physics and chemistry of fire science. Deterministic models can range from a simple straight-line approximation to correlating test data with complex fire models solving hundreds of simultaneous equations.

Mathematical models are usually formulated from interpretations of actual test data. These types of models are usually calculated by hand using formulas and a scientific calculator, a spreadsheet, or a simple computer program. Smoke-filling rates, flame heights, virtual origin, and other approximations can usually be calculated by hand in several minutes. When based on sound mathematical representations and properly applied, fire models can often assure that the scientific method has been satisfied.

The zone and field models are emphasized here. The discussion is limited to a survey of the concepts and is by no means intended to serve as an instruction manual for their use. In fact, most guidance issued with fire models cautions that they are for use only by those having significant competency in the fire engineering field and that the results should supplement the user's professional judgment.

9.2.1 SPREADSHEETS MODELS

One of the better-known spreadsheets for solving simple fire protection engineering relationships emerged from a May 1992 study, "Methods of Quantitative Fire Hazard Analysis," prepared for the Electric Power Research Institute (EPRI) by the University of Maryland, Department of Fire Protection Engineering. The study was distributed through the Society of Fire Protection Engineers (SFPE) (Mowrer 1992).

The study describes fire hazard analysis models used in the Fire-Induced Vulnerability Evaluation (FIVE) methodology, which is used by the Nuclear Regulatory Commission (NRC). The FIVE analysis uses realistic industrial loss histories to evaluate hazards quantitatively, including those losses produced in fires resulting from ignitable liquid spills, cable trays, and electrical cabinets. Many of these examples predict the impact of the fire plumes and ceiling jet temperatures, hot gas layers, thermal radiation to targets, and critical heat fluxes. Many of these concepts are applicable to problems previously posed in fire scene reconstruction and analysis (Mowrer 1992). Spreadsheet models are cited in *NFPA 921* (NFPA 2017, pt. 22.4.8.3.1).

From this study came FiREDSHEETS from the University of Maryland, Department of Fire Protection Engineering (Milke and Mowrer 2001). These spreadsheets concentrated on the specifics of compartment fire analysis and included extensive property tables for typical materials first ignited.

Mowrer has continued to develop spreadsheet templates for fire dynamics calculations, which are presently posted along with ample documentation on the Fire Risk Forum website, www.fireriskforum.com (Mowrer 2003). These templates incorporate a number of enclosure fire dynamics calculations used by FPETool (Nelson 1990) and other suites. Mowrer spreadsheets also include key calculations used in the fire and arson investigation training course for agents of the Bureau of Alcohol, Tobacco, Firearms and Explosives given by the University of Maryland's Department of Fire Protection Engineering.

A later and more industry-oriented set of spreadsheets known as the Fire Dynamics Tools (FDTs) was developed for the NRC fire protection inspection program (Iqbal and Salley 2004). The format of the spreadsheet output is more intuitive in its approach than that of financial spreadsheets. Table 9-2 is a synopsis of the available FDTs spreadsheets.

9.2.2 ZONE MODELS

Two-zone models are based on the concept that a fire in a room or enclosure can be described in terms of two unique zones, and the conditions within each zone can be predicted. The

TABLE 9-2   NRC Fire Dynamics Spreadsheets

CHAPTER	FDTs SPREADSHEET DESCRIPTION
2	Predicting Hot Gas Layer Temperature and Smoke Layer Height in a Room Fire with Natural Ventilation
	Predicting Hot Gas Layer Temperature in a Room Fire with Forced Ventilation
	Predicting Hot Gas Layer Temperature in a Room Fire with Door Closed
3	Estimating Burning Characteristics of Liquid Pool Fire, Heat Release Rate, Burning Duration, and Flame Height
4	Estimating Wall Fire Flame Height
5	Estimating Radiant Heat Flux from Fire to a Target Fuel at Ground Level under Wind-Free Condition Point Source Radiation Model
	Estimating Radiant Heat Flux from Fire to a Target Fuel at Ground Level in Presence of Wind (Tilted Flame) Solid Flame Radiation Model
	Estimating Thermal Radiation from Hydrocarbon Fireballs
6	Estimating the Ignition Time of a Target Fuel Exposed to a Constant Radiative Heat Flux
7	Estimating the Full-Scale Heat Release Rate of a Cable Tray Fire
8	Estimating Burning Duration of Solid Combustibles
9	Estimating Centerline Temperature of a Buoyant Fire Plume
10	Estimating Sprinkler Response Time
13	Calculating Fire Severity
14	Estimating Pressure Rise Due to a Fire in a Closed Compartment
15	Estimating Pressure Increase and Explosive Energy Release Associated with Explosions
16	Calculating the Rate of Hydrogen Gas Generation in Battery Rooms
17	Estimating Thickness of Fire Protection Spray-Applied Coating for Structural Steel Beams (Substitution Correlation)
	Estimating Fire Resistance Time of Steel Beams Protected by Fire Protection Insulation (Quasi-Steady-State Approach)
	Estimating Fire Resistance Time of Unprotected Steel Beams (Quasi-Steady-State Approach)
18	Estimating Visibility Through Smoke

Source: Iqbal and Salley 2004.

zone model ■ A computer fire model based on the assumption that a fire in a room or enclosure can be described in terms of two unique zones known as the upper and the lower zone, or layer, and the conditions within each zone can be predicted. Zone models use a set of differential equations for each zone solving for conditions such as, for example, pressure, temperature, carbon monoxide, oxygen, and soot production.

two zones refer to two individual control volumes known as the upper and lower zone, or layer. The upper zone of heated gases and by-products of combustion is penetrated only by the fire plume. These hot gases and smoke fill the ceiling layer, which then slowly descends. A boundary layer marks the intersection of the upper and the lower areas. The only exchange between the upper and the lower layers is due to the action of the fire plume.

Zone models use a set of differential equations for each zone, solving for pressure, temperature, carbon monoxide, oxygen, and soot production. The accuracy of these calculations varies with not only the model but also the reliability of the input data describing the circumstances and room dimensions and, very importantly, the assumptions as to the heat release rates of the materials burned in the fire. Complex two-zone models of up to 10 rooms typically take a few minutes to run using multi-core-class computer workstations or laptops.

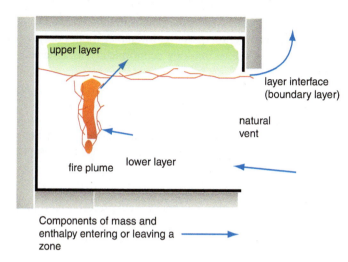

FIGURE 9-1 Representation of the two-zone fire model showing the location of the upper and lower layers, layer interface, fire plume, and compartment vent. *Courtesy of NIST, from Forney and Moss 1991.*

Figure 9-1 shows a schematic representation of the concepts behind a two-zone model. A survey published in 1992 by the SFPE showed ASET-B and DETACT-QS to be the most widely used zone models at that time (Friedman 1992).

Today, CFAST, the Consolidated Model of Fire Growth and Smoke Transport, has become the most widely used zone model. CFAST combines the engineering calculations from the FIREFORM model and the user interface from FASTlite in a unique comprehensive zone modeling and fire analysis tool (Peacock et al. 2008).

9.2.3 FIELD MODELS

Field models, the newest and most sophisticated of all deterministic models, rely on *computational fluid dynamics* (CFD) technology. These models are attractive, especially as a tool in litigation support and fire scene reconstruction, owing to their ability to display the impact of information visually in three dimensions.

However, the downside of field models is that creating input data is typically very time consuming and often requires powerful computer workstations to compute and display the results. The computation time to run field models may be days or weeks depending on the complexity of the model and the relative computational power of the computer system available.

CFD models estimate the fire environment by dividing the compartment into uniform small cells, or control volumes, instead of two zones. The program then simultaneously solves the conservation equations for combustion, radiation, and mass transport to and from each cell surface. The shortcomings include the level of background and training needed to codify a model, particularly for complex layouts.

There are many advantages to using CFD models over zone models such as CFAST. The higher geometric resolution of CFD models makes the solutions more refined. Higher-speed laptops and workstations allow CFD models to be run, whereas, in the past, larger mainframe and minicomputers were required. Multiple workstations have been successfully linked together in parallel processing arrays to perform complex CFD calculations more quickly.

Because CFD models are used in companion areas such as fluid flow, combustion, and heat transfer, their underlying technology is generally more accepted than that of simpler and coarser models. After these models become more broadly validated, they will gain further acceptance in situations where scientifically based testimony is sought, such as in forensic fire scene reconstructions.

CFD has a long history of use in forensic fire scene reconstructions and is gaining in popularity owing to commercially available and intuitive graphical interfaces [e.g.,

field model ■ A computer fire model that uses *computational fluid dynamics* (CFD) to estimate the fire environment by dividing the compartment into uniform small cells, or control volumes. The computer program then attempts to predict conditions in every volume such as, for example, pressure, temperature, carbon monoxide, oxygen, and soot production.

PyroSim (Thunderhead 2012, 2015)]. CFD programs now outpace the capabilities of the zone models, which, for the most part, operate under maintenance modes only. Moreover, CFD programs such as the FDS make the technology economically feasible owing to its wide use, testing, and growing acceptance.

9.3 CFAST Overview

The CFAST two-zone model is a heat and mass-balance model based on not only the physics and chemistry but also the results of experimental and visual observations in actual fires. CFAST computes:

- production of enthalpy and mass by burning objects;
- buoyancy and forced transport of enthalpy and mass through horizontal and vertical vents; and
- temperatures, smoke optical densities, and species concentrations.

CFAST 3.1.7 had a graphical user interface (GUI) that allowed the user to enter and modify characteristics about the physical form of the rooms, the fire signature, and graphics output. An enhancement in CFAST 5.0.1 and, most recently, CFAST 7.1 is that it is linked to Smokeview, the graphical interface of the NIST's Fire Dynamics Simulator (FDS) program. Table 9-3 summarizes the present capabilities of CFAST version 7.1.

TABLE 9-3	Summary of Maximum Numerical Limits in the Software Implementation of the CFAST Model, Version 7.1

FEATURE	MAXIMUM
Maximum simulation time in seconds	86400
Maximum number of compartments	100
Maximum number of horizontal flow (door/window) vent connections that can be included in a single test case	2500
Maximum number of horizontal vent connections between a pair of compartments that can be included in a single test case	25
Maximum number of vertical flow (ceiling/floor) vent connections which can be included in a single test case	200
Maximum number of vertical vent connections between a pair of compartments that can be included in a single test case	1
Maximum total number of connections between compartments and mechanical ventilation systems which can be included in a single test case	200
Maximum number of fans that can be included in a single test case	100
Maximum number of fires which can be included in a single test case	200
Maximum number of data points for a single fire definition	199
Maximum number of data points in a variable cross-sectional area definition for a single compartment	21
Maximum number of material thermal property definitions which can be included in a single thermal database file	125
Maximum number of targets which can be included in a single test case. In addition, the CFAST model includes a target on the floor of each compartment in the simulation and one for each object fire in simulation.	1000
Maximum number of detectors/sprinklers which can be included in a single test case.	1000

Source: (Peacock, Reneke, and Foreny 2016)

Since its first public release in June 1990, CFAST has been enhanced. CFAST version 7.0 includes a newly designed user interface and incorporates improvements in calculating heat transfer, smoke flow through corridors, and more accurate combustion chemistry. NIST added the capability to define a general t^2 growth rate fire that allows the user to select growth rate, peak heat release rate, steady burning time, and decay time, including predefined constants for slow, medium, fast, and ultrafast t^2 fires. The latest CFAST guide for users and documentation follows the guidelines set forth in *ASTM E1355-12: Standard Guide for Evaluating the Predictive Capability of Deterministic Fire Models* (ASTM 2012; Peacock, Reneke, and Forney 2016).

Because CFAST does not have a pyrolysis model to predict fire growth, a fuel source is entered or described by its fire signature (heat release rate). The program converts this fuel information into two characteristics: enthalpy (heat) and mass. In an unconstrained fire, the burning of this fuel takes place within the fire plume. In constrained fires, the pyrolyzed fuel may burn in the fire plume where there is sufficient oxygen, but it may also burn in the upper or lower layer of the room of fire origin, in the plume in the doorway leading to an adjoining room, or even in the layers or plumes in adjacent rooms.

9.3.1 FIRE PLUMES AND LAYERS

As in previous mathematical models in which calculations of heat flux used the fire plume's virtual origin, the CFAST model instructs the fire plume to act as a pump to move enthalpy and mass into the upper layer from the lower layer. Mixed with this enthalpy and mass are inflows and outflows from horizontal or vertical vents like doors and windows, which are modeled as plumes.

Some assumptions about required inputs for the model do not always hold in real fires. Some mixing of the upper and lower layers does take place at their interfaces. At cool wall surfaces, gases will flow downward as they lose heat and buoyancy. Also, heating and air-conditioning systems will cause mixing between the layers.

Horizontal flow of the fire from one room to the next occurs when the upper layer descends below the opening of an open vent. As the upper layer descends, pressure differentials between the connected rooms may cause air to flow into and out of a room or compartment in the opposite direction, resulting in the two flow conditions. Upward vertical flow may occur when the roof or ceiling of a room is opened.

9.3.2 HEAT TRANSFER

In the CFAST model, unique material properties of up to three layers can be defined for surfaces of the room (ceiling, walls, flooring). This design consideration is useful, because, in CFAST, heat transfers to the surface via convective heat transfer and through the surfaces via conductive heat transfer.

Radiative heat transfer takes place among fire plumes, gas layers, and surfaces. In radiative heat transfer, emissivity is dominated primarily by species contributions (smoke, carbon dioxide, and water) within the gas layers. CFAST applies a combustion chemistry scheme that balances carbon, hydrogen, and oxygen in the room of fire origin among the lower-layer portion of the burning fire plume, the upper layer, and air entrained in the lower layer that is absorbed into the upper layer of the next connecting room.

9.3.3 LIMITATIONS

Zone models have their limitations. Six specific aspects of physics and chemistry either are not included or have very limited implementations in zone models: flame spread, heat release rate, fire chemistry, smoke chemistry, realistic layer mixing, and suppression (Babrauskas 1996). Some errors in species concentrations can result in errors in the distribution of enthalpy among the layers, a phenomenon that affects the accuracy of temperature and flow calculations. CFAST has also been known to overpredict the upper-layer temperatures, partly because heat losses due to window radiation are not presently incorporated in the model.

Even with these known limitations, zone models have been extremely successful in forensic fire reconstruction and litigation (Bukowski 1991; DeWitt and Goff 2000) and is cited in *NFPA 921* (NFPA 921, 2014 Ed., pt. 22.4.8.3.2). CFAST zone models have been successfully introduced in state and federal court litigation (*Ledbetter v. Blair Corporation, 2012; Santos v. State Farm Fire and Cas. Co. In Misc. 3d: NY: Supreme Court. 2010; Turner v. Liberty Mutual Fire Insurance Co. Dist. Court, ND Ohio. 2007*). These successes are a result of their correct application by knowledgeable scientists and engineers, continued revalidation in actual fire testing, and applied research efforts, including verification and validation studies by the NRC (Salley and Kassawar 2007a, 2007b, 2007c, 2007d, 2007e, 2007f, 2007g).

9.4 CFD Technology–Based Models

9.4.1 FIRE DYNAMICS SIMULATOR

The recommended field model using CFD technology, owing to its availability at no cost, its focus of research, and its acceptance in the community, is the FDS. This model is available from NIST's Building and Fire Research Laboratory (McGrattan et al. 2010a). The first version of FDS was publicly released in February 2000 and has become a mainstay of the fire research and forensic investigation communities (NFPA 2017, pt. 22.4.8.3.3).

FDS is a fire-driven fluid flow model and numerically solves a form of the Navier-Stokes equations for thermally driven smoke and heat transport. The companion program to FDS is Smokeview, which is a graphical interface that produces a variety of visual records of FDS calculations. These include concentration of species, temperature, and heat flux in various animations. User guides for both FDS (McGrattan et al. 2010b) and Smokeview (Forney 2015) are available at NIST's website, fire.nist.gov.

Traditional use of FDS to date has been divided among the evaluation of smoke-handling systems, sprinkler and detector activation, and fire reconstructions. It is also being used to study fundamental fire dynamics problems encountered in both academic and industrial settings. FDS uses a combination of models to handle the computational problems: a hydrodynamic model to solve the Navier-Stokes equations, a Smagorinsky form of large eddy simulation (LES) for smoke and heat transport, a numerical grid simulation to handle turbulence, a mixture fraction combustion model, and a finite volume method approach for radiation heat transfer.

Unfortunately, FDS uses a rectilinear grid to describe the computational cells. This makes it slightly difficult to model sloping roofs, rounded tunnels, and curved walls without some form of approximation. The boundary conditions for material surfaces consist of assigned thermal constants that include information on their burning behavior. FDS, like other CFD models, breaks up the room (or fire area) into cells and calculates the mass heat energy and species transport (fluxes) into and out of each of the six faces of each cell. Figure 9-2 shows the output grids from a typical FDS problem.

The current version of FDS is version 6.3.2, which offers significant enhancements to previous versions. Subsequent versions with additional enhancements are under development and testing. Enhancements include the ability to evaluate heat transfer through walls and the impact of water suppression and initial conditions, and to add image texturing to solid objects and surfaces. The latest companion release of Smokeview is version 6.3.2. Its enhanced features include controls over viewing the rectilinear mesh used in constructing the FDS model. Scene clipping allows the visualization of obstructed boundary surfaces in complex models having numerous walls. A more robust feature allows more control over the movement and orientation of the scene as rendered by Smokeview.

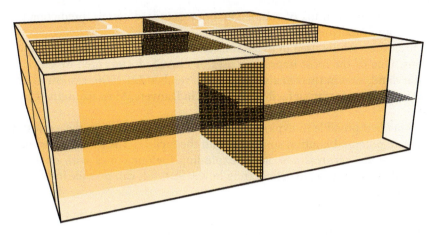

FIGURE 9-2 CFD (field) models break up the room (or fire area) into cells and calculate the mass heat energy and species transport (fluxes) into and out of each of the six faces of each cell. *Courtesy of David J. Icove, University of Tennessee, Knoxville, TN.*

Other features include several visualization modes, such as tracer particle flow, animated contour slices of computed variables such as vector heat flux plots, animated surface data, and multiple isocontours. New visualization tools allow the user to compare fire burn patterns with computed uniform surface contour planes. The option for animated flow vectors and particle animations allows observed heat flow vectors to be compared with computed vectors.

A horizontal time bar displays the duration of the run, and a vertical color-coded bar displays other variables, such as temperature and velocity. Graphics options include the ability to capture the output of the Smokeview program on a screen-by-screen basis. Screens may be exported and made into a movie, but this requires additional (non-NIST) software and can be tedious to produce.

9.4.2 FM GLOBAL CFD FIRE MODELING

FM Global has always served as a leader in the development of many of the fire protection engineering tools, fire dynamics relationships, fire growth and behavior models, and testing protocols cited in this textbook. FM Global maintains a unique center for developing property loss–prevention strategies, conducting scientific research, and product testing at their Research Campus in West Glocester, Rhode Island.

FM Global is presently developing a number of key physical models relating to fluid mechanics, heat transfer, and combustion into a new open-source software package called FireFOAM. This program is a CFD toolbox for fire and explosion modeling applications. To promote outside cooperation, FM Global has released its modeling technologies.

FireFOAM utilizes the finite volume method on arbitrarily unstructured meshes, and is highly scalable on massively parallel computers. The capabilities of FireFOAM include many complex simulations, including fire growth and suppression. For more information about FireFOAM, please refer to FM Global's website, www.fmglobal.com (FireFOAM 2012).

9.4.3 FLACS CFD MODEL

The commercial FLACS CFD model, maintained by CMR GexCon, has historically been used for gas dispersion modeling and explosion calculations within many industries (GexCon 2012). GexCon emphasizes the need for validation of CFD models such as FLACS. The software has many applications, including quantitative risk assessments, investigations into explosion venting of coupled and non-standard vessels, predicting the effect of explosions, and modeling toxic gas dispersion.

FLACS has been successfully used in hypothesis testing during large industrial explosion investigations. One of the most impressive uses of FLACS documented by GexCon US, Bethesda, Maryland, was in their analysis of the November 22, 2006, explosion and fire at an ink and paint manufacturing facility explosion in Danvers, Massachusetts (Davis et al. 2010).

Using FLACS made it possible to explore the chain of events leading to the explosion as well as to evaluate potential ignition sources within the facility. The investigators also compared the calculated overpressures of the exploding fuel/air cloud with observed internal and external blast damage, demonstrating how CFD tools can provide invaluable analyses for explosion investigations.

9.5 Impact of Guidelines and Standards on Fire Models

Within the last decade, the use of fire models created the need to develop guidelines and standards for their use. ASTM Subcommittee E05.33 currently maintains and continues to work on improving four guidelines that standardize the evaluation and use of computer fire models. The Society of Fire Protection Engineers (SFPE) and the *NFPA 921 Committee on Fire and Explosion Investigations* also have professional guidelines for their use. The following is a synopsis of the current standard guides (Janssens and Birk 2000).

9.5.1 ASTM GUIDELINES AND STANDARDS

- *ASTM E1355-12:* Evaluates the predictive capacity of fire models by defining scenarios, validating assumptions, verifying the mathematical underpinnings of the model, and evaluating its accuracy (ASTM 2012).
- *ASTM E1472-07:* Describes how a fire model is to be documented and includes a user's manual, a programmer's guide, mathematical routines, and installation and operation of the software (ASTM 2007a). *Note:* Withdrawn in 2010.
- *ASTM E1591-13:* Covers and documents available literature and data that are beneficial to modelers (ASTM 2013).
- *ASTM E1895-07:* Examines the uses and limitations of fire models and addresses how to choose the most appropriate model for the situation (ASTM 2007b). *Note:* Withdrawn in 2011. The ASTM felt that SFPE would be best suited to maintain this application in the form of a user guide.

9.5.2 SFPE GUIDELINES AND STANDARDS

SFPE (2011) recently published *Guidelines for Substantiating a Fire Model for a Given Application*, Engineering Guide SFPE G.06 2011. This guide supplements the ASTM standards and assists the user of a fire model in defining the problem, selecting a candidate model, interpreting the verification and validation studies for various models, and understanding user effects. An appendix covers fire-related phenomena with guidance as to application to specific models and interpreting the underlying key physics.

9.5.3 NFPA 921 GUIDELINES ON THE USE OF FIRE MODELS

NPFA 921's Chapter 22 on "Failure Analysis and Analytical Tools" devotes a section to the guidance for the use of fire models along with their limitations in forensic fire investigations (NFPA 2017, pt. 22.4.9). The section qualifies the inherent limitations and assumptions, taking care to ensure that the model is being used correctly, and that it is validated using competent data. *NFPA 921* cautions that while fire models can be used to test hypotheses, these models should not be utilized as the sole basis to justify the determination of a fire's origin and cause.

9.6 Verification and Validation

All fire models should pass some form of **verification and validation (V&V)** by comparing their predictions against the results of real fire tests if their results are to be relied on. This testing sometimes reveals flaws or blind spots—where some types of enclosures or conditions can produce predicted values that differ from observed fire behavior. If a model has not been shown to yield valid results for a particular type of fire, its predictions in an unknown scenario should not be accepted without question.

Recent work sponsored in part by the US Nuclear Regulatory Commission (NRC) examined the V&V of fire models, including CFAST and FDS (Salley and Kassawar 2007a, 2007b, 2007c, 2007d, 2007e, 2007f, 2007g). Although the NRC study centered on fire hazards specific to nuclear power plants, it addressed many of the concerns raised by those who think fire models are not accurate or appropriate for forensic fire scene reconstruction, such as in the Dalmarnock tests described in the next section.

These concerns include the ability of the models to accurately predict common features of fires, such as upper-layer temperatures and heat fluxes. One of the features of this report was a comparison between actual fire test results and predictions of hand calculations, zone models, and field models. As shown in Figure 9-3 and in other studies, when the models are applied correctly, there is generally good agreement among them and the variability of real-world fires.

For instance, FDS has been shown to be very accurate in predicting growth of fires in large compartments, but data on how FDS predictions relate to real fires in very small compartments are just now being gathered and published.

It should be noted that FDS was derived from earlier work on modeling the growth and movement of smoke plumes from large stationary fires such as those in oil pools. This work, based on large eddy simulation (LES), focused on atmospheric interaction with the smoke plumes and not on movement of the fire itself. More recently, FDS has been applied to

verification and validation (V&V) ■ A formal process of establishing acceptable uses, suitability, and limitations of fire models. *Verification* determines that a model correctly represents the developer's conceptual description. *Validation* determines that a model is a suitable representation of the real world and is capable of reproducing phenomena of interest (Salley and Kassawar 2007g).

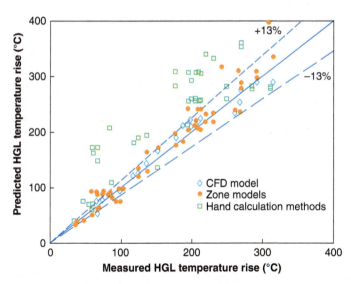

FIGURE 9-3 Comparison of hot gas layer (HGL) temperatures measured in full-scale tests compared with predictions of hand calculations (□), zone models (●), and FDS models (◊). A predicted ±13% variability range is included. Note that the hand calculations tended to overpredict layer temperatures, whereas both zone and field model predictions were generally within variability limits. *Courtesy of US Nuclear Regulatory Commission.*

studying wildland–urban interface (WUI) fires, considering the impact of vegetation fires on nearby structures. These developments depend on validation by comparison with actual incidents, because planned, real-world tests of such fires would be prohibitively expensive and dangerous.

Unfortunately, each year in the United States there are numerous opportunities to collect data from WUI fires after they occur. Because FDS predicts fire growth and spread based on the thermal characteristics of solid fuel surfaces, when fuel masses are porous (i.e., where fire can spread quickly *through* them as well as across them) the physics of heat transfer and ignition for that growth is too complex for FDS to accurately model such fires. The effects of wind-driven fire spread through such porous arrays complicate the process even further.

Wildland fires in heavy brush or timber are almost always crown fires in their most destructive phase; that is, the fire spreads upward and through porous fuel arrays like leaves or needles, often driven by wind—either atmospheric (external) wind or fire-induced drafts. Although FDS has been validated against tests on flat grasslands (no vertical spread factors) with wind-aided spread only, it has not been shown to give accurate predictions for crown fires through heavier brush or timber.

9.6.1 IMPACT OF VERIFICATION AND VALIDATION STUDIES

The V&V reports are presented in seven publications. Volume 1 (Salley and Kassawar 2007g), the main report, provides general background information, programmatic and technical overviews, and project insights and conclusions. Volumes 2 through 6 provide detailed discussions of the V&V of the Fire Dynamics Tools (FDTs) (Salley and Kassawar 2007d); Fire-Induced Vulnerability Evaluation, Revision 1 (FIVE-Rev1) (Salley and Kassawar 2007e); Consolidated Model of Fire Growth and Smoke Transport (CFAST) (Salley and Kassawar 2007a); MAGIC (Salley and Kassawar 2007f); and the Fire Dynamics Simulator (FDS) (Salley and Kassawar 2007c). Volume 7 discusses in detail the uncertainty of the experiments used in the V&V study of these five fire models (Salley and Kassawar 2007b).

9.6.2 THE DALMARNOCK TESTS

In 2006, the Dalmarnock fire tests were conducted in the United Kingdom, coordinated by the BRE Center for Fire Safety Engineering, University of Edinburgh. The tests consisted of a series of large-scale fire experiments conducted in a high-rise 23-story building located in Dalmarnock, Glasgow.

Before the tests, seven teams were given mutual access to the available information on the compartment geometry, fuel packages, ignition source, and ventilation conditions of fire. The teams attempted to build models that would predict the fire scenarios. The primary intent of the tests was to see how accurate the teams' predictions might be. Unfortunately, their results showed a wide range of predictions, emphasizing the difficulties of modeling complex fire scenarios.

Rein et al. (2009) concluded that there was an inherent difficulty in modeling fire dynamics in complex fire scenarios like Dalmarnock, and the modelers' ability to accurately predict fire growth was poor. Several studies and one textbook describe these results in detail (Rein et al. 2009; BRE Center 2012; Abecassis-Empis et al. 2008; Rein, Abecassis-Empis, and Carvel 2007).

However, it is interesting that previous work by Rein et al. (2006) reported that when a combination of a first-order, a zone, and a field model was used, the combined results of these three modeling approaches were in relatively good agreement, particularly in the early stages of the fire. The researchers' work also indicated that this approach to modeling can be used as a first step toward confirming the order of magnitude of the results from more complex models.

9.7 Historical Fire Modeling Case Studies

Science and litigation are two major driving factors behind the evolution of fire modeling as an important tool in both the analysis of building codes and forensic fire scene reconstructions. Fire protection engineering principles developed from correlating tests with actual case histories to stretch the knowledge of fire science. Attorneys seeking answers regarding responsibility and liability for damages due to fires also have a reason to seek the answers to similar questions. Therefore, science and law meet in the courtroom.

Moreover, the public demands to know why and how incidents occur and whether fire codes perform as anticipated during actual fires. People not only are curious but they have a legitimate concern for answers to questions such as the following: Is it safe for my child to live in a non-sprinklered dormitory?

Traditionally, fire models have been used in two separate yet important areas:

- Building fire safety and codes analysis
- Forensic fire scene reconstruction and analysis

Specific fire modeling evaluations have looked at the impact or performance of smoke handling systems, sprinkler and detector activation, and fire/burn patterns in reconstructions. Fire modeling found its way into forensic reconstruction through a long history of applications to real-world events. Table 9-4 gives a partial listing of cases in which NIST-produced fire models provided valuable insight into fire investigation. These and other reports can be obtained from the NIST fire publications website, fire.nist.gov.

TABLE 9-4	Representative Historical NIST Fire Investigations Using Fire Modeling
NIST REPORT NUMBER OR CITATION	**CASE TITLE AND AUTHOR**
NBSIR 87-3560 May 1987	*Engineering Analysis of the Early Stages of Fire Development: The Fire at the Dupont Plaza Hotel and Casino, December 31, 1986* H. E. Nelson
NISTIR 90-4268; August 1990, vol. 1	*Full Scale Simulation of a Fatal Fire and Comparison of Results with Two Multiroom Models* R. S. Levine and H. E. Nelson
NISTIR 4665 September 1991	*Engineering Analysis of the Fire Development in the Hillhaven Nursing Home Fire,* October 5, 1989 H. E. Nelson and K. M. Tu
Journal of Fire Protection Engineering 4, no. 4 (1992): 117–31	*Analysis of the Happyland Social Club Fire With HAZARD I* R. W. Bukowski and R. C. Spetzler
NISTIR 4489 June 1994	*Fire Growth Analysis of the Fire of March 20, 1990, Pulaski Building, 20 Massachusetts Avenue, NW, Washington, DC* H. E. Nelson
Fire Engineers Journal 56, no. 185 (November 1996): 14–17	*Modeling a Backdraft Incident: The 62 Watts Street (New York) Fire* R. W. Bukowski
NISTIR 6030 June 1997	*Fire Investigation: An Analysis of the Waldbaum Fire, Brooklyn, New York, August 3, 1978* J. G. Quintiere
NISTIR 6510 April 2000	*Simulation of the Dynamics of the Fire at 3146 Cherry Road, NE, Washington, DC, May 30, 1999* D. Madrzykowski and R. L. Vettori

(Continued)

TABLE 9-4	Representative Historical NIST Fire Investigations Using Fire Modeling (*Continued*)
NIST REPORT NUMBER OR CITATION	**CASE TITLE AND AUTHOR**
NISTIR 7137 May 2004	*Simulation of the Dynamics of a Fire in the Basement of a Hardware Store, New York, June 17, 2001* N. P. Bryner and S. Kerber
NISTIR 6923 October 2002	*Simulation of the Dynamics of a Fire in a One-Story Restaurant, Texas, February 14, 2000* R. L. Vettori, D. Madrzykowski, and W. D. Walton
NISTIR 6854 January 2002	*Simulation of the Dynamics of a Fire in a Two-Story Duplex, Iowa, December 22, 1999* D. Madrzykowski, G. P. Forney, and W. D. Walton
NIST SP 995 March 2003	*Flame Heights and Heat Release Rates of 1991 Kuwait Oil Field Fires* D. Evans, D. Madrzykowski, and G. A. Haynes
NIST Special Pub. 1021 July 2004	*Cook County Administration Building Fire, 69 West Washington, Chicago, Illinois, October 17, 2003: Heat Release Rate Experiments and FDS Simulations* D. Madrzykowski and W. D. Walton
NISTIR 7137 2004	*Simulation of the Dynamics of a Fire in the Basement of a Hardware Store, New York, June 17, 2001* N. P. Bryner and S. Kerber
NIST NCSTAR September 2005	*Reconstruction of the Fires in the World Trade Center Towers. Federal Building and Fire Safety Investigation of the World Trade Center Disaster* R. G. Gann, A. Hamins, K. B. McGrattan, G. W. Mulholland, H. E. Nelson, T. J. Ohlemiller, W. M. Pitts, and K. R. Prasad
Fire Technology 42, no. 4, (October 2006): 273–81	*Numerical Simulation of the Howard Street Tunnel Fire* K. B. McGrattan and A. Hamins
Fire Protection Engineering 31 (Summer 2006): 34–36	*NIST Station Nightclub Fire Investigation: Physical Simulation of the Fire* D. Madrzykowski, N. P. Bryner, and S. I. Kerber
NIST Special Publication 1118, March 2011	*Technical Study of the Sofa Super Store Fire, South Carolina, June 18, 2007* N. Bryner, S. P. Fuss, B. W. Klein, and A. D. Putorti.
NIST Technical Note 1729, 2012.	*Simulation of the Dynamics of a Wind-Driven Fire in a Ranch-Style House – Texas.* A. Barowy and D. Madrzykowski.
NUREG-1824, US NRC, Supplement 1, 2013.	*Verification and Validation of Selected Fire Models for Nuclear Power Plant Applications for the United States Nuclear Regulatory Commission* D. Stroup and A. Lindeman., Washington, DC,
NIST Technical Note 1838, 2014.	*Simulation of an Attic Fire in a Wood Frame Residential Structure – Chicago, Illinois* C. G. Weinschenk, K. J. Overholt, and D. Madrzykowski.

Note: Many of these and other similar reports can be obtained on the NIST website, fire.nist.gov.

Several keynote case histories are worth mentioning to show the development of fire modeling in forensic evaluations of fire scenes. These historically significant cases are discussed along with the important concepts gleaned from the referenced and published studies.

9.7.1 UK FIRE RESEARCH STATION

The UK government operated the outstanding Fire Research Station (FRS) in Borehamwood, England, until the facility was privatized in 1997 and moved to Garston. Now a modest engineering consultancy, the facility has a history of more than 50 years of assisting with fire investigations for the UK government. FRS investigations and reconstructions have included fire incidents at the Stardust Disco in Dublin, at Windsor Castle, in the Channel Tunnel, and in the King's Cross Underground station. The FRS uses a combination of a statistical database of loss histories, scene investigations, a fire testing laboratory, and fire models to test hypotheses or investigate unusual phenomena (FRS 2012).

Early work at the FRS developed a compartment fire model to address smoke and heat venting, when its researchers examined the similarities of the Livonia, Michigan, and Jaguar auto plant fire losses (Nelson 1991). These fires at two separate parts manufacturing centers had devastating effects on the production of automobiles. What began as a search for a means to vent hot by-products of combustion through the ceiling formed the basis for the zone fire model, which was based on actual fire testing.

9.7.2 DUPONT PLAZA HOTEL AND CASINO FIRE

The December 31, 1986, fire at the Dupont Plaza Hotel and Casino, San Juan, Puerto Rico, killed 98 persons. Owing to the extreme and needless loss of life, this case has become a textbook example of the application of fire reconstruction to the initial development of what became a large, complex fire. The late NIST fire researcher Harold "Bud" Nelson worked in cooperation with ATF investigators to collect and analyze data during the scene investigation. This led to a successful prosecution of the individuals who started the fire simply to harass hotel management.

The analysis combined technical data and fire growth models to explain the dynamics exhibited by the fire (Nelson 1987). The analysis looked at mass burning rate, heat release rate, smoke temperatures, smoke layer, oxygen concentration, visibility, flame extension and spread, sprinkler response, smoke detector response, and fire duration. Fire models used in this analysis included FIRST, ROOMFIR, ASETB, and HOTVENT.

The analysis confirmed the area of origin to be the south ballroom. The fire spread next to a foyer, then to the lobby and casino area. Figure 9-4 documents the conditions at 60 seconds after the fire started.

9.7.3 KING'S CROSS UNDERGROUND STATION FIRE

One of the first important cases using CFD models for fire investigation was the analysis of the King's Cross Underground Station fire on November 18, 1987. The CFD model FLOW3D tracked the fire upward along a 30° incline of the wooden sides and treads of the escalators to the ticket concourse level. The CFD model verified the theory of the trench effect that described this unique phenomenon. Thirty-one people died in the fire, including a senior station officer (Moodie and Jagger 1992, 83-103).

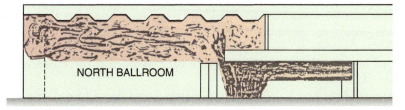

NORTH BALLROOM

FIGURE 9-4 The analysis combined technical data and NIST fire growth models to explain the dynamics exhibited by the fire at the Dupont Plaza. The analysis looked at mass burning rate, heat release rate, smoke temperatures, smoke layer, oxygen concentration, visibility, flame extension and spread, sprinkler response, smoke detector response, and fire duration. *Courtesy of NIST, from Nelson 1987.*

In determining the area of origin for this fire, investigators homed in on the area where the fire first started as observed by witnesses, some 21 m (68 ft) below the top of escalator No. 4. This area was at the lowest point of fire pattern damage to wooden handrails, treads, and risers. An analysis of the paint blistering and ceiling damage was also used to locate the fire origin. Witnesses who saw the fire partway up the escalator from below corroborated physical indicators.

The investigation concluded that the fire started beneath the wooden steps on the moving staircase from discarded smoking materials. The fire consumed much of the available combustible material in the escalator. Fire damage also extended to the other escalators and the upper-level ticket hall. Conditions in the latter were made untenable by the fact that a temporary plywood construction partition had been erected that was able to burn despite a coating of allegedly fire-retardant paint.

In addition to using a CFD model, government health and safety personnel obtained ignition characteristics of the samples taken from near the area of fire origin. Investigators were surprised to determine that escalator lubricating grease could be ignited only if combined with fibrous debris (paper, hair, lint) that acted as a wick.

To assess and validate the results of the CFD model, three types of tests were run. Full-scale fire growth tests determined that the initial fire on the escalator was about 1 MW per meter of escalator burning. Small-scale models implied that above a certain fire size, the flame in the channel of the escalator did not rise vertically but was pushed down into the trench by entrained air, facilitating rapid surface flame spread. Scaled open-channel tests examined the 30° inclined plane and used plywood with various surface coverings to evaluate flame spread. The hot gases moved quickly up the tunnel to fill the ticket lobby. When the gases ignited in a flameover, the fire engulfed the lobby (Moodie and Jagger 1992).

Lessons learned from this fire included the influence of the trench effect on a fire and the speed at which such a fire can develop and spread. Witnesses underestimated the speed of the smoke spread, the growing intensity of the fire, and the need for rapid evacuation. Smoking on underground rail services has since been banned, and combustible escalators, enclosures, and signage have been eliminated.

9.7.4 FIRST INTERSTATE BANK BUILDING FIRE

NIST conducted another engineering analysis on the May 4, 1988, fire at the 62-story, steel-framed high-rise known as the First Interstate Bank Building, in Los Angeles, California (Nelson 1989). The fire involved an after-hours accidental ignition in an office cubicle on the 12th floor that spread across the floor of origin. The fire propagated to the 13th, 14th, and 15th floors and a section of the 16th floor as exterior windows failed, allowing large flame plumes to entrain against the sheer sides of the building, which caused windows above to fail. The fire burned for more than 2 hours before being suppressed by firefighters' hose streams inside the building. One of the maintenance personnel died after taking an elevator to the fire floor.

The NIST analysis of the fire used the Available Safe Egress Time (ASET) program to predict the smoke layer's temperatures, smoke level, and oxygen content after the calculated time for flashover [smoke temperature of 600°C (1150°F)]. The DETACT-QS model was used to estimate the response of smoke detectors and sprinklers to the fire growth. These studies revealed how much damage could have been avoided if there had been sprinklers on the floor of origin.

This analysis was one of the first to evaluate burn patterns and flame spread on combustible furniture, glass breakage, and communication of the fire to upper floors by flame extension from broken windows, and compartment burning rates in reconstructing the fire. The study also advanced the theory of a transfire triangle, which demonstrates the important interdependent relationships among the mass burning (pyrolysis) rate, the heat release rate, and the available air (oxygen) (Nelson 1989).

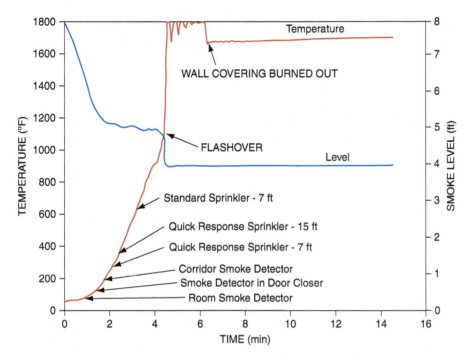

FIGURE 9-5 The impact at the Hillhaven Nursing Home of the "what if" questions that are posed in fire reconstructions, centering on the hypothetical impact of different fire activation devices on fire suppression as well as the predicted time of flashover. *Courtesy of NIST, from Nelson 1991.*

9.7.5 HILLHAVEN NURSING HOME FIRE

A fire just after 10 p.m. on October 5, 1989, at the Hillhaven Rehabilitation and Convalescent Center, Norfolk, Virginia, claimed the lives of 13 persons. None of these individuals were burned, but all breathed sufficient carbon monoxide (CO) to produce fatally high carboxyhemoglobin (COHb) levels.

The late NIST fire researcher Harold E. "Bud" Nelson recognized the importance of evaluating the fire dynamics when reconstructing this incident. His analysis of the room of fire origin in the nursing home showed that the temperature rose to at least 1000°C (1800°F), with a CO concentration of 40,000 ppm (Nelson and Tu 1991).

Using the fire model FIRE SIMULATOR contained in its engineering package, FPE-Tool predicted the smoke temperatures, smoke layer, toxic gas concentrations, and velocity of the smoke front. An important aspect learned in the NIST analysis was the impact of the "what if" questions that are posed in fire reconstructions (Figure 9-5). These questions centered on the hypothetical impact of different fire activation devices on fire suppression as well as the predicted time of flashover.

9.7.6 PULASKI BUILDING FIRE

A fire in Suite 5127 of the Pulaski Building, 20 Massachusetts Avenue, NW, Washington, DC, on March 23, 1990, damaged the offices of the US Army Battlefield Monuments Commission (ABMC). A NIST engineering review of the fire was able to apply sound fire protection engineering principles to estimate the rate of fire growth (Nelson 1994).

At 11:24 a.m., an alert ABMC staff member noticed smoke coming from the open door of the unoccupied audio/visual conference room. The room contained an estimated 4530 kg (10,000 lb) of combustible materials consisting of publications and photos stored in corrugated board boxes and cardboard mailing tubes stacked about 1.5 m (5 ft) high. The fire was thought to have started when cartons of mailing tubes were exposed to a frayed energized electrical lamp cord that passed through a small hole from a podium into the projection room.

FPETool was used to analyze the fire and arrive at a scenario based on witness testimony and observations. FIRE SIMULATOR estimated the environmental conditions, temperature, depth of smoke, thickness of smoke, and energy vented from the room. Also included was the impact of the failure of the suspended ceiling.

The analysis showed that the fire reached flashover approximately 268 seconds into the fire. A unique aspect of this fire engineering analysis was the introduction of a timeline of events (Figure 9-6) that compared the approximate time with the observed fire conditions, behavior of the occupants, impact of existing fire protection systems, and "what if" scenarios of the impact of potential fire protection systems.

FIRE	PEOPLE	APPROXIMATE TIME	EXISTENT PROTECTION SYSTEMS	POTENTIAL PROTECTION SYSTEMS
		11:20		THE ITEMS LISTED IN THIS COLUMN DID NOT EXIST IN THE FIRE AREA. THE ENTRIES REPRESENT THE EXPECTED TIME OF OPERATION HAD THEY BEEN PRESENT.
FIRST FLAME				
		11:21		
FLAME 1 FT. HIGH	PERSONS F & K LEAVE ABMC	11:22		
SMOKE DOWN TO TOP OF DOOR OF CONF. RM.	PERSON L GETS COFFEE	11:23		SMOKE DETECTOR
FLAME 2-3 FT. HIGH				
FLAME TO CEILING	PERSON G SENSES SMOKE	11:24		QUICK RESPONSE SPRINKLER
	PERSONS B & E SEE FLAME IN CONF. RM	11:25		STANDARD SPRINKLER
FLASHOVER IN CONFERENCE ROOM	PERSON SEES SMOKE "BOILING" IN CONF. RM.	11:26		
	EVERYONE OUT OF ABMC SUITE			
CEILING FAILURE IN CONFERENCE RM.	PERSON B RE-ENTERS SUITE TO RETRIEVE BELONGINGS	11:27	FIRE ALARM BOX OPERATED	
		11:28	FIRE DEPT. RECEIVES ALARM	* THERE IS NO RECORD OF THE TIME WHEN THE FIRE DEPARTMENT ACTUALLY ARRIVED AT THE ABMC SUITE. IT PROBABLY OCCURRED BETWEEN 11:35 AND 11:40
		11:29		
		11:30	FIRST FIRE * COMPANY ARRIVES AT BUILDING	

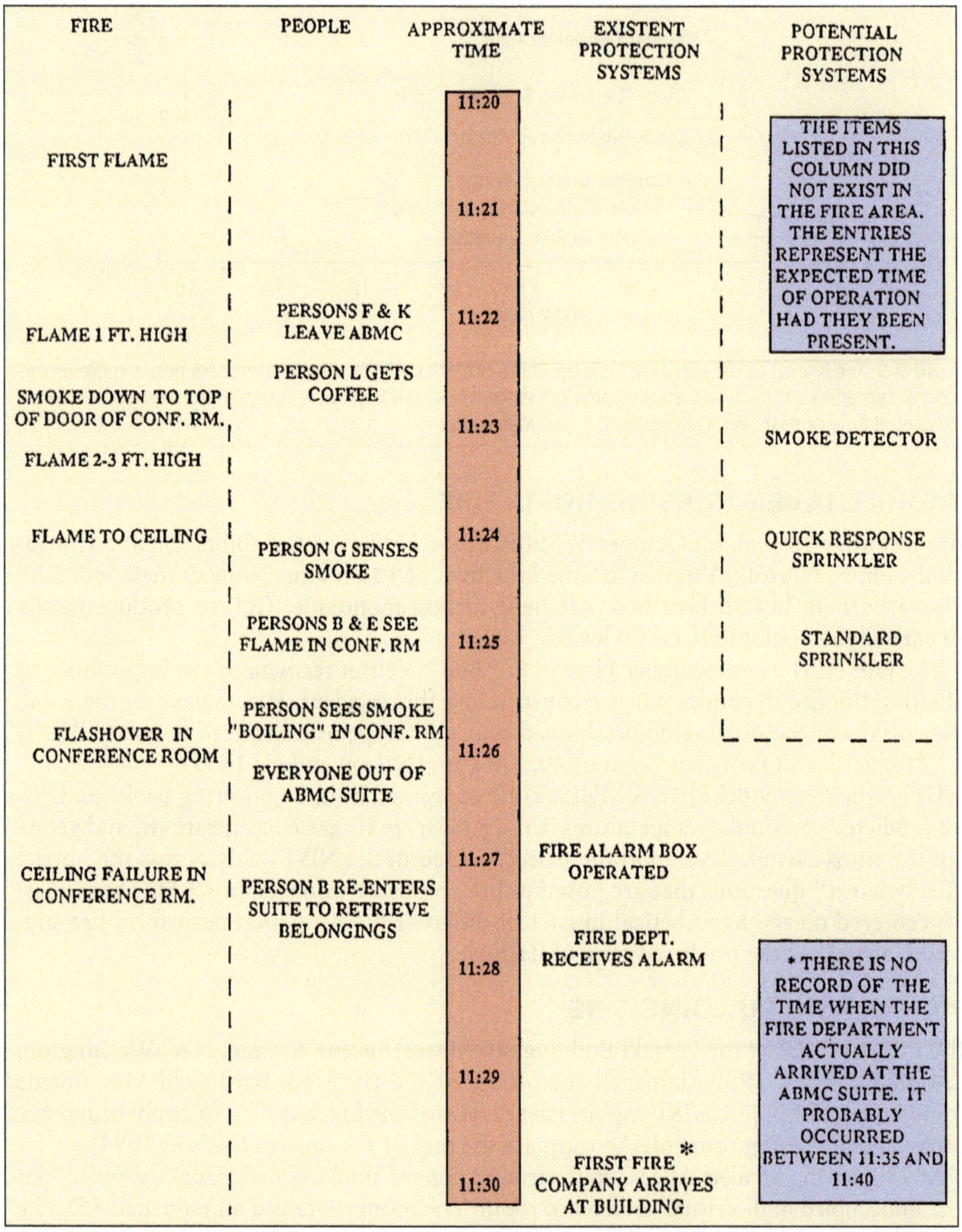

FIGURE 9-6 The timeline of events in the Pulaski Fire, which compares the approximate time with the observed fire conditions, behavior of the occupants, impact of existing fire protection systems, and "what if" scenarios of the impact of potential fire protection systems. *Courtesy of NIST, from Nelson 1989.*

9.7.7 HAPPYLAND SOCIAL CLUB FIRE

On the morning of March 25, 1990, an arsonist set a fire in the entryway of a neighborhood club using 2.8 L (0.75 gal) of gasoline. The fire killed 87 occupants of the two-story club. A NIST fire engineer used the HAZARD I fire model to examine the fire development as well as potential mitigation strategies that could have influenced the outcome of the fire (Bukowski and Spetzler 1992).

These mitigation strategies included the use of automatic sprinkler protection, solid wooden doors at the base of the stairway, a fire escape and enclosed exit stairwell, and a noncombustible interior finish. The analysis also weighed the economic cost estimates to implement these strategies. The study concluded that the combustible wall coverings and the opening of an entry door, which allowed the entry of gasoline-fed flames, caused the fire to grow and combustion gases to spread so rapidly that everyone in the upstairs club was affected within 1 to 2 minutes, precluding their escape.

The NIST analysis also took into account occupant tenability at various locations, based on the output of the HAZARD I fire model (which incorporated CFAST version 2.0). The tenability study looked at heat flux that could cause second-degree burns, temperatures, and fractional exposure doses based on both the NIST and the Purser toxicity models (Bukowski and Spetzler 1992). This analysis showed that a second means of egress could have reduced the number of fatalities, but additional mitigation strategies would have been required to prevent the loss of life.

9.7.8 62 WATTS STREET FIRE

A NIST fire engineer modeled what is now known as the 62 Watts Street Fire, which occurred at 7:36 p.m. on March 28, 1994 (Bukowski 1995, 1996). The fire involved a three-story apartment building in Manhattan, New York. The responding firefighters formed two three-person hose teams. One team planned to enter the first-floor apartments while the second team proceeded up a stairwell to search for fire extension.

Investigation later revealed that the occupant of the first-floor apartment had left at 6:25 p.m. A plastic trash bag inadvertently left on top of the kitchen gas range was ignited by the pilot flame. Several bottles of high-alcohol-content liquid were left close by, on the adjoining countertop, which contributed to the initial fire. The fire burned for approximately an hour, becoming oxygen-deficient as the smoke layer descended to the level of the countertop. Although the fire itself was not large, it produced large quantities of carbon monoxide, smoke, and other unburned fuels trapped in the hot smoke layer in the small, closed apartment.

As the firefighters in the stairwell forced open the door to the first-floor apartment, a *backdraft* occurred, in which warm fire gases flowing out of the burning apartment were replaced by cool outside air. With the ensuing exchange, the combustible gas mixture ignited, creating a large flame in the stairwell for a period of approximately 6 minutes, killing the firefighters on the stairs.

At NIST, Bukowski modeled this event using CFAST, and the analysis has become a classic study in backdrafts and firefighter safety. McGill (2003), at Seneca College, Toronto, Canada, modeled this case using the NIST Fire Dynamics Simulator. A copy of McGill's Smokeview visualization is shown in Figure 9-7. It took approximately 20 hours to define and construct the model.

9.7.9 CHERRY ROAD FIRE

In this case, NIST engineers were requested by Washington, DC, to demonstrate the results of calculations using the NIST FDS to evaluate the thermal and tenability conditions of a fire on May 30, 1999, in a townhouse located at 3146 Cherry Road, NE, Washington, DC, that may have led to the deaths of two firefighters and burned four others (Madrzykowski and Vettori 2000). The fire started in a ceiling electrical fixture on the

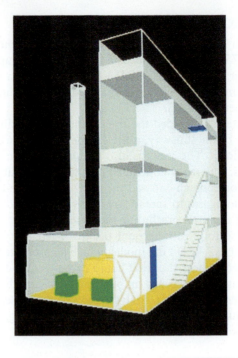

FIGURE 9-7 Model of the 62 Watts Street fire using the NIST Fire Dynamics Simulator. Room of origin at lower left. The fire plume extending from the apartment door (center) into the hallway trapped and killed three firefighters on the stairs. *Courtesy of D. McGill (2003).*

lower level of the townhouse. Responding firefighters entered the first and basement floors of the structure. Both on-scene observations and subsequent modeling showed that the opening of the lower-level sliding glass doors increased the heat release rate of the fire, so that 820°C (1500°F) gases moved up the stairwell. The fire may have smoldered for several hours before flame ignition, producing fuel-rich gases that ignited while firefighters were inside the building searching for the fire and any victims in the heavy smoke.

The Cherry Road fire FDS model may become one of the best examples of application of the NIST FDS. Furthermore, the fire pattern damage observed correlated with the model's predictions. As the technology expands, so does the ability to address harder questions concerning transient heat and ventilation, rapid fire growth, and stratified or localized conditions.

Summary

This chapter introduced the concept and application of fire modeling to forensic fire investigation. Although models have existed since the 1960s, fire modeling centered on explaining the physical phenomena of fires, particularly when applied to verifying existing experimental data.

Through the effort of a few fire scientists and engineers working at NIST and FRS, the acceptability and application of fire modeling moved out of the laboratory and into the world of forensic fire scene reconstruction. As noted at the beginning of this chapter, the purpose of this chapter was not to make the reader an expert in fire modeling, but to allow him or her to gain a better appreciation of its value in an investigation.

As seen in other chapters, fire modeling can be used to explore in more detail the issues of tenability as it applies to the modeling of toxicity of fires.

Review Questions

1. Choose one of the cases mentioned in this chapter and model it using the selected program. Obtain a similar fire modeling program and compare and contrast the results derived using it for the analysis.
2. Many computer fire models contain a database of materials and their burning properties. Examine the databases of two fire models. Compare and contrast the results obtained using each model.
3. Using the Fire Dynamics Tools (FDTs) spreadsheets, conduct a sensitivity analysis of several of its calculations by varying the input data (such as room dimensions or ventilation openings).

References

Abecassis-Empis, C., P. Reszka, T. Steinhaus, A. Cowlard, H. Biteau, S. Welch, G. Rein, and J. L. Torero. 2008. "Characterisation of Dalmarnock Fire Test One." *Experimental Thermal and Fluid Science* 32 (7): 1334–43, doi: 10.1016/j.expthermflusci.2007.11.006.

ASTM. 2007a. *ASTM E1472-07: Standard Guide for Documenting Computer Software for Fire Models* (withdrawn 2011). West Conshohocken, PA: ASTM International.

———. 2007b. *ASTM E1895-07: Standard Guide for Determining Uses and Limitations of Deterministic Fire Models* (withdrawn 2011). West Conshohocken, PA: ASTM International.

———. 2012. *ASTM E1355-12: Standard Guide for Evaluating the Predictive Capability of Deterministic Fire Models.* West Conshohocken, PA: ASTM International.

———. 2013. *ASTM E1591-13: Standard Guide for Obtaining Data for Fire Growth Models.* West Conshohocken, PA: ASTM International.

Babrauskas, V. 1975. *COMPF: A Program for Calculating Post-Flashover Fire Temperatures.* Berkeley, CA: Fire Research Group, University of California, Berkeley.

———. 1996. "Fire Modeling Tools For FSE: Are They Good Enough?" *Journal of Fire Protection Engineering* 8 (2): 87–96.

Bailey, C. 2006. *One Stop Shop in Structural Fire Engineering.* http://www.mace.manchester.ac.uk/project/research/structures/strucfire.

BRE Center. 2012. *The Dalmarnock Fire Tests, 2006, UK.* Retrieved February 5, 2012, from http://www.see.ed.ac.uk/fire/dalmarnock.html.

Bukowski, R. W. 1991. "Fire Models: The Future Is Now!" *Fire Journal* 85 (2): 60–69.

———. 1995. "Modelling a Backdraft Incident: The 62 Watts Street (New York) Fire." *NFPA Journal* November/December: 85–89.

———. 1996. "Modelling a Backdraft Incident: The 62 Watts Street (New York) Fire." *Fire Engineers Journal* 56 (185): 14–17.

Bukowski, R. W., and R. C. Spetzler. 1992. "Analysis of the Happyland Social Club Fire with HAZARD I." *Fire and Arson Investigator* 42 (3): 37–47.

Davis, S. G., D. Engel, F. Gavelli, P. Hinze, and O. R. Hansen. 2010. "Advanced Methods for Determining the Origin of Vapor Cloud Explosions Case Study: 2006 Danvers Explosion Investigation." Paper presented at the International Symposium on Fire Investigation Science and Technology, September 27–29, College Park, MD.

DeHaan, J. D. 2005a. "Reliability of Fire Tests and Computer Modeling in Fire Scene Reconstruction: Part 1." *Fire & Arson Investigator* January: 40–45.

———. 2005b. "Reliability of Fire Tests and Computer Modeling in Fire Scene Reconstruction: Part 2." *Fire & Arson Investigator* April: 35–45.

DeHaan, J. D., and D. J. Icove. 2012. *Kirk's Fire Investigation.* 7th ed. Upper Saddle River, NJ: Pearson-Prentice Hall.

DeWitt, W. E., and D. W. Goff. 2000. "Forensic Engineering Assessment of FAST and FASTLite Fire Modeling Software." *National Academy of Forensic Engineers*, 9–19.

FireFOAM. 2012. *FM Research: Open Source Fire Modeling.* Retrieved May 27, 2012, from http://www.fmglobal.com.

Forney, G. P. 2015. *Smokeview (Version 6): A Tool for Visualizing Fire Dynamics Simulation Data.* Vol. I: *User's Guide.* NIST Special Publication 1017-1, Sixth Edition. Gaithersburg, MD: National Institute of Standards and Technology.

Forney, G. P., and W. F. Moss. 1991. *Analyzing and Exploiting Numerical Characteristic of Zone Models.* NSITIR 4763. Gaithersburg, MD: National Institute of Standards and Technology.

Friedman, R. 1992. "An International Survey of Computer Models for Fire and Smoke." *SFPE Journal of Fire Protection Engineering* 4 (3): 81–92.

FRS. 2012. *Fire Research Station, the Research-Based Consultancy and Testing Company of BRE.* Retrieved January 2012 from www.bre.co.uk/frs.

GexCon. 2012. *GexCon US.* Retrieved February 5, 2012, from http://www.gexcon.com.

Hunt, S. 2000. "Computer Fire Models." *NFPA Section News* 1 (2): 7–9.

Inberg, S. H. 1927. "Fire Tests of Office Occupancies." *NFPA Quarterly* 20 (243).

Iqbal, N., and M. H. Salley. 2004. *Fire Dynamics Tools (FDTs): Quantitative Fire Hazard Analysis Methods for the U.S. Nuclear Regulatory Commission Fire Protection Inspection Program.* Washington, DC.

Janssens, M. L., and D. M. Birk. 2000. *An Introduction to Mathematical Fire Modeling.* 2nd ed. Lancaster, PA: Technomic.

Kawagoe, K. 1958. "Fire Behavior in Rooms. Report No. 27." Tokyo: Building Research Institute.

Madrzykowski, D., and R. L. Vettori. 2000. "Simulation of the Dynamics of the Fire at 3146 Cherry Road, NE, Washington, DC, May 30, 1999." *NISTIR 6510.* Gaithersburg, MD: National Institute of Standards and Technology, Center for Fire Research.

Magnusson, S. E., and S. Thelandersson. 1970. "Temperature–Time Curves of the Complete Process of Fire Development. Theoretical Study of Wood Fuel Fires in Enclosed Spaces." *Civil and Building Construction Series No. 65.* Stockholm: Acta Polytechnica Scandinavia.

McGill, D. 2003. "Fire Dynamics Simulator, FDS 683, Participants' Handbook." Toronto, Ontario, Canada: Seneca College, School of Fire Protection.

McGrattan, K., H. Baum, R. Rehm, W. Mell, R. McDermott, S. Hostikka, and J. Floyd. 2010a. *Fire Dynamics Simulator (Version 5) Technical Reference Guide.* NIST Special Publication 1018-5. Gaithersburg, MD: National Institute of Standards and Technology.

McGrattan, K., R. McDermott, S. Hostikka, and J. Floyd. 2010b. *Fire Dynamics Simulator (Version 5) User's Guide.* NIST Special Publication 1019-5. Gaithersburg, MD: National Institute of Standards and Technology.

Milke, J. A., and F. W. Mowrer. 2001. "Application of Fire Behavior and Compartment Fire Models Seminar." Paper presented at the Tennessee Valley Society of Fire Protection Engineers (TVSFPE), September 27–28, Oak Ridge, TN.

Mitler, H. E. 1991. *Mathematical Modeling of Enclosure Fires.* Gaithersburg, MD: National Institute of Standards and Technology.

Moodie, K., and S. F. Jagger. 1992. "The King's Cross Fire: Results and Analysis from the Scale Model Tests." *Fire Safety Journal* 18 (1): 83–103, doi: 10.1016/0379-7112(92)90049-i.

Mowrer, F. W. 1992. "Methods of Quantitative Fire Hazard Analysis." Boston, MA: Society of Fire Protection Engineers, prepared for Electric Power Research Institute (EPRI).

———. 2003. "Spreadsheet Templates for Fire Dynamics Calculations." College Park, MD: University of Maryland.

Nelson, H. E. 1987. *An Engineering Analysis of the Early Stages of Fire Development: The Fire at the Dupont Plaza Hotel and Casino on December 31, 1986.* Gaithersburg, MD: National Institute of Standards and Technology.

———. 1989. "An Engineering View of the Fire of May 4, 1988, in the First Interstate Bank Building, Los Angeles, California." *NISTIR 89-4061.* Gaithersburg, MD: National Institute of Standards and Technology, Center for Fire Research.

———. 1990. *FPETool: Fire Protection Engineering Tools for Hazard Estimation.* Gaithersburg, MD: National Institute of Standards and Technology.

———. 1991. *History of Fire Technology.* Gaithersburg, MD: National Institute of Standards and Technology.

———. 1994. "Fire Growth Analysis of the Fire of March 20, 1990, Pulaski Building, 20 Massachusetts Avenue, NW, Washington, DC." *NISTIR 4489.* Gaithersburg, MD: National Institute of Standards and Technology, Center for Fire Research.

Nelson, H. E., and K. M. Tu. 1991. "Engineering Analysis of the Fire Development in the Hillhaven Nursing Home Fire, October 5, 1989." *NISTIR 4665.* Gaithersburg, MD: National Institute of Standards and Technology, Center for Fire Research.

NFPA. 2017. *NFPA 921: Guide for Fire and Explosion Investigations.* Quincy, MA: National Fire Protection Association.

Peacock, R. D., W. W. Jones, P. A. Reneke, and G. P. Forney. 2008. *CFAST: Consolidated Model of Fire Growth and Smoke Transport (Version 6) User's Guide.* NIST Special Publication 1041. Gaithersburg, Maryland: National Institute of Standards and Technology.

Peacock, R. D., P. A. Reneke, and G. P. Forney. 2016. *CFAST: Consolidated Model of Fire Growth and Smoke Transport (Version 7) User's Guide.* Volume 2: User's Guide, Special Publication 1041. Gaithersburg, Maryland: National Institute of Standards and Technology.

Rein, G., C. Abecassis-Empis, and R. Carvel. 2007. *The Dalmarnock Fire Tests: Experiments and Modelling.* Edinburgh, Scotland, UK: University of Edinburgh.

Rein, G., A. Bar-Ilan, A. C. Fernandez-Pello, and N. Alvares. 2006. "A Comparison of Three Models for the Simulation of Accidental Fires." *Journal of Fire Protection Engineering* 16 (3): 183–209.

Rein, G., J. L. Torero, W. Jahn, J. Stern-Gottfried, N. L. Ryder, S. Desanghere, M. Lazaaro, F. Mowrer, A. Coles, D. Joyeux, and D. Alvear. 2009. "Round-Robin Study of a Priori Modelling Predictions of the Dalmarnock Fire Test One." *Fire Safety Journal* 44 (4): 590–602, doi: 10.1016/j.firesaf.2008.12.008.

Salley, M. H., and R. P. Kassawar. 2007a. *Verification and Validation of Selected Fire Models for Nuclear Power Plant Applications: Consolidated Fire Growth and Smoke Transport Model (CFAST).* Washington, DC: US Nuclear Regulatory Commission.

———. 2007b. *Verification and Validation of Selected Fire Models for Nuclear Power Plant Applications: Experimental Uncertainty.* Washington, DC: US Nuclear Regulatory Commission.

———. 2007c. *Verification and Validation of Selected Fire Models for Nuclear Power Plant Applications: Fire Dynamics Simulator (FDS).* Washington, DC: US Nuclear Regulatory Commission.

———. 2007d. *Verification and Validation of Selected Fire Models for Nuclear Power Plant Applications: Fire Dynamics Tools (FDTs).* Washington, DC: US Nuclear Regulatory Commission.

———. 2007e. *Verification and Validation of Selected Fire Models for Nuclear Power Plant Applications: Fire-Induced Vulnerability Evaluation (FIVE-Rev1).* Washington, DC: US Nuclear Regulatory Commission.

———. 2007f. *Verification and Validation of Selected Fire Models for Nuclear Power Plant Applications: MAGIC.* Washington, DC: US Nuclear Regulatory Commission.

———. 2007g. *Verification and Validation of Selected Fire Models for Nuclear Power Plant Applications: Main Report.* Washington, DC: US Nuclear Regulatory Commission.

SFPE. 2008. *SFPE Handbook of Fire Protection Engineering.* 4th ed. Quincy, MA: National Fire Protection Association, Society of Fire Protection Engineers.

———. 2011. *Guidelines for Substantiating a Fire Model for a Given Application.* Bethesda, MD: Society of Fire Protection Engineers.

Thunderhead. 2012. *PyroSim Example Guide.* Manhattan, KS: Thunderhead Engineering.

———. 2015. *PyroSim Users Manual.* Manhattan, KS: Thunderhead Engineering.

Legal References

Ledbetter v. Blair Corporation, No. 3: 09-CV-843-WKW [WO] (M.D. Ala. June 27, 2012).

Santos v. State Farm Fire and Cas. Co. In Misc. 3d: NY: Supreme Court. 2010.

Turner v. Liberty Mutual Fire Insurance Co. Dist. Court, ND Ohio. 2007.

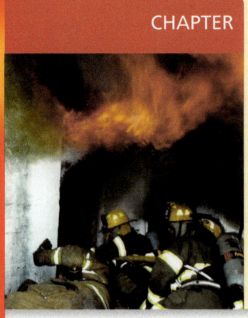

CHAPTER 10

Fire Testing

Courtesy of Greg Lampkin, Knox County Sheriff's Office, Tennessee, Fire Investigation Unit

KEY TERMS

autoignition temperature, *p. 633*

calorimetry, *p. 636*

elastomers, *p. 643*

fire testing, *p. 629*

flash point of a liquid, *p. 636*

furniture calorimeter, *p. 638*

natural fibers, *p. 646*

spontaneous ignition temperature (SIT), *p. 633*

synthetic fibers, *p. 647*

OBJECTIVES

After reading this chapter, you should be able to:

- Recognize the value of fire testing.
- Describe the basic types of fire tests and give examples of each.
- Learn how to interpolate scaled test data to real-world scenarios.
- Appreciate the use of fire test data in the analysis and evaluation of a working hypothesis.
- Identify the common causes of fires in fabrics, upholstered furniture, and mattresses.
- Identify the common types of cloth.
- Explain the basic concepts of the flammability.
- List and explain common tests used to measure cigarette ignition, flame ignition, heat release rate, smoke, and toxicity.
- List and separately describe several flammability tests (examples: clothing, textiles, plastic films, carpets and rugs, mattresses and pads, children's sleepwear, upholstered furniture).
- Search the Internet for current and proposed governmental policies and legislation.

ire testing is a form of physical modeling in which testing or experimentation is conducted using materials related to a case or study. Testing conducted in support of fire reconstruction can span the range from simple field tests requiring no equipment to benchtop flame tests to extensively instrumented, full-scale test burns in real buildings (see Figure 10-1).

NFPA 921 (NFPA 2017, pt. 22.5.1) states, "**Fire testing** is a tool that can provide data that complement data collected at the fire scene (see pt. 4.3.3), or can be used to test hypotheses (see pt. 4.3.6). Such fire testing can range in scope from bench scale testing to full-scale recreations of the entire event" (NFPA 2017).

Fire tests can help confirm or reject hypotheses about the fire's ignition or spread, test and validate the predictions of computational models or those of experienced investigators, or demonstrate the roles of various factors in the fire and its effects on occupants. This chapter explores, in summary form, many of the tests useful in fire investigation.

The criteria for using fire test information in forensic fire scene reconstructions are whether the test was correctly performed, whether the data were accurately collected and reported, and whether the test was appropriate and applicable to the situation under consideration. Fire tests are designed to collect certain data in a reproducible and valid manner. The investigator must ask:

- Did the fuels, conditions, and ignition mechanism reproduce the fire in question?
- Were the tests designed to follow American Society for Testing and Materials (ASTM) or National Fire Protection Association (NFPA) standards? If not, what factors were considered in its design?
- What variables were considered and how were they controlled? Fuel moisture, fuel mass and quantity, physical state, ambient temperature and humidity, heat flux, and oxygen content all play important roles in ignition, flame spread, and heat release.

fire testing ■ A tool that can provide data that complement data collected at the fire scene (see pt. 4.3.3), or can be used to test hypotheses (see pt. 4.3.6). Such fire testing can range in scope from bench scale testing to full-scale recreations of the entire event (NFPA 2017).

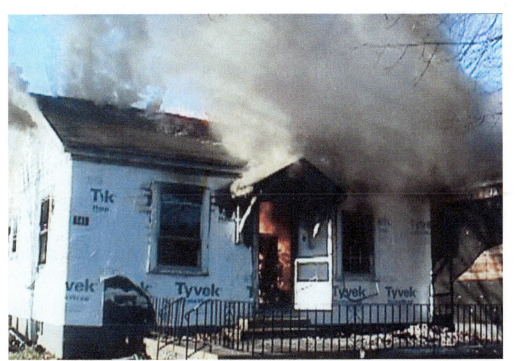

FIGURE 10-1 Testing for fire reconstruction purposes can span the range from simple field tests requiring no equipment to extensively instrumented full-scale test burns on real buildings. *Courtesy of Det. Michael Dalton (ret.), Knox County Sheriff's Office.*

- If it was a custom-designed test, what data could be fairly and accurately collected and analyzed?
- Was there a planned series of tests to examine the sensitivity and reproducibility of the data? Because of the importance of fire test data in both criminal and civil fire investigations, it is imperative that tests be conducted and data be interpreted without misrepresentation in a balanced, impartial, and reproducible manner.

Tests applied to fabrics and finished household goods reflect only the ignitability of the product—its susceptibility to being accidentally ignited. These tests do not determine whether a fabric will burn and contribute to a room's fuel load in a given room fire. All fabrics will burn if the temperature, ventilation, and duration of the fire are sufficient; even highly fire-resistant fabrics of Nomex or PBI will burn under the right conditions. These comments on fabrics and their fire tests are offered to assist the investigator in assessing the logical consequences of ignition from small flames or glowing embers that come in contact with apparel or upholstered furniture.

Although the total number of residential fires in the United States continues to decrease, fires in which upholstered furniture, bedding, mattresses, garments, and draperies were the first fuels to be ignited accounted for 14.3 percent or an estimated 26,900 residential fires (out of 384,100 total) and 1,030 deaths each year in the United States for the period 2004–2006 but were involved in approximately 40 percent of all residential fire deaths (Miller 2015).

The NFPA estimates that from 2002–2005, upholstered furniture alone was the item first ignited in an average of 7,630 home structure fires per year, causing an annual average of 600 civilian fire deaths, 920 civilian fire injuries, and $309 million in direct property damage (Ahrens 2008). Fires beginning with upholstered furniture accounted for only 2 percent of *reported* home fires but 21 percent of home fire deaths. During the same time frame, a mattress or bedding was the first fuel ignited in an average of 11,520 home fires. Such fires accounted for 3 percent of the fires but 13 percent of home fire deaths (378 deaths, 1,286 civilian injuries, and $357 million in direct property damage) (Ahrens 2008).

According to the CPSC, ignition of upholstered furniture was caused by cigarettes or other smoking materials in an estimated 29 percent of home fires and by open flames in about 16 percent. Ignition of mattresses and bedding was caused in about 22 percent of home fires by smoking materials and in 26 percent by open flames (Miller, Chowdhury, and Green 2009). The NFPA estimated (in 2008) that 14 percent of mattress/bedding home fires and 12 percent of upholstered furniture fires were ignited by smoking materials (Hall 2008).

Although garment fires may not frequently go on to cause structural damage, the NFPA estimated that in the years 1999–2000, 120 people died and 150 people were injured (per year) because their clothing caught fire (Rohr 2005). A more recent study by Hoebel et al. used burn injury data from the National Electronic Injury Surveillance System (NEISS) and death data from the National Center for Health Statistics (NCHS) of the Centers for Disease Control and Prevention (CDC). This study revealed that many clothing fires are not reported to the local fire departments and, therefore, do not appear in the NFIRS or NFPA data. This analysis revealed that nearly 4,300 injuries and 120 deaths per year were caused (1997–2006) when peoples' clothes caught fire (Hoebel et al. 2010).

The overall number of upholstered furniture, mattress, and bedding fires in homes has decreased dramatically since the 1980s as fire-retardant materials have become more commonly used in some furnishings and as public awareness of the hazards has improved

(Hall 2001, Krasny, Parker, Babrauskas 2001). Fires in which fabrics are the first materials to be ignited continue to be a common occurrence. The fire investigator should be familiar with the nature of common fabrics and upholstery materials and their contributions to both ignition hazard and fuel load in today's studies.

10.1 ASTM and CFR Flammability Tests

Several of the ASTM tests can be used to assess the ignitability of materials or the nature and speed of flame propagation, and they are discussed briefly here. However, as you will see, there are limitations to the application of results of these tests to an actual case. Many limitations are due mostly to the geometry or size of the sample.

A flame will spread much more quickly upward than it will downward or outward in the same fuel. A fire started at the top edge of a sofa back will spread much more slowly than if the same fabric is ignited at the base of the sofa. A fire ignited at the top of hanging draperies will be much more likely to cause the hooks and drapery rod to fail and collapse with the draperies, possibly resulting in dropdown ignition of materials beneath, whereas draperies ignited at the bottom are often nearly completely consumed before they cause failure of their supports.

Fire resistance properties are sometimes built into a combination of layers of fabrics and backings that result in acceptable ignition resistance. Separating and testing the layers individually may yield very misleading results. The residual moisture in test samples also can affect their ignitability, so specimens are often conditioned for 24 to 48 hours under specific criteria prior to testing.

Most ASTM standard methods include an advisory comment regarding use of the method to compare materials or their performance under controlled conditions to assess the possible contributions a material might make under a specific set of fire conditions, not to predict what a product will do when exposed to different fire conditions.

Tests designed by the National Fire Protection Association (NFPA), American Society for Testing and Materials (ASTM), and the US Consumer Product Safety Commission (CPSC) include the following:

- *Flammability of Clothing Textiles (16 CFR 1610-U.S.):* This test requires that a sample of fabric 50 mm × 150 mm (2 in. × 6 in.) placed in a holder at a 45° angle and exposed to a small flame touching its surface for 1 second not ignite and spread flame up the length of the sample in less than 3.5 seconds for smooth fabrics or 4.0 seconds for napped fabrics. Test sample must be oven dried and cooled prior to the test.

- *ASTM D 1230-10: Standard Test Method for Flammability of Apparel Textiles (ASTM 2010b; not identical with 16 CFR 1610-U.S.):* CPSC requires fabrics introduced into commerce to meet requirements of *16 CFR 1610*. This test is suitable for textile fabrics as they reach the consumer or for apparel other than children's sleepwear or special protective garments. A sample of fabric 50 mm × 150 mm (2 in. × 6 in.) is held at a 45° angle in a metal holder and a controlled flame is applied to the bottom end for 1 second. The time required for the flame to proceed up the fabric a distance of 127 mm (5 in.) is recorded.

- *Flammability of Vinyl Plastic Film (16 CFR 1611-U.S.):* This test requires that vinyl plastic film (for wearing apparel) placed in a holder at a 45° angle and ignited not burn at a rate exceeding 3.0 cm (1.2 in.) per second.

- *Flammability of Carpets and Rugs: 16 CFR 1630-U.S. (Large Carpets) and 16 CFR 1631-U.S. (Small Carpets):* A specimen of carpet is placed under a steel plate with a 20.32-cm (8-in.)-diameter circular hole. A methenamine tablet is placed in the center of the hole and ignited. The duration of burning and heat release rate of the tablet duplicate those of a typical dropped match. If the specimen chars more than 3 in., in any direction, it is considered a fail. The ambient radiant heat flux is minimal, because the sample is tested at room temperature. The ignition source is a modest 50 to 80 W flame of brief duration. Testing has shown that some carpets that pass this test will be readily ignited and spread flames if the radiant heat flux is larger as a result of a larger and more prolonged ignition source. The carpet is tested in the flat, horizontal position, so the same carpet mounted vertically may behave very differently.

- *ASTM D2859-06: Standard Test Method for Ignition Characteristics of Finished Textile Floor Covering Materials* (ASTM 2010c): This method uses a steel plate 22.9 cm (9 in.) square and 0.64 cm (0.25 in.) thick with a 20.32-cm (8-in.)-diameter circular hole. A methenamine tablet is placed in the center and ignited in a draft-free enclosure. Samples are thoroughly oven-dried and cooled in a desiccator before being tested. The product fails if the charred portion reaches within 25 mm (1 in.) of the edge of the hole in the steel plate. Eight specimens are tested. The Flammable Fabrics Act (FFA) regulations require that at least seven of the eight specimens pass this test.

- *Flammability of Mattresses and Pads (16 CFR 1632-U.S.):* A minimum of nine regular tobacco cigarettes are burned at various locations on the bare mattress—quilted and smooth portions, tape edge, tufted pockets, and so forth. The char length of the mattress surface must not be more than 50 mm (2 in.) from any cigarette in any direction. The test is repeated with the cigarettes placed between two sheets covering the mattress.

- *Standard for the Flammability (Open Flame) of Mattress Sets (16 CFR 1633-U.S):* This test method is a full-scale test based on NIST research. The mattress or mattress and foundation set is exposed to a pair of T-shaped propane burners for a short time and allowed to burn freely for 30 minutes. The burners are designed to represent burning bedclothes. Measurements are taken to determine the heat release rate from the specimen and total heat energy generated from the fire. The standard establishes two test criteria, both of which the mattress set must meet to comply with the standard. (1) The peak heat release rate for the specimen must not exceed 200 kW at any time during the 30-minute test. (2) The total heat release must not exceed 15 MJ for the first 10 minutes of the test (*Federal Register* 71 (no. 50), March 15, 2006).

- *Flammability of Children's Sleepwear (16 CFR 1615 and 1616-U.S.):* Each of five 88.9 cm × 25.4 cm (35 in. × 10 in.) specimens is suspended vertically in a holder in a cabinet and exposed to a small gas flame along its bottom edge for 3 seconds. The specimens cannot have an average char length of more than 18 cm (7 in.), no single specimen can have a char length of 25.4 cm (10 in.) (full burn), and no single sample can have flaming material on the bottom of the cabinet 10 seconds after the ignition source is removed. These requirements are for finished items (as produced or after one washing and drying) and after the items have been washed and dried 50 times.

- *ASTM E1352-80a: Standard Test Method for Cigarette Ignition Resistance of Mock-Up Upholstered Furniture Assemblies* (ASTM 2008a): This test uses reduced-scale plywood mock-ups [47 cm × 56 cm (18 in. × 22 in.)] upholstered with simulations of seat, backrest, and armrests to test ignitability of furniture to dropped smoldering cigarettes. The test is employed for furniture to be used in public and private occupancies such as nursing homes and hospitals. The cigarettes are positioned on each of the various surfaces and along crevices between seats, armrest, and back. The distance of char extension from each cigarette or ignition by open flame is recorded for comparison.

- *ASTM E1353-08ae1: Standard Test Method for Cigarette Ignition Resistance of Components of Upholstered Furniture* (ASTM 2008b): This test uses mock-ups to test individual components—cover fabrics, welt cords, interior fabrics, and filling or batting materials in the form, geometry, and combination in which they are used in real furniture. This test uses single cigarettes, but each is covered with a single layer of cotton sheeting that retains more heat and makes it a more severe test than one in open air.

- **ASTM E648-15e1: Standard Test Method for Critical Radiant Flux of Floor-Covering Systems Using a Radiant Heat Energy Source (ASTM 2015d):** This test uses a horizontally mounted floor covering specimen [20 cm × 99 cm (8 in. × 39 in.)] with a gas-fired radiant heater (with a gas pilot burner) mounted at a 30° angle above it that produces a radiant heat flux of 1 to 10 kW/m². The distance the flame propagates along the sample indicates the minimum radiant heat flux for ignition and propagation.

10.1.1 ASTM TEST METHODS FOR OTHER MATERIALS

The ASTM International Committee E05 on Fire Standards identifies methods for testing other materials.

- **ASTM D1929-14: Standard Test Method for Determining Ignition Temperature of Plastics (ASTM 2014b; ISO 871):** This test uses a cylindrical hot-air furnace to heat the test sample in a pan. A thermocouple monitors the temperature of the sample while the temperature is adjusted so that pyrolysis gases venting through the top of the chamber can be ignited by a small pilot flame held near it, which establishes the *flash ignition temperature* (FIT). The same apparatus can be used to establish the **spontaneous ignition temperature (SIT)** by eliminating the pilot flame and observing the sample visually for flaming or glowing combustion (or a rapid rise in the sample temperature). SITs for common plastics are 20°C to 50°C (68°F to 122°F) higher than FITs by this technique. The test requires 3 g of material for each test in the form of pellets, powder, or cut-up solids or films.

- **ASTM E119-15: Standard Test Methods for Fire Tests of Building Construction and Materials (ASTM 2015c):** A specimen (wall assembly, floor, door, etc.) is exposed to a standard fire exposure to evaluate the duration for which those assemblies will contain a fire or retain their integrity. A large furnace (horizontal or vertical) is used to create a standard time–temperature environment. The assembly is exposed to the prescribed conditions, and its surface temperature is measured, its structural integrity is monitored, and the time for penetration of flame through it is determined. The standard time–temperature exposure does not accurately reflect all real-world fire exposures, so the performance rating of tested building components is for comparison only.

- **ASTM E659-15: Standard Test Method for Autoignition Temperature of Liquid Chemicals (ASTM 2015e):** A small sample (100 μL) of liquid is injected into the mouth of a glass flask heated to a predetermined temperature, and the flask is observed for the presence of a flash flame inside the flask and a sudden rise in internal temperature (as monitored by an internal thermocouple). If no ignition is observed, the temperature is increased and the test repeated until the material ignites reliably. This method establishes the *hot-flame* **autoignition temperature** (AIT) in air. Ignition delay times may also be recorded. The temperature at which small sharp rises occur in the internal temperature alone is the *cool-flame autoignition temperature*.

- The method can also be used for solid fuels that melt and vaporize or sublimate completely at the test temperatures, leaving no solid residues. The test conditions are controlled by the heat transfer between the glass flask and the fuel introduced and the confined geometry of the spherical flask. In real-world ignitions, the nature of the surface and the manner of contact will determine the convective heat transfer coefficient and may modify times or temperatures. Any geometry (tube or enclosure) that keeps the fuel in contact with the hot surface is going to produce ignitions at lower temperatures than an open, flat surface, where buoyancy of the heated vapors can transport the fuel away from the heated surface.

- **ASTM D3675-14: Standard Test Method for Surface Flammability of Flexible Cellular Materials Using a Radiant Heat Energy Source (ASTM 2014c):** This method uses a gas-fired radiant heat panel [30 cm × 46 cm (12 in. × 18 in.)] in front of an

spontaneous ignition temperature (SIT) ▪ The lowest temperature at which a combustible material ignites in air without a spark or flame (*NFPA 921*, 2014 ed., pt. 3.3.15).

autoignition temperature ▪ The lowest temperature at which a combustible material ignites in air without a spark or flame (NFPA 2017, pt. 3.3.16).

inclined specimen of material [15 cm × 46 cm (6 in. × 18 in.)], oriented so that ignition with a pilot flame first occurs at the upper edge of the sample and the flame front moves downward. The rate at which the flame moves downward is observed, and a flame spread index is calculated. The test is suitable for any material that may be exposed to fire. At least four specimens must be tested.

■ *ASTM D3659-80e1: Standard Test Method for Flammability of Apparel Fabrics by Semi-restraint Method* (ASTM 1993):   This test simulates the burning characteristics of a garment hanging vertically from the shoulders of a wearer. Test specimens are 15 cm × 38 cm (6 in. × 15 in.) (five specimens required) and are oven-dried and weighed prior to testing. The sample is hung vertically from a crossbar, and the flame of a small gas burner is positioned against the bottom edge of the fabric for 3 seconds and then removed. The weight (percentage area) destroyed by the flame and the time required are the criteria for comparison. (Cross-reference to *FF 3-71: Flammability of Children's Sleepwear, Sizes 0–6X*.)

■ *ASTM E84-15a: Standard Test Method for Surface Burning Characteristics of Building Materials* (ASTM 2015a):   This is the "Steiner Tunnel" test, which mounts specimens on the underside of the top of an insulated tunnel 7.6 m (25 ft) long, 30 cm (12 in.) high, and 45 cm (17.75 in.) wide. A gas burner at one end ignites the sample, and the rate of flame spread along the length of the specimen is observed and recorded. The test specimen must measure at least 51 cm × 7.32 m (20 in. × 24 ft). An optical density measurement system (light source and photocell) is mounted in the vent pipe of the apparatus. Samples of products of combustion can be taken downstream of the photometer. The upside-down configuration of this test apparatus is not often found in real-world situations except with combustible ceiling coverings.

■ *ASTM E1321-13: Standard Test Method for Determining Material Ignition and Flame Spread Properties* (ASTM 2013d):   This method tests for the ignition and flame spread properties of a vertically oriented fuel surface when exposed to an external radiant heat flux. The results can be used to calculate the minimum radiant heat flux and temperature needed for ignition and flame spread. The test configuration is a large, vertically mounted specimen and a gas-fired radiant panel heater mounted at an angle to it. A gas pilot flame is used, and the rate and distance of flame spread along the length of the specimen are recorded (see Figure 10-2).

■ *ASTM E800-14: Standard Guide for Measurement of Gases Present or Generated during Fires* (ASTM 2014d):   This guide describes methods for properly collecting and preserving combustion gas samples during fire tests and analytical methods for O_2, CO, CO_2, N_2, HCl, HCN, NOx, and SOx, using gas chromatography, infrared, or wet chemical methods. As we have seen, some fuels produce high concentrations

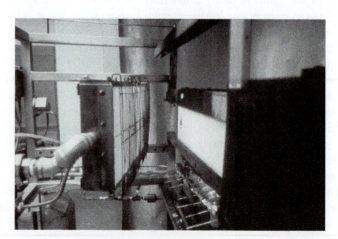

FIGURE 10-2 Surface rate of flame spread test (*ASTM E1321*) uses a radiant heat panel at an angle to the surface being tested. *Courtesy of NIST.*

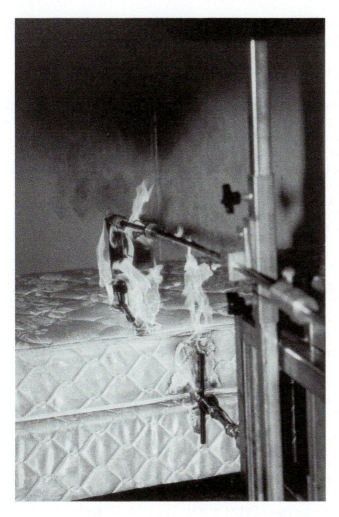

FIGURE 10-3 The *TB 603* test in use on a mattress. All mattresses sold in the United States for residential use after July 1, 2007, must pass the *16 CFR 1633* test, which has a total heat release limit of 15 MJ, compared with the 25 MJ limit of this test. *Courtesy of Bureau of Electronics & Appliance Repair, Home Furnishings.*

of toxic or irritant gases under various fire conditions. Testing materials known to be present in a fatal fire may yield clues as to what role their combustion gases played in the fatality.

■ *California TB 603 Standard for Mattresses, Box Springs, and Futons* (**California Department of Consumer Affairs 2002**): After January 1, 2005, the state of California required that bedding materials sold for residential and commercial use comply with new testing procedures. The test is designed to simulate real-world flaming ignition sources and measure the energy released from burning bedding materials. The top and side of the mattress are exposed to T-shaped gas burners for a period of time (as in Figure 10-3). Failure of the test can be either (1) a peak heat release rate of 200 kW or greater within 30 minutes after ignition or (2) a total heat release of 25 MJ or greater within 10 minutes of ignition. As of July 1, 2007, all mattresses, mattress and foundation in sets, and futons sold for residential use in the United States must pass the *16 CFR 1633* test, which is similar, except it requires that the total heat released must not exceed 15 MJ in the first 10 minutes.

10.1.2 FLASH AND FIRE POINTS OF LIQUIDS

Tests for flash and fire (flame) points of ignitable liquids can be as simple as placing a few drops of the fuel in a petri dish or watch glass at room temperature and waving a lighted match near the surface of the liquid. Ignition will confirm that the material is a Class I A or B flammable liquid with a flash point below room temperature (23°C [73°F]). More reliable testing requires more controlled evaporation and confinement of the vapors with a more reproducible ignition source.

Flash point testing generally involves taking a quantity of liquid fuel and placing it in the cup of a water bath whose temperature is gradually increased. The cup may be open to the atmosphere or closed with a small shutter. A very small flame is introduced periodically, and the cup is observed for the presence of a brief flash of flame. The fire point of many liquids may be established by the open-cup method by increasing the temperature until a self-sustaining flame is established rather than just a flash of flame.

Closed-cup testers retain some of the vapor produced and make it easier to ignite. Closed-cup flash points are typically a few degrees lower than open-cup determinations of the same fuel.

Tests for flash and fire points of liquids include the following:

- *ASTM D56-05: Standard Test Method for Flash Point by Tag Closed Cup Tester* (ASTM 2010a): Applicable to low-viscosity liquids with flash points below 93°C (200°F). Requires 50 mL of liquid for each test. (Sometimes abbreviated TCC.)
- *ASTM D92-12b2: Standard Test Method for Flash and Fire Points by Cleveland Open Cup Tester* (ASTM 2012a): Applicable to all petroleum products with flash points above 79°C (175°F) and below 400°C (752°F) except fuel oils. Requires at least 70 mL for each test. (Sometimes abbreviated COC.)
- *ASTM D93-15b: Standard Test Methods for Flash Point by Pensky-Martens Closed-Cup Tester* (ASTM 2015b): Applicable for petroleum products with a flash point in the range of 40°C to 360°C (104°F to 680°F) including fuel oils, lubricating oils, suspensions, and higher-viscosity liquids. Requires at least 75 mL of fuel for each test.
- *ASTM D1310-14: Standard Test Method for Flash Point and Fire Point of Liquids by Tag Open-Cup Apparatus* (ASTM 2014a): Applicable for liquids with flash points between 218°C and 165°C (0°F and 325°F) and fire points up to 165°C (325°F) will work at subambient temperatures. Fire point criterion: When fuel ignites and burns for at least 5 seconds. Requires 75 mL of sample for each test.
- *ASTM D3278-96: Standard Test Methods for Flash Point of Liquids by Small Scale Closed-Cup Apparatus* (ASTM 2011): Suitable for flash point determination of fuels with a flash point between 0°C and 110°C (32°F to 230°F) in small quantities (2 mL required for each test). Employs a micro-scale apparatus sold as the Setaflash Tester. Test methods similar to those for ISO 3679 and 3680 will work on subambient determinations.
- *ASTM D3828-12a: Standard Test Methods for Flash Point by Small Scale Closed Tester* (ASTM 2012b): Similar to *ASTM D3278*. Employed to establish whether a product will flash at a given temperature, using 2 to 4 mL of sample for each test.

Owing to the multiplicity of flash point test methods, the *ASTM E502-07* offers a *Standard Test Method for Selection and Use of ASTM Standards for the Determination of Flash Points of Chemicals by Closed-Cup Methods* (ASTM 2013b).

10.1.3 CALORIMETRY

Classical bomb **calorimetry** is used to measure the total heat of combustion of fuels [as in *ASTM D4809-13* (ASTM 2013a)]. The term *bomb* refers to a sealed vessel that can withstand internal pressures. The procedure involves burning a weighed specimen in a sealed container with an excess of oxygen until the specimen is completely oxidized. The heat generated by the combustion is determined by measuring the increase in temperature of the sealed vessel and using its specific heat and mass to calculate the heat released in the combustion. This test is unsuitable for fuels comprising multiple substances, as it yields the *total* heat of combustion, not the *effective* heat of combustion, which accounts for losses due to incomplete combustion.

flash point of a liquid ■ The lowest temperature of a liquid, as determined by specific laboratory tests, at which the liquid gives off vapors at a sufficient rate to support a momentary flame across its surface (NFPA 2017, pt. 3.3.82).

calorimetry ■ A test used to measure the total heat of combustion of fuels (as in *ASTM D4809-13*).

Because almost all common fuels yield nearly the same amount of heat per mass of oxygen consumed (13 kJ/g), one could easily calculate the heat generated by measuring the amount of oxygen consumed during the combustion process. This procedure is called *oxygen consumption* (or oxygen depletion) *calorimetry*. If a specimen is burned in air and the waste products are all drawn into a system of ducts, the O_2, CO, and CO_2 concentrations can be measured. If the ventilation rate into the test chamber and through the exhaust duct is measured, the amount of oxygen consumption can be determined. Optical sensors in the ductwork can also monitor the optical density and obscuration of smoke products generated. Note that both the oxygen consumption and the heat release rate are calculated from collected data.

This approach has been refined into four general categories of size and application: cone, furniture, room, and industrial calorimeters. In the *cone calorimeter*, developed by Babrauskas at NIST and described in *ASTM E1354-15a* (ASTM 2015f), a 10 cm × 10 cm (4 in. × 4 in.) specimen in a metal tray is exposed to a uniform incident radiant heat flux from a cone-shaped electric heater mounted above it (as in Figure 10-4).

The radiant flux striking the sample can be controlled by adjusting the temperature of the heater element. A small electric arc source is introduced to ignite the plume of smoke generated by the heating and then removed. The flame and smoke vent upward through the center of the cone heater, and the gases are ducted to where the flow rate; O_2, CO, and CO_2 concentrations; and smoke obscuration are measured. The entire specimen tray is mounted on a sensitive load cell, so the mass loss is continuously measured. The analysis calculates the heat release rate (expressed per unit surface area of fuel), mass loss rate, and effective heat of combustion. Even though the samples tested are reduced scale, testing has shown that the results have a high degree of correlation with real-world fire performance (Babrauskas 1997). The system works with liquid or solid fuels (even low-melting-point thermoplastic materials) in the horizontal configuration. Wood and other rigid fuels can also be tested in the vertical configuration.

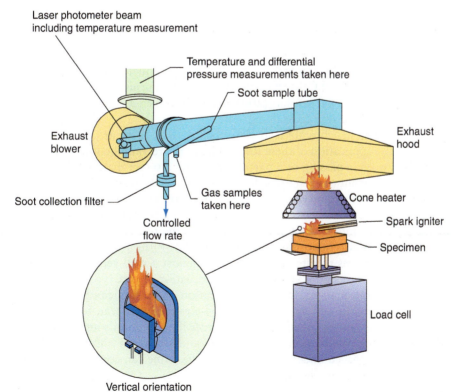

Laser photometer beam including temperature measurement

Temperature and differential pressure measurements taken here

Soot sample tube

Exhaust blower

Exhaust hood

Soot collection filter

Gas samples taken here

Cone heater

Spark igniter

Specimen

Controlled flow rate

Load cell

Vertical orientation

FIGURE 10-4 In the cone calorimeter, developed by Babrauskas at NIST and described in ASTM E1354-11b, a 10 cm × 10 cm (4 in. × 4 in.) specimen in a metal tray is exposed to a uniform incident radiant heat flux from a cone-shaped electric heater mounted above it. *Courtesy of Dr. Vytenis Babrauskas, Fire Science & Technology, San Diego, California.*

furniture calorimeter ■
An instrumental sys-
tem for measuring
the amount of heat
produced by the com-
bustion of a moderate-
sized fuel package, and
the rate at which the
heat is produced.

Furniture calorimeters were developed to test the heat release rate of single items of full-scale real furniture by the same method. Here, the furniture is mounted on a load cell and burned in the open, with all combustion products drawn into a vent hood. The temperature; pressure; and O_2, CO, and CO_2 concentrations are measured in the ductwork. The calculated heat release rate can then be combined with the mass loss data from the load cell to calculate the effective heat of combustion.

When multiple pieces of furniture, along with carpet, wall linings, and other fuels, are to be evaluated as a fuel package, a *room calorimeter* is used. In this case a room is built [often to a standard size of 2.4 m × 3.6 m × 2.4 m (8 ft × 12 ft × 8 ft)], and the entire room becomes the collector for the exhaust vent. The combustion products vent through the door opening and are drawn up into the exhaust hood and measured. This arrangement allows heat release rate to be calculated constantly as fire spreads from one item to another, even culminating in near-flashover conditions.

The largest-scale devices are often called *industrial calorimeters*. These are basically a large exhaust hood with appropriate fans, ducting, and instrumentation. They are generally located in high-bay buildings. Typical measuring capacities are 12 kW (cone calorimeter), 1.5 to 5 MW (furniture calorimeter), 3 to 6 MW (room calorimeter), and 10 to 50 MW (industrial calorimeter). The latter would be most useful for performing fire scene reconstructions; unfortunately, most of these devices are owned by organizations (e.g., UL, ATF) that do not offer commercial testing services for fire reconstruction. Southwest Research Institute (San Antonio, Texas) has 4 to 10 MW calorimeters available for commercial fire reconstruction projects.

Tests for ignitability of upholstered furniture vary widely, from cigarette ignition to small flames to larger gas-fired burners of known heat output (typically 17 to 40 kW). They may be applicable to standardized small-scale mock-ups of furnishings as well as to the actual items taken from the production line. Pass/fail criteria may be based on observable flame spread, penetration, percentage mass loss, peak heat release rate, quantity of smoke produced, or toxicity of fire gases.

10.1.4 TEST METHODS

Various test methods in use today include those described under the US Code of Federal Regulations (CFR), British Standards (BS), International Organization for Standardization (ISO), ASTM, and California Bureau of Home Furnishings Technical Bulletins (TB). Krasny, Parker, and Babrauskas (2001) have assembled a comprehensive description and discussion of the current techniques.

As with the bench-scale tests described earlier, there are limitations and cautions regarding the application of these test results to the reconstruction of real-world fires. For example, the mere passing of a particular test by a target material does not imply that it will be fire resistant or even fire safe in a real-world environment.

Other cautions to be observed include requirements for conditioning samples for 24 to 48 hours at a particular temperature and humidity. The investigator should be aware of the potential influence of such variables on the test result. The geometry of the test compartment is also important. The same piece of furniture may yield different heat outputs or fire patterns if tested in a corner or against a wall versus in the center of a large room that minimizes radiant feedback or ventilation effects.

The location, manner, means, and duration of ignition can play a significant role in the fire performance of furnishings. A vinyl-covered chair seat, for instance, can provide substantial resistance to small ignition sources if an ignition source is placed on the seat. (PVC upholstery tends to char, intumesce, and shield the substrate.) But even a small flaming source placed under the seat, where the flame can contact the polyurethane padding, will readily ignite the chair.

10.1.5 CIGARETTE IGNITION OF UPHOLSTERED FURNITURE

Cigarette ignition of upholstered furniture was a major fire cause for decades owing to the predominant use of cotton or linen upholstery fabrics over cellulosic padding of cotton, coir, kapok, or similar materials, all of which were easily ignited by a glowing cigarette.

Holleyhead (1999) published an extensive review of the literature regarding cigarette ignition of furniture. However, a great deal of misinformation once existed about the time required for such ignition to result in flaming combustion. Investigators erroneously concluded that such ignitions always required 1 to 2 hours, inferring that any flaming ignition in a shorter time must have been the result of deliberate ignition by open flame.

Extensive testing by the California Bureau of Home Furnishings and NIST (then NBS), first reported in the early 1980s, demonstrated that ignition time was variable. Transition to flaming combustion was reported in as little as 22 minutes from the placement of a glowing cigarette between the cushions, or between the cushions and an arm or backrest. Other tests required 1 to 3 hours, and some never transitioned to open flames and smoldered for hours before self-extinguishing. Even identically built mock-ups demonstrated a wide variety of behaviors. A statistical analysis of these results was published by Babrauskas and Krasny (1997).

Tests by the authors have demonstrated similar time and ignition results. If the fabric is torn and the cigarette drops into direct contact with cotton padding that has not been treated to be flame retardant, transition to flame has been observed in as little as 18 minutes in still air. The presence of drafts can influence the progress and increase the heat release rate of smoldering cellulosics. One informal test by DeHaan with a cigarette wrapped loosely in a cotton towel and left outside in a light, variable wind resulted in flames about 15 minutes after placement. Hand-rolled cigarettes present a lower ignition risk because they tend to self-extinguish more often than commercially made tobacco cigarettes. For references and testing of cannabis resin cigarettes on petrol-soaked clothing, see the work by Jewell, Thomas, and Dodds (2011).

According to the NFPA-sponsored website firesafecigarrettes.org, all 50 states have passed legislation mandating what are called self-extinguishing, or fire-safe, cigarettes (FSC). The European Union (EU) established standards for its member countries and required as of November 17, 2011, that all cigarettes sold in the EU be reduced ignition propensity (RIP) cigarettes. The term RIP is a more technically accurate term than fire-safe for these cigarettes, because it means that they have been designed to be less likely than a conventional cigarette to ignite soft furnishings such as a couch or mattress. These redesigned cigarettes will only reduce chances for cigarette ignition of upholstered materials in the future but will not prevent all ignitions. Fire-safe cigarettes typically use a banded paper with alternating high and low porosity in the bands, which causes smoldering to cease.

Latex or natural rubber foam is also easily ignited by contact with a glowing cigarette. A cigarette will be consumed in a maximum of 20 to 25 minutes after being lit, somewhat longer if tucked between seat cushions. Ignition times longer than that result from a self-sustaining smolder in the surrounding fuel initiated by the cigarette, as confirmed by the significant quantity of white smoke that is produced for some minutes prior to flame—far more than can arise from a single cigarette.

10.2 Physical Tests

10.2.1 SCALE MODELS

A great deal of useful information can be obtained from building scaled-down replicas of rooms or furnishings for testing, at reduced cost and complexity compared with full-scale recreations. These models are particularly valuable for testing ignition and incipient fire hypotheses in which the interaction of room surfaces or conditions does not play a major role.

When radiant heat or ventilation factors are involved, the test must take into account that all factors in a fire do not scale down in the same linear fashion as the room dimensions. For instance, ventilation through an opening is controlled by the area of the opening and the square root of its height. It is possible to calculate corrections for such factors, but it is not as simple as building a dollhouse, with all doors and windows in the same proportion as in full scale. Radiant heat flux falls off with the inverse square $(1/r^2)$ of the separation distance, so scale-model builders must keep those relationships in mind as well.

As with all fire investigation tools available to the investigator, a *reduced-scale enclosure* (RSE) can provide a lot of information that may be very helpful and is relatively simple to build and burn. The hot smoke is dynamically a fluid, so its movement through a *full-scale enclosure* (FSE) tends to be similar to that through a RSE. In an early paper, Quintiere evaluated various scaling considerations regarding heat transfer and smoke movement (Quintiere 1989).

Current research in ventilation openings (doors) in RSEs is investigating scaling the vertical dimension but adjusting the width to maintain the entrained air mass flow rate by modifying the ventilation factor $A_0\sqrt{h_0}$, where A_o is the area of the door opening, and h_o is the height of the door opening. For example, if the scale is one-fourth (0.25), then the width of the RSE door is $\sqrt{0.25}$ (or 0.5) times the width of the FSE door. Thus, a 30-in. door opening at one-fourth (0.25) scale would be 7-1/2 in. wide, but with the adjustment of the square root factor, the opening would be 15 in. wide. Note that only the width of the ventilation opening is adjusted (Bryner, Johnsson, and Pitts 1995).

In addition, current research appears to suggest that the scaled furniture constructed does not require precise and intricate construction. The use of standard 1/2-in. oriented-strand board (OSB) as the framework, polyurethane as the padding, and furniture upholstery as the covering appears to provide adequate fuel packages. Overall dimensions are scaled, but the thickness of the furniture is not.

One style of scaled furniture cuts the center out of the OSB to form a frame from which the chairs and couches are made. They are glued or stapled to form the structure. Furniture upholstering is used to wrap the frame and glued in place. The polyurethane is covered with furniture upholstering and placed on the frame. Beds have been made of two layers of polyurethane covered with bed sheets. Simple wood structures are placed under the bed to form the bed frame. See Figure 10-5 for innovative work by Mark Campbell on scale-model demonstrations.

Current testing has shown similarities between FSE, RSE, and FDS models. Some of these similarities include calcination plots, clean-burn areas, ventilation burn patterns, flashover, backdrafts, and thermocouple data. Thermocouple plots in RSEs have shown the growth phase of the fire and the transition to flashover, turbulent mixing that occurs in the enclosure, and decay of the fire. This type of information may be used to help the investigator examine patterns, locations, and intensities.

An RSE will provide information related to fire effects but should not be used to calculate heat release rate, fire spread time, mass loss rate, gas species, or gas concentrations, as these are more difficult to scale. Heat release rate, speed of smoke movement, and time to flashover will also not be linearly correlated. This valuable information is used to help the investigator refine the working hypothesis and should never be the stand-alone research or testing.

Floor or wall materials proportionally reduced in thickness may respond to thermal insult as *thermally thin* targets if they are less than a few millimeters thick and may respond differently than thicker sections of the same material. Special materials may be selected for models of walls and ceiling so their thermal behavior will duplicate, in scale, that of gypsum or plaster walls.

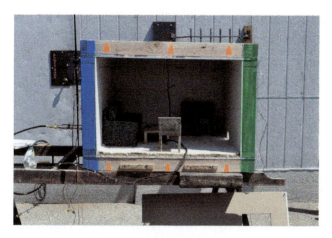

FIGURE 10-5A Quarter-scale room built by Mark Campbell and Dan Hrouda. A front view of the Reduced Scale Enclosure. The drywall front will be added and will face the door opening. Two cameras will be added: one on side A, facing the back of the room, and one on side D, facing the couch. The propane sand burner is in corner B/C. Fifteen thermocouples are located throughout the cell. Mark Campbell, Fire Forensics Research Center, Denver, CO

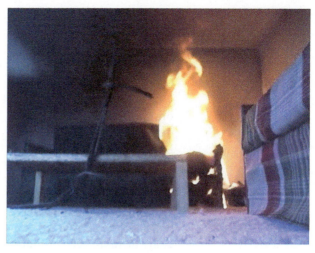

FIGURE 10-5B This is a side view from side D looking toward side B just after the propane sand burner was shot off after 90 seconds. The propane sand burner is located just to the right of the couch. The heat release rate was scaled to be approximately 3 kW so it would scale to the 5/2 scale as required by the scaling laws. A 100 kW fire is used in the Full Scale Enclosure. Mark Campbell, Fire Forensics Research Center, Denver, CO

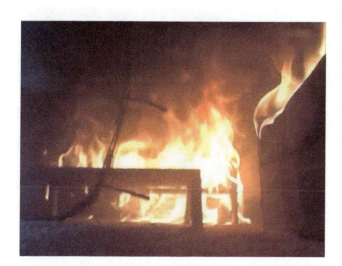

FIGURE 10-5C The fire has spread across the couch, and now the hot ceiling gases have started to pyrolyze the chair and caused it to ignite. The thermocouples in the middle of the room help determine when the room starts the transition through flashover. Mark Campbell, Fire Forensics Research Center, Denver, CO

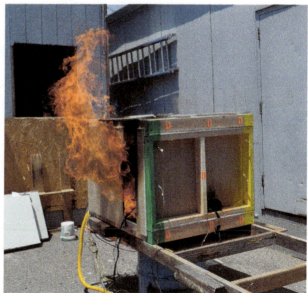

FIGURE 10-5D The fire exits the Reduced Scale Enclosure, as it is now in the postflashover burning stage. The enclosure is burned for 2 minutes post-flashover. The Reduced Scale Enclosure provides the investigator with another tool to help assess the various fire effects and burn patterns. Mark Campbell, Fire Forensics Research Center, Denver, CO

10.2.2 FLUID TANKS

A great deal of the information used to create and test the models of smoke and hot gas movement was developed in *fluid tanks* with no fire or smoke at all. Because the buoyancy of the hot gases relative to normal room air drives the movement of smoke in a building, the same process can be simulated by using two liquids of different densities such as fresh- and saltwater. If one fluid is dyed, its movement and mixing can easily be observed and recorded. See Figure 10-6 for innovative work on fluid tank model demonstrations.

Often, a scale (one-eighth to one-fourth) model of the room(s) is built of clear Plexiglas and immersed and inverted in a large tank of the lighter, less dense, liquid. The heavier liquid is then introduced into the model in a manner to simulate the generation of gases from a fire in the room. Scaling factors are important, and the relative densities and viscosities of the liquids have to be calibrated to simulate the mixing of gases in a buoyant flow, but the technique can provide answers to some investigative problems and confirm or reject computational models and hypotheses (Fleischmann, Pagni, and Williamson 1994).

10.2.3 FIELD TESTS

Identification of the first fuel ignited is critical to the reconstruction process. If the first fuel is more easily susceptible to open-flame ignition than to glowing- or hot-surface ignition (e.g., such fuels as natural gas, gasoline vapors, or polyethylene plastic), the fire scene search can focus on the appropriate type of potential ignition sources. Cellulosic fuels or other natural materials such as wool are much more easily ignited by hot-surface sources like discarded cigarettes or glowing electrical connections. Most such materials can be reliably identified by visual inspection, but information as to their behavior when ignited is much more within the realm of expertise of the fire investigator.

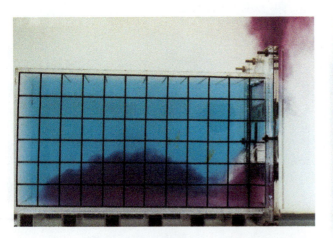

FIGURE 10-6A Side view of one-sixteenth scale fluid tank demonstrating cool denser fluid (representing cool air) entering the chamber through the lower half of the door opening after the door (extreme right) is opened. The buoyant fluid (blue) is venting from the top of the opening. These tests were conducted to evaluate flows and mixing in possible backdraft events in compartment fires. *Courtesy of Dr. Charles Fleischmann, University of Canterbury, Christchurch, New Zealand.*

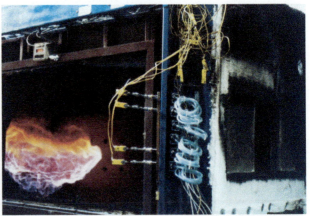

FIGURE 10-6B Quarter view of half-scale fire test chamber. An underventilated burner in the closed chamber has produced a hot, fuel-rich, buoyant smoke layer. When the door (on the right) is opened, the buoyant smoke escapes, and cool fresh air flows in the bottom of the opening to mix with the hot smoke. When ignited by a pilot flame at the far end, the flame progresses quickly along the premixed interface as a backdraft event. This behavior was predicted by the fluid tank tests shown in Figure 10-6A. *Courtesy of Dr. Charles Fleischmann, University of Canterbury, Christchurch, New Zealand.*

A simple *flame* or *ignition susceptibility test* using a match or lighter applied to one corner while the small test sample is held vertically in still air will reveal how readily the material will ignite and whether it will support flaming combustion when the ignition source is removed, as described in *NFPA 705* (NFPA 2013). However, *NFPA 701* (NFPA 2015) is now considered the preferred practice.

Under the *NFPA 705* test conditions, cellulosic materials support a yellow flame with a gray smoke. When the flame is blown out, these materials tend to support glowing combustion. The ash left behind is gray to black in color and powdery or crumbly in texture. There is no droplet of hard-melted residue. Thermoplastic synthetic materials melt as they burn, so melted, burning droplets result. They also tend to shrink and shrivel as they melt and often burn with a blue-based flame, with smoke ranging from negligible to white (polyethylene) to heavy and inky black (polystyrene). These materials do not support smoldering combustion.

Thermosetting resins are usually more difficult to ignite than other fuels. They tend to smolder when flame is removed, produce an aggressive smoke, and leave a hard, semi-porous residue. **Elastomers** (rubbers) can be either natural (latex) or synthetic and can behave like either. Some will burn very readily; others, like silicone rubber, burn much more reluctantly. Silicone rubber leaves a brilliant white, powdery ash, whereas other elastomers leave a hard, dark, porous mass. Samples of any unknown material suspected of being the first fuel ignited should be collected for laboratory analysis if there is doubt concerning their contribution to the ignition or growth of the fire.

elastomers ■ Fibers or materials having elastic properties.

Caution should be exercised in both conducting and interpreting such informal ignition tests. The *NFPA 705* test has been criticized as being subjective and variable owing to the procedures and personnel involved. There is also a risk of injury to personnel and a reported cause of serious accidental fires. A strong suggestion is to use *NFPA 701: Standard Methods of Fire Tests for Flame Propagation of Textiles and Films* (NFPA 2015) when conducting flame or ignition susceptibility tests (as in Figure 10-7).

NFPA 701 is basically a flammability test that applies to typical straight-hanging fabrics such as curtains, draperies, and window treatments. The test determines a fabric's rate of flammability subjected to certain ignition sources. In *NFPA 701* tests, the material is hung vertically and subjected to flame for a prescribed time period; is observed to see

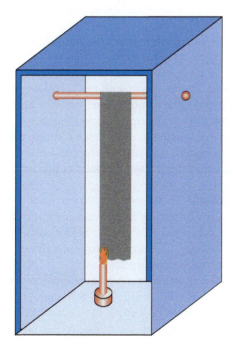

FIGURE 10-7 The *NFPA 701* test is used for small-scale testing of the flammability of fabrics. The *NFPA 701* apparatus uses a free-hanging vertical strip [150 mm × 400 mm (6 in. × 16 in.)] of the fabric to be tested in an enclosed test chamber. The flame from a laboratory burner is applied at the bottom of the strip for 45 seconds and then removed. The flame spread behavior of the fabric is observed, and after extinguishment, the residue is weighed. *Source: Icove, David J.; DeHaan, John D.; Haynes, Gerald A., Forensic Fire Scene Reconstruction, 3rd Ed., ©2013. Reprinted and Electronically reproduced by permission of Pearson Education, Inc., New York, NY.*

whether it self-extinguishes; is measured for char length; and is observed to see whether it does not continue to burn after reaching the floor of the test chamber.

NFPA 701 Test Method No. 1 applies to single-layer fabrics and to multilayer curtain and drapery assemblies. Vinyl-coated fabric blackout linings are tested according to *NFPA 701* Test Method No. 2. *NFPA 701* cautions that materials applied to surfaces of buildings or interior finishes should be tested in accordance with *NFPA 255 2006: Standard Method of Test of Surface Burning Characteristics of Building Materials,* or *NFPA 265: Standard Methods of Fire Tests for Evaluating Room Fire Growth Contribution of Textile Coverings on Full Height Panels and Walls (NFPA 2015).*

The presence of fire retardants may significantly affect ignition and flame spread. Materials like carpet are much more easily ignited from a corner or edge than if the same ignition source is applied to the center of the specimen. Ignition and flame spread are enhanced by vertical sample orientation and may be retarded by draft or moisture in the sample, so the results should be noted but not taken as proof of identity or of actual fire behavior.

10.2.4 FULL-SCALE FIRE TESTS

Considerable knowledge has been gathered from fire tests conducted in real buildings slated for demolition, although the dimensions, ventilation, and construction materials of a test building will not match conditions of a specific fire being studied. Aside from physical suitability, there are often issues of fire exposure to surrounding properties, environmental concerns, logistics of access, and limitation of fire protection services. If a building slated for demolition is used, provisions should be made for multiple video camera viewports and the inclusion of thermocouple arrays and radiometers.

DeHaan found a test house nearly identical to one in which six fire fatalities occurred. The test house was repaired and refurnished to duplicate the initial fire scene. Thermocouples, gas analyzers, and video cameras were used to document fire tests with accelerated and non-accelerated ignitions. The test data revealed that a non-accelerated fire could have been responsible for the structural damage and trapping the victims very quickly on the upper floor (DeHaan 1992).

Because of a number of training-fire deaths in the United States, fire departments have been more reluctant to expose their personnel to the risks of large fires in original buildings. The majority of fire personnel recognize the value of training firefighters in such structures and plan live training burns in accordance with the safety provisions outlined in *NFPA 1403: Standard on Live Fire Training Evolutions* (NFPA 2012).

The investigator should be aware that those provisions include covering floor openings, removing features such as glass windows and doors as well as debris contributing to an unsafe condition, identifying and evaluating all exits, and using only limited fuel loads (i.e., no ignitable liquids or gases). The resulting fire behavior and, most importantly, fire patterns therefore do not generally conform to those features of fires in buildings with normal furnishings, doors, glass windows, and intact ceilings and roofs. It is suggested that fire investigators not attempt to use such firefighting exercises to gather behavior/pattern data. Full-scale rooms that duplicate particular conditions and control other variables can be built for fire tests.

ASTM E603: Standard Guide for Room Fire Experiments (ASTM 2013c) addresses assembling tests to be used for evaluating the fire response of materials, assemblies, or room contents in specific fire situations that cannot be evaluated in small-scale tests. This guide can assist planning full-scale compartment-fire experiments and points out issues that should be resolved before testing commences.

For example, *ASTM E603* suggests that a typical compartment size should be 2.4 m × 3.7 m (8 ft × 12 ft), with allowances for a 2.4-m (8-ft) high ceiling. The standard-size doorway (0.80 m × 2.0 m high) should be located in one wall, and the top of the doorway should be at least 0.4 m (16 in.) down from the ceiling to partially contain smoke and hot gases. The guide also recommends instrumentation having provisions for measuring the optical density of smoke, temperatures, and heat fluxes in the compartment. The documentation and controls necessary are also described.

10.2.5 FULL-SCALE FIRE TESTS CUBICLE CONSTRUCTION

Effective room mock-up cubicles can be assembled at low cost for full-scale tests. Based on a design by Mark Wallace, these are basically four 2.43 m × 2.43 m (8 ft × 8 ft) wood-framed panels [typically wood studs on 61-cm (24-in.) centers with gypsum wallboard], with a similar panel resting on top to form a ceiling. A larger unit can easily be constructed, and designs provide for a knockdown wall that can easily be removed after the test to facilitate documentation.

Doors and windows can be cut as needed. A header must be left above each door 25 to 45 cm (10 to 18 in. deep). Cubicles are easily erected on four wood pallets covered with 13-mm (0.5-in.) sheet plywood or on 2 in. × 4 in. or 4 in. × 4 in. joists. Because these are intended for short-duration (<30 min) tests, lack of insulation will not usually affect the results of interior fires. Electrical outlets can easily be added.

Viewports are easily added by cutting holes approximately 25 cm × 30 cm (10 in. × 12 in.) in size in one or more walls near floor level. An unframed piece of ordinary window glass is then glued to the *interior* surface of the wall using silicone sealant (and allowed to harden for 24 hours before the fire). The absence of a frame means that the entire sheet of glass is exposed to the same heat flux and will not develop the same stresses that cause failure before flashover. Experience reveals that such windows will usually last until flashover. Heat-resistant glass such as that used in fireplace screens or oven doors can ensure integrity post-flashover if that is desired.

A *thermocouple* is a sensor for measuring temperature and consists of two different metal alloys joined together (twisted or welded) at one end. When that junction is exposed to heat, it generates a small voltage somewhat proportional to the temperature. The most common is Type K (Chromel/Alumel) and must be properly connected to extension cables with respect to their polarity to function correctly. Its most useful temperature measurement range is −200°C to 1250°C (−328°F to 2282°F). For a good source of commercial documentation and materials, consult the Omega Engineering Corporation handbooks, which can be requested from their website (www.omega.com).

Thermocouples can easily be added through small holes drilled through the gypsum where desired. A minimum of three thermocouples on one wall is suggested: one near the ceiling, one midlevel, and one approximately 15 cm (6 in.) above the floor at a point well away from the door or other vents. A second set can be installed on the opposite side of the room, or additional thermocouples can be placed inside the door header (to record flameover) or above target fuel packages. They can be shielded with a small-diameter metal, ceramic, or glass tube, leaving only the tip exposed. The smallest-diameter thermocouples that are practicable should be used, because larger wire gauges lead to systematic depression in the measured temperatures. A wire size of 24 AWG is often suitable. Larger AWG numbers indicate a smaller wire diameter; however, thinner thermocouple wires can be more difficult to work with and more prone to breakage under field fire testing conditions. Data are best captured on a digital data logger such as Picolog, although they can also be captured on a video camera monitoring digital outputs of several individual meters at once for later manual transcription.

Such cubicles allow creation of environments that closely simulate real rooms [additional 1 m × 2.5 m (3.3 ft × 8.2 ft) segments can be added for larger rooms] while keeping safety risks to a minimum and reducing hazards for personnel (e.g., toxic material, asbestos exposure, or structural collapse). One entry wall can be framed separately so that it can be easily opened and laid flat on the ground after the fire for ease of examination and photography. Video recordings should be made of all tests, using multiple cameras and synchronized time clocks wherever possible. A visual and audio cue should accompany ignition so that it marks $t = 0$ on all recordings simultaneously. The small size [2.5 m × 2.5 m (8 ft × 8 ft)] will produce flashover in less time (approximately 30 percent less) than a typical 3 m × 4 m (10 ft × 13 ft) room given the same fuel load.

Scientifically valid small-scale tests can be conducted to test flame spread ignitability without special equipment as long as possible roles of the test variables are taken into account. For instance, carpet or furniture can be tested in the open with the realization that it may burn very differently if tested in a compartment because of the radiant heat reflected back from walls and ceiling and changes to ventilation conditions.

Carpets need to be secured to the floor in the same manner as in the actual structure. Synthetic carpets shrink and curl as they burn. If the edges lift, the combustion of the carpet can be significantly enhanced and distort the heat release rate and fire patterns. Carpets must be backed with the same pad as during the fire being duplicated, because interaction between the pad and the carpet can cause self-sustaining combustion, although neither material may sustain flame spread when exposed separately.

The ignition source used should duplicate the one known to be involved, or various kinds should be tested. For instance, polypropylene carpet will resist ignition by a single dropped match at room temperature, as it will pass the required methenamine tablet test (CPSC 1-70 flammability test); however, the carpet will self-sustain combustion if exposed to a slightly larger ignition source such as a burning crumpled sheet of newspaper or any additional external heat flux. After it is ignited, such carpet will sustain combustion at rates up to approximately 0.5 to 1 m²/hr (5 to 11 ft²/hr) with small flames about 5 to 7 cm (2 to 3 in.) tall.

If a fire test is conducted in a compartment, care must be taken that the major fuel packages are located in the same position in each test (or in the same position as in the scene being replicated). Packages in corners will burn differently than packages against the wall or in the middle of the room. A large fire located away from an open door will burn differently than the same fire set near the door. Changes in the compartment vent opening size and location will alter air flow during testing and will influence the resulting fire patterns. Ventilation-effect fire patterns are to be expected if the fire test is allowed to proceed to post-flashover (ventilation-limited) burning.

10.3 Types of Fabrics

Fabrics differ greatly in their properties of combustion, ranging from some that are intrinsically very hazardous to others that cannot be burned at all. The 1953 Flammable Fabrics Act (*16 CFR 1610*) prohibits the use in the United States of a few extremely flammable fabrics; however, fabrics that pass may ignite and burn easily. The most fire-resistant fabrics are, in general, used only for special purposes such as fire-resistant clothing for pilots, firefighters, and drivers of racing cars.

natural fibers ■ Fibers of animal or vegetable origin without chemical manipulation.

The most common types of fabrics include **natural fibers**, petroleum-based synthetic fibers, and non-petroleum based synthetic fibers.

10.3.1 NATURAL FIBERS

Wool

Wool is used in many fabrics utilized for clothing as well as for bedding, upholstery, and miscellaneous purposes. Its fire hazard is minimal because of its high nitrogen and protein content. It can be burned, but with considerable difficulty because it has a high ignition temperature and low heat of combustion. It will not normally sustain a flame. Thus, wool blankets are used to wrap a person whose clothing is on fire and are being tested as a barrier layer in furniture. Exposing wool cloth to a flame will char a hole in it, but it will self-extinguish when the outside heat source is removed. When it does burn, wool generates toxic hydrogen cyanide fumes in addition to other combustion products.

Cotton

Cotton is used extensively in cloth for garments, bedding, and upholstery. It is possibly the most combustible of the common natural fibers. It is cellulosic in composition, like wood and paper. Having a very large surface-to-volume ratio, that is, a large surface for combustion, cotton is ignited with relative ease and will sustain a fire or allow it to increase greatly after ignition as long as it receives adequate ventilation. Cotton's ease of burning is conditioned by several factors, which will be discussed later. Cotton batting was once used universally as padding in garments and furniture and also as filler in cushions. It may still be found in some modern furniture, but it has largely been supplanted by polyester fiberfill or other synthetics.

Linen

Linen is being used much less than formerly, especially in clothing, and only occasionally is it seriously involved in major fires. Its cellulosic fibers are derived from stems (bast) rather than seed pods, as is cotton. Because it is a bast fiber, linen is much more variable than cotton, and this difference is expected to have some influence on combustion rates. Cloth from predominantly fine fibers is expected to burn more freely than that from coarser fibers. Like cotton, linen can be ignited by a smoldering cigarette or contact with a hot surface to support a smoldering or flaming fire.

Kapok

Kapok was once used as a filling for pillows, bedding, and insulated clothing, but is not normally used as a cloth fiber. Kapok is involved in fires with sufficient frequency to make its fire hazards important. Like cotton, kapok is a cellulosic fiber, but because of its cell structure and its fineness, it exceeds cotton significantly in its flammability. It will ignite with ease, and when ventilation is available, kapok will burn with great intensity. It will also support smoldering fire very well. It is fortunate that kapok's uses are limited so that it is not often involved in clothing fires. It can, however, pose a significant hazard in industrial areas, such as life preserver and pillow manufacture, where it is utilized. California's strict upholstered furniture flammability laws do not permit the use of kapok.

Silk

Silk is made by unwinding the cocoon of the silkworm and spinning the filament obtained into thread. It is a proteinaceous material like wool and although not easily ignited in bulk, it is often woven into a thin or sheer fabric that can burn quickly once ignited. It generates toxic gases, including hydrogen cyanide, upon combustion.

10.3.2 PETROLEUM-BASED SYNTHETIC FIBERS

Synthetic fibers, because of their versatility, constitute the largest percentage of fabrics used in upholstery and clothing in the United States today. These fabrics, which bear names such as nylon, Dacron, Orlon, Dynel, and Acrilan, can vary considerably in their ignition properties and burning behavior. Some of these variations are the effect of the chemistry of the fiber itself, but they usually are the result of additives and modifiers used to improve particular properties of the fibers. Most synthetic fibers are made from chemicals that originate from petroleum products. As a class, they tend to be much more susceptible to ignition by open flame than by a hot surface or glowing ember. Nylon, polyester, polyethylene, polystyrene, and polypropylene will ignite when in contact with a flame, especially when in the form of thin fabrics or coatings. Fluffy polyester fiberfill is very commonly found in cushions, pillows, and comforters.

■ **synthetic fibers** Artificial fibers of chemical origin.

Foam Rubber

Butyl, nitrile polybutadiene, and polyurethane rubbers are examples of common synthetic materials used as coatings, padding, and insulation in household goods. They will resist ignition from a glowing source; but without fire-retardant additives, they are easily often ignited with a small open flame and will burn with considerable energy.

Polyurethane foam rubber, because of its widespread use in upholstery (and occasionally clothing), is the most commonly encountered synthetic with a substantial fire hazard. (Today, nearly all upholstered furniture sold in the United States contains some polyurethane rubber padding). More and more of the foam being used today is of the flame-resistant type.

There are many types of flame-retardant foams; most of them are resistant only to small open flames and will burn fiercely when ignited by a larger flame. Others resist ignition even by much larger flame sources. It has been estimated that the percentage of upholstered furniture using flame-retardant grades of flexible urethane foams rose from 1 percent in 1970 to 50 percent in 1994 as those products were improved in strength, durability, and cost (Damant 1996). Flame-retardant grades of foam still remain very underused in residential furniture (Foster and Zicherman 2005).

Not all "foam rubber" is polyurethane. There are other elastomers such as isoprene isobutylene or polyester foams. These may have different ignition and flammability properties than polyurethane and usually require lab identification. Most elastomers do not melt but decompose when heated.

In addition to being flammable, most (but not all) synthetic fabrics have a tendency to melt and flow as they burn. When this occurs, burning droplets may fall into other fuel and start secondary fires. If the fabric is in the form of a garment, the melting material may fall away rapidly with only burning droplets clinging to the skin of the wearer, with their difficult-to-extinguish flames inflicting localized burns (Mehta and Wong 1983).

Interestingly, the fabric of choice for the past 35 years for children's sleepwear has been 100% polyester. Its melting and shrinking behavior actually prevents the propagation of small flames. This permits such fabrics to pass the CPSC sleepwear requirements of *16 CFR 1615* and *16 CFR 1616*. When exposed to large flames, polyester will ignite and melt, possibly causing serious burns. The ignition and burning properties of synthetics change when they are blended with natural fibers. For instance, cotton-polyester blended fabrics cause more injuries than polyester alone because the cotton keeps the burned fabric together to support a rapidly spreading flame, and the fabric remains in contact with the wearer (Holmes 1986). Pure thermoplastic synthetic fibers do not smolder, and burn only in flames.

Nomex

One synthetic fiber, Nomex (an aromatic polyamide), resists all types of ignition and is used to weave fabrics for fire protective gear for firefighters, aircraft pilots, and drivers of racing cars. A single layer of Nomex cloth will protect human tissue from burning in contact with a flame of 600°C (1200°F) for up to 30 seconds. Other fire-retardant fabrics available today include modacrylics, viscose, polybenzimidazole (PBI), Kevlar, Kynol, and some PVC (polyvinyl chloride) fabrics (Bhatnagar 1975; Backer et al. 1976).

10.3.3 NON–PETROLEUM-BASED SYNTHETIC FIBERS

Synthetic fibers that are not petroleum based include rayon and cellulose acetate. Rayon, or regenerated cellulose, is chemically nearly the same as cotton because it is made by dissolving cotton or other cellulosic material and regenerating the cellulose in the form of an extruded fiber by forcing the solution through a spinneret into the regenerating bath. Because of the similarity to cotton, the main difference in fire hazard is due to the different fabric weave and garment configuration and possibly size of the fibers.

Acetate

Acetate (acetylated cellulose) is similar to rayon in its manufacture and appearance, but the chemical modification of the cellulose diminishes its flammability. It melts rather easily but burns with some difficulty, except in lightweight fabrics, where it will burn relatively rapidly.

Glass-Fiber

Other synthetic fibers may be encountered in some unusual fabrics. Glass-fiber cloths are manufactured and used mostly for nonapparel purposes, although clothing has been made from them. Drapery is one of the common uses in which their obvious nonflammability and fire resistance would be of importance. Nearly all draperies sold for residential use, however, are readily ignitable and will support an energetic fire. Curtains for public occupancies are fire resistant and are often required to comply with *NFPA 701*.

Asbestos

Asbestos, a naturally fibrous mineral, has been used in special applications such as theater curtains because of its great fire resistance and absolute nonflammability. Because of the potential carcinogenicity of asbestos, it is no longer permitted in clothing or household textiles.

10.4 Fire Hazards

Few fabrics present an extreme fire hazard, especially those found in garments. The susceptibility of a fabric depends not only on what fibers are used to make it but on how the fabric is woven and the design of the garment in which it is used.

Yarn or thread that is tightly twisted will burn with less intensity than loosely spun yarns. In the manufacture of some cloths, the threads are tightly twisted fibers that are most tightly woven. The degree of tightness in spinning determines the flammability of the fabric. The weight or density of the fabric is also a key factor to ease of ignition. The heavier a fabric is, the more it will resist ignition by flaming sources. However, while heavier fabrics may be harder to ignite, once on fire, the larger fuel load can sustain a fire more likely to cause injuries if the garment cannot be removed or extinguished.

10.4.1 CLOTHING DESIGN

Clothing design affects the likelihood of accidental ignition. Loose-fitting garments such as robes, blouses, and nightgowns, and garments with ruffles, pleats, or loose and flowing sleeves can accidentally come into contact with a heat source. Excesses of material in such loose garments enhance the fuel load as well as the fuel-air ratio and promote rapid burning. From a fire-safety standpoint, the ease with which a burning garment can be removed is also a key design feature that influences the severity of possible injuries.

10.4.2 WEAVE AND FINISH

The weave and finish influence the burning behavior of a fabric because they control the amount of its fuel-air interface. A loosely woven cloth, with spacing between the threads, will always burn much more rapidly than a tightly woven fabric of the same thread. For example, a cotton canvas burns relatively poorly, while cotton gauze is rapidly consumed (but canvas is more easily ignited by a cigarette), although both are made from the same fiber.

10.4.3 FIBER

A tightly woven, heavy fabric like denim will ignite and burn more slowly than a sheer, lightweight cotton fabric such as the broadcloth used in shirts. A fabric with a nap, such as cotton flannel, has air spaces between the loose fibers on the surface and will ignite much more quickly than cotton denim, which is smooth surfaced. Cotton flannel and terry-cloth fabrics are particularly susceptible to ignition. A fluffy high-pile fabric such as that used in some sweaters will ignite and burn faster than a close-knit low-pile fabric of the same fiber.

Similar to other types of fires, clothing fires originate from a variety of sources like cigarette lighters, utility or fireplace lighters, lit matches, burning tobacco, a gas burner, or a heated appliance. Research has shown that it is unlikely that most garment fabrics will be ignited by a smoldering cigarette (Mehta and Wong 1983, 1-30).

10.5 Regulation of Flammable Fabrics

In the United States, the Consumer Product Safety Commission (CPSC) regulates flammability of flammable fabrics on the federal level. Many states and regulatory control agencies have separate and broader-ranging regulations. This is especially true of regulations of carpets, wall coverings, and furnishings used in hotels, theaters, hospitals, and other public buildings. Some local building codes establish strict requirements for flammability of products in high-risk occupancies.

California regulations tend to be the most rigorous. Because manufacturers who sell in California also sell in other states, the California regulations function as de facto national regulations.

10.5.1 OVERVIEW OF FEDERAL JURISDICTION

The Flammable Fabrics Act (FFA) passed in 1953 regulates the manufacture of all highly flammable wearing apparel and fabrics offered for sale on an interstate basis. Under the FFA, regulation rested with the US Department of Commerce (DOC).

The Consumer Product Safety Act of 1972 transferred all enforcement of the FFA to the CPSC, which has broad jurisdiction over household products and their safety and now promulgates standards and enforces them. Since then, a number of important regulations have been enacted with regard to flammable fabric standards. Since 1972 the Department of Health and Human Services (previously the Department of Health, Education, and Welfare) has set the standards for interior finishes and upholstery fabrics used in hospitals and nursing homes. Since 1972, fabrics and cushioning materials used in the interiors of motor vehicles have had to pass tests prescribed by the Department of Transportation (DOT) as required by US Motor Vehicle Safety Standard No. 302. In 1968, the DOT passed FAA Title 14, regulations on the flammability of aircraft interior finishes. The current tests for aircraft upholstery deal with their resistance to radiant heat from a large nearby fire (e.g., a jet fuel spill and smoke emission).

10.5.2 CLOTHING FLAMMABILITY

The first standard published under the FFA, CS-191-53, measured flame spread on fabric after direct flame ignition. This Standard for the Flammability of Clothing Textiles, known as *16 CFR 1610*, is a weak requirement involving only the application of a needlelike flame to the surface of the test specimen for one second and observing fire spread. Because newspaper will pass that test, the standard will exclude only the most dangerous fabrics.

Tests *16 CFR 1615* and *1616* require the application of a larger flame to the exposed edge of the test specimen for 3 seconds. In any such tests, only a fabric specimen is tested. The finished garment may well pose higher ignition risks. In 1967, the act was amended and expanded to include textiles intended for nonclothing uses, such as interior finishes and furnishings. Enforcement responsibilities were divided between DOC and the Federal Trade Commission (FTC).

10.5.3 FLAMMABILITY OF CARPETS AND RUGS

The first standard created under the expanded FFA, known as Standard for the Surface Flammability of Carpets and Rugs (DOC FF 1-70) or *16 CFR 1630*, regulated the flammability of large carpets and rugs. This standard, still mandatory for carpets and rugs sold in the United States, measures horizontal flame spread upon ignition by methenamine tablet, a reproducible ignition source. Created in 1970, DOC FF 2-70, now known as *16 CFR 1631*, regulated the flammability of small area carpets and rugs.

10.5.4 FLAMMABILITY OF CHILDREN'S SLEEPWEAR

In 1971, DOC FF 3-71, now known as *16 CFR 1615*, addressed concerns about the flammability of children's sleepwear, specifically, the smaller sizes (0 to 6X) sold in the United States. DOC FF 5-74, known as *16 CFR 1616*, addressed the flammability of larger sizes (7 to 14). Both standards are fairly stringent, dealing with ignition of vertical fabric surfaces by open flames.

10.5.5 MATTRESS FLAMMABILITY

Because of the frequency and severity of fires started in furniture and mattresses, the most important and most controversial standards have to do with the flammability of mattresses and upholstered furniture sold in the United States. Since 1973 there has been a national standard for the cigarette ignition resistance of all mattresses, futons, and mattress pads sold in the United States (DOC FF 4-72, now *16 CFR 1632*, revised in 1984). This standard mandates that mattresses and mattress pads must not be ignitable by ordinary cigarettes placed directly on the mattress or between sheets covering that mattress.

Before 1973, the standard mattress consisted of coil springs covered with a layer of insulating felt covered by thick batting, protected by a fabric covering or ticking. Although the cotton batting was susceptible to smoldering ignition, it was difficult to ignite by open flame. In compliance with the 1973 law, most manufacturers began using a non-fire-retardant polyurethane pad as a supplement or a complete replacement for the cotton batting. Although the mattresses made between 1973 and 2007 are, indeed, resistant to ignition from cigarettes, they are much more likely to ignite from open flames and to continue to burn than are their predecessors.

Some manufacturers have produced mattresses made with a fire-retardant-treated cotton or flame-resistant polyurethane pad to optimize all forms of fire resistance. These materials are marginally more expensive than the unsafe products, however, and cost-conscious manufacturers have been slow to adopt such materials. Mattresses made for hospitals and prisons generally must meet more stringent standards. Since 1977, the state of California has required all mattresses that do not meet both smoldering and open-flame standards to bear a consumer warning label stating that the mattress is susceptible to open-flame ignition.

In August 2001 the California legislature enacted a law (Assembly Bill 603) requiring all mattresses, futons, and mattress sets manufactured on or after January 1, 2005, and sold in California (including those for residential use) to be resistant to a large open flame. The goal of the legislation was to reduce the incidence of fire deaths, injuries, and property losses associated with bedroom fires.

California *Technical Bulletin (TB) 603: Standard for Mattresses, Box Springs and Futons* required that all mattresses, box springs, and futons comply with new flame-initiated testing procedures. The test was designed to simulate real-world flaming ignition sources and measure the heat released from such items as they burn. This test has been supplanted by CPSC test *16 CFR 1633*, which is described later. Compliance with such standards is almost exclusively achieved by the use of a variety of fire-blocking layers or barriers rather than the use of chemical retardants. These layers involve PVC cloth, metal films, and other passive blocking systems.

California *Technical Bulletin (TB) 117-2013* (California Department of Consumer Affairs 1980b) is the newest regulation that addresses flammability requirement for upholstered furniture and a smolder test requirement for foam for use as uncovered mattress pad products. This regulation now eliminates the open flame test for upholstery components including filling materials, such as flexible polyurethane foam, and revises the smolder resistance requirements. The use of barrier materials is required only if cover fabrics and/or filling materials fail their corresponding tests.

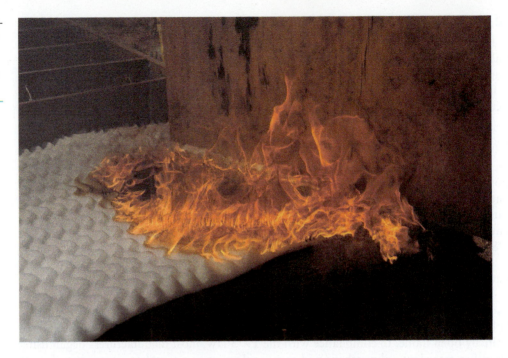

FIGURE 10-8 Foam mattress topper burned readily when ignited by a match flame at its edge. *Courtesy of John Jerome and Jim Albers.*

Flammable bedding materials include such items as aftermarket foam bed-toppers, comforters, pillows, and duvets. Such materials are readily ignited by small flames (as shown in Figures 10-8 and 10-9) and continue to be a threat to life safety despite strenuous efforts to include them in fire standards. The California Bureau of Home Furnishings in 2003 published a draft test standard for such items (denoted as *TB 604*). The CPSC in 2007 published a notice of proposed regulation for bedclothes flammability (*16 CFR 1634*), but it has not progressed further. It would have mandated that such products pass a flame test such as that in Figure 10-9 but was never put into effect.

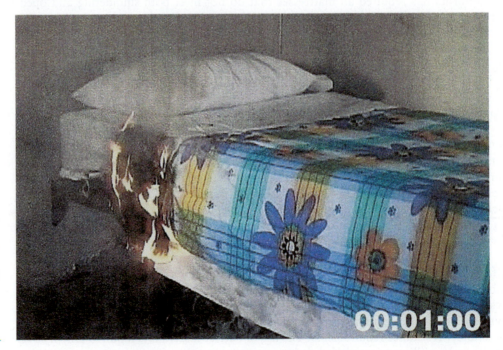

FIGURE 10-9 Comforter built to meet California's proposed safety standard (*TB 604*) resists flaming ignition, and fire spread is dramatically reduced. *Courtesy of Bureau of Electronics & Appliance Repair, Home Furnishings.*

10.6 Upholstered Furniture

Upholstered furniture is subject, to a lesser degree, to the same sorts of regulations. Although there are national industry standards regarding the flammability of upholstered furniture, these are voluntary and aimed at smoldering ignition sources only.

California has developed rigorous standards and flammability test procedures for mattresses and upholstered furniture for use in public buildings such as jails, hospitals, nursing homes, hotels and motels, college dormitories, and public auditoriums. In 1980, California *TB 121: Flammability Test Procedure for Mattresses for Use in High Risk Occupancies*, developed by the California Bureau of Home Furnishings, was adopted by the California Board of Corrections as a mandatory requirement for all California detention facilities (California Department of Consumer Affairs 1980c).

In 1984 the flammability test procedure for seating furniture for use in public occupancies was first developed by the California Bureau of Home Furnishings and Thermal Insulation (Wortman, Williams, and Damant 1984, 55-67). Enacted in 1988, the *Flammability Test Procedure for Seating Furniture for Office and Public Occupancies* is now known as California Technical Bulletin 133 (*TB 133*) (California Department of Consumer Affairs 1988). *TB 133* became a mandatory law in California in 1992 and has been adopted by several other states and a number of local jurisdictions, including Illinois, Ohio, Minnesota, Massachusetts, the city of Boston, and the New York–New Jersey Port Authority. A generic version has been adopted as *ASTM E1537: Standard Test Method for Fire Testing of Upholstered Furniture* (Damant 1994). Finally, *TB 129: Flammability Testing Procedures for Mattresses for Use in Public Buildings* was published in 1992. *TB 129* has also been widely adopted, and a generic version has been published as *ASTM E1590* (California Department of Consumer Affairs 1992).

The California Department of Consumer Affairs maintains a nationally recognized testing laboratory as part of its Bureau of Home Furnishings and Thermal Insulation. This laboratory is responsible for testing fabrics, apparel, and home furnishings to ensure they comply with the stringent state standards. This laboratory reports that there is no way to predict the time frame of smoldering versus flaming combustion in modern upholstered furniture. In its tests, ignition by cigarette may lead to flaming ignition in times ranging from less than 1 hour to 9 or more hours (Babrauskas and Krasny 1997, 1029-31). This variability has been confirmed in a number of full-scale furniture tests conducted by the authors.

The earliest flame-retardant urethane foams demonstrated reduced flame retardance as the foam aged, especially at high temperatures. The additives being used today for the most part are stable under normal living conditions, but a portion of the California law requires that foams meet flammability tests before and after aging. The additives used in some foams to make them more resistant to flaming ignition actually made them more susceptible to smoldering ignition. It appears that manufacturers must be very careful in their choice of flame retardants, adhesives, and even mold release agents to ensure the best fire retardance properties in the finished product.

Combustion-modified, high-resiliency (CMHR) foams supplied by several domestic polyurethane foam manufacturers have exceptional fire resistance but may be less flexible and of much higher density than standard foam. There is also a so-called low-smoke neoprene foam that has excellent flame resistance. The CMHR foam has been useful in high-risk facilities such as jails and other facilities, but until the advent of melamine urethanes manufactured by BASF its physical limitation made it less desirable for regular use. The newest foams promise excellent fire resistance and long life along with light weight, flexibility, and a cost advantage over other fire-retardant foams (Damant 1996). A variety of highly fire resistant foams have been introduced, but except for specialty applications, they have not proven viable in the consumer market.

Laboratory testing of furnishings can provide some general guidance to investigators as to the ignition and flame-spread characteristics involved, but as Krasny, Parker, and Babrauskas (2001) describe, there are many approaches to testing and regulations. Ignition sources vary from radiant sources such as cigarettes or glowing electric heating elements to flaming sources such as matches and methenamine pills to crumpled paper or gas burners of various heat release rates and configurations, depending on the severity of the test. Information can be gathered from rate of heat release (calorimetry), total heat released over a fixed time (typically 180 seconds), rate of mass loss, total mass loss (absolute or percentage), visible charring, smoke production, rate of flame spread, or time to transition to flame. Pass-fail criteria can be based on any one or more of those factors.

The test samples may be individual components, small-scale mock-ups, full-scale mock-ups, prototypes, or real furniture sampled from stores. The small-scale mock-ups have to be tested to demonstrate their correlation to full-scale performance before they can be used in regulatory testing (Babrauskas and Krasny 1985). During the early 1990s, the European Union (EU) sponsored the largest-ever research project on the fire behavior of upholstered furniture [published as Combustion Behavior of Upholstered Furniture (CBUF)]. Of particular interest are the tests that include flame ignition, such as BS 5852 and BS 6807 (UK), *TB 133* and *TB 129*, and some of the ASTM tests. The International Organization for Standardization (ISO) 9705 corner room configuration has also been studied for the information it can provide to modeling real-world performance (Sundstrom 1995). In the United States, the Upholstered Furniture Advisory Council (UFAC) has acted as an adviser to the industry on flammability standards.

The heat release rate of furniture can be measured by bench-scale testing of models or mock-ups of the furniture; however, more accurate results are generally produced by testing in room calorimeters, such as those used in the California Technical Bulletin methods, or an oxygen-depletion furniture calorimeter of the type shown in Figure 10-10. The

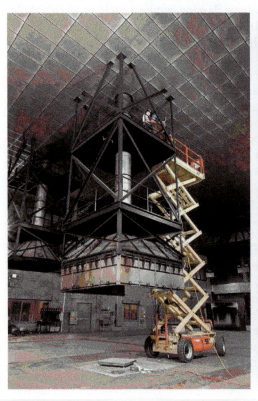
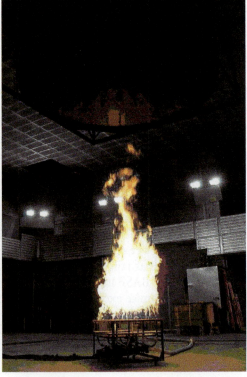

FIGURE 10-10 Furniture calorimeter. Combustion products are drawn into the exhaust hood, where the flow rate, concentration of oxygen, carbon dioxide, and carbon monoxide are measured. The heat produced is then calculated from the rate of oxygen consumption based on the value 13 MJ of heat per 1 kg of oxygen. *Source: Courtesy of Bureau of Alcohol, Tobacco, Firearms and Explosives (ATF).*

maximum heat release rates measured in such devices for upholstered chairs ranged from 370 to 2500 kW; for sofas, 2500 to 3000 kW; for curtains, 150 to 600 kW; and for pillows from 16 kW (feathers) to 35 to 43 kW (urethane foam) to 117 kW (latex foam) (Krasny, Parker, and Babrauskas 2001). The heat release rates of common household furnishings are critical to evaluating the potential for development of the fire. The rates measured in a furniture calorimeter are not directly transferable to predicting their performance in a room fire. The maximum heat release rate of any fuel is dependent on the radiant heat that fuel is receiving from the fire environment. Heat feedback in a room fire may well increase the maximum heat release rate produced over what is recorded in a calorimeter test. At the same time, the furniture calorimeter allows maximum ventilation, while a fire in a room may well reach ventilation limits that reduce the maximum heat release rate.

10.7 Flammability Tests for Federal Regulations

10.7.1 FLAMMABILITY OF CLOTHING TEXTILES (TITLE 16 CFR 1610—U.S.)

Standard *16 CFR 1610* requires that a 10-in. (25-cm) piece of fabric that is placed in a holder at a 45° angle (see Figure 10-11) and whose surface is contacted by a small flame for 1 second not ignite and spread flame up the length of the sample in less than 3.5 seconds for smooth fabrics or 4.0 seconds for napped fabrics (CPSC 1976, 1-5).

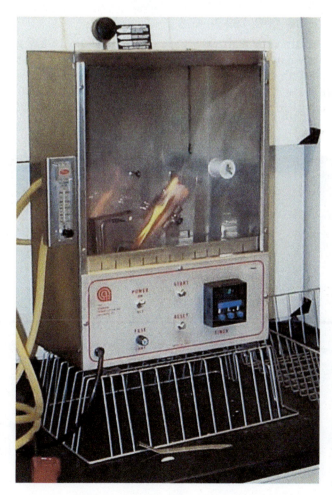

FIGURE 10-11 *16 CFR 1610* fabric test: 6.0-in. (150mm) strip of fabric is held in a metal frame at 45°. Flame is applied to the surface of the fabric slightly above the bottom edge for 1 second. *Photo printed with the permission of Govmark Fire Testing Services.*

10.7.2 FLAMMABILITY OF VINYL PLASTIC FILM (TITLE 16 CFR 1611—U.S.)

Standard *16 CFR 1611* requires that vinyl plastic film (for wearing apparel) placed in a holder at a 45° angle and ignited not burn at a rate exceeding 1.2 in. (3.0 cm) per second.

10.7.3 FLAMMABILITY OF CARPETS AND RUGS [TITLE 16 CFR 1630—U.S. (LARGE CARPETS) AND CFR 1631—U.S. (SMALL CARPETS)]

Standards *16 CFR 1630* and *16 CFR 1631* require that a burning methenamine tablet placed in the center of a specimen not cause a char more than 3 in. (7.6 cm) in any direction. The burning tablet or pill is a reproducible equivalent of a burning match, that is, ~50 W for 1 minute.

10.7.4 FLAMMABILITY OF MATTRESSES AND PADS (TITLE 16 CFR 1632—U.S.)

A minimum of nine regular tobacco cigarettes are burned at various locations on the bare mattress—quilted and smooth portions, tape edge, tufted pockets, and so forth. The char length of the mattress surface must not be more than 2 in. (3 cm) in any direction from any cigarette. The test is repeated with the cigarettes placed between two sheets covering the mattress.

10.7.5 FLAMMABILITY OF MATTRESSES AND BOX SPRINGS (TITLE 16 CFR 1633—U.S.)

The top and side of the mattress or mattress set are exposed to two 18-kW gas burners for a period of time (as shown in Figure 10-12). Failure of the test can be either (1) a peak heat release rate of 200 kW or greater within 30 minutes of ignition or (2) a total heat release of 15 MJ or greater within 10 minutes of ignition. As of July 1, 2007, all mattresses sold for residential use in the United States must have passed the *16 CFR 1633* test.

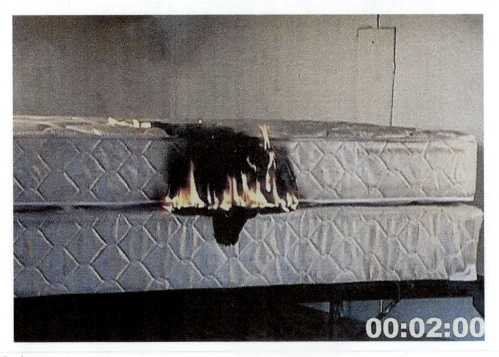

FIGURE 10-12 Mattress and box springs built to meet California's safety standard (*TB 603*) or *16 CFR 1633* are subjected to test burner flames for 70 seconds but meet stringent limits on heat release rate and total heat for 30 minutes. *Courtesy of Bureau of Electronics & Appliance Repair, Home Furnishings.*

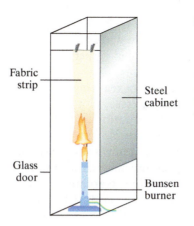

FIGURE 10-13 Test apparatus for 16 CFR 1615 (children's sleepwear): 10 × 3.5-in. (25 × 8.0-cm) strip hung vertically. Flame is applied to bottom edge.

10.7.6 FLAMMABILITY OF CHILDREN'S SLEEPWEAR (TITLE 16 CFR 1615 AND 1616—U.S.)

Each one of five 3.5 × 10-in. (8 × 25-cm) specimens is suspended vertically in holders in a cabinet and exposed to a small gas flame along its bottom edge for 3 seconds (as shown in Figure 10-13). The specimens cannot have an average char length of more than 7 in. (18 cm); no single specimen can have a char length of 10 in. (25 cm) (full burn); and no single sample can have flaming material on the bottom of the cabinet 10 seconds after the ignition source is removed. This test is required for finished items (as produced or after one washing and drying) and after the items have been washed and dried 50 times.

10.8 Considerations for Fire Investigators

Many variables contribute to susceptibility and time factors. These include fuel moisture, ambient temperature, position of the cigarette, and nature of the outer fabric covering(s), thin or thick, cellulosic or synthetic, presence of a barrier layer, and so forth. The presence of external air currents can also affect flame transition, because a draft can increase the combustion rate. As mentioned in the *TB 116* test, a single layer of cloth over a smoldering cigarette can reduce losses by convection and radiation and make ignition more likely.

Holleyhead published an extensive review of the furniture fire test literature and explored a number of the furniture-related variables (Holleyhead 1999, 75-102). The investigator needs to be aware of the variables related to both the furniture and the scene, and what effects they can have on ignitability. Although most accidentally dropped cigarettes are likely to be only partial ones, tests are conducted with full cigarettes. Ignition requires sufficient contact, which may not occur with partial cigarettes or dropped embers. Cigarettes and open flames like candles are competent ignition sources for furniture depending on the nature of the fabrics involved. Open flames will ignite modern fabrics almost on contact (3 to 5 seconds), whereas a smoldering cigarette will require 20 minutes or more, and then only if the other factors are favorable.

Thermoplastic fabrics tend to melt and shrink when exposed to the radiant heat of a growing fire, which can expose the underlying padding to flames and radiant heat, producing very fast fire growth. Polypropylene (polyolefin) and polyvinyl fabrics pose particular hazards in this regard. The inclusion of fire-blocking layers like fiberglass, PBI, coated fabrics, and even neoprene foam bonded to a textile fabric can dramatically reduce the maximum heat release rate demonstrated by these furnishings (Damant 1995).

NIST researchers observed that as polyurethane foams burn they decompose and melt into a semiliquid state that pools under the chair, sofa, or mattress to support a very intense pool fire. Using inert fillers to inhibit the flow of such products resulted in a significantly reduced maximum heat release rate (bfrl.nist.gov). When carpets are involved, the types of face yarn and backing are major factors. Because of its very low melting point, polypropylene fiber carpet melts very readily to expose combustible padding beneath.

Fire investigators today are realizing that the types of fibers, fabrics, and padding involved in furniture, mattresses, clothing, and carpet all can affect ignition, fire spread, fire intensity, and generation of toxic gases. As a result, these items need to be sampled and preserved for possible identification. In the future, fire investigators will have to determine whether the furnishings have met appropriate fire standards. Meeting standards can be accomplished either by design such as barrier layers, chemical structure, or treatment with fire retardants. Tags or labels do not ensure that the product was compliant with fire standards. CPSC and the California Department of Consumer Affairs report numerous failures of consumer products, some complete with false or forged tags.

Summary

Fire testing includes a large range of tests, from simple field flammability tests such as *NFPA 705*, to bench-scale fabric tests such as ASTM and *16 CFR* tests, to full-scale tests in buildings. Useful data from such tests can range from simple observations to temperatures and radiant heat fluxes, and owing to oxygen depletion calorimetry, even heat release rates of large fuel packages. Fire tests are often designed, conducted, and analyzed to collect more information about basic fire processes. This information is then published in peer-reviewed publications and authoritative treatises, or on websites. The data are then available for use in predicting ignition and fire events. Data from such tests can fill a critical role in testing hypotheses about the ignition, spread, and effects of fire.

The criteria for using fire test information in forensic fire scene reconstructions are whether the test was correctly performed, whether the data were accurately collected and reported, and whether the test was appropriate and applicable to the situation under consideration. Fire tests are designed to collect certain data in a reproducible and valid manner.

The investigator must ask whether the fuels, conditions, and ignition mechanism reproduced the fire in question. Was the test designed to follow ASTM or NFPA protocol? If so, did it actually follow that protocol? If not, what factors were considered in its design? What variables were considered and how were they controlled? Fuel moisture, fuel mass and quantity, physical state, ambient temperature and humidity, heat flux, and oxygen content all play important roles in ignition, flame spread, and heat release. If it was a custom-designed test, what data could be fairly and accurately collected and analyzed? Was there a planned series of tests to examine the sensitivity and reproducibility of the data? Because of the importance of fire test data in both criminal and civil fire investigations, it is imperative that tests be conducted and data be interpreted without misrepresentation in a balanced, impartial, and reproducible manner.

In general, tests applied to fabrics and finished household goods reflect only the ignitability of the product—its susceptibility to being accidentally ignited. These tests do not determine whether a fabric will burn and contribute to a room's fuel load in a given room fire. All fabrics will burn if the temperature, ventilation, and duration of the fire are sufficient; even highly fire-resistant fabrics of Nomex or PBI will burn under the right conditions. These comments on fabrics and their fire tests are offered to assist the investigator in assessing the logical consequences of ignition from small flames or glowing embers that come in contact with apparel or upholstered furniture.

One lesson from the extensive tests conducted by the Fire Research Station in the United Kingdom as part of the inquiry into the Stardust Disco disaster (1981) was that even when individual materials and products pass appropriate flammability tests, they may interact in complex ways to create extraordinary fire conditions. In the Stardust Disco fire, the combination of furnishings and wall coverings produced radiative feedback, drop down of flaming residues, and piloted ignition of smoldering upholstery that spread a fire throughout an open seating area much more quickly than anyone could have predicted. It was only through extensive full-scale simulations that the fire could be reenacted. The fire investigator must keep those lessons in mind when evaluating the contributions of individual fuels in any fire (Pigott 1984, 207-12; Morris 1984, 255-65).

Review Questions

1. If the test was intended to replicate an actual event, how closely did the materials, dimensions, and the ventilation match the original conditions?
2. Find an example of a commercial, academic, or governmental fire testing facility in your state. Visit or call this organization and determine what type of testing it performs.
3. Obtain a collection of at least 10 tests involving the use of a calorimeter from published research.
4. Research the methods of conducting field fire testing.
5. Obtain small samples of different clothing or upholstery fabrics from a fabric store (with identified content) and conduct *NFPA 705* ignition

tests on each (in a safe location). Collect data and compare observations with descriptions included in the references.

6. What is the chemical difference between natural fibers and synthetic fibers? Name three examples of each.

7. What fire behavior is peculiar to cellulosic fibers? Why does it not occur with most synthetics?

8. Name three of the US government regulations on flammability of fabrics and describe each application.

9. What is a typical time frame for cigarette ignition of upholstered furniture?

10. What does an oxygen-depletion calorimeter do?

11. What is the California flame resistance standard (*TB 603*) and why is it so different from previous standards?

12. Describe three of the fabric flammability tests used today.

13. What is the methenamine pill test and what is it used for?

14. Why is polypropylene carpet such a special consideration in fire investigations?

References

Ahrens, M. 2008. "Home Fires that Began with Upholstered Furniture" (Quincy, MA: Fire Analysis and Research Division, National Fire Protection Association, 2008).

ASTM. 1993. *ASTM D3659-80e1: Standard Test Method for Flammability of Apparel Fabrics by Semi-restraint Method.* West Conshohocken, PA: ASTM International.

———. 2008a. *ASTM E1352-80a: Standard Test Method for Cigarette Ignition Resistance of Mock-Up Upholstered Furniture Assemblies.* West Conshohocken, PA: ASTM International.

———. 2008b. *ASTM E1353-08ae1: Standard Test Method for Cigarette Ignition Resistance of Components of Upholstered Furniture.* West Conshohocken, PA: ASTM International.

———. 2010a. *ASTM D56-05: Standard Test Method for Flash Point by Tag Closed Cup Tester.* West Conshohocken, PA: ASTM International.

———. 2010b. *ASTM D1230-10: Standard Test Method for Flammability of Apparel Textiles.* West Conshohocken, PA: ASTM International.

———. 2010c. *ASTM D2859-06: Standard Test Method for Ignition Characteristics of Finished Textile Floor Covering Materials.* West Conshohocken, PA: ASTM International.

———. 2011. *ASTM D3278-96: Standard Test Methods for Flash Point of Liquids by Small Scale Closed-Cup Apparatus.* West Conshohocken, PA: ASTM International.

———. 2012a. *ASTM D92-12b: Standard Test Method for Flash and Fire Points by Cleveland Open Cup Tester.* West Conshohocken, PA: ASTM International.

———. 2012b. *ASTM D3828-12a: Standard Test Methods for Flash Point by Small Scale Closed Tester.* West Conshohocken, PA: ASTM International.

———. 2013a. *ASTM D4809-13: Standard Test Method for Heat of Combustion of Liquid Hydrocarbon Fuels by Bomb Calorimeter (Precision Method).* West Conshohocken, PA: ASTM International.

———. 2013b. *ASTM E502-07: Standard Test Method for Selection and Use of ASTM Standards for the Determination of Flash Point of Chemicals by Closed Cup Methods.* West Conshohocken, PA: ASTM International.

———. 2013c. *ASTM E603-13: Standard Guide for Room Fire Experiments.* West Conshohocken, PA: ASTM International.

———. 2013d. *ASTM E1321-13: Standard Test Method for Determining Material Ignition and Flame Spread Properties.* West Conshohocken, PA: ASTM International.

———. 2014a. *ASTM D1310-14: Standard Test Method for* Flash Point *and* Fire Point *of Liquids by Tag Open-Cup Apparatus.* West Conshohocken, PA: ASTM International.

———. 2014b. *ASTM D1929-14: Standard Test Method for Determining Ignition Temperature of Plastics.* West Conshohocken, PA: ASTM International.

———. 2014c. *ASTM D3675-14: Standard Test Method for Surface Flammability of Flexible Cellular Materials Using a Radiant Heat Energy Source.* West Conshohocken, PA: ASTM International.

———. 2014d. *ASTM E800-14: Standard Guide for Measurement of Gases Present or Generated during Fires.* West Conshohocken, PA: ASTM International.

———. 2015a. *ASTM E84-15a: Standard Test Method for Surface Burning Characteristics of Building Materials.* West Conshohocken, PA: ASTM International.

———. 2015b. *ASTM D93-15b: Standard Test Methods for Flash Point by Pensky-Martens Closed-Cup Tester.* West Conshohocken, PA: ASTM International.

———. 2015c. *ASTM E119-15: Standard Test Methods for Fire Tests of Building Construction and Materials.* West Conshohocken, PA: ASTM International.

———. 2015d. *ASTM E648-15e1: Standard Test Method for Critical Radiant Flux of Floor-Covering Systems Using a Radiant Heat Energy Source.* West Conshohocken, PA: ASTM International.

———. 2015e. *ASTM E659-15: Standard Test Method for Autoignition Temperature of Liquid Chemicals*. West Conshohocken, PA: ASTM International.

———. 2015f. *ASTM E1354-15a: Standard Test Method for Heat and Visible Smoke Release Rates for Materials and Products Using an Oxygen Consumption Calorimeter*. West Conshohocken, PA: ASTM International.

Babrauskas, V. 1997. "The Role of Heat Release Rate in Describing Fires." *Fire & Arson Investigator* 47 (June): 54–57.

Babrauskas, V., and J. Krasny. 1985. *Fire Behavior of Upholstered Furniture*. Gaithersburg, MD: US Department of Commerce.

———. 1997. "Upholstered Furniture Transition from Smoldering to Flaming." *Journal of Forensic Sciences* 42: 1029–31.

Backer, S., G. C. Tesoro, T. Y. Yoong, and N. A. Moussa. 1976. *Textile Fabric Flammability*. Cambridge, MA: MIT Press.

Bhatnagar, V. M., ed. 1975. *Advances in Fire Retardant Textiles*. Westport, CT: Technomic, 1975.

Bryner, N. P., E. L. Johnsson, and W. M. Pitts. 1995. "Scaling Compartment Fires: Reduced- and Full-Scale Enclosure Burns." Paper presented at the International Conference on Fire Research and Engineering, September 10–15, Orlando, FL.

California Department of Consumer Affairs. 1980a. *Technical Bulletin 116: Requirements, Test Procedure and Apparatus for Testing the Flame Retardance of Upholstered Furniture*. North Highlands, CA: California Department of Consumer Affairs, January 1980.

———. 1980b. *Technical Bulletin 117: Requirements, Test Procedure and Apparatus for Testing the Flame Retardance of Resilient Filling Materials Used in Upholstered Furniture*. North Highlands, CA: California Department of Consumer Affairs, January 1980.

———. 1980c. *Technical Bulletin 121: Flammability Test Procedure for Mattresses for Use in High Risk Occupancies*. North Highlands, CA: California Department of Consumer Affairs, April 1980.

———. 1988. *Technical Bulletin 133: Flammability Test Procedure for Seating Furniture for Use in Public Occupancies*. North Highlands, CA: California Department of Consumer Affairs.

———. 1992. *Technical Bulletin 129: Flammability Testing Procedures for Mattresses for Use in Public Buildings*. North Highlands, CA: California Department of Consumer Affairs.

———. 2002. *Technical Bulletin 603: Requirements and Test Procedures for Resistance of a Mattress/Box Spring Set to a Large Open Flame* North Highlands, CA: California Department of Consumer Affairs, January 2002.

CPSC. 1976. *Guide to Fabric Flammability*. US Consumer Product Safety Commission.

Damant, G. H. 1994. "Recent United States Developments in Tests and Materials for the Flammability of Furnishings." *Journal of the Textile Institute* 85, no. 4.

———. 1995. "Cigarette Ignition of Upholstered Furniture." Inter-City Testing and Consulting, Sacramento, CA, 1994; also in *Journal of Fire Sciences* September–October 1995.

———. 1996. "The Flexible Polyurethane Foam Industry's Response to Tough Fire Safety Regulations." *Journal of Fire Sciences* 4 (1986). Revised by G. H. Damant, personal communication, January 1996.

DeHaan, J. D. 1992. "Fire: Fatal Intensity; A Third View of the Lime Street Fire." *Fire and Arson Investigator* 43 (1): 5.

Fleischmann, C. M., P. J. Pagni, and R. B. Williamson. 1994. "Salt Water Modeling of Fire Compartment Gravity Currents." Paper presented at Fire Safety Science: Fourth International Symposium, July 13–17, Ottawa, Ontario, Canada.

Foster, R. P., and J. B. Zicherman. 2005. "Is There a Time Bomb in the Sofa?" *Trial* November: 58–63.

Hall, J. R. 2001. "Targeting Upholstered Furniture Fires." *NFPA Journal*, March–April: 57–60.

———. 2008. "The U.S. Smoking Material Fire Problem." Quincy, MA: Fire Analysis and Research Division, National Fire Protection Association.

Hoebel, J. F., G. H. Damant, S. M. Spivak, and G. N. Berlin. 2010. "Clothing Related Burn Casualties: An Overlooked Problem." *Fire Technology* 46 (3), July 2010, 629–649.

Holleyhead, R. 1999. "Ignition of Solid Materials and Furniture by Lighted Cigarettes. A Review." *Science & Justice* 39 (2): 75–102, doi: 10.1016/s1355-0306(99)72027-7.

Holmes, J. 1986. "Some Clothes May Play with Fire." *Insight,* June 9, 1986: 46.

Jewell, R. S., J. D. Thomas, and R. A. Dodds. 2011. "Attempted Ignition of Petrol Vapour By Lit Cigarettes and Lit Cannabis Resin Joints." *Science & Justice* 51 (2): 72–76, doi: 10.1016/j.scijus.2010.10.002.

Krasny, J., W. J. Parker, and V. Babrauskas. 2001. *Fire Behavior of Upholstered Furniture and Mattresses*. Norwich, NY: William Andrew.

Mehta, A. K., and F. Wong. 1983. "Hazards of Burn Injuries from Apparel Fabrics." NTIS COM-73–10960, Fuels Research Laboratory, MIT, February 1983.

Miller, D. 2015. *2010-2012 Residential Fire Loss Estimates: U.S. National Estimates of Fires, Deaths, Injuries, and Property Losses from Unintentional Fires*. Bethesda, MD: US Consumer Product Safety Commission.

Miller, D., R. Chowdury, and M. Greene. 2009. "2004–2006 Residential Fire Loss Estimates." Washington, DC: Consumer Product Safety Commission.

Morris, W. A. 1984. "Stardust Disco Investigation: Some Observations on the Full-Scale Fire Tests." *Fire Safety Journal* 7: 255–65.

NFPA. 2012. *NFPA 1403: Standard on Live Fire Training Evolutions*. Quincy, MA: National Fire Protection Association.

———. 2013. *NFPA 705: Recommended Practice for a Field Flame Test for Textiles and Films*. Quincy, MA: National Fire Protection Association.

———. 2017. *NFPA 921: Guide for Fire and Explosion Investigations*. Quincy, MA: National Fire Protection Association.

———. 2006. NFPA 255: Standard Methods of Test of Surface Burning Characteristics of Building Materials. Quincy, MA: National Fire Protection Association.

———. 2015. NFPA 265: Standard Methods of Fire Tests for Evaluating Room Fire Growth Contribution of Textile on Expanded Vinyl Wall Coverings on Full Height Panels and Walls. Quincy, MA: National Fire Protection Association.

———. 2015. NFPA 701: Standard Methods of Fire Tests for Flame Propagation of Textiles and Films. Quincy, MA: National Fire Protection Association.

Pigott, P. T. 1984. "The Fire at the Stardust, Dublin: The Public Inquiry and Its Findings." *Fire Safety Journal* 7: 207–12.

Quintiere, J. G. 1989. "Scaling Applications in Fire Research." *Fire Safety Journal* 15 (1): 3–29, doi: 10.1016/0379-7112(89)90045-3.

Rohr, K. D. 2005. "Selections for Products First Ignited in U.S. Home Fires: Soft Good and Wearing Apparel." Quincy, MA: Fire Analysis and Research Division, National Fire Protection Association.

Sundstrom, B., ed. 1995. *Fire Safety of Upholstered Furniture: The Full Report of the European Commission Research Programme (CBUF)*. London: Interscience Communications.

Wortman, P. S., S. S. Williams, and G. H. Damant. 1984. "Development of a Fire Test for Furniture for High Risk and Public Occupancies." Pp. 55–67 in *Proceedings of the International Conference on Fire Safety*. Sunnyvale CA: Product Safety Commission.

11

Arson Crime Scene Analysis

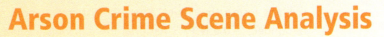

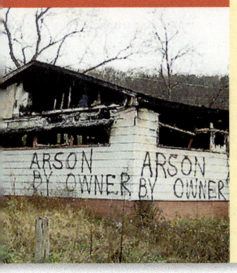

Courtesy of Greg Lampkin, Knox County Sheriff's Office, Tennessee, Fire Investigation Unit.

KEY TERMS

accelerant, *p. 665*
arson, *p. 664*
crime concealment (motive), *p. 676*
excitement (motive), *p. 672*

extremism (motive), *p. 681*
incendiary fire, *p. 664*
motive, *p. 667*
profit (motive), *p. 678*

pyromania, *p. 682*
revenge (motive), *p. 674*
vandalism (motive), *p. 670*

OBJECTIVES

After reading this chapter, you should be able to:

- Describe arson crime scene analysis.
- Define the crime of arson.
- Classify motives.
- Identify indicators of motives.

Based on published statistics from the National Fire Protection Association (NFPA), in 2014, US fire departments responded to an estimated 1,298,000 fires in 2014, which resulted in 3,275 civilian fire fatalities, 15,775 civilian fire injuries, and an estimated $11.6 billion in direct property loss. Home fire losses with deaths are staggering, with 2,745 civilians losing their lives. These statistics were compiled from fire departments that responded to the NFPA's national fire experience survey entitled, "Fire Loss in the United States During 2014" (Haynes 2015).

A leading concern of fire in the United States, arson continues to be an urgent national problem. Often characterized as a clandestine tool for criminals, the true arson picture is not clearly known. The NFPA statistics for 2014 estimate that there were 19,000 intentionally set structure fires resulting in an estimated 157 civilian deaths and $613 million in property losses. There were also an estimated 8,000 intentionally set vehicle fires resulting in $116 million in property loss (Haynes 2015; Campbell, 2014).

Insight into arson statistics is not limited to the United States. In 1999 the UK Home Office provided a view of that country's problems (Home Office 1999). On the other side of the globe, Australia specifically addressed their unique wildland bushfire arson problem with a statistics-driven prevention approach (Willis 2004; Anderson 2010).

Economically, arson affects insurance premium rates, removes taxable property assets, and erodes our communities. Historically, the inner areas of our large cities often are the hardest hit. The result is that much of the costs of this destructive crime falls on those who can least afford it. Historical trends show repeatedly that a decline in the economy results in an increase in arsons (Decker and Ottley 2009).

An understanding of the crime of arson based on its motivations may enhance an investigator's efforts and provide a focus for intervention efforts. Examination of the fire scene and reporting of the findings may facilitate dialogue among the various disciplines and investigative units involved in arson enforcement, investigation, and prevention.

The information in this chapter will assist arson investigators in developing skills for reading and interpreting the characteristics of crime scene evidence and applying that evidence to the arsonist's behavior and patterns of motivation.

11.1 Arson as a Crime

The definitions for arson range widely, owing primarily to differing statutory terminology. The FBI's UCR program defines **arson** as "any willful or malicious burning or attempting to burn, with or without intent to defraud, a dwelling house, public building, motor vehicle or aircraft, or personal property of another" (FBI 2010). In addition, *NFPA 921* (*NFPA 921*, 2014 ed., pt. 3.3.13) defines **arson** as "the crime of maliciously and intentionally, or recklessly, starting a fire or causing an explosion." The most accepted definition is that *arson* is simply the willful and malicious burning of property (Icove et al. 1992).

According to *NFPA 921*, an **incendiary fire** is "a classification of the cause of a fire that is intentionally ignited under circumstances in which the person igniting the fire knows the fire should not be ignited" (see *NFPA 921*, 2014 ed., pt. 3.3.108).

The criminal act of arson is usually divided into three elements (DeHaan and Icove 2012):

1. *There has been a burning of property.* This must be shown to the court to be actual destruction, at least in part, not just scorching or sooting (although some states include any physical or visible impairment of any surface). As used here, "burning" includes destruction by explosion.

arson ■ The crime of maliciously and intentionally, or recklessly, starting a fire or causing an explosion (NFPA 2017, pt. 3.3.14).

arson ■ Any willful or malicious burning or attempting to burn, with or without intent to defraud, a dwelling house, public building, motor vehicle or aircraft, or personal property of another (FBI 2010).

incendiary fire ■ A fire that is intentionally ignited in an area or under circumstances where and when there should not be a fire (NFPA 2017, pt. 3.3.116).

2. **The burning is incendiary in origin.** Proof of the existence of an effective incendiary device, no matter how simple it may be, is adequate. Proof must be established by exhaustively considering all hypotheses, using the scientific method.

3. **The burning is shown to be started with malice.** The fire is started with the intent of destroying property (i.e., a person starts a fire or causes an explosion with the purpose of destroying a building of another or one's own with fire). The "degree" of the arson charge in most jurisdictions has to do with the occupancy: first degree corresponding to an occupied structure, second to an unoccupied structure, and third to other property.

It is the responsibility, per *NFPA 1033* (NFPA 2014, pt. 4.6.4), of the fire investigator to establish evidence as to motive and/or opportunity, given an incendiary fire, so that the evidence is supported by documentation and meets the evidentiary requirements of the jurisdiction.

An arsonist is a person apprehended, charged, and convicted of one or more arsons. Arsonists commonly use **accelerants**, which are any type of material or substance added to the targeted materials to enhance the combustion of those materials and to increase the intensity or speed of the spread (Icove et al. 1992). There are many serial arsonists who set fires to available combustibles without using any accelerants.

accelerant ■ A fuel or oxidizer, often an ignitable liquid, intentionally used to initiate a fire or increase the rate of growth or spread of fire (NFPA 2017, pt. 3.3.2).

11.1.1 DEVELOPING THE WORKING HYPOTHESIS

It is the responsibility of the fire investigator, per *NFPA 1033*, 2014 ed., pt. 4.6.5, to formulate an opinion concerning origin, cause, or responsibility for the fire, given all investigative findings.

Several factors that may contribute to a working hypothesis for an incendiary fire are discussed in *NFPA 921*, 2017 Edition, Chapter 24, "Incendiary Fires" (NFPA 2017). Displayed in Figure 11-1 is a mosaic of several factors that may contribute to a working hypothesis in an incendiary fire or explosion, derived from *NFPA 921*. These factors should not be considered all-inclusive; other indicators may exist. However, investigators should be cautioned that one or more of these factors are not necessarily sufficient to constitute a finding of an incendiary fire.

POST-INCIDENT INVESTIGATION STANDARD: 4.6.5 *NFPA 1033*, 2014 EDITION

TASK:

Formulate an opinion concerning origin, cause, or responsibility for the fire, given all investigative findings, so that the opinion regarding origin, cause, or responsibility for a fire is supported by the data, facts, records, reports, documents, and evidence.

PERFORMANCE OUTCOME:

The investigator will formulate an opinion of the person and/or product responsibility for the fire.

CONDITIONS:

Given a complete fire investigation file, including records, documents, and evidence, the investigator will complete the listed task.

TASK STEPS:

1. Review provided materials
2. Formulate and document an opinion as to the person and/or product responsibility

Source: Derived and updated from Washington State Patrol, Form No. 3000-420-081 (Sept. 2014) Fire Protection Bureau, Standards and Accreditation, Olympia, Washington http://www.wsp.wa.gov/fire/docs/cert/fire_invest.pdf

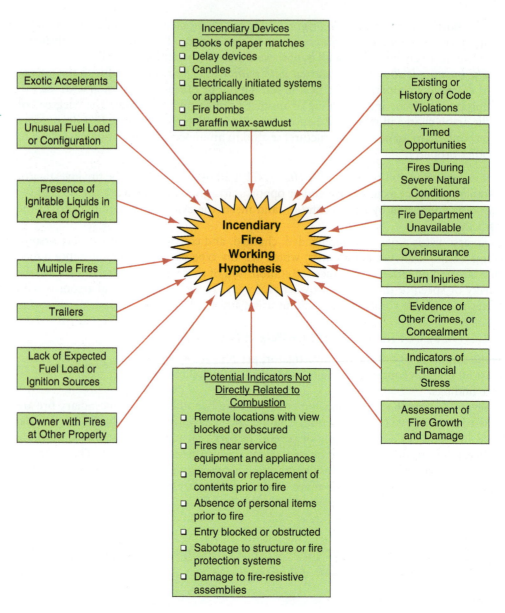

FIGURE 11-1 Several factors that may contribute to a working hypothesis for an incendiary fire or explosion. *Derived from NFPA 921, 2014 ed., Chap. 24.*

Incendiary Devices
- ❏ Books of paper matches
- ❏ Delay devices
- ❏ Candles
- ❏ Electrically initiated systems or appliances
- ❏ Fire bombs
- ❏ Paraffin wax-sawdust

Exotic Accelerants

Unusual Fuel Load or Configuration

Presence of Ignitable Liquids in Area of Origin

Multiple Fires

Trailers

Lack of Expected Fuel Load or Ignition Sources

Owner with Fires at Other Property

Incendiary Fire Working Hypothesis

Existing or History of Code Violations

Timed Opportunities

Fires During Severe Natural Conditions

Fire Department Unavailable

Overinsurance

Burn Injuries

Evidence of Other Crimes, or Concealment

Indicators of Financial Stress

Assessment of Fire Growth and Damage

Potential Indicators Not Directly Related to Combustion
- ❏ Remote locations with view blocked or obscured
- ❏ Fires near service equipment and appliances
- ❏ Removal or replacement of contents prior to fire
- ❏ Absence of personal items prior to fire
- ❏ Entry blocked or obstructed
- ❏ Sabotage to structure or fire protection systems
- ❏ Damage to fire-resistive assemblies

11.1.2 MULTIPLE FIRES

When an offender is involved with three or more fires, particular terminology is used to describe that crime (Icove et al. 1992).

- *Mass arson* involves an offender who sets three or more fires at the same site or location during a limited period of time.
- *Spree arson* involves an arsonist who sets three or more fires at separate locations with no emotional cooling-off or delay period between the fires.
- *Serial arson* involves an offender who sets three or more fires with a cooling-off, or delay, period between the fires.

This chapter includes a detailed discussion of how arson crime scenes are analyzed. Such analysis often leads to the identification of offenders, their method of operation, and their areas of frequent travel.

11.2 Classification of Motive

Juries often want to have a demonstrable motive considered with the evidence so that they can justify the verdict to themselves, even though it is not a legal requirement. Although motive is not essential to establish the crime of arson, and need not be demonstrated in court, the development of a motive frequently leads to the identity of the offender. Establishing motive also provides the prosecution with a vital argument when presented to the judge and jury during trial. It is thought that the motive in an arson case often becomes the mortar that holds together the elements of the crime.

NFPA 921 (NFPA 2017, pt. 24.4.9.2) delineates the distinction between *motive* and *intent*. It states that intent refers to the state of mind, steps, and acts, or failure to act, at the time of the offense. In describing intent, an investigation should show "purposefulness or deliberateness of the person's actions or omissions."

Motive is defined as the "inner drive or impulse that is the cause, reason, or incentive that induces or prompts a specific behavior" (Rider 1980). It may be the reason that an individual or group may decide to act or not to act.

motive ■ An inner drive or impulse that is the cause, reason, or incentive that induces or prompts a specific behavior (Rider 1980).

The job performance requirement listed in *NFPA 1033* (NFPA 2014, pt. 4.6.4) emphasizes the importance of determining motive. It states that the fire investigator shall "establish evidence as to motive and/or opportunity, given an incendiary fire, so that the evidence is supported by documentation and meets the evidentiary requirements of the jurisdiction."

Most of the literature on fire setting and arson concentrates on either psychiatric/psychological or criminological studies (Kocsis and Cooksey 2006). The criminological studies on arson deal with either anecdotal case studies or motive-based classification schemes and typologies. Several of the earlier typologies contributed significantly to the traditional understanding of the motives and psychological profiles of arsonists (Lewis and Yarnell 1951; Robbins and Robbins 1967; Steinmetz 1966; Hurley and Monahan 1969; Inciardi 1970; Vandersall and Wiener 1970; Wolford 1972; Levin 1976; Icove and Estepp 1987).

POST-INCIDENT INVESTIGATION STANDARD: 4.6.4 *NFPA 1033*, 2014 EDITION

TASK:

Establish evidence as to motive and/or opportunity, given an incendiary fire, so that the evidence is supported by documentation and meets the evidentiary requirements of the jurisdiction.

PERFORMANCE OUTCOME:

The investigator will establish motive and/or opportunity of an incendiary fire through the use of prudent and complete investigation files, determining if the evidence meets legal requirements.

CONDITIONS:

Given a complete incendiary fire investigation file and evidence log, the investigator will determine motive and/or opportunity and determine the legal value of provided evidence.

TASK STEPS:

1. Review provided materials
2. Determine and document the motive and/or opportunity of the incendiary fire
3. List supporting documents that establish motive
4. Document evidence used to determine motive
5. Document legal value of evidence provided

Source: Derived and updated from Washington State Patrol, Form No. 3000-420-081 (Sept. 2014) Fire Protection Bureau, Standards and Accreditation, Olympia, Washington http://www.wsp.wa.gov/fire/docs/cert/fire_invest.pdf

The Lewis and Yarnell (1951) study is cited only for historical purposes, since it was an early study and was based on a very limited sample base. However, the focus of research work since that study has examined motive as it relates to arson. Recent comprehensive research by Gannon and Pina (2010) addresses the characteristics of adult fire setters, contemporary research on the theories of fire-setting behavior, and clinical interventions. The researchers suggest that clinical knowledge and practice relating to fire setting is extremely underdeveloped.

11.2.1 CLASSIFICATION

Research on arsonists has historically been conducted largely from the forensic psychiatric viewpoint (Vreeland and Waller 1978). Many forensic researchers do not necessarily assess the crime from the law enforcement perspective. They may have limited access to complete adult and juvenile criminal records and investigative case files and must often rely on the self-reported interviews of the offenders as being totally truthful. Often, these researchers do not have the capabilities and time to validate the information through follow-up investigations. Other researchers have cited that methodological difficulties, including small sample sizes of interviews and skewed databases, may have biased some of the previous studies (Harmon, Rosner, and Wiederlight 1985).

Inciardi's (1970) work deals with a typology of adult fire setters. Geller (1992, 2008) offers exhaustive reviews of that literature and identifies 20 or more attempts to classify arsonists into typologies. Canter and Fritzon (1998) advance the hypothesis that there will be behavioral consistencies in the criminal actions of arsonists that characterize them, which include their target of the attack and the offender's motivation. Doley (2003a) examines the various attempts at classification of typology and motive.

Medical studies suggest several physiological issues, including medical models of fire-setting behaviors. Virkkunen et al. (1987) examined cerebrospinal fluid (CSF) monoamine metabolite levels in 20 arsonists and 20 habitually violent offenders, and 10 healthy inpatient volunteers. Although they found no correlation in CSF concentrations with repeat fire-setting behavior, the researchers did find a tendency for the arsonists to suffer from hypoglycemia. Galliot and Baumeister (2007) also cite that blood glucose is one important part of the energy source of self-control and could be a contributing factor to setting fires.

Studies have looked at various aspects of criminal and psychiatric behavior in convicted arsonists. The study by Repo et al. (1997) examined the medical and criminal records of 282 Finnish arsonists and found that recidivist offenders had common traits of alcohol dependence, antisocial behavior, and a history of long-term enuresis (bed-wetting) during their childhood.

Stewart and Culver (1982), and later Yang and Geller (2009), examined the clinical perspective of dealing with juvenile fire setters. The demographics of female arsonists have been studied by Harmon, Rosner, and Wiederlight (1985) and by Miller and Fritzon (2007). Doley (2003b) along with Fritzon, Doley, and Hollows (2014) trace the research efforts to model the classification of arsonists through their motivations, medical, and behavioral traits.

11.2.2 OFFENDER-BASED MOTIVE CLASSIFICATION

For classification purposes, FBI behavioral science research defines *motive* as an inner drive or impulse that is the cause, reason, or incentive that induces or prompts a specific behavior (Rider 1980). A motive-based method of analysis can be used to identify personal traits and characteristics exhibited by an unknown offender (Icove 1979; Icove and Estepp 1987; Douglas et al. 1986; Douglas et al. 1992, 2006; Icove et al. 1992; Allen 1995). For legal purposes, the motive is often helpful in explaining why an offender committed his or her crime. However, motive is not normally a statutory element of a criminal offense.

General acceptance of this motive-based approach is well-accepted within the fire investigation and legal communities. The motivations discussed in this chapter are also outlined and described in *NFPA 921: Guide for Fire and Explosion Investigations* (NFPA 2017, pt. 24.4.9.3), in the chapter on arson in the FBI's *Crime Classification Manual* (Douglas et al. 1992, 2006; Icove et al. 1992), and the cases cited in the legal reference *Arson Law and Prosecution* (Decker and Ottley 2009).

Santtila, Fritzon, and Tamelander (2004) underscored the importance of linking an arsonist to his or her crime. The arsonist's consistency in offense behavior is linked to motive (Fritzon, Canter, and Wilton 2001). The latter group's research examined 248 arson cases that formed 42 series of arsons and examined 45 variables. The research results statistically confirmed earlier studies suggesting that serial and spree arson cases could be linked based on a consistency of behaviors from one crime scene to another. Woodhams, Bull, and Hollin (2007) underscore the importance for investigators to be familiar with case linkage research.

In the case of criminal investigations and prosecutions, proof of motive, unlike intent, is not required. However, in criminal cases, presenting a plausible motive for a defendant's arson makes it easier for the trier of fact to find that a fire was incendiary and to connect the defendant to the fire. See cited cases *State v. O'Haver*, 33 S.W.3d 555 (Miss. Ct. App. 2001) and *Briggs v. Makowski*, 2000 U.S. Dist. LEXIS 13029 (E.D. Mich. 2000).

Law enforcement–oriented studies on arson motives are *offender-based*; that is, they look at the relationship between the behavioral characteristics exhibited by the offender and the observable crime scene characteristics as it relates to motive. One of the largest offender-based studies consists of 1,016 interviews of both juveniles and adults arrested for arson and fire-related crimes during the years 1980 through 1984 by the Prince George's County Fire Department (PGFD), Fire Investigations Division (Icove and Estepp 1987). These offenses included 504 arrests for arson, 303 for malicious false alarms, 159 for violations of bombing/explosives/fireworks laws, and 50 for miscellaneous fire-related offenses.

The overall purpose of the PGFD study was to create and promote the use of motive-based offender profiles of individuals who commit incendiary and fire-related crimes, to assist in investigations. Prior studies failed to address comprehensively the issues confronting modern law enforcement. Of primary concern were the efforts to provide logical, motive-based investigative leads for incendiary crimes.

The study was conducted primarily because fire and law enforcement professionals were enabled to take on the task of conducting their own independent research into violent incendiary crimes. The PGFD study determined that arrested and incarcerated arsonists most often give the following motives (Icove and Estepp 1987). Since this keynote study, these major motive categories have become accepted in the fire investigation field after first being included in *Kirk's Fire Investigation*. These motive classifications now appear in *NFPA 921* (NFPA 2017, pt. 24.4.9):

- Vandalism
- Excitement
- Revenge
- Crime concealment
- Profit
- Extremist beliefs

This system of classification advances the earlier approach by the FBI to divide criminal offenders, including arsonists, into two groups: organized and disorganized (Douglas et al. 1986). Data in a study by Kocsis, Irwin, and Hayes (1998) supported the presence of an organized/disorganized typology. The researchers analyzed and validated hypotheses about the crime of arson using the crime scene characteristics of profit-motivated and vandalism-motivated arson offenses.

In some cases, there may be several motives. These cases can be classified as *mixed motive*. For example, a businessperson might murder a partner after work, set a fire at their store to cover up the crime, remove valuable merchandise, and file an inflated insurance claim. This hypothetical case would exhibit overlapping motives of revenge, crime concealment, and profit.

11.3 Vandalism-Motivated Arson

Vandalism-motivated arson is defined as malicious or mischievous fire setting that results in damage to property (see Table 11-1 and Figure 11-2). Juvenile arsonists commit some vandalism-motivated arsons, with the most common targets being schools, school property, and educational facilities. Vandals also frequently target abandoned structures and combustible vegetation. The typical vandalism-motivated arsonist will use available materials to set fires with book matches and cigarette lighters as the ignition devices. Time-delay

vandalism (motive) ■ Vandalism-motivated firesetting is defined as mischievous or malicious firesetting that results in damage to property. Common targets include educational facilities and abandoned structures, but also include trash fires and grass fires. Vandalism firesetting categories include willful and malicious mischief and peer or group pressure (NFPA 2017, pt. 24.4.9.3.2).

TABLE 11-1	Vandalism-Motivated Arson
Characteristics Victimology: targeted property	■ Educational facilities common target ■ Residential areas ■ Vegetation (grass, brush, woodland, and timber)
Crime scene indicators frequently noted	■ Multiple offenders acting spontaneously and impulsively ■ Crime scenes reflect spontaneous nature of the offense (disorganized) ■ Offenders use available materials at the scene and leave physical evidence behind (shoeprints, fingerprints, etc.) ■ Flammable liquids occasionally used ■ Entrance may be gained through windows of secured structures ■ Matchbooks, cigarettes, and spray-paint cans (graffiti) often present ■ Materials missing from scene and general destruction of property
Common forensic findings	■ Presence of flammable liquids ■ Presence of fireworks ■ Glass particles on suspect's clothing if entered by breaking a window
Investigative considerations	■ Typical offender is a juvenile male with 7–9 years of formal education ■ Records of poor school performance ■ Not employed ■ Single and lives with one or both parents ■ Alcohol and drug use usually not associated ■ Offender may already be known by police and may have arrest record ■ Majority of offenders live more than 1 mile from the crime scene ■ Most offenders flee from scene immediately and do not return ■ If the offenders return, they view the fire from a safe vantage point ■ Investigators should solicit assistance from school, fire, and police
Search warrant suggestions	■ Spray-paint cans ■ Items from the scene ■ Explosive devices ■ Flammable liquids ■ Clothing: evidence of flammable liquid, glass particles ■ Shoes: shoe prints, flammable liquid traces

Sources: Updated from Icove and Estepp 1987; Icove et al. 1992; Sapp et al. 1995.

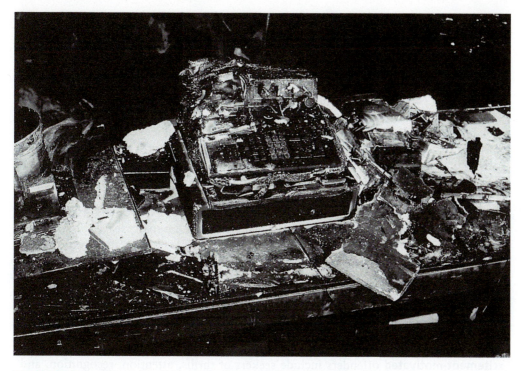

FIGURE 11-2 Vandalism-motivated arson showing a superficially damaged cash register. *Courtesy of David J. Icove, University of Tennessee.*

devices and liquid accelerants are very rarely used. The motive classification for vandalism is referenced in *NFPA 921* (NFPA 2017, pt. 24.4.9.3.2).

Usually, vandalism-motivated arsonists will leave the scene and not return to it. Their interest is in setting the fire, not watching it or the firefighting activities it generates. On average, vandalism arsonists will be questioned twice before being arrested and charged. They will offer no resistance when arrested but will qualify and minimize their responsibility. After an initial not-guilty plea, vandalism-motivated arsonists typically change their plea to guilty before trial.

Several case examples reinforce this motive. In *State v. True*, 190 N.W.2d 405 (Iowa 1971), the defendant and his friends went to a farm with the intent of stealing gasoline for their automobile. While attempting to forcibly remove the padlock and chain off the pump with a tire iron, the defendant ruptured it, allowing gasoline to escape onto the ground. The defendant remarked to his friend while leaving, "You don't have a hair if you don't go back and throw a match on it." The friend then lit a match, throwing it on the pool of gasoline and causing a fire that destroyed some of the buildings on the farm. The defendant was convicted of procuring the arson.

In *Reed v. State*, 326 Ark. 27, 929 S.W.2d 703 (Ark. 1996) a defendant and two companions skipped school and burglarized several homes. At one of the houses, the defendant asked one of his companions if they should burn the house; and then he set fire to curtains. The defendant was convicted of burglary, theft, and arson.

In *People v. Mentzer*, 163 Cal. App. 3d 482, 209 Cal. Rptr. 549 (Cal. Ct. App. 1985) the defendant and friend met in a cemetery, drank several beers, and then decided to set fire to some couches in a mausoleum "for some dumb reason." The fire also discolored, buckled, cracked, and chipped off the marble floor and plaster walls of the mausoleum, resulting in $65,000 in damage. During his trial, the defendant tried to argue that the damage to the mausoleum did not constitute "burning" because it could not be "consumed by fire." The defendant was convicted of attempted arson of a cemetery mausoleum. This argument was also rejected by the California appellate court.

EXAMPLE 11-1 ■ **Vandalism: Case Study of a Vandalism-Motivated Serial Arsonist**

A 19-year-old high-school dropout was responsible for a series of arsons in a northeastern city that were set using available materials and lit by a cigarette lighter. He admitted to setting 31 fires in vacant buildings and garages as well as dumpsters and derelict vehicles. He was questioned twice before being arrested and formally charged with nine of the house fires. When interviewed, he stated, "I just burned them for the hell of it. You know, just to have something to do. Those old houses and that other stuff was not worth anything anyway."

His mother and father had divorced when he was 2 years old. He had lived alternately with his mother and grandmother. He had no contact with his father and said that his mother had remarried several times. After dropping out of school in the 10th grade, he had worked sporadically at unskilled jobs and continued to live with his grandmother.

Several times, he reported just striking a match, tossing it into dry leaves or grass, and walking away without even seeing if it ignited. "I did not care nothing about watching no fire. It was just something to do. There was not much going on most of the time, you know. Just hanging out. It was just kid stuff, just for the hell of it. Half of the guys I knew that hung out would set a fire for the hell of it" (Sapp et al. 1995).

11.4 Excitement-Motivated Arson

Excitement-motivated offenders include seekers of thrills, attention, recognition, and, rarely but importantly, sexual gratification (see Table 11-2 and Figure 11-3). The arsonist who sets fires for sexual gratification is quite rare. The motive classification for excitement is referenced in *NFPA 921* (NFPA 2017, pt. 24.4.9.3.3).

excitement (motive) ■ The excitement-motivated firesetter may enjoy the excitement that is provided by actual firesetting or the activities surrounding the fire suppression efforts, or may have a psychological need for attention. The excitement-motivated offender is often a serial firesetter. This firesetter generally remains at the scene during the fire and will often get in position to respond to, or view the fire and the surrounding activities. The excitement-motivated firesetter's targets range from small trash and grass fires to occupied buildings (NFPA 2017, pt. 24.4.9.3.3).

TABLE 11-2	Excitement-Motivated Arson
Characteristics Victimology: targeted property	■ Dumpsters ■ Vegetation (grass, brush, woodland, timber) ■ Lumber stacks ■ Construction sites ■ Residential property ■ Unoccupied structures ■ Locations that offer a vantage point to observe fire suppression and investigation safely
Crime scene indicators frequently noted	■ Often adjacent to outdoor "hangouts" ■ Often uses available materials on hand to start small fires ■ If incendiary devices are used, they usually have time-delayed triggering mechanisms ■ Offenders in the 18–30 age group more prone to using accelerants ■ Match/cigarette delay device frequently used to ignite vegetation fires ■ Small group of offenders is motivated by sexual perversions, leaving ejaculate, fecal deposits, pornographic material
Common forensic findings	■ Fingerprints, vehicle and bicycle tracks ■ Remnants of incendiary devices ■ Ejaculate or fecal materials

TABLE 11-2	Excitement-Motivated Arson (*Continued*)
Investigative considerations	■ Typical offender is a juvenile or young adult male with 10+ years of formal education ■ Offender unemployed, single, and living with one or both parents from middle- to lower-class bracket ■ Offender generally is socially inadequate, particularly in heterosexual relationships ■ Use of drugs or alcohol limited usually to older offenders ■ History of nuisance offenses ■ Distance offender lives from the crime scene determined through a cluster analysis ■ Some offenders do not leave, mingling in crowds to watch the fire ■ Offenders who leave usually return later to assess the damage and their handiwork
Search warrant suggestions	■ Vehicle: material similar to incendiary devices, floor mats, trunk padding, carpeting, cans, matchbooks, cigarettes, police/fire scanners ■ House: material similar to incendiary devices, clothing, shoes, cans, matchbooks, cigarettes, lighter, diaries, journals, notes, logs, records and maps documenting fires, newspaper articles, souvenirs from the crime scene, police/fire scanners

Sources: Updated from Icove and Estepp 1987; Icove et al. 1992; Sapp et al. 1995.

Potential targets of the excitement-motivated arsonist run the full spectrum from so-called nuisance fires to fires in occupied apartment houses at nighttime. A limited number of firefighters have been known to set fires so they can engage in the suppression effort (Huff 1994; USFA 2003). Security guards have set fires to relieve boredom and gain recognition. Research into this motive category further categorizes excitement-motivated arsonists into several subclassifications, including thrill-, sex-, and recognition/attention-motivated arsonists (Icove et al. 1992). Recent reports on dealing with firefighter arson bring new insight into their prevention by the National Volunteer Fire Council by careful pre-employment screening and criminal records checks (NVFC 2011).

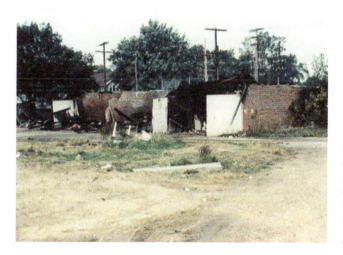

FIGURE 11-3
Excitement-motivated arsonists sometimes target garages, which contain and have easily accessible all the materials and fuels needed for setting the fire. *Courtesy of David J. Icove, University of Tennessee.*

EXAMPLE 11-2 ■ **Excitement: Case History of an Excitement/ Recognition-Motivated Serial Arsonist**

A 23-year-old volunteer firefighter was charged with setting a series of fires shortly after joining the fire department. Initially, he set the fires in trash cans and dumpsters, and then progressed to unoccupied and vacant structures.

The firefighter became a suspect in the fires when he consistently arrived first on the scene and frequently reported the fire. He stated that he set the fires so that he could get practice and others would view him as a good firefighter. He commented that his father was "real proud of his firefighter son" (Sapp et al. 1995).

11.5 Revenge-Motivated Arson

revenge (motive) ■ The revenge-motivated firesetter retaliates for some real or perceived injustice. An important aspect is that a sense of injustice is perceived by the offender. The event or circumstance that is perceived may have occurred months or years before the firesetting activity. A fire by the revenge-motivated offender may be a well-planned, one-time event or may represent serial firesetting, with little or no pre-planning. Serial offenders may direct their retaliation at individuals, institutions, or society in general (NFPA 2017, pt. 24.4.9.3.4.1).

Revenge-motivated fires are set in retaliation for some injustice, real or imagined, perceived by the offender (see Table 11-3 and Figure 11-4). Often, revenge is also an element of other motives. The motive classification for revenge is referenced in *NFPA 921* (NFPA 2017, pt. 24.4.9.3.4). Mixed motives are discussed later in this chapter.

TABLE 11-3	Revenge-Motivated Arson
Characteristics Victimology: targeted property	■ Victim of revenge fire generally has a history of interpersonal or professional conflict with offender (lovers' triangle, landlord/tenant, employer/employee) ■ Tends to be an intraracial offense ■ Female offenders usually target something of significance to victim (vehicle, personal effects) ■ Ex-lover offender frequently burns clothing, bedding, and/or personal effects ■ Societal revenge targets displace aggression to institutions, government facilities, universities, corporations
Crime scene indicators frequently noted	■ Female offenders usually burn an area of personal significance, using victim's clothing or other personal effects ■ Male offenders begin with an area of personal significance, tend to overkill by using more accelerants or incendiary devices than are necessary
Common forensic findings	■ Laboratory tests for accelerants, pieces of incendiary device, cloth, fingerprints
Investigative considerations	■ Offender is predominantly an adult male with 10+ years of formal education ■ If employed, the offender is usually a blue-collar worker of low socioeconomic status ■ Resides in rental property; loner, unstable relationships ■ Event happens months or years after precipitating incident ■ Most often, has some periodic law enforcement contact for burglary, theft, and/or vandalism ■ Use of alcohol more prevalent than drugs, with possible increase after the fire ■ Usually alone at scene and seldom returns after fire started to establish an alibi ■ Lives in affected community, with mobility an important factor ■ Revenge-focused analysis assists in determining true victim ■ Investigative investment significant
Search warrant suggestions	■ If accelerants suspected: shoes, socks, clothing, bottles, flammable liquids, matchbooks

Sources: Updated from Icove and Estepp 1987; Icove et al. 1992; Sapp et al. 1995.

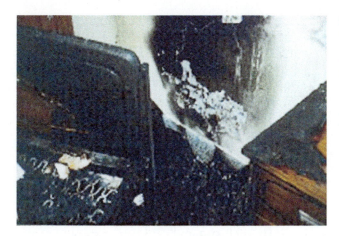

FIGURE 11-4 A revenge-motivated fire set on a bed, which is characteristic of a focused target having personal significance. *Courtesy of David J. Icove, University of Tennessee.*

What may be of concern to investigators is that the event or circumstance that is perceived as unjust may have occurred months or years before the fire-setting activity (Icove and Horbert 1990). For threat assessment purposes, this time delay may not readily be recognized, and investigators are urged to pursue the historical incidents in which a person or property has been targeted.

Revenge- and spite-motivated fires account for more of the serious arson cases, owing to the overkill reflected in the actions of the offender, such as shown in Figure 11-5. In these cases, when one container of a flammable liquid would suffice in setting a building on fire or incinerating a body, the offender may use much larger quantities, reflecting the rage or vengeance of the act.

The broad classification of revenge-motivated arsonists is further divided into subgroups based on the target of the retaliation. Studies show that serial revenge-motivated arsonists are more likely to direct their retaliation at institutions and society than at individuals or groups (Icove et al. 1992).

There are numerous case examples of revenge-motivated arsons by men after disputes with their wives, girlfriends, or former girlfriends. Examples include *Mathews v. State*, 849 N.E.2d 578 (Ind. 2006); *Commonwealth v. Dougherty* [580 Pa.183, 860 A.2d 31 (2004)]; *State v. Curmon*, 171 N.C. App. 697, 615 S.E.2d 417 (N.C. Ct. App. 2005); *State v. Howard*, 2004 Ohio App. LEXIS 385 (Ohio Ct. App. 2004); and *State v. McGinnis*, 2002 N.C. App. LEXIS 2325 (N.C. Ct. App. 2002).

In *State v. Lewis*, 385 N.W.2d 352 (Minn. Ct. App. 1986), the defendant was charged with first-degree arson for setting fire to his ex-girlfriend's apartment, destroying all of her belongings, causing the death of her cat, and resulting in $23,500 of structural damages. The court allowed circumstantial evidence of a witness placing the defendant at the apartment's front door approximately 35 minutes before the fire, as well as evidence of three other fires started by the defendant. This circumstantial evidence was used to show that the defendant's motive, modus operandi, identity, and intent formed a common scheme or plan in that he exhibited a pattern of setting revenge fires to cars of women who had previously rejected him.

In *State v. Bowles*, 754 S.W.2d 902 (Mo. Ct. App. 1988), a defendant was charged with first degree attempted arson when, after an argument with a police officer, the defendant and a friend obtained some gasoline and went to the police officer's house. The officer, hearing a noise, came out of his house to find the defendant "crouched over" next to the house with the gasoline and lighter in his pocket. The officer arrested the defendant before he could light the gasoline, charging him with first degree attempted arson. The Missouri appellate court affirmed the defendant's conviction.

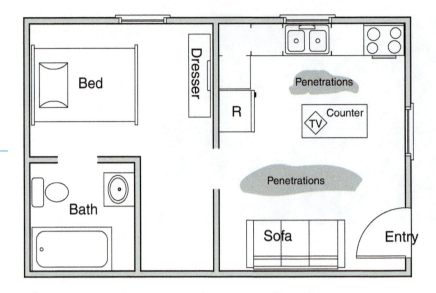

FIGURE 11-5 Example of a revenge-motivated fire where a sofa was ignited for revenge and drove the living room to flashover, which burned holes through the floor. *Courtesy of Det. Michael Dalton (ret.), Knox County Sheriff's Office.*

EXAMPLE 11-3 ■ **Revenge: Case History of an Institutional Retaliation "Revenge" Serial Arsonist**

John (not his real name) is 31 years old and claims to have set more than 60 fires at various local government facilities in the city where he lives. His fire-setting activities have occurred since he was 19 years old.

John started setting fires after he was sentenced to 180 days in the local jail facility for a petty theft. He claims to have set 5 fires while in the jail and then later 20 to 25 trash can fires in the local city hall. His method of operation consisted of simply walking through and dropping lighted matches into the trash containers.

His stated motive for setting the fires was "to cost the city some trouble and money. They did not treat me fair and I will get even." When asked when his revenge against the city would be satisfied, his response was "when the whole damn city hall burns down and the jail too" (Sapp et al. 1995).

crime concealment (motive) ■ This category involves firesetting that is a secondary or a collateral criminal activity, perpetrated for the purpose of concealing the primary criminal activity. In some cases, however, the fire may actually be part of the intended crime, such as revenge. Many people erroneously believe that a fire will destroy all physical evidence at the crime scene. Categories for crime concealment firesetting include murder or burglary concealment and destruction of records or documents (NFPA 2017, pt. 24.4.93.5).

11.6 Crime Concealment–Motivated Arson

Arson is the secondary criminal activity in the category of **crime concealment–motivated arson** (see Table 11-4 and Figure 11-6). Examples of crime concealment–motivated arsons are fires set for the purpose of covering up a murder or burglary or to eliminate evidence left at a crime scene. The motive classification for crime concealment is referenced in *NFPA 921* (NFPA 2017, pt. 24.4.9.3.5).

Other examples include fires set to destroy business records to conceal cases of embezzlement, and fires set to destroy evidence of an auto theft. In these cases, the arsonist may set fire to the structure to destroy the evidence of the initial crime, to obliterate latent fingerprints and shoe prints, and sometimes to attempt to render useless DNA or serological evidence linking him or her to a victim left behind to die in the fire.

In the case *People v. Cvetich*, 73 Ill. App. 3d 580,391 N.E. 2d 1101 (Ill. App. Ct. 1979), the defendant and a co-defendant burglarized a law office. The co-defendant set a fire to the office to cover up the crime. During the appeal of his conviction for burglary and arson, the defendant admitted being present and committing the burglary, but claimed he did not encourage his co-defendant to set the fire. The Illinois appellate court still held the defendant liable for abetting the arson to cover up the burglary even though the co-defendant started the fire.

TABLE 11-4	Crime Concealment–Motivated Arson
Characteristics Victimology: targeted property	■ Dependent on the nature of the concealment
Crime scene indicators frequently noted	■ Murder: attempts to obliterate forensic evidence of potential lead value or conceal victim's identity, commonly using an accelerant in a disorganized manner ■ Burglary: uses available materials to start the fire, characteristic of involvement of multiple offenders ■ Auto theft: strips and burns vehicle to eliminate fingerprints ■ Destruction of records: sets fire in area where records usually kept
Common forensic findings	■ Determine if victim was alive at time of fire and why he/she did not escape ■ Document injuries, particularly if concentrated around genitals
Investigative considerations	■ Common to find alcohol and recreational drug use ■ Offender expected to have history of contacts or arrests by police and fire departments ■ Offender is likely a young adult who lives in the surrounding community and is highly mobile ■ Crime concealment suggests accompanied to scene by coconspirators ■ Murder concealment is usually a one-time event
Search warrant suggestions	■ Refer to other category of primary motive ■ Gasoline containers ■ Clothing, shoes, glass fragments, burned paper documents

Sources: Updated from Icove and Estepp 1987; Icove et al. 1992; Sapp et al. 1995.

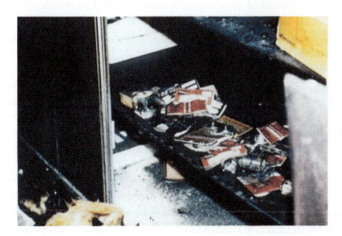

FIGURE 11-6 A crime concealment–motivated arson where valuable inventory was removed prior to the fire. *Courtesy of David J. Icove, University of Tennessee.*

EXAMPLE 11-4 ■ Case History of a Crime-Concealment Serial Arsonist

Three weeks after being released from prison, a 31-year-old unemployed laborer admitted responsibility for burglarizing and setting fires to 12 houses in a residential area over a period of 7 months. All but one of the fires occurred while the owners were out of town.

The offender stated, "I just drove through and looked for newspapers and other things where the people were gone for a while. I just took money and jewelry and stuff that would get lost or burn up in the fire. I would pour gasoline on everything and use a candle to light it off."

The fires were all identified as arson fires because of their rapid development and the detected presence of flammable liquids in the debris. The extensive damage made it difficult for the owners to determine whether valuables in the homes had been removed. The offender stated that he was identified when "one of the ladies spotted a ring in a pawn shop in another town. I would always take stuff somewhere else to sell it. What happened was she recognized the ring and called the cops."

His criminal history record consisted of a burglary conviction when stolen property was recovered and traced back to him. The offender's rationalization was, "I figured it out that if the fire burned everything nobody would know anything was gone. Last time, I got caught on a serial number, so this time I decided I would not leave any way for them to know what was gone" (Sapp et al. 1995).

11.7 Profit-Motivated Arson

profit (motive) ■ Fires set for profit involve those set for material or monetary gain, either directly or indirectly. The direct gain may come from insurance fraud, eliminating or intimidating business competition, extortion, removing unwanted structures to increase property values, or escaping financial obligations (NFPA 2017, pt. 24.4.9.3.6).

Offenders in the category of **profit-motivated** arson expect to profit from their fire setting, either directly from monetary gain or more indirectly to profit from a goal other than money (see Table 11-5 and Figure 11-7). Examples of direct monetary gain include insurance fraud, liquidation of property, dissolution of businesses, destruction of inventory, parcel clearance, and gaining employment. A construction worker's wanting to rebuild an apartment complex he destroyed is one example of getting a job after committing the crime of arson. The motive classification arson-for-profit is referenced in *NFPA 921* (NFPA 2017, pt. 24.4.9.3.6) and in a complete textbook for investigators (Icove, Wherry, and Schroeder 1980).

Arson-for-profit may have interesting twists when the offender benefits directly or indirectly. Arsonists have set fire to western forests to have their equipment rented to support part of the suppression effort. What may be the most disturbing of all are cases in which parents murder their own children for profit, with fire used to cover the intentional death of the child. Although this motive is uncommon, it is by no means rare (Huff 1997, 1999). Cases have been documented in which an insured child is murdered, but more commonly the parents wish to profit from getting rid of a perceived nuisance or hindrance—their own child. This is particularly true in a single-parent or divorce situation in which the child is viewed as an impediment to freedom or marriage. Filicide by fire is further discussed in a later section of this chapter.

Other nonmonetary reasons from which arsonists may profit range from setting brushfires to enhance the availability of animals for hunting, to burning adjacent properties to improve the view. Also, fires have been set to escape an undesirable environment, such as in the case of seamen who do not wish to set sail (Sapp et al. 1993, 1994).

Numerous cases exist that demonstrate profit-motivated arson, particularly for solicitation. In the case *State v. Jovanovic*, 174 N.J.Super, 435, 416A.2d 961 (N.J. Super. Ct. App. Div. 198), the defendant was convicted of solicitation for arson. He confided in an undercover police officer that he was having financial problems with his building that was about to be foreclosed. He told the police officer that if he was unable to sell the building, he wanted to burn it down in order to obtain the $200,000 insurance proceeds.

In the case *People v. Abdetmabi*, 157 ru.App.3d 979.511 N.E.2d 719 (Ill. App. Ct. 1987), two defendants were convicted of conspiracy to commit arson when one of them repeatedly stated his intention to burn down his grocery store and apartment building to collect the fire insurance proceeds. When one of the defendants made this statement to one of the store's employees, the employee reported this information to the police.

Circumstantial evidence can be used to charge and convict in arson-for-profit motivated cases. In *State v. Porter* 454 So.2d 220 (La. Ct. App. 1984), authorities established motive with the introduction of the circumstantial evidence of business and personal financial difficulties. In this case, a husband and wife were convicted of arson with intent to defraud.

TABLE 11-5	Profit-Motivated Arson
Characteristics Victimology: targeted property	■ Property targeted includes residential, business, and transportation (vehicles, boats, etc.)
Crime scene indicators frequently noted	■ Usually well-planned and methodical approach, with crime scene more organized because it contains less physical evidence ■ With large businesses, multiple offenders may be involved ■ Intent is complete destruction, with excessive use of accelerants, incendiary devices, multiple points of fire origin, trailers ■ Lack of forced entry ■ Removal or substitution of items of value prior to fire
Common forensic findings	■ Use of sophisticated accelerants (water-soluble) or mixtures (gasoline and diesel fuel) ■ Components of incendiary devices
Investigative considerations	■ Primary offender is an adult male with 10+ years of formal education ■ Secondary offender is sometimes the "torch," who is usually a male, 25–40 years of age, and unemployed ■ Offender generally lives more than 1 mile from the crime scene, may be accompanied to the scene, leaves, and usually does not return ■ Indicators of financial difficulty ■ Decreasing revenue with increasing and unprofitable production costs ■ Technology outdates processes or equipment ■ Costly lease or rental arrangements ■ Personal expenses paid with corporate funds ■ Hypothetical assets, overstated inventory levels ■ Pending litigation, bankruptcy ■ Prior fire losses and claims ■ Frequent changes in property ownership, back taxes, multiple liens
Search warrant suggestions	■ Check financial records ■ If evidence of fuel/air explosion at scene, check local emergency rooms for patients with burn injuries ■ Determine condition of utilities as soon as possible

Sources: Updated from Icove and Estepp 1987; Icove et al. 1992; Sapp et al. 1995.

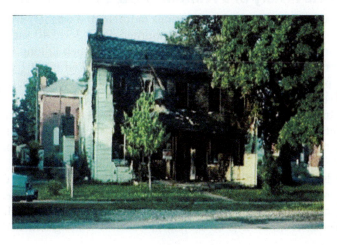

FIGURE 11-7 Profit-motivated arsons to leverage overinflated insurance sometimes involve well-planned fires set in vacant dwellings fueled with excessive amounts of accelerants. *Courtesy of David J. Icove, University of Tennessee.*

Another case involving circumstantial evidence is in *Commonwealth v. Hunter*, 18 Mass. App. 217, 464 N.E.2d 413 (Mass. App. Ct. 1984) where the owner of a discotheque was convicted of attempted arson of insured property with the intent to defraud an insurer. Several business financial difficulties used included that the owner had access to the premises, was experiencing serious financial difficulties, was late in loan repayments and rent payments, and would have derived substantial financial benefit from a fire. Regarding the insurance, circumstantial evidence revealed over-insurance of the property, and the insurance policy was about to be canceled for nonpayment of the premiums.

In some arson-motivated arsons, suspicions have been raised when there is an absence of remains in the fire debris of valuable or sentimental items. In the case *Mountain West Farm Bureau Mutual Insurance Company v. Girton* 697 P.2d 1362 (Mont. 1985), the Montana supreme court held evidence consistent with an arson-for-profit scheme by the defendant when, before the fire, he removed his valuable stamp and coin collections, obtained a rather large insurance policy, and stored a large amount of gasoline on his property.

When inventory of a business is dramatically reduced before a fire, arson is sometimes suspected. This was the fact in the case of *State v. Zayed*, 1997 Ohio App. LEXIS 3518. The defendant was convicted of the arson of his grocery store. Witnesses and vendors noticed the lowered inventory days before the fire. Two weeks before the fire, a vendor making a delivery to the store who was paid with a post-dated and worthless check questioned the defendant, who told the vendor, "Screw you. I'm going to burn my place down and you are going to get nothing."

In a civil case involving an allegation of an arson-for-profit scheme, an expert witness was challenged on whether he could testify based on facts and data along with his professional knowledge and experience. In *State Farm Fire & Casualty Company v. Allied & Associates, Inc., et al.* (United States District Court, Eastern District of Michigan, Case 2:11-cv-10710) the expert witness was prepared to testify that he detected a scheme to commit arson and insurance fraud. The factors documented by the expert witness included the following: a fire occurring a short time after a policy is written; multiple insurance claims and/or losses by the same insured, including related individuals; the building was vacant or unoccupied at the time of the fire; repeated submission of relatively small claims by an individual and/or those associated with him/her; multiple points of origin where a fire started in several different rooms indicate arson because an unintentional fire will not have multiple points of origin; unintentional causes or unidentified causes including cooking, smoking, and lighting candles; and a group of fires in close proximity in an area that is economically depressed and/or the insured is experiencing financial hardship.

EXAMPLE 11-5 ■ Case History of a Profit-Motivated Serial Arsonist

Arnold (not his real name) was a professional arsonist (a torch) and was serving two years in prison for one of his arsons. He admitted having burned down 35 to 40 vacant houses over his career. He became involved in setting fires for profit when talking with a real estate agent who was trying to find him an apartment. "He asked me if I would find somebody to burn a place. Did I know someone who was involved in demolition? I told him yeah and it started from there."

Arnold then partnered with the real estate agent and the demolition specialist. The real estate agent identified the targeted properties and made sure they were vacant. The demolition specialist taught Arnold how to set the fires, even accompanying him on his first job.

Arnold claimed that the fire-setting technique he used never resulted in a confirmed arson. "They could not tell. They would say it is under investigation. When they say it is under investigation, they are pretty sure it is arson but they cannot prove it." His method of operation was to pour 19 to 38 L (5 to 10 gal) of odorless white gas in the attic and leave a time-delayed chemical timer, literally burning the house from the top down. The ignited gasoline resulted in a fast-developing fire that collapsed the roof and overwhelmed the suspicions of the fire investigators, who found it hard to determine that an accelerant was used.

Arnold was concerned that no one would be injured in the fires he set. "I never burned any place where anybody was inside. I made sure I was not hurting anybody. That was important, it really was."

After being implicated with the real estate agent for an attempted arson, Arnold served two years in prison. "It was wrong, but at the time I was making good money and I was not hurting anybody. It was easy, but it is a dangerous job. I was afraid every minute while I was doing it."

As an afterthought, Arnold claimed that he was also a victim of his arsons. "I am the one that got hurt. I was underpaid. I was making $700 or $800 a fire, the real estate man was making about $10,000 on his share of the insurance policy, and I am the one that got sent away and everything" (Sapp et al. 1995).

11.8 Extremist-Motivated Arson

Offenders involved in **extremist-motivated** arson may set fires to further social, political, or religious causes (see Table 11-6). Examples of extremist-motivated targets include abortion clinics, slaughterhouses, animal laboratories, fur farms, furrier outlets, and even, now, sport-utility vehicle (SUV) dealers. The targets of political terrorists reflect the focus of the terrorists' wrath. Random target selection also simply generates fear and confusion. Self-immolation has also been carried out as an extremist act. The motive classification for extremism is referenced in *NFPA 921* (NFPA 2017, pt. 24.4.9.3.7).

extremism (motive) ■ Extremist-motivated firesetting is committed to further a social, political, or religious cause. Fires have been used as a weapon of social protest since revolutions first began. Extremist firesetters may work in groups or as individuals. Also, due to planning aspects and the selection of their targets, extremist firesetters generally have a great degree of organization, as reflected in their use of more elaborate ignition or incendiary devices. Subcategories of extremist firesetting are terrorism and riot/civil disturbance (NFPA 2017, pt. 24.4.9.3.7).

TABLE 11-6	Extremist-Motivated Arson
Characteristics Victimology: targeted property	■ Analysis of targeted property essential in determining specific motive and represents the antithesis of the offender's belief ■ Targets include research laboratories, abortion clinics, businesses, religious institutions
Crime scene indicators frequently noted	■ Crime scene reflects organized and focused attack by the offender(s) ■ Frequently employ incendiary devices, leaving a nonverbal warning or message ■ Overkill when setting fire
Common forensic findings	■ Extremist arsonists are more sophisticated offenders and often use incendiary devices with remote or time-delay ignition
Investigative considerations	■ Offender is frequently identified with cause or group in question ■ May have previous police contact or an arrest record with crimes such as trespassing, criminal mischief, or civil rights violations ■ Post-offense claims should undergo threat assessment examination
Search warrant suggestions	■ Literature: writings, paraphernalia pertaining to a group or cause, manuals, diagrams ■ Incendiary device components, travel records, sales receipts, credit card statements, bank records indicating purchases ■ Flammable materials: materials, liquids

Sources: Updated from Icove and Estepp 1987; Icove et al. 1992; Sapp et al. 1995.

EXAMPLE 11-6 ■ Extremist-Motivated Arson

This is a fictionalized account of an actual extremist-motivated arson targeting a US government agency (ADL 2003).

A federal jury convicted the head of a former anti-government extremist group for setting fire to an Internal Revenue Service office. The jury found the 48-year-old leader guilty of destruction of government property and interference with IRS employees.

Prosecutors said he and two other accomplices used 19 L (5 gal) of gasoline and a timing device to start a fire that destroyed the IRS office. The fire caused $2.5 million in damage, and a firefighter was seriously injured while battling the blaze. The leader was also convicted of witness tampering and suborning perjury for asking a witness to lie when testifying before the federal grand jury. The leader reportedly also threatened a witness to prevent his cooperation with law enforcement officers. Prosecutors stated that the three men were motivated by antigovernment sentiments and set the fire as a protest against paying taxes.

11.9 Other Motive-Related Considerations

Other factors involving motives appear in the literature and are important to address. This information is provided to clarify inaccuracies and misconceptions.

11.9.1 PYROMANIA

pyromania ■ The clinical diagnosis describes this disorder as (1) a compulsion to set fires and (2) a disorder characterized by a fascination with fire and recurrent episodes of fire setting during which the individual experiences a rising subjective sense of tension before the fire setting and a sense of gratification or relief when setting the fire. There is no ulterior motive (such as monetary gain or the expression of political ideology) to the fire setting (2016 ICD-10-CM Diagnosis Code F63.1 ICD-10-CM Medical Diagnosis Codes).

Perhaps most conspicuous by its absence is any mention of **pyromania** in this discussion of motivations. The root derivation of the name of the disorder comes from two Greek words: "pyro," meaning "fire," and "mania," meaning "loss of reason" or "madness."

The US Federal Government's Department of Health and Human Services (DHHS) maintains the Centers for Medicare and Medicaid Services (CMS) and the National Center for Health Statistics (NCHS). The CMS and NCHS provide the following guidelines for coding and reporting using the International Classification of Diseases, 10th Revision, Clinical Modification (ICD-10-CM).

For an authoritative definition of the term, refer to the 2016 ICD-10-CM Diagnosis Code F63.1 ICD-10-CM Medical Diagnosis Codes for pyromania. The clinical diagnosis describes this disorder as (1) a compulsion to set fires and (2) a disorder characterized by a fascination with fire and recurrent episodes of fire setting during which the individual experiences a rising subjective sense of tension before the fire setting and a sense of gratification or relief when setting the fire. There is no ulterior motive (such as monetary gain or the expression of political ideology) to the fire setting.

Researchers ask if the fire-setting impulses—characteristic of the various definitions of pyromania—could be a manifestation of some other disorder. Some report that the "irresistible impulse" to set fires may actually just be an impulse not resisted (Geller, Erlen, and Pinkus 1986). An evaluation of the term *pyromania* has shown that there is no consensus even among mental health professionals and behavioral scientists as to what constitutes pyromania, and, indeed, whether there really is such a disorder (Gardiner 1992). Even the FBI examined (Huff, Gary, and Icove 1997) the "myth of pyromania" at their National Center for the Analysis of Violent Crime in Quantico, Virginia. Doley (2003b) explores the common misperceptions that exist in the literature and attempts to clarify the true magnitude of pyromania as a motive by Australia's arsonists.

Sexual fantasies or desires have often been linked to pyromania in the popular literature, but this is not borne out by the interview research. Sex as a motive is highly overrated. In fact, experiments using penile response as an indicator of sexual arousal showed no correlation between sexual motivation and arson (Quinsey, Chaplin, and Upfold 1989). In the study, the penile responses of 26 fire setters and 15 non–fire setters were recorded and compared when the subjects were exposed to audiotaped narratives of neutral heterosexual activity and of fire-setting activities linked to several motives such as sexual, excitement, insurance, revenge, heroism, and power. There were no significant differences in the responses of fire setters and non–fire setters to any of the narratives they heard.

The so-called motiveless arsonist in many cases knows his or her motive for setting fires, which does not necessarily make sense to normal outsiders. The arsonist may also lack the verbal skills or capacity to express such concerns.

Fire investigators are cautioned not to label a subject a pyromaniac, because this is a diagnosis to be made by a mental health professional. Each practitioner—investigator, criminologist, psychologist, and psychiatrist—has a bias or different view of pyromania; thus, they are working from slightly different definitions.

11.9.2 MIXED MOTIVES

Interviews conducted with incarcerated arsonists underscore the complexity of human behavior, particularly when *mixed motives* arise. When questioned about the motives for their arsons, they gave responses indicating that there were often secondary and supplementary motives in addition to their primary motive (vandalism, excitement, revenge, crime concealment, profit, or extremism).

Arson can be used directly as a weapon, with the intent of killing only the target. Such homicides can be linked to a wide variety of motives, including self-defense. A thorough reconstruction of the entire incident, rather than just the fire-setting event, may reveal the offender's actual intent for the homicide.

Researchers, most notably Lewis and Yarnell (1951), assert that revenge is present as a motive in all arsons to a greater or lesser degree. Motives for arson, like other aspects of human behavior, often defy a structured, unbending definition. Another rationale is that arsonists may lack the social and communicative skills necessary to articulate their motives clearly. Embarrassment about the true motive may also lead to providing an alternative or false motive to investigators or mental health professionals.

Adding the elements of power and revenge reveals the problem with strict, unyielding classification. Fire investigators also should be aware that, because arson is a criminal tool, motivations may change based on the target or situation.

The best examples of many of the factors that arise in a serial arson case are given in an actual account of an arson from an offender's point of view: the well-articulated account by a female serial arsonist who used the pen name Sarah Wheaton (2001). In her published article she included edited excerpts from her discharge summary, which noted a diagnosis of borderline personality disorder. Her treatment therapy included biofeedback, social skills training, and clomipramine, a psychotropic drug. At the time of writing the article, Ms. Wheaton stated that she had been fire-thinking-free for 8 months.

EXAMPLE 11-7 ■ Memoirs of a Serial Fire Setter

Sarah Wheaton (not her real name), a former self-admitted compulsive serial fire setter, is now working on a master's degree in psychology. At the end of her college freshman year, during the summer of 1993, she was involuntarily admitted to a psychiatric hospital for 2 weeks for treatment for fire setting.

The following excerpt is Ms. Wheaton's (2001) from her discharge summary along with a description of her treatment and perception of what she experienced as a serial arsonist.

Reason for admission: This 19-year-old single female was living in a dorm at the University of California at the time of admission. The patient had been involved in bizarre activity, including lighting five fires on campus that did not remain lit.

History of present illness: This young lady is a highly intelligent, highly active young woman who had been the president of her class in her high school for all four years.

She had been going full-time to the university and working full-time at a pizzeria. She had called the police threatening suicide. When she was brought in, she was in absolute and complete denial. Patient claimed that everything was wonderful and she did not need to be here. She was admitted for 72-hour treatment and evaluation.

Hospital course: The hospital course initially was quite tempestuous. It was difficult to determine what the diagnosis was, as the patient was on the one hand very bright and very endearing to the staff and on the other hand was very unpredictable. She jumped over the wall on the patio (AWOL). The police were called and ultimately brought her back. She was subsequently certified to remain in custody for up to 14 days for intensive treatment because she attempted to cut herself with plastic and/or glass. She became more open after this, more tearful and at times more vulnerable. She tended to run from issues, to try to help everyone else, and not look at herself. Her father was seen in family therapy with her by a social worker.

Mother is reported by father to be both an alcoholic and have a history of bipolar illness. The patient herself reported sexual abuse by an older stepbrother when she was about age 9 to age 11.

Initially I intended to use antimanic medication with her, either carbamazepine or lithium, but opted not to as she was adamant against medication. The patient did seem to stabilize without medication. She showed dramatic improvement, although the staff and I still have concern. The stable environment she has been able to pull together may not exist after discharge. She is scheduled to go to Washington, DC, on July 1 to work as an intern in the office of one of the congressional representatives. She had done this two years ago working as a page.

Aftercare instructions: No follow-up appointment is scheduled because she is discharged today and will be leaving for Washington on the first.

Prognosis given by psychiatrist: Prognosis is very guarded given the severity of her condition.

Mental status: She firmly denies . . . destructive ideation, including fire setting at this time.

Discharge diagnosis [33 hospitalizations after the initial hospitalization]: Axis I. Major depressive disorder, recurrent, with psychosis. Axis II. Obsessive-compulsive personality disorder; history of pyromania; Borderline personality disorder. Axis III. Asthma. Axis V. GAF 45.

Because Wheaton was a student of psychology, her article accurately traces many of the traits and characteristics of serial fire setters, particularly those reported in the literature and supported by interviews of law enforcement agents specializing in arson. Quoted next are her observations on how fire dominated her life from preschool to college.

Fire became a part of my vocabulary in my preschool days. During the summers our home would be evacuated because the local mountains were ablaze. I would watch in awe.

Below I have listed some of my thoughts and behaviors eight years after the onset of deviant behavior involving fire. I have also included suggestions for helping a fire setter.

Firesetting behaviors on a continuum: Each summer I look forward to the beginning of fire season as well as the fall—the dry and windy season. I set my fires alone. I am also very impulsive, which makes my behavior unpredictable. I exhibit paranoid characteristics when I am alone, always looking around me to see if someone is following me. I picture everything burnable around me on fire.

I watch the local news broadcasts for fires that have been set each day and read the local newspapers in search of articles dealing with suspicious fires. I read literature about fires, fire setters, pyromania, pyromaniacs, arson, and arsonists. I contact government agencies about fire information and keep up-to-date on the arson detection methods investigators use. I watch movies and listen to music about fires. My dreams are about fires that I have set, want to set, or wish I had set.

I like to investigate fires that are not my own, and I may call to confess to fires that I did not set. I love to drive back and forth in front of fire stations, and I have the desire to pull every fire alarm I see. I am self-critical and defensive, I fear failure, and I sometimes behave suicidally.

Before a fire is set: I may feel abandoned, lonely, or bored, which triggers feelings of anxiety or emotional arousal before the fire. I sometimes experience severe headaches, a rapid heartbeat, uncontrollable motor movements in my hands, and tingling pain in my right arm. I never plan my fire, but typically drive back and forth or around the block or park and walk by the scene I am about to light on fire. I may do this to become familiar with the area and plan escape routes or to wait for the perfect moment to light the fire. This behavior may last anywhere from a few minutes to several hours.

At the time of lighting the fire: I never light a fire in the exact place other fires have occurred. I set fires at random, using material I have just bought or asked for at a gas station—matches, cigarettes, or small amounts of gasoline. I do not leave signatures to claim my fires. I set fires only in places that are secluded, such as roadsides, back canyons, cul-de-sacs, and parking lots. I usually set fires after nightfall because my chances of being caught are much lower then. I may set several small fires or one big fire, depending on my desires and needs at the time. It is at the time of lighting the fire that I experience an intense emotional response like tension release, excitement, or even panic.

Leaving the fire scene: I am well aware of the risks of being at the fire scene. When I leave a fire scene, I drive normally so that I do not look suspicious if another car or other people are nearby. Often I pass in the opposite direction of the fire truck called to the fire.

During the fire: Watching the fire from a perfect vantage point is important to me. I want to see the chaos as well as the destruction that I or others have caused. Talking to authorities on the phone or in person while the action is going on can be part of the thrill. I enjoy hearing about the fire on the radio or watching it on television, learning about all the possible motives and theories that officials have about why and how the fire started.

After the fire is out: At this time I feel sadness and anguish and a desire to set another fire. Overall it seems that the fire has created a temporary solution to a permanent problem.

Within 24 hours after the fire: I revisit the scene of the fire. I may also experience feelings of remorse as well as anger and rage at myself. Fortunately, no one has ever been physically harmed by the fires I have set.

Several days after the fire: I revel in the notoriety of the unknown fire setter, even if I did not set the fire. I also return again to see the damage and note areas of destruction on an area map.

Fire anniversaries: I always revisit the scene on anniversary days of fires that I or others set in the area.

Fires not my own: A fire not my own offers excitement and some tension relief. However, any fire set by someone else is one I wish I had set. The knowledge that there is another fire setter in the area may spark feelings of competition or envy in me and increase my desire to set bigger and better fires. I am just as interested in knowing the other fire setters' interests or motives for lighting their fires.

Suggestions for helping a firesetter. The likelihood of recidivism is high for a fire set-ter. The fire setter should be able to count on someone always being there to talk to about wanting to set fires. Fire setting may be such a big part of the person's life that he or she cannot imagine giving it up. This habit in all aspects fosters many emo-tions that become normal for the fire setter, including love, happiness, excitement, fear, rage, boredom, sadness, and pain.

A fire setter should be taught appropriate problem-solving skills and breath-ing and relaxation techniques. Exposure to burn units and disastrous fire scenes may be therapeutic and may enable the fire setter to talk openly about physical and emotional reactions. Doing so will not only help the fire setter but also give mental health professionals a deeper understanding of the fire setter's obsession.

The self-reported insight of this individual clearly confirms the findings of scientific, psychiatric, and law enforcement research. Of particular note are the pre- and post-offense behaviors at the fire scene, the significance of anniversaries, and the highly suggestive impact of the publicity of fires set by other arsonists. Astute fire investigators can use this information to assist them in identifying and solving cases set by compulsive serial arsonists.

11.9.3 FAKED DEATHS BY FIRE

Insurance fraud by burning a substituted body in an attempt to obliterate the true identity is a crime unique to profit-motivated arson. This form of arson often involves detailed planning, particularly in acquiring the body and evading suspicion by the investigating authorities.

Case studies have shown that the warning signs for *faked deaths* include, but are not limited to, the following (Reardon 2002):

- The death occurs shortly after filing of the insurance application and/or during the contestability period.
- The death occurs abroad.
- The insured has financial problems.
- Large policies or multiple small policies that do not require medical examinations exist. The policies have misrepresentations or omissions.
- The insured uses aliases.
- Previous policies have been canceled.
- The levels of insurance are inappropriate for the actual earned income.
- There is no body, or the body is in an unidentifiable condition.

Reardon emphasizes that the fundamental component in the payment of any life insurance claim is proving that the insured is actually dead. He recommends thorough investigation of these types of claims and litigation when appropriate to reduce the likeli-hood of payment to the claimant.

EXAMPLE 11-8 ■ Out-of-Country Faked Death by Fire Scheme

In 1998, Donny Jones (not his real name) completed an application for a term life policy bearing a face value of $4 million. Jones already had a $3 million policy with another insurer. Six months after the $4 million policy was written, the insurance company received the news that Jones had died in a car accident outside the United States.

The insured prepared his plan carefully. While out of the country with a friend, Jones rented a large SUV, placed his bicycle in the car, and drove away at 10:00 p.m., suppos-edly to take a 3-hour drive through the desert to an adjoining town. Early the next morn-ing, the SUV was found burning at the side of a desert highway. Local authorities found no traces of the mountain bike in the SUV, no signs of collision, and, initially, no body.

Later, a body was found in the vehicle at an impound yard, but the remains were quickly claimed and cremated by the traveling companion of Mr. Jones.

Owing to the unique circumstances, the insurer initiated an immediate investigation into the claim by arranging for a forensic anthropologist to examine the skeletal bones and for a fire protection engineer to document and impartially determine the cause of the vehicle fire. The forensic anthropologist determined that the remains were those of an elderly man of Native American heritage, not those of the insured, who was a 33-year-old Caucasian. The engineer interpreted for the insurance company technical information on the incendiary nature of the fire, the staged accident, and forensic evidence collected during the investigation by the foreign authorities.

The insurance company denied the claim and filed suit in the US District Court for declaratory judgment, seeking rescission of the policy. Initiating the litigation permitted the insurance company to begin to gather and preserve evidence from the authorities, police, and public and private sectors. The investigation outside the United States required the involvement of the US consulate followed by litigation, for which The Hague Convention generally requires approval from a US court and the appropriate foreign authority.

Eventually, the insured was discovered working in the United States through a routine background investigation by a firm for which the insured had been working, under an alias. The insurance policy was rescinded, and the insured later pled guilty in federal court to criminal charges of wire fraud and was ordered to pay full restitution (Reardon 2002).

11.9.4 FILICIDE

Filicide by fire is a crime in which the murderer is the parent of the victim and has used fire to mask the death, often making it appear to be an accident. Even though cases of filicide appear to be rare, these events are becoming more frequently studied by academics (Stanton and Simpson 2006).

Studies by the FBI, although based on limited case samples, provide insight into this crime. This agency speculates that owing to the thoroughness needed to conduct these investigations, this phenomenon may be widespread and underreported (Huff 1997, 1999).

Various motives are found for filicide, as for any crime, including the following:

- *Unwanted child:* Falsely believing that she and her spouse or lover can then live unburdened, a mother commits child murder to remove the perceived obstacle or nuisance child(ren).
- *Acute psychosis:* The parent is psychotic, such as the severely depressed single mother who stabbed her three small children to death and then set their apartment on fire.
- *Spousal revenge:* An estranged husband cruelly decides to deprive his wife of her most cherished treasure, her child.
- *Murder-for-profit:* Parents take out large life insurance policies on their children shortly before killing them by fire. There may be cases in which only a few premiums were paid, and the policy lapsed for nonpayment.

In any of these cases, the authorities may not be suspicious initially, for various reasons, including the lack of a thorough investigation of the fire; the presumption that the fatal fire was accidental, caused by the child's playing with matches; masking by overwhelming compassion for the parents; and sadness for the children. These emotional reactions may override indications (red flags) of suspicion (Huff 1997).

Although there is no single indicator, several common factors appear in cases of filicide, including the following:

Victimology: The children are often young, of preschool age; have little training in how to behave in a fire; and are thus less likely to escape. The perception may be that younger children are more disposable and more easily "replaced" later.

Pre-offense behavior: There is unusual behavior just before the fire, such as preparation of the children's favorite meal or a visit to a special place. For example, in one case a fast-food meal was served to two teenage sons to deliver a dose of common decongestant to make them sleepy when the fire was set (it was identified in the post mortem blood of the decedent and in dried blood stains on the shirt of the survivor). One of the boys died in the fire; the other survived to testify about the pre-fire events. A young daughter was not targeted and was kept out of the fire area of the home.

Temporal: The fires take place at night or early in the morning when the children are most likely to be in bed asleep. This gives the parents time to plan the event and, in some cases, lock the children in their rooms during the fire setting.

Crime scene characteristics: Children are asked to change their sleeping arrangements the night of the fire and sleep in a room not normally used. Sometimes, scenes are staged when the children have already been shot, stabbed, or strangled to death and a fire is set to cover the crime, frequently with a flammable liquid such as gasoline. In some cases escape routes are blocked and doors locked. Drugs may be administered to make the child sleepy or unconscious. A full forensic post mortem including X-ray and toxicology assays is essential on any child victim.

Offender characteristics: Halfhearted rescue attempts by adults are reported, with no appreciable element of danger encountered. Therefore, they do not display smoke-filled clothing, burns, or watery eyes, as would be expected. The parents most commonly live in manufactured housing and are no older than their mid-30s.

Post-offense behavior: After the incident, the adults exhibit inappropriate behavior, such as little or no grief; seldom speak about the victims, favoring the discussion of material losses (including insurance coverage); and are too quick to return to life as usual.

There will be one or a combination of two or more of these indicators. However, investigators are cautioned not to allow one factor alone to raise suspicion. They should move forward in a cautious yet professional manner and not yield to an emotional concern for the parent. As every person deals with trauma differently, investigators should not build a case around or place significant emphasis on lack of expected grief.

EXAMPLE 11-9 ■ Mother Involved in Filicide

Firefighters responding to a late-summer fire found a 22-month-old female hidden under a pile of clothes in a locked bedroom closet, dead from smoke inhalation. The child's mother told firefighters that her young daughter had been known to play with the cigarette lighter, which was found in the kitchen.

Firefighters doubted the story, but it became believable when the deceased child's brother, who was about four years old, demonstrated that he was able to operate the lighter. Investigators then ruled the fire accidental, initially concluding that the deceased girl had lit some paper napkins in the kitchen, taken them into the bedroom, and gone into the closet, with the door locking behind her.

All the facts surrounding this fire were consistent with a child's playing with a cigarette lighter and causing her own death. There was no reason to suspect foul play until 5 years later, when the son, now nine years old, suffered third-degree burns in another fire. When firefighters arrived at the home, they found the child unconscious behind a locked bedroom door. The mother fled immediately after the fire.

One week later, fire investigators located and interviewed the mother, who allegedly confessed to setting both fires, telling them that she was angry with her husband. In each of these fires, individual factors indicated filicide by arson (Huff 1997).

11.10 Geography of Serial Arson

Offender-based classification of arson extends beyond merely identifying the motive. Investigators should also closely examine the *geographic locations* selected by the arsonist. An analysis of these sites may reveal much about the intended target, add insight into the arsonist's motive, and provide a potential surveillance schedule for attempting to identify and apprehend the arsonist.

The results of a joint research effort on the geography of serial violent crime illustrate the patterns found in serial arson cases. Results of the study indicate that criminal offenders who repeatedly set fires exhibit temporal, target-specific, and spatial patterns that are often associated with their modus operandi (method of operation; m.o.) (Icove, Escowitz, and Huff 1993; Fritzon 2001).

Many geographers, criminologists, and law enforcement professionals are concerned with the rising tide of serial violent crimes, including arson, that are plaguing the United States and other Free World countries. Many of these violent offenders purposely use jurisdictional boundaries to evade detection from law enforcement officials.

Serial arsonists often create a climate of fear in entire communities. Community leaders compound this problem by pressuring law enforcement agencies to identify and apprehend the fire setter quickly. Often, the arsonist evades apprehension for months, frustrating even the most experienced investigators. Unpredictable gaps often occur between incidents, leaving law enforcement authorities questioning whether the arsonist has stopped his or her fire setting, left the area, or been apprehended for another offense.

Few studies have been conducted on the geographic distribution of serial violent crimes, including arson. The studies that do exist in the literature focus on specific characteristics found in particular crimes (Icove 1979; Rossmo 2000).

A keynote analysis of violent crime measured it in terms of a spatial and ecological perspective (Georges 1967, 1978). The social-ecological view is that there is a direct relationship between crime and the environment. In this view, an absence of community controls, such as found in inner cities, correlates with high crime rates. Several historical approaches trace methods for interpreting the geography of crime, particularly as it affects arson and fire-related crimes.

11.10.1 TRANSITION ZONES

The Chicago School of Sociology approach first proposed that crime was related to the environment (Park and Burgess 1921). This ecological approach assumed that high crime rates flourish in urban areas called *transition zones*. These zones have mixed land uses and high population fluxes.

In many cities, concentric rings form zones of transition, representing diffusion between the central business district and residential housing. These zones often contain rooming houses, ghettos, red-light districts, and diverse ethnic groups.

The transition zone theory was illustrated in a study of 15 fire bombings in Knoxville, Tennessee, during 1981 (Icove, Keith, and Shipley 1981). An analysis of the fire bombings investigated by the Knoxville Police Department's Arson Task Force showed that 66 percent of the incidents occurred within specific census tracts having significant population decline or growth.

The Knoxville study also examined a census tract in a low-income area where three fire bombings occurred during the reporting period. US census data indicated that this tract had the highest minority population, the highest percentage of poverty, and the second-lowest mean income of all the tracts where bombings occurred.

11.10.2 CENTROGRAPHY

The technique of *centrography* uses descriptive statistics to measure the central tendency of crime on a two-dimensional spatial plane. In certain crimes, the offender's residence may be close to the site of the crime commission. Another hypothesis is that the older the offender, the greater the mean distance from the crime scenes to his or her residence. This mobility is due, in part, to the offender's access to bicycles and other vehicles, as well as being over the curfew age.

A study for the US Department of Justice explored the concept of centrography and described geographic *anchor points* for criminals (Rengert and Wasilchick 1990). Examining the geographic locations of buildings targeted by burglars, the study concluded that criminals select targets close to an anchor point that minimizes the travel and time required to commit their crimes. Often, the dominant anchor point is close to the offender's residence. Other anchor points away from the criminal's residence include bars, schools, and video arcades. Kocsis and Irwin (1997) also examined serial arson cases where the offenders tended to operate from their residence and moved out in various directions to set fires.

Other geographic analysis approaches take place on both the micro and the macro levels. The microlevel approach examines the exact physical location of the crime, such as the type of building, vehicle, or street. The macrolevel approach tends to aggregate the data into zones. These zones can be census tracts, police beats, or other geographic areas. This approach tends to increase the scale of the analysis.

Centrography has been used to examine spatial–temporal relationships of other violent crimes (LeBeau 1987). Observations of the spatial distribution of crime use the *x*- and *y*-axes of a Cartesian coordinate system overlaid on a street-block map. The locations of numerous incidents are analyzed using the *mean center* approach to measure the central tendency by tracking the movement of these mean centers and to determine the standard deviational ellipse to describe the distribution of incidents.

Recent studies on spatiotemporal relationships reconfirm what fire investigators often suspected, that many serial arsonists follow patterns. In a multi-year study of geocoded crime data from the Los Angeles County Sheriff's Office from 2005 to 2012, evidence illustrates that arson generally exhibits enhanced likelihood of near repeat incidents in close spatial and temporal proximity to an initiating event (Grubb and Nobles 2016).

Fritzon (2001) examined the relationship between the distance traveled by an arsonist and his or her motivation. The research used the concept of *smallest space analysis* (SSA) to show the relationships between the distances traveled to set fires, the crime-scene features, and the offender's background characteristics. The research findings demonstrated that expressive crimes occur closer to the arsonist's home, which could be considered an anchor point, than do instrumental crimes. In the case of revenge-motivated attacks, the arsonist will travel the greatest overall distance. Also, arsonists who recently separated from a partner were more likely to travel greater distances. The study certainly adds value to existing research in the field.

11.10.3 SPATIAL AND TEMPORAL TRENDS

The *spatial and temporal trends* of serial arsonists and bombers also have been examined on a local level (Icove 1979; Rossmo 2000). Patterns not previously documented among serial incendiary crimes were found using cluster analysis techniques—individual and group serial arsonists and bombers tend to be geographically bounded by natural and artificial boundaries (see Figure 11-8 for an example.) When the offender moves his or her residence, the cluster of activity normally follows.

Studies on the historical changes of locations of arsons in the city of Buffalo, New York, have also confirmed many of these observations using cluster analysis. The concept of spatial surveillance brought new meaning to the monitoring of the locations of fires over time. The researchers noted that changes in these spatial patterns may occur for many differing reasons, and conclusions should not be reached merely on visual interpretations (Rogerson and Sun 2001).

Using time-based cluster analysis techniques, Icove (1979) examined temporal trends. This form of analysis detects subtle time-of-day and day-of-week trends correlated with geographic changes in the cluster centers. Other temporal trends such as increases in arsons with lunar activity have been documented in New York City (Lieber and Agel 1978). A research thesis at the University of California, Berkeley, School of Criminology, explored the relationship between lunar phenomena (not necessarily full moon) and the crime of arson (Netherwood 1966).

EXAMPLE 11-10 ■ Incendiary Crime Detection

This example demonstrates the application of geographic analysis to detect local clusters of activity of serial arsonists. After plotting the locations of arsons in an eastern city from February through September 1974, researchers detected a major cluster center of activity. Three comparative techniques are shown in Figures 11-8 and 11-9, illustrating the use of two-dimensional gridded incident, and three-dimensional shaded contour maps by Icove (1979).

Further analysis showed that two grids totaling 12 arson fires formed a major cluster center. Investigation revealed that during that time period, a gang of juvenile boys engaged in starting incendiary fires within a section of the large city. Properties targeted by these youths included garages and wooded areas.

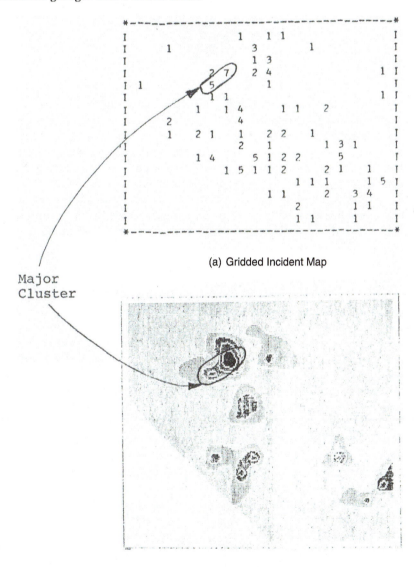

(a) Gridded Incident Map

Major Cluster

(b) Contour Map of Incidents

FIGURE 11-8 Gridded incident and contour maps with major cluster centers of arson fires. *Source: Icove 1979. Courtesy of David J. Icove, University of Tennessee.*

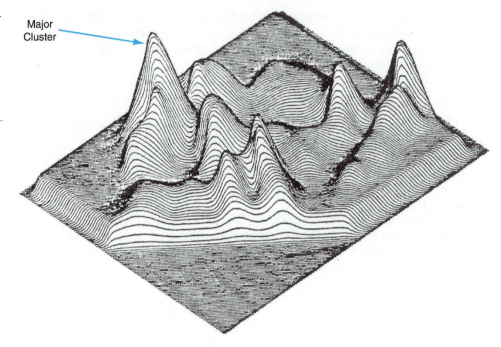

FIGURE 11-9 The detection of geographic clusters of arsons in three dimensions with a 35° counterclockwise rotation. *Source: Icove 1979. Courtesy of David J. Icove, University of Tennessee.*

When plotted on a map along with other arsons in the area, the incidents formed this major cluster. Data from these fires were collected and analyzed to provide a surveillance schedule for local law enforcement. A temporal analysis of the time of day and day of the week for the incidents contained in this major cluster was performed, which revealed that the juveniles set these incendiary fires during breaks in the school day. In the summer months, fires occurred in the evening hours, but the trend reverted to the original pattern at the start of school in the fall. With few exceptions, the fires were on weekdays. During a temporal analysis, lunar patterns are often detected. In this example, 75 percent of the fires occurred within two days of either the new or the full moon phase.

Urban Morphology

Georges (1978) examined the concept of *urban morphology,* which posits that crime tends to concentrate within certain zones or within areas with close access to transportation routes. For example, in Georges' earlier study on the geographic distribution of arsons during the 1967 Newark riots, fires were found to have been set along main commercial routes (Georges 1967). The study further documented earlier theories that as cities grow, crime tends to spread along main transportation routes (Hurd 1903).

Crime pattern analysis is a methodology for detecting recurring patterns, trends, and periodic events in the times, dates, and locations of incidents. After patterns are detected in a serial arson case, much can be learned to help predict the next event and classify the behavioral patterns exhibited by the offender. For a comprehensive discussion, see the National Institute of Justice Web page on crime mapping, which highlights crime reduction projects, geospatial tools, data sources, research, conferences, training, and publications, http://www.nij.gov/maps/.

Authoritative studies continue to reinforce that co-occurrence of offense characteristics also can be tied to both the geographic selection of targeted properties and the residence/workplace of the offender (Canter and Fritzon 1998). A systematic algorithm has been patented that performs crime site analysis in an area of criminal activity to determine a likely center of such activity (Rossmo 2000).

In Australia, the Australian Institute of Criminology, funded by the Bushfire Cooperative Research Centre, produced a handbook that gives a crime analysis-driven approach to detecting, predicting, and preventing arson (Willis 2004; Anderson 2010). The handbook serves as a resource tool for local, fire, and police agencies to develop prevention strategies. The project website contains downloadable manuals, worksheets, and an electronic spreadsheet to assist in capturing geographic and temporal information.

The FBI usually prepares a *criminal investigative analysis*, also referred to as a *profile*, based on exposure to numerous case histories, personal experiences, educational background, and research performed. Suspects developed by crime analysis do not always fit every prediction, because the predictions are made based on similar historical cases, and the offender may often modify his or her modus operandi (m.o.) in response to an active investigation.

The application of computer-assisted geographic profiling systems has been a long-established theme in the crime analysis field. The FBI's work in the 1980s in automated crime profiling (Icove 1986) used many of the concepts derived from incendiary crime analysis (Icove 1979).

Several key points are developed during a criminal investigative analysis involving the geography of serial incidents: temporal analysis, target selection, spatial analysis of the cluster centers, and standard distance.

1. *Temporal analysis.*   The first type of pattern analysis in serial arson cases is temporal analysis, which determines if any time-of-day or day-of-week trends exist. (See Figure 11-9 for an example.) These trends may vary if the offender modifies his or her m.o. in response to an active investigation. This modification may be a conscious act by the suspect.

2. *Target selection.*   Another form of pattern analysis deals with the type and location of the target selected by the offender. A commonly observed characteristic in cases involving serial arsonists is that the offender often escalates the targets selected, and situations become more life-threatening with time. A typical scenario is that the arsonist starts with small grass and brush fires, then moves to outbuildings and vacant structures, and then to occupied structures. Distance traveled is also a factor in target selection (Fritzon 2001).

3. *Spatial analysis.*   Using spatial analysis, an investigator can determine that a series of arson fires set repeatedly within the same geographic area forms a cluster of activity (as in Figure 11-8). Finding this center of activity often reveals information about future target selections or where the offender may live or work. As indicated previously, serial arsonists and bombers often tend to be geographically bounded by natural and artificial constraints. Therefore, the offenders either consciously or unknowingly maintain their activities within a bounded area, not often crossing major highways, rivers, or railroad tracks. Spatial monitoring of geographic patterns of arsons in Buffalo, New York, showed the value of searching for changes in spatial patterns (Rogerson and Sun 2001).

4. *Geographic profiling.*   The use of geographic profiling has proven to be a trainable and heuristic talent. In a recent research study on geographic profiling, 215 individuals participated in an experiment to predict the residential locations of serial offenders based on information about where their crimes were committed. In the study, these individuals were pre- and post-tested when given formal training on one actuarial profiling technique (Snook, Taylor, and Bennell 2004). Analysis of the study participants' performance showed that 50 percent of them used heuristics that led to accurate predictions before receiving the formal training. Almost 75 percent of the study participants improved in their predictive ability after receiving the formal training. Bennell and Corey (2007) propose the use of geographic profiling in the context of detecting and predicting terrorist attacks. See also work by Canter and Fritzon (1998) and Rossmo (2000) in geographic profiling.

5. **Cluster centers.** The *mean center* is the primary measurement of a spatial distribution of a cluster of data points. Given that the columns on a map equate to *x*-values on a Cartesian coordinate system, and the rows to *y*-values, the equations for calculating the mean center (Ebdon 1983) are

$$\bar{x} = \frac{1}{n}\sum_{i=1}^{n} x_i,$$

$$\bar{y} = \frac{1}{n}\sum_{i=1}^{n} y_i.$$

For the general case of cluster center *z*, the formula is

$$z_i = \frac{1}{n}\sum_{i=1}^{n} x.$$

Long-term analysis of these *cluster centers* is useful for determining whether the offender has changed his or her residence or place of work. In cases spanning 3 years or more, a cluster center should be calculated for each year and plotted on a map (Icove 1979). If the cluster centers do not move significantly, or if they hover in a specific area, the offender has not likely changed residence or job. When a marked change is detected, this information is conveyed to the law enforcement agency, which compares this knowledge with the potential movement of the suspects.

Studies suggest a correlation between motivation and distance traveled by arsonists (Fritzon 2001). Offenders whose behavior had a strong emotional component, such as a revenge motivation, tended to travel greater distances.

A more suitable center of activity for crime pattern analysis is known as the *center of minimum travel*, or what is often referred to as the *centroid*. This center is the point or coordinate at which the total sum of the squared Euclidean distances to all other points on the map is the lowest.

The centroid is more meaningful than a mean center when examining the geographic locations of crimes committed by a single offender. The reasoning behind this assumption is that an offender who walks to his or her crime scenes will choose the minimum travel distance. The mean center does not always coincide with the centroid.

The calculation of the centroid is not a simple formula, but requires an iterative process of minimizing a performance index. The best clustering procedure using this technique is referred to as the *K-means algorithm* (MacQueen 1967). The application of this algorithm (Tou and Gonzalez 1974) is best broken down into logical steps.

6. **Standard distance.** Once a cluster center is calculated for the geographic locations of a series of crimes, law enforcement officials can use this knowledge to concentrate their investigative and surveillance efforts within that neighborhood. This search radius from the cluster center is useful in focusing a criminal investigation within a reasonable distance from the cluster center of activity. For example, in a detailed crime analysis of a serial arson case, profilers often recommend a surveillance schedule and area of concentration within the area bounded by a radius of one standard deviation from the cluster center (Icove 1979). This area is known as the *standard distance*.

The following cases illustrating the importance of the geography of the crime were submitted for crime pattern analysis after an intensive investigation by a local law enforcement agency had exhausted all logical leads (Icove, Escowitz, and Huff 1993).

EXAMPLE 11-11 ■ Shifting Cluster Centers

During the fall and winter months in a southwestern state, an unknown arsonist was suspected of setting 24 fires involving fields, vehicles, mobile homes, residences, and

VARIABLE	AUG.	SEPT.	OCT.	NOV.	DEC.	TOTAL
8 a.m.–4 p.m.					1	1
4 p.m.–12 a.m.	1		4	3		8
12 a.m.–8 a.m.		1	4	6	3	14
Unknown			1			1
Monday					1	1
Tuesday	1					1
Wednesday					2	2
Thursday			1	2	1	4
Friday				2		2
Saturday		1	4	6		11
Sunday				2	1	3
Field				1	1	2
Vehicle			2			2
Mobile home				2	1	3
House, vacant	1	1	1			3
House, occupied					1	1
Structure		1	3	5	2	11
Total	**1**	**1**	**9**	**9**	**4**	**24**

Source: Icove, Escowitz, and Huff 1993.

TABLE 11-7 Temporal and Target Analysis of Geographically Shifting Cluster Centers

other structures. Some of the fires were set after the offender broke into the structures.

A temporal analysis of the 24 incidents revealed that the arsonist favored the late evening and early morning hours. The majority of the fires occurred on the weekends, as shown in Table 11-7. An analysis of the targets selected by the arsonist showed that the structures were either unoccupied, vacant, or closed for business. Over a period of time, the arsonist escalated the severity of his fire setting, first using available materials, and later turning to flammable liquids to accelerate the fires.

A geographic cluster analysis showed that the first three fires clustered tightly on the west side of the town. The remaining fires concentrated in a larger cluster of activity on the east side (Figure 11-10).

A crime analysis of this case was conducted, and the results were forwarded to the agency that requested the assistance. The investigators were told to concentrate their efforts on any suspects who first lived near the west cluster and then changed their residence to close to the center of the east-side cluster.

Armed with this information, the law enforcement agency later charged and convicted a 19-year-old single white male who matched the characteristics determined by the crime analysis. A key element in the case was that the offender lived near both cluster centers of the arsons. The geographic center of the activity shifted when the offender moved from the west to the east side of town (Icove, Escowitz, and Huff 1993).

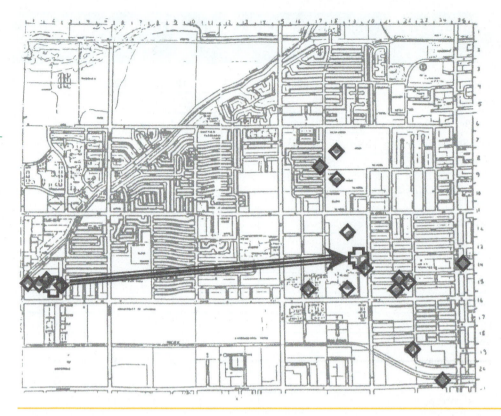

EXAMPLE 11-12 ■ Temporal Clustering

A southeastern city was plagued with 52 arson fires in vacant buildings, vehicles, commercial businesses, residences, and garages over a 2-year period. The law enforcement agency investigating the case was stumped and turned to crime analysis after exhausting all traditional leads.

A crime analysis revealed temporal and geographic patterns in the time and locations of the arsons. The majority of the fires were set during the afternoon and evening weekday hours. There were two 6-month gaps in activity. An overwhelming majority of the arsons occurred within a 1-mile radius of the downtown area of the city, with two additional clusters adjacent to two lakes. The crime analysis returned to the agency stated that the offender lived close to the cluster center of activity of his fires. When later apprehended, the arsonist admitted in most cases walking to the scenes of his fires and using available materials and matches or a lighter carried to the scenes. Even though it is a high-risk scenario for the offender to set a fire in the afternoon and evening hours, his intimate knowledge of the geographic area diminished the possibility of his being detected and followed.

Four months after the department received the crime analysis, a 29-year-old white male was arrested after fleeing the scene of a fire he had just set. The suspect later told police that he first started setting fires when his relationship with a girlfriend failed. The different clusters of fires were the result of the subject's changing his residence. Periods of inactivity in his fire setting correlated directly with times when the offender had ongoing social relationships. Only when these relationships failed did the offender return to setting fires. His motive appeared to be revenge.

When arrested, the suspect had in his possession a map that marked the locations of the fires he had set. The offender's prior arrest history included charges for disorderly conduct, criminal mischief, harassment, and filing a false report to law enforcement (Icove, Escowitz, and Huff 1993).

CHAPTER REVIEW

Summary

Arson is defined as the willful and deliberate destruction of property by fire. Although establishing a motive for fire setting is not a legal requirement of the elements of the criminal offense, it can help focus investigative efforts and aid in the prosecution of the arsonist. Motives for fire setting usually include one or more of the following general categories: vandalism, excitement, revenge, crime concealment, profit, and political terrorism. Motiveless arson or pyromania is not considered an identifiable classification.

Arson crime scene analysis is still in its infancy. Problems associated with its use and applications include the broad degree of knowledge required to assess and interpret the crime scenes, particularly using a motive-based approach.

A combined background in the principles of fire protection engineering as well as in behavioral and forensic sciences can certainly enhance the analysis. Clearly, the concept that the "ashes can speak" is paramount in the application of arson crime scene analysis.

Future work in this area should combine the knowledge of fire pattern analysis with comprehensive photographic techniques to assist in the visualization of fire scenes long after they occur and deteriorate.

Review Questions

1. Research a local serial arson case that appears in the media. Plot the locations of these fires and conduct a temporal analysis. What can you learn from this analysis?
2. For the case from problem 1, determine what motive was developed. Is the assessment by the media correct? What was the motive stated by the prosecution? By the defense?
3. What published studies support the popular notion that sex is a major motive for arson? What is the reliability of such conclusions today?

Suggested Readings

Canter, David. 2003. *Mapping Murder: The Secrets of Geographical Profiling*. London: Virgin Books.

Icove, D. J., V. B. Wherry, and J. D. Schroeder. 1980. *Combating Arson-for-Profit: Advanced Techniques for Investigators*. Columbus, OH: Battelle Press.

Nordskog, E. 2011. *"Torchered" Minds: Case Histories of Notorious Serial Arsonists*. Xlibris.

References

ADL. 2003. *Anti-Government Extremist Convicted in Colorado IRS Arson*. Anti-Defamation League.

Allen, D. H. 1995. "The Multiple Fire Setter." Paper presented at the International Association of Arson Investigators, Los Angeles, CA.

Anderson, J. 2010. "Bushfire Arson Prevention Handbook." *Handbook No. 10*. Canberra: Australian Institute of Criminology.

Bennell, C., and S. Corey. 2007. "Geographic Profiling of Terrorist Attacks." Chap. 9 in *Criminal Profiling: International Theory, Research, and Practice*, ed. R. N. Kocsis. Totowa, NJ: Humana Press.

Campbell, R. 2014. *Intentional Fires*, ed. National Fire Protection Association. Quincy, MA, USA.

Canter, D., and K. Fritzon. 1998. "Differentiating Arsonists: A Model of Firesetting Actions and Characteristics." *Legal and Criminological Psychology* 3 (1): 73–96, doi: 10.1111/j.2044-8333.1998.tb00352.x.

Decker, J. F., and Ottley, B. L. 2009. *Arson Law and Prosecution*. Durham, NC: Carolina Academic Press.

DeHaan, J. D., and D. J. Icove. 2012. *Kirk's Fire Investigation*. 7th ed. Upper Saddle River, NJ: Pearson-Prentice Hall.

Doley, R. 2003a. "Making Sense of Arson Through Classification." *Psychiatry, Psychology and Law* 10 (2): 346–52, doi: 10.1375/pplt.2003.10.2.346.

———. 2003b. "Pyromania: Fact or Fiction?" *British Journal of Criminology* 43 (4): 797–807, doi: 10.1093/bjc/43.4.797.

Douglas, J. E., A.W. Burgess, A. G. Burgess, and R. K. Ressler. 1992. *Crime Classification Manual: A Standard System for Investigating and Classifying Violent Crimes*. San Francisco, CA: Jossey-Bass.

———. 2006. *Crime Classification Manual: A Standard System for Investigating and Classifying Violent Crimes*. 2nd ed. New York: Wiley.

Douglas, J. E., R. K. Ressler, A. W. Burgess, and C. R. Hartman. 1986. "Criminal Profiling from Crime Scene Analysis." *Behavioral Sciences & the Law* 4 (4): 401–21, doi: 10.1002/bsl.2370040405.

Ebdon, D. 1983. *Statistics in Geography*. Oxford: Blackwell.

FBI. 2010. *Crime in the United States, 2010: Arson*. Washington, DC: Federal Bureau of Investigation.

Fritzon, K. 2001. "An Examination of the Relationship Between Distance Travelled and Motivational Aspects of Firesetting Behaviour." *Journal of Environmental Psychology* 21 (1): 45–60, doi: 10.1006/jevp.2000.0197.

Fritzon, K., D. Canter, and Z. Wilton. 2001. "The Application of an Action System Model to Destructive Behaviour: The Examples of Arson and Terrorism." *Behavioral Sciences & the Law* 19 (5–6): 657–90, doi: 10.1002/bsl.464.

Fritzon, K., R. Doley, and K. Hollows. 2014. "Variations in the Offence Actions of Deliberate Firesetters: A Cross-National Analysis." *International Journal of Offender Therapy and Comparative Criminology* 58(10), 1150–1165.

Gailliot, M. T., and R. F. Baumeister. 2007. "The Physiology of Willpower: Linking Blood Glucose to Self-Control." *Personality and Social Psychology Review* 11(4), 303–27.

Gannon, T. A., and A. Pina. 2010. "Firesetting: Psychopathology, Theory and Treatment." *Aggression and Violent Behavior* 15 (3): 224–38, doi: 10.1016/j.avb.2010.01.001.

Gardiner, M. 1992. "Arson and the Arsonist: A Need for Further Research." *Project Report*. London, UK: Polytechnic of Central London.

Geller, J. L. 1992. "Arson in Review: From Profit to Pathology." *Psychiatric Clinics of North America* 15: 623–46.

———. 2008. "Firesetting: A Burning Issue." Pp. 141–77 in *Serial Murder and the Psychology of Violent Crimes*, ed. R. N. Kocsis. Totowa, NJ: Humana Press.

Geller, J. L., J. Erlen, and R. L. Pinkus. 1986. "A Historical Appraisal of America's Experience with "Pyromania": A Diagnosis in Search of a Disorder." *International Journal of Law and Psychiatry* 9 (2): 201–29.

Georges, D. E. 1967. "The Ecology of Urban Unrest in the City of Newark, New Jersey, During the July 1967 Riots." *Journal of Environmental Systems* 5 (3): 203–28.

———. 1978. "The Geography of Crime and Violence: A Spatial and Ecological Perspective." Resource Paper for College Geography. No. 78-1. Washington, DC: Association of American Geographers.

Grubb, J. A., and M. R. Nobles. 2016. "A Spatiotemporal Analysis of Arson." *Journal of Research in Crime and Delinquency* 53 (1), 66–92.

Harmon, R. B., R. Rosner, and M. Wiederlight. 1985. "Women and Arson: A Demographic Study." *Journal of Forensic Science* 30 (2): 467–77.

Haynes, H. J. G. 2015. *Fire Loss in the United States During 2014*. Quincy, MA: National Fire Protection Association.

Home Office. 1999. *Safer Communities: Towards Effective Arson Control; The Report of the Arson Scoping Study*. London, UK: Home Office.

Huff, T. G. 1994. *Fire-Setting Fire Fighters: Arsonists in the Fire Department; Identification and Prevention*. Quantico, VA: Federal Bureau of Investigation, National Center for the Analysis of Violent Crime.

———. 1997. *Killing Children by Fire. Filicide: A Preliminary Analysis*. Quantico, VA: Federal Bureau of Investigation, National Center for the Analysis of Violent Crime.

———. 1999. "Filicide by Fire." *Fire Chief* 43 (7): 66.

Huff, T. G., G. P. Gary, and D. J. Icove. 1997. *The Myth of Pyromania*. Quantico, VA: National Center for the Analysis of Violent Crime, FBI Academy.

Hurd, R. M. 1903. *Principles of City Land Values*. New York: Record and Guide.

Hurley, W., and Monahan, T. M. 1969. "Arson: The Criminal and the Crime." *British Journal of Criminology* 9 (1): 4–21.

Icove, D. J. 1979. *Principles of Incendiary Crime Analysis*. PhD diss., University of Tennessee, Knoxville, TN.

———. 1986. "Automated Crime Profiling." *FBI Law Enforcement Bulletin* 55 (12): 27–30.

Icove, D. J., J. E. Douglas, G. Gary, T. G. Huff, and P. A. Smerick. 1992. "Arson." Chap. 4 in *Crime Classification Manual*, ed. J. E. Douglas, A. W. Burgess, A. G. Burgess, and R. K. Ressler. San Francisco, CA: Jossey-Bass.

Icove, D. J., E. C. Escowitz, and T. G. Huff. 1993. "The Geography of Violent Crime: Serial Arsonists." Paper presented at the 8th Annual Geographic Resources Analysis Support System (GRASS) Users Conference, March 14–19, Reston, VA.

Icove, D. J., and M. H. Estepp. 1987. "Motive-Based Offender Profiles of Arson and Fire Related Crimes." *FBI Law Enforcement Bulletin* 56 (4): 17–23.

Icove, D. J., and P. R. Horbert. 1990. "Serial Arsonists: An Introduction." *Police Chief* (Arlington, VA), December: 46–48.

Icove, D. J., P. E. Keith, and H. L. Shipley. 1981. *An Analysis of Fire Bombings in Knoxville, Tennessee.* US Fire Administration, Grant EMW-R-0599. Knoxville, TN: Knoxville Police Department, Arson Task Force.

Icove, D. J., V. B. Wherry, and J. D. Schroeder. 1980. *Combating Arson-For-Profit: Advanced Techniques for Investigators.* Columbus, OH: Battelle Press.

Inciardi, J. A. 1970. "The Adult Firesetter: A Typology." *Criminology* 8 (2): 141–55, doi: 10.1111/j.1745-9125.1970.tb00736.x.

Kocsis, R. N., and R. W. Cooksey. 2006. "Criminal Profiling of Serial Arson Offenses." Chap. 9 in *Criminal Profiling: Principles and Practice,* ed. R. N. Kocsis. Totowa, NJ: Humana Press.

Kocsis, R. N., and H. J. Irwin. 1997. "An Analysis of Spatial Patterns in Serial Rape, Arson, and Burglary: The Utility of the Circle Theory of Environmental Range for Psychological Profiling." *Psychiatry, Psychology and Law* 4 (2): 195–206, doi: 10.1080/13218719709524910.

Kocsis, R. N., H. J. Irwin, and A. F. Hayes. 1998. "Organised and Disorganised Criminal Behaviour Syndromes in Arsonists: A Validation Study of a Psychological Profiling Concept." *Psychiatry, Psychology and Law* 5 (1): 117–31, doi: 10.1080/13218719809524925.

LeBeau, J. L. 1987. "The Methods and Measures of Centrography and the Spatial Dynamics of Rape." *Journal of Quantitative Criminology* 3 (2): 125–41.

Levin, B. 1976. "Psychological Characteristics of Firesetters." *Fire Journal* (March): 36–41.

Lewis, N. D. C., and H. Yarnell. 1951. *Pathological Firesetting: Pyromania.* New York: Nervous and Mental Disease Monographs.

Lieber, A. L., and J. Agel. 1978. *The Lunar Effect: Biological Tides and Human Emotions.* Garden City, NY: Anchor Press.

MacQueen, J. B. 1967. "Some Methods for Classification and Analysis of Multivariate Observations." Paper presented at the Fifth Berkeley Symposium on Mathematical Statistics and Probability.

Miller, S., and K. Fritzon. 2007. "Functional Consistency Across Two Behavioural Modalities: Fire-Setting and Self-Harm in Female Special Hospital Patients." *Criminal Behaviour & Mental Health* 17 (1): 31–44.

Netherwood, R. E. 1966. "The Relationship Between Lunar Phenomena and the Crime of Arson." Master's thesis, University of California, Berkeley.

NFPA. 2014. *NFPA 1033: Professional Qualifications for Fire Investigator.* 2014 Edition. Quincy, MA: National Fire Protection Association.

———. 2017. *NFPA 921: Guide for Fire and Explosion Investigations.* 2017 Edition. Quincy, MA: National Fire Protection Association.

NVFC. 2011. "Report on the Firefighter Arson Problem: Context, Considerations, and Best Practices." Greenbelt, MD: National Volunteer Fire Council.

Park, R. E., and E. W. Burgess. 1921. *Introduction to the Science of Sociology.* Chicago, IL: The University of Chicago Press.

Quinsey, V. L., T. C. Chaplin, and D. Upfold. 1989. "Arsonists and Sexual Arousal to Fire Setting: Correlation Unsupported." *Journal of Behavioral and Experimental Psychiatry* 20 (no. 3): 203–8.

Reardon, J. J. 2002. "The Warning Signs of a Faked Death: Life Insurance Beneficiaries Can't Recover Without Providing 'Due Proof' of Death." *Connecticut Law Tribune* 5.

Rengert, G., and J. Wasilchick. 1990. *Space, Time, and Crime: Ethnographic Insights into Residential Burglary.* Final Report to the US Department of Justice. Philadelphia, PA: Temple University, Department of Criminal Justice.

Repo, E., M. Virkkunen, R. Rawlings, and M. Linnoila. 1997. "Criminal and Psychiatric Histories of Finnish Arsonists." *Acta Psychiatrica Scandinavica* 95 (4): 318–23, doi: 10.1111/j.1600-0447.1997.tb09638.x.

Rider, A. O. 1980. "The Firesetter: A Psychological Profile." *FBI Law Enforcement Bulletin* 49 (June, July, August): 7–23.

Robbins, E., and L. Robbins. 1967. "Arson with Special Reference to Pyromania." *New York State Journal of Medicine* 67: 795–98.

Rogerson, P., and Y. Sun. 2001. "Spatial Monitoring of Geographic Patterns: An Application to Crime Analysis." *Computers, Environment and Urban Systems* 25 (6): 539–56, doi: 10.1016/s0198-9715(00)00030-2.

Rossmo, D. K. 2000. *Geographic Profiling.* Boca Raton, FL: CRC Press.

Santtila, P., K. Fritzon, and A. Tamelander. 2004. "Linking Arson Incidents on the Basis of Crime Scene Behavior." *Journal of Police and Criminal Psychology* 19 (1): 1–16, doi: 10.1007/bf02802570.

Sapp, A. D., G. P. Gary, T. G. Huff, D. J. Icove, and P. R. Horbett. 1994. *Motives of Serial Arsonists: Investigative Implications.* Monograph. Quantico, VA: Federal Bureau of Investigation.

Sapp, A. D., G. P. Gary, T. G. Huff, and S. James. 1993. *Characteristics of Arsons Aboard Naval Ships.* Monograph. Quantico, VA: Federal Bureau of Investigation.

Sapp, A. D., T. G. Huff, G. P. Gary, D. J. Icove, and P. Horbett. 1995. *Report of Essential Findings from a Study of Serial Arsonists.* Monograph. Quantico, VA: Federal Bureau of Investigation.

Snook, B., P. J. Taylor, and C. Bennell. 2004. "Geographic Profiling: The Fast, Frugal, and Accurate Way." *Applied Cognitive Psychology* 18 (1): 105–21, doi: 10.1002/acp.956.

Stanton, J., and A. I. F. Simpson. 2006. "The Aftermath: Aspects of Recovery Described by Perpetrators of Maternal Filicide Committed in the Context of Severe Mental Illness." *Behavioral Sciences & the Law* 24 (1): 103–12, doi: 10.1002/bsl.688.

Steinmetz, R. C. 1966. "Current Arson Problems." *Fire Journal* 60 (no. 5): 23–31.

Stewart, M. A., and K. W. Culver. 1982. "Children Who Set Fires: The Clinical Picture and a Follow-Up." *British Journal of Psychiatry* 140:357–63, doi: 10.1192/bjp.140.4.357.

Tou, J. T., and R. C. Gonzalez. 1974. *Pattern Recognition Principles*. Reading, MA: Addison-Wesley.

USFA. 2003. "Special Report: Firefighter Arson." *Technical Report Series*. Emmitsburg, MD: US Fire Administration.

Vandersall, T. A., and J. M. Wiener. 1970. "Children Who Set Fires." *Archives of General Psychiatry* 22 (January).

Virkkunen, M., A. Nuutila, F. K. Goodwin, and M. Linnoila. 1987. "Cerebrospinal Fluid Monoamine Metabolite Levels in Male Arsonists." *Archives of General Psychiatry* 44 (March): 241–47.

Vreeland, R. G., and M. B. Waller. 1978. *The Psychology of Firesetting: A Review and Appraisal*. Chapel Hill, NC: University of North Carolina.

Wheaton, S. 2001. "Personal Accounts: Memoirs of a Compulsive Firesetter." *Psychiatric Services,* 52 (8), doi: 10.1176/appi.ps.52.8.1035.

Willis, M. 2004. "Bushfire Arson: A Review of the Literature." *Research and Public Policy Series No. 61.* Canberra, Australia: Australian Institute of Criminology.

Wolford, M. R. 1972. "Some Attitudinal, Psychological and Sociological Characteristics of Incarcerated Arsonists." *Fire and Arson Investigator* 22.

Woodhams, J., R. Bull, and C. R. Hollin. 2007. "Case Linkage: Identifying Crimes Committed by the Same Offender." Chapter 6 in *Criminal Profiling: Principles and Practice,* ed. R. N. Kocsis. Totowa, NJ: Humana Press.

Yang, S., and J. L. Geller. 2009. "Firesetting." In *Wiley Encyclopedia of Forensic Science*. Chichester, UK: Wiley. (See online edition at www.wiley.com.)

Legal References

Briggs v. Makowski, 2000 U.S. Dist. LEXIS 13029 (E.D. Mich. 2000).

Commonwealth v. Dougherty, 580 Pa.183, 860 A.2d 31 (2004).

Commonwealth v. Hunter, 18 Mass. App. 217, 464 N.E.2d 413 (Mass. App. Ct. 1984).

Mathews v. State, 849 N.E.2d 578 (Ind. 2006).

Mountain West Farm Bureau Mutual Insurance Company v Girton 697 P.2d 1362 (Mont. 1985).

People v. Abdetmabi, 157 ru. App.3d 979.511 N.E.2d 719 (Ill. App. Ct. 1987).

People v. Cvetich, 73 Ill.App.3d 580,391 N.E.2d 1101 (Ill. App. Ct. 1979).

People v. Mentzer, 163 Cal.App.3d 482, 209 Cal.Rptr. 549 (Cal. Ct. App. 1985).

Reed v. State, 326 Ark. 27,929 S.W.2d 703 (Ark. 1996).

State Farm Fire & Casualty Company v. Allied & Associates, Inc., et al., United States District Court, Eastern District of Michigan, Case 2:11-cv-10710.

State v. Bowles, 754 S.W.2d 902 (Mo. Ct. App. 1988).

State v. Curmon, 171 N.C. App. 697, 615 S.E.2d 417 (N.C. Ct. App. 2005).

State v. Howard, 2004 Ohio App. LEXIS 385 (Ohio Ct. App. 2004).

State v. Jovanovic, 174 N.J. Super. 435, 416A.2d 961 (N.J. Super. Ct. App. Div. 198).

State v. Lewis, 385 N.W.2d 352 (Minn. Ct. App. 1986).

State v. McGinnis, 2002 N.C.App. LEXIS 2325 (N.C. Ct. App. 2002).

State v. O'Haver, 33 S.W.3d 555 (Miss. Ct. App. 2001).

State v. Porter, 454 So.2d 220 (La. Ct. App. 1984).

State v. True, 190 N.W.2d 405 (Iowa 1971).

State v. Zayed, 1997 Ohio App. LEXIS 3518.

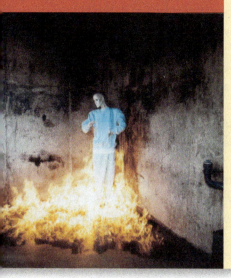

Courtesy of Ross Brogan (ret.), NSW Fire Brigades, Greenacre, NSW, Australia.

OBJECTIVES

After reading this chapter, you should be able to:

- Recognize problems and pitfalls of death or injury scenes.
- Interpret the various contributions to human injuries and deaths at fire scenes.
- Compare case histories and their outcomes.
- Evaluate scenes and the cooperation of investigators.

I n every country, particularly in highly industrialized ones, fire kills a significant number of people. In the United States, it is one of the five leading causes of accidental death. Fire investigators should evaluate the common problems and pitfalls when conducting forensic reconstructions, particularly when death occurs. The purpose of this chapter is to review these human tenability factors, present some analytical approaches, and provide illustrative case histories.

Most fatalities in fires are not directly the result of the effects of the flames but rather of the asphyxiation caused by the replacement of breathable air by toxic gases. In fact, about three times as many victims die from asphyxiation as from the thermal or physical impact of a fire or explosion-caused injuries (Purser 2002). Subsequent exposure to fire then causes the destruction of the body. No matter what the actual cause of death, the finding of a victim amid the ashes initiates a new series of investigative steps. Deaths from fires are not always instantaneous; they may occur hours, days, or weeks after the fire. For this reason, every fire that produces a serious injury to an occupant or emergency responder (serious enough to warrant hospitalization) should be considered a potentially fatal fire and should be treated accordingly.

The involvement of the fire investigator or forensic specialist in fatal fires can come in any form, from any sector, and challenge his or her talents and knowledge to come to just and accurate conclusions. These cases require the highest degree of cooperation among the investigators, all of whom have contributions to make toward a successful investigation. When deaths occur in a fire, the event becomes the focus of the press and the public, as well as police, fire, insurance, and forensic professionals. When problems occur, they can have far-reaching consequences.

12.1 The Team Effort

Every fire investigation involving a death becomes a team effort, and properly so. The fire investigator, pathologist, toxicologist, radiologist, and odontologist all play vital roles in the investigation, each to a greater or lesser degree depending on the exact circumstances. Without their combined expertise, the cause and manner of death cannot be determined, and the failure of a fire investigator to appreciate the value of forensic medical contributions will seriously compromise the success of the entire investigation.

Whenever human, or suspected human, remains are discovered at a fire scene, the investigator must consider six questions:

1. Are the remains human?
2. Who is the victim?
3. What was the cause of death?
4. What was the manner of death?
5. Was the person alive and conscious at the time of the fire? If so, why did he or she not escape?
6. Was the death due to the fire or only associated with it?

We shall examine each of these points in order.

12.1.1 SPECIES OF REMAINS

Unless the remains can be conclusively identified as those of an animal, they should be presumed to be human. A coroner, medical examiner, or sheriff should be contacted before anything else is disturbed. One investigator who used a pocket knife to slice into what was thought to be a pig carcass in a farm building fire was horrified to learn later that the remains were, indeed, human. The reverse is not unusual. Seriously burned remains of pigs, deer, even those of large dogs, have been mistaken for human remains. In many areas, human remains are the sole province of the coroner or medical examiner by statute, and it is a violation of the law to disturb them.

Crime laboratory personnel can be called upon to make a preliminary assessment, but a physical or forensic anthropologist from a local college or university may be required to identify badly charred or fragmentary remains. Even fragmentary remains can be identified as to species if any unburned tissue is present to allow serological tests in the crime laboratory. DNA has been found to be quite resistant to degradation. Even badly burned bones and teeth have yielded some DNA of use in establishing species. The investigator should also consider having the remains of any pets found in the fire examined. The presence of injuries or bullets or the presence of carbon monoxide (CO) or drugs in the body of the pet has sometimes been an important clue in the reconstruction of equivocal fire deaths.

12.1.2 IDENTITY OF THE VICTIM

If the remains are human, it is important to determine the identity of the victim. Because the identification will usually have great bearing on the motive or opportunity in an incendiary fire, such identification is essential to any thorough fire investigation. It is also possible that remains have been substituted for purposes of insurance fraud or homicide. In instances of homicide, there must be a positive identification in order to prosecute the responsible party. The identification offered by personal effects such as jewelry or documents such as a driver's license or credit cards should not be relied on except under special circumstances (such as airplane crashes where the identities of a fixed number of possible victims are already suspected) and then *only* if there are *no* disparities between known facts and the remains.

Although in some rare cases friends or relatives of the decedent can correctly make personal visual identification, the effects of fire and putrefaction usually make these identifications of limited reliability. Edema can bloat faces, and heat shrink skin, tightening facial features and sometimes taking years off the estimated age. Heat and soot can also dramatically change the appearance of hair color and skin color, making misidentifications of even basic factors like age, race, or hair color more likely. The emotional trauma of dealing with a relative killed in a fire makes personal visual identification even more unreliable.

For the purpose of identification then, the services of a qualified forensic pathologist, forensic odontologist, and radiologist may be required. Identifying characteristics may include the pathological signs left by illness or previously suffered injuries, unique tattoos, surgical scars, or reconstruction of height and weight by measurement of the long bones of the limbs.

The best form of conclusive identification is often provided by comparison of the teeth of the remains with dental charts and X-rays. The teeth, fillings, replacements (prosthetics), bridges, and similar features can survive even extensive incineration and offer conclusive identification in most cases if there are adequate antemortem records (such as X-rays, impressions, and photographs) (Delattre 2000). Porcelain crowns can resist temperatures up to 1100°C (2000°F), and dental amalgam resists temperatures up to 870°C (1600°F). Some of the newer generations of restorative dental materials degrade at temperatures of 300°C to 500°C (575°F to 930°F) (Robinson, Rueggeberg, and Lockwood 1998). Composite resins have been identified as to manufacturer by scanning electron microscopy/energy dispersive x-ray spectrometry (SEM/EDS) even after thermal damage (Bush, Bush, and Miller 2006). Resins and metal fillings can be damaged by direct fire-exposure heat, but the teeth themselves will withstand more severe fire exposure (eventually shattering from failure of the dentin).

Other evidence revealed by the x-rays may lead to an identification, since pacemakers, orthopedic plates, screws, pins, artificial joints, implants, and heart valves may be custom made for a patient and may be traceable. Dentures may be identified by a numbered tag, microchip, or other feature imbedded in the resin when the plate is made. Previous fractures or unusual skeletal features revealed by radiography have been used to substantiate identifications of seriously burned bodies. The internal structural features of sinus cavities, roots of teeth, and other bones have been used to make identifications if the jaws and exposed teeth are missing and if antemortem x-rays are available (Kirk et al. 2002; Schmidt 2008).

In addition to providing information of value in the identification of the victim, the radiologist is essential to a fire death investigation, for he or she can see beyond the char and destruction and detect both injuries and weapons. Fires may be set to conceal evidence of foul play, so a careful x-ray examination for the presence of injuries, bullets, broken bones, or even knife blades is essential. More than one investigator has been convinced that he or she was dealing with an accidental death until moving the body onto the stretcher revealed a knife still protruding from its fatal wound, or x-rays revealed shotgun pellets in the torso.

Fingerprints should not be discounted as a means of identification if any of the skin tissue of the fingers remains. If the identity of the victim is suspected, even a small portion of fingertip skin may bear sufficient detail for comparison. The epidermis of finger skin can be released by heat-caused skin slippage and may be found in the debris adjacent to the body. The analysis of remaining tissue for its DNA profile is becoming a practical reality for identification, particularly when immediate family members are available to provide blood or tissue samples for comparison with the unknown body. DNA analysis has been shown to provide accurate identifications even after extreme fire exposure and post-fire decomposition (di Zinno et al. 1994; Owsley et al. 1995). DNA identifications were made even from fragmentary remains after the 2001 World Trade Center attack (Mundorff, Bartelink, and Mar-Casslh 2009).

12.1.3 CAUSE OF DEATH

cause of death ■ The injury or disease that triggers the sequence of events leading to death.

The establishment of cause and manner of death is almost always the province of the medical examiner, coroner, or equivalent official (Hickman et al. 2007). The **cause of death** is the injury or disease that triggers the sequence of events leading to death. In addition to the entire range of homicidal and accidental causes of death, in a fire, cause of death may include the following:

- Asphyxiation by carbon monoxide or other toxic gases (the most common)
- Burns (incineration)
- Anoxia due to oxygen depletion
- Internal edema caused by the inhalation of hot gases
- Hyperthermia from exposure to high temperatures alone
- Falls
- Electrocution
- Trauma from being struck by falling structural members of the building

Because of the importance of asphyxia and burns, these topics will be treated in greater depth later in this chapter.

In general terms, fire-related causes of death can be linked to the time elapsed between the fire and time of death. If death ensues very rapidly (seconds to minutes to a few hours), the cause is often related to heat, smoke, or carbon monoxide. Deaths in the first day or so are more often associated with shock, fluid loss, or electrolyte imbalance, while those occurring many days or weeks after the fire are usually precipitated by infections or organ failures. It is in this last set of cases that the link between the death and the actual cause may be lost. Here the cause of death may be listed as an infection, kidney failure, respiratory failure, toxemia, or even cardiac arrest, but these are mechanisms of death, not causes. The mechanism of death is the immediate medical event that brought about the cessation of life. The erroneous listing of one of these mechanisms as the cause of death obscures the involvement of fire as the actual causal event.

12.1.4 MANNER OF DEATH

The **manner of death** may be defined as the way or circumstances in which the cause of death occurred. This is determined by pathological and toxicological findings supported by a reconstruction of the fire scene and the victim's activities there. This reconstruction requires the fullest cooperation between the fire investigator, the pathologist, and, sometimes, the criminalist.

manner of death ▪ The way or circumstances in which the cause of death occurred.

There are five generally accepted manners of death in the United States: (1) natural, (2) homicidal, (3) suicidal, (4) accidental, and (5) undetermined. In some jurisdictions, a finding of death by misadventure or medical intervention is accepted. Although the largest percentage of deaths at fire scenes will be accidental, investigators should never prejudge the manner of death any more than they should prejudge the cause of the fire itself.

12.1.5 VICTIM STATUS AT TIME OF DEATH

Carbon monoxide levels, indications of asphyxiation and the degree of inhalation of flaming gases, and the presence of toxic combustion products in the blood or tissues and soot in the airways all play important parts in establishing the manner of death, because they can help reconstruct the circumstances at the time of the fire. These indicators help answer two questions: Was the victim alive and conscious during the fire? If the victim was conscious, what circumstances prevented escape?

Additionally, barred windows; inadequately marked exits; mental confusion due to drugs, alcohol, age, or partial asphyxiation; incapacitation by irritant smoke; obscuration of exits by heavy smoke; physical restraints; or physical disability all are possibilities that the investigator must consider. The clothing worn by the victim and the position and location of the body may also be clues to his or her activities at the time of the fire. Items found near the body—a fire extinguisher, flashlight, telephone, purse, car keys, and the like—may provide a clue as to what the victim was doing or attempting to do when overcome.

12.1.6 DEATH DUE TO FIRE VERSUS DEATH ASSOCIATED WITH FIRE

Only a comprehensive investigation including a full pathological and toxicological examination can determine if the death was due to the fire, as we will see shortly. But fire can be part of a ritual or retaliative crime, in which case the victim is already dead due to other causes, or it may be the result of a completely accidental sequence of events. The cause of the fire and the cause of death may or may not be related. The relationship between the victim and the fire may be determined by assessing both in terms of the spread of fire and its heat and smoke. Accidental fires may occur whether the death is accidental, suicidal, natural, or homicidal. Similarly, an arson fire may trigger an accidental or natural death or be part of a homicide. Factors such as smoke detector activation (or, usually, lack thereof) may play a major role in the reconstruction (Flemming 2004).

12.1.7 PROBLEMS AND PITFALLS

There are several problem areas that can complicate investigations of fires involving fatalities and compromise the accuracy and reliability of the conclusions reached.

▪ *Linkage between the fire and death investigations:* Prejudging the fire and its attendant death as an accident and automatically treating the scene investigation accordingly is a major problem. Fires can be intentional, natural, or accidental in their cause, and deaths can be accidental, homicidal, suicidal, or natural. The linkage between the two events can be direct, indirect, or simple coincidence. The responsibility of the fire investigation team in these cases is to establish the cause of the fire and assist the medical examiner in the death investigation and to determine the connection (if any) between the two.

- **Time interval to death:**   Sudden violent deaths are assumed to be due to an instantaneous exposure to insult followed by immediate collapse and death of a victim (e.g., a shot is fired, and the victim collapses to die shortly afterward). Many forensic investigations are considered (and successfully concluded) in this light. Fires, however, occur over a period of time, creating dangerous environments that vary greatly with time and can kill by a variety of mechanisms. A person may be killed nearly instantaneously by exposure to a flash fire or only after hours of exposure to toxic gases. Investigators must have an appreciation for the nature of fire, its lethal products, and variables that must be considered, and must not treat the event as a single exposure to a single set of conditions at a precise moment in time that results in instant collapse.

- **Heat intensity and duration:**   There is little accurate information available to detectives, pathologists, and medical examiners about the temperatures and intensities of heat exposure that occur in a fire as it develops. Misunderstandings and misapprehensions can lead investigators seriously astray in their interpretations when they try to assess injuries or postmortem damage resulting from fires.

- **Fire-related human behavior:**   In most violent deaths, the victim responds with what is often referred to as a fight-or-flight response to a threat, then suffers an injury, collapses, and dies. In fires, the potential responses of victims often include going to investigate; simply observing; failing to notice or appreciate the danger; failing to respond due to incapacitation from drugs or alcohol or infirmity; returning to the fire or delaying escape to rescue pets, family, or personal or valuable property; as well as fighting or attempting to fight the fire. This variability of responses can vastly complicate the process of solving critical problems of why the victim failed to escape the fire (and perhaps why other people escaped).

- **Time interval between fire and death:**   Fires can kill in seconds, or death can occur minutes, hours, days, or even months after the victim is removed from the scene. The longer the time interval between the fire and the death, the harder it is to keep track of the link between the actual cause (the fire) and its result (the death). Evidence is lost when a living victim is removed from a scene and dies later, away from the scene; it may be too late to recover or document that evidence. Fatalities that occur after a victim is hospitalized are inevitably omitted from the NFIRS statistics and may also be omitted from the national vital statistics.

- **Conflicts among investigating agencies:**   Conflicts can arise regarding the perceived or mandated responsibilities of police, fire, medicolegal, and forensic personnel who are often involved in fire scene deaths.

- **Postmortem effects:**   After death, severe postmortem fire effects on the body can complicate the investigation by obliterating evidence. The body can bear fire patterns of heat effects and smoke deposits that can be masked by exposure to fire after death. The body can be incinerated by exposure to flames, so that evidence of pre-fire wounds or even clinical evidence such as blood samples is destroyed. Structural collapse and effects of firefighting hose streams and overhaul can cause additional damage to the scene and to the body.

- **Premature removal of the body:**   The premature removal of a deceased victim from the fire scene is a major problem. The compulsion to rescue and remove every fire victim is a very strong one, particularly among firefighters. However, once the fire is under control and unable to inflict further damage to the body of a confirmed deceased, there is nothing to be gained by the undocumented and hurried removal of the remains and much to be lost in the way of burn pattern analysis, recovery of body fragments (especially dental evidence), projectiles, clothing and associated artifacts (e.g., keys, flashlight, dog leash), and even trace evidence.

12.2 Tenability: What Kills People in Fires?

Structural fires can achieve their deadly result in a number of ways—heat, smoke, flames, soot, and others—but fire conditions change continually as a fire grows and evolves, and the conditions of victim exposure can vary from conditions involving little or no threat of injury to almost instant lethality. Lethal agents of fires can and usually do act in combination and include heat, smoke, and inhalation of smoke or toxic gases, hypoxia, flames, and blunt trauma. These lethal agents of fires are discussed in further detail later in this chapter.

The ability of humans to escape a fire, **tenability**, is measured by the time frame during which their environment remains survivable. Fires can produce incapacitating effects on humans when they are exposed to heat and smoke. The causes of these physiological effects are generally categorized into the following areas (Purser 2008):

- **Toxic gases and irritants:**   Depending on the chemical compositions in the toxic gases, toxic gas inhalation can cause mental confusion, respiratory tract injuries, loss of consciousness, asphyxiation, and skin reactions.
- **Heat transfer:**   Excessive heat irritates exposed skin and the respiratory tract, causing severe pain as well as varying degrees of burn injuries, hyperthermia, or heat stroke.
- **Visibility:**   Optical opacity of the smoke and irritants from a fire produces impaired vision as the distribution of thick smoke descends toward the floor through rooms, stairwells, and hallways.

tenability ■ An assessment of the potential for harm that may be imposed from a fire based on (1) an analysis of the source, heat release rates, and rates of production of the combustion products; (2) when occupants might become exposed to these harmful conditions; and (3) the effects on the occupants from this exposure.

Fire investigators should also consider the synergistic effects of two or more of these factors when conducting a forensic analysis. Of primary concern is assessing the point at which exposure to one or more of the preceding variables would cause injury or block the individual from successfully escaping the fire, resulting in death. The psychological behavior of people in fires when exposed and reacting to these variables affects their decisions and the time required to travel via safe escape routes.

Critical limits to human tenability include a limit of visibility to 5 m (16.4 ft), an accumulated exposure rate of carbon monoxide of 30,000 parts per million minute (ppm-min), and a critical temperature of approximately 120°C (240°F). The synergistic effects of two or more of these critical factors may override an individual's limits (Jensen 1998).

The major goal of the investigator when conducting a *tenability analysis* is to determine how an individual attempting to escape a burning structure becomes impaired and how the fire changes his or her environment and perceptions. These tenability analysis techniques are grounded in both experimental and forensic data, giving the investigator a balanced and practical approach.

The physiological and toxicological effects of heat transfer and toxic smoke on animals and humans are based on scientifically valid experiments. For example, studies correlating carbon monoxide exposure to carboxyhemoglobin levels in the bloodstream used individual subjects ranging from laboratory rats to volunteer medical students (Nelson 1998). Some of these data were extrapolated to model the results at higher levels of exposure to carbon monoxide. These models must take into account variations in age, health, and stature of the individual, because an individual's height affects exposure when he or she is standing upright in the stratified upper smoke layer, where nearly all the toxic gases normally reside. See Figure 12-1 for a graphic illustration of the exposure of humans walking upright through smoke layers (Bukowski 1995).

Forensic evaluations of incapacitation of a fire victim also come from forensic data derived from actual case histories and investigations. The major studies of the behavior of people in fires come from subject interviews of people surviving large fires and explosions (Bryan and Icove 1977).

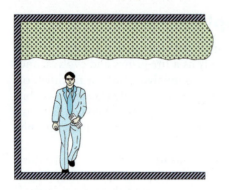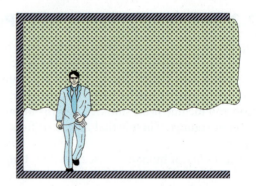

FIGURE 12-1 Illustration of human tenability in varying smoke layer levels. *R. W. Bukowski, "Predicting the Fire Performance of Buildings: Establishing Appropriate Calculation Methods of Regulatory Applications," National Institute of Standards and Technology, Gaithersburg, MD, 1995.*

12.3 Toxic Gases

The previous section on tenability discussed visibility and irritant effects on humans as they try to navigate and survive fires. *Toxic gases* contained within smoke can also have a narcotic effect that asphyxiates victims. The dominant narcotic gases in smoke that affect the nervous and cardiovascular systems are carbon monoxide (CO) and hydrogen cyanide (HCN). Carbon dioxide and reduced oxygen levels (hypoxia) that are not toxic individually may have severe synergistic effects on tenability.

Increased exposure to toxic gases may cause confusion, loss of consciousness, and eventually asphyxial death. The prediction of asphyxiation resulting in incapacitation and death in fires can be modeled (Purser 2008). Toxic products of combustion can include a wide variety of chemicals depending on what is burning and how efficiently it is burning (temperature, mixing, and oxygen concentration are all important variables in determining what chemical species are created).

Toxic gases can generally be classified into three basic categories:

- *Nonirritant gases:* (sometimes referred to as "narcotic gases"): CO, HCN, H_2S (hydrogen sulfide), and phosgene (CCl_2O).
- *Acidic irritants:* HCl (hydrogen chloride)—produced during the combustion of polyvinyl chloride (PVC) plastics; sulfur oxides (SO_x), which form H_2SO_3 (sulfurous acid) and H_2SO_4 (sulfuric acid)—produced by oxidation of sulfur-containing fuels; and nitrogen oxides (NO_x), which form HNO_2 (nitrous acid) and HNO_3 (nitric acid)—from nitrogen-containing fuels.
- *Organic irritants:* Formaldehyde (CH_2O) and acrolein (2-propenal, C_3H_4O) are produced by the combustion of cellulosic fuels. Isocyanates are produced by the combustion of polyurethanes.

Acidic irritant gases dissolve in the water of the mucous membranes and generate the corrosive acids listed. These acids disrupt the epithelial cell membranes and cause the cells to lyse, releasing fluids and producing edema, as evidenced by extreme watering of the eyes, coughing, and inability to breathe. Sulfur dioxide combines with water to form sulfurous acid, a strong irritant. These reactions can all result in incapacitation, preventing escape from lethal gases such as hydrogen cyanide and carbon monoxide. Exposure to hydrogen chloride (HCl) starting at concentrations of 50 ppm usually causes respiratory or visual impairment sufficient to affect walking movement. Total cessation of movement occurs at a concentration of hydrogen chloride gas approaching 300 ppm. The effects of concentrations of HCl above the 1000 ppm level are most likely severe enough to prevent escape (Purser 2001).

Table 12-1 shows the effects of various fire gases on both the escape and the incapacitation of humans. Most fires present occupants with a complex mixture of toxic and

TABLE 12-1	Irritant Concentrations of Fire Gases Predicted to Cause 50 Percent Impaired Escape or Incapacitation in the Human Population	
COMMON FIRE GASES	**IMPAIRED ESCAPE (ppm)**	**INCAPACITATION (ppm)**
Hydrogen chloride (HCl)	200	900
Hydrogen bromine (HBr)	200	900
Hydrogen fluoride (HF)	200	900
Sulfur dioxide (SO_2)	24	120
Nitrogen dioxide (NO_2)	70	350
Formaldehyde (CH_2O)	6	30
Acrolein (C_3H_4O)	4	20

Source: Derived from Purser 2001.

irritant gases and vapors combined with high carbon dioxide and *hypoxic* (low-oxygen) conditions. The fire investigator must assess what fuels were burning, under what conditions (smoldering, open flame, underventilated), and where the occupants would have been exposed to the toxic gases and vapors when assessing the tenability of the fire exposure.

HCl is a major combustion/decomposition product of vinyl plastics, in both the flaming and the smoldering modes. Hydrogen bromide (HBr) or hydrogen fluoride (HF) is produced when some synthetic rubbers are burned. Acrolein is created when wood or cardboard or cellulosic materials are burned.

The term **fractional effective concentration (FEC)** was developed to assess the impact of toxic smoke and by-products of combustion on a subject (Purser 2001). The use of the concept of FECs by fire investigators will give them a greater appreciation and understanding of what tools in combustion toxicology are available to calculate the impact of lethal toxic products as hazardous to humans (Purser 2008).

fractional effective concentration ■ A measurement that assesses the impact of toxic smoke and by-products of combustion on a subject. The FEC depends on the concentration of particular toxins within the fire gases, and the duration of exposure.

The FEC is expressed in general terms as

$$\text{FEC} = \frac{\text{dose received at time } t(C_t)}{\text{effective } C_t \text{ dose to cause in capacitation or death}}. \qquad (12.1)$$

The FEC, in special situations, is also referred to as the *fractional incapacitation dose* (FID) or the *fractional lethal dose* (FLD).

12.3.1 CARBON MONOXIDE

Carbon monoxide (CO) is produced in fires by the incomplete combustion of any carbon-containing fuel; however, it is not produced at the same rate in all fires. In free-burning (well-ventilated) fires, the CO concentration can be as little as 0.02 percent (200 ppm) of the total gaseous products of the fire. The CO concentrations in smoldering, post-flashover, or underventilated fires range from 1 to 10 percent in the smoke stream.

Sources of CO can vary and are elusive at times to investigators. These sources include, but are not limited to, the following examples:

- Fires involving structures, clothing, or furnishings
- Defective heating equipment (including charcoal grills used indoors), the primary cause of non-fire fatalities involving CO (Flynn 2008; Mah 2000)
- Automobile or other internal combustion motor exhaust, especially in tightly sealed garages (deRoux 2006; Suchard 2006)

- Industrial processes in which CO is intentionally generated as a fuel or as part of a manufacturing process or in which it is produced as an unintentional product by incomplete combustion of some fuel

CO must be inhaled into a living human to be transferred to the bloodstream. Thus, there is no measurable diffusion from an external atmosphere rich in CO into the blood or tissues of a dead body, owing to the lack of respiration. Similarly, CO content is stable in the blood of a dead body and is not lost until postmortem decomposition.

When inhaled and absorbed into the bloodstream, CO combines with the hemoglobin molecules and forms the complex carboxyhemoglobin (COHb) in the red blood cells. The binding affinity of CO for the heme portion of the hemoglobin is 200 to 300 times stronger than that of O_2. CO also binds with the heme group in myoglobin, which is the "red" in red muscle tissue. The affinity of CO for myoglobin is about 60 times that of O_2. Myoglobin stores and transports O_2 in muscle tissue, particularly in cardiac muscle. Under hypoxic conditions, CO can shift from the blood into the muscle and has a higher affinity for cardiac muscle than for striated muscle (Myers, Linberg, and Cowley 1979). This may explain why low concentrations of COHb are sometimes found in the blood of deceased victims with heart conditions.

Carbon monoxide also affects Cya_3 oxidase, an enzyme that catalyzes the production of ATP in the cell (Feld 2002). The stability of the COHb complex reduces the O_2-carrying capacity of the blood. Without O_2 and water, ATP cannot be produced in the mitochondria of the cell, and the cell dies (Feld 2002). CO also impairs cellular tissue respiration by combining with cytochromes b and aa3 (Purser 2010).

Goldbaum, Orellano, and Dergal (1976) reported that experimentally reducing the hematocrit (the blood-carrying capacity) of dogs by as much as 75 percent did not result in death. Even replacing blood with blood containing 60 percent COHb by transfusion or infusion of CO through the peritoneal cavity did not result in death. Only when these experimental animals inhaled the CO did deaths occur. This suggests that respiration of CO and its interference with metabolism plays a critical role in causing death (Goldbaum, Orellano, and Dergal 1976).

The mere presence of CO in the blood is not a sign of breathing fire gases. The normal human body has COHb saturations of 0.5 to 1 percent as a result of degradation of heme in the blood. Higher concentrations (up to 3 percent) may be found in non-fire victims with anemia or other blood disorders (Penney 2000, 2008, 2010). Smokers can have levels of 4 to 10 percent, as tobacco smoke contains a high concentration of CO. People in confined spaces with emergency generators, pumps, fuel-burning heaters, and compressors can have elevated—sometimes dangerous—blood COHb concentrations.

When a victim is removed from a CO-rich environment to fresh air, the CO is gradually eliminated from the blood. The higher the partial pressure of O_2 (such as administered by medical personnel), the faster CO is eliminated. In fresh air the initial concentration of COHb will be reduced by 50 percent in 250 to 320 minutes (approx. 4 to 5 hr). In 100 percent O_2 via mask, a 50 percent reduction can be achieved in 65 to 85 minutes (approx. 1 to 1.5 hr). In O_2 at hyperbaric pressures (3 to 4 atm), there is a 50 percent reduction of COHb in 20 minutes (Penney 2000, 2008, 2010). Treatment for high concentrations of CO or nitrogen gases in the blood may include time in a hyperbaric chamber to reduce the effects of CO or nitrogen gas poisoning.

The time at which a blood sample is drawn from a fire victim must be noted, as well as the nature of any medical treatment (such as the antemortem administration of O_2). The COHb saturation of blood in a dead body is very stable, even after decomposition has begun. CO poisoning kills many fire victims before they are ever exposed to fire. Because CO gas is colorless and odorless, it may go undetected by the victim. It can kill victims even some distance away from a fire when they are not exposed to any heat or flames, but it is not the only factor in many fire deaths.

Carbon dioxide is a product of nearly all fires. Levels of 4 to 5 percent CO_2 in air cause the adult respiratory rate to double (Purser 2010). Levels of 10 percent cause it to quadruple and possibly cause unconsciousness (Purser 2010). This increase in respiration increases the rate at which CO and other toxic gases are inhaled. High concentrations of CO_2 may also dilute the concentration of breathable oxygen to the point of inducing hypoxic collapse. Carbon dioxide concentration in the blood can be measured in living subjects, but blood chemistry begins to change after death. As a result, accurate CO_2 (and O_2) saturation measurements are difficult to obtain postmortem, because postmortem decomposition can also contribute to the CO_2 measured.

12.3.2 PREDICTING THE TIME TO INCAPACITATION BY CARBON MONOXIDE

It is well recognized that all individuals show different tolerances to the influence of toxic gases and other environmental influences. Certainly, such variations must exist with carbon monoxide as well. It remains to be explained how the death of one person from carbon monoxide at 40 percent saturation can be consistent with that of another who had accumulated a 90 percent saturation. The relevant factors appear to be as follows:

- Rate of inhalation of the gas
- Activity or its lack, which changes the requirements for oxygen
- Individual variations in susceptibility

The first two factors are firmly linked. The more physical activity, the faster the breathing will be, and the faster a lethal level will be reached. Physical activity increases the demand for oxygen from the voluntary muscles, and oxygen starvation of those issues will tend to incapacitate a person and reduce his or her chances of escape. Case histories reveal that persons at rest (asleep or unconscious) tend to have the highest COHb saturations because they make no demands on their heart.

The role of CO interaction with heart muscle may be the strongest factor in human variability. If a person is relatively inactive, the need for oxygen is diminished, the breathing is slower and more shallow, and carbon monoxide in the air will accumulate more slowly than if breathing is faster and deeper. Carbon monoxide in the air will rapidly be accumulated if breathing is deep and at a high rate, as would be required in performing physical work. Thus, it can be stated that if a person suspects that carbon monoxide is present in significant amounts in the ambient air, he or she is better off resting quietly, breathing as little and as shallowly as possible, and avoiding all activity that will increase the breathing rate. These considerations are often important for firefighters who must exert themselves in fighting a fire and rescuing trapped persons, because the high degree of activity will inevitably increase the hazard considerably. This is one of the reasons firefighters use self-contained breathing apparatus during interior firefighting efforts.

Physical activity also increases the body's demand for oxygen, and a sudden increase in demand when 40 or 50 percent of the blood is already saturated may bring about collapse (Hazucha 2000). Variations in individual tolerance lie in the area of physiological differences, concentrations of hemoglobin in the blood, and related factors that are generally not under the control of the individual. Many of the toxicological studies cited previously dealt with healthy adult males as test subjects.

Effects on the elderly men and women along with small children have not been studied, but it would be expected that CO would have a negative effect on these victims at lower levels than for healthy adults. Elderly victims, whose heart and lung functions may already be impaired as a result of age or illness, are most probably more likely to die when less than 40 percent of their blood is bound up with CO. Infants have a faster respiration rate, and their uptake of CO may be faster than that evidenced in adults. There are also indications that the effects of CO are combined with or even enhanced by the effects of other toxic gases (such as CN or formaldehyde) from the fire, and by the CO_2 and low O_2 levels present (Purser 2000).

The estimation of dosage levels for predicting times to incapacitation is an important concept. Under **Haber's rule**, the dosage of toxic gases assimilated by an individual is assumed to be equivalent to the concentration times the duration of exposure. For example, a 1-hour exposure to a toxic gas at one concentration would be equivalent to a 2-hour exposure to half that concentration.

The Coburn-Forster-Kane (CFK) Equation

In certain cases, Haber's rule does not hold exactly true for exposure to CO. The relationship between concentration and uptake is linear only for high CO concentrations and is not valid at extremely high concentrations. For lower concentrations, the time to incapacitation is an exponential relationship and is described by the CFK equation. The CFK equation (12.2) also predicts that the half-time elimination of CO is a hyperbolic function of the ventilation rate (Peterson and Stewart 1975).

$$\frac{A[COHb]_t - BV_{CO} - PI_{CO}}{A[COHb]_0 - BV_{CO} - PI_{CO}} = e^{-tAV_bB}, \tag{12.2}$$

where

$[COHB]_t$ = concentration of CO in blood at time t (mL/mL),
$[COHb]_0$ = concentration of CO in blood at beginning of exposure (mL/mL),
PI_{CO} = partial pressure of CO in inhaled air (mm Hg),
V_{CO} = rate of CO production (mL/min),
A = derived constant,
B = derived constant, and
V_b = derived constant.

An obvious disadvantage of using the CFK equation is the number of variables needed. The CFK equation is appropriately used for exposure to CO concentrations of less than 2000 ppm (0.2 percent), exposure durations greater than 1 hour, or estimation of time to death where COHb is 50 percent (Purser 2008). The CFK equation is of limited value in reconstructing most fire death cases where the CO concentration is greater than 0.2 percent, and the COHb saturations are often much greater than 50 percent.

The Stewart Equation

When predictions of time to incapacitation deal with atmospheric CO concentrations higher than 2000 ppm (0.2 percent), and COHb in the blood is determined to be less than 50 percent saturation, a simpler equation known as the *Stewart equation* (12.3) applies:

$$\%COHb = (3.317 \times 10^{-5})(ppm\ CO)^{1.036}(RMV)(t), \tag{12.3}$$

where

CO   = CO concentration (ppm),
RMV = respirations per minute of volume of air breathed (L/min), and
t = exposure time (min).

Solving the Stewart equation for exposure time gives

$$t = \frac{(3.015 \times 10^4)(\%COHb)}{(ppm\ CO)^{1.036}(RMV)}. \tag{12.4}$$

The standard inhalation values (RMV) are listed in Table 12-2, providing typical data for a man, woman, child, infant, and newborn. For additional information on RMVs, see Health Canada 1995; SFPE 2008; and Bide, Armour, and Yee 1997.

TABLE 12-2	Standard Inhalation Values (RMV; L/min)				
ACTIVITY	MAN	WOMAN	CHILD	INFANT	NEWBORN
Resting	7.5	6.0	4.8	1.5	0.5
Light activity	20.0	19.0	13.0	4.2	1.5

Sources: Derived from Health Canada 1995; SFPE 2008, 2-102; Bide, Armour, and Yee 1997.

According to Stewart, a few breaths of CO in concentrations of 1 to 10 percent (10,000 to 100,000 ppm) rapidly elevate the COHb saturation in the blood. For example, a 120-second exposure at 1 percent (10,000 ppm) CO results in a 30 percent COHb saturation, and a 30-second exposure at 10 percent (100,000 ppm) CO results in a 75 percent COHb saturation (Spitz and Spitz 2006).

The standard approach for evaluating incapacitation from CO is to calculate the fraction of the CO inhaled per minute in 1 hour. During moderate activity, human RMV value is approximately 25 L/min, and loss of consciousness occurs at 30 percent COHb in the blood (Purser in SFPE 2008). The formula for the fractional incapacitating dose (FID) valid for up to 1 hour is

$$F_{I_{CO}} = \frac{3.317 \times 10^{-5}[CO]1.036(V)(t)}{D},$$ (12.5)

where

$$F_{I_{CO}} = \text{fractional incapacitating dose (FID)} = \frac{\text{concentration of irritant to which subject is exposed at time } t}{\text{concentration of irritant required to cause impairment of escape efficiency}},$$ (12.6)

$[CO]$ = carbon monoxide concentration (ppm v/v $20°C$)
t = exposure time (min), and
D = exposure dose (percent COHb) for incapacitation.

Resting or sleeping $V = 8.3$ L/min and $D = 40\%$ COHb
Light work: walking to escape $V = 25$ L/min and $D = 30\%$ COHb
Heavy work: slow running, walking up stairs $V = 50$ L/min and $D = 20\%$ COHb

---

EXAMPLE 12-1 ■ CO Incapacitation

Problem. Rescuers found an adult female unconscious in her bed at the scene of a house fire. Assume that rough estimates suggest that she was exposed to a CO concentration of approximately 5000 ppm. Calculate the time to incapacitation and fractional incapacitating dose, assuming that the victim was at rest.

Suggested Solution. Use Table 12-2 for RMV data.

Volume of air breathed   RMV = 6.0 L/min (resting)

Loss of consciousness   COHb = 40% (resting)

CO concentration   CO = 5000 ppm

Time to incapacitation (eq. 12.4) $t = \dfrac{(3.015 \times 10^4)(40)}{(5000)^{1.036}(6.0)} = 30$ min

Fractional incapacitating dose (eq. 12.6) $F_{I_{CO}} = \dfrac{(8.2925 \times 10^{-4})(5000^{1.036})}{30} = 0.188$

EXAMPLE 12-2 ■ CO Incapacitation and Death of Firefighters

Problem. Computer fire modeling was used to reevaluate a US Fire Administration investigation (Routley 1995) into a reported Pittsburgh fire that killed three firefighters (Christensen and Icove 2004). NIST's Fire Dynamics Simulator (FDS) was employed to model the fire and estimate the concentration of carbon monoxide present in the dwelling, which was the immediate cause of death of two of the firefighters, who were unable to escape the interior of a burning dwelling.

The fire occurred in a four-story townhouse when an arson fire was ignited using gasoline in a room on the ground floor. Firefighters entered on the street level and were attempting to locate the seat of the smoky fire. Details of the minutes before the deaths of the firefighters were unclear, but it appeared that at some point they realized they were running short of air in their SCBA, needed to leave, were unable to find an exit, and exhausted their air supplies. Two of the firefighters were believed to have removed or loosened their face pieces and made attempts to share the air that was available by buddy breathing, involving the alternating use of a single breathing apparatus. It was concluded that both had been rendered unconscious owing to toxic gas inhalation. They were found to have COHb saturations of 44 percent and 49 percent, respectively, at autopsy. A third firefighter was found with his face piece in place, and his COHb was 10 percent, indicating death from oxygen deficiency.

Solution. This estimate, along with an assumed respiration volume and known blood COHb levels, was used with the Stewart equation to estimate the time of exposure. The FDS model, as shown in Figure 12-2, indicated that 27 minutes into the fire, the CO concentration in the atmosphere at the location where the firefighters were found had already reached approximately 3600 ppm. At this concentration and a respiration rate of 70 L/min, an estimated 3 to 8 minutes of exposure would have been required to accumulate the average 47 percent COHb measured in two of the firefighter's blood at autopsy.

Solution of this problem with the Stewart equation using the CO value from the FDS model calculation gives

$$\%COHb = \left(3.317 \times 10^{-5}\right)(ppm\ CO)^{1.036}(RMV)(t),$$

where

CO = CO concentration = 3600 ppm
%COHb = carboxyhemoglobin saturation = 47%
RMV = respirations per minute of volume of air breathed = 70 L/min
t = exposure time (min).

Solving for time of exposure, we obtain

$$47\% = \left(3.317 \times 10^{-5}\right)(3600)^{1.036}(70)(t)$$
$$t = 4.2\ min$$

Estimated range for t = 3 to 8 min

A total exposure time of 4.2 minutes suggests that following the removal of the firefighters' face pieces, only a few minutes of exposure to CO with no air from the SCBA would have been required to produce the lethal concentrations of COHb observed at autopsy.

12.3.3 HYDROGEN CYANIDE

Hydrogen cyanide (HCN) is readily soluble in the aqueous phase of blood plasma, cells, and organs, where it forms the CN radical. The main effect of HCN or CN in the cell is to inhibit the use of oxygen by the cell so that oxygen in the blood cannot be properly used by the cells (Purser 2010). The CN radical also combines with Cya_3 oxidase,

EAST SIDE OF DWELLING - 8361 Bricelyn Street

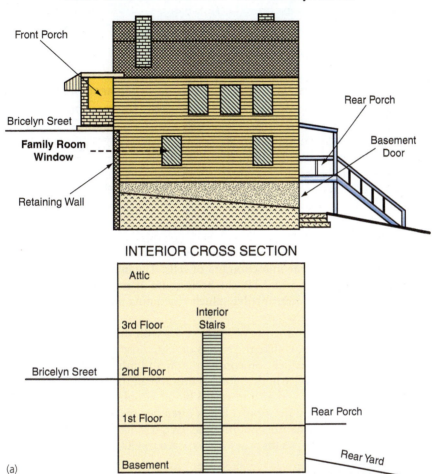

Front Porch

Bricelyn Sreet

**Family Room
Window**

Retaining Wall

Rear Porch

Basement
Door

INTERIOR CROSS SECTION

Attic		
3rd Floor	Interior Stairs	
2nd Floor		
1st Floor		
Basement		

Bricelyn Sreet

Rear Porch

Rear Yard

(a)

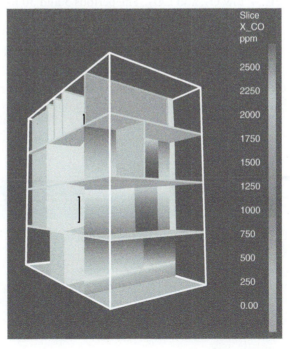

Slice
X_CO
ppm

2500
2250
2000
1750
1500
1250
1000
750
500
250
0.00

(b)

FIGURE 12-2 (a) Plan of town house where three firefighters were trapped. (b) FDS model of the distribution of carbon monoxide in a town house at 27 minutes. *Courtesy of David J. Icove, University of Tennessee.*

TABLE 12-3 — Tenability Limits for Incapacitation or Death from Exposures to Common Toxic Products of Combustion

	5 MIN		30 MIN	
	INCAPACITATION	DEATH	INCAPACITATION	DEATH
CO (ppm)	6000–8000	12,000–16,000	1400–1700	2500–4000
HCN (ppm)	150–200	250–400	90–120	170–230
Low O_2 (%)	10–13	<5	<12	6–7
CO_2 (%)	7–8	>10	6–7	>9

Source: SFPE 2008, Table 2.6.B1, 2-185, Courtesy of the Society of Fire Protection Engineers, © 2008, reprinted with permission.

inhibiting its action in the mitochondria of cells. The inhibition of Cya_3 oxidase prevents the formation of water and ATP, the basic route of respiration in the cell (Feld 2002). HCN is produced in all fires involving fuels containing nitrogen, especially acrylic rubber, ABS plastics, and polyurethane.

As with CO, the production of HCN varies with the temperature and oxygen supply in the combustion zone. Unlike the effects of CO, those of HCN are immediate but complex and are often dependent on concentration and inhalation rate. Unlike with COHb, the concentration of HCN in the blood is unstable in the body, decreasing by 50 percent in 24 hours after death and also in stored blood samples (Purser 2010). CN is suspected of contributing to many fire deaths but is often not measured immediately. Because it is produced under the same fire conditions as CO, it is likely to act quickly at low doses to incapacitate the victims, so that they are exposed to CO and other fire gases longer, causing their deaths.

Table 12-3 lists the tenability limits for incapacitation or death from exposure to CO, HCN, low O_2, and CO_2. The periods 5 and 30 minutes are common benchmarks for narcotic products of combustion.

12.3.4 PREDICTING THE TIME TO INCAPACITATION BY HYDROGEN CYANIDE

As discussed earlier, hydrogen cyanide (HCN) is another toxic gas in fires that incapacitates through biochemical asphyxiation. As with CO, the time to incapacitation depends on the uptake rate and dosage (Purser 2008). Typical effects of HCN exposure are listed in Table 12-4.

TABLE 12-4 — Typical Effects of HCN Exposure

REPORTED EFFECTS ON HEALTHY ADULTS

Extremely toxic
  170—230 ppm = death in 30 minutes
  250—400 ppm = death in 5 minutes (SFPE)

Produced by any fuel that contains nitrogen (hair, wool, fur, leather, polyurethane, nylon).

Absorbed through inhalation and ingestion.

Exposure to less than 80 ppm is expected to have minimal effect on a healthy adult (Purser 2010). The effect of concentrations greater than 80 ppm can be calculated (Purser in SFPE 2008). The formula for time to incapacitation for inhalation of 80 to 180 ppm HCN concentrations is

$$t_{I_{CN}}(\text{min}) = \frac{185 - \text{ppm HCN}}{4.4}; \tag{12.7}$$

the formula for time to incapacitation for HCN exposure concentrations above 180 ppm is

$$t_{I_{CN}}(\text{min}) = \exp[5.396 - (0.023)(\text{ppm HCN})]; \tag{12.8}$$

and the fractional incapacitating dose per minute (FID/min) is

$$F_{I_{CN}} = \frac{1}{\exp[5.396 - (0.023)(\text{ppm HCN})]}. \tag{12.9}$$

Note that "exp" in equations (12.8) and (12.9) denotes the exponential form. As shown in Table 12-3, the HCN dosages required for incapacitation are much lower than the CO dosages. The lowest blood concentration associated with adult death by acute cyanide poisoning is 1 to 2 mg/ml. More typical levels are 2.4 to 2.5 at death (Purser 2010). A case study using these equations is illustrated in Example 12-3.

EXAMPLE 12-3 ■ HCN Incapacitation

Problem. An adult male was found unconscious in the waiting room after being exposed to toxic by-products from the fire in Example 12-1. Fire modeling estimated that a burning polyurethane plastic mattress cushion had produced an HCN concentration of approximately 200 ppm in the air being breathed.

Solution. Calculate the time to incapacitation and the fractional incapacitating dose per minute (FID/min).

HCN concentration	HCN = 200 ppm
Time to incapacitation	$t = \exp[5.396 - (0.023)(200)] = 2.2\,\text{min}$
Fractional incapacitating dose per minute	$F_{I_{CN}} = \left(\dfrac{1}{\exp[5.396 - (0.023)(200)]}\right) = 0.45\,\text{FID/min}$

12.3.5 INCAPACITATION BY LOW OXYGEN LEVELS

Anoxia (absence of oxygen) or **hypoxia** (low concentration of oxygen) is the condition of inadequate oxygen to support life. This situation can occur when oxygen is displaced by another inert gas, such as nitrogen or carbon dioxide; by a fuel gas such as methane; or even by benign products of combustion, such as CO_2 and water vapor. Normal air contains 20.9 percent O_2. At concentrations down to 15 percent O_2, there are no readily observable effects in humans owing to decreased oxygen concentrations. At concentrations between 10 and 15 percent, disorientation (similar to intoxication) occurs, and judgment is affected. At levels below 10 percent, unconsciousness and death may occur. Hypoxia is aggravated by high levels of CO_2, which accelerate breathing rates. The effects of hypoxia include cerebral depression, causing lethargy; problems with memory and mental concentration; loss of consciousness; and death (Purser 2010) (see Table 12-5).

anoxia ■ Condition relating to an absence of oxygen.

hypoxia ■ Condition relating to low concentrations of oxygen.

TABLE 12-5	The Effects of Exposure to Low Oxygen Levels

PERCENT OXYGEN	REPORTED EFFECTS ON HEALTHY ADULTS
14.14–20.9	No significant effects, slight loss of exercise tolerance
11.18–14.14	Slight effects on memory and mental task performance, reduced exercise tolerance
9.6–11.8	Severe incapacitation, lethargy, euphoria, loss of consciousness
7.8–9.6	Loss of consciousness, death

Source: Derived from SFPE 2008.

The time to loss of consciousness for an adult exposed to a hypoxia equivalent is

$$(t_{lo}) = \exp[\,8.13 - 0.54(20.9 - \%O_2)\,], \tag{12.10}$$

where

t_{lo} = exposure time in minutes
$\%O_2$ = concentration at $20°C$ in the air being inhaled

12.3.6 PREDICTING THE TIME TO INCAPACITATION BY CARBON DIOXIDE

Exposure to carbon dioxide can produce a wide range of effects, ranging from respiratory distress to loss of consciousness (SFPE 2008, 2-119) (see Table 12-6).

Along with being an asphyxiant capable of displacing oxygen, carbon dioxide also increases the RMV, which in turn causes the individual to increase the uptake of the other toxic gases (Purser 2008). This formula for the multiplication factor VCO_2 is

$$VCO_2 = \exp\left(\frac{CO_2}{5}\right), \tag{12.11}$$

$$VCO_2 = \left(\frac{\exp[\,(1.903)(\%CO_2) + 2.0004\,]}{7.1}\right). \tag{12.12}$$

The formula for the time to unconsciousness (incapacitation) from carbon dioxide is

$$t_{I_{CO_2}} = \exp[\,6.1623 - (0.5189)(\%CO_2)\,], \tag{12.13}$$

and the fractional incapacitating dose per minute (FID/min) is

$$F_{I_{CO_2}} = \left(\frac{1}{\exp[\,6.1623 - (0.5189)(\%CO_2)\,]}\right). \tag{12.14}$$

TABLE 12-6	The Effects of Exposure to Carbon Dioxide

PERCENT CARBON DIOXIDE	REPORTED EFFECT(S)
7–10	Loss of consciousness
6–7	Severe respiratory distress, dizziness, possible loss of consciousness
3–6	Respiratory distress increasing with concentration

Source: Derived from SFPE 2008.

12.4 Heat

The human body is capable of surviving exposure to external heat as long as it can moderate its core temperature by radiant cooling of the blood through the skin and, more importantly, by evaporative cooling. This process occurs internally via evaporation of water from the mucosal linings of the mouth, nose, throat, and lungs and externally via evaporation of sweat from the skin. If the core body temperature exceeds 43°C (109°F), death is likely to occur.

Prolonged exposure to high external temperatures, 80 to 120°C (175 to 250°F), with low humidity can trigger fatal hyperthermia. Exposure to elevated temperatures accompanied by high humidity (which reduces the cooling evaporation rate of the water from the skin or mucosa) can also be lethal. Fire victims can die of exposure to heat alone even if they are protected from CO, smoke, and flames. These victims may have minimal postmortem changes, although skin blistering and sloughing can occur after death owing to heat denaturation of collagen and other proteins in the connective tissue and skin.

12.4.1 PREDICTING THE TIME TO INCAPACITATION BY HEAT

For exposure to convected heat in a fire environment, the fractional incapacitating dose per minute (FID/min) is calculated as follows:

$$F_{I_h} = \left(\frac{1}{\exp\left[5.1849 - (0.0273)\left(T[°C] \right) \right]} \right). \tag{12.15}$$

Assimilation of various data formed the basis for the *Toxic and Physical Hazard Assessment Model* (Purser in SFPE 2008). Data such as toxic chemical and physical species concentration levels generated by fire models can serve as input to this hazard assessment model. According to this model, the normally accepted threshold for tolerance of radiant heat is 2.5 kW/m² for only a few minutes. Besides the burns to the skin (from both radiant and convected heat), thermal damage to the upper respiratory tract can also occur when dry gases at temperatures over 120°C (250°F) are inhaled.

Information needed to evaluate this hazard model is derived from two sets of information: concentration and time profiles of major toxic products, including time, concentration, and toxicity relationships. The estimated toxic products within the victim's breathing zone include concentrations of gases such as carbon monoxide, hydrogen cyanide, carbon dioxide, and factors such as radiant heat flux, and air temperature. Some of these values can be calculated by sophisticated computer models discussed previously.

12.4.2 INHALATION OF HOT GASES

Inhalation of very hot gases causes edema (swelling and inflammation) of mucosal tissues. This edema can be severe enough to cause blockage of the trachea and physical asphyxia. Inhalation of hot gases may also trigger *laryngospasm,* in which the larynx involuntarily closes up to prevent entry of foreign material, and *vagal inhibition,* in which the breathing stops, and the heart rate drops.

Rapid cooling of the inhaled hot gases occurs on inhalation as the water evaporates from mucosal tissues, so thermal damage usually does not extend below the larynx if the inhaled gases are dry. If the hot gases include steam or are otherwise water saturated, evaporative cooling is minimized, and burns/edema can extend to the major bronchi and alveoli, which are tiny air sacs in the lungs. If inhaled gases are hot enough to damage the trachea and internal lung infrastructures, they will usually be hot enough to burn the facial skin and mouth as well as singe the facial or nasal hair.

12.4.3 EFFECTS OF HEAT AND FLAME

The human body is a complex target when being affected by heat from a fire. The skin consists of two basic layers. A thin outer layer of *epidermis* (dead, keratinized skin cells) overlies a thicker inner dermal layer of actively growing cells in which are embedded the nerve endings, hair follicles, and blood capillaries that supply nutrients to the growing skin. Beneath the dermal layer is a layer of tough elastic connective tissue, subcutaneous fat, and, finally, muscle and bone.

Each of these components is affected differently by heat and flames. Application of heat can cause the epidermis to separate from the underlying *dermis* and form blisters in much the way paint or wallpaper blisters away from the wood or plaster beneath when heated. Blistering of the skin occurs when the tissue reaches temperatures in excess of 54°C (130°F). The raised epidermal layer is very thin and is more easily affected by continuing heat, which can cause the epidermal layer to char and turn black if the temperature is high enough. The epidermis can also separate in larger areas and form generalized skin slippage. Exposure of the denuded dermal layer to heat can cause extreme pain when its temperature exceeds 43°C to 44°C (110°F to 112°F) (Purser in SFPE 2008).

More prolonged exposure can destroy the proteins of the dermal layer and cause further desiccation and discoloration. Higher heat fluxes can cause higher temperatures that cook and even char the tissues. As the skin desiccates, it shrinks, eliminating wrinkles and changing facial contours (making visual identifications of victims very risky). If the skin continues to shrink, it can split open, leaving jagged, irregular, torn surfaces (as opposed to the sharply defined surfaces of knife cuts) (Pope and Smith 2003). Heat-split skin often exhibits subcutaneous bridging of underlying tissue, whereas cut skin does not.

If a victim survives for some time, shrinkage can constrict blood vessels, so incisions (called *escharotomies*) are made through the damaged dermal layer to relieve the pressure and maintain circulation. If a fire victim survived for some time after the fire and underwent medical interventions such as an escharotomy or skin graft harvesting, the investigator must recognize the effects of these and distinguish them from fire effects.

Owing to its small individual dimensions and low thermal mass, hair is affected very quickly by heat. Colors will change (typically changing to darker or redder colors or completely to a gray, ashen color). The hair shaft will bubble, shrink, and fracture as it singes from heat. This shrinkage causes the curling of hair shafts seen as singeing. The microscopic appearance of singed hair shafts is very distinctive (as compared with cut or broken hair shafts). If the hair is burned in large masses, it can form a black, puffy, entangled mass.

If the body continues to be exposed to heat, the shrinkage can affect muscles. When the skin and muscles of the neck shrink, they can force the tongue out of the mouth. Shrinkage of muscle and tendons can cause the joints to flex, causing what is called *pugilistic posturing*. This flexing and posturing can cause bodies to move during fire exposure. If the body is on an irregular or unstable surface, this movement can cause the body to fall from a bed or chair and, possibly, change the direction of heat application, eliminating or obscuring previously protected areas. Pugilistic posturing has been observed during legal cremations after 10 minutes of exposure to flames at temperatures of 670°C to 810°C (1240°F to 1490°F) (Bohnert, Rost, and Pollak 1998; Pope 2007).

Direct flame impingement, with its high-temperature gases of 500°C to 900°C (930°F to 1650°F) and high heat fluxes (55 kW/m^2), produces responses from the human body very quickly. Blisters will form in about 5 seconds, with charring following seconds later. Skin can be charred completely away in 5 to 10 minutes of direct flame contact, especially where stretched over the bone (joints, nose, forehead, skull) (Pope and Smith 2003, 2004; Pope 2007). Very short but intense (flash) fire exposure can cause blistering of the epidermal layer without the sensation of pain (because the pain sensors are in the dermal layer beneath), and the heat takes longer to penetrate deeply.

Even in the absence of fire, prolonged exposure of the body to high temperatures [over 50°C (122°F)] causes desiccation and shrinkage of muscle tissue, which causes pugilistic posturing. Exposure to flames can cause muscles to combust and major limb bones to fracture as they degrade where the bone is exposed to flames. Extreme heat causes bones to twist and fracture, and continued flame exposure (30 minutes or longer in observed cremations) causes calcination (in which the charred organic matter is burned away). As the bones become calcined, they become very fragile and may disintegrate of their own accord. The lower-density major bones from elderly victims of osteoporosis have been seen to disintegrate under fire exposure more quickly and completely than bones with normal densities (Christensen 2002).

Tests have revealed that fire exposure can cause fluid that cushions the brain as well as the brain cell fluids to leak through fissures in the exposed skull, but does not cause the skull to explode. Internal organs that are exposed to the fire desiccate and char, thus requiring at least 30 to 40 minutes of cremation to burn away (Bohnert, Rost, and Pollak 1998). The adult torso will require longer exposure to a normal structure fire before the organs are affected. Bones exposed to fire can also shrink in length, thus giving rise to potential errors in the estimation of antemortem height.

The thin bones of the skull may delaminate, with the inner and outer layers failing separately. This delamination has given rise to thermally caused holes in the skull that have beveled edges similar to those produced by gunshots (Pope and Smith 2003). Recent experiments have demonstrated that failure of the skull can occur from fire damage whether or not there was preexisting mechanical or blunt force trauma. Some thermally induced failures can mimic bullet wounds, requiring extreme care in casework investigative interpretations (Pope and Smith 2004).

Heat exposure to the head can cause blood and fluids to accumulate and form a hematoma in the *extradural* or *epidural* space between the skull and the tough bag of tissue (the *dura mater*) that surrounds the brain. With further heating, these fluids boil, desiccate, and then char, producing a rigid, foamy, blackened mass. Physical trauma to the brain as a result of the impact from falling structures overhead also can cause *subdural* hematomas. However, fractures at the base of the skull have not been observed to be produced by fire exposure (Bohnert, Rost, and Pollak 1998; Pope 2007). Fire exposure chars and seals exposed tissues, so as a rule, bodies exposed to an enveloping fire do not bleed. When the body is moved, however, the fragile layer of char covering the tissues can be broken, allowing body fluids to seep out. Thus, great care must be taken when moving a charred body with exposed charred tissues, and its condition prior to being moved must be carefully documented.

Within certain considerations, the amount of fire damage on a body can be related to the duration of exposure if the intensity of the fire can be estimated from the fuel, ventilation, and distribution factors described elsewhere in this text. In recent studies DeHaan, Campbell, and Nurbakhsh (1999) have explored factors such as combustion rates, thermal inertia, and relative combustibility of body components. Some aspects of postmortem fire damage to the human body are discussed later in this chapter.

Clothing is not often completely destroyed by a fire. What the victim was wearing may indicate his or her activity just prior to the fire. Consideration must be given here to the time of the fire relative to the state of dress. Was the victim normally fully clothed at 3 A.M. or in pajamas until noon? If the fire occurred at 3 P.M. and the victim was dressed for bed, was he or she ill or incapacitated prior to the fire? More traditional time of death markers such as rigor mortis and body temperature are seriously skewed by fire exposure, and environmental indicators take on additional importance.

Dark hair may lighten and turn reddish with some fire exposure. Artificial dyes can react differently than natural pigments. This may be due to ventilation effects, with an oxidizing atmosphere having one effect, while a fuel-rich reducing atmosphere has quite another. In severely charred bodies, computed tomography (CT) and magnetic resonance imaging (MRI) have been used successfully to document injuries caused by burns, as well as vital reactions in soft tissues caused by mechanical trauma (Thali et al. 2002).

12.4.4 FLAMES (INCINERATION)

When heat is applied to a surface, the rate at which it penetrates that surface is determined by the thermal inertia of the material (the numerical product of thermal capacity, density, and thermal conductivity). The thermal inertia of skin is not much different from that of a block of wood or polyethylene plastic (see Table 12-4). The pain sensors for human skin are in the dermis, about 2 mm (0.1 in.) below the surface. If heat is applied very briefly, there may not be any sensation of discomfort or pain. The longer the heat is applied, the deeper it will penetrate into the skin. The higher the intensity of the heat applied, the faster it will penetrate into the skin. Pain is triggered when skin cells reach a temperature of about 48°C (120°F), and cells are damaged if their temperature exceeds 54°C (130°F) (Stoll and Greene 1959).

Exposing skin to 2 to 4 kW/m^2 radiant heat for 30 seconds causes pain but no permanent cellular damage. Higher heat fluxes trigger damage such as blisters and skin slippage. Exposing skin to 4 to 6 kW/m^2 radiant heat for 8 seconds produces blisters (second-degree burns). Exposing skin to 10 kW/m^2 radiant heat for 5 seconds causes deeper, partial-thickness injuries. Exposing skin to 50 to 60 kW/m^2 radiant heat for 5 seconds produces third-degree burns with the destruction of the dermis (Stoll and Greene 1959).

The investigator should not presume that the condition of the body as recovered from the fire is in the same condition as it was at the time of death. The body represents a fuel package and will undergo changes postmortem if it continues to be exposed to fire. It is very rare to encounter heat of sufficient intensity and duration that it destroys all anatomical features. Complete legal incineration (cremation) of an adult human body requires temperatures on the order of 950°C to 1100°C (1800°F to 2100°F) for destruction to be completed within 1 to 2 hours (Eckert, James, and Katchis 1988; Bohnert, Rost, and Pollak 1998). Even then, identifiable portions of the skull, pelvic bones, and dentition usually survive. A fully involved, wood-frame structure fire lasting one hour resulted in a reduction of an adult male body to large bone fragments (Pope 2004). Identifiable portions of the skeletal structures still remained.

Often furnishings, bedding, or carpets provide not only a continuous source of fuel for an external fire but also a supply of char to act as a wick. This phenomenon, termed the candle effect, or wick effect, describes a fire in which fuel, in the form of clothing or bedding as the first fuel, ignited as well as the body fat to feed later stages; an ignition source—smoking materials or cooking or heating appliances; and finally, the dynamics of heat, fuel, and ventilation to promote a slow, steady flaming fire that may generate only small open flames and insufficient radiant heat to encourage fire growth. In these circumstances, the fat rendered from a burning body will act in the same manner as the fuel in an oil lamp or candle. If the body is positioned so that fats rendered from it can seep into a porous wicking material or drip or drain onto an ignition source, it will continue to fuel the flames. This effect is dramatically enhanced if there are combustible fuels—carpet padding, bedding, upholstery stuffing—that form a rigid, carbonaceous char that can absorb the rendered fat and act as a wick (Ettling 1968; Gee 1965; DeHaan, Campbell, and Nurbakhsh 1999). Under appropriate conditions, an adult body can sustain a flaming fire for 6 to 7 hours (DeHaan et al. 1999, 2001).

12.4.5 BURNS

Burns may appear in the absence of fire or flames as a result of prolonged exposure of the body or body parts to heat that raises their overall temperature above 54°C (130°F) and causes desiccation, sloughing, and blistering. These effects can also be caused by exposure of the body to caustic chemicals. It is often very difficult, if not impossible, to distinguish between these types of burns suffered near the time of death (*perimortem*) and those inflicted after death (*postmortem*). Fluid-filled blisters can result from fire exposure both antemortem and postmortem as well as from postmortem decomposition.

Most, but not all, medical personnel agree that *first-degree burns* involve only reddening of the skin. *Second-degree burns*, sometimes referred to as *partial-thickness burns*, involve damage to the epidermis with blistering and sloughing. Because the germinative layer of the dermis remains, the entire surface of such burns will usually heal, most often without grafts. *Third-degree burns* are called *full-thickness burns* because the dermis is damaged, and the wound heals from the edges only and requires grafting. *Fourth-degree burns,* sometimes also referred to as full-thickness burns, can include those in which the skin is destroyed, exposing subcutaneous fat and muscle and the bones beneath the muscles. *Fifth-degree burns* involve underlying muscle and bone.

When gasoline or a similar volatile liquid fuel with low viscosity and low surface tension is poured on bare skin, some is absorbed into the epidermis, but the bulk of the fuel runs off, leaving a very thin film of liquid, particularly on vertical surfaces. This thin film burns off very quickly (less than 10 seconds). The skin beneath may be spared completely or reddened (first-degree burns), except where folds of the skin or clothing retain enough fuel to sustain longer burning, producing severe blistering, and even charring of the epidermis in extreme cases. Deep penetrating burns exposing the subcutaneous fat or muscle below require flame exposures of several minutes, much longer than the typical thin-film gasoline fire. On horizontal skin surfaces, a deeper pool may be retained long enough to produce a halo or ring of blisters (second-degree burns) around the circumference of the pool (DeHaan and Icove 2012).

12.4.6 BLUNT FORCE TRAUMA

Blunt force trauma can also cause or contribute to the death of fire victims. Structural collapse or explosions can cause solid materials to strike victims. Falls or impacts with stationary surfaces (furniture or door frames) during escape attempts can induce blunt trauma that only a careful medical examination can distinguish from an assault. Wound patterns, bloodstains, or even trace evidence can be used to interpret blunt trauma injuries and establish whether they resulted from assault or from some fire-related event. The fire investigator should consider consulting with the pathologist and the criminalist to help evaluate blunt trauma injuries and possibly link them to features at the fire scene.

12.5 Visibility

The optical opacity of dense smoke and its irritants impairs the vision and respiration of normal-sighted people who may find their ability to travel impaired by the smoke. This optically dense smoke affects:

- Exit choice and escape decisions,
- Speed of movement, and
- Wayfinding ability.

During structure fires, the occupants often depend on their ability to seek out exit signs, doors, and windows (Jin 1976; Jin and Yamada 1985). Visibility of an object depends on several factors such as the smoke's ability to scatter or absorb the ambient light, the wavelength of the light, whether the item viewed (e.g., an exit sign) is light emitting or light reflecting, and the individual's visual acuity (Mulholland 2008).

Studies by the US Naval Medical Research Laboratory, Bureau of Medicine and Surgery provide an insight into the underlying principles on the first use of red exit signs. The studies examined the detectability of colored field targets at sea. Colors that were distinguishable at the greatest distances were the red fluorescents (yellow-red and orange-red)

(USN 1955). Later research by the US Air Force (Miller and Tredici 1992) on night vision expanded these findings when it was determined that the sensitivity of the eye changes from the red end of the visible spectrum toward the blue end when shifting the *photopic* vision (high illumination levels) to *scotopic* vision (reduced illumination levels, typically at night).

The naval study on the ability of the eye to perceive the color red at greater distances gives credence to the logic of using the color red for fire exit signs, whether they be passive fluorescent or illuminated. OSHA regulations state that exit signs, when required, shall be lettered in legible red letters, not less than 6 inches high, on a white field [*OSHA 29 CFR 126-200(d)*].

12.5.1 OPTICAL DENSITY

Visibility can be estimated regarding the *optical density* per meter. The calculation involves a collateral term known as the extinction coefficient, K, which is the product of an *extinction coefficient* per unit mass, K_m, and the mass concentration of the smoke aerosol, m:

$$K = K_m m; \qquad (12.16)$$

$$D = \frac{K}{2.3}, \qquad (12.17)$$

where

K = extinction coefficient (m^{-1})
K_m = specific extinction coefficient (m^2/g),
m = mass concentration of smoke (g/m^3), and
D = optical density per meter (m^{-1})

The values for K_m are typically 7.6 m^2/g for smoke produced during flaming combustion of wood or plastics, and 4.4 m^2/g for smoke produced during pyrolysis (SFPE 2008).

Regarding the extinction coefficient K, one problem at a fire is determining the visibility, S, of light-emitting and light-reflecting exit signs to occupants. The value S is a measure of how well an individual can see through the smoke. Light-emitting signs are two to four times more visible than light-reflecting signs (Mulholland in SFPE 2008, 2-297), as the values for KS reveal in equations (12.18) and (12.19),

$$KS = 8 \text{ for light-emitting signs}, \qquad (12.18)$$

$$KS = 3 \text{ for light-reflecting signs}, \qquad (12.19)$$

where

K = extinction coefficient (m^{-1}) and
S = visibility (m).

Methods for estimating visibility based on the mass optical density are considered realistic because they are based on actual human studies. In these studies, the optical density at which people turned back from a smoke-filled area was a visibility distance of 3 m (9.84 ft) (Bryan 1983). The study also showed a tendency for women to be more likely to turn back than men. Other factors include the ability of the persons to see exit signs directing them to safe egress from the building. The height of exit signs as well as the height of the viewer may be critical to visibility.

Estimates of visibility are based on mass optical densities, D_m, derived from test data (Babrauskas 1981). Typical values of mass optical density produced by mattresses in flaming combustion are listed in Table 12-7.

TABLE 12-7	Mass Optical Density (D_m) for Flaming Mattresses

TYPE OF MATERIAL	MASS OPTICAL DENSITY (m²/g)
Polyurethane	0.22
Cotton	0.12
Latex	0.44
Neoprene	0.20

Source: Derived from Babrauskas 1981.

The following equation is used to estimate the density, D, of the visible smoke:

$$D = \frac{D_m \Delta M}{V_C}, \tag{12.20}$$

where

D = optical density per meter (m^{-1}),
D_m = mass optical density (m^2/g),
ΔM = total mass loss of sample (g), and
V_c = total volume of compartment or chamber (m^3).

EXAMPLE 12-4 ■ Visibility

Problem. A small, 300-g (0.66-lb), polyurethane mattress cushion on a waiting-room bench is set afire by a juvenile arsonist and is undergoing flaming combustion. The bench is located in a 6-m-square (20-ft-square) waiting room with a ceiling height of 2.5 m (8.2 ft). Determine the closest visibility of both light-emitting and light-reflecting signs leading to the exit door.

Solution. Assume that the smoke filling the waiting room is uniformly mixed.

Total mass loss of mattress	ΔM	= 300 g
Mass optical density	D_m	= (from Table 12-7) = 0.22 m²/g
Volume of compartment	V_c	= (6 m)(6 m)(2.5 m) = 90.0 m³
Optical density	D	= $(0.22^2/g)(300\ g)/(90.0\ m^3)$ = 0.733 m⁻¹
Extinction coefficient	K	= 2.3 D = $(2.3)(0.733\ m^{-1})$ = 1.687 m⁻¹
Visibility (light emitting)	S	= 8/K = $(8)/(1.687\ m^{-1})$ = 4.74 m
Visibility (light reflecting)	S	= 3/K = $(3)/(1.687\ m^{-1})$ = 1.77 m

The calculations indicate that a light-emitting sign can be seen in this fire at a distance of up to 4.74 m (15.5 ft), compared with 1.7 m (5.58 ft) for an unlit sign. In real rooms, the buoyancy of the hot smoke layer makes it harder to see signs in the upper half of the room than this example indicates. Exit signs are being placed at knee level or lower today to make them more visible longer.

12.5.2 FRACTIONAL EQUIVALENT CONCENTRATIONS OF SMOKE

The following formulas relate to enclosed spaces. As the value of FEC_{smoke} approaches 1, the level of visual obscuration increases, and the chance of escape decreases significantly.

$$\text{FEC}_{\text{smoke}} = \frac{D}{0.2} \text{ for small enclosures;} \tag{12.21}$$

$$\text{FEC}_{\text{smoke}} = \frac{D}{0.1} \text{ for large enclosures,} \tag{12.22}$$

where

D = optical density per meter of the smoke being encountered.

12.5.3 WALKING SPEED

As previously summarized, the optical density of the smoke affects a person's decision to choose the closest exit and ability to make proper escape decisions, as well as wayfinding ability and speed of movement. Normal adult walking speed is about 2 m/s in clear areas and with normal visibility. During smoky conditions furniture and other occupants impeding the escape will reduce walking speed. The fire investigator should take this factor into consideration when assessing witness statements as to egress times from structures during fires.

Experiments with human subjects navigating through nonirritant smoke–filled corridors indicated that speed of movement decreases with increased smoke density (Jin 1976; Jin and Yamada 1985).

Based on Jin's (1976) research, equation (12.23) provides an expression of this relationship:

$$\text{FWS} = (-1.738)(D) + 1.236 \text{ for the range } 0.13 \text{ m}^{-1} \le D \le 0.30 \text{ m}^{-1}, \tag{12.23}$$

where

FWS = fractional walking speed (m/s), and
D = optical density per meter (m^{-1}).

For this equation, the optical smoke density ranges between 0.13/m (below normal walking speed) and 0.56/m (above walking speed of 0.3 m/s in darkness). The limits of the equation do not allow for delays such as erratic walking and sensory irritation. Jin used wood smoke in his experiments.

12.5.4 WAYFINDING

Jin's expression does not correlate midcourse corrections in wayfinding, reduced visibility, and irritability of the smoke. Studies have shown that the average density of smoke at which persons turn back is a visibility distance of 3 m (9.84 ft) ($D = 0.33 \text{ m}^{-1}$ and $K = 0.76$). Poor visibility and irritation of the eyes are the leading factors in reduced wayfinding, followed by irritation of the respiratory system (Jensen 1998).

12.5.5 SMOKE

Smoke contains water vapor, CO, CO_2, inorganic ash, toxic gases, and chemicals in aerosol form as well as soot. Soot is agglomerations of carbon from incomplete combustion large enough to produce visible particles. These particles may be very hot and are not cooled readily as they are inhaled, so they may induce edema and burns where they lodge in the mucosal tissue of the respiratory system. Soot particles are active adsorbents, so they may carry toxic chemicals and permit their ingestion or inhalation (with direct absorption by the mucosal tissues). Soot can be inhaled in quantities sufficient to physically block airways and cause mechanical asphyxiation. Soot, water vapor, ash, and aerosols in smoke can also obscure the vision of victims and prevent their escape.

12.6 Scene Investigation

The reconstruction of the activities of a fire victim may depend on finding and documenting bloodstains (from impact with a wall or door jamb), or handprints on a wall, mechanical (blunt trauma) injuries, or artifacts found with the body. The nature of dress (street clothes, robe, nightgown) or objects (dog leash, jewelry, flashlight, fire extinguisher, house keys, phone, keepsakes, etc.) can provide clues as to what the person was doing prior to collapse.

The position of the victim (face up or face down) is not usually significant, as people known to have died during a fire have been found in all positions. Because of pugilistic posturing, the attitude of the body bears little reliable relation to antemortem actions. As mentioned earlier, pugilistic posturing occurs as a physical reaction of the body to the heat and can occur whether the person was dead before the fire or died during the fire. It can cause bodies to shift position, sometimes to the point where they roll off unstable surfaces like chairs or mattresses. Young children may hide under beds or in closets, but finding them in other locations is not proof that they did not have the time or physical capacity to seek safety.

12.6.1 POSTMORTEM DESTRUCTION

A body exposed to fire can support combustion, the rate and thoroughness of which depend on the nature and condition of exposure of the body to the flames. The skin, fat, muscles, and connective tissues will shrink as they dehydrate and char. If exposed to enough flame, they will burn and yield some heat of combustion. The relatively water-logged tissues of the internal organs must be dried by heat exposure before they can combust, and that dehydration step increases their fire resistance and delays their consumption.

Bones have moisture and a high fat content, especially in the marrow, so they will shrink, crack, and split and contribute fuel to an external fire. The subcutaneous fat of the human body provides the best fuel, having an effective heat of combustion on the order of 32 to 36 kJ/g (DeHaan, Campbell, and Nurbakhsh 1999). Like candle wax, however, it will not self-ignite or smolder and will not normally support flaming combustion unless the rendered fat is absorbed into a suitable wick. The material for the wick can be charred clothing, bedding, carpet, upholstery, or wood in the vicinity (as long as it forms a porous, rigid mass). The size of the fire that can be supported by such a process is controlled by the size (surface area) of the wick. Depending on the position of the body and its available wick area, fires supported by the combustion of a body will be of the order of 20 to 120 kW, similar to a small wastebasket fire. Such a fire will affect only items close to it, and fire damage will often be very confined.

Flame temperatures produced by combustion of body fat range from 800°C to 900°C (1475°F to 1650°F), and if flames impinge on the body surface, they can aid the destruction of the body. The process, if unaided by an external fire, is quite slow, with a fuel consumption rate on the order of 3.6 to 10.8 kg/hr (7 to 25 lb/hr). It is possible, given a long enough time (5 to 10 hr), for a great deal of the body to be reduced to bone fragments (DeHaan 2001; DeHaan, Campbell, and Nurbakhsh 1999; DeHaan and Pope 2007).

If a body is exposed to a fully developed room or vehicle fire, however, the rate of destruction is much closer to that observed in a commercial crematorium. In those cases, flames of 700°C to 900°C (1300°F to 1650°F) and a heat intensity of 100 kW/m^2 envelop the body and can reduce it to ash and fragments of the larger bones in 1.5 to 3 hours (Bohnert, Rost, and Pollak 1998; DeHaan and Fisher 2003; DeHaan 2012).

12.6.2 INTERVAL BETWEEN FIRE AND DEATH

One of the problems outlined earlier is the time interval between exposure to a fire and its fatal aftermath. Death can occur nearly instantaneously or within minutes or hours later. Under these conditions, it is not difficult to connect the death to its actual cause. When a person dies weeks or even months after a fire, the cause can still be the fire, but the linkage can be obscured by extensive medical interventions.

There is a range of effects that can determine the time interval between the fire and death. Death can occur within seconds to minutes from *hyperthermia,* exposure to very hot gases or steam, or from anoxia, a lack of oxygen. With *instantaneous death,* vagal inhibition or laryngospasm can occur on inhalation of flames and hot gases, causing cessation of breathing followed very quickly by death. Explosion trauma and incineration from exposure to a fully developed fire, often resulting in structural collapse, result in nearly instantaneous death.

Inhalation of toxic gases such as hydrogen cyanide, carbon monoxide, or other pyrolysis products; blockage of airways by soot or exposure to flames; physical trauma (with the loss of blood); internal injuries; and brain injuries can cause death within minutes.

Death can occur within hours of carbon monoxide exposure, edema from inhalation of hot gases, burns, and brain or other internal injuries. Dehydration and shock from burns cause death days after the fire. Even weeks or months after the fire, deaths can occur owing to infections or organ failure triggered by fire injuries.

The *cause of death* is defined as the injury or disease that triggers the sequence of events leading to death. In a fire, the cause of death may include inhalation of hot gases, CO, or other toxic gases, heat, burns, anoxia, asphyxia, structural collapse, or blunt trauma. The *mechanism of death* is the biological or biochemical derangement incompatible with life. Mechanisms of death can be respiratory failure, exsanguination, infection, organ failure, and cardiac arrest. The *manner of death* is a medicolegal assessment and classification of the circumstances in which the cause of death was brought about. In the United States, these classifications are most often *homicide, suicide, accident, natural,* or *undetermined.*

The longer the interval between the cause (the fire) and the onset of the mechanism of death (organ failure, septicemia, etc.), the more likely it is that the connection will be lost. This is especially true when victims are moved from trauma care hospitals to long-term care facilities, sometimes in other geographic areas. The investigator must be diligent to ensure that the cause of death is not listed on the final death certificate as some generic mechanism term such as respiratory failure, cardiac arrest, or septicemia.

12.6.3 POSTMORTEM TESTS DESIRABLE IN FIRE DEATH CASES

The complexity of many fire death cases may necessitate finding the answers to questions that were not apparent earlier. Having comprehensive forensic samples and data is the best route to a successful and accurate investigation. Although not all forensic tests and data may be needed in all fire death cases, once the body is released for burial or cremation, it will be too late for forensic examination.

Postmortem tests include:

- *Blood:* (taken from a major blood vessel or chamber of the heart, not from the body cavity): tested for COHb saturation, HCN, drugs (therapeutic and abuse), alcohol, and volatile hydrocarbons.
- *Tissue (brain, kidney, liver, lung):* Tested for drugs, poisons, volatile hydrocarbons, combustion by-products, CO (as a backup for insufficient blood).
- *Tissue (skin near burns):* Tested for vital chemical or cellular response to burns.
- *Stomach contents:* Tested for establishment of activities before death and possible time of death.
- *Eye fluid:* An uncontaminated source of drugs and metabolites.
- *Airways:* Full longitudinal transection of airways from mouth to lungs to examine and document the extent and distribution of edema, scorching/dehydration, and soot.

- **X-rays:** Full-body (including associated debris in body bag) and details of teeth and any unusual features discovered (fractures, implants).
- **Clothing:** All clothing remnants and associated artifacts removed and preserved.
- **Photographs:** General (overall), with close-ups of any burns or wounds, in color, with scale.
- **Postmortem Multidetector Computed Tomography (MDCT):** Experimentally has been found to be a valuable tool, should this resource be available (see Levy and Harcke 2011).
- **Postmortem weight:** Postmortem weight of the body with organs determined, *not* including the fire debris or body bag.

It is very useful for the fire investigator to be present when the postmortem examination and autopsy are conducted, not only to ensure that all appropriate observations are made, but also to be on hand to answer any questions that arise during the examination. Few pathologists have extensive knowledge of fire chemistry or fire dynamics, or can interpret the effects of fire on the body, so the investigator is in a good position to advise the pathologist as to the fire conditions in the vicinity of the body.

Summary

In a fatal fire, the cause of death and the cause of the fire are independent but linked by circumstances. Each must be established, and only then can the link between them be determined.

Accidental fires can accompany deaths by accident, suicide, homicide, or even natural causes. Incendiary fires can be associated with homicide (as a direct cause of death or simply as part of the crime event) but also with accidental or natural-cause deaths. For a fire death investigation to be successful (i.e., accurate and defensible), the following guidelines must be observed.

- *Treat the scene as a crime scene.* Every fire with a death or major injury should be treated as a potential crime scene and not prejudged as accidental. The scene should be secured, preserved, documented, and searched by qualified personnel acting as a cooperative team.
- *Document all critical features.* Documentation includes accurate floor plans, with dimensions and major fuel packages included, and comprehensive photographic coverage. Photos must include pre-search survey photos, photos during search and layering, and photos of all views of the body before removal, during removal, and during postmortem examination by a medical examiner. This documentation is essential to proper forensic fire scene reconstruction.
- *Avoid moving the body.* The body must not be moved until it has been properly examined by the fire investigator and the pathologist or coroner's representative and documented by photos and diagrams. The debris under and within 0.9 m (3 ft) of the body should be carefully layered and sifted. All clothing or fragments should be preserved. Artifacts (jewelry, weapons, etc.) must be documented and collected.
- *Assess the fuels.* The fire investigator has to assess the fuels already at the scene (structure as well as furnishings), and the role fuels may or may not have played in ignition, flame spread, heat release rates, time of development, and the creation of flashover conditions.
- *Perform full forensic exams.* Every fire death deserves a full forensic postmortem examination including toxicology and X-rays. Toxicology samples should be tested for alcohol and drugs, as well as COHb and HCN, and should include both blood and tissue. The clothing should remain with the body and be documented and evaluated in situ before removal, if possible, then properly preserved. The internal (liver) body temperature should be taken as soon as possible (preferably at the scene).
- *Examine pets.* Deceased pets should be X-rayed and necropsied. Injuries to living pets should be noted and documented. Blood from deceased pets should also be tested for COHb saturation and drugs.
- *Examine living victims.* Fire victims who are survivors, whether burned or not, should be visually examined during interviews and, when possible, be photographed. Blood samples should be taken from them for analysis later if needed. External clothing (pants, shoes, shirt) should be saved and properly preserved.
- *Fully appreciate the fire environment.* Pathologists and homicide detectives must appreciate the fire environment—temperatures, heat and its transfer, flames, and smoke—and the distribution of fire products and the variables in human response to those conditions. In best practice, the medical examiner and/or pathologist visits the scene and sees the body in situ to appreciate its conditions of exposure (to flame, heat, and smoke), the nature of debris, and its location and the position.
- *Carry out forensic reconstructions.* A full reconstruction may involve criminalistics evidence such as blood spatter, blood transfers, fingerprints, tool marks, shoe prints, and trace evidence. The criminalist should be part of the scene investigation team along with the homicide detective, fire investigator, and pathologist.

As we have seen, a death involving fire is not just a simple exposure to a static set of conditions at a single moment in time. Fire is a very complex event, and a fire death investigation is even more complex and challenging. A coalition of talents and knowledge working together as a team is the only way to get the right answers to the three big questions: What killed the victim? Was the fire accidental or deliberate? And how did those two events interact?

Review Questions

1. Discuss the common problems and pitfalls associated with fatal fire investigations. Compare them with a recent ongoing case in the national media. What parallels can you find?
2. Referring to Example 12-4, determine the visibility of the same fire in an enclosed hallway measuring 3 m × 15 m (9.84 ft × 49.2 ft) with a ceiling height of 2.5 m (8.2 ft).
3. Referring to Example 12-3, calculate the fractional incapacitating dose for a male, a child, and an infant in the same scenario.
4. Review the newspaper coverage of a recent fatal fire in your community. Determine who investigated it, what the conclusions were, and whether criminal charges resulted.

References

Babrauskas, V. 1981. "Applications of Predictive Smoke Measurements." *Journal of Fire and Flammability* 12: 51–66.

Bide, R. W., S. J. Armour, and E. Yee. 1997. *Estimation of Human Toxicity from Animal Inhalation Toxicity Data: 1. Minute Volume–Body Weight Relationships Between Animals and Man*. Ralston, Alberta, Canada: Defence Research Establishment Suffield (DRES).

Bohnert, M., T. Rost, and S. Pollak. 1998. "The Degree of Destruction of Human Bodies in Relation to the Duration of the Fire." *Forensic Science International* 95 (1): 11–21, doi: 10.1016/s0379-0738(98)00076-0.

Bryan, J. L. 1983. *An Examination and Analysis of the Dynamics of the Human Behavior in the Westchase Hilton Hotel Fire, Houston, Texas, on March 6, 1982*. Quincy, MA: National Fire Protection Association.

Bryan, J. L., and D. J. Icove. 1977. Recent Advances in Computer-Assisted Arson Investigation. *Fire Journal* 71 (1): 20–23.

Bukowski, R. W. 1995. "Predicting the Fire Performance of Buildings: Establishing Appropriate Calculation Methods for Regulatory Applications." Pp. 9–18 in *Proceedings of ASIAFLAM95 International Conference on Fire Science and Engineering*, Kowloon, Hong Kong, March 15–16.

Bush, M.A., P. J. Bush, and R. G. Miller. 2006. "Detection of Classification of Composite Resins in Incinerated Teeth for Forensic Purposes." *Journal of Forensic Sciences* 51, no. 3 (May): 636–42.

Christensen, A. M. 2002. "Experiments in the Combustibility of the Human Body." *Journal of Forensic Sciences* 47 (3): 466–70.

Christensen, A. M., and D. J. Icove. 2004. "The Application of NIST's Fire Dynamics Simulator to the Investigation of Carbon Monoxide Exposure in the Deaths of Three Pittsburgh Fire Fighters." *Journal of Forensic Sciences* 49 (1): 104–7.

DeHaan, J. D. 2001. "Full-Scale Compartment Fire Tests." *CAC News* Second Quarter: 14–21.

———. 2012. "Sustained Combustion of Bodies: Some Observations." *Journal of Forensic Sciences,* doi: 10.1111/j.1556-4029.2012.02190.x.

DeHaan, J. D., S. J. Campbell, and S. Nurbakhsh. 1999. "Combustion of Animal Fat and Its Implications for the Consumption of Human Bodies in Fires." *Science & Justice* 39 (1): 27–38, doi: 10.1016/s1355-0306(99)72011-3.

DeHaan, J. D., and F. L. Fisher. 2003. "Reconstruction of a Fatal Fire in a Parked Motor Vehicle." *Fire & Arson Investigator* 53 (2): 42–46.

DeHaan, J. D., and D. J. Icove. 2012. *Kirk's Fire Investigation*. 7th ed. Upper Saddle River, NJ: Pearson-Prentice Hall.

DeHaan, J. D., and E. J. Pope. 2007. "Combustion Properties of Human and Large Animal Remains." Paper presented at Interflam, July 3–5, London, UK.

Delattre, V. F. 2000. "Burned Beyond Recognition: Systematic Approach to the Dental Identification of Charred Human Remains." *Journal of Forensic Sciences* 45, no. 3 (July): 589–96.

deRoux, S. J. 2006. "Suicidal Asphyxiation of Automobile Emission without Carbon Monoxide Poisoning." *Journal of Forensic Sciences* 51, no. 5 (September): 1158–59.

di Zinno, J., et al. 1994. "The Waco Texas Incident: The Use of DNA Analysis in the Identification of Human Remains." Paper presented at *Fifth International Symposium on Human Identification*, London, England.

Eckert, W. G., S. James, and S. Katchis. 1988. "Investigation of Cremations and Severely Burned Bodies." *American Journal of Forensic Medicine and Pathology* 9, no. 3 (1988): 188–200.

Ettling, B. V. 1968. "Consumption of an Animal Carcass in a Fire." *Fire and Arson Investigator* April–June.

Feld, J. M. 2002. "The Physiology and Biochemistry of Combustion Toxicology." Paper presented at Fire Risk and Hazard Assessment Research Applications Symposium, July 24–26, Baltimore, Md.

Flemming, D. 2004. *Explosion in Halifax Harbour: The Illustrated Account of a Disaster that Shook the World*. Nova Scotia: Formac Publishing Company.

Flynn, J. 2008. "CO Deaths." *NFPA Journal* January–February: 33–35.

Gee, D. J. 1965. "A Case of Spontaneous Combustion." *Medicine, Science and Law* 5 (January): 37–38.

Goldbaum, L. R., T. Orellano, and E. Dergal. 1976. "Mechanism of the Toxic Action of Carbon Monoxide." *Annals of Clinical and Laboratory Science* 6 (4): 372–76.

Hazucha, M. J. 2000. "Effect of Carbon Monoxide on Work and Exercise Capacity in Homes." Chapter 5, pp. 102–7 in *Carbon Monoxide Toxicity*, ed. D. G. Penney. Boca Raton, FL: CRC Press.

Health Canada. 1995. "Investigating Human Exposure to Contaminants in the Environment: A Handbook for Exposure Calculations." Ottawa, Ontario, Canada: Ministry of National Health and Welfare, H. C. Health Protection Branch.

Hickman, M. J., et al. 2007. "Medical Examiners' and Coroners' Offices, 2004." Washington, DC: US Department of Justice, Bureau of Justice Statistics, June 2007.

Jensen, G. 1998. "Wayfinding in Heavy Smoke: Decisive Factors and Safety Products; Findings Related to Full-Scale Tests." IGPAS: InterConsult Group.

Jin, T. 1976. "Visibility Through Fire Smoke: Part 5, Allowable Smoke Density for Escape from Fire." *Report No. 42*. Fire Research Institute of Japan.

Jin, T., and T. Yamada. 1985. "Irritating Effects of Fire Smoke on Visibility." *Fire Science and Technology* 5 (1): 79–90.

Kirk, N. J., et al. 2002. "Skeletal Identification Using the Frontal Sinus Region." *Journal of Forensic Science*s 47, no. 2 (March): 318–23.

Levy, A. D., and H. T. Harcke Jr. 2011. *Essentials of Forensic Imaging*. Baton Rouge, LA: CRC Press.

Mah, J. C. 2000. "Non-Fire Carbon Monoxide Deaths and Injuries Associated with the Use of Consumer Products." Bethesda, MD: CPSC.

Miller, R. E., and T. J. Tredici. 1992. "Night Vision Manual for the Flight Surgeon." *Special Report AL-SR-1992-0002*. Brooks Air Force Base, TX: Armstrong Laboratory.

Mulholland, G. W. 2008. "Smoke Production and Properties." In *SFPE Handbook of Fire Protection Engineering*, 4th ed., ed. P. J. DiNenno, pt. 2, chap. 13, 12–297. Quincy, MA: National Fire Protection Association.

Mundorff, A. Z., E. J. Bartelink, and E. Mar-Casslh. 2009. "DNA Preservation in Skeletal Elements from the World Trade Center Disaster." *Journal of Forensic Sciences* 54, no. 4 (July): 739–45.

Myers, R. A. M., S. E. Linberg, and R. A. Cowley. 1979. "Carbon Monoxide Poisoning: The Injury and Its Treatment." *Journal of the American College of Emergency Physicians* 8 (11): 479–84.

Nelson, G. L. 1998. "Carbon Monoxide and Fire Toxicity: A Review and Analysis of Recent Work." *Fire Technology* 34 (1): 39–58, doi: 10.1023/a:1015308915032.

Owsley, D. W., et al. 1995. "The Role of Forensic Anthropology in the Recovery and Analysis of Branch Davidian Compound Victims: Techniques of Analysis." *Journal of Forensic Sciences* 40, no. 3 (May): 341–48.

Penney, D. G. 2000. *Carbon Monoxide Toxicity*. Boca Raton, FL: CRC Press.

———. 2008. *Carbon Monoxide Poisoning*. Boca Raton, FL: CRC Press.

———. 2010. "Hazards from Smoke and Irritants." In *Fire Toxicity*, ed. A. A. Stec and T. R. Hull. Boca Raton, FL: CRC Press.

Peterson, J. E., and R. D. Stewart. 1975. "Predicting the Carboxyhemoglobin Levels Resulting from Carbon Monoxide Exposure." *Journal of Applied Physiology* 39: 633–38.

Pope, E. J. 2007. "The Effects of Fire on Human Remains: Characteristics of Taphonomy and Trauma." PhD diss., University of Arkansas, Fayetteville, Arkansas.

Pope, E. J., and O. C. Smith. 2003. "Features of Preexisting Trauma and Burned Cranial Bone." Presentation lecture, American Academy of Forensic Sciences (AAFS) 55th Annual Meeting, Chicago, February 17–22.

———. 2004. "Identification of Traumatic Injury in Burned Cranial Bone: An Experimental Approach." *Journal of Forensic Sciences* 49 (3): 431–40.

Pope, E. J., O. C. Smith, and T. G. Huff. 2004. "Exploding Skulls and Other Myths about How the Human Body Burns." *Fire and Arson Investigator* (April): 23–28.

Purser, D.A. 2000. "Interactions among Carbon Monoxide, Hydrogen Cyanide, Low Oxygen Hypoxia, Carbon Dioxide, and Inhaled Irritant Gases." Chap. 7 in *Carbon Monoxide Toxicity*, ed. D. G. Penney. Boca Raton, FL: CRC Press.

———. 2001. "Human Tenability. The Technical Basis for Performance-Based Fire Regulations." Paper presented at the United Engineering Foundation Conference, January 7–11, San Diego, CA.

———. 2002. "Toxicity Assessment of Combustion Products." Chap. 2–6 in *SFPE Handbook of Fire Protection Engineering*, 3rd ed. Bethesda, MD: Society of Fire Protection Engineers.

———. 2008. "Assessment of Hazards to Occupants from Smoke, Toxic Gases and Heat." In *SFPE Handbook of Fire Protection Engineering*, 4th ed., ed. P. J. DiNenno, pt. 2, chap. 6, 96–193. Quincy, MA: National Fire Protection Association.

———. 2010. "Asphyxiant Components of Fire Effluents." Pp. 118–98 in *Fire Toxicity*. Boca Raton, FL: CRC Press.

Robinson, F. G., F. A. Rueggeberg, and P. E. Lockwood. 1998. "Thermal Stability of Direct Dental Esthetic Restorative Materials at Elevated Temperatures." *Journal of Forensic Sciences* 43, no. 6 (November): 1163–67.

Routley, J. G. 1995. "Three Firefighters Die in Pittsburgh House Fire, Pittsburgh, Pennsylvania." In *Major Fires Investigation Project*. Emmitsburg, PA: US Fire Administration.

Schmidt, C. W. 2008. "The Recovery and Study of Burned Human Teeth." Pp. 55–74 in *The Analysis of Burned Human Remains*, ed. C. W. Schmidt and S. A. Symes. New York: Academic Press.

SFPE. 2008. *SFPE Handbook of Fire Protection Engineering*. 4th ed. Quincy, MA: National Fire Protection Association, Society of Fire Protection Engineers.

Smith, O.B.C., and E. J. Pope. 2003. "Burning Extremities: Patterns of Arms, Legs, and Preexisting Trauma." Paper presented at the 55th Annual Meeting of the American Academy of Forensic Sciences, Chicago, IL.

Spitz, W. U., and D. J. Spitz, eds. 2006. *Spitz and Fisher's Medicolegal Investigation of Death: Guidelines for the Application of Pathology to Crime Investigation,* 4th ed. Springfield, IL: Charles C. Thomas.

Stoll, A. M., and L. C. Greene. 1959. "Relationship Between Pain and Tissue Damage Due to Thermal Radiation." *Journal of Applied Physiology* 14 (3): 373–82.

Suchard, J. R. 2006. "Motor-Vehicle Related Toxicology." *Topics in Emergency Medicine* 28, no. 1 (2006): 76–84.

Thali, M. J., K. Yen, T. Plattner, W. Schweitzer, P. Vock, C. Ozdoba, and R. Dirnhofer. 2002. "Charred Body: Virtual Autopsy with Multi-Slice Computed Tomography and Magnetic Resonance Imaging." *Journal of Forensic Science* 47 (6): 1326–31.

USN. 1955. "Field Study of Detectability of Colored Targets at Sea." *Medical Research Laboratory Report No. 265* (vol. 14, no. 5). New London, CT: US Naval Medical Research Laboratory.

Conversion of Units

Pressure

1 atm = 101.3 kpa = 14.7 psi = 760 mmHg = 406.7 in. w.c.
1 psi = 0.068 atm = 6.89 kPa (kilopascals)
1 bar = 100 kPa = 0.987 atm = 100 kN/m^2 (kilonewtons/m^2)
1 psi = 27.67 in. w.c. = 51.7 mmHg = 70 mbar
1 mbar = 0.014 psi
1 kN/m^2 = 10 mbar = 0.14 psi

Length

1 ft = 0.3048 m
1 in. = 25.4 mm
1 m = 39.6 in.

Area

1 ft^2 = 0.092 m^2
1 m^2 = 10.87 ft^2

Volume

1 ft^3 = 0.028 m^3
1 m^3 = 35.7 ft^3
1 L = 61 in.^{3} = 0.001 m^3
1 fl oz = 30.2 cc
1 gal = 3.8 L

Mass (Weight)

1 kg = 2.2 lb
1 lb = 454.5 g
1 oz = 28.4 g

Temperature

1°F = 5/9°C
°F = (9/5°C) + 32
°C = (°F − 32)5/9
°R = (°F) + 460 (absolute temperature)
K = (°C) + 273 (absolute temperature)

Energy

1 Btu = 1055 J = 1.055 kJ = 252 cal

Energy Flow Rate

1 W = 1 J/s = 3.412 Btu/hr
1 kW = 1,000 J/s = 3,412 Btu/hr = 0.95 Btu/s

Mathematics Refresher

When a number (or value) is followed by a superscript number or fraction, such as X^n, it means that the number (X) is raised to a power (n). If the power is 2, the number is squared (multiplied by itself) ($3^2 = 3 \times 3 = 9$). If the power is 3, the number is cubed (multiplied by itself and then by itself again) ($3^3 = 3 \times 3 \times 3 = 27$).

The number n can be a fraction, such as $\frac{1}{2}$.

$$X^{1/2} \quad \text{or} \quad X^{0.5} = \sqrt{X} \qquad \text{(the square root of } X\text{).} \qquad \text{(A.1)}$$

The number n can be any value: $n = 2/5$, $5/2$, and $3/2$ are common calculations in fire dynamics. Such values must be calculated using a "scientific notation" pocket calculator with a y^x or y^n function (where $y = X$, and x [or n] is the power to which y is raised). If n is a negative number, then X^{-n} denotes $1/X^n$ (X^n is put in the denominator of a fraction).

The following are general examples of mathematical equations using powers:

$$Q^x Q^y = Q^{x+y} \qquad \text{(A.2)}$$

$$\frac{Q^x}{Q^y} = Q^{x-y} \qquad \text{(A.3)}$$

$$(Q^x)^y = Q^{xy} \qquad \text{(A.4)}$$

Logarithms

Logarithms are numerical equivalents calculated by raising 10 to a power, where $\log_{10}$ = the value to which the number 10 must be raised to be equal to the original number.
Thus,

$$\log_{10} \text{ of } 100 = 2, \qquad \text{(A.5)}$$

because

$$10^2 = 100. \qquad \text{(A.6)}$$

Also,

$$\log_{10} \text{ of } 10 = 1, \qquad \text{(A.7)}$$

because

$$10^1 = 10. \qquad \text{(A.8)}$$

This value can be found using a pocket calculator or mathematical tables. For instance,

$$\log_{10} 3.5 = 0.54, \qquad \text{(A.9)}$$

and

$$\log_{10} 2330 = 3.3673. \tag{A.10}$$

The inverse function is sometimes called the *antilog*:

$$\text{antilog}_{10}(2) = 10^2 = 100. \tag{A.11}$$

When the base unit e is used ($e = 2.71$), the value is called the *natural log* (ln). For example,

$$\log_e 5 = \ln 5 = 1.6094, \tag{A.12}$$

and

$$\ln 10 = 2.3025. \tag{A.13}$$

The antilog e^x is the value calculated by raising e to that power:

$$e^5 = 148.413, \tag{A.14}$$

and

$$e^{10} = 22{,}026.5. \tag{A.15}$$

A modified "power of 10" notation is used as shorthand for very large or very small numbers. For example,

$$3.40\text{E} - 05 = 3.4 \times 10^{-5} = 0.000034,$$
$$2.88\text{E} + 00 = 2.88 \times 10^0 = 2.88,$$
$$5.00\text{E} + 02 = 5.0 \times 10^2 = 500.$$

Dimensional Analysis

A useful concept for checking calculations is called *dimensional analysis*. If one keeps track of the units used for variables and constants and applies the rules of canceling units when they appear in both the numerator and the denominator of a function, for instance, one can verify that the correct relationship was used.

For example

$$\dot{Q} = \dot{m}'' A \Delta H_c, \tag{A.16}$$

where

$\dot{m}'' = $ mass flux $[\text{kg}/(\text{m}^2 \cdot \text{s})]$,
$A = $ area of burning surface (m^2), and
$\Delta H_c = $ heat of combustion (kJ/Kg).

Multiplication gives

$$\left(\frac{\text{kg}}{\text{m}^2 \cdot \text{s}}\right)(\text{m}^2)\left(\frac{\text{kJ}}{\text{kg}}\right) = \frac{\text{kJ}}{\text{s}} = \text{kW}, \tag{A.17}$$

which is the correct unit for $\dot{Q}$.

For conduction calculations,

$$\dot{Q} = k\frac{T_2 - T_1}{l}A, \tag{A.18}$$

where

$$k = \frac{\text{W}}{\text{m} \cdot \text{K}},$$
$l = $ lengh (m),
$T_2 - T_1 = \Delta T(\text{K})$, and
$A = $ area (m^2).

Carrying out the calculation, we obtain

$$\dot{Q} = \frac{\left(\dfrac{\text{W}}{\text{m} \cdot \text{K}}\right)(\text{K})\left(\text{m}^2\right)}{\text{m}} = \text{W}, \qquad (A.19)$$

which is the correct unit for $\dot{Q}$.

Selected Material Properties

TABLE 1	Flammability (Explosive) Limits and Ignition Temperatures of Common Gases

Fuel	EXPLOSIVE LIMITS (IN AIR)		IGNITION TEMPERATURE (MINIMUM)		MINIMUM IGNITION ENERGY
	Lower	Upper	°C	°F	mJ
Natural gas	4.5	15	482–632	900–1,170	0.25
Propane (commercial)	2.15	9.6	493–604	920–1,120	0.25
Butane (commercial)	1.9	8.5	482–538	900–1,000	0.25
Acetylene	2.5	81[a]	305	581	0.02
Hydrogen	4	75	500	932	0.01
Ammonia (NH_3)	16	25	651	1,204	—
Carbon monoxide	12.5	74	609	1,128	—
Ethylene	2.7	36	490	914	0.07
Ethylene oxide	3	100	429	8041	0.06

Sources: NFPA. 2003. *Fire Protection Handbook.* 19th ed. Quincy, MA: National Fire Protection Association, Table 8-9.2; and SFPE. 2008. *SFPE Handbook of Fire Protection Engineering.* 4th ed. Quincy, MA: Society of Fire Protection Engineers and the National Fire Protection Association, Table 3-18.1.
[a]Higher concentrations (up to 100) may detonate.

Also Table 2-3 in Chapter 2

	TABLE 2	Flash Points and Flame (Fire) Points of Some Ignitable Liquids					

	FLASH POINT (CLOSED CUP)[*]		FLASH POINT (OPEN CUP)		FIRE POINT	
FUEL	**°C**	**°F**	**°C**	**°F**	**°C**	**°F**
Gasoline (auto, low octane)	−43	−45	—	—	—	—
Gasoline (100 octane)	−38	−38				
Petroleum naphtha[a]	−29	−20				
JP-4 (jet aviation fuel)	−23 to −1	−10 to −30				
Acetone	−20	−4				
Petroleum ether	<−18	<0				
Benzene	−11	−12				
Toluene	4	40				
Methanol	11	52	1(13.5)[†]	34(56)	1(13.5)	34(56)
Ethanol	12	54				
n-Octane	13	56				
Turpentine (gum)	35	95				
Fuel oil (kerosene)	38[b]	100				
Mineral spirits	40	104				
n-Decane	46	115	52[†]	125	61.5[†]	143
Fuel oil #2 (diesel)	52 (min.)	126				
Fuel oil (unspecified)	—	—	133[a]	271	164[a]	327
Jet A	43–66	110–150				
p-Xylene	25[§]	77[§]	29[§]	84[§]	—	—
JP-5 (Jet aviation fuel)	66	151				

Sources: [*]NFPA. 2001. *Fire Protection Guide to Hazardous Materials.* Quincy, MA: National Fire Protection Association, except as noted.
[†]Calculated minimum limit for open-cup tests with flame igniter. Higher values in parentheses are for spark source ignition. *Source:* Glassman, I., and Dryer, F. L. 1980–1981. "Flame Spreading across Liquid Fuels." *Fire Safety Journal* 3: 123–38.
[‡]SFPE. 2008. *SFPE Handbook of Fire Protection Engineering.* 4th ed. Quincy, MA: NFPA, Table 2-8.5.
[§]www.ScienceLab.com, MSDS *p*-xylene, 2008.
[a]Generic name for miscellaneous light petroleum fractions used in such consumer products as cigarette lighter fuels and fuels for camping stoves and lanterns.
[b]The flash point of kerosene is set by law in many jurisdictions and may be higher in compliance with local laws.

Also Table 2-4 in Chapter 2

TABLE 3	Minimum Autoignition Temperatures, Flammable Ranges, and Specific Gravities of Some Common Ignitable Liquids				
FUEL	**IGNITION TEMPERATURE (°C)**	**(°F)**	**MINIMUM IGNITION ENERGY (MJ)**	**FLAMMABLE RANGE (% IN AIR @ 20°C)**	**SPECIFIC GRAVITY**
Acetone	465	869	1.15	2.6–12.8	0.8
Benzene	498	928	0.2	1.4–7.1	0.9
Diethyl ether	160	320	—	1.9–36.0	0.7
Ethanol (100 percent)	363	685	—	—	0.8
Ethylene glycol	398	748	—	—	1.1
Fuel oil #1 (kerosene)	210	410	—	—	
Fuel oil #2	257	495	—	—	
Gasoline (low octane)	280	536	—	1.4–7.6	0.8
Gasoline (100 octane)	456	853	—	1.5–7.6	0.8
Jet fuel (JP-6)	230	446	—	—	
Linseed oil (boiled)	206	403	—	—	
Methanol	464	867	0.14	6.7–36.0	0.8
n-Pentane	260	500	0.22	1.5–7.8	0.6
n-Hexane	225	437	0.24	1.2–7.5	0.7
n-Heptane	204	399	0.24	—	0.7
n-Octane	206	403	—	1.0–7.0	0.7
n-Decane	210	410	—	—	0.7
Petroleum ether	288	550	—	1.1–5.9	0.6
Pinene (alpha)	255	491	—	—	
Turpentine (spirits)	253	488	—	—	<1

Sources: Data taken from NFPA. 2001. *Fire Protection Guide to Hazardous Materials.* Quincy, MA: National Fire Protection Association; Turner, C. F., and J. W. McCreery. 1981. *The Chemistry of Fire and Hazardous Materials.* Boston: Allyn and Bacon.

Also Table 2-5 in Chapter 2

	THERMAL CONDUCTIVITY k [W/(m · K)]	DENSITY ρ (kg/m^3)	SPECIFIC HEAT c_p [J/(kg · K)]	THERMAL INERTIA $k\rho c_p$ [W^2 · s/(m^4 · K^2)]
TABLE 4	\multicolumn{4}{l}{**Thermal Characteristics of Common Materials Found at Fire Scenes**}
MATERIAL				
Copper	387	8940	380	1.30×10^9
Steel	45.8	7850	460	1.65×10^8
Brick	0.69	1600	840	9.27×10^5
Concrete	0.8–1.4	1900–2300	880	2×10^6
Glass	0.76	2700	840	1.72×10^6
Gypsum plaster	0.48	1440	840	5.81×10^5
PPMA	0.19	1190	1420	3.21×10^5
Oak	0.17	800	2380	3.24×10^5
Yellow pine	0.14	640	2850	2.55×10^5
Asbestos	0.15	577	1050	9.09×10^4
Fiberboard	0.041	229	2090	1.96×10^4
Polyurethane foam	0.034	20	1400	9.52×10^2
Air	0.026	1.1	1040	2.97×10^1

Sources: Data derived from Drysdale 2011, 37.

Also Table 2-11 in Chapter 2

TABLE 5 — Heat Release Rates and Burn Times of Common Ignition Sources

	TYPICAL OUTPUT (kW)	TYPICAL BURN TIME (s)[a]	MAXIMUM FLAME HEIGHT FLAME (mm)	MAXIMUM HEAT FLUX (kW/m^2)
Cigarette 1.1 g (not puffed, laid on solid surface) bone dry	0.005	1,200	—	42
Cigarette 1.1 g (not puffed, laid on solid surface) conditioned to 50% R.H.	0.005	1,200	—	35
Methenamine pill, 0.15 g	0.045	90		4
Candle (21 mm, wax)*	0.075	—	42	70[b]
Wood cribs, BS 5852 Part 2				
No. 4 crib, 8.5 g	1	190		15[c]
No. 5 crib, 17 g	1.9	200		17[c]
No. 6 crib, 60 g	2.6	190		20[c]
No. 7 crib, 126 g	6.4	350		25[c]
(Crumpled) brown lunch bag, 6 g	1.2	80		
(Crumpled) wax paper, 4.5 g (tight)	1.8	25		
Newspaper—folded double sheet, 22 g (bottom ignition)	4	100		
(Crumpled) wax paper, 4.5 g (loose)	5.3	20		
Newspaper—crumpled double sheet, 22 g (top ignition)	7.4	40		
Newspaper double sheet newspaper, 22 g (bottom ignition)	17	20		
Polyethylene wastebasket, 285 g, filled with 12 milk cartons (390 g)	50	200[d]	550	35[e]
Plastic trash bags, filled with cellulosic trash (1.2–14 kg)[f]	120–350	200[d]		
Small upholstered chair	150–250	—	—	—
Upholstered (modern foam) easy chair	350–750	—	—	—
Recliner (PU foam, synthetic upholstery)	500–1000	—	—	—
Gasoline pool on concrete (2 L) (1/m^2 area)	1000	30–60	—	—
Sofa	1000–3000	—	—	—

Sources: V. Babrauskas and J. Krasny, *Fire Behavior of Upholstered Furniture*, NBS Monograph 173 (Gaithersburg, MD: US Department of Commerce, National Bureau of Standards, 1985).

*From S. E. Dillon and A. Hamins, "Ignition Propensity and Heat Flux Profiles of Candle Flames for Fire Investigation" in *Proceedings: Fire and Materials 2003* (London: Interscience Communications), 363–76.

[a]Time duration of significant flaming.

[b]Centerline—immediately above flame; <4 kW/m^2 outside.

[c]Measured from 25 mm away.

[d]Total burn time in excess of 1800 s.

[e]As measured on simulation burner.

[f]Results vary greatly with packing density.

Also Table 4-1 in Chapter 4

GLOSSARY

A

abductive reasoning The process of reasoning to the best explanations for a phenomenon.

absolute temperature A temperature measured in Kelvins (K) or Rankines (R) (*NFPA 921,* 2017 ed., pt. 3.3.1).

accelerant A fuel or oxidizer, often an ignitable liquid, intentionally used to initiate a fire or increase the rate of growth or spread of fire (*NFPA 921,* 2017 ed., pt. 3.3.2).

accident An unplanned event that interrupts an activity and sometimes causes injury or damage or a chance occurrence arising from unknown causes; an unexpected happening due to carelessness, ignorance, and the like (*NFPA 921,* 2017 ed., pt. 3.3.3).

accidental fire cause classification Accidental fires involve all those for which the proven cause does not involve an intentional human act to ignite or spread fire into an area where the fire should not be (*NFPA 921,* 2017 ed., pt. 20.1.1).

adiabatic The ideal conditions of equilibrium of temperature and pressure. The actual flame temperature of wood has been measured and reported as being some 500°C less (estimated to be 1040°C, or 1900°F) (Lightsey and Henderson 1985).

adiabatic heating The heating of a gas caused by its compression (*NFPA 99,* 2015 ed.).

adsorption Trapping of gaseous materials on the surface of a solid substrate.

aliphatic Relating to, or being an organic compound (such as an alkane) having an open-chain structure. Source: Merriam-Webster dictionary. https://www.merriam-webster.com/dictionary/aromatic. Last retrieved April 26, 2017

alligatoring Rectangular patterns of char formed on burned wood.

ambient Someone's or something's surroundings, especially as they pertain to the local environment; for example, ambient air and ambient temperature (*NFPA 921,* 2017 ed., pt. 3.3.5).

ambient temperature The temperature of the surrounding medium; usually used to refer to the temperature of the air in which a structure is situated or a device operates (*NFPA 414,* 2017 ed.).

ampacity The maximum current, in amperes, that a conductor can carry continuously under the conditions of use without exceeding its temperature rating (*NFPA 921,* 2017 ed., pt. 3.3.6; *see also NFPA 70,* 2014 ed., Article 100).

ampere The unit of electric current that is equivalent to a flow of one coulomb per second; one coulomb is defined as 6.24×10^{18} electrons (*NFPA 921,* 2017 ed., pt. 3.3.7).

annealing Loss of temper in metal caused by heating.

anoxia Condition relating to an absence of oxygen.

appliance Utilization equipment, generally other than industrial, that is normally built in standardized sizes or types and is installed or connected as a unit to perform one or more functions such as clothes washing, air-conditioning, food mixing, deep frying, and so forth (*NFPA 70,* 2014 ed., Article 100).

arc A high-temperature luminous electric discharge across a gap or through a medium such as charred insulation (*NFPA 921,* 2017 ed., pt. 3.3.8).

arc-fault circuit interrupter (AFCI) A device intended to provide protection from the effects of arc faults by recognizing characteristics unique to arcing and by functioning to de-energize the circuit when an arc fault is detected (*NFPA 70,* 2014 ed., Article 100).

arc-fault mapping The systematic evaluation of the electrical circuit configuration, spatial relationship of the circuit components, and identification of electrical arc sites to assist in the identification of the area of origin and analysis of the fire's spread (*NFPA 921,* 2017 ed., pt. 3.3.9).

arc site The location on a conductor with localized damage that resulted from an electrical arc (*NFPA 921,* 2017 ed., pt. 3.3.10).

arcing through char Arcing associated with a matrix of charred material (e.g., charred conductor insulation) that acts as a semi-conductive medium (*NFPA 921,* 2017 ed., pt. 3.3.11).

arc tracking A deflagration resulting from the sudden introduction of air into a confined space containing oxygen-deficient products of incomplete combustion (*NFPA 921,* 2017 ed., pt. 3.3.16).

area of origin A structure, part of a structure, or general geographic location within a fire scene, in which the "point of origin" of a fire or explosion is reasonably believed to be located (*NFPA 921,* 2017 ed., pt. 3.3.12; *see also* Point of Origin, pt. 3.3.142)

area of transition Mixture of fire directional indicators in a wildlands fire.

aromatic An organic compound characterized by increased chemical stability resulting from the delocalization of electrons in a ring system (such as benzene) containing usually multiple conjugated double bonds. Source: Merriam-Webster dictionary. https://www.merriam-webster.com/dictionary/aromatic. Last retrieved April 26, 2017

arrow pattern A fire pattern displayed on the cross-section of a burned wooden structural member (*NFPA 921,* 2017 ed., pt. 3.3.13).

arson The crime of maliciously and intentionally, or recklessly, starting a fire or causing an explosion (*NFPA 921,* 2017 ed., pt. 3.3.14).

arson Any willful or malicious burning or attempting to burn, with or without intent to defraud, a dwelling house, public building, motor vehicle or aircraft, or personal property of another (FBI 2010).

atom The smallest particle of an element that can exist either alone or in combination such as an atom of hydrogen.

autoignition Initiation of combustion by heat but without a spark or flame (*NFPA 921,* 2017 ed., pt. 3.3.15).

autoignition temperature The lowest temperature at which a combustible material ignites in air without a spark or flame (*NFPA 921,* 2017 ed., pt. 3.3.16).

B

backdraft A deflagration resulting from the sudden introduction of air into a confined space containing oxygen-deficient products of incomplete combustion (*NFPA 921,* 2017 ed., pt. 3.3.17).

backing Slow extension of a fire down-slope or into wind in the opposite direction of its main spread.

bead A rounded globule of re-solidified metal at the end of the remains of an electrical conductor that was caused by arcing and is characterized by a sharp line of demarcation between the melted and unmelted conductor surfaces (*NFPA 921,* 2017 ed., pt. 3.3.18).

blast pressure front The expanding leading edge of an explosion reaction that separates a major difference in pressure between normal ambient pressure ahead of the front and potentially damaging high pressure at and behind the front (*NFPA 921,* 2017 ed., pt. 3.3.19).

BLEVE Boiling liquid expanding vapor explosion (*NFPA 921,* 2017 ed., pt. 3.3.20).

boiling point The temperature at which the vapor pressure of a liquid equals the surrounding atmospheric pressure. For purposes of defining the boiling point, atmospheric pressure shall be considered to be 14.7 psia (760 mm Hg or 101.4 kPa). For mixtures that do not have a constant boiling point, the 20 percent evaporated point of a distillation performed in accordance with ASTM D86, Standard Test Method for Distillation of Petroleum Products at Atmospheric Pressure, shall be considered to be the boiling point (*NFPA 35,* 2016 ed.).

bonding The permanent joining of metallic parts to form an electrically conductive path that ensures electrical continuity and the capacity to conduct safely any current likely to be imposed (*NFPA 921,* 2017 ed., pt. 3.3.21).

branch circuit The circuit conductors between the final overcurrent device protecting the circuit and the outlet(s) (*NFPA 70,* 2014 ed., Article 100).

brisance The shattering effect or power of an explosion or explosive.

British thermal unit (Btu) The quantity of heat required to raise the temperature of one pound of water 1°F at the pressure of 1 atmosphere and temperature of 60°F; a British thermal unit is equal to 1055 joules, 1.055 kilojoules, and 252.15 calories (*NFPA 921,* 2017 ed., pt. 3.3.22).

C

calcination of gypsum A fire effect realized in gypsum products, including wallboard, as a result of exposure to heat that drives off free and chemically bound water (*NFPA 921,* 2017 ed., pt. 3.3.24).

calorie The amount of heat necessary to raise 1 gram of water 1°C at the pressure of 1 atmosphere and temperature of 15°C; a calorie is 4.184 joules, and there are 252.15 calories in a British thermal unit (Btu) (*NFPA 921,* 2017 ed., pt. 3.3.25).

calorimetry A test used to measure the total heat of combustion of fuels (as in *ASTM D4809-13*).

cause The circumstances, conditions, or agencies that brought about or resulted in the fire or explosion incident, damage to property resulting from the fire or explosion incident, or bodily injury or loss of life resulting from the fire or explosion incident (*NFPA 921,* 2017 ed., pt. 3.3.26).

cause of death The injury or disease that triggers the sequence of events leading to death.

ceiling jet A relatively thin layer of flowing hot gases that develops under a horizontal surface (e.g., ceiling) as a result of plume impingement and the flowing gas being forced to move horizontally (*NFPA 921,* 2017 ed., pt. 3.3.27).

ceiling layer A buoyant layer of hot gases and smoke produced by a fire in a compartment (*NFPA 921,* 2017 ed., pt. 3.3.28).

cellulosic Plant-based materials based on a natural polymer of sugars.

chain of evidence (chain of custody) The chronological documentation or paper trail, showing the seizure, custody, control, transfer, analysis, and disposition of physical or electronic evidence.

char Carbonaceous material that has been burned or pyrolyzed and has a blackened appearance (*NFPA 921,* 2017 ed., pt. 3.3.29).

char depth The measurement of pyrolytic or combustion damage to a wood surface compared with its original surface height.

chromatography Chemical procedure that allows the separation of compounds based on differences in their chemical affinities for two materials in different physical states (e.g., gas/liquid, liquid/solid).

circuit breaker A device designed to open and close a circuit by nonautomatic means and to open the circuit automatically on a predetermined overcurrent without damage to itself when properly applied within its rating (*NFPA 70*, 2014 ed., Article 100).

clean burn   A distinct and visible fire effect generally apparent on noncombustible surfaces after combustible layer(s) (such as soot, paint, and paper) have been burned away. The effect may also appear where soot has failed to be deposited because of high surface temperatures (*NFPA 921*, 2017 ed., pt. 3.3.31).

combustible   Capable of undergoing combustion (*NFPA 921*, 2017 ed., pt. 3.3.32).

combustible liquid   Any liquid that has a closed-cup flash point at or above 37.8°C (100°F) (*NFPA 921*, 2017 ed., pt. 3.3.34; *see also* pt. 3.3.85, Flammable Liquid).

combustion   A chemical process of oxidation that occurs at a rate fast enough to produce heat and usually light in the form of either a glow or flame (*NFPA 921*, 2017 ed., pt. 3.3.35).

combustion efficiency   The ratio of a substance's effective heat of combustion to the complete heat of combustion

combustion products   The heat, gases, volatilized liquids and solids, particulate matter, and ash generated by combustion (*NFPA 921*, 2017 ed., pt. 3.3.36).

competent ignition source   An ignition source that has sufficient energy and is capable of transferring that energy to the fuel long enough to raise the fuel to its ignition temperature (*NFPA 921*, 2017 ed., pt. 3.3.37; *see also* pt. 19.4.2).

conduction   Heat transfer to another body or within a body by direct contact (*NFPA 921*, 2017 ed., pt. 3.3.38).

conductor   A material or object that allows an electric charge to flow easily through it. (1) bare—a conductor having no covering or electrical insulation whatsoever; (2) insulated—a conductor encased within material of composition and thickness that is recognized by this Code as electrical insulation; (3) covered—a conductor encased within material of composition or thickness that is not recognized by this Code as electrical insulation (*NFPA 70*, 2014 ed., Article 100).

consumer fireworks   Small fireworks devices containing restricted amounts of pyrotechnic composition, designed primarily to produce visible or audible effects by combustion, that comply with the construction, chemical composition, and labelling regulations of the US Consumer Product Safety Commission (CPSC), as set forth in *CPSC 16 CFR 1500* and *1507*, *49 CFR 172*, and *APA Standard 87-1, Standard for the Construction and Approval for Transportation of Fireworks, Novelties, and Theatrical Pyrotechnics* (*NFPA 1123*, 2014 ed.).

convection   Heat transfer by circulation within a medium such as a gas or a liquid (*NFPA 921*, 2017 ed., pt. 3.3.39).

corpus delicti   Literally, the body of the crime. The fundamental facts necessary to prove the commission of a crime.

craze   The appearance of fine cracks in the surface of a helmet shell or other smooth surface of an ensemble element.

crazing   Stress cracks in glass as the result of rapid cooling.

creep   The tendency of a material to move or deform permanently to relieve stresses (*NFPA 921*, 2017 ed., pt. 3.3.40).

crime concealment (motive)   This category involves fire setting that is a secondary or a collateral criminal activity, perpetrated for the purpose of concealing the primary criminal activity. In some cases, however, the fire may actually be part of the intended crime, such as revenge. Many people erroneously believe that a fire will destroy all physical evidence at the crime scene. Categories for crime concealment firesetting include murder or burglary concealment and destruction of records or documents (*NFPA 921*, 2017 ed., pt. 24.4.9.3.5).

crowning   Rapid extension of fire through the porous array of leaves, needles, and fine fuels above 2 m.

current   A flow of electric charge (*NFPA 921*, 2017 ed., pt. 3.3.41).

D

data   Facts or information to be used as a basis for a discussion or decision (*ASTM E1138-89*, 1989 ed.).

deductive reasoning   The process by which conclusions are drawn by logical inference from given premises (*NFPA 921*, 2017 ed., pt. 3.3.44).

deflagration   Propagation of a combustion zone at a velocity that is less than the speed of sound in the unreacted medium (*NFPA 921*, 2017 ed., pt. 3.3.43; *see also NFPA 68*, 2013 ed.).

density   The mass of a substance per unit volume, usually specified at standard temperature and pressure. The density of water is approximately one gram per cubic centimeter. The density of air is approximately 1.275 grams per cubic meter (*NFPA 921*, 2017 ed., pt. 3.3.44).

detection   (1) Sensing the existence of a fire, especially by a detector from one or more products of the fire, such as smoke, heat, infrared radiation, and the like. (2) The act or process of discovering and locating a fire (*NFPA 921*, 2017 ed., pt. 3.3.45).

detonation   Propagation of a combustion zone at a velocity greater than the speed of sound in the unreacted medium (*NFPA 921*, 2017 ed., pt. 3.3.46; *see also NFPA 68*, 2013 ed.).

diatomic   Molecules made up of two atoms.

diffuse fuel   A gas, vapor, dust, particulate, aerosol, mist, fog, or hybrid mixture of these, suspended in the atmosphere, which is capable of being ignited and propagating a flame front (*NFPA 921*, 2017 ed., pt. 3.3.47).

diffusion flame   A flame in which fuel and air mix or diffuse together at the region of combustion (*NFPA 921,* 2017 ed., pt. 3.3.48).

drop down   The spread of fire by the dropping or falling of burning materials. Synonymous with "fall down" (*NFPA 921,* 2017 ed., pt. 3.3.49).

due process   The compliance with the criminal and civil laws and procedures within the jurisdiction where the incident occurred (*NFPA 1033,* 2014 ed., pt. 3.3.1).

duty, continuous   Operation at a substantially constant load for an indefinitely long time. (*NFPA 70,* 2014 ed., Article 100).

E

elastomers   Fibers or materials having elastic properties.

electric spark   A small, incandescent particle created by some arcs (*NFPA 921,* 2017 ed., pt. 3.3.51).

entrainment   The process of air or gases being drawn into a fire, plume, or jet (*NFPA 921,* 2017 ed., pt. 3.3.54).

excitement (motive)   The excitement-motivated fire setter may enjoy the excitement that is provided by actual firesetting or the activities surrounding the fire suppression efforts, or may have a psychological need for attention. The excitement-motivated offender is often a serial firesetter. This firesetter will generally remain at the scene during the fire and will often get in position to respond to, or view the fire and the surrounding activities. The excitement-motivated fire setter's targets range from small trash and grass fires to occupied buildings (*NFPA 921,* 2017 ed., pt. 24.4.9.3.3).

eutectic melting   Eutectic melting (alloying) involves damage that occurs when a metal of different composition contacts the subject metal. The original melting may or may not be electrically related, but the damage to the subject metal caused by deposition of the second does not involve an electrical current and is not a form of electrical damage (*NFPA 921,* 2017 ed., pt. 9.11.3).

exothermic   A reaction or process accompanied by the release of heat.

explosion   The sudden conversion of potential energy (chemical or mechanical) into kinetic energy with the production and release of gases under pressure, or the release of gas under pressure. These high-pressure gases then do mechanical work such as moving, changing, or shattering nearby materials (*NFPA 921,* 2017 ed., pt. 3.3.56).

explosive   Any chemical compound, mixture, or device that functions by explosion (*NFPA 921,* 2017 ed., pt. 3.3.58).

explosive material   Any material that can act as fuel for an explosion (*NFPA 921,* 2017 ed., pt. 3.3.59).

extremism (motive)   Extremist-motivated firesetting is committed to further a social, political, or religious cause. Fires have been used as a weapon of social protest since revolutions first began. Extremist fire setters may work in groups or as individuals. Also, due to planning aspects and the selection of their targets, extremist firesetters generally have a great degree of organization, as reflected in their use of more elaborate ignition or incendiary devices. Subcategories of extremist firesetting are terrorism and riot/civil disturbance (*NFPA 921,* 2017 ed., pt. 24.4.9.3.7).

F

field model   A computer fire model that uses *computational fluid dynamics* (CFD) to estimate the fire environment by dividing the compartment into uniform small cells, or control volumes. The computer program then attempts to predict conditions in every volume such as, for example, pressure, temperature, carbon monoxide, oxygen, and soot production.

fire   A rapid oxidation process, which is a chemical reaction resulting in the evolution of light and heat in varying intensities (*NFPA 921,* 2017 ed., pt. 3.3.66).

fire analysis   The process of determining the origin, cause, development, responsibility, and, when required, a failure analysis of a fire or explosion (*NFPA 921,* 2017 ed., pt. 3.3.67).

fire cause   The circumstances, conditions, or agencies that bring together a fuel, ignition source, and oxidizer (such as air or oxygen) resulting in a fire or a combustion explosion (*NFPA 921,* 2017 ed., pt. 3.3.69).

fire dynamics   The detailed study of how chemistry, fire science, and the engineering disciplines of fluid mechanics and heat transfer interact to influence fire behavior (*NFPA 921,* 2017 ed., pt. 3.3.70).

fire effects   The observable or measurable changes in or on a material as a result of a fire (*NFPA 921,* 2017 ed., pt. 3.3.71).

fire hazard   Any situation, process, material, or condition that can cause a fire or explosion or that can provide a ready fuel supply to augment the spread or intensity of a fire or explosion, all of which pose a threat to life or property (*NFPA 921,* 2017 ed., pt. 3.3.72).

fire investigation   The process of determining the origin, cause, and development of a fire or explosion (*NFPA 921,* 2017 ed., pt. 3.3.73).

fire investigator   An individual who has demonstrated the skills and knowledge necessary to conduct, coordinate, and complete a fire investigation (*NFPA 1033,* 2014 ed., pt. 3.3.7).

fire model   A method using mathematical or computer calculations that describes a system or process related to fire development, including fire dynamics, fire spread, occupant exposure, and the effects of fire. The results produced by fire models can be compared with physical and eyewitness evidence to test working hypotheses.

fire patterns   The visible or measurable physical changes, or identifiable shapes, formed by a fire effect or group of fire effects (*NFPA 921,* 2017 ed., pt. 3.3.74).

fire point The lowest temperature at which a liquid ignites and achieves sustained burning when exposed to a test flame.

fire scene reconstruction The process of recreating the physical scene during fire scene analysis investigation or through the removal of debris and the placement of contents or structural elements in their pre-fire positions (*NFPA 921*, 2017 ed., pt. 3.3.76).

fire signature A fire development curve of time versus heat release rate typically having four phases of incipient ignition, growth, fully developed, and decay.

fire spread The movement of fire from one place to another (*NFPA 921*, 2017 ed., pt. 3.3.78).

fire testing A tool that can provide data that complement data collected at the fire scene (see pt. 4.3.3), or can be used to test hypotheses (see pt. 4.3.6). Such fire testing can range in scope from bench scale testing to full-scale recreations of the entire event (*NFPA 921*, 2017 ed.).

fire tetrahedron A geometric representation of the four factors necessary for fire: fuel, heat, an oxidizing agent, and an uninhibited chemical chain reaction.

flame A body or stream of gaseous material involved in the combustion process and emitting radiant energy at specific wavelength bands determined by the combustion chemistry of the fuel. In most cases, some portion of the emitted radiant energy is visible to the human eye (*NFPA 921*, 2017 ed., pt. 3.3.80; *see also NFPA 72*, 2016 ed.).

flame front The flaming leading edge of a propagating combustion reaction zone (*NFPA 921*, 2017 ed., pt. 3.3.81).

flame resistant Materials that are inherently nonflammable. These materials have flame resistance built into their chemical structures.

flame retardant Materials that are chemically treated to be slow burning or self-extinguishing when exposed to an open flame.

flameover The condition where unburned fuel (pyrolysate) from the originating fire has accumulated in the ceiling layer to a sufficient concentration (i.e., at or above the lower flammable limit) that it ignites and burns; can occur without ignition of, or prior to, the ignition of other fuels separate from the origin (*NFPA 921*, 2017 ed., pt. 3.3.82).

flaming combustion Combustion of the gaseous vapors produced from pyrolysis.

flammable Capable of burning with a flame (*NFPA 921*, 2017 ed., pt. 3.3.83).

flammable limit The upper or lower concentration limit at a specified temperature and pressure of a flammable gas or a vapor of an ignitable liquid and air, expressed as a percentage of fuel by volume that can be ignited (*NFPA 921*, 2017 ed., pt. 3.3.84).

flammable liquid A liquid that has a closed-cup flash point that is below 37.8°C (100°F) and a maximum vapor pressure of 2068 mm Hg (40 psia) at 37.8°C (100°F) (*NFPA 921*, 2017 ed., pt. 3.3.85; *see also* pt. 3.3.343, Combustible Liquid).

flammable range The range of concentrations between the lower and upper flammable limits (*NFPA 921*, 2017 ed., pt. 3.3.86; *see also NFPA 68*, 2013 ed.).

flanking Lateral spread of fire in a direction at right angles to the main direction of fire growth.

flash fire A fire that spreads by means of a flame front rapidly through a diffuse fuel, such as dust, gas, or the vapors of an ignitable liquid, without the production of damaging pressure (*NFPA 921*, 2017 ed., pt. 3.3.87).

flash point The lowest temperature of a liquid, as determined by specific laboratory tests, at which the liquid gives off vapors at a sufficient rate to support a momentary flame across its surface (*NFPA 921*, 2017 ed., pt. 3.3.88).

flashover A transition phase in the development of a compartment fire in which surfaces exposed to thermal radiation reach ignition temperature more or less simultaneously and fire spreads rapidly throughout the space, resulting in full room involvement or total involvement of the compartment or enclosed space (*NFPA 921*, 2017 ed., pt. 3.3.89).

forensic (forensic science) The application of science to answer questions of interest to the legal system (*NFPA 921*, 2017 ed., pt. 3.3.90).

fractional effective concentration A measurement that assesses the impact of toxic smoke and by-products of combustion on a subject. The FEC depends on the concentration of particular toxins within the fire gases, and the duration of exposure.

fragmentation The process by which the casing of an artillery shell, bomb, grenade, etc., is shattered by the detonation of the *explosive* filler.

fuel A material that will maintain combustion under specified environmental conditions (*NFPA 921*, 2017 ed., pt. 3.3.91; *see also NFPA 53*, 2016 ed.).

fuel gas Natural gas, manufactured gas, LP gas, and similar gases commonly used for commercial or residential purposes such as heating, cooling, or cooking (*NFPA 921*, 2017 ed., pt. 3.3.92).

fuel load The total quantity of combustible contents of a building, space, or fire area, including interior finish and trim, expressed in heat units or the equivalent weight in wood (*NFPA 921*, 2017 ed., pt. 3.3.93).

fuel-controlled fire A fire in which the heat release rate and growth rate are controlled by the characteristics of the fuel, such as quantity and geometry, and in which adequate air for combustion is available (*NFPA 921*, 2017 ed., pt. 3.3.94).

full room involvement Condition in a compartment fire in which the entire volume is involved in combustion of varying intensities (*NFPA 921*, 2017 ed., pt. 3.3.95).

furniture calorimeter An instrumental system for measuring the amount of heat produced by the combustion of a moderate-sized fuel package, and the rate at which the heat is produced.

fuse An overcurrent protective device with a circuit-opening fusible part that is heated and severed by the passage of overcurrent through it (*NFPA 70,* 2014 ed., Article 100).

G

gas   The physical state of a substance that has no shape or volume of its own and will expand to take the shape and volume of the container or enclosure it occupies (*NFPA 921,* 2017 ed., pt. 3.3.96).

ghost marks   Stained outlines of floor tiles produced on non-combustible floors by the dissolution and combustion of tile adhesive.

glowing combustion   Luminous burning of solid material without a visible flame (*NFPA 921,* 2017 ed., pt. 3.3.97).

ground   A conducting connection, whether intentional or accidental, between an electrical circuit or equipment and earth or to some conducting body that serves in place of the earth (*NFPA 921,* 2017 ed., pt. 3.3.98).

ground fault   An unintended current that flows outside the normal circuit path, such as (a) through the equipment grounding conductor; (b) through conductive material in contact with lower potential (such as earth), other than the electrical system ground (metal water or plumbing pipes, etc.); or (c) through a combination of these ground return paths (*NFPA 921,* 2017 ed., pt. 3.3.99).

ground-fault circuit interrupter (GFCI)   A device intended for the protection of personnel that functions to de-energize a circuit or portion thereof within an established period of time when a current to ground exceeds the values established for a Class A device (*NFPA 70,* 2014 ed., Article 100).

H

Haber's rule   The dosage of toxic gases assimilated by an individual is assumed to be equivalent to the concentration times the duration of exposure.

hazard   Any arrangement of materials that presents the potential for harm (*NFPA 921,* 2017 ed., pt. 3.3.100).

heat   A form of energy characterized by vibration of molecules and capable of initiating and supporting chemical changes and changes of state (*NFPA 921,* 2017 ed., pt. 3.3.101).

heat and flame vector   An arrow used in a fire scene drawing to show the direction of heat, smoke, or flame flow (*NFPA 921,* 2017 ed., pt. 3.3.102).

heat flux   The measure of the rate of heat transfer to a surface, expressed in kilowatts/m^2, kilojoules/m$^2 \cdot$ sec, or Btu/ft$^2 \cdot$ sec (*NFPA 921,* 2017 ed., pt. 3.3.103).

heat horizon   The demarcation (usually horizontal) of fire damage revealed by the charring, burning, or discoloration of paint or wall coverings.

heat of combustion   The total energy released as heat when a substance undergoes complete combustion with oxygen under standard conditions.

heat of ignition   The heat energy that brings about ignition (*NFPA 921,* 2017 ed., pt. 3.3.104).

heat release rate (HRR)   The rate at which heat energy is generated by burning (*NFPA 921,* 2017 ed., pt. 3.3.105).

heat transfer   The exchange of thermal energy between materials through conduction, convection, and/or radiation (*NFPA 921,* 2017 ed., pt. 3.3.106).

high explosive   A material that is capable of sustaining a reaction front that moves through the unreacted material at a speed equal to or greater than that of sound in that medium [typically 1000 m/sec (3000 ft/sec)]; a material capable of sustaining a detonation (*NFPA 921,* 2017 ed., pt. 3.3.107; *see also* pt.3.3.46, Detonation.)

high-order damage   A rapid pressure rise or high-force explosion characterized by a shattering effect on the confining structure or container and long missile distances (*NFPA 921,* 2017 ed., pt. 3.3.108).

high-resistance connection   A condition resulting from loose or poor connections in traditional electrical accessories and switchgear in which high resistance can cause heat to develop which may be capable of starting a fire.

hot-plate ignition (hot surface ignition)   Temperature of a metal test plate at which liquid fuel ignites on contact.

hot set   Direct ignition of available fuels with an open flame (match or lighter).

hydrocarbon   An organic compound consisting entirely of hydrogen and carbon.

hypothesis   A supposition or conjecture put forward to account for certain facts, and used as a basis for further investigation by which it may be proved or disproved (*ASTM E1138-89,* 1989 ed.).

hypoxia   Condition relating to low concentrations of oxygen.

I

ignitable liquid   Any liquid or the liquid phase of any material that is capable of fueling a fire, including a flammable liquid, combustible liquid, or any other material that can be liquefied and burned (*NFPA 921,* 2017 ed., pt. 3.3.111).

ignition   The process of initiating self-sustained combustion (*NFPA 921,* 2017 ed., pt. 3.3.112).

ignition energy   The quantity of heat energy that should be absorbed by a substance to ignite and burn (*NFPA 921,* 2017 ed., pt. 3.3.113).

ignition temperature   Minimum temperature a substance should attain in order to ignite under specific test conditions (*NFPA 921,* 2017 ed., pt. 3.3.114).

ignition time   The time between the application of an ignition source to a material and the onset of self-sustained combustion (*NFPA 921,* 2017 ed., pt. 3.3.115).

incendiary fire   A fire that is intentionally ignited in an area or under circumstances where and when there should not be a fire (*NFPA 921,* 2017 ed., pt. 3.3.116).

indicators   Observable (and usually measurable) changes in appearance caused by heat, flame or smoke.

inductive logic or reasoning   The process by which a person starts from a particular experience and proceeds to generalizations. The process by which hypotheses are developed based upon observable or known facts and the training, experience, knowledge, and expertise of the observer (*NFPA 921,* 2017 ed., pt. 3.3.117).

inorganic   A material made from or containing material that does not come from plants or animals.

interested party   Any person, entity, or organization, including their representatives, with statutory obligations or whose legal rights or interests may be affected by the investigation of a specific incident (*NFPA 921,* 2017 ed., pt. 3.3.118).

intumescent coatings   A coating used to increase the fire endurance of structural steel or other materials. These coatings appear as paints during normal conditions, but when heated intumesce, or swell, forming an insulation around the steel (see *NFPA 921,* 2017 ed., pt. 7.5.1.4).

iodine number   A measure of the unsaturation of a substance (as an oil or fat) expressed as the number of grams of iodine or equivalent halogen absorbed by 100 grams of the substance. ("Iodine Number." Merriam-Webster.com. Accessed January 10, 2017. https://www.merriam-webster.com/dictionary/iodine number.)

isochar   A line on a diagram connecting points of equal char depth (*NFPA 921,* 2017 ed., pt. 3.3.121).

J

job performance requirement (JPR)   A statement that describes a specific job task, lists the items necessary to complete the task, and defines measurable or observable outcomes and evaluation areas for the specific task (*NFPA 1033,* 2014 ed., pt. 3.3.9).

joule   The preferred SI unit of heat, energy, or work. A joule is the heat produced when one ampere is passed through a resistance of one ohm for one second, or it is the work required to move a distance of one meter against a force of one newton. There are 4.184 joules in a calorie, and 1055 joules in a British thermal unit (Btu). A watt is a joule/second (*NFPA 921,* 2017 ed., pt. 3.3.122; *see also* pt. 3.3.22, British Thermal Unit (Btu), and pt. 3.3.25, Calorie].

K

kilowatt   A measurement of energy release rate (*NFPA 921,* 2017 ed., pt. 3.3.123).

kindling temperature   See 3.3.114, Ignition Temperature (*NFPA 921,* 2017 ed., pt. 3.3.124).

L

ladder fuels   Intermediate height fuels between the ground litter and the crowns of trees overhead.

layering   The systematic process of removing debris from the top down and observing the relative location of artifacts at the fire scene (*NFPA 921,* 2017 ed., pt. 3.3.125).

low explosive   An explosive that has a reaction velocity of less than 1000 m/sec (3000 ft/sec) (*NFPA 921,* 2017 ed., pt. 3.3.126).

low-order damage   A slow rate of pressure rise or low-force explosion characterized by a pushing or dislodging effect on the confining structure or container and by short missile distances (*NFPA 921,* 2017 ed., pt. 3.3.127).

M

manner of death   The way or circumstances in which the cause of death occurred.

mass spectrometry   Analysis of organic molecules by fragmenting them and separating them by size.

material first ignited   The fuel that is first set on fire by the heat of ignition; to be meaningful, both a type of material and a form of material should be identified (*NFPA 921,* 2017 ed., pt. 3.3.128).

mechanical explosion   An explosion where a container, vessel, or pipe bursts when internal gas or liquid pressures exceed the tensile strength of the container.

motive   An inner drive or impulse that is the cause, reason, or incentive that induces or prompts a specific behavior (Rider 1980).

N

naphthenics   Relating to or derived from naphthene.

natural fibers   Fibers of animal or vegetable origin without chemical manipulation.

negative corpus   The process of determining what caused a fire by eliminating each possible cause, one by one, until only one possible cause remains.

neutral conductor   The conductor connected to the neutral point of a system that is intended to carry current under normal conditions (*NFPA 70,* 2014 ed., Article 100).

noncombustible material   A material that, in the form in which it is used and under the condition anticipated, will not ignite, burn, support combustion, or release flammable vapors when subjected to fire or heat (*NFPA 921,* 2017 ed., pt. 3.3.130).

nonflammable   (1) Not readily capable of burning with a flame. (2) Not liable to ignite and burn when exposed to flame. Its antonym is *flammable* (*NFPA 921, 2017* ed., pt. 3.3.131).

O

odorant   A chemical compound that has a smell or odor.

ohm   The SI unit of electrical impedance or, in the direct current case, electrical resistance (*NFPA 921, 2017* ed., pt. 3.3.132).

olefinic   Characteristic of, or containing olefins.

open neutral condition   In an American single-phase, 120/240 V residential system, the neutral return leg is not connected to the service ground (*NFPA 70, 2014* ed., Article 100).

opinion   A belief or judgment based on facts and logic, but without absolute proof of its truth (*ASTM E1138-89, 1989* ed.).

organic   Of, relating to, or derived from living organisms.

origin   The general location where a fire or explosion began (*NFPA 921, 2017* ed., pt. 3.3.133; *see also* pt. 3.3.142, Point of Origin, or pt. 3.3.12, Area of Origin).

overcurrent   Any current in excess of the rated current of equipment or the ampacity of a conductor; it may result from an overload (*NFPA 921, 2017* ed., pt. 3.3.135; *see also* pt. 3.3.167, short circuit, or pt. 3.3.99, ground fault; *NFPA 70, 2014* ed., Article 100).

overhaul   A fire fighting term involving the process of final extinguishment after the main body of the fire has been knocked down. All traces of fire must be extinguished at this time (*NFPA 921, 2017* ed., pt. 3.3.135).

overload   Operation of equipment in excess of normal, full-load rating or of a conductor in excess of rated ampacity that when it persists for a sufficient length of time would cause damage or dangerous overheating. A fault, such as a short circuit or ground fault, is not an overload (*NFPA 921, 2017* ed., pt. 3.3.136).

oxidation   Reaction with oxygen either in the form of the element or in the form of one of its compounds (*NFPA 53, 2016* ed.).

P

paraffinic   Characteristic of paraffin wax or a paraffin hydrocarbon.

peer review   Peer review is a formal procedure generally employed in prepublication review of scientific or technical documents and screening of grant applications by research-sponsoring agencies. Peer review carries with it connotations of both independence and objectivity. Peer reviewers should not have any interest in the outcome of the review. The author does not select the reviewers, and reviews are often conducted anonymously. As such, the term "peer review" should not be applied to reviews of an investigator's work by coworkers, supervisors, or investigators from agencies conducting investigations of the same incident. Such reviews are more appropriately characterized as "technical reviews" (*NFPA 921, 2017* ed., pt. 4.6.3).

physical hazard material   A chemical or substance classified as a combustible liquid, explosive, flammable cryogen, flammable gas, flammable liquid, flammable solid, organic peroxide, oxidizer, oxidizing cryogen, pyrophoric, unstable (reactive), or water-reactive material.

piloted ignition   The initiation of combustion by means of contact of gaseous material with an external high-energy source, such as a flame, spark, electrical arc, or glowing wire.

piloted ignition temperature   (*NFPA 921, 2017* ed., pt. 3.3.139; *see also* pt. 3.3.114, Ignition Temperature).

plastic   Any of a wide range of natural or synthetic organic materials of high molecular weight that can be formed by pressure, heat, extrusion, and other methods into desired shapes (*NFPA 921, 2017* ed., pt. 3.3.140).

plume   The column of hot gases, flames, and smoke rising above a fire; also called *convection column*, *thermal updraft*, or *thermal column* (*NFPA 921, 2017* ed., pt. 3.3.141).

point of origin   The exact physical location within the area of origin where a heat source and the fuel interact, resulting in a fire or explosion (*NFPA 921, 2017* ed., pt. 3.3.142).

possible   At this level of certainty, the hypothesis can be demonstrated to be feasible but cannot be declared probable (*NFPA 921, 2017* ed., pt. 4.5.1).

premixed flame   A flame for which the fuel and oxidizer are mixed prior to combustion, as in a laboratory Bunsen burner or a gas cooking range; propagation of the flame is governed by the interaction between flow rate, transport processes, and chemical reaction (*NFPA 921, 2017* ed., pt. 3.3.144).

probable   This level of certainty corresponds to being more likely true than not. At this level of certainty, the likelihood of the hypothesis being true is greater than 50 percent (*NFPA 921, 2017* ed., pt. 4.5.1).

products of combustion   See 3.3.35, Combustion Products (*NFPA 921, 2017* ed., pt. 3.3.146).

profit (motive)   Fires set for profit involve those set for material or monetary gain, either directly or indirectly. The direct gain may come from insurance fraud, eliminating or intimidating business competition, extortion, removing unwanted structures to increase property values, or escaping financial obligations (*NFPA 921, 2017* ed., pt. 24.4.9.3.6).

pyrolysis   A process in which material is decomposed, or broken down, into simpler molecular compounds by the effects of heat alone; pyrolysis often precedes combustion (*NFPA 921, 2017* ed., pt. 3.3.150).

pyromania   The clinical diagnosis describes this disorder as (1) A compulsion to set fires and (2) A disorder characterized by a fascination with fire and recurrent episodes of fire setting during which the individual experiences a rising subjective sense of tension before the fire setting and a sense of gratification or relief when setting the fire. There is no ulterior motive (such as monetary gain or the expression of political ideology) to the fire setting (2016 ICD-10-CM Diagnosis Code F63.1 ICD-10-CM Medical Diagnosis Codes).

pyrophoric material   Any substance that spontaneously ignites upon exposure to atmospheric oxygen (*NFPA 921*, 2017 ed., pt. 3.3.151).

R

radiant heat   Heat energy carried by electromagnetic waves that are longer than light waves and shorter than radio waves; radiant heat (electromagnetic radiation) increases the sensible temperature of any substance capable of absorbing the radiation, especially solid and opaque objects (*NFPA 921*, 2017 ed., pt. 3.3.152).

radiation   Heat transfer by way of electromagnetic energy (*NFPA 921*, 2017 ed., pt. 3.3.153).

rate of heat release   See 3.3.99, Heat Release Rate (HRR) (*NFPA 921*, 2017 ed., pt. 3.3.154).

receptacle/socket   A receptacle is a contact device installed at the outlet for the connection of an attachment plug. A single receptacle is a single contact device with no other contact device on the same yoke. A multiple receptacle is two or more contact devices on the same yoke (*NFPA 70*, 2014 ed., Article 100).

rekindle   A return to flaming combustion after apparent but incomplete extinguishment (*NFPA 921*, 2017 ed., pt. 3.3.155).

requisite knowledge   Fundamental knowledge one must have in order to perform a specific task (*NFPA 1033*, 2014 ed., pt.3.3.10).

requisite skills   The essential skills one must have in order to perform a specific task (*NFPA 1033*, 2014 ed., pt. 3.3.11).

responsibility   The accountability of a person or other entity for the event or sequence of events that caused the fire or explosion, spread of the fire, bodily injuries, loss of life, or property damage (*NFPA 921*, 2017 ed., pt. 3.3.156).

revenge (motive)   The revenge-motivated firesetter retaliates for some real or perceived injustice. An important aspect is that a sense of injustice is perceived by the offender. The event or circumstance that is perceived may have occurred months or years before the firesetting activity. A fire by the revenge motivated offender may be a well-planned, one-time event or may represent serial firesetting, with little or no preplanning. Serial offenders may direct their retaliation at individuals, institutions, or society in general (*NFPA 921*, 2017 ed., pt. 24.4.9.3.4.1).

risk   The degree of peril; the possible harm that might occur that is represented by the statistical probability or quantitative estimate of the frequency or severity of injury or loss (*NFPA 921*, 2017 ed., pt. 3.3.157).

rollout   Exiting of burner flames in an appliance due to massive overfueling.

rollover   See 3.3.82, Flameover (*NFPA 921*, 2017 ed., pt. 3.3.158).

S

salvage   Procedures to reduce incidental losses from smoke, water, and weather following fires, generally by removal or covering of contents.

saturated   A hydrocarbon which has no double or triple bonds, and containing the greatest possible number of hydrogen atoms.

scene   The general physical location of a fire or explosion incident (geographic area, structure or portion of a structure, vehicle, boat, piece of equipment, etc.) designated as important to the investigation because it may contain physical damage or debris, evidence, victims, or incident-related hazards (*NFPA 921*, 2017 ed., pt. 3.3.159).

scientific method   The systematic pursuit of knowledge involving the recognition and definition of a problem; the collection of data through observation and experimentation; analysis of the data; the formulation, evaluation and testing of hypotheses; and, where possible, the selection of a final hypothesis (*NFPA 921*, 2017 ed., pt. 3.3.160).

seat of explosion   A craterlike indentation created at the point of origin of some explosions (*NFPA 921*, 2017 ed., pt. 3.3.161).

self-heating   The result of exothermic reactions, occurring spontaneously in some materials under certain conditions, whereby heat is generated at a rate sufficient to raise the temperature of the material (*NFPA 921*, 2017 ed., pt. 3.3.164).

self-ignition   Ignition resulting from self-heating, synonymous with *spontaneous ignition* (*NFPA 921*, 2017 ed., pt. 3.3.165).

self-ignition temperature   The minimum temperature at which the self-heating properties of a material lead to ignition (*NFPA 921*, 2017 ed., pt. 3.3.166).

service   The conductors and equipment for delivering electricity from the supply system to the equipment of the premises served (*NFPA 70*, 2014 ed., Article 100).

service conductors   The conductors from the service point to the service disconnecting means (*NFPA 70*, 2014 ed., Article 100).

service conductors, overhead   The overhead conductors between the service point and the first point of connection to the service-entrance conductors at the building or other structure (*NFPA 70*, 2014 ed., Article 100).

service conductors, underground   The underground conductors between the service point and the first point of connection to the service-entrance conductors in a terminal box, meter, or other enclosure, inside or outside the building wall (*NFPA 70*, 2014 ed., Article 100).

service drop   The overhead conductors between the utility electric supply system and the service point (*NFPA 70*, 2014 ed., Article 100).

short circuit   An abnormal connection of low resistance between normal circuit conductors where the resistance is normally much greater; this is an overcurrent situation but it is not an overload (*NFPA 921*, 2017 ed., pt. 3.3.167).

site   The general physical location of the incident, including the scene and the surrounding area deemed significant to the process of the investigation and support areas (*NFPA 921*, 2017 ed., pt. 3.3.168).

smoke   The airborne solid and liquid particulates and gases evolved when a material undergoes pyrolysis or combustion, together with the quantity of air that is entrained or otherwise mixed into the mass (*NFPA 921*, 2017 ed., pt. 3.3.169; *see also NFPA 318*, 2012 ed.).

smoke horizon   Surface deposits that reveal the height at which smoke and soot stained the walls and windows of a room without thermal damage.

smoldering   Combustion without flame, usually with incandescence and smoke (*NFPA 921*, 2017 ed., pt. 3.3.172).

soot   Black particles of carbon produced in a flame (*NFPA 921*, 2017 ed., pt. 3.3.173).

spalling   Chipping or pitting of concrete or masonry surfaces (*NFPA 921*, 2017 ed., pt. 3.3.174).

spark   A moving particle of solid material that emits radiant energy due either to its temperature or the process of combustion on its surface (*NFPA 921*, 2017 ed., pt. 3.3.175; *see also NFPA 654*, 2013 ed.).

specific gravity (air) (vapor density)   The ratio of the average molecular weight of a gas or vapor to the average molecular weight of air (*NFPA 921*, 2017 ed., pt. 3.3.176).

specific gravity (of a liquid or solid)   The ratio of the mass of a given volume of a substance to the mass of an equal volume of water at a temperature of 4°C (*NFPA 921*, 2017 ed., pt. 3.3.177).

spoliation   Loss, destruction, or material alteration of an object or document that is evidence or potential evidence in a legal proceeding by one who has the responsibility for its preservation (*NFPA 921*, 2017 ed., pt. 3.3.178).

spontaneous combustion   Due to self-heating is a special form of smoldering ignition that does not involve an external heating process. An exothermic reaction within the material is the source of the energy that leads to ignition and burning (*NFPA 921*, 2017 ed., pt. 5.7.4.1.1.5).

spontaneous heating   Process whereby a material increases in temperature without drawing heat from its surroundings (*NFPA 921*, 2017 ed., pt. 3.3.179).

spontaneous ignition   Initiation of combustion of a material by an internal chemical or biological reaction that has produced sufficient heat to ignite the material (*NFPA 921*, 2017 ed., pt. 3.3.180).

spontaneous ignition temperature (SIT)   Also called autoignition temperature; the lowest temperature at which a combustible material ignites in air without a spark or flame (*NFPA 921*, 2017 ed., pt. 3.3.16).

spot fires   Fires started by airborne embers some distance away from the main body of the fire.

stoichiometric   Every fuel–air mixture has an optimum ratio at which point the combustion will be most efficient. This ratio occurs at or near the mixture known by chemists as the stoichiometric ratio. When the amount of air is in balance with the amount of fuel (i.e., after burning there is neither unused fuel nor unused air), the burning is referred to as stoichiometric. This condition rarely occurs in fires except in certain types of gas fires (*NFPA 921*, 2017 ed., pt. 5.1.2.2: *see also* pt. 23.8.2.1.3.)

superposition   The combined effects of two or more fires or heat transfer effects, a phenomenon that may generate confusing fire damage indicators.

suppression   The sum of all the work done to extinguish a fire, beginning at the time of its discovery (*NFPA 921*, 2017 ed., pt. 3.3.181).

suspicious   Fire cause has not been determined, but there are indications that the fire was deliberately set and all accidental fire causes have been eliminated.

synthetic   A material or chemical, especially a textile fiber, not made of natural origin.

synthetic fibers   Manmade fibers of chemical origin.

T

target fuel   A fuel that is subject to ignition by thermal radiation such as from a flame or a hot gas layer (*NFPA 921*, 2017 ed., pt. 3.3.182).

technical expert   A person educated, skilled, or experienced in the mechanical arts, applied sciences, or related crafts (*ASTM E1138-89*, 1989 ed.).

temperature   The degree of sensible heat of a body as measured by a thermometer or similar instrument (*NFPA 921*, 2017 ed., pt. 3.3.183).

tenability   An assessment of the potential for harm that may be imposed from a fire based on (1) an analysis of the source, heat release rates, and rates of production of the combustion products; (2) when occupants might become exposed to these harmful conditions; and (3) the effects on the occupants to this exposure.

thermal column   See 3.3.141, Plume (*NFPA 921*, 2017 ed., pt. 3.3.184).

thermal cutoff (TCO)   An electrical safety device that interrupts electric current when exposed to heat at a specific temperature.

thermal expansion The increase in length, volume, or surface area of a body with rise in temperature (*NFPA 921,* 2017 ed., pt. 3.3.185).

thermal inertia The properties of a material that characterize its rate of surface temperature rise when exposed to heat; related to the product of the material's thermal conductivity (k), its density (ρ), and its heat capacity (c) (*NFPA 921,* 2017 ed., pt. 3.3.186).

thermal protection device An inherent device against overheating that is responsive to temperature or current and will protect the equipment against overheating due to overload or failure to start (*NFPA 70,* 2014 ed., Article 100).

thermal runaway An unstable condition when the heat generated exceeds the heat losses within the material to the environment. The temperature rise is so large that stable conditions no longer exist (*NFPA 921,* 2017 ed., pt. 5.7.4.1.3).

thermodynamics The branch of physics that deals with the relationship between heat and other forms of energy (*NFPA 921,* 2017 ed., pt. 3.3.187).

thermometry The study of the science, methodology, and practice of temperature measurement (*NFPA 921,* 2017 ed., pt. 3.3.188).

thermoplastic Plastic materials that soften and melt under exposure to heat and can reach a flowable state (*NFPA 921,* 2017 ed., pt. 3.3.189).

thermoset plastics Plastic materials that are hardened into a permanent shape in the manufacturing process and are not commonly subject to softening when heated; typically form char in a fire (*NFPA 921,* 2017 ed., pt. 3.3.190).

thermosetting resin Polymer that decomposes or degrades as it is heated rather than melts.

time line Graphic representation of the events in a fire incident displayed in chronological order (*NFPA 921,* 2017 ed., pt. 3.3.191).

total burn A fire scene where a fire continued to burn until most combustibles were consumed and the fire self-extinguished due to a lack of fuel or was extinguished when the fuel load was reduced by burning and there was sufficient suppression agent application to extinguish the fire (*NFPA 921,* 2017 ed., pt. 3.3.192).

trailer Solid or liquid fuel used to intentionally spread or accelerate the spread of a fire from one area to another (*NFPA 921,* 2017 ed., pt. 3.3.193).

trench effect A phenomenon, also known as the Coanda effect, in which there is a tendency for a fast-moving stream of air to deflect itself toward and along nearby surfaces.

U

unconfined vapor cloud explosion (UCVE) When a flammable vapor is released, its mixture with air will form a flammable vapor cloud. If ignited, the flame speed may accelerate to high velocities and produce significant blast overpressure (American Institute of Chemical Engineers (AIChE), Glossary of Terms, 2017).

undetermined fire cause The final opinion is only as good as the quality of the data used in reaching that opinion. If the level of certainty of the opinion is only "possible" or "suspected," the fire cause is unresolved and should be classified as "undetermined." This decision as to the level of certainty in data collected in the investigation or of any hypothesis drawn from an analysis of the data rests with the investigator (*NFPA 921,* 2017 ed., pt. 19.7.4).

V

vandalism (motive) Vandalism-motivated firesetting is defined as mischievous or malicious firesetting that results in damage to property. Common targets include educational facilities and abandoned structures, but also include trash fires and grass fires. Vandalism firesetting categories include willful and malicious mischief and peer or group pressure (*NFPA 921,* 2017 ed., pt. 24.4.9.3.2).

vapor The gas phase of a substance, particularly of those that are normally liquids or solids at ordinary temperatures (*NFPA 921,* 2017 ed., pt. 3.3.196; see also pt. 3.3.96, Gas).

vapor density See 3.3.176, Specific Gravity (air) (vapor density) (*NFPA 921,* 2017 ed., pt. 3.3.197).

vent An opening for the passage of, or dissipation of, fluids, such as gases, fumes, smoke, and the like (*NFPA 921,* 2017 ed., pt. 3.3.198).

ventilation Circulation of air in any space by natural wind or convection or by fans blowing air into or exhausting air out of a building; a fire-fighting operation of removing smoke and heat from the structure by opening windows and doors or making holes in the roof (*NFPA 921,* 2017 ed., pt. 3.3.199).

ventilation-controlled fire A fire in which the heat release rate or growth is controlled by the amount of air available to the fire (*NFPA 921,* 2017 ed., pt. 3.3.200).

venting The escape of smoke and heat through openings in a building (*NFPA 921,* 2017 ed., pt. 3.3.201).

verification and validation (V&V) A formal process of establishing acceptable uses, suitability, and limitations of fire models. *Verification* determines that a model correctly represents the developer's conceptual description. *Validation* determines that a model is a suitable representation of the real world and is capable of reproducing phenomena of interest (Salley and Kassawar 2007g).

volatile A liquid having a low boiling point typically less than 68°F (20°C) that is readily evaporated into the vapor state.

volt (V) The unit of electrical pressure (electromotive force) represented by the symbol "E"; the difference in potential required to make a current of one ampere flow through a resistance of one ohm (*NFPA 921,* 2017 ed., pt. 3.3.202).

voltage, nominal   A nominal value assigned to a circuit or system for the purpose of conveniently designating its voltage class (e.g., 120/240 volts, 480Y/277 volts, 600 volts).

W

watt (W)   Unit of power, or rate of work, equal to one joule per second, or the rate of work represented by a current of one ampere under the potential of one volt (*NFPA 921,* 2017 ed., pt. 3.3.203).

Z

zone model   A computer fire model based on the assumption that a fire in a room or enclosure can be described in terms of two unique zones known as the upper and the lower zone or layer, and the conditions within each zone can be predicted. Zone models use a set of differential equations for each zone, solving for conditions such as, for example, pressure, temperature, carbon monoxide, oxygen, and soot production.

References

ASTME E1138-89, 1989 ed. Terminology of Technical Aspects of Product Liability Litigation. West Conshohocken, PA: ASTM International.

Henderson, R.W. and G.R. Lightsey. 1985. "Theoretical Combustion Temperature of Wood Charcoal." National Fire and Arson Report 3:7.

ICD 10, 2008. International Statistical Classification of Diseases and Related Health Problems, 10th rev. World Health Organization, New York.

NFPA 35, 2016 ed. Standard for the Manufacture of Organic Coatings. Quincy, MA: National Fire Protection Association.

NFPA 53, 2016 ed. Recommended Practice on Materials, Equipment, and Systems Used on Oxygen-Enriched Atmospheres. Quincy, MA: National Fire Protection Association.

NFPA 68, 2013 ed. Standard on Explosion Protection by Deflagration Venting. Quincy, MA: National Fire Protection Association.

NFPA 70, 2014 ed. Article in National Electric Code. Quincy, MA: National Fire Protection Association.

NFPA 72, 2016 ed. National Fire Alarm and Signaling Code. Quincy, MA: National Fire Protection Association.

NFPA 921, 2017 ed. Guide for Fire and Explosion Investigations. Quincy, MA: National Fire Protection Association.

NFPA 1033, 2014 ed. Standard for Professional Qualifications for Fire Investigator. Quincy, MA: National Fire Protection Association.

NFPA 1123, 2014 ed. Code for Fireworks Display. Quincy, MA: National Fire Protection Association.

Rider, A.O., 1980. "The Firesetter: A Psychological Profile." FBI Law Enforcement Bulletin 49 (June, July, August): 7–23.

INDEX

Investigative information during
  suppression
    minimization of post-fire damage,
      297–298
    overhaul, 297
    responsibility of firefighters, 296–297
    salvage and security concerns,
      297–298
Investigative protocols, 38–39
*Investors I, L.P. v. Square D
  Company*, 43
Iodine number, 276
Isochar lines, 327, 428
Isolated burns, 478

J

*Jacob J. Booth and Kathleen Booth
  v. Black and Decker, Inc.*, 40
James B. McCoy v. Whirlpool Corp.,
  39
*John Witten Tunnell v. Ford Motor
  Company*, 38
Joiner case, 32–33
Joule, 67
*Journal of Fire Protection
  Engineering*, 294
Journal of Forensic Science, 294

K

Kapok, 647
Kelly-Frye test, 30
Kerosene, as hydrocarbon fuel, 117
Kerosene heaters, 252–253
King's Cross Underground Station
  fire case study, 619–620
Kumbo Tire Co. Ltd. v. Carmichael,
  30

L

Laboratory services
  accreditation, 563–565
  appliances and wiring evaluation,
    584–589
  availability of, 563
  blood, 592–594
  burned documents, 582–583
  charred/burned materials
    identification, 582
  chemical incendiaries, 579–581
  in explosion investigation,
    205–206
  failure analysis, 583–584
  fingerprints, 590–592
  fire evidence analysis, 581–590
  fire testing laboratories, 563
  gas chromatography (GC),
    565–578

impression evidence, 594–596
non-fire-related physical evidence,
  590
overview, 563
physical matches, 596
smoke alarms, 589–590
spoliation, 590
trace evidence, 596–598
volatile accelerants, 565–578
Ladder fuels, 500
Laminar flame, 509
Laryngospasm, 719
Laser measurement techniques, 390
Laser scanning systems, 395–398
Latent fingerprints, 408, 591, 592
Lateral flame spread, 342
Latex, 86
Layering, 402, 403–407
Leaks, gas line, 124–125
Lean mixture, 178
Legal opinions, 23
Leuco crystal violet (LCV), 594
LIDAR (Light Detection And
  Ranging) technology, 395
Life cycle, fire, 454
Lighters, 237–239
Lighting, photography, 422
Lightning
  detection services, 280
  as ignition source, 278–280
  strike illustrations, 279
  strike locations, 365
  trees and, 280
  as wildland fire ignition source,
    515–516
Line plumes. *See also* Fire plumes
  defined, 308
  entrainment of air, 309
  flame height, 308–309
  illustrated, 308
Linen, 647
Liquefied petroleum gas (LPG). *See*
  LP gas
Liquid fuels
  boiling points, 108–109
  combustion of, 118–120
  defined, 68
  flame point, 101, 106
  flammable ranges, 107
  flash point, 98, 101, 104–106, 242
  heat of combustion, 114, 115
  hydrocarbon, 116–118
  ignition energy, 107–108
  ignition temperature, 106–107
  ignition test, 103
  minimum autoignition
    temperature, 105
  nonhydrocarbon, 120–121

physical properties of, 98–115
pyrolysis and, 114–115
specific gravities, 105
vapor pressure, 98–99
Liquids
  collection and preservation, 455,
    458
  combustible, 106
  decomposition of, 114–115
  flammable, 106
  flash point and fire point testing
    of, 635–636
  hazardous, 217–221
  ignitable, 84, 456
  ignition behavior of, 148
Liquified petroleum gas (LPG), 68
Logarithms, 735–736
Logical winds, 503
Long-term heating, 259–264
Loss histories, 20
Loss of material. *See also* Fire
  patterns
  defined, 322, 336
  examples, 322
  mass, 337
  variables, 322
Low burns and penetration
  causes of, 475
  fire behavior and indicator,
    471–477
  illustrated, 479
Low explosives
  black powder, 186–188
  smokeless powder, 186, 187–188
  traces of, 205
Low-order damage, 192
Low-order detonation, 192
Low-order explosions, 192
Low-temperature ignition sources.
  See also Ignition sources
  bonfires, 261
  exploding ammunition, 263–264
  firearms residues, 263
  hot metals, 261–262
  mechanical sparks, 262–263
  military ammunition, 264
  overview, 259–260
  trash burners and incinerators,
    260–261
Low-yield explosion, 185
LP gas. *See also* Gases
  characteristics of, 122–124
  containers, 215
  containers illustrations, 123
  defined, 116
  delivery pressure, 124
  gas lines, 124–128
  leaks, 124–125